Administrative
MEDICAL
ASSISTING

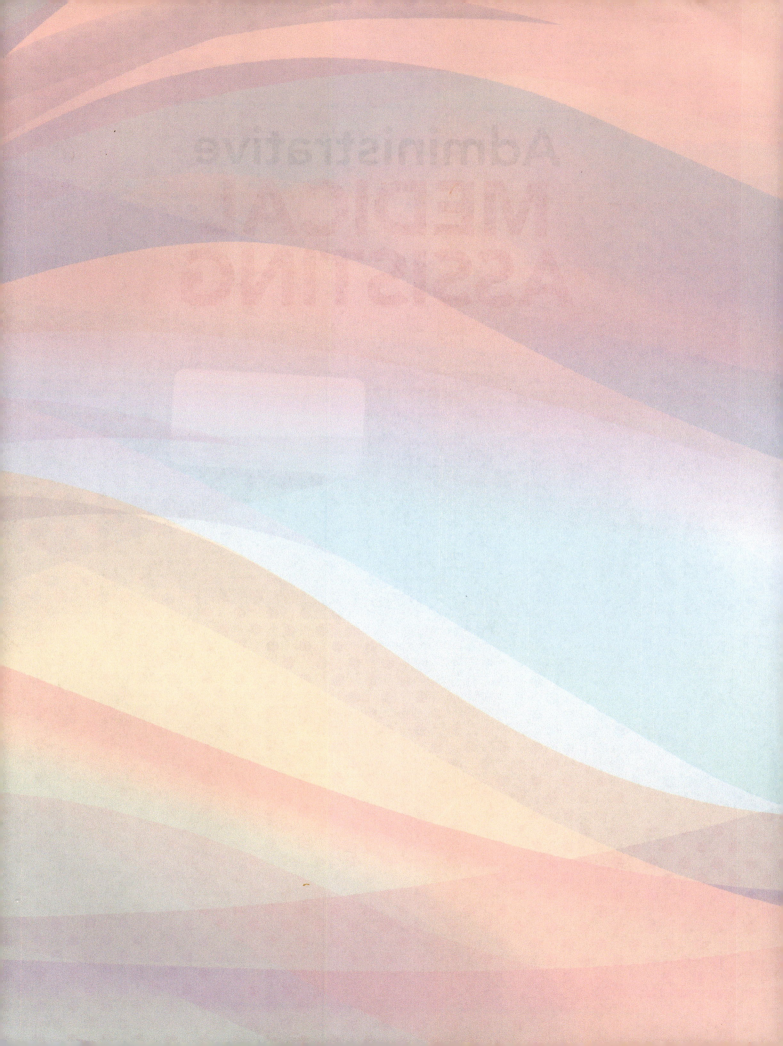

Administrative
MEDICAL ASSISTING

Eighth Edition

Linda L. French, CMA-C (AAMA), NCICS, CPC

Formerly, Instructor and Business Consultant,
Administrative Medical Assisting,
Medical Terminology, and Medical Insurance Billing and Coding
Simi Valley Adult School and Career Institute, Simi Valley, California
Ventura College, Ventura, California
Oxnard College, Oxnard, California
Santa Barbara Business College, Ventura, California
Harbor College of Court Reporting, Ventura, California
University of California Santa Barbara Extension, Ventura, California

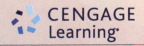

Australia • Brazil • Mexico • Singapore • United Kingdom • United States

**Administrative Medical Assisting,
Eighth Edition**
Linda L. French

SVP, GM Skills & Global Product Management:
Jonathan Lau

Product Director: Matthew Seeley

Product Team Manager: Stephen Smith

Senior Director, Development:
Marah Bellegarde

Product Development Manager: Juliet Steiner

Product Assistant: Mark Turner

Vice President, Marketing Services:
Jennifer Ann Baker

Senior Production Director: Wendy Troeger

Production Director: Andrew Crouth

Senior Content Project Manager:
Thomas Heffernan

Managing Art Director: Jack Pendleton

Cover image(s): antishock/Shutterstock.com

For product information and technology assistance, contact us at
Cengage Learning Customer & Sales Support, 1-800-354-9706

For permission to use material from this text or product,
submit all requests online at **www.cengage.com/permissions.**
Further permissions questions can be e-mailed to
permissionrequest@cengage.com

Library of Congress Control Number: 2016950837

ISBN: 978-1-305-85917-3

Cengage Learning
20 Channel Center Street
Boston, MA 02210
USA

Cengage Learning is a leading provider of customized learning solutions with employees residing in nearly 40 different countries and sales in more than 125 countries around the world. Find your local representative at **www.cengage.com**

Cengage Learning products are represented in Canada by Nelson Education, Ltd.

To learn more about Cengage Learning, visit **www.cengage.com**

Purchase any of our products at your local college store or at our preferred online store **www.cengagebrain.com**

Notice to the Reader

Printed in Mexico
Print Number: 07   Print Year: 2022

Money doesn't make people rich—knowledge makes people rich.
                                                    —Author unknown

We all need a *sounding board*; someone to run ideas by, help absorb the bumps in the road, and encourage us along life's journey. This edition is dedicated to my husband Dick, who has been my sounding board for the past 50 years. Without his words of encouragement, practical help, and hours of patient listening, I could not have completed this edition. My love and gratitude are eternal.

—Linda L. French, CMA (AAMA), NCICS, CPC

Always remember what you have learned.
Your education is your life—guard it well.
                                                    —Proverbs 4:13

BRIEF CONTENTS

UNIT 5
FINANCIAL ADMINISTRATION 409

UNIT 6
MANAGING THE OFFICE 605

CONTENTS

1 PROFESSIONAL AND CAREER RESPONSIBILITIES   1

Chapter 1 A CAREER AS AN ADMINISTRATIVE MEDICAL ASSISTANT   2

Chapter 2 THE HEALTH CARE ENVIRONMENT: PAST, PRESENT, AND FUTURE   26

Chapter 6

TELEPHONE PROCEDURES / 178

Chapter 7

APPOINTMENTS / 204

4 WRITTEN COMMUNICATION / 339

Chapter 11 WRITTEN CORRESPONDENCE / 340

Chapter 12 PROCESSING MAIL AND ELECTRONIC CORRESPONDENCE / 374

6 MANAGING THE OFFICE / 605

COMPREHENSIVE LIST OF PROCEDURES AND JOB SKILLS

The following Procedures appear in the *textbook* and Job Skills appear in the *Workbook*:

CHAPTER 1

A CAREER AS AN ADMINISTRATIVE MEDICAL ASSISTANT

Performance Objectives (Procedures) in This Textbook

- Procedure 1-1 Interpret and accurately spell medical terms and abbreviations

Performance Objectives (Job Skills) in the Workbook

- Job Skill 1-1 Interpret and accurately spell medical terms and abbreviations
- Job Skill 1-2 Use the Internet to look up key terms and hear pronunciations
- Job Skill 1-3 Prioritize a task list to practice time management skills
- Job Skill 1-4 Use the Internet to obtain information on certification or registration
- Job Skill 1-5 Use the Internet to test your knowledge of anatomy and physiology or medical terminology
- Job Skill 1-6 Develop a medical practice survey

CHAPTER 2

THE HEALTH CARE ENVIRONMENT: PAST, PRESENT, AND FUTURE

Performance Objectives (Procedures) in This Textbook

- Procedure 2-1 Direct patients to specific hospital departments
- Procedure 2-2 Refer patients to the correct physician specialist

Performance Objectives (Job Skills) in the Workbook

- Job Skill 2-1 Use the Internet to research and write an essay about a medical pioneer
- Job Skill 2-2 Direct patients to specific hospital departments
- Job Skill 2-3 Refer patients to the correct physician specialist
- Job Skill 2-4 Define abbreviations for health care professionals
- Job Skill 2-5 Determine basic skills needed by the administrative medical assistant

CHAPTER 3

MEDICOLEGAL AND ETHICAL RESPONSIBILITIES

Performance Objectives (Procedures) in This Textbook

- Procedure 3-1 Release patient information

Performance Objectives (Job Skills) in the Workbook

- Job Skill 3-1 List personal ethics and set professional ethical goals
- Job Skill 3-2 Complete an authorization form to release medical records
- Job Skill 3-3 Download state-specific scope of practice laws and determine parameters for a medical assistant
- Job Skill 3-4 Compose a letter of withdrawal
- Job Skill 3-5 View a MedWatch online form and learn submitting requirements
- Job Skill 3-6 Print the *Patient Care Partnership* online brochure and apply it to the medical office setting
- Job Skill 3-7 Download and compare state-specific advance directives

CHAPTER 4

The Art of Communication

Performance Objectives (Procedures) in This Textbook

- Procedure 4-1 Demonstrate active listening by following guidelines
- Procedure 4-2 Communicate with children
- Procedure 4-3 Communicate with older adults
- Procedure 4-4 Communicate with hearing-impaired patients
- Procedure 4-5 Communicate with visually impaired patients
- Procedure 4-6 Communicate with speech-impaired patients
- Procedure 4-7 Communicate with patients who have an impaired level of understanding
- Procedure 4-8 Communicate with anxious patients
- Procedure 4-9 Communicate with angry patients
- Procedure 4-10 Communicate with patients and their family members and friends
- Procedure 4-11 Communicate with the health care team

Performance Objectives (Job Skills) in the Workbook

- Job Skill 4-1 Demonstrate body language
- Job Skill 4-2 Use the Internet to research active listening skills and write a report
- Job Skill 4-3 Communicate with a child via role-playing
- Job Skill 4-4 Communicate with an older adult via role-playing
- Job Skill 4-5 Name unique qualities of other cultures
- Job Skill 4-6 Communicate with a hearing-impaired patient via role-playing
- Job Skill 4-7 Communicate with a visually impaired patient via role-playing
- Job Skill 4-8 Communicate with a speech-impaired patient via role-playing
- Job Skill 4-9 Communicate with a patient who has an impaired level of understanding via role-playing
- Job Skill 4-10 Communicate with an anxious patient via role-playing
- Job Skill 4-11 Communicate with an angry patient via role-playing
- Job Skill 4-12 Communicate with a patient and his or her family members and friends via role-playing
- Job Skill 4-13 Communicate with a coworker on the health care team via role-playing

CHAPTER 5

RECEPTIONIST AND THE MEDICAL OFFICE ENVIRONMENT

Performance Objectives (Procedures) in This Textbook

- Procedure 5-1 Open the medical office
- Procedure 5-2 Assist patients with in-office registration procedures
- Procedure 5-3 Assist patient in preparing an application form for a disabled person placard
- Procedure 5-4 Develop a list of community resources
- Procedure 5-5 Develop a patient education plan for diseases or injuries related to the medical specialty
- Procedure 5-6 Work at a computer station and comply with ergonomic standards
- Procedure 5-7 Prevent and prepare for fires in the workplace
- Procedure 5-8 Learn how and when to use a fire extinguisher
- Procedure 5-9 Develop an emergency disaster plan
- Procedure 5-10 Close the medical office

Performance Objectives (Job Skills) in the Workbook

- Job Skill 5-1 Prepare a patient registration form
- Job Skill 5-2 Prepare an application form for a disabled person placard
- Job Skill 5-3 Research community resources for patient referrals and patient education
- Job Skill 5-4 Assess and use proper body mechanics
- Job Skill 5-5 Evaluate the work or school environment and develop a safety plan
- Job Skill 5-6 Take steps to prevent and prepare for fires in a health care setting
- Job Skill 5-7 Demonstrate proper use of a fire extinguisher
- Job Skill 5-8 Determine potential disaster hazards in your local community
- Job Skill 5-9 Develop an emergency response template with an evacuation plan

CHAPTER 6

TELEPHONE PROCEDURES

Performance Objectives (Procedures) in This Textbook

- Procedure 6-1 Prepare and leave a voice mail message
- Procedure 6-2 Take messages from an answering service

- Procedure 6-3 Answer incoming telephone calls
- Procedure 6-4 Place outgoing telephone calls
- Procedure 6-5 Screen telephone calls
- Procedure 6-6 Identify and manage emergency calls
- Procedure 6-7 Handle a complaint from an angry caller

Performance Objectives (Job Skills) in the Workbook

- Job Skill 6-1 Screen incoming telephone calls
- Job Skill 6-2 Prepare telephone message forms
- Job Skill 6-3 Document telephone messages and physician responses
- Job Skill 6-4 Role-play emergency telephone scenario(s)

CHAPTER 7

APPOINTMENTS

Performance Objectives (Procedures) in This Textbook

- Procedure 7-1 Prepare an appointment matrix
- Procedure 7-2 Execute appointment procedures
- Procedure 7-3 Schedule appointments in a paper-based system
- Procedure 7-4 Schedule electronic appointments
- Procedure 7-5 Reorganize patients in an emergency situation
- Procedure 7-6 Schedule surgery, complete form, and notify the patient
- Procedure 7-7 Schedule an outpatient diagnostic test

Performance Objectives (Job Skills) in the Workbook

- Job Skill 7-1 Set up appointment matrix
- Job Skill 7-2 Schedule appointments
- Job Skill 7-3 Prepare an appointment reference sheet
- Job Skill 7-4 Complete appointment cards
- Job Skill 7-5 Abstract information and complete a hospital/surgery scheduling form
- Job Skill 7-6 Transfer surgery scheduling information to a form letter
- Job Skill 7-7 Complete requisition forms to schedule outpatient diagnostic tests

CHAPTER 8

FILING PROCEDURES

Performance Objectives (Procedures) in This Textbook

- Procedure 8-1 Set up an email filing system
- Procedure 8-2 File using a subject filing system
- Procedure 8-3 Organize a tickler file
- Procedure 8-4 Determine filing units and indexing order to alphabetically file a patient's medical record
- Procedure 8-5 Label and color-code patient charts
- Procedure 8-6 Prepare, sort, and file documents in patient records
- Procedure 8-7 Locate a misfiled medical record file folder

Performance Objectives (Job Skills) in the Workbook

- Job Skill 8-1 Determine filing units
- Job Skill 8-2 Index and file names alphabetically
- Job Skill 8-3 File patient and business names alphabetically
- Job Skill 8-4 Index names on file folder labels and arrange file cards in alphabetical order
- Job Skill 8-5 Color-code file cards

CHAPTER 9

MEDICAL RECORDS

Performance Objectives (Procedures) in This Textbook

- Procedure 9-1 Prepare and compile a medical record for a new patient
- Procedure 9-2 Follow documentation guidelines to record information in a medical record
- Procedure 9-3 Correct a medical record
- Procedure 9-4 Abstract data from a medical record

Performance Objectives (Job Skills) in the Workbook

- Job Skill 9-1 Prepare a patient record and insert progress notes
- Job Skill 9-2 Prepare a patient record and format chart notes
- Job Skill 9-3 Correct a medical record
- Job Skill 9-4 Abstract from a medical record
- Job Skill 9-5 Prepare a history and physical (H & P) report
- Job Skill 9-6 Record test results on a flow sheet

CHAPTER 10

DRUG AND PRESCRIPTION RECORDS

Performance Objectives (Procedures) in This Textbook

- Procedure 10-1 Use a drug reference book to spell and locate drug information
- Procedure 10-2 Read and interpret a written prescription
- Procedure 10-3 Record medication in a patient's medical record and on a medication log

Performance Objectives (Job Skills) in the Workbook

- Job Skill 13-1 Use a physician's fee schedule to determine correct fees
- Job Skill 13-2 Complete cash receipts
- Job Skill 13-3 Interpret an explanation of benefits form
- Job Skill 13-4 Role-play collection scenarios
- Job Skill 13-5 Compose a collection letter and prepare an envelope
- Job Skill 13-6 Complete a financial agreement

CHAPTER 14
BANKING

Performance Objectives (Procedures) in This Textbook

- Procedure 14-1 Prepare a bank deposit
- Procedure 14-2 Write a check using proper format and calculate a running balance
- Procedure 14-3 Reconcile a bank statement

Performance Objectives (Job Skills) in the Workbook

- Job Skill 14-1 Prepare a bank deposit
- Job Skill 14-2 Write checks
- Job Skill 14-3 Endorse a check
- Job Skill 14-4 Inspect a check
- Job Skill 14-5 Reconcile a bank statement

CHAPTER 15
BOOKKEEPING

Performance Objectives (Procedures) in This Textbook

- Procedure 15-1 Prepare and post to a patient's account
- Procedure 15-2 Prepare the pegboard; post charges, payments, and adjustments; and balance the day sheet
- Procedure 15-3 Establish, record, balance, and replenish the petty cash fund

Performance Objectives (Job Skills) in the Workbook

- Job Skill 15-1 Post entries to ledger cards and calculate balances
- Job Skill 15-2 Prepare ledger cards
- Job Skill 15-3 Bookkeeping Day 1—Post to patient ledger cards and prepare cash receipts
- Job Skill 15-4 Bookkeeping Day 1—Prepare the daily journal
- Job Skill 15-5 Bookkeeping Day 1—Post charges, payments, and adjustments using a daily journal

- Job Skill 15-6 Bookkeeping Day 1—Balance the day sheet
- Job Skill 15-7 Bookkeeping Day 2—Prepare the daily journal
- Job Skill 15-8 Bookkeeping Day 2—Post charges, payments, and adjustments to patient ledger cards and to the daily journal; prepare cash receipts and the bank deposit
- Job Skill 15-9 Bookkeeping Day 2—Balance the day sheet
- Job Skill 15-10 Bookkeeping Day 3—Prepare the daily journal
- Job Skill 15-11 Bookkeeping Day 3—Post charges, payments, and adjustments to patient ledger cards and to the daily journal; prepare cash receipts and the bank deposit
- Job Skill 15-12 Bookkeeping Day 3—Balance the day sheet
- Job Skill 15-13 Set up the day sheet for a new month

CHAPTER 16
PROCEDURE CODING

Performance Objectives (Procedures) in This Textbook

- Procedure 16-1 Select correct procedure codes
- Procedure 16-2 Determine code selection from an operative report

Performance Objectives (Job Skills) in the Workbook

- Job Skill 16-1 Review *Current Procedural Terminology* codebook sections
- Job Skill 16-2 Code evaluation and management services
- Job Skill 16-3 Code surgical services and procedures
- Job Skill 16-4 Code radiology and laboratory services and procedures
- Job Skill 16-5 Code procedures and services in the Medicine section
- Job Skill 16-6 Code clinical examples

CHAPTER 17
DIAGNOSTIC CODING

Performance Objectives (Procedures) in This Textbook

- Procedure 17-1 Select correct diagnostic codes using *ICD-10-CM*
- Procedure 17-2 Select burn and corrosion codes
- Procedure 17-3 Select diagnostic codes from the Table of Drugs and Chemicals

Performance Objectives (Job Skills) in the Workbook

- Job Skill 17-1 Code diagnoses from Chapters 1, 2, 3, 4, and 5 in *ICD-10-CM*
- Job Skill 17-2 Code diagnoses from Chapters 6, 7, 8, 9, and 10 in *ICD-10-CM*
- Job Skill 17-3 Code diagnoses from Chapters 11, 12, 13, 14, and 15 in *ICD-10-CM*
- Job Skill 17-4 Code diagnoses from Chapters 16, 17, 18, 19, and 20 in *ICD-10-CM*
- Job Skill 17-5 Code diagnoses from Chapter 21 and the Table of Drugs and Chemicals in *ICD-10-CM*
- Job Skill 17-6 Code diagnoses from chart notes using *ICD-10-CM*

CHAPTER 18

HEALTH INSURANCE SYSTEMS AND CLAIM SUBMISSION

Performance Objectives (Procedures) in This Textbook

- Procedure 18-1 Verify insurance coverage
- Procedure 18-2 Complete the CMS-1500 Health Insurance Claim Form using OCR guidelines
- Procedure 18-3 Complete an Advance Beneficiary Notice form (ABN)

Performance Objectives (Job Skills) in the Workbook

- Job Skill 18-1 Complete a managed care authorization form
- Job Skill 18-2 Complete a health insurance claim form for a commercial case
- Job Skill 18-3 Complete a health insurance claim form for a Medicare case
- Job Skill 18-4 Complete a health insurance claim form for a TRICARE case

CHAPTER 19

OFFICE MANAGERIAL RESPONSIBILITIES

Performance Objectives (Procedures) in This Textbook

- Procedure 19-1 Develop a complaint protocol
- Procedure 19-2 Setup a staff meeting
- Procedure 19-3 Prepare a staff meeting agenda
- Procedure 19-4 Develop and maintain an employee handbook
- Procedure 19-5 Prepare an incident report
- Procedure 19-6 Compile and maintain an office policies and procedures manual
- Procedure 19-7 Recruit an employee

- Procedure 19-8 Orient a new employee
- Procedure 19-9 Manage equipment maintenance
- Procedure 19-10 Prepare an order form
- Procedure 19-11 Pay an invoice
- Procedure 19-12 Establish and maintain inventory
- Procedure 19-13 Prepare a travel expense report

Performance Objectives (Job Skills) in the Workbook

- Job Skill 19-1 Document patient complaints and determine actions to resolve problems
- Job Skill 19-2 Write an agenda for an office meeting
- Job Skill 19-3 Prepare material for an office procedures manual
- Job Skill 19-4 Perform inventory control and keep an equipment maintenance log
- Job Skill 19-5 Abstract data from a catalogue and key an order form
- Job Skill 19-6 Complete an order form for office supplies
- Job Skill 19-7 Perform mathematic calculations of an office manager
- Job Skill 19-8 Prepare two order forms
- Job Skill 19-9 Prepare a travel expense report

CHAPTER 20

FINANCIAL MANAGEMENT OF THE MEDICAL PRACTICE

Performance Objectives (Procedures) in This Textbook

- Procedure 20-1 Create headings and post entries in an accounts payable system; write checks
- Procedure 20-2 Create category headings, determine deductions, calculate payroll, and make entries to a payroll register

Performance Objectives (Job Skills) in the Workbook

- Job Skill 20-1 Perform accounts payable functions: write checks and record disbursements
- Job Skill 20-2 Pay bills and record expenditures
- Job Skill 20-3 Replenish and balance the petty cash fund
- Job Skill 20-4 Balance a check register
- Job Skill 20-5 Reconcile a bank statement
- Job Skill 20-6 Prepare payroll
- Job Skill 20-7 Complete a payroll register
- Job Skill 20-8 Complete an employee earning record
- Job Skill 20-9 Complete an employee's withholding allowance certificate
- Job Skill 20-10 Complete an employee benefit form

PREFACE

When I started preparations for the revision of *Administrative Medical Assisting*, eighth edition, I adopted the following quote by William Arthur Ward:

> ### Four Steps to Achievement
> *Plan purposefully*
> *Prepare prayerfully*
> *Proceed positively*
> *Pursue persistently*

I read this quote every morning and took to heart each step as I worked to make this edition the very best! My goals were to streamline the content in order to simplify the learning path, highlight electronic components that are now a part of the medical office, and include all skills needed by an administrative medical assistant—all while focusing on the "heart of the health care professional" who works with compassion and sensitivity while tending to the needs of patients.

In the eighth edition, an emphasis has been placed on the **electronic health record** (EHR) and a new icon has been added to identify chapter-specific content. The **health care reform** (HCR) icon remains throughout the text with updated legislative actions and implementation dates. The continued development of additional critical thinking presented in real-life scenarios helps cultivate problem-solving skills. Materials needed and referred to for Job Skills in the *Workbook* are now presented in a concise easy-to-follow list.

DEVELOPMENT OF THIS TEXT

The longevity of this award-winning *textbook*, which has been in publication for 34 years, speaks of the excellence of its founding authors, Marilyn T. Fordney and Joan J. Follis, whose great dedication, perseverance, and vision for the future role of the medical assistant helped create a working tool out of a classroom syllabus at Ventura College, California. This book has been used to expand knowledge and understanding, teach practical skills used by medical assistants all across America, as well as increase productivity in medical offices. While being mentored by these two great authors, my role has grown from a contributing author in the fourth edition, to coauthor in the fifth edition, and then becoming a primary author in the sixth, seventh, and eighth editions.

COMPETENCY-BASED LEARNING

Curriculum competencies and standards define the role and responsibilities of an administrative medical assistant, and certification tasks and test parameters help students understand topics and areas to study. Educational components for each of the following are presented in Appendix B of the *textbook* where cross-reference tables may be found that refer individual competencies to chapters and assignments within the text:

- American Medical Technologists (AMT) Medical Assisting Task List for the Registered Medical Assistant (RMA)
- Commission on Allied Health Education Programs (CAAHEP) Educational Competencies
- Accrediting Bureau of Health Education Schools (ABHES) Curriculum Competencies

xxiii

- Certified Medical Assistants (CMA [AAMA]) Certification Examination Content
- Registered Medical Assistants (RMA [AMT]) Certification Examination Competencies
- Certified Medical Administrative Specialist (CMAS [AMT]) Examination Specifications

WHO IS THIS TEXT DESIGNED FOR?

The *textbook* material is designed for the learner who plans to work as an administrative (front-office) medical assistant in a private physician's office, single- or multiple-specialty clinic, or hospital setting; however, the skills presented also apply to other technicians and assistants who perform clerical functions similar to those of an administrative medical assistant.

The book can be used in community colleges, vocational and commercial educational institutions, welfare-to-work programs, and in-service training in the private medical office. It is an appropriate textbook for a one- or two-semester course. It may be used for self-study if no formal classes are available in the community or if a medical assistant wants to increase his or her skills but is unable to attend classes. Finally, the book serves as a reference for the working medical assistant, featuring the most up-to-date methods of performing medical office tasks.

ORGANIZATION OF THE TEXT

The *textbook* and *Workbook* chapters are arranged to better facilitate learning with legal and electronic health record information integrated throughout. The chapters are divided into seven units that progress from professional and career responsibilities, interpersonal communications, records management, written communications, financial administration, and managing the medical office to the final unit, where the learner prepares for employment.

NEW TO THIS EDITION

- **Chapter 1**, *A Career as an Administrative Medial Assistant,* now includes content about job outlook and externship folded in from Chapter 21.

- **Chapter 2**, *The Health Care Environment: Past, Present, and Future,* contains new content on electronic laboratory reports, medial pioneers, and telemedicine. Content has been moved from Chapter 16 that encompasses types of managed care organizations; precertification, predetermination, and preauthorization; as well as patient referrals, medical review, and nonphysician providers. Content moved from Chapter 21 includes global influences on health care and goals to improve health care internationally.

- **Chapter 8**, *Filing Procedures,* has been simplified and rearranged to decrease information on paper-based filing and includes the following new sections on an electronic filing system: Creating electronic documents, preserving computerized reports, maintaining email files, backing up computer files, and electronic confidentiality guidelines, security, and tickler files, along with a record retention schedule.

- **Chapter 9**, *Medical Records,* has been reorganized with the paper-based system de-emphasized and the EMR system brought to the forefront. Computerized provider order entry (CPOE), cloning of medical records, and meaningful use sections are expanded and new content appears on medical scribes, various types of medical reports, medical record access and backup, Medicare documentation guidelines, as well as outside tests and test results. There are new compliance boxes, examples, figures, and exam-style review questions.

- **Chapter 13**, *The Revenue Cycle: Fees, Credit and Collection,* has been renamed to emphasize features of the revenue cycle and reorganized to include all items that address "fees" (e.g., assignment, coinsurance payment, and participating/nonparticipating physicians); these have been relocated from Chapter 16. New sections include the sliding fee schedule, online payment, receiving payment, and explanation of benefits including the Medicare Remittance Advice and Medicare Summary Notice. The section on "Billing" has been renamed to "Patient Billing" in order to differentiate it from "Insurance Billing" in Chapter 18. All content having to do with posting procedures has been moved to Chapter 15, *Bookkeeping.* The "History of Credit" has been moved to the end of the chapter, prior to "History of Credit Laws."

- **Chapter 15**, *Bookkeeping*, now includes all related posting content (moved from Chapters 13 and 14) with five new examples, a new figure, and two new exam-style questions.

- **Chapter 16**, *Procedure Coding*, has been split off from Chapter 17—*Diagnostic Coding*. New items include: Learning objectives, procedure (Determine Code Selections from an Operative Report), 13 key terms, table on observation status, six examples, stop and think scenario, and six exam-style questions. New sections include: Encoders, hospital admits and observation status, and how to code from an operative report. The table on modifiers has been reconfigured, reduced, and updated.

- **Chapter 17**, *Diagnostic Coding*, has been reorganized with a focus on coding all chapters in *ICD-10-CM*. It has the following new items: Five objectives, a procedure (Select Diagnostic Codes from the Table of Drugs and Chemicals), six key terms, nine codebook terms, two compliance boxes, two examples, and new sections that include: The encounter form, encoders and computer-assisted coding, codebook official guidelines, principal versus primary diagnosis, linking codes for medical necessity, code edits and audits, combination codes, the alphabetic index (Volume II), the tabular list (Volume I), chapter-specific coding guidelines, and myocardial infarction.

- **Chapter 18**, *Health Insurance Systems and Claim Submission*, has five new figures depicting insurance cards for private insurance, Medicaid, Part D prescription drugs, TRICARE, and CHAMPVA. It also includes a new table on the type of health insurance coverage in the United States, a major update on Health Care Reform, and two new procedures (18-1, Verify Insurance Coverage and 18-3, Complete an Advance Beneficiary Notice). The bulk of information on managed care has been moved to Chapter 2, and information on methods of payment, the physician's fee schedule, UCR payments, relative value studies, the physician's fee profile, and capitation has been moved to Chapter 13. New sections include: Health insurance identification card, provider contracts, Genetic Information Nondiscrimination Act, Medicare National and Local Coverage Determinations, Physician Quality Reporting System, senior-assisted programs, insurance-related identification numbers, claim adjudication and payment, comprehensive error rate testing program, recovery audit contractor review, unprocessed claims, missing and incorrect information, and unpaid or denied claims.

CONTENT FEATURES

New features are preceded by an asterisk (*).

- *****Chapter content** is updated in all chapters to reflect changes in competency requirements, technology, job responsibilities, insurance regulations, legal directives, and compliance mandates.

- **Objectives** are divided into (1) Learning Objectives that state chapter goals, (2) Performance Objectives in the *textbook* that contain a numbered list of step-by-step procedures, and (3) Performance Objectives for the *Workbook* containing a numbered list of Job Skills, provided as an opportunity for practice.

- **Customer service** is emphasized at the beginning of each chapter in a section titled *Heart of the Health Care Professional*.

- *****Key terms** introduce the student to basic terminology at the beginning of each chapter and are listed throughout the chapter in bold, colored type, with expanded definitions in the glossary at the end of the textbook. Multiple key terms have been added to reflect current trends in terminology.

- *****Italicized terms* have been included throughout the text to emphasize additional terms that are routinely used in today's health care profession and competency language. These terms are also listed in the index to help ease finding key topics.

- *****Photographs** visually support textual content and give the learner a better perspective of the office duties and situations mentioned. New photos are found in Chapters 1, 2, 4, 8 and 13.

- *****Icons** give quick reference to Customer Service applications, Compliance issues, Health Care Reform, Patient Education boxes, Procedures, Stop and Think Case Scenarios, Summary of Certification Topics, Exam-Style Review Questions, Workbook Assignments, and Resources. An icon for the Electronic Health Record (EHR) has been added within the chapter material for this edition to help the reader locate content related to today's electronic medical office.

- *****Compliance issues** mandated by the federal government are emphasized by a color-screened box with an icon for quick identification. New boxes occur in Chapters 9, 12, 13, and 17. Each is titled and many cite HIPAA regulations.

- *****Patient Education boxes** describe how the medical assistant should keep the patient informed. New boxes occur in Chapters 3 and 4; each is titled and indexed to help locate various types of educational situations.

- *****Figures, tables,** and **examples**, enhanced in full color, present information in a succinct, easy-to-understand format.

New Figures may be found in Chapter 9, (sample letter from a medical clinic advising patients about a new EHR system) and Chapter 15 (practice management software system screenshot).

New or Enhanced Tables may be found throughout the *textbook*, which provide an orderly arrangement of detailed data.

New Examples (#18) are titled and indexed and each of these components is numbered for easy reference. These aids are referred to throughout each chapter to clarify concepts, illustrate graphics, and depict realistic scenarios.

INSTRUCTIONAL FEATURES

New features are preceded by an asterisk (*).

- *****Procedures** include step-by-step directions for completing tasks in the medical office. Each is numbered and listed at the beginning of each chapter, and many are cross-referenced to be referred to while completing Job Skills in the *Workbook*. New procedures have been added to Chapters 7, 15, 16, 17, and 18; others have been enhanced totaling over 100 procedures.

- *****Critical Thinking Component** is presented in Stop and Think Case Scenarios, which appear at the end of each chapter. These questions help stimulate the thought process and exercise reasoning skills. New scenarios may be found in Chapters 2, 5, 6, 7, and 16. (Answers are found in the *Instructor Resources*.)

- **Focus on Certification** summarizes the key areas of study for students who are preparing to take the CMA (AAMA), RMA (AMT), or CMAS (AMT) certification exams.

- *****Exam-Style Review Questions** offer a quick review of key points in the same multiple-choice format as seen on certification examinations. New questions have been added and others revised. (Answers are found in the *Instructor Resources*.)

- *****Workbook Assignments** are divided into:

(1) *Review Questions*, which include all major topics. New questions have been added to multiple chapters and others have been rewritten and/or reordered to follow chapter material.

(2) *Critical Thinking Exercises*, which stimulate reasoning capabilities. Ten new telephone role-playing scenarios have been added to Chapter 6; other new questions appear in Chapters 2 and 3.

(3) *Job Skills*, which offer step-by-step directions and hands-on practice for all major tasks an administrative medical assistant performs. The materials needed and referred to under "Conditions" now appear in a bulleted list for easy reference. (Answers are found in the *Instructor Resources*.)

- *****Resources,** listed at the end of each chapter, have been updated and include booklets, books, medical directives, newsletters, professional magazines, and organizations pertinent to each chapter topic. Most Internet site addresses have been eliminated due to frequent changes and instead "Search for" suggestions have been added.

- *****CMS-1500 Claim Form Instructions and Templates**, found in Appendix A, offer a quick reference. A template of the new CMS-1500 form (02/12) is shown as well as each field, with updated instructions for commercial payers, Medicare (Medicare/Medicaid, Medicare/Medigap, MSP), and TRICARE.

LEARNING PACKAGE

Workbook ISBN 978-1-305-85918-0

There is great synergy between the *textbook* and the *Workbook*, which is an essential resource available for use. A realistic approach is experienced as the student assumes that he or she is employed by two physicians who are married to each other and who share a professional corporation. Through job skill exercises, the student, assuming the role of the administrative medical assistant, performs a variety of duties that are a realistic part of the day-by-day activities in the joint office of a general practitioner and a family practitioner. Following, major changes are listed in a brief section on "What is new to this edition" and a list of features. New features are preceded by an asterisk (*).

New to This Edition of the *Workbook*

- **Chapter 13**, *The Revenue Cycle: Fees, Credit, and Collection,* has been modified so that all posting exercises are now located in Chapter 15, *Bookkeeping.*
- **Chapter 16**, *Procedure Coding,* contains new review questions to reinforce new material.
- **Chapter 17**, *Diagnostic Coding,* has 18 new review questions and a new job skill—Code from Chart Notes.
- **Editable PDFs of the *Blank Forms*** are now found exclusively online. These Blank Forms are realistic and similar to those found in medical offices; they are necessary to complete a variety of job skill exercises found in the *Workbook.* They can be found on the free Student Companion site accompanying this *textbook* by going to www.cengagebrain.com and searching either by author and title (French *Administrative Medical Assistant,* eighth edition) or by ISBN (9781305859173). Once accessed, the forms can be downloaded and completed electronically or printed and filled out manually.

Part I

- **Abbreviation and Spelling Review** incorporates medical terminology into a short chart note for each chapter, giving learners an opportunity to write definitions for abbreviations and spell medical terms. (Answers are found in the online *Instructor Resources.*)
- ***Review Questions*** cover key points in chapters, address areas not covered in the Exam-Style Review Questions in the text, and are presented in various formats to increase learning. New questions have been added and others reordered to follow the content. (Answers are found in the online *Instructor Resources.*)
- ***Critical Thinking Exercises*** offer learners an opportunity to address situations and solve problems that are realistic to an office setting. New questions have been added to various chapters. (Answers are found in the online *Instructor Resources.*)

- ***Job Skill*** exercises offer students experience as they practice tasks realistic to the medical office. Step-by-step directions incorporate *Performance Evaluation Checklists* so students and instructors have both detailed directions and the checklist in the same area. The student has three attempts to complete each job skill and points have been assigned proportionate to the time and effort the student spends completing the exercise and performing the skill. Job Skill interactive forms are now located on the student/instructor companion website at www.cengagebrain.com. There are over 150 job skills and each one is cross-referenced to CAAHEP and ABHES competencies. (Answers are found in the online *Instructor Resources.*)

Appendices

- **Appendix A** for Practon Medical Group, Inc., lists references for the simulated medical practice and states office policies to be followed while completing exercises and making decisions that relate to the operations of a medical office. A **mock fee schedule** with procedure codes that are organized according to sections in the *CPT* codebook include descriptions of services and fees followed by *CPT* modifiers and a small selection of *HCPCS Level II* codes with descriptions and fees.
- **Appendix B: List of Abbreviations** includes all abbreviation tables found in the text in one location.

Student Companion Website

(www.cengagebrain.com)

This student website provides students with the editable *PDF Blank Forms* needed to complete many of the activities in the *Workbook.* Chapter 21: Seeking a Position as an Administrative Medical Assistant is provided as a valuable online supplement to the text. Students can also access comprehensive support slides created in Microsoft PowerPoint to use in study and review.

MindTap to Accompany *Administrative Medical Assisting*, Eighth Edition

MindTap is a fully online, interactive learning experience built upon authoritative Cengage Learning content. By combining readings, multimedia, activities, and assessments into a singular learning path, MindTap elevates learning by providing real-world application to better engage students. Instructors customize the learning path by selecting Cengage Learning resources and adding their own content via apps that integrate into the MindTap framework seamlessly with many learning management systems.

The guided learning path demonstrates the importance of the medical assistant through engagement activities and interactive exercises. Learners can apply their understanding of the material through interactive activities taken from Critical Thinking Challenge 3.0 and the Medical Assisting Learning Lab, in addition to quizzing, certification-style assessments, and case studies. These simulations elevate the study of medical assisting by challenging students to apply concepts to practice. Videos from the Medical Assisting Video series are incorporated to demonstrate key skills correctly in a dynamic and engaging way. Additional resources including Online Job Skills, flashcards, transcription tapes, and self-review make MindTap the most comprehensive package for Administrative Medical Assisting instruction and learning.

To learn more, visit www.cengage.com/mindtap.

INSTRUCTIONAL PACKAGE

Instructor Companion Site

Deliver powerful lectures, create lesson plans, customize exams, and monitor student progress throughout the course with the tools provided on the online *Instructor Companion Site*. Access the *Instructor Companion Site* at www.cengagebrain.com, and use your Cengage Learning faculty account to log in. Once inside, add the *textbook* to your dashboard to view these resources:

- Customize the **electronic Instructor Manual files** to individual class needs.
- Deliver effective presentations with chapter **presentations in Microsoft PowerPoint**.
- Create quizzes and tests to monitor student progress with the **Computerized Test Bank**, which can be delivered through your school's learning management system, provided as paper tests, or integrated and delivered right through MindTap.
- Complete *Curriculum* with detailed lesson outlines for each Unit.
- Access to all Student Resources.

Electronic Instructor's Manual

An Electronic Instructors Manual is available on the Instructor Companion Site for use with this *textbook*, offering the following features. New features are preceded by an asterisk (*).

- **General Instructions** cover materials and equipment, audiovisual aids, instructor resources, online companion website features, competency-based learning, job skill competency checklists with automated grading and correcting using grading software programs,* updated competency tables, outline and contents of the course, student evaluation, and evaluation of course and instructor.

Section I: Textbook and Workbook Answer Key

Each chapter contains:

- *CAAHEP Areas of Competence listed according to the Cognitive, Psychomotor, and Affective domains that pertain to each chapter.
- *ABHES Areas of Competence that pertain to each chapter.
- **Lesson Plan** Suggestions offer ideas for topics to discuss with a list of activities to assign.
- **Additional Activities** are suggested for each chapter and could be adopted to enhance class time and motivate students or assigned as extra credit.
- **Abbreviation and Spelling Review** chart note answers appear for *Workbook* chapters.
- **Stop-and-Think Case Scenarios and Answers** are included to aid the instructor with discussion of possible answers to problems presented in realistic office situations.
- **Exam-Style Review Question Answers** are included for the *textbook's* end-of-chapter multiple-choice questions.
- **Review Questions and Answers** provide an easy reference source during class discussion or independent assignment correction.
- **Critical Thinking Exercises and Answers** are listed for easy reference during class discussion or independent assignment correction.
- **Job Skill Answer Keys** are listed with rationales and various forms are illustrated to assist the instructor with correction.

Section II: Medical Terminology and Abbreviation Tests

- **Review Tests** provide a review of terms and abbreviation definitions.

Instructors' feedback and comments on the *textbook* and all ancillary materials are welcome and should be emailed or addressed to the publisher or author using the addresses listed in the *Instructor Resources*.

Section III: Educational Competencies

Competency-Based Learning

- AMT Medical Assisting Task List for the RMA

Competency Tables for:

- CAAHEP Educational Competencies
- ABHES Competencies
- CMA (AAMA) Certification Examination Content
- RMA (AMT) Certification Examination Competencies
- CMAS (AMT) Examination Specifications

SUMMARY

One of the things that makes medical assisting such an exciting field is its ever-changing nature; nothing stays the same. Thus, it is essential that all medical personnel attend workshops and continue to update their knowledge by reading current notices such as those listed in the expanded *Resources* section at the end of each chapter. It is my hope that this learning package will assist in patient care by helping to educate competent, service-oriented medical assistants and will be a stepping stone to new knowledge, understanding, appreciation, and advancement in the medical assisting profession.

Linda L. French, CMA-C (AAMA), NCICS, CPC
Email: Frenchmedical@aol.com

ACKNOWLEDGMENTS

I would like to thank the founding authors, Marilyn T. Fordney and Joan J. Follis, who had a vision and pursued their dream with great dedication, perseverance, an abundance of hope, and plenty of enthusiasm, which made this textbook what it is today. I feel blessed to have grown from a contributing author, to a coauthor, and now a primary author. It is my desire to continue this vision into the future. Many students, physicians, friends, colleagues, and instructors have contributed valuable suggestions and interesting material throughout the years and I wish to express my thanks to all of them.

I am indebted to many individuals on the staff of Delmar Cengage Learning for encouragement and guidance. I express particular appreciation to Juliet Steiner and Patty Gaworecki, content developers who worked with me day-by-day, answered questions, and helped motivate me along the way. I want to thank Stephen G. Smith, product team manager—health care, who added a fresh voice and insight to this project. Special thanks go to, senior content project manager, Thomas Heffernan, for overseeing the production process, and, managing art director, Jack Pendleton, for the beautiful color and unique design. I would also like to thank the staff of Publishing Services, especially, project editor, and, copyeditors, who did an excellent job of tending to all the details a book of this magnitude presents while moving it through the production process.

Special thanks are extended to Carolyn Talesfore, advertising and promotion manager of Bibbero Systems, Inc., and her staff in Petaluma, California, for designing the new multipurpose billing form with *ICD-10-CM* codes and for all of their products that have been used in the text throughout the years so that students can see and work with realistic forms. Several other medical office supply companies were kind enough to cooperate by providing forms and descriptive literature of their products and their names will be found throughout the text and *Workbook* figures.

Connie Allen
Wallace State Community College
Hanceville, AL

Janet Booth
Tyler Junior College
Tyler, TX

Jean Brown
Wake Technical Community College
Raleigh, NC

Sybil Burrell
Jefferson State Community College
Homewood, AL

Rhoda Cooper
Piedmont Virginia Community College
Rice, VA

Louise Corcoran
Springfield Technical Community College
Palmer, MA

Cynthia Imber
Delaware County Community College
Ford, PA

Lindsey Klimek
Alexandria Technical and Community College
Alexandria, MN

Kathy Locke
Spartanburg Community College
Alsip, IL

Michelle McClatchey
Westwood College
Hammond, IN

Tracey McKethan
Springfield Technical Community College
Westfield, MA

Nancy Measell
Ivy Tech Community College
South Bend, IN

Tanya Ocampo
Meridian Community College
Meridian, MS

Diana Reeder
Maysville Community and Technical College
Morehead, KY

Becky Rodenbaugh
Baker College
Cadillac, MI

Linda Scarborough
Lanier Technical College
Gainesville, GA

Debra Tymcio
National College
Atwater, OH

Rebecca Voelker
Baker College of Cadillac
McBain, MI

Maria Washington
Bryant Stratton College
Rochester, NY

ABOUT THE AUTHOR

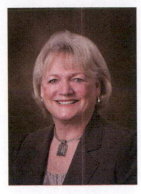

LINDA L. FRENCH,
CMA-C (AAMA), NCICS, CPC

Linda French worked in a physician office setting for 15 years performing administrative and clinical duties including medical insurance billing and was then promoted to office manager. She became a Certified Medical Assistant-Clinical Specialist through the American Association of Medical Assistants in 1982. The practices included obstetrics and gynecology, internal medicine-cardiology, orthopedics, and chiropractic medicine.

In 1995, she began her teaching career at Simi Valley Adult School where she expanded medical insurance billing-related classes and developed a coding program. In 1999, she became certified as a National Certified Insurance Coding Specialist through the National Center for Competency Testing and in 2002 received her Certified Professional Coding certificate through the American Academy of Professional Coders. In addition to teaching at the Adult School for 10 years, she also taught medically related classes at two community colleges, several private post-secondary institutions, and private corporations through the University of California at Santa Barbara's UCSB-Extend program.

She is a member of several national professional organizations and has contributed to a number of textbooks, including *Understanding Medical Coding: A Comprehensive Guide* (by Sandra L. Johnson, Delmar, 2000), and coauthored *Medical Insurance Billing and Coding: An Essentials Worktext* (W. B. Saunders, 2003). She lectures on occasion, has done private consulting work for physicians, and has performed customized employee training for a private billing service.

Unit 1

PROFESSIONAL AND CAREER RESPONSIBILITIES

CHAPTER 1

A CAREER AS AN ADMINISTRATIVE MEDICAL ASSISTANT

LEARNING OBJECTIVES

After reading this chapter and learning step-by-step procedures to gain job skills,* you should be able to:

- Demonstrate how customer service skills are applied in the medical office.
- Describe the variety of career advantages, employment opportunities, areas of specialization, and job prospects for those trained as administrative medical assistants.
- Itemize 10 job responsibilities of an administrative medical assistant.
- List interpersonal skills needed to be an administrative medical assistant.
- Establish priorities and implement time management principles to organize and perform clerical duties.
- Compare and contrast assertive and aggressive behavior.
- Discuss patient reactions to health problems and your role when interacting with a distressed patient or family member.
- Explain various patient reactions to death and name the stages of dying.
- Define stress and identify strategies to reduce stress and burnout.
- State various components in professionalism.
- Understand the importance of and opportunities for certification or registration in your area of study.
- Relate how a health care professional can keep current in medical knowledge, policies, procedures, and the latest trends in the medical community.

PERFORMANCE OBJECTIVES (PROCEDURES) IN THIS TEXTBOOK

- Interpret and accurately spell medical terms and abbreviations (Procedure 1-1).

PERFORMANCE OBJECTIVES (JOB SKILLS) IN THE WORKBOOK

- Interpret and accurately spell medical terms and abbreviations (Job Skill 1-1).
- Use the Internet to look up key terms and hear pronunciations (Job Skill 1-2).
- Prioritize a task list to practice time management skills (Job Skill 1-3).

---

*This textbook *and the accompanying* Workbook *meet the educational components for entry-level administrative and general competencies outlined by CAAHEP and ABHES.*

- Use the Internet to obtain information on certification or registration (Job Skill 1-4).
- Use the Internet to test your knowledge of anatomy and physiology or medical terminology (Job Skill 1-5).
- Develop a medical practice survey (Job Skill 1-6).

KEY TERMS

accreditation

administrative medical assistant

aggressive

American Association of Medical Assistants (AAMA)

American Medical Technologists (AMT)

assertive

burnout

certification

Certified Clinical Medical Assistant (CCMA)

Certified Medical Administrative Assistant (CMAA)

Certified Medical Administrative Specialist (CMAS [AMT])

Certified Medical Assistant (CMA [AAMA])

clinical medical assistant

continuing education units (CEUs)

empathy

flextime

hospice

interpersonal skills

licensure

multiskilled health practitioner (MSHP)

National Center for Competency Testing (NCCT)

National Certified Medical Assistant (NCMA)

National Certified Medical Office Assistant (NCMOA)

National Healthcareer Association (NHA)

patient navigator

professionalism

recertification

Registered Medical Assistant (RMA [AMT])

registration

stress

sympathy

HEART OF THE HEALTH CARE PROFESSIONAL

Service

Motto: *Think with empathy, act through service.*

The heart of the health care professional should be directed at serving patients. Regardless of your duties, service is woven into all areas of medical assisting. You have the ability to make this world a better place by becoming a vital part of a health care team and serving patients' needs. Believe in yourself, always do your best, and remember—there is no goal you cannot achieve.

WELCOME TO ADMINISTRATIVE MEDICAL ASSISTING

Welcome to *Administrative Medical Assisting*. You have taken the first step into a world that will stimulate your mind, motivate your curiosity, energize your work ethic, and enliven your spirit so that you will want to learn and contribute something good to today's society.

A typical day in a medical office might include expediting an appointment so that an anxious mother can bring in her ill infant, building rapport with a teenager who is afraid to tell the doctor about her promiscuous behavior, calming a patient who is angry about a bill, reassuring a pregnant mother who is experiencing morning sickness for the first time, or offering a listening ear to a patient who has just received a problematic diagnosis. Every day is different and exciting, and each day offers challenges and opportunities for personal growth and advancement. It is an ever-changing, dynamic field, one where fascinating breakthroughs are taking place in patient care and technology and one in which the rewards always outweigh the task at hand.

Whether you are learning clerical skills to perform as an administrative medical assistant, pharmacy technician, massage therapist, or other type of health care professional, this book will help you learn step-by-step procedures needed to perform a full range of activities to master job skills that will enable you to demonstrate customer service, educate patients, and call upon your newly learned knowledge. As you become proficient in medical terminology and learn guidelines and laws, they will help you manage patient care and create a safe environment to promote healing. You will play an integral role in a medical office as you work closely with physicians or pharmacists and become a lifeline to many patients who rely upon you to educate and assist them. "The versatility of a well prepared medical assistant is what the physician practices are looking for and need to stay afloat in today's global market."*

CUSTOMER SERVICE-ORIENTED PRACTICE

A vibrant medical practice is a service-oriented practice where the elements of customer service are demonstrated by the physician, management team, and all employees. Satisfied patients are the key to a health care provider's success. A willingness to serve patients is an attribute that all health care professionals need—those who do not have this attitude are in the wrong career. Serving means putting someone else's needs before your own. Patients often interrupt daily work routines, so it is imperative to continually remind yourself that serving the needs of patients is the reason for going into this profession (Figure 1-1).

Within the "Heart of the Health Care Professional," as shown at the beginning of each chapter, is a variety of ways to serve patients. As you work your way through this text and study the step-by-step procedures that will help you perform new job skills, you will be able to determine different ways that you can provide good customer service. Remember, each employee and patient may have a different idea about what "good" service means. All employees are customer service personnel at the same time they are performing other duties. Any time you have contact with a patient, it has an effect. Always put the patient above your own needs and routine duties. The following questions will help you determine where customer service occurs:

- Has the patient's confidentiality been protected and physical safety ensured?
- Has the patient been dealt with in a courteous, respectful, and caring manner?
- How is the task that you are performing beneficial to the patient?

*Medical Assisting Education Review Board (MAERB) 2009 report on administrative competencies.

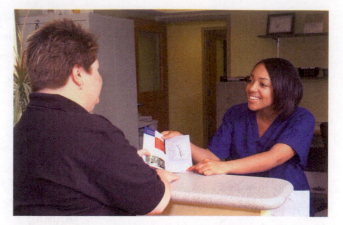

FIGURE 1-1 An administrative medical assistant serving a patient by explaining office policies

- How can this task be accomplished efficiently?
- Are you observing patient interactions, and are you aware if there is patient involvement or problems?
- What is the desired outcome for the patient?
- Have the patient's expectations been met?
- Have you seized every opportunity to educate the patient?

Another way to serve the patient is by taking on the role of a **patient navigator**. A patient navigator provides emotional support and helps coordinate patient care by connecting patients with resources and guiding them through the health care system so that timely care is provided. Trained, culturally sensitive patient navigators are frequently used when a chronic disease, such as cancer, heart disease, or diabetes, exists so that informed medical decisions can be made and the treatment plan is understood and followed.

The medical assistant is in a prime position to orient the patient to office policies so that information is gathered, schedules are kept, and treatment is

Patient Education

The physician may ask you, as a competent and knowledgeable medical assistant, to educate patients. The doctor should provide guidelines and give you parameters on the information or instructions he or she would like you to share. You will see Patient Education boxes with this icon throughout this text. These boxes can be used to gain insight regarding a variety of ways to instruct patients.

uninterrupted. Information about treatment and medications, test results, pre- and postoperative care, personal and physical safety, and community services may also be relayed.

He or she may help the physician educate patients to take better care of themselves with respect to smoking cessation, eating a balanced diet, maintaining optimal weight, increasing exercise, good hygiene, body mechanics, and learning methods for stress management. Patient education is ongoing and takes many forms. In some medical practices, the medical assistant may teach the patient using health-related educational materials, such as brochures, DVDs, or other visual aids. The Internet is also available for research, and a technical-savvy physician can help you direct patients to approved sites. Or, it can be as simple as answering a question, explaining a procedure, assisting with paperwork, or demonstrating as you give instruction. If you give patients new information and they indicate they understand, access their understanding by having them summarize the new information. No matter which method is used, the goal is to inform and teach patients on their level, so they can understand how to take an active part in their medical care (Figure 1-2).

CAREER ADVANTAGES

Medical assisting, both clinical and administrative, attracts individuals with an interest in people and medicine. The skills and knowledge required for this career will last a lifetime, and work is available anywhere in the world that medicine is practiced. A training

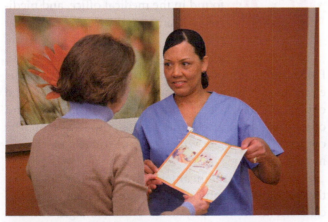

FIGURE 1-2 Patient education requires skill in communicating instructions to patients in language appropriate to their needs

program prepares the individual for a variety of employment opportunities. It may be combined with further education and can result in both certification or registration and a college degree. The work is rewarding and challenging because of its variety and ever-changing nature. Part-time, **flextime**, and full-time employment are available in a variety of medical settings, as described in Chapter 2.

Flextime offers the employee a range of hours (instead of fixed hours), which may include a split shift, coming in early, leaving late, or working different times on different days to maximize the efficient running of the office.

EMPLOYMENT OPPORTUNITIES

According to experts in career outlook, a variety of positions in the health care field are estimated to grow much faster than the average. The health care industry will continue to expand because of technological advances in medicine and the growth and aging of the population. Among those are clerical or administrative jobs in medical assisting and specialty career options such as bookkeeper, insurance and coding specialist, managed care coordinator, medication assistant, patient care technician, patient navigator, pharmacy technician, physical therapist aid, and pediatric medical assistant. Some of these career options offer specialized certifications. Although the terms *medical assistant* and *administrative medical assistant* are used primarily in this text, many of the job functions are similar to the clerical duties performed by other allied health professionals specializing in these areas.

Job Outlook

According to the U.S. Department of Labor *Occupational Outlook Handbook* (2012 edition), a 29% growth rate is predicted for medical assistants from 2012 to 2022. The *Handbook* also states that, "Medical assistants with formal training or experience—particularly those with certification—should have the best job opportunities, since employers generally prefer to hire these workers" (see Table 1-1).

Administrative Medical Assistant

Employment opportunities for those with clerical skills are available in physicians' offices (both solo and group practices), clinics, hospitals, dental offices, foundations, research institutes, public school health service

TABLE 1-1 Job Projection Data*

Occupational Title	2014 Employment	2024 Projected Employment
Medical assistants	591,300	730,200

*U.S. Department of Labor *Occupational Outlook Handbook*, 2014–2015 edition.

departments, prisons, the armed services, insurance companies, public health departments, medical departments of large companies, Medicare agencies, managed care organizations, offices of nurse practitioners, outpatient facility centers, laboratories, pharmaceutical companies, and medical instrument and supply firms. Employment opportunities are also available in the fields of manufacturing, publishing, and teaching; and in freelancing, for example, as a self-employed insurance biller or medical transcriptionist, now known as a *medical language specialist* (MLS) or *speech recognition technician* (SRT).

Clinical Medical Assistant

The clinical medical assistant performs back-office or clinical duties, such as assisting during physical examinations, maintaining treatment rooms, sterilizing instruments, assisting with minor surgery, giving injections, performing electrocardiograms (ECGs), obtaining vital signs, performing phlebotomy, and doing laboratory procedures.

Those who want active involvement and a great variety of duties can become medical assistants performing both administrative and clinical duties. (Online Chapter 21 has information on finding a job.)

The clinical duties mentioned, however, are beyond the scope of this book.

ADMINISTRATIVE MEDICAL ASSISTANT JOB RESPONSIBILITIES

The position of administrative medical assistant requires medical knowledge, organizational and business skills, and the ability to meet accepted performance standards of health care workers. Managed care has had an impact on the way in which medical assistants perform their jobs, and additional documents must be completed for preauthorization of tests or surgeries. Patients must be greeted, either on the telephone or on their arrival at the office. Appointments must be

carefully scheduled for efficient use of every working moment. Written correspondence involves composing or transcribing dictated letters, and a medical assistant should have a good command of the English language—and sometimes additional languages. Insurance forms need to be completed and submitted, and the mail must be screened for security, opened, sorted, and acted on. Patients' chart notes must be keyed into an electronic medical record (EMR) system to record the progress of the patient. Medical documents must be scanned and filed or transmitted electronically or photocopied and faxed to other facilities. Medical and office supplies have to be ordered and an inventory kept. The medical assistant oversees the reception room, making certain that furniture and magazines are in order and plants are fed and watered.

The administrative medical assistant is also in charge of collecting fees, billing patients, maintaining records on accounts receivable, and collecting overdue accounts, so basic mathematic skills are necessary. When invoices arrive, there are checks to be written for payment and records to be maintained on accounts payable. Banking and payroll may be two more of the medical assistant's functions.

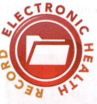

Electronic Health Record

Computer technology is now routinely found in the medical office, and medical assistants need to know computer programs to operate an electronic health record (EHR) system, maintain EMRs and patient accounts, transmit insurance claims electronically, obtain information from the Internet, and communicate via electronic mail with patients and other businesses. Each time you see the EHR icon, the content following it will focus on today's electronic medical office.

A fluency in medical terminology is imperative so that communication can take place between the medical assistant and the physician, office manager, coworkers, patients, and outside professionals. Medicolegal knowledge is vital in avoiding medical professional liability suits.

When the physician attends a convention or delivers a lecture, the assistant may be responsible for preparing the manuscript and setting up travel arrangements. Hospital admissions need to be arranged as well as surgeries scheduled. Telephone calls come in from patients, laboratories, physicians, representatives of pharmaceutical companies, equipment manufacturers, and the physician's family, and all require expertise and tact. As you have read, the administrative medical assistant performs a multitude of job skills and is responsible for the smooth functioning of the medical office.

A generic job description for an entry-level administrative medical assistant is presented in Figure 1-3. Although this is not a complete list of job responsibilities or performance standards, it provides an overview of what an individual does on the job when working in this career. It may also serve as a guideline for an employer who is developing a job description. Subsequent chapters and job skills in the *Workbook* that accompanies this text will help you achieve the many skills outlined in this job description.

INTERPERSONAL SKILLS

Being a medical assistant is more than a job—it is a career. The career of medical assisting requires many office and **interpersonal skills** often referred to as "soft skills." These are positive behavior traits and exemplary personality characteristics. They include business etiquette, commitment, consideration and respect for others, creativity, critical thinking, dedication, drive, enthusiasm, friendliness, genuineness, initiative, integrity, negotiation skills, openness, oral communication skills, social grace, team spirit, a sense of warmth and sensitivity, a positive attitude, and a willingness to learn and take on responsibility. However, the most important personality traits are liking people and being able to get along with other individuals.

The ability to keep information confidential honors patients' rights and instills trust. Patients need to know they can count on health care workers to be discreet. Everything a medical assistant sees, hears, or reads in the office is privileged information.

Listen and Observe

Listening and *observing* are important skills to use when trying to understand a viewpoint or evaluating a patient's behavior. They allow you to decide what response is best (see Chapter 4).

Interest and Concern

Patients expect the assistant to act toward them with a sincere desire to help. To show *interest* and *concern* for their welfare acknowledges patients as individuals with special needs. Tone of voice can convey this concern in person or over the telephone.

Respect

Respect is something we each desire. Following are some ways to gain and give respect, but we must first love and respect ourselves. Always keep an open mind and try to understand another's viewpoint. Listen without interrupting and take others' feelings into consideration. Do not pressure others into agreeing with you; instead agree to disagree. Be a friend and build your coworkers up instead of tearing them down. Be honest, communicate directly, and build trust by fulfilling obligations and completing work projects in a timely manner. Respect is holding a special regard for someone and it can be obtained and shown by following the Golden Rule: *Do to others as you would have them do to you.*

Sensitivity to Others

It is important to be *sensitive* to a patient's feelings; pretending that feelings do not exist does not serve the patient's best interest. Dealing with ill people who are often cranky, depressed, or angry at their situation makes it even more important to always be pleasant. It requires the use of discretion and tact to know what to say in a variety of situations.

Empathetic and Positive Attitude

When an emergency arises, the ability to follow instructions is imperative, as is using sound judgment, maintaining a calm demeanor, and displaying **empathy**. Being able to put yourself in the patient's situation or understanding his or her point of view (Example 1-1) is the basis of empathy; you need not agree with the

EXAMPLE 1-1

Empathetic Phrases

"You seem to be upset."

"That must have been painful."

"How disturbing."

"What a frustration."

ADMINISTRATIVE MEDICAL ASSISTANT JOB DESCRIPTION

Knowledge, skills, and abilities

1. Minimum education level consists of high school graduation or equivalent and (a) a certificate from a 1- or 2-year medical assisting program emphasizing administrative procedures, (b) an associate degree, or (c) the equivalent in work experience and continuing education.

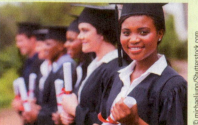

2. Knowledge of basic medical terminology, math skills, and insurance claims completion; anatomy and physiology, diseases, surgeries, medical specialties, and various administrative procedures as required in areas of responsibility.
3. Ability to operate computer, scanner, photocopy, facsimile, and calculator equipment.
4. Understand commercial medical software programs, electronic medical record management, and telemedicine.
5. Written and oral communication skills, including grammar, punctuation, and style.
6. Knowledge of and the ability to use procedure and diagnostic codebooks as well as an understanding of computerized coding programs.
7. Ability to key or type a minimum of 45 wpm.
8. Ability to follow directions, participate as part of a team, as well as work independently.

Working conditions

Medical office setting. Sufficient lighting and work space, adjustable chair, and adequate office supplies.

Physical demands

Prolonged sitting, standing, and walking, using computer equipment. Some stooping, reaching, climbing, and bending. Occasional lifting of several pounds to a height of 5 feet. Hearing and speech capabilities necessary to communicate with patients and staff in person and on telephone. Vision capable of viewing computer monitors, calculators, charts, forms, text, and numbers for prolonged periods.

Salary

Employer would list range of remuneration for the position.

Job responsibilities	Performance standards
1. Exhibits an understanding of ethical and business.	1.1 Observes policies and procedures related to medicolegal responsibilities related to confidentiality, medical records, and all professional liability matters in a physician's office practice. 1.2 Meets standards of professional etiquette and ethical conduct. 1.3 Recognizes and reports potential medicolegal problems to appropriate individuals.
2. Receives incoming telephone calls, places calls, and documents certain types of calls.	2.1 Screens incoming telephone calls properly. 2.2 Logs telephone calls and documents certain types of phone calls in patients' medical records.
3. Schedules and reschedules appointments.	3.1 Maintains appointments accurately. 3.2 Obtains precertification, predetermination, and/or preauthorization for services and procedures when necessary.

FIGURE 1-3 A generic job description for an entry-level administrative medical assistant. This is a practical, useful compilation of the basic job responsibilities. It is not a complete list of duties and responsibilities but may be used as a guideline when developing a job description.

ADMINISTRATIVE MEDICAL ASSISTANT JOB DESCRIPTION (continued)

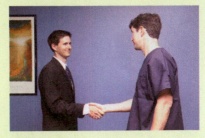

Job responsibilities

4. Greets and receives patients and visitors.

5. Registers new patients and updates existing records.

6. Screens for security, opens, sorts, and distributes mail, electronic mail, and faxed communications.

7. Maintains reception room and business office.

8. Maintains inventory and orders supplies.

9. Documents prescription refills.

10. Prepares electronic records or charts.

11. Files and refiles patient charts and documents.

12. Operates computer and calculator equipment.

13. Keys correspondence and/or transcribes patients' chart notes.

14. Prepares and posts transactions in computer or on daysheets.

15. Posts transactions in computer or on ledgers (accounts).

16. Executes banking responsibilities.

Performance standards

4.1 Receives each patient in a professional manner.

4.2 Makes eye contact with patients to acknowledge them when otherwise occupied by various duties.

5.1 Issues proper forms to new and established patient files for good recordkeeping.

5.2 Reviews documents for accurate and complete information.

5.3 Collects, scans or photocopies, and returns insurance cards to patients.

6.1 Handles daily mail using proper screening techniques, carefully sorting and distributing it.

6.2 Electronically transmits or faxes documents using legal guidelines to maintain confidentiality.

6.3 Communicates by email using proper format and etiquette.

7.1 Keeps reception room and business office clean and organized so it presents a professional image at all times.

8.1 Reviews inventory and orders office and medical supplies at proper time intervals.

9.1 Logs prescription refills made via telephone, fax, or electronic mail.

10.1 Obtains patient information data and scans into EMR or assembles into a chart using required labels.

11.1 Organizes and maintains files efficiently using appropriate filing systems for ease in retrieval.

12.1 Operates equipment skillfully and efficiently.

12.2 Evaluates condition of equipment and reports need for repair or replacement.

13.1 Formats and keys correspondence and medical records according to employer's guidelines.

14.1 Posts entries into computer or daysheet with appropriate bookkeeping expertise, bringing totals forward.

15.1 Posts charges, payments, and adjustments in computer or by hand, calculating a running balance, to patient accounts/ledgers with appropriate accounting expertise as professional services are rendered.

16.1 Writes and posts checks correctly.

16.2 Makes timely bank deposits.

16.3 Reconciles bank statements using proper bookkeeping procedures.

16.4 Maintains petty cash fund daily.

FIGURE 1-3 (Continues)

ADMINISTRATIVE MEDICAL ASSISTANT JOB DESCRIPTION   (*continued*)

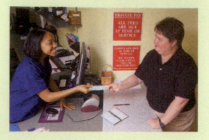

Job responsibilities	Performance standards
17. Collects payments from patients and/or bills patients.	17.1 Communicates effectively with patients to collect payments. 17.2 Prints and sends statements at proper intervals using appropriate reminder (dun) messages.
18. Follows up on delinquent accounts and insurance claims.	18.1 Telephones patients for payment of monies owed and traces insurance claims in a timely manner.
19. Reconciles daily receipts received.	19.1 Reconciles daily monies with appropriate financial expertise.
20. Processes managed-care forms and paperwork.	20.1 Completes appropriate managed-care paperwork with accuracy according to each plan's guidelines.
21. Follows employer's policies and procedures.	21.1 Arrives punctually for work and is dependable. 21.2 Answers routine inquiries related to the medical practice, insurance, and so forth.
22. Enhances knowledge and skills to keep up-to-date.	22.1 Attends continuing education activities on an ongoing basis. 22.2 Obtains current knowledge applicable to all administrative medical assisting duties.
23. Employs interpersonal expertise to provide good working relationships with patients, employer, employees, and individuals contacting the medical office.	23.1 Works with employer and employees cooperatively as a team. 23.2 Communicates effectively with patients and individuals who come in contact with the medical practice. 23.3 Executes job assignments with diligence and skill. 23.4 Assists other employees when needed.
24. Optional: Makes travel arrangements for physician's medical conferences.	24.1 Telephones travel agent to arrange for physician's business trips in a timely manner.
25. Optional: Prepares employee payroll.	25.1 Calculates payroll deductions, writes checks, and maintains financial business records accurately. 25.2 Prepares federal and state forms within time limits.
26. Optional: Completes insurance claim forms.	26.1 Inserts and reviews data on insurance claims for accuracy. 26.2 Codes procedures and diagnoses correctly. 26.3 Transmits claims electronically.
27. Optional: Performs library research responsibilities and prepares manuscripts.	27.1 Formats and keys manuscripts according to guidelines of professional association or publication. 27.2 Researches information using the library or Internet.

FIGURE 1-3

patient's point of view. **Sympathy**, on the other hand, is displaying feelings that are so close to the person affected that you are similarly affected. This can inhibit you from helping.

A patient's mental state has a strong influence on his or her overall health. A *positive attitude* plays an important role in wellness. A medical assistant with a positive attitude may act as a role model and may help encourage patients who are naturally negative or *pessimistic*.

Initiative and Motivation

Initiative and high *motivation* indicate job satisfaction to the employer, who is, of course, pleased with employees who are content and productive. An ambitious medical assistant also impresses patients. It is easy to spot a medical assistant who takes pleasure in performing office tasks and serving patient needs.

Time Management

Being able to manage time well is an attribute that can be learned while in the classroom. With effective time management, an efficient medical assistant with good organizational abilities can often take over chores that free the physician to spend more time with patients. The medical assistant should be able to prioritize and perform multiple tasks. Each day a task list should be created, and every job that needs to be done prioritized. Using self-discipline by self-imposing deadlines aids in overcoming indecision, vacillation, and procrastination. Remembering that patients come first will help set goals for the day instead of doing each task as it appears. The physician or office manager can help by giving an outline of priorities in the office setting.

Medical Assistant's Creed

Perhaps nothing states personal qualifications better than the Medical Assistant's Creed, which was adopted in 1996 by the American Association of Medical Assistants House of Delegates. It reads:

I believe in the principles and purposes of the profession of medical assisting. I endeavor to be more effective. I aspire to render greater service. I protect the confidence entrusted to me. I am dedicated to the care and well-being of all people. I am loyal to my employer. I am true to the ethics of my profession. I am strengthened by compassion, courage, and faith.

Team Interaction

Working as a medical assistant requires a *team effort*. The assistant should view every task as important and no job as too small or insignificant to do. You should establish a good working relationship with coworkers, treating them with respect and support. It is also important to get along with supervisors, accept criticism, and show regard for their authority. Those who can join in doing their part, no matter how small, are viewed as a vital part of a team. An assistant should reinforce effective rather than ineffective behavior and, instead of complaining about problems, focus on finding solutions. More staff members lose their positions because of an inability to get along with coworkers than because of an inability to perform office duties. Positive relations are further fostered by handling the special needs of people who are disabled with kindness and courtesy and by remaining composed when dealing with people who are unruly or inconsiderate.

UNDERSTANDING WORK-RELATED EMOTIONAL AND PSYCHOLOGICAL PROBLEMS

Even though there is a spirit of interdependence and teamwork among medical office staff, some frictions and irritations may arise. The medical assistant who is aware of types of behavior and conditions that may cause negative reactions, stress, and burnout, and who understands those reactions can attempt to head off problems before they become a matter of concern and affect productivity.

Work Relationships

Coworkers come in many shapes with a variety of personalities. As you strive to build good working relationships, you will discover that some behaviors require action and some do not. For instance, the office *gossip* may distract you while conveying personal secrets or talking about others. The rule is to never tell anything that you do not want repeated. The *disruptor* may interrupt you with something trivial. Try to tell them politely but directly that you are busy and need to get your work done. The *credit hog* wants to take all the glory and usually does so in front of the supervisor. Most likely, you will not have to do or say a thing because the credit hog's behavior will become transparent. The worker with the *one-track mind* may be annoying because he or she will not stop to do a prioritized task but instead will work diligently to complete what was started. It is usually best to let this worker finish the task. Perhaps the most bothersome personality trait is the *know-it-all*. You cannot tell them anything, correct them, or train them—they know it all! It may be necessary to speak to the office manager if you encounter such a person. It is wise to examine yourself to see if you display any of the above traits—and if so, once you recognize it you will be more successful at discarding that behavior.

Aggressive versus Assertive Behavior

Sometimes there is a fine line between being aggressive and assertive. **Aggressive** people are forward, pushy, and overbearing. They may not intend to behave this way as they try to convince or manipulate others, but they often depict a righteous attitude that can lead to confrontation. They come across as if they think they are superior and often make derogative remarks. They may have underlying resentment or anger, which leads to a defensive attitude and behavior. They are usually more concerned with their own agenda than another person's needs.

Being **assertive** reflects professional confidence. The assertive health care worker shows respect for others and does not feel threatened. To be assertive, you need to trust your instincts, feelings, and opinions when you are communicating with coworkers and patients. An example of acting assertively based on your instincts (instead of being *passive* and doing nothing) is when you see a coworker or patient who looks fatigued, speaking up and saying something like, "You look tired. Are you getting enough rest or is something bothering you that I can help you with?" Being assertive takes practice but will help you develop leadership ability and resolve conflicts peacefully.

Grieving or Distressed Patients

Unstable health, a poor diagnosis, or a terminal illness will cause a variety of emotions in patients and families. It is important to understand emotional behavior such as being subdued or quiet, talkative or inquisitive, loud or volatile, and distraught. The patient may go into emotional shock from being told bad news. People in shock react differently and may cry loudly, sit quietly, or talk incessantly. They may feel like they want to leave the office abruptly or have a sense that they are outside their bodies hearing and watching all of the events.

Physically, the patient may start crying uncontrollably (hysteria), have increased breathing, begin trembling, experience a change in skin color, or sit with a blank stare. These are all normal and understandable reactions to upsetting news.

When patients receive unfortunate news about themselves or loved ones, it is important to demonstrate empathy, offer assistance, and provide follow-up support. Patients may be so upset or shocked that they are unable to remember anything said during such times. Written instructions, health care pamphlets, or other materials about the patient's particular diagnosis should be offered. These should include cause of illness, treatment options, prognosis, and contact sources in the community or on the Internet where additional information may be found. Follow-up appointments should be arranged to further discuss the situation after the patient and family have time to digest the news. When dealing with a distressed patient, follow these guidelines:

1. Be open and honest by asking what they would like to know about the situation.
2. Treat every problem with concern no matter how small it may seem.
3. Offer support through words, actions, and resources.
4. Do not give false reassurances.

Death and Dying

The rights of patients who are terminally ill and their families must be considered and honored when making decisions regarding family issues, quality of life, and quantity of life. The assistant should become familiar with *living will* and *durable power of attorney* documents and help the patient complete these, especially in regard to decisions about life support, resuscitation, and artificial feeding. These advance directives are further discussed in Chapter 3 *Medicolegal and Ethical Responsibilities*.

The way people face death may include extreme responses, and the health care worker needs to be aware of and respect each patient's reactions. Each person should be allowed the freedom and dignity to have an active part in the choices made. The dying patient should retain some control over financial decisions as well as his or her treatment.

If survivors of the deceased come to your office, you may want to give them a list of support groups that offer grief counseling. The listing should contain both religious and secular groups. Demonstrate kindness by sending a sympathy card—your thoughtfulness will be appreciated. Reassure survivors that they do not need to worry about the medical bill right now, and that the billing department will work with them.

Elisabeth Kubler-Ross introduced several stages typical of someone diagnosed with a terminal illness in her book *Death: The Final Stage of Growth*. Each stage takes varying amounts of time and may or may not occur in the order shown. The medical assistant needs to accept the various emotions expressed by patients and their families. Experiencing a loss is painful, and each person must be allowed to grieve. There is no standard as to how long grief, the readjustment period, or the recovery time lasts. Demonstrating sincere concern with a warm smile and an expression of sympathy will provide comfort to grieving family members.

Stages of Dying

Denial—In the first stage, denial appears to be a defense mechanism and may recur at other times during the dying process. The patient refuses to believe that life is coming to an end and may continue to go about daily activities as if nothing were wrong.

Anger—During the second stage, anger may be directed at anyone and everyone. A common question the patient asks is, "Why me?" This is a difficult time for family, friends, and the health care worker.

Bargaining—While experiencing the third stage, the patient may keep information private, so others may or may not be aware of any problem. The patient pleads and tries to negotiate his or her life for a period of time. There may be an upcoming event that the patient may want to experience, expressing, "If I can only last until . . . ." The bargaining may be with God, with fate, or with other people.

Depression—At the fourth stage as the illness progresses, so do the pain, weakness, and other symptoms. The patient has trouble denying what is happening. Bargaining is futile and anger begins to give way to sorrow. The patient may slip into a depression over the impending loss and separation that are about to be experienced.

Acceptance—During the last stage, it is hoped that the patient has had enough time and has been able to work through the other stages. Being able to *accept* what is *inevitable* will help the patient be at peace while awaiting what is about to happen.

Death with Dignity Act

The *Death with Dignity Act* became law in the state of Oregon in 1997. More recently, a similar act went into effect in the states of California, Montana, New Mexico, and Washington. This act allows licensed physicians (MDs or DOs) to prescribe lethal medications for voluntary self-administration by state residents who are mentally competent, terminally ill adults.

This act does not cover *euthanasia*, in which a doctor injects a patient with a lethal dose of medication; euthanasia is illegal in every state. Health care workers should take a neutral position when dealing with patients who request "death with dignity." They should respect individual patient decisions and not offer opinions or reflect personal judgment.

Hospice

The **Hospice** Foundation of America is a national program that offers medical care and support to patients and family members dealing with a terminal illness and the loss of a loved one. The hospice staff consists of an interdisciplinary team comprising physicians, nurses, social workers, home health aids, counselors, therapists, chaplains, and trained volunteers on call 24 hours a day, 7 days a week.

The earlier the hospice team enters a terminal case, the more help they can provide. All members of the team are trained in dealing with the various aspects a patient and the family face during a life-threatening illness and the dying process. They provide medical

---

PATIENT EDUCATION

The Dying Process

An administrative assistant trained in patient education can help motivate patients and extend the physician's reach and effectiveness. The medical assistant may need to help family members of a patient who is dying by educating them about the stages Kubler-Ross describes in the dying process, that is, denial, anger, bargaining, and depression, before being able to accept the situation. Being open, answering questions, and rendering support will show care and concern. Supplying information about community services and contacting a hospice agency makes evident your regard for their situation.

PATIENT EDUCATION
Hospice

Hospice, a term used in the Middle Ages to signify a place where weary pilgrims could stop, rest, and refresh themselves before continuing on with their journey, has become a worldwide movement symbolizing a new kind of care for the terminally ill. In 1967, a British physician, Cicely Saunders, founded St. Christopher's Hospice in a London suburb and in 2014, in the United States alone, between 1.6 and 1.7 million patients received services from hospice. Hospice information pamphlets are available for educational purposes, and the professional staff promotes comfort, safety, meaningful living, and closure for patients and families.

equipment, medicine, and pain management; answer questions; acknowledge emotional and psychological needs; promote independence at home; assist with funeral arrangements; and help with the transition that both patients and family members are faced with. Their primary focus is on the quality of life and the dignity of the dying patient.

Stress and the Health Care Worker

Stress is a condition comprising physical, psychological, and emotional reactions to time constraints and frightening, exciting, confusing, endangering, or irritating circumstances. Coping with illness, life and death issues, and emotionally upset patients on a daily basis can cause stress for the health care worker. A fast-paced office, demands of the physician, emergency situations, lack of private time or space, and interactions with coworkers and other professionals can all add to the pressure and tension that are felt by the medical assistant. Also, personal circumstances such as financial obligations, relationship problems, or the illness or death of a loved one contribute to the emotional overload that sometimes occurs. Even positive events such as marriage, pregnancy, moving, or a promotion can add stress to the mix.

Ongoing stress can be overwhelming and a barrier to communication. As mentioned, events and situations, both positive and negative, can cause physical and psychological tension. The less control you have over the event or situation, the more you feel stress.

Both physical and mental changes occur when stress levels increase. Symptoms such as aching muscles, difficulty concentrating, forgetfulness, loss of appetite, restless sleep, stomach pain, shortness of breath, a nervous tic, or a complete sense of exhaustion can appear. It is considered a contributing factor to many disorders society experiences today such as depression, headaches, hormonal changes, hypertension, and lowered resistance to disease. Some emotional components that occur when stress is not managed are crying, shouting, drinking alcohol, taking drugs, sleeping more than necessary, and becoming angry. Such negative responses are referred to as *nonadaptive* or *maladaptive* coping mechanisms.

Coping with Stress

Occasionally people say, "a little bit of stress is good for you" or "there is good stress and bad stress." However, stress is often confused with challenges. A challenge will energize you, both physically and psychologically, as it motivates and pushes you to perform at a high level. A relaxed and satisfied feeling is realized once the challenge is met. Stress, on the other hand, can cause tension and create negative physical and emotional responses. Different people can cope with different amounts of stress in different ways.

To deal with stress, you first need to be aware of what causes it. When the requirements of a job do not match the capabilities, resources, or needs of the worker, stress occurs. The multiple duties of the health care worker and changes in the work environment or home situation are common causes. Frustration may build, anger sets in, and before you know it, you are stressed out. After you identify its root, evaluate the situation to see if you can eliminate some of the sources that are the cause. Confront the problem directly and work toward a solution, so you feel as if you have some control over the situation. Cultivate healthy relationships, take regular breaks at work, and schedule fun outings to help take your mind off the more serious side of life. Another way to cope with stress is to *adapt* (change) your behavior in response to stress. Use the following guidelines to practice positive *adaptive coping mechanisms* and help manage stress in the workplace:

- Go to bed and get up early to allow yourself plenty of sleep and more time before going to work.
- Notice what kind of day it is. Enjoy the environment, whether it is a bird singing, rain cleansing the earth, or a beautiful flower in the garden.

- Take your full lunch break and avoid discussing business. Eat slowly and enjoy your food by dining with an enthusiastic, good-natured staff member.
- Prepare to handle the responsibilities of your job by practicing skills. Accept your limitations and do not be afraid to acknowledge when you do not know how to do something. Instead, ask for help, get adequate instruction, and accept advice.
- Learn organizational skills, plan ahead, and prioritize tasks.
- Set realistic goals and remember there are always choices even when you feel otherwise.
- Practice relaxation techniques, such as deep breathing or focusing on something entirely different.
- Exercise your sense of humor; laughter is the best cure for tension (Figure 1-4).

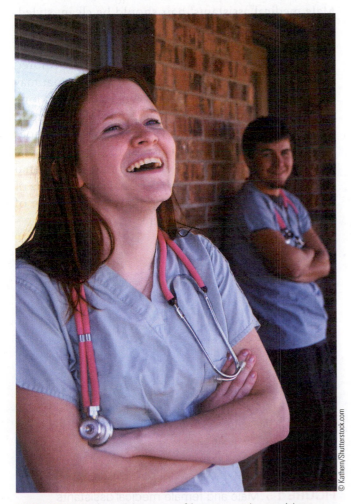

FIGURE 1-4 A good sense of humor and a positive support system can help you cope with stress

- Do not overreact to problematic situations, instead be creative in exercising problem-solving skills and talk over difficult work situations with your supervisor. Always be open to share ideas and receive suggestions.
- Create and rely on a good support system. Whether it be family, friends, or coworkers, share your feelings and talk over your problems without complaining.
- Think positive and strive for a wholesome balance in your life. Monitor your own health by getting regular checkups, eating a balanced diet, resting adequately, exercising consistently, and relaxing regularly. Take quiet time to be alone, reflect, and reenergize your batteries.
- If you are not able to adapt, seek help from professionals or support groups.

By recognizing stress, understanding its common causes, and learning to apply techniques to reduce it, you can learn to cope with it, reduce its effects on your life, and live a healthier, happier life. You can also help educate patients about stress management.

Burnout

Burnout is a condition that results from too much or too little stress. It may occur suddenly or develop slowly over months. Burnout occurs most often in the "helping" professions where there may be erratic hours and emergencies involving critically ill people and death. In attempting to cope, a person withdraws from interaction with others and experiences fear, anxiety, and depression, with resulting decreased energy and productivity.

The medical assistant who has a voice in the decision-making process in an office is less likely to experience burnout. Routines might be rearranged to relieve boredom or slowed down to limit physical and mental pressure. Assignments could be varied to ensure skillful backup when an employee is absent. Remember the preceding suggestions and follow the guidelines to help relieve stress from your life and avoid burnout.

PROFESSIONALISM

It is important for a medical assistant to develop and maintain a professional image and attitude while performing assigned tasks. The ability to make independent decisions, to take initiative, to respect confidentiality, and to carefully follow the physician's advice will project **professionalism** and establish the assistant as an efficient administrator. Professionals have a positive work ethic and demonstrate confidence because they are well trained and have mastered the skills of a given profession. All the personal attributes previously discussed are connected to professionalism. Other important attributes are punctuality, having the ability to adapt to new situations, being dependable and responsible in the workplace, and being emotionally stable. A professional aspires to be a better person, to reach a higher standard, to demonstrate personal integrity, and to behave according to the ethical standards of the profession. A professional uses diplomacy in dealing with difficult patients and situations and is honest and trustworthy—always respecting the patient's dignity. The term *professionalism* projects an image in the minds of all those who interact with the health care worker. This image includes both how the people present themselves and how they conduct themselves.

Personal Image

A well-groomed medical assistant conveys a professional image and creates the impression that the office procedures and medical care are of good quality, whereas a disheveled appearance suggests the office may be run carelessly. Basically, the image should be that of a professional business executive, conservative and stylish but not trendy. The dress code is usually set by the physician-employer. Medical assistants should observe other health care professionals at the top of their career ladders, and then upgrade their image to that level.

Female Grooming

Most medical offices prefer medical assistants wear uniforms. In some office settings, it is all right to wear surgical scrub suits (scrubs). If a medical facility, such as a pediatrician's office, prefers the staff to wear colors other than white, choose jewel-tone colors or deeper muted colors (Figure 1-5).

One study found that when the physician's staff dressed professionally, like the physician, there was less discrepancy in salaries. The same was true about how physicians and staff addressed one another. For instance, if the staff called the physician "Doctor" or "Practon," instead of "Doctor Practon," and the physician called the staff by their first name, there was a greater discrepancy in salary. Keep this in mind when going for a job interview.

Female medical assistants' hair should be clean and neatly styled. Makeup should be subdued for the day.

Fingernails should be carefully manicured. Do not wear long artificial nails, and do not paint on designs or have rhinestones glued to fingernails. It has been found that long nails not only interfere with various job tasks but also become a hiding place for dangerous bacteria. Nail polish may be considered as part of a professional image if a clear or light color polish is selected.

Jewelry is also considered part of the professional image for women, but it must be kept simple; earrings should not be the dangling type. A professional emblem, certification pin, or identification pin worn on the laboratory coat or uniform further identifies the medical assistant as a staff member. A certification pin should also be worn at professional functions. Consult the employer for office policy regarding body piercing and tattoos. Although perfume can be worn, use it in small amounts because it can be offensive and cause allergic reactions in some patients.

Male Grooming

Male medical assistants' hair should be clean, styled, and off the collar. Beards, mustaches, or sideburns should be neatly trimmed. A uniform may consist of white or colored slacks with a white or light-colored shirt worn with optional tie. Over this, a lab coat may be worn. If preferred, a medium-length or classic-long laboratory coat may be worn over street clothes, and in some offices scrubs may be worn (Figure 1-5). Shoes should be unsoiled and polished, with clean shoelaces. Limit jewelry to a ring or wedding band, professional pin, and identification badge. Personal cleanliness is of utmost importance, including daily bathing, use of deodorant, and good oral hygiene.

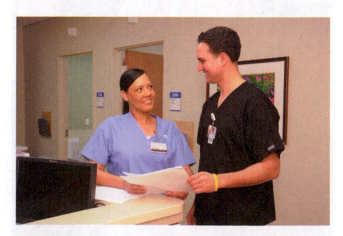

FIGURE 1-5 Male and female medical assistants projecting a clean, fresh, and professional image with hairstyling in good taste

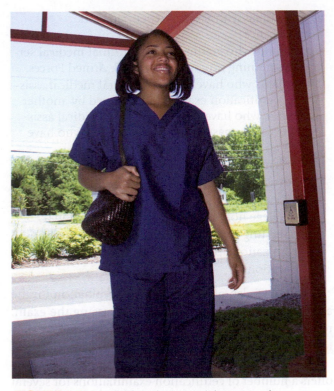

FIGURE 1-6 Medical assistant arriving at work

Health and Physical Fitness

The medical assistant should exemplify health and physical fitness (Figure 1-6). Some employers avoid hiring smokers and those who are extremely overweight because this would appear as a contradiction to what the physician advocates. A certain amount of physical exercise (walking, jogging, biking, swimming) is necessary to diminish stress and keep physically fit for those who have sedentary jobs.

LICENSURE, ACCREDITATION, CERTIFICATION, AND REGISTRATION

Licensure is credentialing sanctioned by a state's legislature (the government), which passes laws making it illegal for an individual who is not licensed to engage in activities of a licensed occupation. For example, Registered Nurses take state boards to become licensed in the state in which they would like to practice nursing. There are no states that require a license to work as a medical assistant, although limited permits are issued in some states for invasive procedures such as injections and venipuncture or limited radiology services. Check with your local Department of Health or the State Medical

Examiner's Office to determine if there is a current law or pending legislation in your state regarding your profession.

Accreditation can mean either meeting a state standard or being evaluated and recognized by a national organization. Usually the minimum education requirement for the position of a medical assistant is high school graduate.

Most physicians prefer to hire a person with some education in medical terminology. Vocational and commercial schools offer 6 to 18 months of training in a variety of areas that are required in medical assisting. Many community colleges offer an associate-degree program that provides a broad foundation of clinical and administrative skills either separately or combined.

Certification is not controlled by the government. It implies that an individual has met either minimum competency requirements or a level of excellence in the area defined. It is based on voluntary action by a professional organization that develops a system to grant recognition to those practitioners who meet a stated level of training and experience. Once certification is attained, most organizations require **recertification** through a continuing education process in which the health care professional is awarded **continuing education units (CEUs)**. One hour of continuing education (1 CEU) equals 1 hour of activity (contact hour).

Because a medical assistant is a **multiskilled health practitioner (MSHP)** cross-trained to provide more than one function, often in more than one discipline, it is possible to gain certification in more than one area (e.g., phlebotomist, ECG technician, medical insurance billing specialist, or professional coder).

The **American Association of Medical Assistants (AAMA)** offers a national certification examination to graduates of medical assisting programs trained in both administrative and clinical areas that are accredited by the Commission on Accreditation of Allied Health Education Programs (CAAHEP) or the Accrediting Bureau of Health Education Schools (ABHES). By passing this examination, the examinee receives the title **Certified Medical Assistant (CMA [AAMA])**. The content of the examination is based on a scientifically grounded occupational analysis, that is, what medical assistants are actually doing on their job. A 2012–2013 survey shows that the 12 most frequently performed responsibilities are:

1. Abide by principles and laws related to confidentiality.
2. Adapt communications to an individual's understanding.

3. Demonstrate respect for individual diversity (culture, ethnicity, gender, race, religion, age, economic status).
4. Employ professional techniques during verbal, nonverbal, and text-based interactions.
5. Comply with risk management and safety procedures.
6. Interact with staff and patients to optimize workflow efficiency.
7. Maintain patient records.
8. Provide care within legal and ethical boundaries.
9. Practice standard precautions.
10. Document patient communication, observations, and clinical treatments.
11. Identify potential consequences of failing to operate within the scope of practice of a medical assistant.
12. Transmit information electronically.

The **National Center for Competency Testing (NCCT)** is an independent certifying agency that validates the competence of a person's knowledge in different areas of the medical profession through examination. The NCCT assesses a candidate's performance against predetermined standards that are created by a job analysis survey. Either graduation from an NCCT-approved medical assisting program, 2 years of full-time employment, or equivalent part-time employment in the last 10 years is required. Medical assistants who pass the competency test receive the designation **National Certified Medical Assistant (NCMA)**. Students who focus on the administrative side of medical assisting can sit for a specialized exam, and after passing it they receive the designation **National Certified Medical Office Assistant (NCMOA)**. Following are some of the other areas of certification offered:

- National Certified ECG Technician (NCET)
- National Certified Pharmacy Technician (NCPhT)
- National Certified Phlebotomy Technician (NCPT)
- National Certified Insurance and Coding Specialist (NCICS)
- National Certified Patient Care Technician (NCPCT)

Registration is similar to certification and may be done on a state or national level. The **American Medical Technologists (AMT)** offers a **Registered Medical Assistant (RMA [AMT])** certification examination to high school graduates in any one of the following categories:

1. Students who graduate from a medical assisting program at a school accredited by either ABHES or CAAHEP.

2. Individual with 5 years of verified work experience.
3. Students who graduate from a formal medical services training program of the U.S. Armed Forces.
4. Students who have passed a general medical assistant certification examination offered by another agency, who have been working as medical assistants for the past 3 out of 5 years, and who have met all other AMT requirements.
5. Students who complete a medical assisting course with a minimum of 720 clock-hours (including 160 externship hours) in a post-secondary school or college holding accreditation by a regional accrediting commission or a national accrediting organization approved by the U.S. Department of Education.

The AMT also offers a national examination for the administrative assistant who, when passing the exam, receives the credential of **Certified Medical Administrative Specialist (CMAS [AMT])**.

The **National Healthcareer Association (NHA)** offers a number of certification examinations for several allied health care areas including **Certified Medical Administrative Assistant (CMAA)** and **Certified Clinical Medical Assistant (CCMA)**. Eligibility requirements include high school graduation or equivalent and successful completion of a training program or the minimum of 1-year work experience.

The *National Association for Health Professionals (NAHP)* also offers certification for the following nationally registered credentials: medical assistant (NRCMA), administrative health assistant (NRCAHA), and coding specialist (NRCCS), among others.

In addition, a number of specialty certifications are available on a national level, for example, medical transcription, diagnostic and procedural coding, office management, and so on. Table 1-2 provides a list of certified and registered titles with abbreviations, a brief description of how to obtain the certification or registration, and the professional organizations to contact in order to obtain more information.

Credentialing is another way to portray a professional image. When a health care worker receives such accreditation, employers and the public can be assured that an academic standard is met and that the person holds a certain body of knowledge. It also advances the profession, meets the requirements of government regulators, and demonstrates an individual's commitment to a profession. The medical assistant receives a sense of pride and professional accomplishment when obtaining a credential.

Many of these organizations offer student membership and may have regional chapters.

TABLE 1-2 Certification and Registration

Title and Abbreviation	Description to Obtain Certification or Registration	Professional Association
Certified Bookkeeper (CB)	Self-study program and employment experience; pass national examination	American Institute of Professional Bookkeepers (AIPB)
Certified Coding: • Associate (CCA) • Specialist (CCS) • Specialist—Physician based (CCS-P)	Self-study program; pass certification examination	American Health Information Management Association (AHIMA)
Certified in Health Care Compliance (CHC)	Work experience, continuing education, and pass examination	Health Care Compliance Association (HCCA)
Certified Medical Assistant (CMA [AAMA])	Graduate from accredited medical assisting program; apply to take national certifying examination	American Association of Medical Assistants (AAMA)
Certified Medical Billing Specialist (CMBS)	Take six online courses and pass test	Medical Association of Billers (MAB)
Certified Medical Manager (CMM)	Minimum of 3 years' experience Twelve college credit hours 200 multiple-choice questions	Professional Association of Health Care (PAHC)
Certified Medical Practice Executive (CMPE)	Two years' experience managing a medical practice	Medical Group Management Association (MGMA)
Medical Transcriptionist Level 1: Registered Healthcare Documentation Specialist (RHDS) Level 2: Certified Healthcare Documentation Specialist (CHDS) Level 3: AHDI Fellow	Level 1: Graduate of MT program Level 2: Two years' transcription experience Level 3: Earn 50 fellowship points in five of eight categories	Association for Healthcare Documentation Integrity (AHDI)
Certified Professional Biller (CPB) Certified Professional Coder (CPC) Certified Professional Coder—Hospital Outpatient (CPC-H) Certified Professional Coder-Payer (CPC-P) Other Specialty Certifications Available	Independent study program; examination approximately 5 hours and 40 minutes in length	American Academy of Professional Coders (AAPC)
National Certified Insurance and Coding Specialist (NCICS) National Certified Medical Assistant (NCMA) National Certified Medical Office Assistant (NCMOA) National Certified Patient Care Technician (NCPCT)	Qualify to sit for certification examination given by independent testing agency at many school sites across the nation with one of the following criteria: 1. Current student or graduate from an authorized school or military institution 2. One-year experience 3. Recognition of related credential	National Center for Competency Testing (NCCT)

(continues)

TABLE 1-2 **Certification and Registration** (*continued*)

Title and Abbreviation	Description to Obtain Certification or Registration	Professional Association
Registered Medical Assistant (RMA [AMT]) Certified Medical Administrative Specialist (CMAS [AMT])	Graduate from accredited medical assisting program or 5 years' experience; sit for certification exam	American Medical Technologists (AMT)

Externship

After completing most or all of your classroom education in medical assisting, you may be serving as an extern to gain experience in the "real world." Before beginning this training program, you will have to demonstrate your ability to perform entry-level medical assisting skills in both clinical and administrative competencies. For the employer, this offers a free preview of qualifications and skill levels.

Take advantage of this opportunity to demonstrate your professionalism, work ethic, technical skills, business savvy, and team-oriented attitude. Make the most of your externship experience, learn from each person you are assigned to, and ask questions regarding why things are done the way they are. Prior to your extern assignment, you may have an interview with the office manager. While working as an extern, you will have your work performance evaluated; this will help you improve. Make use of this valued experience to help you obtain confidence and a future position in health care.

Remember, a medical assistant is the most versatile health care worker—one who has the opportunity to serve as a bridge between sickness and wellness, disease and good health, and misery and quality of life.

KEEPING CURRENT

A job in a medical office is never static, always stimulating, and constantly challenging. You must be able to adapt to change. To succeed both professionally and personally, effective lifelong learning is the key. To keep up with technology and current practices, it is important for the administrative medical assistant to read professional publications, attend educational seminars, and research information on the Internet. Some publications currently of value to the administrative medical assistant are listed in the *Resources* section at the end of this chapter.

Another way to keep up to date in medical matters is through membership in a professional organization, such as one of those listed in Table 1-2. State and local membership is usually automatic with national membership; there are monthly meetings, bulletins and newsletters, educational seminars and workshops, and national and state conventions.

Networking with peers at workshops and conventions is an additional way to keep in tune with the medical environment outside your office. By building relationships with other office personnel, you can share ideas, increase your knowledge, and receive support when implementing new laws and regulations that are mandated by the government.

HEALTH CARE REFORM*

The government has been trying to reform our health care system for decades. Health care reform was listed as a priority in the Truman, Nixon, and Carter administrations—but no reforms were passed. During the Clinton administration, legislation for the Health Security Act of 1993 was introduced but also failed to pass.

---

*Current information on Health Care Reform may be located on the following website managed by the U.S. Department of Health & Human Services: http://www.whitehouse.gov /healthreform

With health care spending in the trillions of dollars per year and millions of Americans lacking insurance, health care reform became a top priority for the Obama administration and the 111th Congress. The Patient Protection and Affordable Care Act (PPACA) was passed into law in 2010 and implementation dates for various areas of the law have been staggered throughout several years. Each time you see the above icon you will find a snippet on health care reform directed at the chapter material. The $940 billion plan is projected to extend insurance coverage to 32 million additional Americans and enrollment started in 2014. Besides helping moderate- or low-income citizens gain insurance, it affects employers (especially small businesses), taxes, private insurance companies, Medicaid, Medicare, flexible spending accounts, health savings accounts, illegal immigrants, doctors, hospitals, and physician offices. The adoption of Health Information Technology (Health IT), the electronic health information exchange (HIE), is another focus of the reform.

Just For Today

So, just for today . . .
Show a little kindness to everyone you meet,
Be loving and smile to all whom you greet.
Demonstrate patience if someone's upset,
You don't want to say any words you'll regret.
Be joyful and offer a glimmer of hope,
Your positive attitude can help someone cope.
Have faith and be humble in all that you do,
Show gentleness, goodness, and empathy too.
Hold your head high at the end of the day,
Even when thankfulness does not come your way.
You'll be at peace, with your spirit at rest,
In knowing you've done your very best!

by Linda French

PROCEDURE 1-1

Interpret and Accurately Spell Medical Terms and Abbreviations

OBJECTIVES: Enhance knowledge of medical terminology, interpret abbreviations, and accurately spell medical terms while reading patients' chart notes.

EQUIPMENT/SUPPLIES: One sheet of white 8½" by 11" paper and pen or pencil.

DIRECTIONS: Follow these step-by-step directions, which include rationales, to learn this procedure. Job Skill 1-1 and additional exercises entitled "Abbreviation and Spelling Review" are presented at the beginning of each chapter of the *Workbook* to practice this skill.

1. Read a patient's medical record.
2. Identify unfamiliar medical terms.
3. Use a medical dictionary to locate and learn the meanings of each medical term.
4. Break the term apart into word components (i.e., root, prefix, suffix) and memorize the spelling of each medical term.
5. Find abbreviations in each chart or progress note that you do not understand or appear unfamiliar to you.
6. Decode and define each abbreviation (see Appendix B of the *Workbook*).

STOP AND THINK CASE SCENARIO

Listen and Observe

SCENARIO: A patient who is usually cheerful comes into the office and sits in the corner not talking to anyone. She looks grumpy and her posture is one of dejection.

CRITICAL THINKING: What would you think and say to her?

_____
_____
_____
_____
_____

STOP AND THINK CASE SCENARIO
Positive Attitude

SCENARIO: A patient arrives and you ask him how he is. He responds, "Well, I won't know until I find out my test results." He also says, "The numbers probably haven't changed and I'll have to continue taking all of these pills."

CRITICAL THINKING: Think about each statement and tell how you would respond, considering whether his statement(s) and your responses are positive, negative, or neutral.

_____
_____
_____
_____

STOP AND THINK CASE SCENARIO
Patient Education

SCENARIO: Mary Lou is a 3-year-old whose mother has brought her in to see the doctor for an earache. She is crying softly and wiggling around in her mother's arms. Her mother tells her to hold still and stop crying, that the doctor is going to fix her, and that there is nothing to cry about.

CRITICAL THINKING:

a. How can you tactfully educate Mary Lou's mother about her daughter's reactions?

_____
_____

b. How would you inform the mother and Mary Lou about what the physician will be doing?

_____
_____

STOP AND THINK CASE SCENARIO
Aggressive versus Assertive Response

SCENARIO: You have been given the assignment of directing Mrs. Hartley, a very angry and upset patient, to the laboratory to have a test done and telling her that the results will not be ready until tomorrow afternoon. You feel like saying, "You need to go to ABC Laboratory to have this test done. You will not be able to find out the results until tomorrow afternoon; someone will probably call you then."

CRITICAL THINKING: Try to reword what you would say to the patient so that it is assertive instead of aggressive.

_____
_____
_____
_____
_____
_____
_____
_____
_____
_____
_____

FOCUS ON CERTIFICATION*

CMA (AAMA) Content Summary

- Medical terminology
- Death and dying
- Defense mechanisms
- Professionalism
- Empathy/sympathy
- Understanding emotional behavior
- Time management

RMA (AMT) Content Summary

- Medical terminology
- Abbreviations and symbols

- Licensure, certification, registration
- Credentialing requirements
- Professional development and conduct
- Interpersonal skills and relations
- Instructing patients

CMAS (AMT) Content Summary

- Medical terminology
- Professionalism
- Continuing education

REVIEW EXAM-STYLE QUESTIONS

1. Among a medical assistant's interpersonal skills, the most important personality trait is:
   a. dedication
   b. consideration and respect for others
   c. displaying a sense of warmth and sensitivity
   d. liking people and being able to get along with other individuals
   e. dedication to the profession of medical assisting

2. Being able to put yourself in the patient's situation is commonly referred to as:
   a. sympathy
   b. empathy
   c. having a positive attitude
   d. identification
   e. commiseration

3. The Medical Assistant's Creed was adopted in:
   a. 1954
   b. 1966
   c. 1996
   d. 1998
   e. 2000

4. Being assertive means to:
   a. respect others and reflect professional confidence
   b. be aggressive in your approach with people
   c. convince and manipulate
   d. concentrate on your own agenda
   e. confront with a righteous attitude

5. Grieving or distressed patients tend to be:
   a. subdued or quiet
   b. talkative or inquisitive
   c. loud and volatile
   d. distraught
   e. all of the above

6. Although patients do not always go through the stages of dying in the order presented, the fourth stage is usually:
   a. anger
   b. bargaining
   c. depression
   d. acceptance
   e. denial

*This textbook and the accompanying Workbook meet the entry-level administrative and general competencies for the CMA outlined by the AAMA Examination Content Outline and Occupational Analysis and for the RMA and CMAS outlined by the AMT Competencies, Construction Parameters, and Examination Specifications (see Competency Grid in Appendix B).

7. The first thing you need to do in order to deal with stress is to:
    a. act out anger so it does not bottle up inside you
    b. become aware of what causes it
    c. take time off work
    d. not take your job so seriously
    e. tell the office manager, so he or she can lighten your workload

8. Using diplomacy in dealing with difficult patients is a/an:
    a. sign of professionalism
    b. personal characteristic
    c. personal attribute
    d. interpersonal skill
    e. sign of having a high intellect

9. Determine the correct statement regarding the medical assistant's personal image and grooming.
    a. The dress code in a medical office is usually set by a consensus of the employees.

b. No jewelry should be worn by men or women in the health care field.
c. There is *no* connection between the medical assistant's personal image and the way the patient perceives how the office is run.
d. There *is* a connection between the medical assistant's personal image and the way the patient perceives how the office is run.
e. No beards, mustaches, or sideburns should be worn by men in the health care field.

10. Select the correct statement regarding licensure, accreditation, certification, and registration.
    a. Licensure, accreditation, certification, and registration all mean the same thing.
    b. Certification is controlled by the government.
    c. Standardized testing is a way of portraying a professional image.
    d. Licensure is required of medical assistants in all states.
    e. Certification is typically obtained on the state level.

WORKBOOK ASSIGNMENT

To develop competency-based job skills, refer to the *Workbook* and complete the:
- Abbreviations and Spelling Review
- Review Questions

- Critical Thinking Exercises
- Job Skill activities, which are listed at the beginning of the chapter under *Performance Objectives in the Workbook*

RESOURCES

To obtain answers to questions related to certification and become a member of a professional organization, refer to the data listed in Table 1-2.

Certification Review Books

American Association of Medical Assistants CMA Practice Exams
  Go to: CMA (AAMA) Exam, Study for the Exam, select Practice Tests:
- Anatomy and Physiology
- Medical Terminology
Website: http://aama-ntl.org/

Comprehensive Medical Assisting Exam Review: Preparation for the CMA, RMA, and CMAS Exams, 3rd edition
  Cody, J.P. Delmar Cengage Learning, 2011
  Website: http://www.cengagebrain.com

Delmar's Medical Assisting Exam Review; Preparation for the CMA, RMA, and CMAS Exams, 2nd edition
  Cody/Kelley-Arney
  Delmar Cengage Learning, 2006
  Website: http://www.cengagebrain.com

Medical Assisting Exam Review Online, 1st edition
  Delmar Cengage Learning, 2010
  Website: http://www.cengagebrain.com

Internet

AAMA E-Learning Center
  Go to: Continuing Education, E-Learning Center
  View list of articles
  Website: http://www.aama-ntl.org
Center for Professional Well Being
  View multitude of services
Death with Dignity National Center
  History and mission
National Center for Health Statistics
  Diseases and Conditions
Online Dictionary
  - Abbreviations and Acronyms Dictionary
    Acronym Finder
    Website: http://www.acronymfinder.com
  - Funk & Wagnalls Standard Dictionary
    English language
  - Merriam-Webster Collegiate Dictionary
    Medical, regular, Spanish/English, and thesaurus
    Website: http://www.m-w.com (Merriam-Webster)
  - Taber's Online Medical Dictionary
    Definitions and audio pronunciations

Newsletters

HCPro Newsletter
  Select category (e.g., physician practice)
National Institutes of Health
  Newsletter

Professional Magazines

Advance News Magazine
  Biweekly-free—Select area of interest
Advanstar Healthcare (online)
  Select area of interest
American Medical Technologist Journal of Continuing Education
  Select area of interest
CMA Today (Certified Medical Assistant) (bimonthly)
  Website: http://www.ama_ntl.org/
Compassion and Choices
  End of life choices
e-Perspectives on the Medical Transcription Profession
(periodical)
  Health Professional Institute
For the Record
  Magazine for Health Information Professionals
  Great Valley Publishing Company, Inc.
Plexus (medical transcription publication)
  Association for Healthcare Documentation Integrity

CHAPTER 2

THE HEALTH CARE ENVIRONMENT: PAST, PRESENT, AND FUTURE

LEARNING OBJECTIVES

After reading this chapter and learning step-by-step procedures to gain job skills,* you should be able to:

- Describe the history of medicine and some of the changes that have taken place in health care.
- Discuss cultural, environmental, political, and socioeconomic influences that affect peoples' health and health care in the United States.
- State current and future trends in health care.
- Explain how health care reform will help primary care physicians.
- List four indicators of a population's health.
- Identify goals to improve health care internationally.
- Understand how managed care functions; contrast and compare types of managed care organizations.
- Define precertification, predetermination, and preauthorization.
- Analyze health care settings and compare their similarities and differences.
- Determine employment opportunities in a variety of health care settings.
- Name different types of medical specialties.
- Compare the administrative medical assistant's job responsibilities among medical specialties.
- Learn the abbreviations for various physician specialists and health care organizations.

PERFORMANCE OBJECTIVES (PROCEDURES) IN THIS TEXTBOOK

- Direct patients to specific hospital departments (Procedure 2-1).
- Refer patients to the correct physician specialist (Procedure 2-2).

PERFORMANCE OBJECTIVES (JOB SKILLS) IN THE WORKBOOK

- Use the Internet to research and write an essay about a medical pioneer (Job Skill 2-1).
- Direct patients to specific hospital departments (Job Skill 2-2).

---

*This textbook and the accompanying Workbook meet the educational components for entry-level administrative and general competencies outlined by CAAHEP and ABHES.

- Refer patients to the correct physician specialist (Job Skill 2-3).
- Define abbreviations for health care professionals (Job Skill 2-4).
- Determine basic skills needed by the administrative medical assistant (Job Skill 2-5).

KEY TERMS

associate practice

caduceus

capitation

clinics

consumer-directed health plans (CDHPs)

exclusive provider organization (EPO)

fee-for-service (FFS)

group practice

health maintenance organization (HMO)

hospital

independent practice association (IPA)

laboratories

managed care organization (MCO)

medical assistant

medical center

medical necessity

MinuteClinic

multispecialty practice

partnership

patient advocate

patient-centered medical home (PCMH)

point-of-service (POS) plan

preauthorization

precertification

predetermination

preferred provider organization (PPO)

primary care physician (PCP)

professional corporation

referral

solo physician practice

specialized care centers

telemedicine

urgent care centers

utilization review

HEART OF THE HEALTH CARE PROFESSIONAL

Service

Patients can become confused with the various types of managed care organizations, authorization requirements, copayments, and so forth. As you interact with patients, you may be responsible for navigating them through the maze of managed care. By taking the time to explain plan requirements with cheerfulness and patience, you will be helping the medical practice and serving patients at the same time.

HISTORY OF MEDICINE

Sculptured artifacts, drawings, and hieroglyphics from prehistoric times indicate that humans have long tried to cure their illnesses. Medicine was closely connected to religion in early times, and people felt that illness was punishment indicating the gods' anger. Priests came to be the healers of illness, using magical formulas, sacrifices, and the application of herbs and other natural substances. Some of these remedies were successful and became part of folklore medicine; others have not proven so. Preventive medicine dates back to Biblical times when "clean" (healthy) and "unclean" (unhealthy) foods were listed in the Hebrew religion.

The first prescription (Figure 2-1) was discovered in the tomb of an Egyptian pharaoh. This first written record, from about 3000 B.C., was made by a physician, Imhotep, who attended the pharaohs and was known as the god of healing. Hippocrates, "the father of medicine," was the first to describe disease, and his descriptions were so accurate that some remain valid even today. The Oath of Hippocrates is the oath of medicine that physicians pledge to their patients and profession on graduation from medical school (see Chapter 3).*

---

*All medical schools use some form of oath, although many have moved away from reciting the ancient Hippocratic oath.

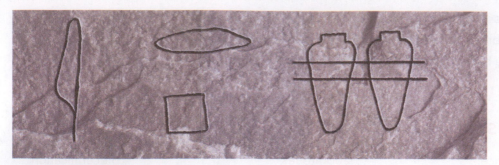

FIGURE 2-1 Ancient Egyptian prescription: "Six senna (pods) and fruit of colocynth are ground fine, put in honey, and eaten by the man, swallowed with sweet wine 5 ro"

In Greek legend, the god of healing, Aesculapius (Asclepius), was represented as a serpent coiled around a staff, which was a symbol of power. Today the caduceus, as this symbol is called, represents the medical profession. Its modern form is a winged staff with two snakes twined around it (Figure 2-2).

During the Middle Ages, universities in France and England started up medical schools, and down through the ages, many people have developed medical instruments and techniques, conducted research resulting in remedies for disease, and contributed to medical knowledge and practice. Some of these highlights in medical history appear in Table 2-1.

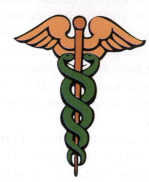

FIGURE 2-2 Caduceus, the symbol of the medical profession

EVOLUTION OF THE MEDICAL ASSISTING CAREER

In the early 1900s, the administrative side of medical practice was still relatively simple. Administrative duties were often handled by the physician or the office secretary. During World War II when office nurses were needed in hospitals, physicians began to train their secretaries to perform this function. Since then, medical assistants have performed both administrative and clinical duties to capably manage the outpatient medical practice.

In recent years, the role of the medical assistant has been radically changed by the increasing number of patients seen, the tremendous volume of paperwork, and government mandates for electronic recordkeeping. Physicians now devote most of their time to taking care of patients, leaving the administrative and clinical work to one or more medical assistants. Medical assistants have greater responsibility and are given more authority than their counterparts of earlier years; therefore, they must approach this challenge with dedication and creativity. Today, the administrative assistant is an essential part of every ambulatory practice and the support functions they offer are critical, ensuring the productivity of the medical practice.

Global Influences on Health Care

As we look into the future and note the influences that affect health care—cultural, environmental, political, and socioeconomic—we can learn more about the global effect of health care, not only in the United States but throughout the world.

Cultural Influences

Beliefs and practices related to health, illness, and healing are influenced by culture, religion, and ethnicity. Cultural influences on health care can be seen by the global spread of communicable diseases from country to country. The *World Health Organization (WHO)* reports that since 1967, at least 39 new pathogens have been identified, including human immunodeficiency virus (HIV), acquired immunodeficiency syndrome

TABLE 2-1 Highlights of Medical History

Medical Notable	Nationality and Accomplishment
Ambroise Paré (1510–1590)	A French surgeon, called "the father of modern surgery," who introduced advanced surgical techniques
Andreas Vesalius (1514–1564)	A Flemish anatomist, sometimes called "the father of modern anatomy," who wrote the first complete description of the human body and dissected bodies to prove his theories
William Harvey (1578–1657)	An English physician and anatomist who demonstrated the exact circulation of the blood
Anton van Leeuwenhoek (1623–1723)	A Dutch lens maker who developed the first lens strong enough to allow bacteria to be seen
John Hunter (1728–1793)	A British practitioner known as "the founder of scientific surgery"
Edward Jenner (1749–1823)	An Englishman who developed the process of vaccination and the smallpox vaccine
James Marion Sims (1813–1883)	An American gynecologist who invented the vaginal speculum and originated Sims' position
John Snow (1813–1858)	A legendary figure in the history of public health, epidemiology, and anesthesiology who determined how cholera was transmitted
Crawford Williamson Long (1815–1878)	An American physician, the first to employ ether as an anesthetic agent
Ignaz Philipp Semmelweis (1818–1865)	A Hungarian physician called "the savior of mothers," who first used antiseptic methods extensively in childbirth to prevent puerperal fever
Florence Nightingale (1820–1910)	An English hospital reformer and the founder of nursing
Clara Barton (1821–1912)	Founder of the American Red Cross
Elizabeth Blackwell (1821–1910)	First woman physician in the United States who helped open a New York medical college for women in 1853 and a hospital exclusively for women in 1857
Louis Pasteur (1822–1895) Courtesy of Parke Davis and Company, copyright 1957	A French chemist, known as "the father of bacteriology" and "the father of preventive medicine," who developed the process called pasteurization and was involved in the prevention of anthrax (in cattle and sheep), rabies, chicken cholera, and swine erysipelas

(continues)

TABLE 2-1 Highlights of Medical History (continued)

Medical Notable	Nationality and Accomplishment
Joseph Lister (1827–1912) Courtesy of Parke Davis and Company, copyright 1957	A British surgeon, known as "the father of sterile surgery," who used carbolic acid as an antiseptic in the operating room
Robert Koch (1843–1910)	A German scientist who discovered the cause of cholera and discovered tuberculin while working with tuberculosis
Wilhelm C. Roentgen (1845–1923)	A German physicist who discovered the x-ray, which is used in diagnosing diseases and treating cancer
Walter Reed (1851–1902)	An American physician who discovered that yellow fever is caused by a virus that is carried from one person to another by a particular kind of mosquito
Paul Ehrlich (1854–1915)	A German physician known for the drug he developed to fight syphilis; also for developing chemotherapy
Pierre Curie (1859–1906) and Marie Curie (1867–1934)	French researchers known for their discovery of/and work with radium
Alexander Fleming (1881–1955)	An English bacteriologist who discovered penicillin, the first antibiotic drug
George Papanicolaou (1883–1962)	Discovered cancer cells in 1928 and developed the Pap test, which has become a routine preventive medicine procedure
Frederick Banting (1891–1941)	A Canadian physician who discovered insulin
Albert Sabin (1906–1993)	An American scientist who developed an effective oral polio vaccine
Michael Ellis DeBakey (1908–2008)	An American surgeon who contributed to techniques used to replace blood vessels including the coronary artery bypass operation; developed artificial blood vessels made of Dacron
Jonas Edward Salk (1914–1995)	An American scientist who developed an injection vaccine against poliomyelitis in 1954
Francis H. C. Crick (1916–2004), James D. Watson (1928–), and Maurice Wilkins (1916—2004)	In 1953, Crick, from England, Watson, an American, and Wilkins, from New Zealand, received the Nobel Prize for their contribution to the basic understanding of deoxyribonucleic acid (DNA). DNA makes possible the transmission of inherited characteristics.
Christiaan Neethling Barnard (1922–2001)	A South African surgeon who performed the world's first human heart transplant in 1967
Thomas Earl Starzl (1926–)	An American surgeon who performed the first liver transplant and became known as the "Dean of Transplantation"

(AIDS), and Ebola hemorrhagic fever. These and other diseases such as Marburg fever, tuberculosis, H1N1 influenza, and severe acute respiratory syndrome (SARS) are noticed in populations that have large groups immigrating to other countries. They continue to pose a health threat through a combination of mutation, rising resistance to antimicrobial medicines, weak health systems, and poor adherence to medical regimens. Human migration and the increase in travel in our now "borderless" world make cultural health issues an international concern.

Environmental Influences

A wide range of environmental factors influence health; the work environment is one. Workers are healthiest when they believe their jobs are secure, when their workplace is safe, and when they feel their work is important and of value. Work-related injury, illness, and disease affect the long-term health of employees.

Climate also has an impact on health, from overexposure to the sun in warm climates to frostbite, pneumonia, and vitamin D deficiency in cold climates. Air pollution increases the risk of cardiovascular and respiratory diseases. And, weather changes that occur across the globe (e.g., global warming) and natural disasters affect individual health and the well-being of entire populations.

Political Influences

Political forces affect health care and result in federal regulations and state laws that are implemented by government agencies, private insurers, and institutions. Many of these beneficial programs affect the poor. Smoking bans in public places and advertising campaigns on binge drinking, AIDS, driving after drinking alcohol, and the effects of smoking have been supported by the government to help improve the health of young people. To raise revenue and discourage items that are deemed as unhealthy, taxes have been placed on such things as alcohol, tobacco, and fast food.

Socioeconomic Influences

The social and economic conditions in which people live affect their health because there is a direct relationship between the quantity and quality of health resources that are available for various socioeconomic groups. The economically disadvantaged face an increase in disease and are more likely than other groups to be employed in hazardous work conditions.

Financial factors influence whether people live in safe, clean housing; whether they eat nutritionally balanced meals; and if they can afford central heating and air conditioning. People with low-income levels tend to live in areas with high crime rates, so their children often stay indoors because of neighborhood dangers. They do not get out in the fresh air or exercise properly—they cannot afford to join a gym or travel to areas with good facilities. An increased sedentary lifestyle promotes the risk of obesity, which leads to illness and disease (e.g., type 2 diabetes). The lack of education that exists in poverty results in decreased knowledge about the dangers of smoking and sexually transmitted diseases as well as the benefits of eating a well-balanced diet and exercising properly. This all contributes to the state of mental health and manifests in stress indicators, such as depression and suicide. People are healthiest when they feel safe and secure, and when they are supported and connected to their family, workplace, and community.

CHANGES IN HEALTH CARE

It was not that long ago that country doctors traded their services for chickens, eggs, or produce. This was followed by a time when families went to physicians and opened an account, paying for services monthly or whenever they were able. As time passed, medical school costs increased, physicians' knowledge base and expertise expanded, and the cost of health care began to rise. Soon insurance companies were arriving on the scene to pick up the price tag. At this time, there were few limitations on the costs of services with minimal expense to patients while most employers paid the insurance premiums. Health care was rapidly changing from personal payments to third-party reimbursement.

As medicine advanced, so did the life expectancy of the American population. Life support measures, including quicker and better resuscitation, feeding tubes, respirators, and new drugs, helped keep individuals alive beyond normal years. More and more older adults entered convalescent hospitals to live out the remainder of their lives when unable to care for themselves at home. Babies weighing less than 2 pounds made medical history when they survived the trauma of premature delivery and the complications of underdeveloped lungs. The general population began to expect the highest level of medical attention regardless of an ability to pay. Malpractice insurance soared as lawsuits increased. Physicians tried to protect themselves by ordering more, and sometimes unnecessary, tests and procedures. Hospitals and outpatient centers started competing with each other by buying the largest, most advanced equipment and began investing hundreds of thousands of dollars in marketing campaigns to lure patients to their facilities. Women especially were being targeted, after a survey showed that women make 85% of the medical decisions in nonemergency cases. All of these factors combined to increase health care costs and necessitated the need for health care reform.

Current and Future Trends

Today, with the discovery of new diseases, the increase in existing illnesses (e.g., diabetes and obesity), and the explosion in clinical knowledge, there are increased demands on physicians' time. Health care reimbursement is declining while the cost of living and operating a medical practice is increasing. High rents, climbing malpractice and health insurance rates, and utilization of the electronic health system all contribute to the increase in the overhead of medical practices.

The health care delivery system continues to change to try to accommodate a diverse population, comply with federal regulations, and make a profit. It is an exciting and challenging time for physicians and health care workers who must diligently work to tend to patient needs as well as focus on the future of medicine.

Following are some current and future trends in health care:

- Aging of the baby boomer generation adds to the need for medical attention and their retirement in the workforce is being replaced by a less experienced millennial generation that will affect management and personnel in medical offices. A major turnover of employees is expected due to lack of salary increases and a decrease in the loyalty of workers.
- The "Big Data Revolution" at present is experiencing a shortage of skilled health IT professionals evidenced by the increased need to manage electronic health systems and transport or share data with other health care organizations.
- New forms of health care employment are emerging, such as a health coach who knows the patient on a one-on-one basis and functions much like a personal trainer—listening, motivating, challenging, and inspiring patients.

- *Evidence-based medicine*, which emphasizes the use of reliable research, is being used in health care decision-making.
- *Accountable Care Organizations (ACOs)* are increasing, which integrate physicians, clinics, and hospitals together to pool resources and trim expenses while focusing on quality of care.
- Independent physicians and stand-alone hospitals will become a thing of the past as payers, hospitals, health systems, and pharmaceutical suppliers consolidate into super-sized organizations.
- "Hospital at Home" programs will provide acute care services in the homes of patients who might otherwise be hospitalized.
- *Intensive Care Units Without Walls* or *Ambulatory Intensive Care Units (A-ICUs)* will spring up to offer intensive care wherever beds are available.
- The focus on whole person care, aging gracefully, and living longer will be evidenced by more naturopathic doctors, holistic medicine approaches, herbal supplements, and natural antiaging techniques.
- Patients are starting to take more control of their own care and there will be a growth in self-monitoring techniques and the use of interoperable electronic health records, cloud-based computing, data storage, and smartphones. Health portals for individuals will allow patients to easily connect with their providers as well as compile data from their health and fitness devices.
- Employers will increase the value of wellness incentives and offer free health tools (e.g., pedometers), subscriptions to wellness websites, gift cards, extra paid days off, or gym memberships. Some employers are focusing on cost issues by addressing employee's lifestyle choices that lead to higher health care consumption including tobacco use and obesity, which are reflected in higher premiums.
- More employers are considering private insurance exchanges where employees can compare benefits from dozens of insurers. Patients will become informed consumers as the cost and quality of care, as well as expected outcomes become more transparent.
- Managing care for those with multiple chronic conditions, who are the biggest health care consumers, has become a primary focus. New ways to deal with this will resort in lower hospital utilization as inpatient bed days, length of stay, admissions, readmissions, and emergency room visits are shortened.

- Health insurance companies are looking for more innovative ways to motivate and monitor the health of their members. Behavior tools, like mobile wellness apps, will give members ways to improve their sleep patterns, nutrition, and exercise routines and will eventually lead to lower premiums.

Today there is a shortage of primary care physicians in the United States and one question being asked is "How is health care reform affecting doctors?" The American Medical Association states that new laws passed in the reform have helped improve the situation even though more people are insured. Following are some ways in which the reform has helped physicians:

- New measures have attracted more doctors, nurses, and physician assistants to primary care.
- Doctors now have more time with patients as paperwork is simplified.
- Physicians and nurses who provide primary care to Medicare patients in areas with doctor shortages are receiving extra payments.
- Health professionals seeing Medicare patients are starting to be paid according to the quality of care they provide instead of the number of services they perform.
- Physicians seeing Medicaid patients are realizing increased payments.
- Community health centers are receiving billions of dollars, allowing for an expected 20 million new patients.

Goals to Improve Health Care Internationally

There are four indicators of a population's health:

1. Life expectancy (number of years lived)
2. Healthy life expectancy (HLE), that is, quality of life
3. Mortality (deaths)
4. Disability

The following goals are broadly supported throughout the world:

- *Achieving universal primary education*—Links literacy to good health practices.
- *Combating diseases, such as HIV/AIDS, malaria, and obesity*—Will reduce the number of overweight people who are prone to chronic illness; the United States has the highest number of obese people in the entire world.
- *Developing a global partnership with pharmaceutical companies*—Provides access to affordable drugs in developing countries.
- *Ensuring environmental sustainability*—Helps provide clean water and the riddance of air pollution and land erosion, which affects our basic needs (air, water, and food).
- *Eradicating poverty and hunger*—Directly influences health.
- *Improving maternal health*—Decreases the number of mothers who are still dying in childbirth due to unskilled birth attendants, infection, and hemorrhage.
- *Reducing the child mortality rate*—A major indicator of health structure, which shows a great disparity between different ethnic groups (see Table 2-2).

TABLE 2-2 Disparity in Infant Mortality Rate in the United States

Infant Mortality Rates*	1998	2005	2010	2013
U.S. average	7.20	6.86	6.14	5.96
American Indian/Alaska Native	9.3	8.06	8.28	unavailable
Black/African American	13.8	13.63	11.46	11.22
Hispanic/Latino	5.8	5.62	5.25	unavailable
White	6.0	5.76	5.18	5.07

*Per 1000 live births. Information gathered from U.S. Center for National Vital Statistics, Centers for Disease Control and Prevention (CDC), December 2013, published February 16, 2016.

Although the United States spends more on health care than any other nation in the world, we do not have the highest longevity rate or the lowest infant mortality rate. The American health care system is not cost-effective for the amount of money spent. The poorest countries with weak health care systems have the greatest risk—the most vulnerable are women, children, and older adults. With doctors and nurses leaving the rural areas of Africa, Asia, and Latin America for cities, and leaving their home countries to relocate in developing nations, many areas are left without health care practitioners. The number one concern of the surgeon general is that which was stated by Nelson Mandela, "The greatest single challenge facing our globalized world is to combat and eradicate its disparities." Some have very much, while others do not.

TODAY'S HEALTH CARE DELIVERY SYSTEM

Beginning in the mid- to late 1970s, many managed care plans began to make their appearance throughout the United States. By the early 1980s, health maintenance organizations (HMOs) had entered the picture in an effort to curb skyrocketing health costs. To control increased spending, a process called **utilization review** started to be used to monitor and control testing, medication, surgeries, and other areas where overuse occurred. However, this utilization process often created delays in medical care. Doctors who were once allowed to make all decisions regarding their patient's health care soon found these decisions placed in the hands of HMO personnel. Current health care delivery systems include both traditional and managed care.

Traditional Care

In traditional health care, patients may select their own **primary care physician (PCP)** who assumes the ongoing responsibility for the overall treatment of a patient, usually a general or family practitioner, internist, gynecologist, or pediatrician. They may choose to see a specialist whenever necessary, go to the hospital they prefer, and choose the facility where laboratory tests are performed. Because there is no authorization process, testing and referrals can be done immediately.

Physicians charge on a **fee-for-service (FFS)** arrangement in which either the physician's office or the patient submits a claim to the insurance company and the full amount allowed by the insurance company is collected.

Consumer-Directed Health Plan

A popular alternative to traditional health care, **consumer-directed health plans (CDHPs)**, also referred to as *consumer-driven health care (CDHC)*, offers lower premiums, higher deductibles, higher out-of-pocket maximum costs, and a tiered benefit structure. The plan provides 100% coverage for preventive benefits with no deductible. Plan participants have more responsibility in making health care decisions and are motivated to control the cost of health benefits while experiencing greater freedom in spending health care dollars. Typically, an Internet site is available to track medical expenses and obtain other useful information.

Members are allowed to use health savings accounts (HSAs), health reimbursement accounts (HRAs), or similar prefunded spending accounts to pay medical expenses directly, while a high-deductible health plan protects them from catastrophic medical expenses. When money in the savings account has been spent-down, the deductible is applied and when met the catastrophic plan goes into effect. Any money left over in the account may be rolled-over to the following year.

Managed Care

A **managed care organization (MCO)** is a type of health care delivery system that strives to manage the cost, quality, and delivery of health care by emphasizing preventive medicine, utilization of services, and a network of providers.

MCOs usually have no deductible, a small co-payment at the time of each visit, and 100% coverage of medical expenses, including preventive services, most medications, and medical supplies. Patients pay monthly medical insurance premiums individually or through their employer. The reduced cost to patients makes MCOs a popular choice. Patients, however, have limitations in their choice of PCPs and specialty care. Often patients may have to wait for medical services to be approved. At every visit, verify insurance coverage with the patient because patients change plans frequently. Collect the copayment when the patient arrives for his or her appointment, because it is easy to forget to ask for payment when the patient is leaving the office and billing for copays is not cost-effective.

Many plans require patients to have laboratory and x-ray tests performed at plan-specified *network facilities*. Always direct patients to in-network facilities and allow enough time to receive test results before scheduling a patient's return appointment. Most MCOs require prior approval or preauthorization for diagnostic services, some procedures, hospitalization, and specialist care. Such referrals may be formal, direct, verbal, or self-directed.

Precertification, Predetermination, and Preauthorization

Precertification refers to finding out if a service or procedure is covered under a patient's insurance policy. **Predetermination** means finding out the maximum dollar amount that the insurance company will pay for a professional service.

Most managed care programs and some private insurance plans require **preauthorization** for certain services, hospital admissions, inpatient or outpatient surgeries, elective procedures, or when the patient must be seen by someone other than the PCP, also known as the *gatekeeper*. Preauthorization, also referred to as *prior authorization* or *prior approval*, relates to whether a service or procedure is covered and whether the insurance plan approves it as medically necessary. The definition of **medical necessity** varies by insurance carrier or program. The American Medical Association defines it as "Health care services or products that a prudent physician would provide to a patient for the purpose of preventing, diagnosing or treating an illness, injury, disease or its symptoms in a manner that is in accordance with generally accepted standards of medical practice; clinically appropriate in terms of type, frequency, extent, site and duration; not primarily for the convenience of the patient, physician or other healthcare provider." The Medicare Claims Processing Manual defines it as ". . . the overarching criterion for payment in addition to the individual requirements of a *Current Procedural Terminology (CPT)* code."

If the preauthorization is not obtained when required, the insurance company may refuse to pay part or the entire fee. Patients may not be aware of this stipulation, so be sure to check on preauthorization requirements.

If the patient has received authorization for a service, obtain the authorization number and verify that the authorization form has been approved prior to the time of the scheduled visit. If the authorization is delayed and the patient comes in for the appointment, telephone the plan and obtain oral authorization documenting the date, time, and name of the authorizing person; otherwise, the patient's appointment may have to be rescheduled.

Patient Referrals—When a PCP recommends and sends the patient to another physician for further medical treatment, it is referred to as a **referral**. All referrals must be documented in the patient's record and if a specialist is the referring physician, a copy needs to be sent to the PCP. An organized office keeps a referral-tracking log and does a weekly or biweekly follow-up.

Following are several types of referrals that a plan may use for different levels of prior approval:

- *Formal referral*—An authorization request is required by the managed care plan to determine medical necessity. This preauthorization may sometimes be obtained via telephone, but usually a completed authorization form is electronically transmitted, mailed, or faxed (Figure 2-3).
- *Direct referral*—A simplified authorization request form is completed and signed by the physician and handed to the patient at the time of referral. Certain services may not require a formal referral (e.g., obstetrical care, dermatology).
- *Verbal referral*—The PCP informs the patient that he or she would like to refer the patient to a specialist. The physician telephones the specialist and indicates that the patient is being referred for an appointment.
- *Self-referral*—The patient refers himself or herself to a specialist. The patient may be required to inform the PCP.

If a patient refuses to be referred, this must be documented. If an authorization form is required, a letter may be written but only to supplement the mandatory form. When authorization is approved, be sure you have a copy of the form for each approved service. The form may be electronically or manually attached to the claim when billing for the services. Some referral forms authorize several office visits or multiple procedures to be done by one provider. If additional services are needed, a new authorization request must be made.

Medical Review

MCOs must follow general federal guidelines when they are established, and the government requires that the quality of care be assessed. Regional *professional review organizations (PROs)* have been set up and are composed of physicians who evaluate the quality of professional care. They also settle disputes on fees and examine evidence for admission and discharge of hospital patients. PROs play an important role in Medicare inpatient cases.

MANAGED CARE PLAN
TREATMENT AUTHORIZATION REQUEST

TO BE COMPLETED BY PRIMARY CARE PHYSICIAN OR OUTSIDE PROVIDER

Health Net	☐	Met Life	☐
Pacificare	☒	Travelers	☐
Secure Horizons	☐	Pru Care	☐

Patient Name: *Terisita Blanco* Date: *6/13/xx*

M___ F *X* Birthdate *10/23/47* Home telephone number *(555) 487-7870*

Address *29 Seaview Lane, Woodland Hills, XY 12345-0439*

Primary Care Physician *Fran Practon, MD* Member ID# *C 15038*

Referring Physician *Fran Practon, MD* Member ID# *C15038*

Referred to *George Hansevoda MD* Address *2000 Broad Avenue*

Woodland Hills, XY 12345-0001 Office telephone no. *(555) 486-7000*

Diagnosis Code *N73.9** Diagnosis *Chronic pelvic inflammatory disease*

Diagnosis Code *R19.04** Diagnosis *LLQ pelvic mass*

Treatment Plan: *Gynecology consultation for chronic pelvic inflammatory disease, left lower quadrant pain and palpable mass*

Authorization requested for procedures/tests/visits:

Procedure Code *99244*** Description *New patient consultation*

Procedure Code *76856* Description *Pelvic ultrasound*

Facility to be used: *College Hospital* Estimated length of stay *0*

Office ☒ Outpatient ☒ Inpatient ☐ Other ☐

List of potential consultants (i.e., anesthetists, assistants, or medical/surgical):

George Hansevoda, MD - Gynecologist

Physician's signature *Fran Practon, MD*

TO BE COMPLETED BY PRIMARY CARE PHYSICIAN

PCP Recommendations: *See above* PCP Initials *FP MD*

Eligibility checked *6/13/XX* Effective date *1/1/XX*

TO BE COMPLETED BY UTILIZATION MANAGEMENT

Authorized________ Not authorized________

Deferred________ Modified________

Authorization Request #________

Comments:________

FIGURE 2-3 Example of a managed care plan treatment authorization request form completed by a primary care physician for preauthorization of consultation services and pelvic ultrasound

Types of Managed Care Organizations

There are many types of MCOs. They vary from plans that restrict patients from going outside the MCO group to plans that offer great flexibility. The definitions of such plans have changed throughout the years as plan guidelines have adjusted to patient demands and medical costs.

Plans are often referred to by their abbreviations, for example, HMOs, PPOs, and IPAs, and plans that take the place of Medicare are often called "Senior Medicare." Following are some basic types of MCO plans.

Health Maintenance Organization*—A health maintenance organization (HMO) is a prepaid health plan that has been in existence the longest of all managed care plans. It is a comprehensive health care financing and delivery organization where medical services are rendered by *member physicians* to a group of enrolled people in a designated geographic area. Members select, or are assigned, to a *PCP*, who typically collects a copayment and is paid by capitation, a fixed fee paid monthly by the plan per enrolled patient, regardless of the number of services actually used.

HMOs stress preventive care. Enrollees under government programs, such as TRICARE, Medicaid, and Medicare may also join HMOs if desired, and may assign their benefits to these prepaid health plans. The Blue Plans also have enrollees from large companies serviced by managed care plans. The following are three types of HMO plans (Figure 2-4):

1. *Group practice model*—Physicians form an independent group and contract with an HMO plan to provide medical treatment to members. The physicians are paid a salary by their own independent group, not by the administrators of the health plan. Health services are available at one or more locations from a group of physicians contracting with the HMO or from physicians who are employees of the HMO.
2. *Staff model*—This HMO plan hires physicians and pays them a salary instead of contracting with a medical group.
3. *Network model*—This plan contracts with two or more group practices to provide health services.

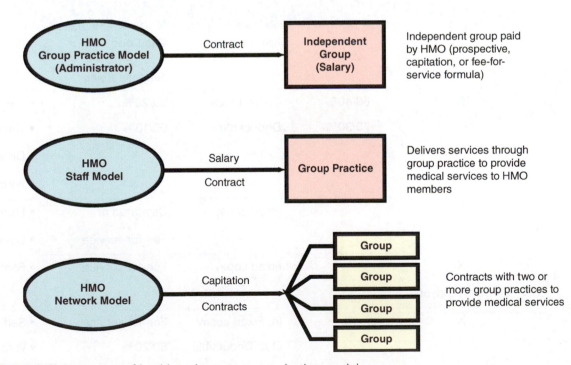

FIGURE 2-4 Different types of health maintenance organization models

---

*More than 70 million Americans participate in health maintenance organization (HMO) plans (CMA Today Sept/Oct 2012).

Preferred Provider Organization*—A variation of the HMO, a preferred provider organization (PPO) contracts with health care providers (called preferred providers) and employers, insurance carriers, or third-party administrators to provide health care service at a discounted rate. A PPO allows the subscriber more freedom of choice than does an HMO. Patients are given the incentive of lower copayments and deductibles when they go to a preferred provider within the network of contracted physicians. Patients may go to non-participating physicians, but the fee will be covered at a lesser rate (Table 2-3).

Independent Practice Association—An independent (or individual) practice association (IPA) is a type of MCO in which a program administrator contracts with several physicians who agree to provide treatment to subscribers in their own offices for a fixed capitation payment per month. Providers are placed on the organization's approved list (physician network) and

guaranteed a patient base. Besides rendering services to subscribers of the IPA, the physician also sees private-pay patients. The physicians are not employees and are not paid salaries. They are paid for their services on a capitation or fee-for-service basis from a fund drawn from the premiums collected from the subscriber, union, or corporation by the organization that markets the plan. A discount of up to 30% is withheld to cover operating costs. At the end of the year, the physicians share in any surplus or they must contribute if there is any deficit.

Physician Provider Group—*Physician provider groups (PPGs)* are physician-owned businesses, which have flexibility built into them. One division may function as an IPA under contract to an HMO. A second division may act as the provider in a PPO that contracts with hospitals as well as with other physicians to market services or medical supplies to employers and other third parties. A third division might be involved in joint ventures with hospitals, such as purchasing diagnostic equipment. The difference

TABLE 2-3 Summary of Managed Care Plan Requirements Including In- and Out-of-Network Physician Stipulations, Copayment versus Deductible Options, Payment Methods, and Authorization Requirements

Managed Care Plan	In Network	Out of Network	Copay Deductible	Payment Method	Authorization Required
HMO	X		Fixed copay	Capitated Some fee-for-service	• Formal
PPO	X	60/40% 70/30%	Coinsurance Deductible	80/20% 90/10%	• Self • Verbal • Direct • Formal
IPA	X		Fixed copay	Capitated or Fee-for-service	• Formal • Direct
EPO	X Large employers		Fixed copay	Fee-for-service	• Formal
POS	X	X	In: Fixed copay Out: Deductible	Fee-for-service 80/20% 70/30%	• Self • Verbal • Direct • Formal

*More than 90 million Americans participate in preferred provider organization (PPO) plans (CMA Today Sept/Oct 2012).

between an IPA and a PPG is that a PPG is physician owned, whereas an IPA is not owned by its member physicians. PPGs contain costs by combining services and by purchasing in bulk; appointments are made and billing is done at a central location. The member physicians give a small percentage of their income to the PPG for expenses.

Exclusive Provider Organization—An **exclusive provider organization (EPO)**, very similar to an HMO, requires members to have a designated PCP. It is called exclusive because it is offered to large employers who agree not to contract with any other plan. Members must choose care from providers offered within a limited physician network. State health insurance laws control such plans instead of federal and state HMO regulations.

Point-of-Service Plan—A managed care organization that combines elements of an HMO and a PPO and in addition offers some unique features is a **point-of-service (POS) plan**. It is basically an HMO consisting of a network of physicians and hospitals that provides an insurance company or an employer with discounts on its services. Members choose a PCP who manages specialty care and referrals. At the time of service (i.e., point of service), members have the flexibility to go out of network and can self-refer himself or herself to a specialist or see a nonnetwork provider for a higher coinsurance payment.

Accountable Care Organization—Medicare has recently launched *ACOs*, which are made up of voluntary networks of physicians, hospitals, and other health care providers who pool their resources and share joint accountability. The goal is to coordinate quality care and ensure that patients, especially the chronically ill, "get the right care at the right time" and avoid duplication of services and medical errors. Patients are allowed to choose their physician and a primary care-led clinical

team oversees patient care; cost savings are redirected back to ACO providers.

ACOs are part of a *Clinically Integrated Network*, which must share electronic data sets and meet 33 quality measures (metrics) across the following four domains: (1) patient/caregiver experience, (2) preventive health, (3) care coordination/patient safety, and (4) at-risk populations. Some examples from the first domain are "getting timely care," "patient rating of provider," and "shared decision-making."

Innovative new payment models are used, such as the *Bundled Payments for Care Improvement* (BPCI) initiative, which is made up of four broadly defined models in which a bundled payment is made for multiple services in a single episode of care.

Coordinated Care Organization—Another new model, similar to the ACO model, *coordinated care organizations (CCOs)*, serves the Medicaid population. Quality of care is emphasized and a flat fee is paid by Medicaid for services rendered.

Patient-Centered Medical Home

The **patient-centered medical home (PCMH)** is an approach to care for children, youth, and adults in which a PCP heads up a team of medical professionals who deliver comprehensive care. Although the term patient-centered medical home sounds like a medical setting or location, it is not; it is a delivery system. A team of qualified professionals is formed and the PCP and allied health care team arrange for the delivery of services (e.g., nurse evaluator, dietitian, counselor, physical therapist, occupational therapist, social worker). The physician directs and oversees all services provided, which routinely includes (1) acute care for minor injuries and illnesses, (2) ongoing management of chronic diseases, (3) office-based procedures and diagnostic tests, and (4) patient education and self-management support. Each team member takes responsibility for the ongoing care of the patient and, rather than making separate appointments for patients to see a variety of specialists, the delivery of these services is coordinated to occur right in the home. The *triple aim* of PCMH is to (1) improve patient experience, (2) reduce healthcare costs, and (3) produce healthier populations.

As a member of a multidisciplinary team, the medical assistant acts as the **patient advocate**, promoting and supporting the interest of the patient. Patients are encouraged to participate in the decision-making process and feedback is encouraged to ensure that the patient's expectations are being met. The medical assistant also enters data in an electronic medical record system and makes sure that follow-up care is provided. The team-based care approach enhances patient monitoring of chronic ailments and access to specialized care.

Employment opportunities for the medical assistant working in PCMH situations are becoming more prevalent. They serve as vital and important allied health professionals who are needed for the successful implementation of this approach. Therefore, the medical assistant will not just perform tasks but will be required to explain to patients why various questions regarding meaningful use are being asked and to think critically as he or she performs patient assessment and care.

Concierge Medical Care

A unique type of medical delivery system that allows physicians to control different aspects of their practice is referred to as *boutique* or *concierge medicine*, also known as a cash-only practice, direct care, innovative medical practice design, membership medicine, personalized medicine, or retainer-based medicine. All concierge medical practices have similarities but they vary widely in their form of operation and payment structure. With this type of practice, physicians usually limit the size of their practice from 100 to 1000 patients per year instead of 3000 or 4000. This enables the physician to offer same-day or next-day appointments, little or no waiting times, exceptional service, a relaxed atmosphere, and a customized wellness program designed for each patient. Physician access is typically offered 24 hours a day, 7 days a week via cellular telephone or email.

The physician usually "opts out" of participating in all insurance plans including Medicare. Instead, a monthly or yearly fee or retainer that varies from $500 to $5000 is charged depending on the service structure, and a flat, per-visit fee may be charged as well. If out-of-network physicians are included in the patient's insurance plan, patients can bill their insurance carrier.

Employment opportunities for the medical assistant who wishes to work for a PCP are available anywhere boutique medicine is practiced. Most concierge physicians are internal medicine specialists. Typically, in such a practice, overhead and administrative costs are kept low. Working for a concierge medical practice would appeal to a medical assistant with strong interpersonal skills because customer service is what attracts patients to this type of practice. On the negative side, complaints have been registered regarding the exclusiveness of such a practice because not everyone can afford these services; they are viewed as being for the elite.

THE MEDICAL PRACTICE SETTING

The setting in which the physician works has changed as much as the medicine he or she practices. In this section, a description of the different settings in which a physician practices as well as the employment opportunities for an administrative medical assistant are discussed.

Solo Physician Practice

The standard practice for many years was the single physician practice. In the **solo physician practice**, one physician works alone in a small office with a limited staff. The physician is either on call 24 hours a day or shares calls with another solo practitioner. Typically, the charges are based on a fee-for-service arrangement. Although solo practices still exist in some areas, this setting is beginning to be the exception, not the rule. In most areas, a solo practitioner cannot compete with large group practices and large group insurance contracts. The physician has been forced to join a group, relocate, or close the practice. Patients reap the benefits of a single physician practice in terms of a physician and staff who know them by name, treat them like family, and offer individual attention and care. The trust and loyalty that form between the physician and the patient are hard to obtain in any other medical setting.

Employment in a solo practice offers the medical assistant diverse responsibilities. In a very small practice, the medical assistant might handle both clinical and administrative duties. In an established practice, the medical assistant might be responsible for all administrative duties ranging from appointment scheduling to payroll and housekeeping. In a large solo practice, two or three medical assistants may share the administrative duties.

Associate Practice

In an **associate practice**, two or more practitioners share office expenses, employees, and the on-call schedule. Physicians practice at the same office location or at different sites, but bill under separate tax identification numbers and do not share the revenue. Such an arrangement allows a decrease in expenses and an increase in productivity.

Employment in an associate practice offers the administrative medical assistant a unique challenge. There may be two to five physicians who need to be regarded as "the boss." Duties may need to be performed for each physician in a different manner according to their specific orders, for example, keeping separate appointment schedules with varying time slots for patient treatment, lunch hours, meeting schedules, and days off. The sharing of ideas and medical decision-making can create a stimulating environment and offer patients the benefits of more sophisticated diagnosis and treatment.

Group Practice

In a **group practice**, three or more physicians agree to practice using the same office space, sharing office expenses, employees, income, and the on-call schedule. The physicians may be incorporated or in a legal partnership. A medical group is legally recognized by the American Group Practice Association. The physicians share one tax identification number and bill all claims under a group name. Three to seven physicians would be considered a small group (Figures 2-5 and 2-6). A medium group might involve 8 to 30 physicians, and any group over 30 would be considered large. Most small group practices are composed of physicians of the same specialty. A variety of specialties are called a **multispecialty practice**.

Employment in a group practice offers a variety of job duties. In a larger group, the departments become more subdivided. With more specific duties, the knowledge and job skills become more specialized, making the medical assistant a true specialist in a particular field. For example, in a large group, the assistant might work in the billing department and be the Medicare specialist, while another employee might be the managed care specialist.

Partnership

In a **partnership**, two or more physicians associate in the practice of medicine under a legal partnership agreement. The agreement specifies the responsibilities, rights, and obligations of each partner. Each physician in the partnership becomes liable for the other partner's actions and conduct, making lawsuits a great disadvantage.

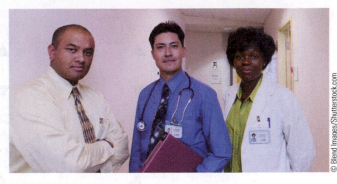

FIGURE 2-5 Three physicians working together in a group medical practice

Employment in a partnership would be similar to working in an association or group, depending on the number of physicians.

Professional Corporation

A **professional corporation** is an entity unto itself. It has a legal and business status that is independent of its shareholders. The physician shareholders are employees in the corporation and are regulated by individual state statutes. Current laws make the financial advantages of a corporation less beneficial to the physician, so as a result, fewer doctors incorporate.

Employment in a corporation is similar to working in any of the previously mentioned practice settings. A solo physician, as well as a large group, can incorporate. There may be differences in the bookkeeping aspects of the corporate practice because corporations operate under a *fiscal year*, which may involve preparing budget projections and closing their books at different times during the calendar year.

Urgent Care Center

Urgent care centers, also known as *freestanding emergency centers* or *ambulatory centers*, are available in most large and midsize cities throughout the country. Some centers provide extended hours to accommodate patients who have problems getting to the doctor weekdays between 8 a.m. and 5 p.m. and others are open 24 hours a day, 7 days a week, including holidays. They also provide a walk-in capability for minor emergencies and urgent health problems. Prior to the formulation of urgent care centers, many hospital emergency departments were overcrowded with patients requesting services for minor complaints, resulting in the staff having less time to handle major emergencies. Most patients

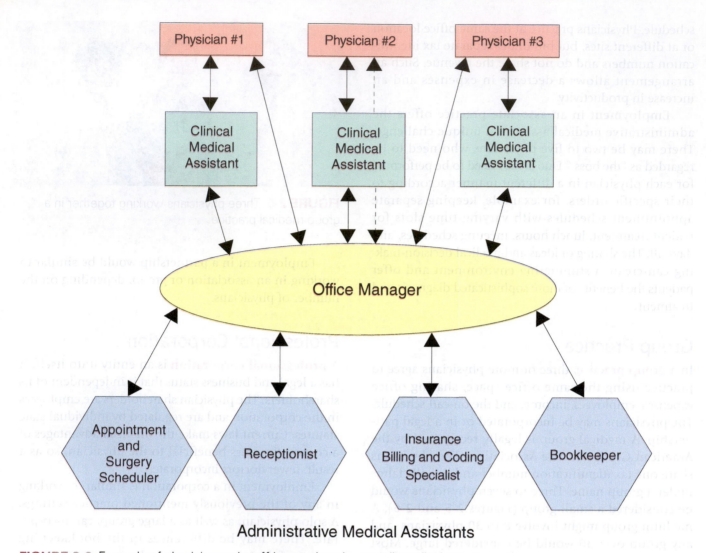

FIGURE 2-6 Example of physician and staff interactions in a small medical group practice

with minor complaints had insurance contracts that were paying for their emergency room services, thus contributing to the overutilization of insurance monies and increased medical costs.

An advantage of urgent care centers is the one-stop-shopping feature, because many centers have full laboratories, x-ray equipment, and physical therapy on-site.

Most urgent care centers are private, for-profit centers that employ salaried physicians who compete directly with private physician practices. After delivering primary emergency care, some centers refer patients to private physicians. Because of the competition from urgent care centers, many private physicians have added walk-in hours to their regularly scheduled appointment hours.

Employment with an urgent care center offers one of the most varied experiences in a health care setting because the medical assistant sees a variety of medical problems. Many centers contract with a large number of managed care plans and private insurance companies, so an insurance billing specialist is needed. A center can be an exciting, fast-paced working environment offering many challenges. It is often the first choice of a medical assistant extern after completion of training.

Clinic

Clinics are often hard to distinguish from large group practices. Patients can be admitted for special studies and treatment by a group of health care professionals practicing medicine together. Clinics usually offer a broad range of specialties and sophisticated testing equipment. The doctors can bring a complicated case to a panel of physicians for discussion and treatment options. This approach offers patients the most advanced medical decision-making available, so patients often travel great distances to seek clinics with prestigious reputations.

A clinic may also be a department of a hospital where patients who do not have to be admitted may be treated. *Satellite clinics*, also known as outpatient clinics, are usually owned by a hospital, a large medical group, or a managed care organization. They are located off-site from the main facility and are strategically placed to serve the needs of a different geographic area. These clinics usually employ physicians practicing a specialty, so advanced care can be provided to patients who have similar physical problems. Examples of *specialty clinics* are abortion clinics, family planning clinics, industrial clinics, sleep diagnostic clinics, and eye clinics.

Employment in a large clinic offers a broad range of benefits to medical assistants including job versatility and career advancement opportunities. The disadvantages of employment in such a setting are less personal contact with patients and having to cope with bureaucratic management.

In-Store Clinic

Found in chain stores is the MinuteClinic, which offers a limited range of basic tests and treatments at a lower cost than most doctors' offices. In-store clinics are operated by an outside company and generally staffed by physician assistants or nurse practitioners. These clinics may also partner with local hospitals and health care systems that staff and operate the facilities. In addition to the "Get Well" services mentioned, affordably priced "Stay Well" preventive care may be offered. Pharmacies may also offer limited health care services such as immunizations, simple blood tests (e.g., cholesterol screening), and equipment, so patients can self-monitor their blood pressure. They are typically patronized by people who do not have a PCP, do not have health insurance, and do not like waiting. In-store clinics promote quick care on a walk-in basis during normal business hours.

Employment opportunities in an in-store clinic would depend on the volume of patients seen. A multiskilled assistant performing both clinical and administrative functions would be an asset to the doctor, physician assistant, or nurse practitioner.

Hospital

Hospitals are facilities that provide 24-hour acute care and treatment for the sick and injured. They also provide emergency medical care. Patients are divided into units, formerly called wards, according to the type of illness or injuries incurred. In larger hospitals, these units may occupy complete floors or wings of a building. See Figures 2-7A and 2-7B for some common unit divisions and Figure 2-8 for a hospital organizational chart. By dividing the patient load in this manner, the nursing staff can better care for patients with similar ailments because units call for similar skills, diagnostic testing, procedures, and treatment. Larger hospitals have specialized units to serve the needs of patients who are medically unstable. See Figure 2-8 for examples of *specialized care units*. Intensive care units offer 24-hour monitoring by the nursing staff for patients whose conditions are considered critical, guarded, and unstable.

It is wise for medical assistants to meet hospital personnel that they interact with by telephone. Developing a relationship with admitting clerks, billing specialists, and laboratory personnel is prudent, because establishing a relationship paves the way for good communication.

Another major function of a hospital is its surgical unit. A hospital may have several surgical suites and a delivery room in addition to an outpatient or same-day surgery unit. A major portion of a hospital's revenue and expenses is generated through its surgical cases, so a considerable amount of thought and investigation goes into the hospital's choice of staff surgeons. The prestige of the hospital and its credibility are often measured by its staff physicians. The public image of a hospital is greatly affected by having satisfied patients in the community who have had successful surgeries and hospital stays. For online hospital ratings, refer to the *Resources* section at the end of this chapter.

Hospital Categories

Hospitals can be either government owned or non–government owned. Government-owned hospitals are subsidized by federal, state, county, or city government. An example of a federal hospital is a Veterans Administration hospital. The federal government also finances hospitals and health care facilities for Native Americans, Alaskans, merchant marines, and other groups. A state hospital can be a facility for individuals who are chronically ill or developmentally disabled, whereas county, district, and city hospitals are established primarily to meet the needs of a particular community.

Non–government-owned hospitals can be either "for profit" or "not for profit." General and community hospitals are usually nonprofit and serve a specific geographic area and need in the community. Other nonprofit hospitals include those owned by industries, unions, churches, and religious orders.

HOSPITAL ADMINISTRATIVE DEPARTMENTS

Administration department

- Oversees the management and operations of the hospital
- The Chief Executive Officer (CEO) or President works in this department
- The Board of Directors establishes bylaws outlining duties and responsibilities for the governing body, administrator, and all hospital committees

Admitting department

Handles:

- Admittance/discharge of patients
- Insurance verification
- Precertification of insurance
- Preauthorization for hospitalization and procedures

Business department

- Provides cashiers and patient statements (bills)
- Submits insurance claims
- Collects accounts receivable

Financial department

Oversees and controls:

- Business department
- Accounts receivable/payable
- Budgets and financial reports
- Insurance contracts
- Payroll

Human resource department

Manages:

- Employee benefits
- Hiring
- Orientation and training
- Job evaluations

Medical records department

Provides:

- Coding diagnoses and procedures
- In- and outpatient medical records
- Medical transcription
- Registries

Medical staff department

- Processes credentialing of all allied health professionals
- Schedules and monitors department meetings

Nursing administration department

Supervises:

- Nursing care, staffing, and education
- Nursing care of patients in specialized medical care units
- Utilization review nurses who may report to this department

FIGURE 2-7A Comprehensive listing of hospital administrative departments and their services

For-profit hospitals, also called private or investor-owned hospitals, are controlled by the individual, partnership, or corporation that owns them. A teaching or research hospital affiliated with a university utilizes the services of doctors who continue training after medical school.

Hospital sizes are measured by the number of beds provided, with state licenses issued on that basis. Physicians apply for staff privileges at the hospitals of their choice. This involves a credentialing process with a review of the physician's curriculum vitae, practice history, hospital references, and peer references, and usually includes an oral interview. Credentials are reevaluated yearly after checking on licensure and continuing medical education via the accrual of continuing education units (CEUs).

Hospital Types

Hospitals may be named for the types of patients they serve. *Acute care hospitals* treat the severely ill or injured patient. *Specialty hospitals*, such as burn centers, cancer institutes, or eye foundations, treat a specific type of patient. *Mental health hospitals* serve patients with psychiatric problems. *Substance abuse hospitals* deal with patients recovering from drug and alcohol abuse, and *convalescent hospitals*, for example, skilled nursing facilities, long-term-care facilities, or nursing homes, serve the needs of patients, usually older adults, who can no longer care for themselves at home. Many acute care hospitals have separate units to serve the needs of long-term-care patients. They may refer to these as extended care units or transitional care units. Convalescent

HOSPITAL ADJUNCT DEPARTMENTS

Dietetic/nutrition department

Furnishes:
- Dietitian and diet preparation
- Nutritional assessment and education
- Therapy

Emergency department

Physician and staff on duty 24 hours a day to handle trauma and emergencies and observe and monitor patients while collecting data to make decisions regarding admissions. Sections include:
- Casting room
- Examination room
- Observation room
- Trauma room

Gastrointestinal laboratory (GI lab)

Performs endoscopic procedures such as:
- Colonoscopy
- Proctoscopy
- Sigmoidoscopy

Intensive care units

- Coronary care
- Manage critically ill patients
- Neonatal care

Laboratory department

Offers inpatient and outpatient services such as:
- Blood bank
- Chemistry
- Cytology
- Hematology
- Histopathology
- Microbiology
- Organ bank
- Pathology
- Urinalysis

Magnetic resonance imaging department (MRI)

Performs:
- MRI scans with and without contrast Agents

Nuclear medicine department

Handles radioactive materials used in tests such as:
- Bone scans
- Liver scans
- Radioimmunoassays
- Thyroid testing

One-day surgery department

Takes care of patients who do not require overnight stay for procedures such as:
- Angiography
- Blood transfusion
- Heart catheterization
- Myelogram

Pharmacy department

Supplies medication to inpatients such as:
- Injectable medications
- Intravenous solutions
- Oral medications
- Topicals, suppositories and inhalers

Physical therapy department

Provides:
- Inpatient physical therapy
- Outpatient physical therapy
- Occupational therapy
- Speech therapy

Physiology department

Offers a variety of services such as:
- Cardiology (ECG, treadmill, 2-D echocardiogram)
- Electrophysiology (EMG, EEG, nerve conduction studies)
- Vascular medicine (deep vein Doppler)
- Myelogram

Radiology department

Performs the following procedures:
- Barium enema
- Barium swallow
- Computed tomography
- Diagnostic x-ray
- Mammograpy
- Therapeutic radiation
- Ultrasound

(continues)

FIGURE 2-7B Comprehensive listing of hospital adjunct departments and their services

HOSPITAL ADJUNCT DEPARTMENTS (continued)

Respiratory care department

Provides diagnostic and therapeutic services including the administration of:
- Bronchodilators
- Oxygen

Performs:
- Arterial blood gases
- Pulmonary function studies
- Spirometry

Sets up and assists with:
- Cardiopulmonary resuscitation
- Mechanical ventilators

Social services department

Employs medical and psychiatric social workers to work with patients and families regarding:
- Community services
- Discharge planning
- Economic factors
- Emotional situations
- Social issues
- Medical resources

FIGURE 2-7B (Continued)

PROCEDURE 2-1

Direct Patients to Specific Hospital Departments

OBJECTIVES: Use critical thinking skills and deductive reasoning to determine a specific hospital department when directing patients.

EQUIPMENT/SUPPLIES: Comprehensive list of hospital departments and their services (see Figures 2-7A and 2-7B), paper, and pen or pencil.

DIRECTIONS: Follow these step-by-step directions, which include rationales, to learn this procedure. Job Skill 2-2 in the *Workbook* is presented to practice this skill.

1. Read the physician's instructions carefully or listen attentively to the patient's question or request.
2. Record the patient's request or question stating his or her need.
3. Think about what each hospital department offers and determine what department the patient needs to be directed to according to the physician's order, patient request, or patient question.
4. Jot down the department where the patient needs to be directed to.
5. Determine if services from more than one department are needed.
6. Write the department name on the requisition slip or inform the patient of the hospital department that they are to go to.
7. Hand the patient a map of the hospital if available, or explain where to park and which entrance to use.

---

hospitals also serve the needs of short-term patients rehabilitating from illness or injury. Stroke victims and hip fracture patients are two examples of patients frequently taken care of in a transitional care unit until they have recovered sufficiently to care for themselves.

Rehabilitation hospitals provide 24-hour care for patients who have been declared medically stable, but who need acute and subacute rehabilitation. Doctors on staff direct the patient's care through a multidisciplinary team of health care professionals, including physical therapists, occupational therapists, speech pathologists, recreation therapists, dietitians, nutritionists, psychologists, pulmonary specialists, and a case manager. In addition to medical care units, surgical

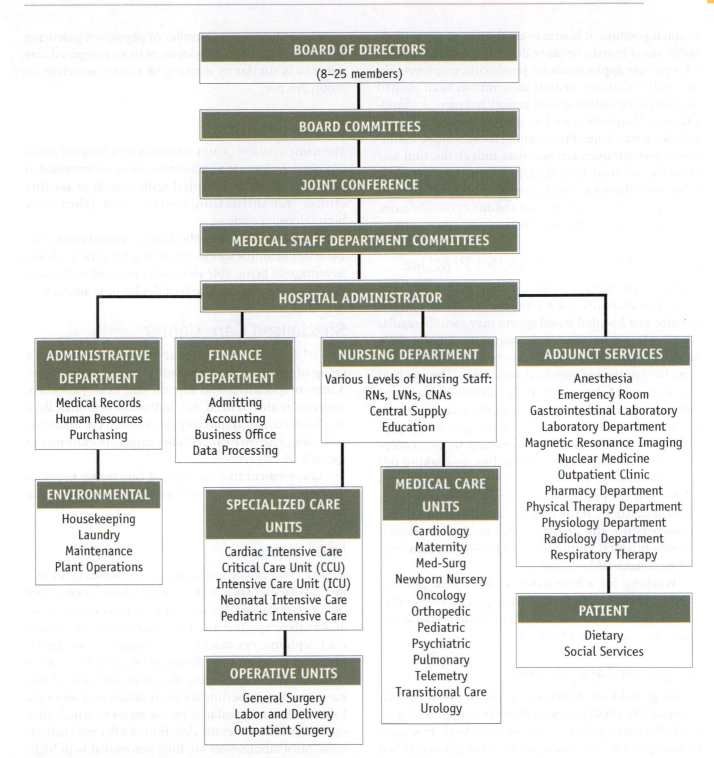

FIGURE 2-8 Hospital organizational chart showing administration and departments

suites, and delivery rooms, hospitals have many other units offering additional services. These services are essential to good medical care; they are referred to as adjunct services instead of ancillary or auxiliary as they were once called. See Figure 2-7B for a listing of adjunct departments.

The business portion of the hospital is handled in many administrative departments. For a listing and explanation of these departments, see Figures 2-7A and 2-7B.

Employment in a hospital provides a variety of administrative opportunities and employment benefits for the medical assistant. When one is applying for a hospital position, it is wise to emphasize administrative skills. Many human resource department staff members who process applications for prospective employees do not realize that the medical assistant has been trained in most of the skills required to work in hospital administration. Hospitals often hire medical assistants for the following positions: Preadmitting coordinators, admitting representatives, receptionists, unit clerks, unit secretaries, medical record technicians, clerk typists, insurance billing specialists, insurance verification coordinators, insurance coders, bed condition coordinators, cashiers, collectors, and file clerks.

Hospital-Owned Physician Practice

Physician practices are being bought by hospital systems. The incentive for a physician to sell his or her practice to a hospital-based system may include regular working hours for the doctor, payment of malpractice insurance premiums, a salary plus bonus, and more free time for family and personal endeavors. The medical assistant and other employee positions will change depending on the legal structure of the arrangement. If the practice continues to operate independently (i.e., renting space from the hospital, owning its own equipment, purchasing drugs and supplies, and taking full responsibility for employees), the medical assistant's role within the practice will be similar to that of other medical practices. If the practice operates under hospital ownership, the physician and medical assistants become hospital employees and business operations will be considerably different.

Working for a hospital-owned medical practice would offer a strong benefit package as well as other work opportunities; it would be similar to working in a medical center or for a hospital.

Integrated Care Network

An *Integrated Care Network* is a "big network" of private-practice small and solo physicians (e.g., 250 doctors) who ban together to compete with large, expansive health systems. Physicians practice independently but pool their resources to advertise and have more negotiating power with insurance carriers. Doctors in the network commit to meeting national quality standards of care to keep patients out of hospitals, drive down costs, and trigger reimbursement bonuses. The loosely affiliated network is typically run by physicians but funded by local hospitals in which they serve as partners. In the network arrangement, hospitals receive part of the reimbursement from insurance companies.

Depending on the number of physicians practicing in the same location, employment in an integrated care network is similar to working in a solo, associate, or group practice.

Medical Center

The name **medical center** written after a hospital name usually denotes that additional services are provided at sites other than the hospital setting, such as satellite clinics, rehabilitation centers, and laboratory blood-drawing stations.

Employment in a medical center would render the same opportunities as working in a hospital with the advantage of being able to transfer to another location as positions at the satellite facilities become available.

Specialized Care Center

Specialized care centers exist to serve the needs of a group of patients who have similar medical conditions. A team of specialists with support staff treats patients in a particular area of need. Rehabilitation institutes, drug treatment centers, respiratory care centers, eye institutes, and comprehensive cancer care centers are examples of specialized care centers.

Employment in a specialized care center provides the opportunity to work in a specialized area, with one particular type of patient.

Laboratory

Laboratories can be independent, freestanding, or in a medical facility such as a hospital, clinic, urgent care center, or research institute. Laboratories collect, receive, and analyze specimens. They disseminate test results via telephone, fax machine, computer transmission, and mailing of reports. Research laboratories seeking information leading to the diagnosis and cure of diseases conduct experiments on humans and animals. Laboratories are regulated by the states in which they operate and are under the direction of a licensed pathologist. Most laboratories are fully automated with high-tech computers, thereby eliminating manual analysis. In many states, regulations have become so strict that doctors have closed *physician office laboratories* (POLs) and instead send specimens to outside laboratories.

Physicians are very dependent on laboratory results to expedite the diagnosis and treatment of their patients. The quality control standards of the laboratory, the turn-around time (speed of testing specimens and sending results to physicians), and the cost to the patient are three very important factors in choosing a dependable laboratory.

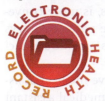

Electronic Lab Reporting (ELR) is the distribution of laboratory test results using electronic transmission rather than paper for fax. It is part of the "Meaningful Use" requirements outlined by the Centers for Medicare and Medicaid Services for reporting communicable and environmental diseases to public health departments. Physician offices, hospitals, and free-standing laboratories are using electronic transmission of laboratory orders and results to reduce errors, improve timelines, and for the completeness of reports.

Employment in a laboratory requires precision and accuracy. Articulating and recording exact test results are skills both the clinical and administrative medical assistant should have. One transposed or misunderstood number could change the course of treatment for a patient. Other administrative skills include scheduling appointments; laboratory data entry; filing; bookkeeping; keying autopsy, forensic, coroner, and statistical reports; maintaining tumor and autopsy logs; labeling and filing specimens; and being familiar with diagnostic codes for laboratory and pathology procedures, more commonly referred to as SNOMED.

Managed Care Organization

MCOs operate under the concept of prepaid group health care. As mentioned earlier in this chapter there are many different types of prepaid health plans, usually administered by HMOs, IPAs, and PPOs.

The setting of these practices usually consists of a group of doctors who act as PCPs for one or more of the previously mentioned plans. There may also be specialists at the facility. Because increased efficiency and decreased costs are primary goals, the physicians may have increased patient loads resulting in less time spent with each patient. The PCP gatekeeper strives to avoid unnecessary tests or referrals to specialists. The concept is to make the best utilization of time and money. Employment in a managed care setting offers many of the same opportunities as a large group practice, such as benefit plans, a variety of job duties, seeing health care dollars well spent, and opportunities for advancement.

Holistic Health Environment

The holistic approach to health care evolved from the philosophy that the physical, mental, and social well-being of the "whole" person is as important as the treatment of a separate medical problem. Investigation is made into the cause of the disease instead of just treating symptoms. The patient is trained to take total responsibility for his or her health from birth to death and to develop a lifestyle that produces wellness.

Complementary and alternative medicine (CAM) physicians are used by 30% to 50% of the adult population according to the National Institutes of Health (NIH). Although still not considered a part of conventional medical care, this group of diverse medical and health care systems, practices, and products is used in conjunction with traditional health care and includes the following:

- Acupressure, acupuncture, and hypnosis therapy
- Biofield and bioelectromagnetic-based therapies
- Chiropractic medicine and massage therapy
- Dietary supplements and herbal products
- Homeopathic, naturopathic, and traditional Chinese medicine
- Meditation, prayer, yoga, and mental healing

See the *Resources* section at the end of the chapter for website listings of licensed CAM practitioners.

Employment in a holistic health care setting would involve the medical assistant in patient education by ordering educational literature and communicating holistic principles to the patient. The medical assistant would have duties similar to those of other health care settings, but would need to display the optimistic attitude toward parenting, aging, and death that is characteristic of holistic thinking. The medical assistant would also be expected to encourage the patient to improve all aspects of health, including exercise; proper nutrition and diet; freedom from substances such as prescription medications, drugs, and alcohol; and a positive approach to mental health that includes freedom from stress and depression.

Telemedicine

Telemedicine is the wireless transfer of medical information via electronic technology to provide health care when there is a separation between the health care professional and the patient. Innovative complex technologies may be used such as satellite technology, videoconferencing equipment, or a computer, which can process data and be programmed to monitor data and sound alerts to early warning signs. *Remote monitoring*, also called self-monitoring, allows a clinician to monitor a patient with a chronic disease (e.g., asthma, diabetes, heart disease) remotely using various technological devices such as biotelemetry, which monitors the heart rate, heart rhythm, body temperature, and produces a single-line ECG rhythm. A clinician at a host site who provides clinical consultation to a patient at a remote site can use interactive telemedicine applications, such as the digital stethoscope.

Care at a distance, also called *absentia* care, has been around for years; however, new technology has propelled this type of medicine into new areas. For example, today, in remote locations found in Alaska and Hawaii, medical data (e.g., x-rays, pathology slides, biosignals) can be transferred to a specialist for interpretation offline; this is called "store-and-forward" telemedicine. Physicians who frequently use this method include dermatologists (teledermatology), pathologists (telepathology), and radiologists (teleradiology). When online communication or videoconferencing is used, this is called *interactive telemedicine services*. A "centralized hub" (Tele-Hub) with a call center is another type of telemedicine used to monitor patients 24/7 in an intensive care unit, or a decentralized "e-hub" may be used to provide consultations from anywhere.

When the term *telehealth* is used, it most likely refers to nonclinical services such as administration, medical education, and research. The term *e-health* is used as an umbrella term encompassing telemedicine, telehealth, electronic medical records, and other components of electronic media.

Clinical applications of telemedicine may be used as a substitute for transportation of patients or health care professionals when it is impractical, expensive, or complicated for the patient to be moved. People who live in remote locations, prisoners with infectious diseases, people who are homebound and cannot drive, and medical emergencies where immediate treatment is of the utmost importance are all circumstances where this technology can be applied.

The Telecommunications Bill of 1996 provided key legislation to ensure that rural, high-cost, or low-income areas would have access to telecommunication services at affordable rates. The Comprehensive Telehealth Act of 1999 articulated new reimbursement policies for consultative telemedicine services performed in underserved areas by Medicare providers. These are referred to as rural Health Professional Shortage Areas (HPSA). The originating site for a Medicare patient must be in some type of health care facility or office as opposed to their home; however, some providers are still offering home services and absorbing the cost. Individual states have taken different approaches, which vary greatly, to providing telemedicine to Medicaid patients.

With a shortage of physicians, telemedicine is a good alternative to bring health care into or close to the patient's home. It offers better access, is more convenient, and reduces travel costs while patient surveys indicate that that telemedicine services provide satisfactory medical care.

Employment for an administrative medical assistant in telemedicine varies greatly. A medical assistant may be employed at the host site as a "telepresenter" who ensures an efficient telehealth exchange, or at the remote site, delivering and setting up equipment and providing patient support. Cutting-edge technology is being applied to this field of medicine making it an exciting new frontier to work in.

THE PHYSICIAN SPECIALIST

Another aspect of the medical assistant's decision about what type of practice to choose is what type of doctor to work with. A variety of specialty practices offer a broad range of patient types and job duties. Table 2-4 lists medical specialties with a brief description and job responsibilities for each specialty. All specialized areas would require the administrative medial assistant to have knowledge in medical terminology, medical coding, and claims processing unique to each area.

The physician who is certified in a medical specialty must fulfill educational and internship requirements and pass an examination beyond the standard medical degree (see Chapter 3). When a physician has been certified in a field of specialization, he or she is known as a *diplomat.*

Nonphysician Providers

Many busy medical practices have found the need to free the physician's time to handle complex clinical problems. Nonphysician providers (NPPs) with advanced education, specialized clinical training, and the ability to diagnose and treat patients with a variety of medical problems may be on staff. These *physician extenders* might be a physician assistant (PA), a nurse practitioner (NP), a clinical nurse specialist (CNS), or a nurse midwife (NMW). Always address these individuals using their correct professional title. Be sure to correct patients who refer to a nonphysician practitioner as "doctor" or to a medical assistant as "nurse." If the patient is led to believe that the medical assistant is a nurse and a lawsuit develops, the assistant may be held to standards to which nurses are held.

PROCEDURE 2-2

Refer Patients to the Correct Physician Specialist

OBJECTIVE: Use critical thinking skills and deductive reasoning to determine what physician specialist the patient needs.

EQUIPMENT/SUPPLIES: Comprehensive list of physician specialists (see Table 2-4), paper, and pen or pencil. *Note: Most primary care physicians have a list of specialists in the community that they refer to and may collect appointment cards from those doctors, so appointments may be scheduled from your office. Do not refer patients without the physician's direction.*

DIRECTIONS: Follow these step-by-step directions, which include rationales, to learn this procedure. Job Skill 2-3 in the *Workbook* is presented to practice this skill.

1. Read the physician's instructions carefully or listen attentively to the request or question from the patient, family member, or other party. Allowing the party to fully verbalize his or her request will give you more information to determine the person's needs.

2. Record the patient's request or question stating his or her need. Writing a note you can refer back to will help if there is more than one request or a lengthy conversation.

3. Think about what services each type of physician specialty offers and determine if the services requested are handled by your physician or another specialist.

4. Jot down the type of specialist the patient needs to be referred to.

5. Determine if services from more than one specialist are needed.

6. Write the physician's name and specialty on an appointment card or inform the patient of the specialist's name.

7. Offer to call and arrange the appointment and explain how to get to the office location.

TABLE 2-4 Medical Specialties and Administrative Medical Assisting Job Requirements

Medical Specialties	Administrative Medical Assistant Must ...
Allergy and Immunology (All. and immun.)—Diagnosis and treatment of allergic conditions	Handle numerous referrals from other physicians Determine time required for tests and schedule appointments efficiently Have excellent transcription skills
Anesthesiology (Anes.)—Administration of anesthesia for major surgery	Schedule surgery and calculate anesthesia time into units to bill insurance carriers Know types and routes of anesthesia
Bariatric medicine—Management and control of obesity	Receive referrals and obtain medical histories Schedule tests and surgery Verify insurance coverage Be sensitive to the problem of obesity while referring patients for psychological evaluations Encourage and support patients
Dermatology (Derm.)—Treatment of diseases affecting the skin; proper care of the skin	Obtain accurate, detailed case histories Be comfortable in the presence of unsightly skin disorders
Emergency medicine (Emerg. Med.)—Treatment of trauma and sudden emergent medical conditions	Handle emergent situations Be able to prioritize incoming calls and walk-in patients Calm patients and visitors

(continues)

TABLE 2-4 Medical Specialties and Administrative Medical Assisting Job Requirements (*continued*)

Medical Specialties	Administrative Medical Assistant Must ...
Family practice (FP)—Comprehensive medical care for individuals of all ages, often entire families	Manage multiple appointments Handle frequent telephone calls and deal well with emergencies Enjoy people and be expert in public relations Be able to relate to children
Gerontology (Ger. or geriat.)—Study of the aging process; geriatricians diagnose and treat problems and diseases of the older adult	Communicate resourcefully with patients who have hearing impairments Attend to older adult patients who have mobility problems Interact well with patients suffering visual loss or blindness Be diplomatic with older adult patients who suffer memory loss
Internal medicine (I.M.)—Consultations on and diagnosis of complex diseases, such as cardiovascular disease, endocrinology, gastroenterology, hematology, infectious disease, oncology, nephrology, pulmonary disease, rheumatology, proctology, and epidemiology	Key letters to referring physicians and transcribe reports Skillfully handle telephone when physician is away from office Interact with older adult patients who have hearing and sight problems Maintain detailed flow sheets for multiple medical conditions
Medical genetics—Diagnosis and treatment of genetic-linked diseases	Be detail oriented and like research Process referrals and schedule tests Understand molecules, genes, and chromosomes Be sensitive to patient anxieties while undergoing testing and empathetic to those suffering from genetic abnormalities
Neonatology (Neonat.)—Dealing with disorders of the newborn, from birth to 28 days (subspecialty of pediatrics)	Calm parents skillfully in telephone conversations Use empathy with parents who are dealing with sick newborns Transmit records to primary care physicians
Neurology/Neurosurgery (Neuro.)—Disorders of the nervous system that may be hereditary or caused by injuries, disease, or infection	Record physician's findings during examinations Be familiar with problems of people with physical handicaps Deal with patients with emotional and abnormal behavior
Nuclear medicine (Nuc. med.)—Diagnosis and treatment of disease by radionuclear methods	Understand radioisotopes and malignant diseases
Obstetrics and gynecology (OB-GYN)—Combined specialty of the study and treatment of the female reproductive system: OB—medical care of women during pregnancy and childbirth; GYN—diagnosis and treatment of female disorders	Have a mature and dignified personality Be competent in managing appointment schedules when frequent interruptions and delays occur
Subspecialty: Female pelvic medicine and reconstructive surgery (also subspecialty of urology). Treats urogynecological problems (e.g., pelvic floor disorders [PFDs])	Arrange appointments with hospital for baby delivery; transmit patient records Explain patient fees and reasons for regularly scheduled visits Be sensitive to patients with infertility problems Arrange for surgical scheduling of patients Interrelate well with babies in the office

(continues)

TABLE 2-4 **Medical Specialties and Administrative Medical Assisting Job Requirements** (*continued*)

Medical Specialties	Administrative Medical Assistant Must ...
Ophthalmology (Ophth.)—Treat disorders of the eye	Schedule patients to be seen when others are waiting for refraction drops to take effect Interact well with patients who are sight impaired or blind
Orthopedic surgery (Orth. surg.)—Treat various parts of skeletal and muscular systems, including bones and joints	Maintain a flexible appointment schedule involving emergency appointments Schedule x-rays, MRIs, CTs, bone scans, and various tests Schedule supplementary treatments with physical therapist Handle a large volume of industrial accident cases Maintain separate records for workers' compensation and liability cases
Otolaryngology (ENT)—Treat disorders of the ear, nose, and throat (also called otorhinolaryngology)	Key case histories and pre- and postoperative reports Schedule office and hospital surgery Communicate resourcefully with patients who have a hearing loss Work allergy testing and injections into daily schedule
Pathology (Path.)—Hematology, medical microbiology, neuropathology, and forensic medicine; determine causes and nature of diseases and contribute to diagnosis, prognosis, and treatment	Possess accurate transcription skills Telephone oral reports accurately
Pediatrics (Ped.) **and adolescent medicine**—Medical treatment of children and adolescents	Enjoy children and understand child psychology Calm upset parents skillfully on telephone and in office Follow office protocol when giving information to parents over the telephone
Pediatric subspecialties: Adolescent medicine Hematology-oncology Cardiology Infectious diseases Critical care Nephrology Development-behavioral Neurodevelopmental disabilities Emergency medicine Pulmonology Endocrinology Rheumatology Gastroenterology Sports medicine	Screen calls and merge emergency appointments into a full schedule Schedule appointments with a minimum of waiting time Handle teenagers diplomatically when they have nervous or drug-related disorders
Perinatology—Specializes in maternal-fetal medicine; consultations on complications of pregnancy, genetic counseling, prematurity prevention, fetal echocardiography, and antenatal testing	Check health insurance to verify covered and noncovered services Handle high-risk perinatal referrals from OB-GYN specialists Communicate results of ultrasound and amniocentesis procedures according to office protocol
Physiatrist (Phys. med. rehab.)—Physical medicine and rehabilitation; treatment of an ill or injured patient by massage, electrotherapy, and exercise; specializes in pain management	Deal with patients who are in continual pain Encourage patients on long rehabilitation programs Schedule epidural appointments and communicate pre- and postoperative guidelines

(*continues*)

TABLE 2-4 Medical Specialties and Administrative Medical Assisting Job Requirements (continued)

Medical Specialties	Administrative Medical Assistant Must ...
Plastic surgery (P. surgery)—Repair or rebuild imperfect or damaged body parts	Obtain accurate, detailed case histories Handle emergency situations well Be comfortable dealing with patients who are disfigured
Podiatry (DPM)—Diagnosis and treatment of conditions affecting the human foot	Schedule surgery Assist older adult patients with mobility problems Take a vascular evaluation history
Preventive medicine (PM)—Protect, promote, and maintain health and well-being; prevent disease, disability, and premature death	Understand and interact with managed care plan providers Send recall and reminder notices to patients Know preventive medicine procedures Understand insurance rules regarding preventive medicine
Psychiatry (Psy.)—Treatment, diagnosis, and prevention of mental disorders of a functional nature, such as stress	Deal calmly with disturbed patients Screen patients on the telephone Empathize with patients having varied mental disorders Like people and convey a welcoming attitude Guard confidential patient records and maintain office security
Radiology (Rad.)—Diagnosis and treatment of disease using x-rays and radium	Handle referrals from physicians Understand requirements for various x-rays and radiology procedures Telephone oral reports accurately
Surgery (Surg.)—Treatment of injuries, deformities, or disease by operation **Specific surgery disciplines:** Cardiovascular Oral Colon and rectal Orthopedic General Pediatric Hand Plastic Head and neck Thoracic Neurologic Urologic Ophthalmic Vascular	Handle manage care authorizations for procedures Schedule in-office and hospital surgeries Schedule pre-op and post-op appointments Be able to discern and handle surgical emergencies and complications
Urology (Urol.)—Disorders of the genitourinary tract: bladder, kidney, and prostate surgery	Schedule surgery with hospital personnel Have good telephone skills Be tactful when dealing with patients who have sensitive health concerns

Health Care Professionals' Abbreviations

Table 2-5 contains a list of abbreviations of assorted common professional positions in the field of medicine. An administrative medical assistant will interact with various health care professionals when employed in the medical field and should be familiar with these abbreviations.

TABLE 2-5 Abbreviations for Physician Specialists and Health Care Professionals

Physician Specialist	Abbreviation	Health Care Professional	Abbreviation
Doctor of Chiropractic	DC	Certified Coding Specialist; certified by the American Health Information Management Association (AHIMA)	CCS
Doctor of Dental Science	DD Sc	Certified First Assistant (surgical)	CFA
Doctor of Dental Surgery	DDS	Certified Laboratory Assistant; certified by Registry of American Society for Clinical Pathologists	CLA (ASCP)
Doctor of Emergency Medicine	DEM	Certified Medical Transcriptionist	CMT
Doctor of Hygiene	D Hy	Certified Nurse Midwife	CNM
Doctor of Medical Dentistry	DMD	Certified Professional Coder; certified by AAPC (formerly the American Academy of Professional Coders)	CPC
Doctor of Medicine	MD	Certified Registered Nurse Anesthetist	CRNA
Doctor of Ophthalmology	OphD	Certified Surgical Technician (2nd surgical asst.)	CST
Doctor of Optometry	OD	Emergency Medical Technician	EMT
Doctor of Osteopathy	DO	Health Information Management professional	HIM
Doctor of Pharmacy	Pharm D	Inhalation Therapist	IT
Doctor of Podiatry	DPM	Laboratory Technician Assistant	LTA
Doctor of Public Health	DPH	Licensed Practical Nurse	LPN
Doctor of Tropical Medicine	DTM	Licensed Vocational Nurse	LVN
Doctor of Veterinary Medicine	DVM	Master of Public Health	MPH
Doctor of Veterinary Surgery	DVS	Medical Technologist; certified by the American Society for Clinical Pathology	MT (ASCP)
Fellow of the American Academy of Pediatrics	FAAP	Physician's Assistant—Certified	PA-C
Fellow of the American College of Obstetricians and Gynecologists	FACOG	Public Health Nurse	PHN
Fellow of the American College of Surgery	FACS	Registered Dietitian	RD
Senior Fellow	SF	Registered Nurse	RN
		Registered Nurse First Assistant (surgical)	RNFA
		Registered Nurse Practitioner	RNP
		Registered Occupational Therapist	ROT
		Registered Physical Therapist	RPT
		Registered Respiratory Therapist	RRT
		Registered Technologist (Radiology)	RT (R)
		Registered Technologist (Therapy)	RT (T)
		Visiting Nurse	VN

STOP AND THINK CASE SCENARIO
Traditional versus Managed Care

SCENARIO: Janet takes her two grandmothers to see the same physician who accepts Medicare and Senior Medicare. She arranges both of their appointments for Tuesday morning. Granny needs to write a check for her yearly deductible and Nana pays a $10 copayment. After they have both seen the doctor, the medical assistant appears with directions regarding their treatment plans. Granny needs to see a urologist and an appointment is made for the following day. Nana needs to have an x-ray and an authorization will be processed. The medical assistant will call when it is approved.

CRITICAL THINKING:

1. What type of Medicare plan is Granny on?

_____

_____

_____

2. What type of Medicare plan is Nana on?

_____

_____

_____

3. What type of MCO does the physician belong to that enables him or her to see both of these types of patients in the office?

_____

_____

_____

_____

_____

_____

STOP AND THINK CASE SCENARIO
Determination of Benefits

SCENARIO: A patient is seen in the office and the physician determines that a bronchoscopy is needed. You are asked to make sure the procedure is a covered benefit, determine what the payment will be, and find out whether prior approval is necessary.

CRITICAL THINKING: Consider which process is necessary to determine the following:

1. What process will you go through to determine whether a bronchoscopy is a covered benefit?

_____

_____

2. What process will you go through to determine the maximum dollar amount that the insurance company will pay for this procedure?

_____

_____

3. What process will you go through to determine if prior approval is necessary?

_____

_____

STOP AND THINK CASE SCENARIO
Types of Medical Practice Settings

SCENARIO 1: You have a desire to go to a physician who will know you by name and treat you like family.

CRITICAL THINKING 1: What type of practice setting will you look for?

_____

_____

SCENARIO 2: You would like to walk into a physician's office without having to make an appointment.

CRITICAL THINKING 2: What type of practice setting will you look for?

_____

_____

SCENARIO 3: You are looking for a job as an administrative medical assistant and benefits are more important to you than high pay.

CRITICAL THINKING 3: What type of practice setting will you look for?

_____

_____

CRITICAL THINKING 4: What type of practice setting will you look for?

_____

_____

SCENARIO 4: You have a friend who is a burn victim and you want to work in a setting that treats such patients.

CRITICAL THINKING 5: What type of practice setting will you look for?

_____

_____

SCENARIO 5: You believe that the physician should treat the body, mind, and soul, not just the physical ailment.

_____

_____

FOCUS ON CERTIFICATION*

CMA (AAMA) Content Summary

- Medical terminology
- Working as a team
- Patient advocate
- Patient instruction
- Appropriate referrals
- Prepaid HMO, PPO, POS
- Applying managed care policies and procedures
- Referrals
- Precertification

RMA (AMT) Content Summary

- Medical terminology
- Patient instruction
- Insurance terminology
- Insurance plans: HMO, PPO, EPO
- Identify and comply with contractual requirements of insurance plans
- Identify and apply plan policies and regulations for HMO, PPO, EPO, indemnity, and open programs

*This textbook and the accompanying Workbook meet the entry-level administrative and general competencies for the CMA outlined by the AAMA Examination Content Outline and Occupational Analysis and for the RMA and CMAS outlined by the AMT Competencies, Construction Parameters, and Examination Specifications (see Competency Grid in Appendix B)

CMAS (AMT) Content Summary

- Medical terminology
- Prepare information for referrals
- Private/commercial insurance plans
- Understand health care insurance terminology (deductible, copayment, preauthorization, capitation, coinsurance)
- Understand requirements for health care insurance plans

REVIEW EXAM-STYLE QUESTIONS

1. What is the name of the medical profession symbol, which is represented by a serpent coiled around a staff, and according to Greek legend, represents a Greek god of healing?
   a. Twin snakes
   b. Aesculapius
   c. Caduceus
   d. Asclepius
   e. Serpent

2. The "father of medicine" was:
   a. Imhotep
   b. Hippocrates
   c. Pasteur
   d. Lister
   e. Salk

3. The "father of modern surgery" was:
   a. Pierre Curie
   b. Francis Crick
   c. Ambroise Paré
   d. Walter Reed
   e. William Harvey

4. The founder of the American Red Cross was:
   a. Clara Barton
   b. Florence Nightingale
   c. Ignaz P. Semmelweis
   d. John Hunter
   e. Edward Jenner

5. Managed care started the practice of "utilization review" to:
   a. review physicians' diagnostic skills
   b. review all aspects of the medical practice
   c. utilize HMO personnel more efficiently
   d. monitor and control areas in medicine where overuse occurs
   e. control doctors' decision-making

6. The managed care organization that has been in existence the longest is a/an:
   a. PPO
   b. IPA
   c. HMO
   d. EPO
   e. POS

7. The type of managed care organization that offers the patient flexibility when making a choice of going to a contracted or noncontracted physician at the time services are needed is a/an:
   a. PPO
   b. HMO
   c. IPA
   d. EPO
   e. POS

8. A freestanding practice center that provides extended hours and walk-in appointments is a/an:
   a. medical center
   b. family practice
   c. medical clinic
   d. specialized care center
   e. urgent care center

9. A specialty that deals with the management and control of obesity is called:
   a. a weight control clinic
   b. bariatric medicine
   c. gerontology
   d. nuclear medicine
   e. medical genetics

10. A medical specialty that determines the causes and nature of diseases and contributes to diagnosis, prognosis, and treatment is called:
    a. gerontology
    b. family practice
    c. internal medicine
    d. surgery
    e. pathology

11. The abbreviation for a doctor of ophthalmology is:
    a. OD
    b. OP
    c. OphD
    d. DO
    e. MD

WORKBOOK ASSIGNMENT

To develop competency-based job skills, refer to the *Workbook* and complete the:
- Abbreviation and Spelling Review
- Review Questions

- Critical Thinking Exercises
- Job Skill activities, which are listed at the beginning of the chapter under *Performance Objectives in the Workbook.*

RESOURCES

Books

Essentials of Managed Health Care, 5th edition
> Kungstvedt, MD, Peter
> Jones and Bartlett Publishers

Health Care Careers
> American Medical Association Store, 2012–2013
> Website: http://www.ama-assn.org

The Merck Manual for Health Care Professionals, 19th edition
> The Merck Publishing Group, 2011
> Springhouse, PA

Hospital Ratings

> Individual states: Search key terms—"compare hospitals" or "rate hospitals"

Internet: Health Care and Diseases

Agency for Healthcare Research and Quality (AHRQ)
> Safe Practices for Better Healthcare: Summary

American Association of Naturopathic Physicians
> Natural health insights

American Medical Association
> Resources, publications, education
> Locate physicians: See "DoctorFinder"

Association of American Medical Colleges
> Health care news and publications

Healthfinder®
> Search: Health topics

National Institutes of Health
> Health information

Priory Medical Journals (free)
> Online medical journals/articles

TRIP Database (five free searches per week)
> Evidence-based medical resources: Look up diseases

U.S. National Library of Medicine
> Databases

White House Commission on Complementary and Alternative Medicine Policy
> Search: Complementary and Alternative Medicine Policy

Medical Specialties

Select type of specialty and search:
> Example: American Academy of Dermatology
> American Association of Naturopathic Physicians
> American Board of Medical Specialties
> American College of Physicians

CHAPTER 3

MEDICOLEGAL AND ETHICAL RESPONSIBILITIES

LEARNING OBJECTIVES

After reading this chapter and learning step-by-step procedures to gain job skills,* you should be able to:

- Define legal terminology used in the chapter.
- Compare medical ethics and medical etiquette.
- Outline the purpose and provisions of the Health Insurance Portability and Accountability Act.
- Articulate the purpose for obtaining a signed consent.
- Determine reasons for disclosure that need an authorization to release medical information.
- State the licensing requirements for a physician.
- Describe the medical assistants' scope of practice.
- Indicate two types of medical professional liability insurance.
- Understand various types of contracts.
- Explain instances when a minor is emancipated.
- List prevention measures for medicolegal claims.
- Distinguish three alternatives to the litigation process.
- Cite components of an informed consent for a procedure or service.
- Identify statutes governing subpoena of records.
- Learn about various types of advance directives.
- Name the provisions of the Uniform Anatomical Gift Act.

PERFORMANCE OBJECTIVES (PROCEDURES) IN THIS TEXTBOOK

- Release patient information (Procedure 3-1).

PERFORMANCE OBJECTIVES (JOB SKILLS) IN THIS WORKBOOK

- List personal ethics and set professional ethical goals (Job Skill 3-1).
- Complete an authorization form to release medical records (Job Skill 3-2).

---

*This textbook and the accompanying Workbook meet the educational components for entry-level administrative and general competencies outlined by CAAHEP and ABHES.

- Download state-specific scope of practice laws and determine parameters for a medical assistant (Job Skill 3-3).
- Compose a letter of withdrawal (Job Skill 3-4).
- View a MedWatch online form and learn submitting requirements (Job Skill 3-5).
- Print the Patient Care Partnership online brochure and apply it to the medical office setting (Job Skill 3-6).
- Download and compare state-specific advance directives (Job Skill 3-7).

KEY TERMS*

administrative law	emancipated minors	living will
advance directive	ethics	minimum necessary standard
authorization form	etiquette	plaintiff
bioethics	expert testimony	portability
bonding	grievance committee	privileged information
civil law	health care power of attorney	protected health information (PHI)
complaint	Health Information Technology for Economic and Clinical Health Act (HITECH)	*respondeat superior*
compliance plan		risk management
consent form	Health Insurance Portability and Accountability Act (HIPAA)	scope of practice
contract law		subpoena
covered entities	implied contract	*subpoena duces tecum*
criminal law	litigation	tort
defendant		

HEART OF THE HEALTH CARE PROFESSIONAL

Service

The health care professional has the responsibility to conduct business in a legal and ethical manner. Serving patients' needs presents the perfect opportunity to exhibit high values and principles. It is through service-oriented duties that your moral character will stand out, be noticed, and be appreciated.

MEDICAL ETHICS

Before entering the profession of administrative medical assisting, it is advisable to have some basic knowledge of ethical and legal responsibilities as they pertain to the medical profession. Professional medical **ethics** are not laws but are standards of conduct generally accepted as a moral guide for behavior. Ethical principles should be reflected in administrative procedures. For example, the principle of the patient's right to privacy is guaranteed by an administrative rule against discussing a patient's condition with others. These moral principles and related professional standards of conduct apply equally to

*All key terms and italicized terms may be found online in Chapter 3 table "Legal Terms at a Glance" with definitions and examples (see www.cengagebrain.com for student website resources or go to MindTap).

relationships with patients, other physicians, members of allied professions, and the public.

The focus in this chapter is on professional ethics and medicolegal responsibilities with which a medical assistant needs to be concerned. For specific questions beyond the scope of this chapter, medical assistants should seek legal advice and the counsel of an attorney; each state has its own laws pertaining to medical practice. Ethical and legal considerations relating to drugs, prescriptions, and the Controlled Substances Act of 1970 are discussed in Chapter 10.

Principles of Medical Ethics for the Physician

The first standards of *medical conduct and ethics* are those set down in the Oath of Hippocrates (Figure 3-1). Included in this famous affirmation, which some doctors graduating from medical school still swear to, are many of the basics of medical ethics. This oath was updated by Dr. Louis Lasagna and appears in Figure 3-2.

In 1980, the American Medical Association (AMA) adopted a modern code of ethics called the Principles of Medical Ethics. This code benefits health professionals and meets the needs of changing times. Refer to Figure 3-3, listing these principles, which guide a physician's standards of conduct for honorable behavior in the practice of medicine.

A physician must also adhere to a body of generally accepted practice procedures, such as the following:

- A physician may ethically receive payments from patients for medical services but cannot accept a rebate of any kind from anyone.
- A physician may accept small gifts (e.g., plastic anatomic models, stethoscopes, booklets) but may not ethically accept large "gifts" from manufacturers or distributors of pharmaceuticals, remedies, or equipment. This practice could influence the physician to prescribe a particular product.
- A physician may employ a collection agency to try to collect overdue bills but may not sell delinquent accounts to the agency.

OATH OF HIPPOCRATES

I swear by Apollo, the physician, and Aesculapius and health and all-heal and all the Gods and Goddesses that, according to my ability and judgment, I will keep this oath and stipulation:

TO RECKON him who taught me this art equally dear to me as my parents, to share my substance with him and relieve his necessities if required; to regard his offspring as on the same footing with my own brothers, and to teach them this art if they should wish to learn it, without fee or stipulation, and that by precept, lecture and every other mode of instruction, I will impart a knowledge of the art to my own sons and to those of my teachers, and to disciples bound by a stipulation and oath, according to the law of medicine, but to none others.

I WILL FOLLOW that method of treatment which, according to my ability and judgment, I consider for the benefit of my patients, and abstain from whatever is deleterious and mischievous. I will give no deadly medicine to anyone if asked, nor suggest any such counsel; furthermore, I will not give to a woman an instrument to produce abortion.

WITH PURITY AND WITH HOLINESS I will pass my life and practice my art. I will not cut a person who is suffering from a stone, but will leave this to be done by practitioners of this work. Into whatever houses I enter I will go into them for the benefit of the sick and will abstain from every voluntary act of mischief and corruption; and further from the seduction of females or males, bond or free.

WHATEVER, in connection with my professional practice, or not in connection with it, I may see or hear in the lives of men which ought not to be spoken broad I will not divulge, as reckoning that all such should be kept secret.

WHILE I CONTINUE to keep this oath unviolated may it be granted to me to enjoy life and the practice of the art, respected by all men at all times but should I trespass and violate this oath, may the reverse be my lot.

FIGURE 3-1 Hippocrates (c. 460 b.c.–377 b.c.), a Greek physician known as the "father of medicine," developed a code, the Oath of Hippocrates, based on the golden rule that to be a good physician one must first be a good and kind person

A MODERN HIPPOCRATIC OATH

I swear to fulfill, to the best of my ability and judgment, this covenant:

I will respect the hard-won scientific gains of those physicians in whose steps I walk, and gladly share such knowledge as is mine with those who are to follow.

I will apply, for the benefit of the sick, all measures which are required, avoiding those twin traps of overtreatment and therapeutic nihilism.

I will remember that there is art to medicine as well as science, and that warmth, sympathy and understanding may outweigh the surgeon's knife or the chemist's drug.

I will not be ashamed to say, "I know not," nor will I fail to call in my colleague when the skills of another are needed for a patient's recovery.

I will respect the privacy of my patients, for their problems are not disclosed to me that the world may know. Most especially must I tread with care in matters of life and death. If it is given me to save a life, all thanks. But it may also be within my power to take a life; this awesome responsibility must be faced with great humbleness and awareness of my own frailty. Above all, I must not play God.

I will remember that I do not treat a fever chart, or a cancerous growth, but a sick human being, whose illness may affect the person's family and economic stability. My responsibility includes these related problems, if I am to care adequately for the sick.

I will prevent disease whenever I can, for prevention is preferable to cure.

I will remember that I remain a member of society, with special obligations to all my fellow human beings, those sound of mind and body, as well as the infirm.

If I do not violate this oath, may I enjoy life and art, respected while I live and remembered with affection thereafter. May I always act so as to preserve the finest traditions of my calling and may I long experience the joy of healing those who seek my help.

FIGURE 3-2 The Modern Hippocratic Oath

PRINCIPLES OF MEDICAL ETHICS FOR THE PHYSICIAN

Preamble

The medical profession has long subscribed to a body of ethical statements developed primarily for the benefit of the patient. As a member of this profession, a physician must recognize responsibility to patients first and foremost, as well as to society, to other health professionals, and to self. The following Principles adopted by the American Medical Association are not laws, but standards of conduct which define the essentials of honorable behavior for the physician.

I. A physician shall be dedicated to providing competent medical care with compassion and respect for human dignity and rights.

II. A physician shall uphold the standards of professionalism, be honest in all professional interactions, and strive to report physicians deficient in character or competence, or engaging in fraud or deception, to appropriate entities.

III. A physician shall respect the law and also recognize a responsibility to seek changes in those requirements which are contrary to the best interests of the patient.

IV. A physician shall respect the rights of patients, of colleagues, and of other health professionals, and shall safeguard patient confidences within the constraints of the law.

V. A physician shall continue to study, apply and advance scientific knowledge, maintain a commitment to medical education, make relevant information available to patients, colleagues, and the public, obtain consultation, and use the talents of other health professionals when indicated.

VI. A physician shall, in the provision of appropriate patient care, except in emergencies, be free to choose whom to serve, with whom to associate, and the environment in which to provide medical care.

VII. A physician shall recognize a responsibility to participate in activities contributing to an improvement of the community and the betterment of public health.

VIII. A physician shall, while caring for a patient, regard responsibility to the patient as paramount.

IX. A physician shall support access to medical care for all people.

FIGURE 3-3 Principles of Medical Ethics for the Physician

PATIENT EDUCATION

Office Policy Booklet

Office policies should be printed in a booklet or handout so that patients will be informed about charges for missed appointments, telephone calls, insurance form completion, and so forth. The AMA considers it ethical for a physician to charge a fee for such services only if the patient has been informed of the policies beforehand. Chapter 5 covers preparation of patient information booklets.

Bioethics

Because technology has brought more sophistication to the medical profession, there is increased concern about ethical and moral issues among those in the field of medicine and the lay public. Bioethics is the branch of ethics dealing with issues, questions, and problems that arise in the practice of medicine and in biomedical research. It is a very complex field that draws on medical, scientific, philosophic, sociologic, and theological knowledge. The term bioethics emerged as a result of issues about the transplantation of organs, genetic engineering or manipulation, maintaining life with life-sustaining equipment, physician-assisted suicide, cloning, abortion, fetal tissue research, artificial insemination, in vitro fertilization, surrogate motherhood, stem cell research, and so on. Examples 3-1 and 3-2 describe some bioethical issues.

EXAMPLE 3-1

Quality of Life versus Length of Life

An infant is born with severe deformities and many medical problems. The decision-making process may involve whether to provide or withhold treatment, what type of treatment should or should not be used, and who will bear the expense of the treatment, which may be costly.

EXAMPLE 3-2

Physician-Assisted Suicide

An 82-year-old, terminally ill patient is requesting physician-assisted suicide because the patient is completely dependent on others for daily care, is in continual pain, and is experiencing total loss of dignity. Questions that arise include: What if this patient is a relative of yours? How long will this pain and suffering last? How do you feel about the patient's request?

Principles of Medical Ethics for the Medical Assistant

Before learning the principles of medical ethics, it is good to look at our individual "code of ethics." This is human behavior that comes into play in our personal lives, at work, and anytime we interact with others. Simply put, it is about our character (being a good person) and doing the right thing. As small children, we began to develop a sense of right and wrong. While growing up, the influence of family, culture, and society helped us develop a code of ethics that can vary for different people based on what the surroundings were. However, despite the environment in which you were raised, you can continue to mature and redevelop your moral code as you practice ethical behavior. First, you need to establish what ethical behavior is. Individual character reveals itself through the choices we make, the wisdom displayed behind those choices, and standards of acceptable behavior used to live by. To help discern where you are on an ethical scale, ask yourself the following questions:

- Can you discern right from wrong and act accordingly? Do you?
- Do you avoid unethical temptations? Frequently?
- Do you act with temperance and self-control?
- Do you treat people fairly, thinking of others before yourself?
- Do you have the courage to make ethical decisions in tough situations?
- When making decisions, have you ever broken the law or a company policy?

- Have you ever caused harm or embarrassed the company you worked for, or the customers or patients?
- Are you accountable for your actions, or do you blame others?
- Do you feel good about yourself and what you have done at the end of each day?
- Did what you have done match what you felt, what you said, or what others believe is good or right?
- Do you strive to be consistently ethical in your professional life as well as your personal life?

Example 3-3 illustrates some ethical situations that help you make decisions.

One of the most common unethical acts that occur in an office is theft—in the form of misuse of office equipment, such as using the copy machine to copy your taxes, using the fax machine to send something personal, using company time to send emails or look at Facebook, or taking office supplies home. Most of the time it is small-value items, a pen or pencil, sticky note pads, file folders, and so forth. Theft or improper use of company assets is not acceptable in any form. Following are some questions

regarding ethics that may come up frequently in a physician's office: What would you do if you received too much change from a patient? If you would like a day off work, will you take a vacation day or call in sick? If a supervisor compliments you for something your coworker did, will you accept the compliment? We read in our daily newspapers of unethical behavior, questionable business practices, and outright law violations that occur in our communities and throughout our country. Following high ethical standards is not easy, but it is more important than ever to strive for and maintain in the business environment.

To maintain a high degree of ethical conduct in relating to patients, physicians, and coworkers, a medical assistant should:

1. Remember that everything seen, heard, or read about a patient is confidential and should not leave the office (Figures 3-4 and 3-5). Before information about a patient may be released, the patient must sign an authorization form for release of information unless subpoenaed by the court. This is discussed and illustrated later in this chapter.
2. Apply discretion when speaking and using an intercom or voice pager, as there may be others in the room that may hear the information being relayed. If the system permits storing the messages, the user should try to receive messages only in private areas.
3. Avoid talking about anything of a private nature when speaking to a physician via cellular or cordless telephone because it is possible for other parties to overhear conversations electronically, thus breaching a patient's confidentiality.
4. Never discuss a patient's condition within hearing distance of others.

EXAMPLE 3-3

Ethical Situations

Lying: It is against the law to lie in a courtroom.

It is NOT against the law to lie to an acquaintance.

IT IS UNETHICAL BEHAVIOR TO LIE, AT ANY TIME.

Cheating: It is against the law to cheat on your taxes.

It is NOT against the law to cheat while playing a game with your family.

IT IS UNETHICAL BEHAVIOR TO CHEAT, AT ANY TIME.

Stealing: It is against the law to steal something from a store.

It is NOT against the law to steal something from your mother's purse.

IT IS UNETHICAL BEHAVIOR TO STEAL, AT ANY TIME.

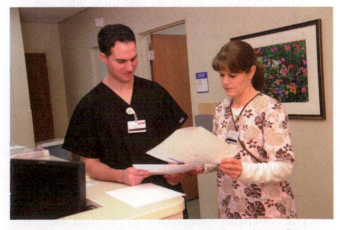

FIGURE 3-4 All information about patients is confidential

PRACTON MEDICAL GROUP, INC.

4567 BROAD AVENUE • WOODLAND HILLS, XY 12345-4700
OFFICE: (555) 486-9002 • FAX: (555) 486-7815

Fran Practon, M.D.
Gerald Practon, M.D.

EMPLOYEE CONFIDENTIALITY STATEMENT

As an employee of _____*Practon Medical Group*_____ (employer), and having been trained as an (administrative) / clinical medical assistant with employee responsibilities and authorization to access personal medical and health information, I recognize that violation of confidentiality statutes and rules may lead to immediate dismissal from employment and, depending on state laws, criminal prosecution. I understand that such violation may cause irreparable damage to my employer, and the employer and any other injured party may seek legal action against me. I acknowledge that this signed document will be placed in my personnel file at this facility.

Constance Gutierrez
Signature

JoAnne Bonet   Office Manager
Witness signature

Constance Gutierrez
Print Name

June 12, 20XX
Date

FIGURE 3-5 Example of an employee confidentiality agreement that may be used by an employer when hiring a new employee

5. Sidestep discussing a patient with acquaintances or the patient's friends.
6. Never leave a patient's records lying exposed.
7. Remain loyal to your employer; do not criticize the physician to a patient.
8. Communicate in a dignified, courteous manner with everyone in the office and those who telephone or visit; never degrade or malign a patient.
9. Notify the physician if you learn that a patient is being treated by another physician for the same ailment. (A consultation does not constitute treatment.)
10. Support physicians in your community. Never make critical statements about the treatment given to a patient by another physician.
11. Avoid dishonest or unethical coworkers. Do not allow them to steer you into questionable practices. Keep the physician fully informed of your own work, so it will be clear to everyone that any misdeeds are not yours.

The American Association of Medical Assistants (AAMA) has established a code of ethics and a creed appropriate for medical assistants whether they are members of this association or not (Figure 3-6). Other ethical issues about using computers are addressed in Chapter 9.

MEDICAL ETIQUETTE

Etiquette should not be confused with ethics. Medical **etiquette** is the customary code of conduct, courtesy, and manners in the medical profession. Courtesy in medical offices is more important than ever since customer service is emphasized and medical practices try to maximize productivity and work flow.

The medical assistant should immediately acknowledge people when they enter the office, even if he or she is on the telephone. The assistant should look up, smile, and convey a signal that says, "I'll be with you in a moment" (Figure 3-7). When other physicians visit the office to discuss a patient, it is customary to usher them into the inner office as soon as possible and not keep them waiting. Likewise, when another physician telephones, the medical assistant should connect him or her immediately without interrogation. When the physician is calling about a mutual patient, the medical assistant should take a moment to verify the patient's name, look up the electronic medical record, or pull the paper chart and then transfer the call.

Medical assistants should always identify themselves when answering the telephone. Never leave patients on

AAMA CODE OF ETHICS

The Code of Ethics of AAMA shall set forth principles of ethical and moral conduct as they relate to the medical profession and the particular practice of medical assisting.

Members of AAMA dedicated to the conscientious pursuit of their profession, and thus desiring to merit the high regard of the entire medical profession and the respect of the general public which they serve, do pledge themselves to strive always to:

A. render service with full respect for the dignity of humanity;
B. respect confidential information obtained through employment unless legally authorized or required by responsible performance of duty to divulge such information;
C. uphold the honor and high principles of the profession and accept its disciplines;
D. seek to continually improve the knowledge and skills of medical assistants for the benefit of patients and professional colleagues;
E. participate in additional service activities aimed toward improving the health and well-being of the community.

AAMA CREED

I believe in the principles and purposes of the profession of medical assisting.

I endeavor to be more effective.

I aspire to render greater service.

I protect the confidence entrusted to me.

I am dedicated to the care and well-being of all people.

I am loyal to my employer.

I am true to the ethics of my profession.

I am strengthened by compassion, courage and faith.

Reprinted with permission of the American Association of Medical Assistants, Chicago, Illinois

FIGURE 3-6 Code of medical ethics and creed for medical assistants as established by the American Association of Medical Assistants

hold longer than 1 minute. When making a call, identify yourself and give the reason why you are telephoning.

Etiquette among coworkers is dictated by common sense. Those in the workplace must be careful of how they act in their place of employment. It is always courteous to say, "Good morning" and "Good night" to everyone whether or not you know them personally. Use of first names is common in an informal atmosphere, but the physician should always be addressed formally (e.g., "Doctor Practon"). Respect the office's customs; for example, if everyone pitches in to handle meeting a deadline or assisting in an emergency, this might mean working late or coming in on a Saturday.

When working as a new employee or as an extern in a medical office, never gossip and remember to use all ethical and etiquette guidelines of common courtesy presented here.

Etiquette is a vast subject and numerous additional instances are discussed throughout this text. Etiquette in

communications is discussed in Chapter 4, *The Art of Communication*. Etiquette guidelines on greeting the patient are found in Chapter 5, *Receptionist and the Medical Office Environment*. Additional rules of etiquette for telephone, voice mail, cell phone, and so forth are found in Chapter 6, *Telephone Procedures*. When sending documents via facsimile there are both etiquette and legal confidentiality issues to be considered, which are described in Chapter 12, *Processing Mail and Electronic Correspondence*.

HEALTH INSURANCE PORTABILITY AND ACCOUNTABILITY ACT OF 1996

The **Health Insurance Portability and Accountability Act**, commonly referred to as **HIPAA** (pronounced hĭpăh), became a federal law in 1996. The purpose of

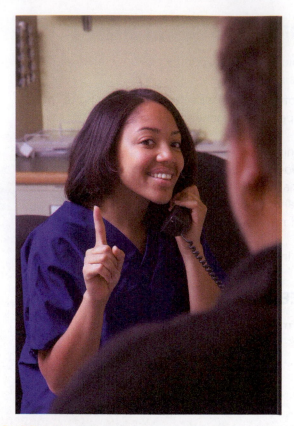

FIGURE 3-7 Medical assistant acknowledging a patient with a smile and gesturing that it will only be one moment before she will be able to help

HIPAA is to provide a standardized framework within which all insurance companies and providers work to:

- Enhance the **portability** (transferability) of health care coverage
- Increase accuracy of data
- Protect private health information and the rights of patients
- Reduce fraud, abuse, and waste in the health care delivery system
- Upgrade efficiency and financial management
- Expedite claim processing
- Lower administrative costs and simplify implementation
- Promote medical savings accounts
- Avail better access to long-term care coverage
- Improve customer satisfaction to restore trust in the health care system.

The act is divided into sections that address different issues of health care. The two main provisions are addressed in Title I and Title II; however,

additional titles are listed and briefly described to provide an overview of all provisions that affect the medical office. If state laws offer protection greater than HIPAA laws, then state laws prevail. Information pertaining to HIPAA appears throughout chapters in this text where the subject matter is addressed. "Compliance" boxes are used to alert the reader to key legal issues.

- *Title I: Health Insurance Access, Portability, and Renewal*—Increases the portability of health insurance by protecting coverage when employees change jobs. It does this by prohibiting preexisting condition exclusions, disallowing discrimination of health insurance coverage based on health status and guaranteeing renewability for certain group health plans.
- *Title II: Health Care Fraud, Abuse, Prevention, and Administrative Simplification*—Prevents fraud and abuse in health care delivery and payment for services, establishes guidelines to simplify administrative procedures, provides national standards to protect privacy, and mandates electronic transmission of certain health information.
- *Title III: Medical Savings Account (MSA) Benefits*—Addresses the MSA, increases deductions, adds consumer protection, and addresses income tax refund payments.
- *Title IV: Group Health Plan Directives*—Details how group health plans must allow for portability, access, and renewability for members.
- *Title V: Internal Revenue Code Amendments*—Explains changes in the Internal Revenue Code of 1986 so that more revenue is generated to offset costs of implementing HIPAA.
- *Title XI: General Provisions*—Focuses on Medicare-related plans and addresses the coordination of general provisions, peer review, and administration simplification.
- *Title XXVII: Portability Assurance*—Speaks to the carryover of health insurance plans from one plan to another.

The implementation of HIPAA has changed administrative policies and procedures and affects patients seen in both in- and outpatient facilities as well as everyone who works in allied health careers. Knowing HIPAA law and how to work within its boundaries is critical for medical assistants. Compliance to HIPAA standards affects all **covered entities** such as health care professionals, health plans, health care clearinghouses, and hospitals that either provide health care or send data that are protected under HIPAA law.

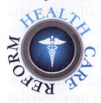

Health care reform laws may address and overlap HIPAA law, so it is important to have a basic understanding of what is covered under HIPAA.

Protected Health Information

Protected health information (PHI), * under HIPAA, is defined as information about the patient's past, present, or future health condition that contains personal identifying data. This includes patient demographic information (i.e., name, date of birth, address, telephone/fax number, sex), Social Security number, diagnosis, email address, and medical record account number. It can be maintained or transmitted in any form—oral, written, or electronic. Under the *Privacy Rule*, strong federal protection is provided for the privacy of patients without interfering with the quality of health care or its access. The rule sets boundaries, defines safeguards, holds violators accountable, and gives patients more control over their health information. The use (sharing, utilizing, examining) and disclosure (releasing, transferring, or providing access) of PHI is protected under the rule.

The medical practice must have and implement written policies and procedures that comply with HIPAA standards, which include developing privacy policies; adopting electronic medical record, email, and mobile device policies; conducting regular risk assessment; initiating employee training sessions; and providing a notice of privacy practices to all patients. A policy and procedures manual may be used both as a resource and to train employees and physicians. Revisions need to be made as necessary and documentation retained a minimum of 6 years.

Under HIPAA's privacy rules for PHI, patients have the right to:

1. Receive *notices* of privacy practices.
   Example: A written policy describing how the practice uses PHI and informing patients about their rights should be posted in the office and be available in a handout or booklet kept at the front desk with a signature page signed by the patient acknowledging receipt.

---

*The acronym PHI has been erroneously referred to as personal, privileged, or private health information.

2. Access medical and financial records.
   Example: If patients want to inspect or obtain a copy of their medical record, the request must be acted on within 5 days and a fee may be charged although certain information may be exempt (e.g., psychotherapy notes).
3. Request an amendment to the medical record.
   Example: A patient requests that changes, additions, or deletions be made to correct information. The health care provider needs to be the creator of the information and must act on the request within 60 days.
4. Receive an accounting of disclosures made. Excluded are disclosures for treatment, payment, and health care operation (TPO).
   Example: A disclosure is made to the health authority reporting a disease for public purposes. The log of disclosures should include the current date, name of individual, medical record number, purpose, date(s) of service, and brief description of PHI disclosed.
5. Request restrictions on disclosures for certain uses, not for TPO (to treat the patient, to receive payment, or for normal business operations).
   Example: A patient asks her gynecologist not to share positive test results indicating a sexually transmitted disease with her primary care physician.
6. Ask that all communication be confidential.
   Example: A patient may not want to approach the front desk and talk about the reason for the visit in front of other patients, or may want to receive test results at an alternative location.

If a friend or family member is involved in a patient's care, you can disclose PHI that is relevant;

however, the patient may need to agree to such a disclosure, depending on whether he or she is present and competent. The disclosure should be related only to the patient's current condition and should not include past medical history.

Health Information Technology for Economic and Clinical Health Act

The **Health Information Technology for Economic and Clinical Health Act (HITECH)** is part of the American Reinvestment and Recovery Act (ARRA) that was passed in February 2009. HITECH "promotes the adoption of meaningful use of health information technology" by offering financial incentives to providers who demonstrate *meaningful use* of electronic health record (EHR) systems. The law sets standards to manage the incentive program. The hope is that these incentives will accelerate the adoption of EHR systems to help achieve efficiency goals that show EHR technology is being used in ways that can be measured significantly in both quality and quantity (1) in a meaningful way, such as e-prescribing, (2) for electronic exchange of health information to improve quality of care, and (3) to submit clinical quality reports, procedure and diagnostic codes, and other measures. Incentives are categorized as follows:

- Engage patients and their families
- Ensure adequate privacy and security
- Enhance care coordination
- Improve population and public health
- Reduce health care disparities

The law provides enforcement to encourage physicians and health care entities to comply with HIPAA regulations by increasing the potential legal liability for noncompliance and by enacting stiff penalties.

HITECH also imposes data breach notification requirements that apply to unauthorized uses and disclosures of unsecured private health information. According to present HIPAA privacy rules, an individual can ask a covered entity to restrict disclosures for the purpose of treatment, receiving payment, or day-to-day operations (TPO); however, the covered entity is not required to agree to the request. With the HITECH Act, "A covered entity must grant a request for a restriction if: (1) The disclosure is to a health plan for purposes of either payment or health care operations, and (2) the personal health information pertains to a service for which the patient paid in full, out-of-pocket." The provider has to honor the patient's request because the patient paid for the service and now has the right not to

use his or her insurance benefit. This requirement does not apply to disclosures for treatment.

HITECH applies universally—for all health care plans (i.e., Medicare, Medicaid, TRICARE, state commercial insurance plans, and the Employee Retirement Income Security Act). The medical record must be flagged so that records are not disclosed to the health plan, should a record request be received. You must also flag the record when sending it to another provider so that the receiving physician knows not to disclose the information to the health plan. Meaningful use requirements are discussed in detail in Chapter 9, *Medical Records*.

Compliance Plan

A **compliance plan** is a written document that includes office policies and procedures, rules to follow, and practice standards that are monitored through internal auditing. It is an ever-changing program that recognizes challenges, addresses problem areas, and identifies risk to the medical practice. It ensures compliance not only with HIPAA law but also with all federal, state, and local laws that affect the medical practice. As problems are identified, investigated, and corrected, it helps prevent repeated violations as well as fraud and abuse.

A *compliance officer*, who may also be the *security* and *privacy officer*, needs to be named as the professional who oversees internal monitoring and auditing, conducts ongoing educational training sessions, identifies offenses, responds appropriately to detected offences, and develops corrective action. Open communication is essential and written guidelines need to be publicized in order to enforce disciplinary standards. Compliance reporting may be found in Chapter 19, *Office Managerial Responsibilities*.

COMPLIANCE
Identity Theft

The health care industry is at special risk for identity theft because it accumulates and retains large volumes of PHI. *Phishers* masquerade as legitimate companies to try to obtain sensitive and personal information. Email requests or telephone calls are used to falsely verify accounts or request resubmission of certain information stating records were lost. Employees should be trained to be alert to *phishing* expeditions and verify all suspect requests.

HIPAA Walkthrough

Following are items that a compliance officer might look for when performing a walkthrough in the medical office to identify HIPAA violations:

- Privacy Practices
  - not given to every patient upon registration
- Protected Health Information
  - discarded in regular trash
  - left unattended on computer screen
  - transported in an unsecured fashion
  - discussed openly with no regard to privacy
- Medication
  - stored in unsecure place
  - charts left open and unattended
  - printouts in regular trash
- Patient diagnosis
  - recorded on sign-in sheet
  - referred to openly
- Identification badges
  - not worn by employees
  - contain incorrect job title

Security Rule

HIPAA's *security rule* has detailed instructions (see *Resources* section at end of chapter) for implementing safeguard standards that interact with the privacy rule as well as covering physical and technical safeguards; policies, procedures, and documentation requirements; risk analysis and risk management; and administrative safeguards to secure electronic PHI. The rule applies to all covered entities.

HIPAA violators may be subjected to fines, prison, or both. A breach of HIPAA regulations carries a maximum civil monetary penalty of $100 per violation. There is a maximum fine of $25,000 per calendar year for all identical violations. HIPAA information as it relates to insurance and coding is further explained in Chapters 16, 17, and 18. In this chapter, PHI, confidentiality, and release of patient information are detailed.

CONFIDENTIALITY

The first policy that should be mentioned to a new employee in a medical setting is to keep information about patients confidential. Refrain from talking about patients and their problems where outsiders may overhear. A medical record contains **privileged information,** which includes data or a confidential exchange between a professional (e.g., physician, attorney) and the patient related to the treatment and progress of the patient; therefore, it must not be overheard or mislaid, so other individuals can see it or leaf through it.

Procedures on how to retain confidentiality when using voice mail, facsimile equipment, or electronic mail are discussed in subsequent chapters.

Release of Medical Information

The medical record is the property of the physician who created it, and he or she is legally and ethically obligated to keep it confidential. The patient has the right to access the information but does not own the physical record. Medical assistants must become familiar with individual state laws regarding release of information as these may vary from federal law.

Consent

A signed patient consent for the use and disclosure of *PHI for treatment, payment, and health care operations (TPO)* is NOT required under the privacy rule. However, covered entities may design a process to obtain this voluntarily and if doing so, a **consent form** should be obtained at the patient's first encounter (Figure 3-8).

HIPAA regulations state that patients have the right to know how their health information is used and may exercise control over the content of the information disclosed.

Authorization

Under HIPAA, it is necessary to obtain a signed **authorization form** for use and disclosure of PHI for specific purposes, other than TPO (Figure 3-9). In an authorization, a minimum set of elements must be included, outlining the purpose for which the health care information is to be used and disclosed. A physician is bound by the statements on the authorization and can only use or disclose the specific information listed. Requests from physicians, insurance companies, and

COMPLIANCE

Medical Record Disclosure

Disclosure of data from a medical record is allowed only after written permission is given by the patient or by the guardian in the case of a minor, or if subpoenaed by a court.

PRACTON MEDICAL GROUP, INC.

4567 BROAD AVENUE • WOODLAND HILLS, XY 12345-4700
OFFICE: (555) 486-9002 • FAX: (555) 486-7815

Fran Practon, M.D.
Gerald Practon, M.D.

CONSENT TO THE USE AND DISCLOSURE OF HEALTH INFORMATION

I understand that this organization originates and maintains health records which describe my health history, symptoms, examination, test results, diagnoses, treatment, and any plans for future care or treatment. I understand that this information is used to:

- plan my care and treatment
- communicate among health professionals who contribute to my care
- apply my diagnosis and services, procedures, and surgical information to my bill
- verify services billed by third-party payers
- assess quality of care and review the competence of health care professionals in routine health care operations

I further understand that:

- a complete description of information uses and disclosures is included in a *Notice of Information Practices* which has been provided to me
- I have a right to review the notice prior to signing this consent
- the organization reserves the right to change their notice and practices
- any revised notice will be mailed to the address I have provided prior to implementation
- I have the right to object to the use of my health information for directory purposes
- I have the right to request restrictions as to how my health information may be used or disclosed to carry out treatment, payment, or health care operations
- the organization is not required to agree to the restrictions requested
- I may revoke this consent in writing, except to the extent that the organization has already taken action in reliance thereon.

☑ I request the following restrictions to the use or disclosure of my health information.
All information may be shared with my husband, Ernesto Hernandez

June 29, 20XX	_June 29, 20XX_
Date	Notice Effective Date
Consuelo Hernandez	_Melody Day_
Signature of Patient or Legal Representative	Witness
	Office Manager
Signature	Title
	✓ Accepted _____ Rejected
Date	

FIGURE 3-8 Example of a voluntary consent form for the use and disclosure of health information for treatment, payment, and routine health care operations (TPO)

AUTHORIZATION FOR RELEASE OF INFORMATION

Section A: Must be completed for all authorizations.

I hereby authorize the use or disclosure of my individually identifiable health information as described below.
I understand that this authorization is voluntary. I understand that if the organization authorized to receive the information is not a health plan or health care provider, the released information may no longer be protected by federal privacy regulations.

Identity of person/ organization disclosing protected health information

Patient name: _Hilda F. Goodman_   **ID Number:** _4309_

Persons/organizations providing information: **Persons/organizations receiving information:**
Practon Medical Group, Inc.   _Jennifer P. Lee, MD_
4567 Broad Avenue   _400 North M Street_
Woodland Hills, XY 12345-4700   _Anytown, XY 54098-1235_

Specific description of information [including from and to date(s)]:
Complete medical records from 4-22-XX to 9-15-XX

Identity of those authorized to use protected health information

Specific description of information to be used or disclosed with dates

Examples:
• HIV status
• Drug or alcohol use/abuse statements
• Physical or mental abuse statements
• Psychiatric notes

Section B: Must be completed only if a health plan or a heath care provider has requested the authorization.

Purpose for disclosure

1. The health plan or health care provider must complete the following:
   a. What is the purpose of the use or disclosure?_____ _Patient relocating to another city_ _____

   b. Will the health plan or health care provider requesting the authorization receive financial or in-kind compensation in exchange for using or disclosing the health information described above? Yes___ No _X_

2. The patient or the patient's representative must read and initial the following statements:
   a. I understand that my health care and the payment for my health care will not be affected if I do not sign this form.
      Initials: _hfg_

   b. I understand that I may see and copy the information described on this form if I ask for it, and that I get a copy of this form after I sign it.
      Initials: _hfg_

Section C: Must be completed for all authorizations.

The patient or the patient's representative must read and initial the following statements:

Expiration date

1. I understand that this authorization will expire on _12_ / _31_ / _20XX_ (DD/MM/YR).
      Initials: _hfg_

Individual's right to revoke this authorization in writing

2. I understand that I may revoke this authorization at any time by notifying the providing organization in writing, but if I do not it will not have any effect on any actions they took before they received the revocation.
      Initials: _hfg_

Rediscloure conditions

3. I understand that any disclosure of information carries with it the potential for an unauthorized redisclosure and the information may not be protected by federal confidentiality rules.
      Initials: _hfg_

Individual's signature

Hilda F. Goodman   _September 15, 20XX_
Signature of patient or patient's representative   **Date**
(Form MUST be completed before signing)

Date of signature

Printed name of patient's representative:_____

Relationship to the patient:_____

YOU MAY REFUSE TO SIGN THIS AUTHORIZATION
You may not use this form to release information for treatment or payment except
when the information to be released is psychotherapy notes or certain research information.

FIGURE 3-9 Example of an authorization form for the release of information

attorneys may be honored when a patient has signed the authorization form for release of information. For cases involving continuity of patient care when requests are received to move records from hospital to hospital, physician to physician, or hospital to nursing home, it is not necessary to have the authorization form signed by the patient.

Mandated Reporting and Exceptions to Disclosure Rules—Although public health statutes may differ among states, the principal occurrences that require mandated reporting to the Department of Health are:

- Births, stillbirths, and deaths
- Certain communicable, infectious, or contagious diseases

COMPLIANCE
Disclosure Accountings

Patients have a right to ask for an accounting of all health information disclosures using the authorization form, which have been made by a provider in the past 6 years. This request must be answered within 60 days. In some situations, a fee may be charged, but the majority of requests are provided at no charge.

- Abuse, neglect, or exploitation of vulnerable individuals (child, spouse, older adults, disabled)
- Incest
- Spousal rape
- Suspicious wounds
- Injuries inflicted by oneself or by the acts of another by means of a knife, gun, pistol, or other deadly weapon
- Assaultive or abusive conduct
- Injuries inflicted in violation of any penal law
- Known or suspected drug abuse
- Epileptic seizures and related disorders

These are exceptions to the right of privacy and privileged communication that do not need consent or authorization because state laws require disclosure to protect the public. Other situations include the release of information to coroners, medical examiners, and funeral directors; for cadaver organ and tissue donation purposes; and for certain public health activities and specialized government functions.

An exception also occurs in workers' compensation cases as the contract is between the physician and the insurance company. If a patient is given advance notice and an opportunity to object to the use of disclosure, limited information may be provided to family members, used in facility directories, and disclosed to disaster relief organizations. Children's immunization records may be shared directly with the school.

Restricted Record Access—State laws may set a higher standard for sharing certain sensitive health information, such as HIV status, psychiatric notes, drug or alcohol use, and physical or mental abuse statements. For example, if a patient has a positive human immunodeficiency virus (HIV) test for acquired immune deficiency syndrome (AIDS), applies for life or health insurance, and signs an authorization form to release

this information to the insurance company, the medical assistant should seek counsel from a supervisor or the proper authorities before processing the request. Some state laws allow AIDS information to be given only to the patient's spouse. Authorization for release of information in states with restricted access about HIV test results must be carefully handled as results may appear in many sections of the health record. Use of *ICD-10-CM* codes R75, B20, or Z21 indicates positive HIV test results, and this information must be considered confidential. The authorization form must list the specific description of particularly sensitive information to be disclosed including inclusive dates of treatment. The signed form should be retained in the health record. All information released and sent for such a request should contain a statement prohibiting redisclosure of the information to another party without the prior authorization of the patient. The individual receiving the information should be requested to destroy the information after the stated need is fulfilled.

A physician caring for a patient who has had psychiatric care should always be consulted before any information is divulged, even with a signed authorization form from the patient. Physicians can prevent psychiatric patients from gaining access to privileged information by noting on a chart, prior to the patient's request, that they believe knowledge of its contents would be detrimental to the patient's best interests. Usually the courts will uphold a physician's judgment in these circumstances. Many states allow for authorization for release of information to a representative of a patient if the physician determines that the release of information to the patient may not be in the patient's best interests.

Patients Receiving Records—If patients request to access, read, or copy their medical records, the request must be honored, generally within 30 days. However, caution should be taken because a patient may not understand technical or medical terms used within the record and become emotionally upset. For this reason, some providers prefer not to release records directly to a patient or allow the patient to hand-carry the records to a consultant without the opportunity to sit down with the patient and ask if anything in the record needs interpretation. In an urgent situation, electronic transmission can be used or photocopies of the records can be sealed in an envelope or sent via facsimile using a special authorization form. The patient should sign a receipt for any radiographic films removed from the office. Consultation reports from other physicians, even if stamped "confidential," as well as accounting records may be released to a patient.

Medical Litigation Records—In the event of litigation (lawsuit), the patient waives the right to confidentiality and the physician's lawyer has access to the patient's medical record. The attorney would then limit authorizations to disclose medical information to those conditions that are relevant to the injuries claimed in the given lawsuit and not release information to any other party unless it is subpoenaed. For example, in the case of a subpoena for a mother's obstetric records and sealed records of an adopted child, you would release only the portion of the mother's record that applies to the situation in order to honor that part of the subpoena.

The patient's attorney must subpoena medical records and if he or she cannot read the physician's handwriting, *the medical assistant should not try to interpret it.* If interpretation is needed, it can be done at a *deposition,* when the involved physician would have legal representation and a court reporter would be present to record the testimony.

If a photocopying service visits the office to copy a record for the attorney, the medical assistant should either number the pages released or observe the photocopying process to ensure that pages are not missing when the copying is completed. It is preferable for the physician's staff to photocopy the record and charge the attorney a fee for this service.

Medicare, Medicaid, and TRICARE Records—The Privacy Act of 1974 guarantees the right of those receiving Medicare and TRICARE benefits to have access to their records. Federal and state agencies may also have access to medical records pertaining to federal- and state-sponsored programs, such as Medicaid.

Medicaid rules permit members of a state attorney general's staff or the department of public welfare to review Medicaid records without the patient's signed authorization form to verify billing information and determine whether the services provided were medically necessary. The information in the medical records can be used only for the audit and may not be released.

Employers Receiving Records—Special attention is required when information is to be released to an employer even with the patient's signed authorization. The exception is in workers' compensation cases.

Publications Release—If a patient's medical record or photograph is requested for publication, the authorization form must contain wording that indicates the information or photograph is to be used in this manner.

Whenever disclosing PHI, it is prudent to consider the minimum necessary standard in which you make a reasonable effort to limit the information to the minimum necessary to accomplish the intended purpose of the use, disclosure, or request (see Procedure 3-1).

PROCEDURE 3-1

Release Patient Information

OBJECTIVE: Determine reason for disclosure, dates of disclosure, and authorization form used to legally disclose medical information. Process authorization request and document in medical record.

EQUIPMENT/SUPPLIES: Consent form, authorization form, pen or pencil.

DIRECTIONS: Follow these step-by-step directions, which include rationales, to learn this procedure. Job Skill 3-2 in the *Workbook* is presented to practice this skill.

1. Determine the reason for disclosure of the personally identifiable health information and the specific dates of service being requested.

2. Verify the request.

3. Access the electronic medical record or locate and retrieve the chart.

4. Identify and validate the requester.

5. Mark specific areas or pages of the document requested.

6. Select one of the following categories and continue to follow the instructions:

   a. *Disclosure for treatment, payment, or routine health care operations.* Prepare a voluntary consent form if the office uses one.

   b. *Transfer of medical record to a physician for consultation.* Continuity of care rules apply; no authorization needed.

(continues)

c. *Transfer of medical record to a physician who will be taking over care of a specific problem.* Continuity of care rules apply; no authorization needed.

d. *Transfer of medical record to an acute or convalescent hospital for inpatient treatment.* Continuity of care rules apply; no authorization needed.

e. *Transfer of medical record for therapeutic purposes (e.g., to a physical therapist, occupational therapist, radiation treatment center).* Continuity of care rules apply; no authorization needed.

f. *Transfer of diagnostic information from the medical record for diagnostic purposes (e.g., to a laboratory, radiology center, physiology department).* Continuity of care rules apply; no authorization needed.

g. *Permanent transfer of medical record to a physician who will be taking over care (e.g., patient dissatisfied with physician's care or moving to another area).* Prepare an authorization form.

h. *Transfer of sensitive information (e.g., positive HIV or AIDS test, alcohol or drug dependency, psychiatric problems, physical/mental abuse).* Prepare an authorization form outlining the specific information to be disclosed including dates of treatment. Note: Redisclosure not allowed without patient's prior authorization.

i. *Transfer of medical record to a court of law by way of a subpoena.* Refer to guidelines under "Medical Litigation." Carefully read the subpoena, give it to the custodian of medical records, prepare only dates outlined in the subpoena for copy and remove to a separate record jacket, have the record reviewed by the physician, and send or make an appointment for the copy service to copy.

j. *Transfer of medical record by court order.* Certain sensitive medical records may be legally sealed for confidentiality purposes. In such cases, a court order is necessary to transfer the record, and identifying and nonidentifying information may be separated and treated differently. State laws vary and should be referred to regarding sealed records.

k. *Transfer of medical record requested by law enforcement officials.* Under the HIPAA privacy rule, PHI may be disclosed to law enforcement officials without written authorization under the following special circumstances: (1) in response to an administrative request, (2) to comply with a court order or court-ordered warrant, or (3) for the purpose of identifying or locating a suspect, fugitive, material witness, or missing person.

l. *Transfer of medical record into the patient's personal possession.* Try to determine the reason the patient wants the records. If it is for one of the above stated reasons, offer to send the records without charge to the physician or facility in an expedient manner. If the patient states he or she "just wants to have a copy," advise the physician and have the physician go over the record with the patient prior to releasing it so no misunderstandings occur due to medical terminology, abbreviations, or other language. Charge the patient according to your state's guidelines.

7. Copy only requested material.

8. Mark all transfer details in the patient's medical record and in a disclosure log.

9. File a copy of the request in the patient's medical record.

10. Select a method to send or deliver the documents, and send or deliver them.

11. Generate an invoice, if billable.

12. Return a paper chart to the medical record file cabinet.

13. Receive and post payment.

MEDICAL PRACTICE ACTS

By the 1800s, there was a prevalence of individuals across the United States who falsely represented having medical skills and offered cures of diseases by selling appliances and medicinal elixirs. This was known as quackery. By the early 1900s, it became necessary to protect citizens from such unqualified medical personnel, so Medical Practice Acts were passed in all states. Their purpose was for each state to establish licensure requirements for individuals to practice medicine. Each state has different requirements, but some of the basic conditions that must be met are premedical training, graduation from an approved medical school, internship approved by the State Board of Medical Examiners, and good moral character. In some states, requirements are placed on age and residency, and the State Board of Medical Examiners gives written and oral examinations. A physician who comes from a foreign country must pass examinations and satisfy state laws before receiving permission to practice medicine in the United States.

Physician Licensure

Physicians' medical licenses are renewed either annually or every 2 years by payment of a licensing fee and acquiring the required continuing education units. It may be a responsibility of the administrative medical assistant to provide the medical staff office secretary at the local hospital or a health care organization with whom the physician wishes to contract with such information. See Table 3-1 for a listing of licensing requirements for new physicians. The original license and annual renewal certificate should be displayed in the office of the medical practice. The State Board of Medical Examiners can revoke a license for conviction of a crime, unprofessional conduct, or personal or professional incapacity, such as drug addiction, alcoholism, or mental illness.

Medical Assistants' Scope of Practice

Health care professionals should become familiar with state medical practice acts and policies of state board of medical examiners to know the **scope of practice** for their job description and whether those duties require certificates of competency or licensure. The scope of practice is the range of education, training, ability, and skills a health care professional is expected to have and operate within according to the law and within the *standard of care*, that is, what an individual is expected to do or not to do in a given situation. The law states that you have a legal or moral obligation to act in certain circumstances on the patient's behalf.

TABLE 3-1 New Physician Licensing Requirements

Licensing Requirement	Requirement Details
Board certifications	Current with expiration date
Criminal background check	Date it was done
Data bank information	National Practitioner Data Bank (NPDB), Healthcare Integrity and Protection Data Bank (HIPDB)
Drug Enforcement Administration (DEA) or Controlled Drug Substance (CDS) registration	Current with expiration date
Federation of State Medical Boards (FSMB) information	Current and past
Hospital privileges	Current and past with description of privileges
Malpractice insurance	Current and previous with litigation history if applicable
National Provider Identifier (NPI) number	Needed to contract with health care plans
State licenses	Include expiration dates
Work history	Curriculum vitae with education, awards, references, and sanctions

In most states, medical assistants work under the "direct supervision" of the physician who is to be on the premises and available; however, this responsibility may be delegated to a physician extender (e.g., nurse practitioner). Legal responsibility falls on the physician for any negligent acts by the medical assistant.

There are several states whose laws contain specific language for medical assistants and the standard of care may vary from state to state. Some states require medical assistants to have certificates of competency if their duties include taking x-rays, performing laboratory tests, giving injections, performing venipunctures, or distributing medication. In addition, some states require that a medical assistant be a graduate from an accredited medical assisting program. Certain state laws do not permit a medical assistant to perform arterial punctures, administer intravenous medication, insert urinary catheters, administer physical therapy modalities, analyze test results, advise patients about their condition, make assessments, or perform medical care decision-making. Failure to act, as the law obligates you to act within the scope of practice and according to the standard of care, results in a *breach of duty* (see Example 3-4).

Refer to the following references for a listing of, or specific language pertaining to, the scope of practice for medical assistants: (1) Occupational Analysis of the CMA (AAMA) in Appendix B of this *textbook*, (2) Medical Assisting Task List (AMT) in Appendix B of this *textbook*, and (3) Key State Scope of Practice Laws (AAMA) in the *Resources* section at the end of this chapter.

EXAMPLE 3-4

Scope of Practice

- Know your state regulations.
- Do only that which you are trained to do and do not perform duties restricted in state law to other health professionals.
- If questions arise regarding health care, answer with facts. Do not offer your opinion; exercise independent professional judgment; or make clinical assessments, evaluations, or interpretations—this may constitute the practice of medicine.
- Do not answer to a wrong title (e.g., office nurse)—you may be held for misrepresentation.

MEDICAL PROFESSIONAL LIABILITY

The term *medical malpractice* is defined by *Black's Law Dictionary* (10th edition, 2014, West) as "a doctor's failure to exercise the degree of care and skill that a physician or surgeon of the same medical specialty would use under similar circumstances." It literally means "bad medical practice." This may also be referred to as *medical professional liability*.

Liability Insurance

A physician may carry two types of medical professional liability insurance. The first type is called *claims-incurred* or *occurrence insurance*; in this type, the insured is covered for any claims arising from an incident that occurred or is alleged to have occurred during the policy period regardless of when the claim is made.

The second type is called *claims-made insurance*, in which the insured is covered for any claim made rather than any injury occurring while the policy is in force. Such policies offer extended discovery options that can be purchased 30 to 60 days after purchase of the policy. This "tail" coverage allows the physician to report claims for events that occurred before the policy expiration date. When a new policy is purchased, the physician may elect to obtain "nose" coverage, which gives the doctor the privilege of reporting claims for medical incidents that occurred before that policy's effective date, under certain conditions. Medical incidents reported previously are not covered, nor are incidents of which the physician is aware, should be aware, or should have been aware.

Respondeat Superior

The doctrine of *respondeat superior*, which means, "Let the master answer" (also known as vicarious liability), applies to the relationship between the physician and the medical assistant. In other words, physicians are legally responsible for their own conduct and for any actions that a medical assistant might take while in their employ. This does not mean, however, that a medical assistant cannot be sued. Generally, the physician would purchase a master insurance policy that provides coverage for the medical office staff and the medical assistant would be covered under such a policy. If medical assistants want to purchase individual protection, they would purchase medical professional liability insurance. It should be noted that this type of insurance offers coverage only in civil matters, such as malpractice and wrongful death suits; it does not provide coverage for state law violations.

CRIMINAL AND CIVIL LAW

Two main divisions of law that affect health care are criminal law and civil law. Criminal laws are most familiar. They are made to protect the public against the harmful acts of others. These laws regulate crimes against the state such as arson, burglary, rape, robbery, and murder. Criminal law is divided into two categories, depending on the severity of the crime: felonies and misdemeanors. Some examples of *felonies* are embezzlement, fraud, homicide, manslaughter, tax evasion, theft (more than $500), and practicing medicine without a license. Punishment for a criminal act is incarceration in a state or federal prison for more than 1 year or death. *Misdemeanors* are less serious crimes such as attempted burglary, battery, disturbing the peace, petty theft, traffic violations, and vandalism. Punishment varies for the type of misdemeanor but may include monetary fines, incarceration for less than 12 months in the county jail, community service, or probation.

Civil law is the statute that enforces private rights and liabilities. It typically involves relations between individuals, corporations, government entities, and other organizations. Most actions encountered in the health care industry are based on civil law. Some examples are contract violations, copyright violations, libel, trespassing, slander, and family law matters such as child custody, child support, and divorce. Civil judgments involve payment to the injured party. There are several categories of civil law: administrative law, contract law, and tort law.

Administrative Law

Administrative law governs the activities of government agencies such as the Internal Revenue Service, Medicare, and Medicaid. Administrative hearings are executive hearings, not judicial. Some of the administrative acts (laws) are listed and described in this chapter such as the Health Insurance Portability and Accountability Act, Medical Practice Act, and Uniform Anatomical Gift Act. Others are presented throughout this textbook, such as the Controlled Substance Act (Chapter 10), the Federal Truth in Lending Act (Chapter 13), and the Occupational Safety and Health Act (Chapter 18).

Contract Law

Contract law addresses legally binding contracts. *Black's Law Dictionary* (10th edition, 2014, West) defines a contract as "an agreement between two or more parties creating obligations that are enforceable or otherwise recognizable as law." The existence of a contract requires an offer, an acceptance, and a promise to perform.

Physician-Patient Contract

Patients often seek a physician who they have researched and whom they believe delivers a certain standard of care. Legally, this would be interpreted to mean that the physician has a certain amount of knowledge and skill comparable to other physicians who practice in the same specialty in the community. It does not necessarily mean the physician can provide a cure to an illness. A medical assistant should never encourage false expectations on the outcome of an injury or illness. When necessary, the medical assistant should help the patient understand the course of treatment, encourage willingness to comply with the treatment advised, and help navigate the patient through the treatment plan.

A medical contract exists when a physician performs a service after a patient has requested it. The patient can *express consent*, therefore this request can be bound by an *express contract* as in a direct verbal or written statement, or it can be implied. An implied contract means not expressed by direct words but gathered by implication (*implied consent*) or necessary deduction from the situation, the general language, or the conduct of the patient. If the patient goes to the physician's office and the physician renders professional services that the patient accepts, this is an implied contract. Although a patient has medical insurance, the contract for treatment is between the physician and the patient, and the patient is thus liable for the physician's fee.

Physicians treating patients whose medical services are paid from federal or state funds (Medicare or Medicaid cases) are contractually obligated to the government and may not receive payment if they fail to follow federal or state guidelines; however, their treatment falls under a physician-patient contract.

When a physician is under contract to a managed care plan, the contract for treatment is between the physician and the enrolled patient and occurs when the patient is first seen. If the physician no longer wishes to treat an individual, termination is handled the same as with patients insured under private insurance or state or government programs.

Third-Party Contracts

There are exceptions to the physician-patient contract. Sometimes the physician's contract is with a third party. Industrial injuries without third-party litigation are covered by a contract between the physician and the employer's industrial insurance company. Such cases do not require an authorization to release information. However, when an insurance company adjuster calls for information on a workers' compensation case, verify the caller before providing medical information.

Another instance might be if a patient is brought in suffering a bite from a neighbor's dog and the neighbor says he will pay the bill. After treatment, what happens if the neighbor decides not to pay? In an implied contractual agreement, the assumption is the patient is responsible for the bill. Although this is a third-party liability case, it may be difficult to collect the fee. In such cases, always obtain a written agreement from the third party promising to pay for the services the patient receives prior to the patient being seen. The agreement should be signed and witnessed. If an agreement is not obtained, there is no legal right to seek payment from the third party.

Contracts and Emergency Care

In emergency situations, when a patient may be unconscious and unable to give valid consent, the consent is implied. A medical assistant may render first aid if a physician is not present but should do no more than is absolutely essential. General procedure is to telephone 911 and try to get emergency personnel on the premises in the interim. If the state law covers the medical assistant and he or she is certified in cardiopulmonary resuscitation (CPR), it may be rendered. The staff should attempt to contact a physician immediately after emergency measures have been taken. The office procedure manual should contain information on how the physician wishes the medical assistant to act in an office emergency. Often office policies state that the office should be locked if a physician is not present, and any patients who telephone indicating an emergent situation should be directed to a hospital emergency department. Refer to Chapter 5 for information on emergency preparedness.

Good Samaritan Law—The *Good Samaritan Law* is designed to encourage physicians to provide care in circumstances where they have no legal obligation to do so, without fear of being sued should things not turn out well. Generally, this statute applies to instances of emergencies outside the office, such as highway accidents. In such situations, a legal patient-physician contract relationship is not created, and the physician cannot be charged with neglect or abandonment for not providing follow-up care. However, a physician may be held liable for injuries that result if it can be shown the physician did not provide an acceptable standard of care under the circumstances in which care was given.

Contracts with Minors

Many states have different ages of majority. In some instances, it is necessary for a parent to authorize (in writing) surgery or treatment for a child. If the child has a guardian, this information should be recorded in the patient's medical record. A nonemancipated minor (i.e., a minor under parental control) over 14 years of age *can almost always* consent to medical and surgical treatment under the *mature minor rule*. Parental consent is never mandatory in a medical emergency that is interpreted as a life-threatening situation.

If a minor has a communicable disease that by law must be reported to the Department of Health (i.e., infectious hepatitis, tuberculosis, measles, mumps, venereal disease, AIDS), the physician may treat the minor without parental consent.

If an unmarried pregnant minor requires hospitalization or medical care for the pregnancy, the laws of the state determine whether parental consent is necessary. If a minor requests an abortion, some states will allow it without parental consent. The medical assistant should keep up to date on the changing legalities and illegalities of abortion. In some states, it would be unwise for a physician to sterilize an unmarried minor in the absence of parental consent because of the irreversible nature of the procedure. To determine the age of majority and the various types of medical care available to minors in your state, refer to "Minors' Access to Health Care," in the *Resources* section at the end of this chapter.

Emancipated Minors—Children of any age who fall outside the jurisdiction and custody of their parents or guardians are called **emancipated minors.** They may personally consent to medical, surgical, or hospital treatment. Parents are not liable for the medical expenses incurred. A minor is considered emancipated when he or she is:

1. Living apart from parents or guardians and managing his or her own financial affairs
2. Married or divorced at any age
3. On active duty in the military service
4. A college student living away from home even when financially dependent on his or her parents
5. A parent (even if not married)

To avoid disagreements with parents, the patient's records should include some evidence of emancipation, such as a minor's signed statement acknowledging the fact (Figure 3-10).

In summary, when treating minors, it is advisable to:

1. Seek parental approval in cases that are not sensitive or confidential.
2. Encourage minors to involve their parents in medical decisions that are of a sensitive nature.

3. Become familiar with state laws concerning treatment of minors.
4. Obtain another medical opinion before proceeding in cases where there is any doubt about a minor's ability to consent or about the urgency or appropriateness of therapy.
5. Make sure that minors who consent to their own care are clearly aware of the nature and consequences of the procedure and obtain a signed consent form to this effect.

Terminating a Contract

A physician who wishes to terminate a contract must do so legally so as not to be accused of abandoning a case. First, the physician may want to send an "at risk" letter to warn the patient that he or she could experience serious negative health effects if he or she remains noncompliant. The letter should (1) specify the area in which the patient is noncompliant, (2) state the risk of remaining noncompliant, (3) describe how the patient

Documentation Of Self-Sufficient Minor Status

For the purposes of obtaining medical, dental or surgical diagnosis or treatment, pursuant to Family Code §6922, I hereby certify that the following is true:

1. I am fifteen years of age or older, having been born on ___4-21-9X___, at ___Woodland Hills, XY___ .
   (date) _(location)_

2. I am living separate and apart from my parents or legal guardian.

   ___2011 Edgehill Drive, Woodland Hills, XY 12345___   ___555-476-0215___
   (Residence)   (Phone)

   ___459 Temecula Way, Woodland Hills, XY 12345___   ___(555) 476-5120___
   (Residence of parents/guardians)   (Phone)

3. I am managing my own financial affairs.

   ___Hi Ho Burger, 20 Main, Woodland Hills, XY___
   (Name and Address of Employer)

   ___None___
   (Other Source(s) of Income)

   ___College Bank, Woodland Hills, XY___
   (Location of Bank Account)

4. I understand that, under the law, I will be financially responsible for my medical, dental, or surgical care and treatment.

   ___Brett Hayward___   ___July 10, 20XX___
   (Signed)   (Date)

FIGURE 3-10 Documentation of Self-Sufficient Minor Status form

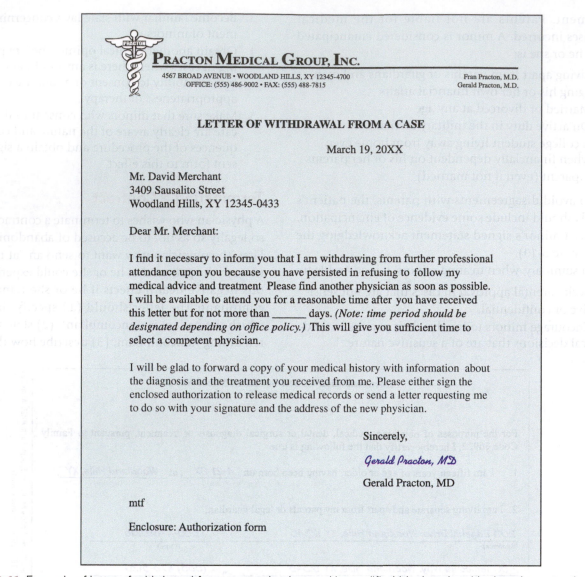

PRACTON MEDICAL GROUP, INC.

4567 BROAD AVENUE • WOODLAND HILLS, XY 12345-4700
OFFICE: (555) 486-9002 • FAX: (555) 488-7815

Fran Practon, M.D.
Gerald Practon, M.D.

LETTER OF WITHDRAWAL FROM A CASE

March 19, 20XX

Mr. David Merchant
3409 Sausalito Street
Woodland Hills, XY 12345-0433

Dear Mr. Merchant:

I find it necessary to inform you that I am withdrawing from further professional attendance upon you because you have persisted in refusing to follow my medical advice and treatment Please find another physician as soon as possible. I will be available to attend you for a reasonable time after you have received this letter but for not more than _____ days. *(Note: time period should be designated depending on office policy.)* This will give you sufficient time to select a competent physician.

I will be glad to forward a copy of your medical history with information about the diagnosis and the treatment you received from me. Please either sign the enclosed authorization to release medical records or send a letter requesting me to do so with your signature and the address of the new physician.

Sincerely,

Gerald Practon, MD

Gerald Practon, MD

mtf

Enclosure: Authorization form

FIGURE 3-11 Example of letter of withdrawal from a case that is typed in modified-block style with closed punctuation. This letter should be sent certified mail with return receipt requested.

can become compliant, and (4) end with a positive statement to encourage the patient to achieve the desired result. If the patient fails to become compliant, a letter should be written to the patient explaining the withdrawal of the physician from the case and sent by registered or certified mail with return receipt requested (Figure 3-11).

When terminating a contract, it is important to allow a transition period (e.g., 30 days) so that the patient can obtain a new physician before care terminates. The letter should clearly state the reason for termination.

Reasons for Terminating a Contract—A patient may fail to keep an appointment, fail to follow medical advice, or fail to pay the balance due on an account. If the patient continues to disregard a recommended plan or if the patient is not to be seen again, it is recommended that an appropriate letter be written to document the action (Figure 3-12). Copies of the correspondence as well as the mail receipts are placed with the patient's medical record.

Abandonment—Abandonment is when a physician terminates supervision of a patient without notifying the patient in writing. Many instances may present when abandonment becomes an issue, and this is an area where litigation frequently occurs. The physician may move out of town, or if the physician goes on vacation and does not arrange for coverage by another

PRACTON MEDICAL GROUP, INC.

4567 BROAD AVENUE • WOODLAND HILLS, XY 12345-4700
OFFICE: (555) 486-9002 • FAX: (555) 488-7815

Fran Practon, M.D.
Gerald Practon, M.D.

LETTER TO PATIENT WHO FAILS TO KEEP APPOINTMENT

June 25, 20XX

Mr. Jonathan Reed
50 Maryland Street
Woodland Hills, XY 12345-0432

Dear Mr. Reed:

On June 24, 20XX, you failed to keep your appointment at my office.

In my opinion, your condition requires continued medical treatment. If you so desire, you may telephone me for another appointment, but if you prefer to have another physician attend you, I suggest that you arrange to do so without delay.

You may be assured that, upon your authorization, I will make available my knowledge of your case to the physician of your choice.

I trust that you will understand that my purpose in writing this letter is out of concern for your health and well-being.

Sincerely,

Gerald Practon, MD

Gerald Practon, MD

mtf

FIGURE 3-12 Letter sent on patient's failure to keep an appointment

physician of equal competence in the same specialty, the physician can be liable for negligence and abandonment, as this becomes an issue of continuity of care. If an established patient telephones indicating an emergency and an appointment is denied, the physician also can be charged with abandonment and neglect.

It is equally important that the physician's answering service be contacted by the medical assistant and given accurate information as to where the physician can be reached when the office is closed. If this is not done, a physician can be sued for patient abandonment. If the practice uses an answering machine instead of a live answering service, the prerecorded message should give information to the caller about where to telephone to obtain help in the event of an emergency.

When a patient is admitted to the hospital and the physician does not see the patient within a reasonable amount of time to check on the condition and order treatment, the physician can be charged with abandoning the patient.

A written office policy should be established to include protocols for contacting patients who have canceled or failed to keep appointments, particularly when test results are involved and a follow-up plan has been communicated. It is important to show that the physician has taken reasonable steps to reach the patient, and more than one attempt may need to be documented in the medical record.

Confirmation of Discharge—If a patient discharges a physician by telephone or discharges him- or herself from a hospital setting, the physician sends a letter similar to that in Figure 3-13. If there is a signed statement in the patient's hospital records in the latter case, it is not necessary for the physician to send the patient a letter.

Tort Law

A **tort** is an action brought when one person believes that another person conducted a wrongful act and caused harm, and the party bringing action is seeking compensation for the damage or injury. The action may also be brought to discourage the wrongdoer from committing further improper acts. In a type of tort lawsuit that alleges negligence-caused *personal injury*, damages would include bodily injury as well as intentional or negligent infliction of emotional distress.

When a tort is being considered, an evaluation of the circumstances must be made to determine whether there is *proximate cause*. To establish proximate cause, the "cause" must be considered legally sufficient to result in damage or injury. Questions to ask when trying to establish this might be:

1. Did the physician or medical assistant act in an expedient fashion?
2. Was the patient left unattended?
3. Could the damage or injury be foreseen?
4. Was there intention to hurt or injure?

The three categories of tort liability are intentional torts, negligent torts, and liability without fault, which will not be expanded on here because it most commonly occurs in cases of manufactured products that are found to be unsafe or cause harm. Medical products such as pacemakers or orthopedic instrumentation could fall into this last category, but litigation would most likely be directed at the manufacturer, not the physician. Most health care incidents arise in the negligent tort category.

PRACTON MEDICAL GROUP, INC.

4567 BROAD AVENUE • WOODLAND HILLS, XY 12345-4700
OFFICE: (555) 486-9002 • FAX: (555) 488-7815

Fran Practon, M.D.
Gerald Practon, M.D.

LETTER TO CONFIRM DISCHARGE BY PATIENT

April 2, 20XX

Mrs. Moo McDermott
439 Nordstrom Road
Woodland Hills, XY 12345-0432

Dear Mrs. McDermott:

This will confirm our telephone conversation today during which you discharged me from attending you as your physician in your present illness.

In my opinion, your condition requires continued medical treatment by a physician. If you have not already obtained the services of another physician, I suggest that you do so without delay.

You may be assured that, upon your authorization, I will furnish that physician with information regarding the diagnosis and treatment that you have received from me.

Sincerely,

Gerald Practon, MD

Gerald Practon, MD

mtf

FIGURE 3-13 Letter confirming discharge

Intentional Torts

An intentional tort is an injury or wrong intentionally committed, with or without force, to another person or to another's property. In the medical field, intentional torts are rare, but they occur. Usually, standard medical malpractice insurance policies do not cover intentional torts on the grounds that the physician could have avoided them. Policies are usually written to protect the physician from accidents and good-faith mistakes and errors of judgment. Intentional torts are:

1. *Assault and battery*—Assault is the intentional and unlawful attempt to do bodily harm to another person.
   Example: Forcing a patient to take medication when the patient has refused to take it is an assault. Battery is a deliberate physical attack on another person. Any surgical operation is technically a "battery" regardless of the result and is excusable only when express or implied consent is given by the patient.

2. *Invasion of privacy and breach of confidential communication*—The invasion of privacy is the unwarranted appropriation or exploitation of another's personality, the publicizing of another's private affairs with which the public has no legitimate concern, or the wrongful intrusion into another's private activities, in such a manner as to cause mental anguish, shame, or humiliation. Breach of confidential communication is the unauthorized release of information.
   Example: Publicizing a patient's medical case or showing a photograph or video from which the identity of a patient can be determined without the knowledge and authorization of the patient.

3. *Defamation of character, libel, and slander*—This is an attack on a person's reputation or subjecting a person to ridicule. It is called libel when written and slander when spoken.
   Example: Referring to a patient as a "malingerer" (one who pretends to be ill or incapacitated) in medical records or in correspondence about the patient.

4. *False imprisonment or personal restraint of the patient*—This is the unlawful detention of a person by another, for any length of time, whereby that person is deprived of personal liberty.
   Example: Wrongfully refusing a patient permission to leave a hospital and using physical restraint to prevent a patient's departure.

5. *Intentional infliction of emotional distress*—This is an action that is so offensive as to cause great emotional upset.
   Example: Intentionally telling a patient that a terminal illness has been diagnosed even though this is not true.

6. *Fraud or deceit*—This is an intentional perversion of truth for the purpose of inducing another (in reliance on it) to part with some valuable thing belonging to that person or to surrender a legal right.
   Example: Intentionally telling a patient that the injuries are minor when they are serious.

Negligent Torts

The health care professional, whether it be a physician or medical assistant, is expected to behave in the way a prudent person who is similarly educated and trained would behave under comparable circumstances. *Negligence* is "failure to exercise reasonable care" or careless conduct outside the accepted standard of care for the health care professional.

Example: Overexposing a patient to x-rays or leaving a surgical instrument in a patient. The "four Ds" must be present for a judgment of negligence to be obtained against the physician. They are:

- *Duty*—Duty of care is when a moral obligation to treat is owed to the patient or when a contract has been established between the patient and physician.
- *Derelict*—When the physician did not comply with the duty that was needed, according to the situation (the patient has to show proof).
- *Direct cause**—Proof that the injury that resulted from the physician's breach of duty was a direct result of the breach, and nothing else interfered that could have caused the damage.
- *Damages*—Injuries suffered by the patient; also called compensatory damages. There are two types:
  - *General damages* provide for compensation for pain and suffering and loss of bodily members.
  - *Special compensation* replaces loss of earnings and cost of medical care.

---

*In some jurisdictions, the verbiage "direct cause" is not used. Instead, it is required to prove that the conduct of the physician be a substantial factor in producing the injury for which the lawsuit has been brought.

Negligent torts can be categorized as:

- *Malfeasance*—Unlawful or improper treatment of the patient.
- *Misfeasance*—Lawful treatment that has been done in the wrong way.
- *Nonfeasance*—Failure to act when the physician has a duty to do so.
- *Malpractice*—Carelessness or negligence of a professional person.
- *Criminal negligence*—Reckless disregard for the safety of another; being indifferent to an injury that could occur.

Liability for the acts of others can also occur, which refers to damage or injury suffered by the patient when someone other than the physician renders a medical service, for example, injection of the wrong dosage of medication by the medical assistant at the direction of the physician.

Principal Defenses

If a patient (plaintiff) institutes a lawsuit against a physician, three principal defenses are available. They are:

- *Contributory negligence*—The defense that applies when patients act in such a manner as to contribute to their own injury, disability, or disfigurement. If the negligence is strongly inferred and very obvious, it is referred to as, *res ipsa loquitur*—Latin for "the things speaks for itself." If a patient does not cooperate with the physician by following all reasonable instructions and this failure contributes to the harm he or she suffered, the patient may not be able to collect damages. In most states, the concept of contributory negligence has been replaced with *comparative negligence*, which means in essence that even if a patient contributes to his or her own injury or loss, the extent of the patient's negligence is compared to that of the physician; instead of being prevented from collecting damages, any monetary recovery is reduced by a percentage equal to the percentage of the patient's negligence.
- *Assumption of risk*—Not used as an affirmative defense in most states, the assumption of risk refers to a patient voluntarily participating in an activity with the knowledge that the activity entails some level of risk for which the patient has signed a document giving informed consent. This document can be used in the physician's defense as long as the physician has complied with the standard of care. A patient, however, never assumes the risk of negligent medical treatment. Informed consent is explained later in this chapter.
- *Statute of limitations*—The defense that applies when the time limit for legal action on medical negligence has been exceeded. This time limit varies among states, 2 years being the most common. In some states, a statutory policy involved in establishing the time limit is called the rule of discovery. This means that the statutory period does not begin until the patient discovers or should discover the negligence. The discovery date is the day a reasonable person would have known of the negligence. In the case of a minor, state laws vary. Lawsuits on behalf of injured minors may have to be filed within a specific time period (e.g., 3 years) of the discovery of the event giving rise to the injury. Or, in other states, the statute of limitations may begin when the minor reaches the age of majority. For information on state statutes of limitations, refer to the *Resources* section at the end of this chapter.

LITIGATION PREVENTION

There are a number of ways to reduce a medical practice's malpractice exposure. The medical assistant can be involved in the process and needs to be familiar with legal terms and guidelines.

The medical assistant is expected to represent and be loyal to the physician and to execute reasonable orders; nevertheless, the assistant should never support, aid, protect, or encourage the physician or any staff member in the performance of an unlawful act even if instructed to do so.

Such unsafe activities and behaviors that affect the health, safety, and welfare of others, as well as any conflict of interest, should be reported to the proper authorities (see MedWatch online report form in the *Resources* section at the end of this chapter and refer to Chapter 19 for *incident reporting*). Medical assistants should execute only duties and responsibilities that are within the scope of their training; if asked to do something they cannot competently perform or have no knowledge of how to handle, they should inform the physician-employer.

Risk Management

Risk management involves identifying problem practices or behaviors, then taking action to control or eliminate them. This reduces the likelihood of a malpractice lawsuit. Providing written job descriptions for each employee, an office procedure manual, an employee handbook, and a compliance plan can help avoid misunderstanding and mistakes that lead to liability risks. Identifying poor practices such as breach of confidentiality, substandard documentation or recordkeeping, absence of emergent appointment slots, lack of follow-up for patient care, and ineffective communication with patients can help reduce the risk of malpractice claims. Environmental issues (e.g., wet floors, poor security) also need to be addressed. After identifying problem areas, determine a plan of action. Practicing risk management makes the medical assistant and physician less vulnerable to litigation. Identify potential problems before they arise and take steps to prevent them; recognize when you need an attorney.

Guidelines to Prevent Medicolegal Claims

Patients may have unrealistic expectations and perceive that they are not receiving quality medical care. Remember, "Every lawsuit is the consequence of a bad result."* To prevent medicolegal claims with up-to-date knowledge of federal and state statutes, follow these guidelines:

1. Communicate with patients. Explain, encourage, ask their opinion, spend time, and listen. Build a relationship of honesty and trust.

2. Document information accurately and assist the physician in keeping up-to-date and comprehensive medical records. Avoid entering wrong diagnoses on claim forms, on requisition slips, or in the EHR.

3. Encourage the physician to identify the 20 most common clinical questions, write protocols, and develop a matrix for the office staff to follow. Refer to the matrix, office procedure manual, and compliance plan often.

4. Make sure patients have proper medication and after-care instructions. Consult with the physician if there are any doubts or confusion regarding a prescription or order.

5. Lock up all medical records pertaining to a lawsuit. Types of ink may be verified by the court as well as "ink dry time" and "imprints" left on other records. Always keep original documentation and follow correct protocol when making late entries.

6. Refrain from discussing another physician with a patient. Sometimes patients invite criticism of methods or results of former physicians by presenting only one side of the story.

7. Follow up on patients who have no-showed their appointments, schedule tests and make follow-up appointments, and make sure all test results are acted on.

8. Avoid making any statements that might be construed as an admission of fault on the part of the physician-employer. The medical assistant's position in lawsuits is to say nothing to anyone except as required by an attorney or by the court of law.

9. Never compare the respective merits of various forms of treatment or discuss the patient's ailments. The medical assistant should avoid rendering an opinion as this may contradict the physician's recommendations.

10. Inform patients who call the practice when the physician is absent that a qualified substitute is available—referred to as a *locum tenens*. Make sure the on-call physician has been briefed on patients with acute problems and has access to all medical records. The patient must not be abandoned.

11. Avoid referring to "authorization for release of information" forms as "releases." The word release may give the wrong impression to the patient.

12. Keep well informed and up-to-date by reading newsletters and medical office publications and by attending seminars. Knowledge obtained may prevent legal problems from developing and enhance financial operations.

13. Watch for various hazards that might cause injury to the physician, patients, or yourself.

14. Make sure patients understand which services they will receive and any fees for "extras." If a patient is to be hospitalized, explain that the fee the physician charges is for his or her services only and that there will be additional charges for the operating room, laboratory tests, anesthesia, the bed charge, and so forth.

15. Never leave drug samples out or prescription pads lying on the desk. They should be locked in a safe location. Never recommend (prescribe) a medication, even though you may have a feeling of confidence of what the physician would order.

16. Perform only those tasks that are within your scope of knowledge and training. Leave other tasks to individuals who are certified or licensed to perform them.

17. Create a medical disclaimer and post it and all legal policies in your office or on a website for the

*Stephen G. Reuter, Attorney at Law, Lashly & Baer, P.C., Saint Louis, Missouri

medical practice. If materials on health care are handed out or posted on the website, make sure patients understand that the content is not intended to be used in lieu of medical advice; it is for general informational purposes and educational use only.

18. Compose a website privacy policy that cautions patients that whatever they post becomes public information, that the practice cannot control the privacy policies of links to different sites, and that files (cookies) may be automatically downloaded to the visitor's computer and used in the future to establish identification.

If you become involved in a malpractice claim, inform the physician immediately, advise your supervisor, contact the insurance carrier, notify a lawyer, and determine a defense.

Bonding

Another preventive measure for the medical assistant who handles cash is to be bonded. A *fidelity bond* is insurance against theft or embezzlement, which unfortunately can occur in any business or medical office that handles cash. In **bonding** an employee, an insurance or bonding company guarantees payment of a specified amount to the physician in the event of financial loss caused by an employee or by some contingency over which an employee handling money has no control. Three effective bonding methods are:

1. *Position-schedule bonding*—Also known as a "name schedule" or umbrella bond, offers coverage for a specific job, such as a bookkeeper or receptionist, rather than a named individual. If an employee in a specified category leaves, the newly employed replacement is automatically covered. This bond generally requires little, if any, personal background investigation.
2. Blanket-position bonding—Coverage for all employees regardless of job title.
3. Personal bonding—Coverage for those who handle large amounts of money; a thorough background investigation is required.

Bond coverage should be reviewed periodically with the insurance agent to make sure coverage is keeping pace with expansion of the medical practice.

To further remove any temptations for embezzlement, the physician should sign checks, periodically review bills, examine records, and scan the mail to get an idea of what payments are coming in. All encounter forms should be numbered, and a copy of the deposit slip should always be retained and stapled to the computer printout or day sheet so that the physician can review it at frequent but irregular intervals.

Patients' Bill of Rights

On February 6, 1973, the House of Delegates of the American Hospital Association (AHA) approved a *Patients' Bill of Rights* to provide a remedy for some recurring complaints about attitudes of and treatment by physicians and administrators. It has also helped to reduce malpractice suits as these often result from misunderstandings between the patient and physician or hospital.

In 2003, the AHA's Patients' Bill of Rights was changed into a plain language brochure, *The Patient Care Partnership.* It outlines what to expect during a hospital stay, how to prepare when going home, what information will be needed from the patient, and rights and responsibilities regarding privacy, medical bills, and insurance claims.

In 2010, a new Patient's Bill of Rights was created along with the Affordable Care Act, which focuses on patients' rights in the private health insurance market. It helps Americans with preexisting conditions gain coverage, protects choice of doctors, and ends lifetime limits on the care consumers receive.

Today's physicians are urged to include patients in medical decision-making and inform patients of their rights regarding choice of treatment, consent for treatment, and refusal of treatment. Refer to the *Resources* section at the end of this chapter for information on where to obtain the new Patient's Bill of Rights and the Patient Care Partnership booklet.

ALTERNATIVES TO THE LITIGATION PROCESS

Litigation is *trial by jury* following a plaintiff's filing of a **complaint** or petition. Before trial, the **defendant** who is the opposing side may file a motion called a "demurrer" to have the case dismissed if there are not sufficient grounds for action. If not dismissed, the case goes to a trial judge or pretrial conference and then to a jury trial, resulting in a verdict and the possibility of an appeal. Following are several alternative methods to resolve a malpractice dispute.

Screening Panel

One alternative to litigation is a *screening panel*, or physician review panel, that hears cases outside the courtroom in the hope of solving them without the expense, publicity, and difficulty of court proceedings. In states where these panels have been established, review may or may not be a prerequisite for going to court. These panels issue advisory opinions but cannot legally bar litigation. Through this review process, some nuisance suits can be avoided.

Arbitration

Another method of resolving malpractice disputes is *arbitration*. This process is used when a patient and physician have agreed before treatment (*preclaim agreement*) that both will waive the right to a court trial in case of a dispute. This legal method is provided by statute in some states and helps resolve any patient-physician controversy before an impartial panel or **grievance committee**. It saves time, is less expensive, may be fairer, and allows greater privacy for the parties involved in disagreements. For such an agreement to be binding, the patient must have plain and clear notification of all terms, which must be specifically explained. Patients are free not to sign the agreement, and signing is not a requirement for being seen by a doctor or receiving continuing medical treatment.

Usually this is the medical assistant who must explain and present the arbitration agreement to patients for signature. Using tact and answering the patient's questions are most important in making the initial request for signature. If a lawsuit is instituted against the physician, it is the medical assistant's job to notify the physician's insurance carrier promptly and include a copy of the arbitration agreement. Not invoking arbitration at the outset can result in a waiver of the arbitration agreement. Some managed care plans and some insurance programs have preclaim agreements as a requirement or option of the policy.

A second type of arbitration agreement is a *postclaim agreement* that is transacted after a dispute occurs and both sides must agree to arbitrate rather than litigate.

Mediation

Mediation is an attempt to settle a legal dispute out of court and is frequently ordered by a judge. It is similar to arbitration; however, an arbitrator acts much like a judge while a mediator is a neutral third-party facilitator that guides the opposing parties to work mutually toward a resolution. Mediation increases the control the parties have while coming to an agreement, takes less time than a court hearing, and is less expensive. Compliance with a mediated agreement is usually high.

No-Fault Malpractice Insurance

The last and most far-reaching approach to resolution of the medical malpractice problem is *no-fault malpractice insurance.* No-fault systems eliminate the requirement of proving negligence, so the injured person is compensated without regard to fault. This system allows the physician to come forward when an error occurs, without the threat of a law suite, and join forces with the patient to ensure appropriate compensation. The workers' compensation system is an example of a no-fault model.

MEDICAL RECORDS

It is essential that medical records be accurate, complete, up-to-date, and readable, reflecting the history, physical examination, assessment, and treatment plan. This documentation is necessary to provide the best medical care, justify services billed to the insurance company, and defend a physician in the event of a lawsuit. Detailed information on patients' medical records is found in Chapter 9.

Informed Consent

When a physician recommends a procedure to enhance making a diagnosis or for treatment, it is the obligation of the physician to inform the patient of all significant risks and alternatives to the suggested procedure. The patient then must decide whether to accept the physician's recommendation. If the patient decides to accept the risks, a consent form is signed acknowledging the assumed risks. This is called *informed consent*. This process is important when dealing with minor or major surgical cases whether in an office or hospital setting. When witnessing the consent form, the medical assistant is witnessing the signature and not the consent (Figure 3-14). For proper wording of informed consent forms, see Figure 3-15. If a patient who does not speak English is being treated, an interpreter should be present and the forms should also be written in the patient's primary language.

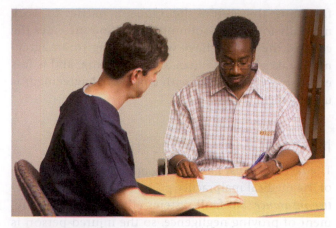

FIGURE 3-14 Patient signing an informed consent with a medical assistant witnessing the signature

Subpoena

Subpoena literally means "under penalty," and it is an order by the court for a witness to appear at a designated place to give testimony. In medical malpractice cases, the physician or other health care professional are not obligated to state opinions and give **expert testimony** in which they are considered an authority on the subject matter and provide a statement that is scientific, technical, or professional in nature. The physician or health care professional may instead be a "percipient witness" who merely describes what he or she did, said, and observed about a given set of circumstances.

A *subpoena duces tecum*, which literally means, "under penalty you shall bring with you," is a court order for the appearance of a witness with the subpoenaed medical records. However, the medical record might be all that is required, as is the typical scenario experienced in most medical practices.

A physician-employer may authorize the medical assistant to receive a subpoena in his or her name (Figure 3-16). Although a subpoena must generally be personally served to the person named in it, the medical

COMPLIANCE

Informed Consent

In 38 states, minors under the age of 18 need parental permission for abortion procedures. To determine if your state requires permission, refer to "Planned Parenthood" in the *Resources* section at the end of this chapter.

assistant's receipt of the subpoena as the physician's representative is considered the equivalent of personal service. A witness or mileage fee should accompany the subpoena and be requested from the deputy when the subpoena is served. Neither civil nor criminal subpoenas can be served via electronic mail or fax transmission. The medical records may be delivered or mailed to the court in a sealed envelope. Some states provide for a substitute service by mail or through newspaper publication if efforts to effect personal service have failed.

If the physician is on vacation or at a medical meeting, do not accept the subpoena in the physician's absence. Suggest to the deputy that it be served after the physician returns or that the physician's attorney be contacted; then, inform the attorney. The assistant may also ask one of the other physicians in the office for advice.

The physician or office manager will review the subpoena and verify the exact dates covered; the entire medical record should not be released. The "custodian of the medical record" will be advised regarding which sections of the medical record need to be copied.

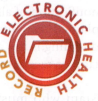 Medical records that are to be released via subpoena, records of high-profile patients, and records that contain highly sensitive health data (e.g., mental health statements, HIV/AIDS status, substance abuse, or chemical dependency) may be categorized as "high-risk data" in the electronic medical record system, which restricts and limits access. This type of special security feature offers a higher degree of protection to sensitive documents. Hard copy medical records of this nature should be stored under lock and key.

Do not permit the representative from the copy service to take possession of an original medical record, unless he or she is being supervised during the photocopying process. And, do not allow an original chart to be removed from the office for photocopying, even if someone promises to promptly return it. When a subpoena is served, a patient's signed authorization for release of information form is not required.

ADVANCE DIRECTIVES

Congress passed a law known as the *Patient Self-Determination Act (PSDA)*, also known as the Danforth Bill or Medical Miranda Rights for Patients Act. It requires hospitals, hospices, physicians' offices, skilled

Procedure: VULVAR BIOPSY

You and your doctor are considering a biopsy of your vulva. This is a type of examination in which the doctor will take a specimen of the tissue of the vulva or private area and have it examined further. Specimens may be taken from different areas of the vulva after local anesthesia has "numbed" the area. The purpose of the test is to detect cancer or other abnormal cells. This biopsy is not treatment for any disease; it is just an examination. It is possible that an area of cancer or other abnormality may not be sampled and therefore go undetected. Because of this fact, your doctor can make no guarantee as to the accuracy of the test.

This test is quite safe and complications from it are very unusual. The possibility of complications is greater in patients who have other disease or who take steroids or certain herbs or medications that affect blood clotting. Bleeding and infection are uncommon complications. In very rare cases, bleeding and infection from the test have resulted in the need for surgery and blood transfusions. General pain, discomfort or pain with urination, pain during sexual intercourse, and scarring may also occur. Allergic reactions to one or more of the substances used in the test are very uncommon. In very, very rare instances allergic reactions have caused death.

The vulvar biopsy is a reasonably safe and accurate method of diagnosing abnormal cells or cancer of the vulva. In those women in which the test is indicated, this procedure may provide the best chance of successful diagnosis and the lowest risk of complications.

ADDITIONAL RISKS AND ALTERNATIVES:
(To be filled here and on reverse
side by doctor as necessary)

_____

_____

_____

I CERTIFY: I have read or had read to me the contents of this form; I understand the risks and alternatives involved in this procedure; I have had the opportunity to ask any questions which I had and all of my questions have been answered.

DATE: _____ TIME: _____   SIGNED: _____
                                                          (Signed by patient or person legally
                                                           authorized to consent for patient)

WITNESS: _____   PHYSICIAN: _____
                                                          (Signed by physician)

(A GENERAL CONSENT FORM MUST ALSO BE SIGNED BY THE PATIENT.)

Prepared by In-Forms No. 1494

FIGURE 3-15 A risk disclosure form (informed consent). Procedure: Vulvar Biopsy, prepared for the patient's signature giving permission to have the procedure performed in the physician's office

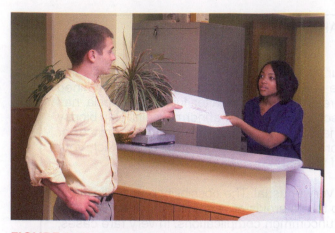

FIGURE 3-16 Representative of the court serving a subpoena to a medical assistant, the physician's representative

nursing facilities, and home health providers who participate in the Medicare or Medicaid programs to ask each patient whether he or she has drawn up an **advance directive** (living will or health care power of attorney) and to document the response in the patient's chart. This law took effect in 1991 and requires that institutions supply patients with written information about state laws concerning advance directives and a patient's right to reject end-of-life treatment. Such documents conform to state laws and detail in legal form the desires for procedures to be performed or withheld when death is imminent, or if the patient becomes *incompetent*. Incompetence is a legal status, not a medical condition; however, a physician generally accesses the patients' competence—sometimes a court order is necessary. In such cases, a surrogate, who has been named on the advance directive, sees that the patient's wishes are carried out and, if necessary, makes medical decisions. The surrogate is typically a relative, friend, or physician who knows the patient.

Although the legal definition of competence varies from state to state, generally it refers to the patient having the ability to understand the nature of his illness, the choices of treatments available, and the risks and benefits of accepting or declining the treatment. Some of the more common conditions in which incompetence is declared are neurological brain impairments, such as an unconscious patient in a coma, a patient with dementia from Alzheimer's disease, a patient with an acute delirium from a metabolic disorder, or one under the influence or suffering from withdrawal from alcohol or drugs. Advance directives take different forms; many are simply titled "Declarations" and several other types are mentioned here.

Living Will

Basically, a **living will** is a document stating the desires of a person should he or she become incompetent because of injury or illness and death is imminent. Living wills are not legally binding, but more than 40 states have *right-to-die laws* that often recognize living wills as evidence of intent. Living wills have become popular as a result of medical situations in which use of equipment assists a person to live for an undeterminable amount of time even when comatose. A living will can be revoked (usually by a simple oral statement) at any time.

Health Care Power of Attorney

Another document called a **health care power of attorney** is legally binding and is more flexible than a living will. It allows the individual to detail precise wishes about treatment. This document can be used for all medical decisions, not just those about life-prolonging treatment, and by all people, not just those who are terminally ill. Some states recognize a combination living will with a durable power of attorney for health care that allows the person to appoint another person to withhold or consent to medical care.

Medical Directive

Ezekiel and Linda Emanuel, a husband-and-wife physician team in Boston, developed a detailed document called a *medical directive*. It allows patients to specify what they would and would not want done in four specific dire situations by answering 48 questions. It can be used by itself or in conjunction with other state-authorized documents.

Values History Form

Another advance directive, a *values history form*, was developed to try to uncover a patient's value system and to guide a physician's decisions about treatment. It asks questions such as, "How important is independence and self-sufficiency in your life?" It is not a legal document, but it may be used to supplement a living will or durable power of attorney for health care.

Health Care Proxy

In Massachusetts, after many years of deliberation, legislation was enacted for a *health care proxy*, which is a type of advance directive. The patient has the responsibility to communicate his or her decisions about various forms of life support to the surrogate. If this does not occur, the surrogate is left to make decisions without direction. The responsibilities need to be explained to the patient. A physician or medical assistant can be valuable in aiding the patient in the choice of a surrogate.

Do Not Resuscitate Form

Some states have developed a *do not resuscitate form* for use in prehospital settings, for example, in a patient's home, in a long-term care facility, during transport to or from a health care facility, and in other locations outside acute care hospitals. In some regions, emergency responders and hospitals are encouraged to honor the form when a patient is transported to an emergency department. When signed by the patient, it protects health care providers from criminal prosecution, civil liability, and discipline for unprofessional conduct, administrative sanction, or any other sanction. Copies of the form are retained by the patient and physician and made part of the patient's permanent medical record. In certain regions, some ambulance companies require a copy of the form to be retained in their files. In some states, a specific organization may issue a wrist or neck medallion for identification purposes. In an emergency when a patient's heart has stopped and emergency medical services (EMS) are called, EMS providers forgo resuscitation attempts if a form is present or if the individual is wearing such a medallion. For information pertaining to laws in your region, contact the local Department of Health Services.

Uniform Anatomical Gift Act

It is the right of a competent adult to make disposition of all or part of his or her body for transplant or research purposes. The Uniform Anatomical Gift Act was approved by the National Conference of Commissioners on Uniform State Laws in July 1968. It has been

PATIENT EDUCATION
Organ Donations

Patients may need to be informed about the many uses of donor tissue and organs. Donor hearts or kidneys are vitally needed and many potential recipients are on waiting lists. Best results for a match occur when a donor is closely related to the recipient. Corneal transplants for individuals with scarred or opaque corneas are successful because the cornea has no blood supply and antibodies responsible for rejection of foreign tissue do not reach it. Livers, lungs, and pancreases have also been transplanted but the longevity of such transplants is not as successful. Materials may be ordered for your office from your state registry. To find your local contact, go to "Donate Life America" homepage, and search "Get Involved locally." Inform patients about organ donations when advising them about advance directives.

adopted in all states. The act provides that a person 18 years of age or over may give all or any part of his or her body after death for research, transplant, or placement in a tissue bank.

Donor Registration

While donated organs and tissues are shared at a national level, laws that govern donations vary from state to state. A coalition on donation called Donate Life has a website (see the *Resources* section at the end of the chapter) that offers a state-by-state guide to donation registration. On the website, select "Commit to Donation," then click on the map of the United States and select your state. Directions will appear instructing you how to sign up. At present, 40 states have electronic registries. For other states, you are directed to sign up by applying for a form from a state organization by downloading a donation card, or signing up at the state's Department of Motor Vehicles (Figure 3-17). Advance directives may also have questions regarding whether you would like body parts donated.

Although the trend is to use online registration services because databases can be quickly accessed

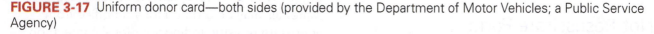

```
Uniform Donor Card—Front
THIS IS A LEGALLY BINDING DOCUMENT

According to the guidelines of the Uniform Anatomical Gift Act. I
choose, upon my death to:
A ___   Donate any of my organs, tissues, or parts
B ___   Donate a pacemaker (date implanted_____)
C ___   Donate parts, tissues, or organs listed _____
        _____
D ___   Donate my entire body
E ___   ☐ Transplantation   ☐ Medical Research   ☐ Both
F ___   Not donate any organs, parts, tissues or pacemaker
        _____
     SIGNATURE                          DATE

        _____
     WITNESS SIGNATURE                  DATE
☐ Discussed with affected parties
                                        _____
                                        DOCTOR'S INITIALS

DMV                        ●
A Public Service Agency   DONOR
```

```
Uniform Donor Card—Back

IMPORTANT INSTRUCTION
If you wish to make a donation, ÿll out this card and put the "DONOR" dot on the
front of your license or I.D. card next to the photo where indicated. Keep the card
with your license or I.D. card. If you change your mind, complete a new card and
remove the dot.

To refuse to donate, ÿll out part "F" of this card and carry it with your license or
I.D. card. Do not use the dot.

NOTICE
If you are at least 18, you may choose to donate any needed organs, tissues, a pace-
maker or whole body for medical transplantation or research or both, and indicate
this decision on your driver license or I.D. card. According to the Uniform Anatomical
Gift Act (Section 7150, Health & Safety Code), your donation will take effect on your
death. (Entering the name of your next of kin below is optional)

Name _____
Address _____
Telephone No. _____
          Keep this card with your driver license or I.D. card
```

FIGURE 3-17 Uniform donor card—both sides (provided by the Department of Motor Vehicles; a Public Service Agency)

and donor registration confirmed, donor cards, which are legal documents, may also be distributed to patients by physicians. If cards are used, the patient and one or more witnesses must sign the card and it should be kept with the patient at all times near a driver's license or identification card. It is important for patients to inform family members of their decision to donate.

Advance Directive Guidelines

The various types of advance directives are signed by the individual and two witnesses (preferably not relatives) and in some states must be notarized. When a patient has signed such a document, a copy of it should be filed in the patient's medical record (a colored label may be placed on the outside of the chart). It is recommended that copies be given to the patient's clergy, lawyer, a close friend, relatives, and anyone to whom the patient gives the power of attorney. An advance directive should be periodically reviewed and revised. It is essential that a form be used that will be upheld by state law. Medical assistants can informally educate the patient concerning advance directives by obtaining booklets and forms and by becoming knowledgeable of the laws in the states in which they are working. Refer to the *Resources* section at the end of this chapter to download state-specific advance directive documents or to contact organizations for information.

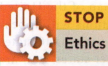

STOP AND THINK CASE SCENARIO

Ethics

SCENARIO: An older patient has severe osteoporosis and has a collapsed vertebra. She is in constant pain and receives relief only from taking a narcotic painkiller, four times a day, which is addictive.

CRITICAL THINKING: Should the physician supply enough medication to provide relief or only enough pills for the patient to take when she is experiencing pain that she absolutely cannot bear? Think this through and formulate questions that might help you decide what stance to take.

_____

_____

_____

STOP AND THINK CASE SCENARIO
Bioethics

SCENARIO: You have a child who is diagnosed with cystic fibrosis and have heard that a cloning research project is progressing that holds the key to curing this disease.

CRITICAL THINKING:

1. Would you want your child to benefit from this method of treatment if the research proves successful?

_____

_____

_____

2. Would you advocate cloning research for other scientific breakthroughs?

_____

_____

STOP AND THINK CASE SCENARIO
Stem Cell Research

SCENARIO: There are three main sources for obtaining stem cells: (1) adult stem cells are found in bone marrow and the peripheral system, (2) umbilical cord cells are extracted during pregnancy, and (3) human embryonic stem cells are naturally created in the first days after conception. They each can develop into all different types of cells, have the ability to continually renew themselves, and give rise to all organs and tissues in the human body. By fusing a stem cell to an adult human skin cell, researchers report that they can create a hybrid cell that acts like a stem cell. Stem cells are also cultivated from embryos frozen in test tubes after being created by couples using in vitro fertilization and from embryos cloned from patients seeking treatment such as abortion. They hold the potential to be genetically programmed to treat various diseases by replacing diseased tissue, including the following:

- Brain tissue for use in patients with Parkinson's or Alzheimer's disease
- Liver tissue for use in patients with liver disease
- Nerve tissue for use in patients with spinal cord injury

CRITICAL THINKING: Stem cell research is fighting for its life. Think through this complex scenario. You may want to do additional research on your own or your instructor may assign this as a research or writing project. Be prepared to take a stance and debate various types of stem cell research with your classmates. Formulate your response here.

_____

_____

_____

_____

_____

_____

_____

- Pancreatic cells for use in patients with diabetes
- Blood cells to repair ailing hearts or blocked arteries

Advocacy groups oppose the research of embryonic stem cells because human embryos are destroyed during research and some consider that human life starts at the point of conception—to destroy a cell would be considered murder. Research done on a state level has been opposed by lawyers on the grounds that it violates the state constitution because taxpayer money is being given to an organization not sufficiently controlled by the state government

STOP AND THINK CASE SCENARIO
Confidential Information

SCENARIO: Abigail Snyder hobbles into the medical office suffering from a broken right foot. The receptionist greets her and begins asking her personal questions that everyone in the waiting room can hear the answers to. Abigail tries talking softly, but the receptionist repeats her answers loud enough so all can hear them. Abigail feels compelled to answer the questions because they pertain to her medical case.

CRITICAL THINKING:

1. How do you think Abigail feels?

_____

_____

2. What are the dangers of obtaining information in such a manner?

_____

_____

3. How could the receptionist handle the situation to obtain the information without jeopardizing patient confidentiality?

_____

_____

STOP AND THINK CASE SCENARIO
HIPAA: Verbal Permission

SCENARIO: You receive a telephone call from Mrs. Wiltfang who has been a patient for several years; you recognize her voice. She says she is very ill and would like to give permission for a neighbor to pick up her medication, which she needs to begin immediately. You view Mrs. Wiltfang's electronic medical record, and then document the call noting that verbal permission was given. When the neighbor arrives she asks what is wrong with Mrs. Wiltfang and wants to know whether she is going to be OK. You realize that the medication itself might tell the neighbor something about the patient's condition.

CRITICAL THINKING: Refer to HIPAA guidelines and determine what you would do.

_____

_____

_____

_____

_____

_____

_____

_____

_____

_____

_____

_____

_____

_____

_____

_____

_____

STOP AND THINK CASE SCENARIO

HIPAA: Written Permission

SCENARIO: Written permission is received from a cancer patient stating that the physician and office staff may discuss his medical condition with his sons; their names are not given. You receive a telephone call from someone claiming to be the patient's youngest son in another state who asks for an update on his father's condition. You have met the patient's two sons who live in town but are not familiar with the person on the telephone.

CRITICAL THINKING: Refer to HIPAA guidelines and determine what you would do.

_____
_____
_____
_____
_____
_____
_____
_____
_____
_____
_____

FOCUS ON CERTIFICATION*

CMA (AAMA) Content Summary

- Medical practice acts (physician license)
- Advance directives
- Anatomical gifts
- Reportable incidences
- Public health statutes
- HIPAA
- Consent/authorization
- Right to privacy
- Drug and alcohol rehabilitation records
- HIV-related issues
- _Subpoena duces tecum_
- Physician-patient relationship (contract/noncompliance)
- Responsibility and rights (physician/patient/medical assistant)
- Third-party agreements
- Professional liability
- Standard of care
- Arbitration
- Affirmative defenses
- Comparative/contributory negligence

- Termination of care
- Medicolegal terms and doctrines
- Releasing information
- Tort law
- Ethical standards (AAMA/AMA)
- Bioethics
- Liability coverage

RMA (AMT) Content Summary

- Types of consents
- Federal and state laws
- HIPAA
- Privacy acts
- Scope of practice
- Patient Bill of Rights
- Licensure
- Legal terminology
- Medical ethics (AMA)
- Legal responsibilities
- Good Samaritan Act
- Emergency first aid
- Mandatory reporting guidelines

*This textbook _and the accompanying_ Workbook _meet the entry-level administrative and general competencies for the CMA outlined by the AAMA Examination Content Outline and Occupational Analysis and for the RMA and CMAS outlined by the AMT Competencies, Construction Parameters, and Examination Specifications (see Competency Grid in Appendix B)._

CMAS (AMT Content Summary)

- Principles of medical laws and ethics (AMA)
- Scope of practice
- Disclosure laws
- Unethical practices
- Confidentiality
- Protected health information

REVIEW EXAM-STYLE QUESTIONS

1. Standards of conduct generally accepted as a moral guide for behavior are referred to as:
   a. laws
   b. bioethics
   c. professional medical etiquette
   d. professional medical ethics
   e. rules for medical professionals

2. The modern code of ethics adopted by the American Medical Association to guide physicians' standards of conduct is the:
   a. Oath of Hippocrates
   b. Modern Hippocratic Oath
   c. Principles of Medical Ethics for the Physician
   d. AAMA Code of Ethics
   e. AAMA Creed

3. The Health Insurance Portability and Accountability Act became federal law in:
   a. 1996
   b. 1998
   c. 1976
   d. 1956
   e. 2001

4. The correct meaning for the acronym PHI is:
   a. private health information
   b. personal health information
   c. protected health information
   d. portability of health information
   e. privileged health information

5. The "consent form" is:
   a. another term for the "authorization form"
   b. mandated by HIPAA for the release of personally identifiable health information for treatment, payment, and routine health care operations
   c. used for the release of personally identifiable health information for reasons other than treatment, payment, and routine health care operations
   d. used voluntarily for the release of personally identifiable health information for treatment, payment, and routine health care operations
   e. used to release sensitive information such as HIV or AIDS status

6. If a patient requests copies of his or her medical records and signs the proper authorization, you should:
   a. honor the request
   b. seal them in an envelope before handing them to the patient
   c. take caution before complying with the request
   d. not honor the request; instead send them directly to another physician
   e. a, b, and c are all correct

7. An exception to the right to privacy (privileged communication) that does not need an authorization form because it must be reported to the Department of Health is information about a:
   a. patient with multiple sclerosis
   b. patient with amyotrophic lateral sclerosis (ALS)
   c. patient experiencing epileptic seizures
   d. patient with diabetes mellitus
   e. patient with a skin rash on the genital area

8. The most common torts in health care incidents are:
   a. assault and battery torts
   b. liability without fault torts
   c. intentional torts
   d. negligent torts
   e. fraud or deceit torts

9. Unlawful treatment that has been done in the wrong way is:
   a. misfeasance
   b. malfeasance
   c. nonfeasance
   d. malpractice
   e. criminal negligence

10. Arbitration is:
   a. a physician review panel that hears cases outside the courtroom
   b. a type of no-fault insurance
   c. an alternative way of resolving malpractice disputes out of court
   d. litigation
   e. a type of lawsuit

11. When a physician recommends a surgical procedure and the patient decides to accept the risks and have the procedure, the patient must sign a/an:
    a. authorization to release medical records
    b. informed consent
    c. consent to release personally identifiable health information for treatment
    d. HIPAA consent
    e. health care power of attorney

12. With a *subpoena duces tecum*:
    a. a witness must appear
    b. a witness must appear with the medical record
    c. the physician must personally accept it
    d. the medical record may be all that is required
    e. the physician never needs to appear

13. A living will:
    a. is not legally binding
    b. is not recognized in the majority of states
    c. cannot be revoked orally
    d. can only be revoked in writing
    e. is more legally binding than a durable power of attorney for health care

14. Under HIPAA law, what is the best description of PHI?
    a. Pertinent health information related to the patient's current treatment at your facility.
    b. Personal health information such as mental illness and sexually transmitted diseases.
    c. Protected health information about the patient's past, present, or future health condition that could identify the person.
    d. Private health information any reasonable person would not want disclosed without permission.

WORKBOOK ASSIGNMENT

To develop competency-based job skills, refer to the *Workbook* and complete the:
- Abbreviation and Spelling Review
- Review Questions

- Critical Thinking Exercises
- Job Skill activities, which are listed at the beginning of the chapter under *Performance Objectives in the Workbook.*

RESOURCES

Some state and local medical societies and consumer organizations can provide appropriate forms and information for advance directives. It is important to keep well informed on legal issues affecting responsibilities of the medical assistant, and there are many publications available. The following are resources to assist you.

Books

Black's Law Dictionary, 10th edition
  Legal terms—online version available
  Garner, Bryan A. Thomson West, 2014
Code of Medical Ethics: Current Opinions with Annotations
  American Medical Association, 2012–2013

Ethical Challenges in the Management of Health Information, 2nd edition
  Harman, L.
  Jones & Bartlett, 2006
Health Care Law and Ethics
  American Association of Medical Assistants
  Self-study course
Law, Liability, and Ethics for Medical Office Professionals, 5th edition
  Flight, Myrtle
  Cengage Learning, 2011
  Website: http://www.cengagebrain.com
The Power of Ethical Management
  Blanchard/Peale
  William Morrow and Company, Inc., 1988

Compliance

Compliance program guidance for individual and small group physician practices, third-party medical billing companies, and home health agencies:

Office of Inspector General (OIG)

Search: Fraud, compliance

Donor Cards

Donate Life

Online tissue donor registry service

Select your state

National Kidney Foundation

Kidney donation

Internet

Accreditation of Healthcare Organizations

Public Policy Reports and Safety Standards

Acronym Finder

Legal acronym and abbreviation locator

Code of Federal Regulations

U.S. Government Printing Office

Elder Justice Act

Elder abuse protections

Expert Law

State-by-state overview for lawsuits to be filed

Search: State statute of limitations

Health Care Compliance Association

Website: http://www.hcca-info.org

HIPAA Law

U. S. Department of Health and Human Services

Medicolegal Forms with Legal Analysis

Search: Medicolegal forms

MedWatch

U.S. Food and Drug Administration Information

Adverse Event Reporting Program

Minors' Access to Health Care in the United States

Age of majority

Available types of medical care for minors

National Committee for Quality Assurance

Consumer reports (feature articles)

Patient Care Partnership

American Hospital Association

Patient's Bill of Rights

Search: New Patient's Bill of Rights

Planned Parenthood

Search: Parental Consent and Notification Laws

Individual state requirements for minors

The Secretarial and Office Professional Ethics

Ethic list with definitions

The Security Rule

Search: HIPAA, Administrative Safeguard Standards

U.S. Department of Health and Human Services

HIPAA updates

U.S. Department of Justice

Featured articles and resources

Medical Directives

American Medical Association

Advance care directives

Caring Connections

State-specific advance directives

National Healthcare Decisions Day

Listing of where to get advance directives

Values History Form

Center for Health Law and Ethics

Institute of Public Law

University of New Mexico School of Law

Search the Internet for the following organizations' advanced directives:

- Aging with Dignity—Five Wishes
- American Association of Retired Persons (AARP)— End of life resources
- American Bar Association—Tool Kit for Advance Planning
- American Hospital Association—Create and register a living will

Physician Credentials

Federation of State Medical Boards

Verifying physician credentials

Verify and Comply: A Quick Reference Guide to Credentialing Standards, 5th edition

Cairns, Carol

HCPro, 2009

Scope of Practice

American Association of Medical Assistants

Key State Scope of Practice Laws

Select: Employers, Key State Scope of Practice Laws—select your state

Unit 2

INTERPERSONAL COMMUNICATIONS

CHAPTER 4

THE ART OF COMMUNICATION

LEARNING OBJECTIVES

After reading this chapter and learning step-by-step procedures to gain job skills,* you should be able to:

- Recognize the importance of effective communication in the medical office.
- List and define the basic elements of the communication cycle.
- Name three primary modes of communication.
- Communicate accurately and succinctly showing empathy and sensitivity.
- Differentiate between subjective and objective information.
- State and define five types of defensive mechanisms.
- Understand the five levels of human needs described by Maslow's hierarchy theory.
- Summarize the eight stages of development in Erickson's Human Life Cycle.
- Explain what the comfort zone is.
- Describe how nonverbal communication occurs.
- Give examples of components used in active listening.
- Recall three types of feedback used to evaluate whether the message sent is the message received.
- Indicate things to avoid when communicating.
- Adapt methods of communication to meet the needs of patients in different age groups.
- Discuss how to handle communication problems caused by language barriers.
- Outline four common biases in today's society and define stereotyping, prejudice, and discrimination.
- Demonstrate ways to adapt communication when barriers are present such as sight impairment, hearing impairment, and impaired level of understanding.
- Determine ways to establish positive communication with patients, coworkers, and superiors.

PERFORMANCE OBJECTIVES (PROCEDURES) IN THIS TEXTBOOK

- Demonstrate active listening by following guidelines (Procedure 4-1).
- Communicate with children (Procedure 4-2).

---

*This textbook and the accompanying Workbook meet the educational components for entry-level administrative and general competencies outlined by CAAHEP and ABHES.

- Communicate with older adults (Procedure 4-3).
- Communicate with hearing-impaired patients (Procedure 4-4).
- Communicate with visually impaired patients (Procedure 4-5).
- Communicate with speech-impaired patients (Procedure 4-6).
- Communicate with patients who have an impaired level of understanding (Procedure 4-7).
- Communicate with anxious patients (Procedure 4-8).
- Communicate with angry patients (Procedure 4-9).
- Communicate with patients and their family members and friends (Procedure 4-10).
- Communicate with the health care team (Procedure 4-11).

PERFORMANCE OBJECTIVES (JOB SKILLS) IN THE WORKBOOK

- Demonstrate body language (Job Skill 4-1).
- Use the Internet to research active listening skills and write a report (Job Skill 4-2).
- Communicate with a child via role-playing (Job Skill 4-3).
- Communicate with an older adult via role-playing (Job Skill 4-4).
- Name unique qualities of other cultures (Job Skill 4-5).
- Communicate with a hearing-impaired patient via role-playing (Job Skill 4-6).
- Communicate with a visually impaired patient via role-playing (Job Skill 4-7).
- Communicate with a speech-impaired patient via role-playing (Job Skill 4-8).
- Communicate with a patient who has an impaired level of understanding via role-playing (Job Skill 4-9).
- Communicate with an anxious patient via role-playing (Job Skill 4-10).
- Communicate with an angry patient via role-playing (Job Skill 4-11).
- Communicate with a patient and his or her family members and friends via role-playing (Job Skill 4-12).
- Communicate with a coworker on the health care team via role-playing (Job Skill 4-13).

KEY TERMS

active listening	discrimination	open-ended questions
bias	displaced anger	perceptions
body language	enunciate	prejudice
colloquialisms	ethnic	reflective listening
communicate	feedback	stereotype
communication cycle	noncompliant	subjective information
defensive	nonverbal communication	verbal communication
demeanor	objective information	

ESSENTIAL COMMUNICATION

Good interpersonal and communication skills are essential traits that should accompany the technical administrative and clinical skills each medical assistant obtains. As mentioned in Chapter 1, these are referred to as *soft skills* and they complement the "hard skills" that you will learn. Of all the professionals who make up a health care team, the medical assistant will have the most interaction with the patient; therefore, the art

Service

Communication is the foundation of every action taken as a health care professional serves and cares for patients, regardless of the task. In good times and in times of illness, you may be the lifeline that connects patients with the physician so that they can get the help they need. Accurate communication is vital to helping maintain this connection, but is often a silent component not readily seen as a way of serving patients' needs.

of *patient-centered communication* must be learned, developed, and practiced. As with other skills, it may seem easy for some and difficult for others.

The health care professional who learns how to communicate effectively will be an asset to the medical practice and an important cog in the **communication cycle** (Figure 4-1). Effective communication is highly valued because it affects office interactions, patient understanding of office policies, and various aspects of health care delivery as well as public relations. It is perhaps the most important aspect of customer service. Employers are looking for potential employees who balance their technical knowledge with effective communication skills. Those who communicate well are trusted and respected; they have the best job security.

What Is Communication?

To **communicate** is to transfer information from one party to another. The information being shared is facts, feelings, ideas, opinions, and thoughts. This exchange process takes place between two individuals—a sender and a receiver. Basic elements of the communication cycle include:

- *Sender*—Person who has an idea or information and wants to convey it.
- *Message*—Content that needs to be communicated.
- *Channel*—Method of sending the message to the receiver.

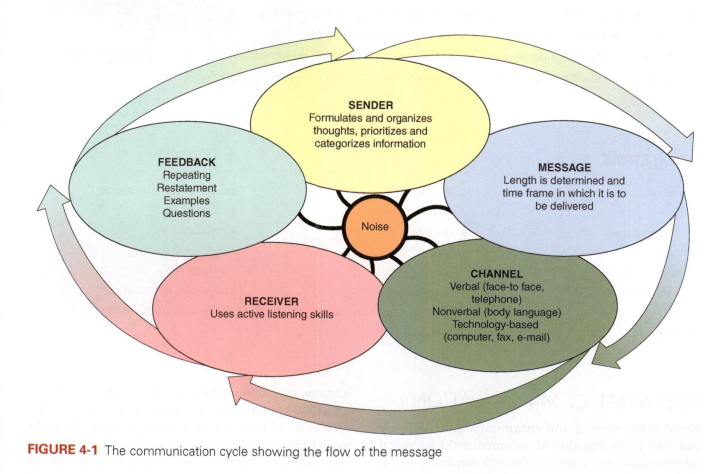

FIGURE 4-1 The communication cycle showing the flow of the message

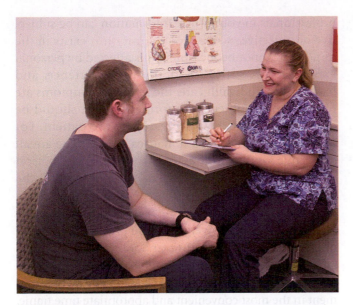

FIGURE 4-2 Positive communication is demonstrated by an open posture and a friendly smile

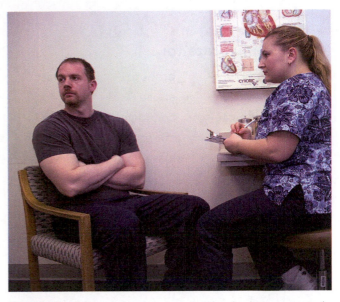

FIGURE 4-3 Negative communication is demonstrated by a closed posture, lack of eye contact, and a bored or disgruntled appearance

- *Receiver*—Recipient getting the message and interpreting it.
- *Feedback*—Response from the receiver used to decide whether clarification is necessary and to determine whether the message sent is the message received.

The top three ways humans communicate messages are (1) body language; (2) tonality (voice tone, tempo, volume, inflection, projection); and (3) spoken word. One would think that words are the most important element in communication; however, some experts* indicate that more information is communicated by body language than words and the tone in which they are spoken. This chapter will inform you of the various components involved in each element of communication and their usefulness. Other topics covered include methods of communication, elements that influence and interfere with communication, and professional communication with others.

Communication can be *positive* or *negative* (Figures 4-2 and 4-3). When you are attentive, encouraging, friendly, and show concern, you are demonstrating a positive attitude. Acting bored, avoiding eye contact, being impatient, finishing another person's sentences, forgetting common courtesies,

---

*Mehrabian, A. (1981). *Silent Messages: Implicit Communication of Emotions and Attitudes* (2nd ed.). Belmont, California: Wadsworth.

EXAMPLE 4-1

Positive versus Negative Communicators

Use Your Eyes, Ears, Hearts, and Minds to Be Receptive

Poor communicators focus on themselves—their own thoughts, feelings, experiences, and ideas.

Good communicators focus on others, paying attention to everything the other person is trying to communicate.

Poor communicators speak their part and think that the communication is finished.

Good communicators know that what they have said is only the beginning of the communication cycle.

interrupting, mumbling, rushing, speaking sharply, and even doing two things at the same time when trying to communicate are received as negative communication. Observe other service industry professionals, such as a waitress in a restaurant, a clerk in a store, or a teller at the bank to assess whether they have a positive or negative communication style (Example 4-1).

Take charge of your communication style, because it is a part of almost everything you do. It may be intentional, accidental, or even involuntary, but you

EXAMPLE 4-2

We Communicate to:

achieve credibility	greet	motivate
pass the time	abuse	help
improve self-esteem	complain	reassure
earn respect	inform	socialize
form friendships	learn	survive

cannot help communicating. You can, however, choose the way in which you would like to communicate; your choice will affect you and your career path (Example 4-2).

Elements and Goals of Communication

As a health care worker, communication will take on many forms. Talking on the telephone, composing office memos or letters, sending messages by computer or facsimile machine, texting, and interacting on Facebook and Twitter are all ways of communicating. The most productive communication takes place in face-to-face conversations. For example, if you are trying to collect on an account, you can send a statement or call the patient, but if the patient comes into the office you have the best chance of collecting by having a conversation with the patient. Also, if you are trying to convey to the patient the risks of a surgical procedure, you can give the patient an information pamphlet; however, if you sit down and outline the risks of the procedure and allow time for questions, you will have a much better chance of being sure the patient is fully informed.

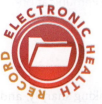

Physicians and medical assistants need to remain patient centered while using electronic health records. Although EHRs assist face-to-face communication by supplying immediate access to patient information, sometimes it is a distraction during visits.

Obtaining Information

As a health care professional, much of the communication you will be involved in will be centered on gathering information. You will use informal interviewing techniques, and your goal will be to obtain accurate data that can be used by the physician and all of the professionals in your office. Information can be subjective or objective. **Subjective information** exists in the mind but cannot be measured; it is affected by personal views, moods, attitudes, opinions, experience, and background. In health care, the patient's symptoms are referred to as subjective information and should be documented exactly as expressed by the patient. For example, a headache, pain, nausea, and fatigue are all subjective symptoms that vary from person to person according to the above. They may also vary within the individual depending on the type of day he or she is having. **Objective information,** on the other hand, can be measured. Height, weight, blood pressure, pulse, respiration, swelling, vomiting, and a lump or bump are all examples of objective information.

You may be communicating to schedule an appointment in the most convenient and appropriate time frame, gather insurance information to process a claim efficiently, or transfer a call to the correct staff member. Regardless of what you are communicating, first consider the area of the office in which you will be speaking to the patient, and be sure it matches the type of information you will receive. For instance, always use a private area when obtaining confidential information. Also, you will want to organize your thoughts prior to speaking. Remember to introduce yourself, wear a name badge, and let the patient know why you are trying to obtain information. You should always document the patient's responses accurately.

Building Patient Relationships

When selecting a physician, patients often ask, "Will the doctor take time with me, speak to me in a way that I can understand, and treat me with respect?" Have you ever heard someone say that they changed physicians because they could not stand the receptionist? Although patients do not often ask about the office staff, they expect the same respectful treatment from staff members as they do from the physician. Effective communication takes time and builds good relationships. Negative or poor communication damages relationships because it causes defensive reactions, misunderstandings, and a breakdown of the communication cycle. In fact, failure to communicate is the number one reason for the failure of relationships.

As a medical assistant, your goal should be to present the physician and medical practice in a positive light and to establish rapport and maintain positive relationships with patients. How you present yourself communicates a message about who you are and the medical practice in which you work. As an administrative medical assistant, you can be the friendly voice, the face

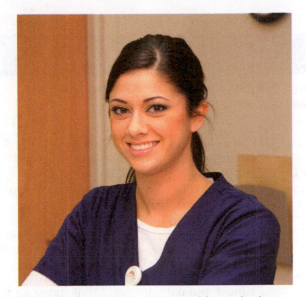

FIGURE 4-4 Smiling conveys a positive attitude

with the smile, or the helpful assistant to patients who are going through times of illness or distress (see Figure 4-4). Each patient is unique, so treat all patients individually and with respect. When you do so, they will respond positively.

Trust begins to develop between the physician and the patient long before the patient ever meets the physician—it begins with the relationship that is established upon first contact. This relationship between the patient and the health care professional is not equal. The power and control belongs to the person on the health care team, therefore it is important to try to equalize the relationship as much as possible. This is accomplished by showing concern and building an atmosphere of trust. Patients often open up to a medical assistant easier than to the physician. Even if a patient asks you to not tell the physician something, you should never withhold any information that relates to health care. Encourage patients to talk to the physician freely and openly, reminding them that all things discussed are confidential.

Generally, people do not feel in control while being examined by a physician, especially when they have an illness. They often must do things they do not want to do in order to get well. It is not uncommon for patients to become impatient, and they want the physician to help them get better immediately, so they can get on with their lives with minimal interruption of their normal routine. Patients may feel guilty and think that even though the illness is out of their control, they could have done something different to avoid it. All of this may make people become anxious, and in order to cope

they behave in a **defensive** manner. Defensive behavior is usually unconscious and is a response designed to protect oneself from a perceived threat. The threat may stem from anxiety, guilt, loss of self-esteem, or an injured ego. Understanding defense mechanisms will help you cope with patients who use them. They may become **noncompliant** and refuse to follow the doctor's treatment plan. Refer to Table 4-1 for a brief description of the various types of defense mechanisms and examples that apply to the physician's office.

Maslow's Hierarchy of Needs

An American psychologist, Abraham Maslow, studied human behavior and developed a theory that states people are motivated by needs and that their basic needs must be met before they can progress to fulfill other needs. Maslow's hierarchy pyramid (Figure 4-5) groups human needs into five levels. Basic needs are at the bottom of the pyramid, and it progresses to higher needs at each tier. The importance of understanding this concept is to be able to apply it to patients' needs. Health care professionals must realize that patients must fulfill their basic needs before expecting them to actually take on responsibility for their own health care. That ability is obtained only through self-actualization, the highest level of the pyramid. Following are brief descriptions of the various levels of needs.

Physiological Needs—Basic needs, or survival needs that include water, air, sleep, hygiene, and sexual activity, fall into the physiological need category and must be met before a patient can move on to consider other types of needs. Physiological needs can control thoughts and behaviors, and if not met, people can feel sick and uncomfortable. Each person has a different

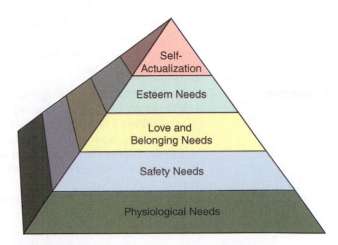

FIGURE 4-5 Maslow's hierarchy of needs

TABLE 4-1 Types of Defense Mechanisms

Type of Defense Mechanism	Description	Example
Apathy	Demonstrating disinterest or indifference to what is happening. The patient may appear to have a lack of emotion or feeling and display a flippant attitude.	"Who cares what the diagnosis is, we're all going to die sometime."
Aggression	Belligerent, combative attitude, such as lashing out by verbally attacking in order to avoid or diminish their role in wrongdoing.	A patient arrives late for an appointment and the waiting room is full. The medical assistant calls the patient from the waiting room and says, "Would you like to come with me to the treatment room?" The patient responds, "Does the physician think we are all puppy dogs, at his beck and call?"
Avoidance	Not seeing someone or not going to a place that evokes bad memories or pain.	After a physician diagnoses a patient with cancer, the patient says, "I will never go to that doctor again because he gave me cancer."
Compensation	Consciously or unconsciously overemphasizing something to make up for a real or imagined deficiency. This is also known as substituting a strength for a weakness and may be considered healthy in some cases.	"I know I haven't stopped smoking, Dr. Practon, but I have lost five pounds."
Denial	Refusing to accept painful information or an unpleasant situation; disbelieving reality. It is often the first response after a traumatic event.	A patient is told that she has pancreatic cancer and has only 3 months to live. The person or a family member hears what the physician says but goes about her business as if she was never told about the serious disease and that she is going to die. A loved one's response may be, "My wife can't have cancer, she plays tennis three times a week, eats a healthy diet, and gets a checkup every year."
Displacement	Unconscious transfer or redirection of unacceptable emotions, feelings, or thoughts from self to someone or something else. Channeling negative feelings to an unrelated area in order to feel a sense of control in situations that are not controllable.	A patient who is upset with the physician makes a rude remark to the receptionist on the way out of the office.
Projection	Taking unacceptable desires, thoughts, or impulses and falsely attributing them to others instead of admitting that they are connected to how the person feels. This defense mechanism comes out when people have feelings or urges that they do not want to admit they are experiencing. This is a sign of mental illness.	A child is fussing during an examination, and the father, who has been abusing this child, accuses the health care professional of being rough with the child in order to hide his feelings of wanting to hit the child.

(continues)

TABLE 4-1 Types of Defense Mechanisms (*continued*)

Type of Defense Mechanism	Description	Example
Rationalization	Making up a reason to justify unacceptable actions, behavior, or events. This is sometimes done to avoid obeying instructions or because the person knows that he or she is wrong and wants to avoid embarrassment or guilt. The reason used is usually a stretch of the truth; most people rationalize to some extent.	The patient tells the physician that he did not get his blood drawn as ordered because the line was too long and he did not have time to wait. Of course, he could have made an appointment and avoided the wait.
Regression	Withdrawing from an unpleasant circumstance by reverting to an earlier, more secure time in life either mentally or behaviorally. Usually this is done when a person feels desperate and powerless over whatever is causing the pain.	A 4-year-old reverts to baby talk after the arrival of a new baby sister.
Repression	An unconscious reaction in which the person seems to experience amnesia in order to block the problem from the mind. It could manifest as forgetfulness and is the mind's way of defending against mental trauma. This is not the same as outright lying. Severe cases may be associated with mental illness.	A rape victim unconsciously forgets to tell her parents that the reason she cannot go to a movie is because she was leaving a movie theater when the rapist followed her.
Sarcasm	Speaking with a sharp edge; usually intended to cause pain or anger. Sometimes it is used for humor, but it is not always amusing.	The medical assistant comments on how good the patient looks. The patient, who is not feeling well, responds, "I guess I'll go to my grave looking great." Or children have been left in the waiting room and made a mess, and a medical assistant comments sarcastically, "I hope your children enjoyed destroying the waiting room."
Undoing	Actions taken to cancel or make up for inappropriate behavior.	Mrs. Clark brings the physician a gift, because the last time she was in the office she was very rude and spoke unkind words.

point of view regarding the satisfaction of these basic needs that may arise from his or her background or upbringing. One person may think he needs three square meals per day, while another has only a cup of coffee in the morning and soup in the afternoon. These are individual perceptions and should be accepted, not judged. Once these needs have been satisfied, the body recognizes a state of balance (*homeostasis*), and our minds are freed to think about other things.

Safety Needs—Once the physiological needs have been met, the need for safety will emerge. These needs include having a safe environment, feeling secure, and living without fear or anxiety. Patients who are injured or facing a battle with disease are often anxious and fearful. They may become preoccupied with thoughts of dying and no longer feel safe. Safety also has to do with law, order, structure, and feeling protected.

Love and Belonging Needs—After physiological and safety needs have been met, social needs emerge. This involves emotionally based relationships such as feelings of belonging and being connected to our roots, friends, family, neighborhood, and so forth. To give and be shown affection and love are essential elements, and in the absence of these people feel lonely and/or depressed.

Esteem Needs—Maslow describes self-esteem as the need for respect from others (recognition, acceptance, status, appreciation) and the need for self-respect. People need to engage in activities that give a sense of contribution and self-value. The less self-assured we are, the less likely we are to place importance on our own health, and elements such as inferiority complexes, an inflated sense of self-importance, or snobbishness can occur.

Self-Actualization Needs—The highest level of need is that of self-actualization, or a person reaching his or her potential by making the most of unique abilities. At this level, people are free to be creative, spontaneous, interested, and objective, and they have a general appreciation of life. Patients who reach this level strive to control their state of wellness and are involved in their health care decisions. All other basic needs must be satisfied before one can reach this level.

Erikson's Human Development Life Cycle

Erik Erikson, a German psychiatrist, was the first child analyst in the United Sates and developed a theory involving eight different stages in which a healthy developing human should pass through from infancy to end-of-life. Each stage is characterized by a psychosocial crisis of two conflicting forces, as well as demands put on the individual by parents and/or society. If an individual successfully reconciles these forces, he or she emerges favorably from the stage with the corresponding virtue (see Table 4-2). Each stage builds on the proceeding stage and paves the way for subsequent stages and healthy growth.

PATIENT EDUCATION

Sensitive Medical Assistant

It is important to realize where on Maslow's hierarchy pyramid patients are so that you can understand how to help educate and communicate with them effectively. We all do not start at the bottom of the pyramid, and we all do not reach the top. Sometimes circumstances cause us to go up a level but slide back down. Encourage patients to verbalize their concerns and ask questions. Listen carefully and be sensitive to where they are in life's circumstances.

METHODS OF COMMUNICATION

In this section, we look at the two parties involved in the communication cycle—the sender and the receiver. How does the sender get his or her message across? Does he or she use verbal or nonverbal communication channels? How does the recipient receive the intended information?

Verbal Communication

Verbal communication involves the use of language or spoken words to transmit messages. This is the most common form of communication, and as we talk and listen throughout the day we are sending and receiving oral messages. Select your words carefully and be aware of the power behind them. Each of us can remember a time when our feelings were hurt due to unkind words or thoughtless remarks. The meaning of some spoken words can vary depending on the settings in which they are spoken. **Perceptions**, cultural or ethic backgrounds, and a variety of other factors also impact the meanings of some words. Perceptions are based on awareness or assumptions that people make and on their point of view as they discern what is being said. Proper English, grammar, and medical terminology are necessary to communicate succinctly, accurately, and professionally. Speak clearly and **enunciate** (pronounce) words properly. Do not use **colloquialisms**, which are slang or informal words such as "you know" or "gonna," or phrases such as "I'm fixin' to get your chart." To avoid misconceptions or miscommunications, be sure that the words used match the voice tone and body language communicated. In other words, say what you mean clearly and use positive body language that is nonthreatening and presents a professional, compassionate tone.

Communicate according to the patient's level of education and understanding. For example, when speaking to a physician or other health care professional about a referral, it would be proper to use medical terms; however, when speaking to the patient who is being referred you may need to use nontechnical language (*layman's terms*) instead.

Voice Tone

Voice tone is very important. The pitch, quality, and range within which you speak determine the overall tone. Voice tone and other nonlanguage sounds such as laughing, sobbing, sighing, and grunting often provide more information than words themselves. Remember

TABLE 4-2 Erikson's Human Development Life Cycle

Stage	Age	Virtues and Conflicting Forces	Development Theory
1	Birth to 1 year (infancy)	Trust versus Mistrust	Experiences familiarity with surroundings and develops the ability to distinguish between trust and mistrust
2	1 to 3 years (early childhood)	Autonomy versus Shame and Doubt	Explores the environment and develops independence (autonomy) and a sense of self-control; shame about self-consciousness and doubt about abilities occur as rules are encountered
3	3 to 6 years (play age)	Initiative versus Guilt	Begins to discover what kind of person he or she is going to be and develops a sense of responsibility, which increases initiative; guilt is compensated by a sense of accomplishment
4	5 to 12 years (school age)	Industry versus Inferiority	Desires to enter the larger world and interact with more people as he or she enters school and is exposed to technology and society; successful experiences give the child a sense of competence while failure gives a sense of inadequacy and inferiority
5	9 to 18 years (adolescence)	Identity versus Confusion	Seeks to discover who they are and how they appear to others as identity concern reaches a climax
6	18 to 40 years (young adult)	Intimacy versus Isolation	Cultivates intimacy with others if a reasonable identity emerges from stage five, otherwise isolation occurs leading to severe character problems
7	30 to 65 years (adulthood)	Generosity versus Stagnation	Develops generosity and socially valued work that contributes to the next generation and leads to a useful life; if nothing is accomplished, then stagnation occurs
8	50+ older (mature age)	Integrity versus Despair	Looks back and evaluates life; if previous stages have developed properly, then development is primarily qualitative; loss of self-sufficiency and love among partners leads to despair

the old saying, "It's not *what* you say, but *how* you say it." The way the message is delivered affects the way it is received.

The speaker's articulation, pronunciation, and grammatical structure also offer nonlanguage clues to understanding, and can vary from region to region and can indicate the person's level of education and cultural background.

Nonverbal Communication

Nonverbal communication is the sending of a message without words. It is important for us to be aware of what we communicate nonverbally. Body movements, also called nonverbal communication, accompany oral messages and are commonly referred to as **body language**. These movements are sometimes unconscious and

unintentional, or they can be natural responses to the way we feel. Nonverbal communication begins in infancy, prior to speech development. We realize this when we watch how a baby communicates. Some motions and gestures are instinctive while others may be imitated or taught. The culture in which a person is raised and the home environment greatly influence body language.

A boss's head-nod typically indicates approval. But such things as eye contact, facial movement, gestures, posture, touch, mannerisms, position, stance, gait, and attention to personal space are all nonverbal signals that can send specific messages (Figure 4-6). These expressions can be used by the medical assistant to set a professional but compassionate tone, and they can be "read" in order to better understand what patients are trying to communicate verbally. When communicating, maintain an open, relaxed body posture. See how the

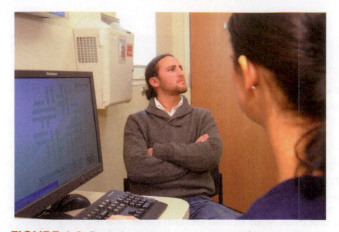

FIGURE 4-6 Body language can communicate more than spoken words

person is receiving the message by noticing his or her facial expressions. Following are various parts of the body and some messages that may be communicated while using them.

- *Eyes*—It is often said that the eyes are the window to a person's soul. What does that mean? The expression of anxiety, happiness, grief, joy, sorrow, and worry is reflected through the eyes. The eyes may also show interest or disinterest. Downcast eyes may indicate that you are not interested or that you are trying to avoid the person speaking; it can also be a sign of submission or avoidance. An eye-wink can communicate that you are kidding and not serious. Note that these interpretations are typical in Western culture and that other cultures may not view eye contact in the same way.
- *Mouth*—The mouth can be used to offer a smile, opened wide in surprise, puckered to show dissatisfaction, or it can be set in a firm grimace to indicate impatience or anger.
- *Face*—The face is the most expressive part of the body. Laugh lines around the eyes, worry lines in the forehead, or an inquisitive eyebrow all help to convey nonverbal clues.
- *Gait*—Walking briskly can mean the person is in a hurry or energized; it also demonstrates confidence. Walking slowly suggests fatigue or demonstrates a laid-back attitude. Problems with the gait, such as stiffness or limping, can be signs of illness or injury.
- *Gestures*—Gestures are used to enhance storytelling, add drama, or clarify the size and shape of objects. Avoid informal gestures such as a

clenched fist, fingers pointing upward to indicate victory, or even pointing, because these can be misinterpreted.

- *Hands*—Hands may be offered as a greeting (e.g., handshake) used to demonstrate size or to make a gesture to emphasize something said. Fingers may be used to point, to indicate that all is "OK," or to snap to get someone's attention. Be aware that pointing a finger can be interpreted as very rude and "OK" signs are considered obscene in some cultures. Other mannerisms such as doodling, tapping the finger, wringing of hands, and so forth may be interpreted as indications of wandering thoughts, boredom, or anxiety. A military salute typically says "Yes, sir" or "You have my attention" without any spoken words.
- *Posture*—How people hold themselves may be a sign of how a message is being received or how someone is feeling. Shoulders held back with head held high indicates confidence, whereas slumped shoulders and head held down indicates tiredness or defeat. Shrugging shoulders often means "I don't know." Arms crossed over the chest may indicate a closed demeanor.
- *Touch*—Touch is perceived in different ways among different cultures, but in America a light touch on the arm, shoulder, or back usually communicates interest or concern and can be beneficial to some patients. Like words, touch is a powerful tool and can indicate emotional support. Being touched by a stranger can have a negative effect and can make some patients uncomfortable, while hugging is usually reserved for close relationships. Reading the patient's demeanor is important when assessing a patient's response to touch. To evaluate patients' **demeanor**, notice how they appear, what their expressions are, and try to read their body language. Learn about other cultures common to your medical practice and be sensitive to their perception of touch.*

Double Messages

Patients may say one thing but show a completely different response with their body language; this is referred to as a double message. For example, a patient might say, "I'd like the doctor to check my foot but it really isn't that bad"; however, her face is grimacing in pain with each step she

---

*To read more about cultural gestures, refer to the Resource Section at the end of this chapter.

takes. In this case, the nonverbal clues demonstrate an inconsistent message. Patients may hide their feelings, so you need to read the nonverbal clues in addition to listening to what they tell you. As a rule, when the words spoken and the body language do not match, the body language usually depicts the true feelings of the person and his or her emotional state.

The Comfort Zone

The type of communication and the distance between two people communicating vary depending on how emotionally involved they are. For instance, a husband and wife communicate more intimately than two friends and would be comfortable standing or sitting very close to one another. When conversing in a health care setting, the appropriate space, or "comfort zone," is usually about an arm's length, or 3 to 4 feet. This professional distance is not to be invaded and varies with individuals, circumstances, and cultures. Be aware of where patients physically place themselves in relation to others. This can be another nonverbal clue and can affect the communication process.

In a medical office, it may be necessary to enter a patient's personal space, especially when delivering care. Using a professional manner, explaining what is being done, and being sensitive to patients' reactions are important when you have to work in close proximity. If you notice a patient or coworker sitting back in the chair or stepping back, you may have invaded his or her *territorial boundary*. Personal boundaries will vary among different people and cultures, so be respectful and ask if you are unsure. For example, "Would you like to take my arm for support while I escort you to the physician's office?" is a simple way to establish a patient's sense of personal space.

Also keep a professional distance, so you can be objective. Do not become too personally involved with patients and resist the temptation to tell patients intimate information about yourself, such as financial troubles or marital problems. Do not compare or offer reassurance by telling patients about similar health care situations you or your family may have experienced. For instance, "My husband has diabetes and is doing fine." The patient may misread your intentions and think that their diagnosis of diabetes is not very important, but to them it is.

The Receiver

When preparing to convey a message, consider the timing so that you have the best possible chance of having your message received accurately. The receiver is not always receptive and communication can be hampered if you try to send a message regardless of the receiver's mood or circumstances. For instance, if you want to talk to the physician about a raise but there is an office emergency, it would be best to wait until another time. Or if you have been meaning to talk to your supervisor about a problem with a coworker but this is her first day back from vacation, select another day. To receive a message clearly, you must be a good listener, respond to body language, and maintain eye contact.

Active Listening

Listening is not the same as hearing. In an office setting, we hear many sounds throughout the day—the copy machine running, the phone ringing, traffic outside—but we do not listen to them. We filter out these sounds and can do the same thing when someone is speaking. A wandering mind, due to anxiety or boredom, causes inattention or imprecise listening as you hear roughly what the person says but do not get the details of the message. The person who talks all the time or the one who appears to be listening but is not does not really want to understand the message that the other person is expressing.

Active listening involves being patient while the message is spoken and giving the speaker your undivided attention (Figure 4-7). We all want to feel that we

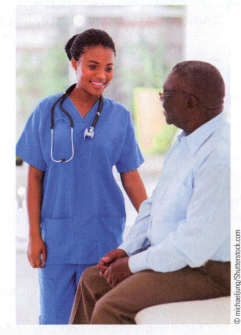

FIGURE 4-7 Active listening means giving your undivided attention to your patients

are listened to—it makes us feel understood, validated, and safe. Focus on the person with whom you are speaking and concentrate on the message being relayed. Do not think about anything else or let your mind wander. As the speaker talks, responses will come to mind, and it may be difficult to let go of the urge to respond immediately. However, that is exactly what you should do in order to continue listening actively. This practice is an exercise that moves your mental focus from yourself to the speaker. It should be practiced over and over; otherwise, you will continue to think about how you want to respond, and you will not be able to focus on what the speaker is saying. You must recognize your own attitudes and feelings so that you can put aside anything that may interfere with your ability to concentrate on the speaker's message.

Both active and **reflective listening** help you to hear the message precisely. To listen reflectively you need to dwell on, mull over, and even study or weigh what has been said. Listen not only to the words spoken, but notice the speaker's tone of voice and body language in order to receive the complete message. Be observant. When practicing active listening, try to keep interruptions to a minimum. Your response to interruptions is interpreted either positively or negatively by the other person (see Procedure 4-1).

Feedback

The oral or nonverbal response, referred to as **feedback**, is the best indicator of whether the message sent was the message received. As the speaker, the medical assistant should periodically verify that the person is receiving the message by being a careful observer and watching for body language as well as oral responses. Asking whether the patient understands does not always produce an honest answer. As the listener, the assistant should use feedback to verify that the message was heard correctly. Following are various techniques used to obtain feedback.

Repeating

Asking the patient to repeat back to you what was said can help verify that all the information was received. This echoing helps clarify feedback. You can prompt a patient to repeat the message by saying, "We have been talking for a while and I want to make sure you understand all of the instructions the physician has asked me to convey to you. Could you please tell me what you heard in your own words?"

Restatement or Paraphrasing

To ensure you have accurately heard what was said, you may want to restate or paraphrase the information

---

PROCEDURE 4-1

Demonstrate Active Listening by Following Guidelines

OBJECTIVE: Practice active listening to develop better listening skills.

EQUIPMENT/SUPPLIES: Two people in conversation.

DIRECTIONS: Follow these step-by-step directions when someone else is speaking to learn to listen actively and attentively.

1. Prepare yourself by leaning forward in your chair or tilting your head so that you can receive all that is said.

2. Give your full attention to the speaker. Do not pretend to listen.

3. Maintain eye contact and be sensitive to the other person's personal space.

4. Notice facial expressions, posture, and other signs of body language.

5. Remove all distractions, do not look at other things in the room, try to hear other conversations, or think about other tasks you have to accomplish.

6. Offer vocal responses, for example "mm-hmm" or "I understand," or an occasional nod to let the speaker know you are listening but do not talk over or interrupt the speaker.

7. Think before you respond and consider the other person's viewpoint.

8. Offer feedback so that the sender knows you have received the message.

9. Ask questions or have the sender repeat the message if it is not understood.

received. Use your own words or phrases and begin with statements such as "I understood you to say that ..." or "You are saying that...." Paraphrasing tells the patient that you have listened and helps clarify what was said.

Requesting Examples

Requesting examples may help clarify information being communicated. For instance, if the doctor referred a patient and she starts describing a rude receptionist at the specialist's office, ask the patient to give you an example of what happened. The patient's example should give you an insight into how the patient perceives the situation and help you better understand exactly what she is saying.

Questioning

Asking good questions is the key to receiving accurate information. Closed-ended questions that frequently begin with the words *did* or *do* often result in a "yes" or "no" answer and should be avoided when you are trying to gather information. Such questions can be used for obtaining specific information, such as a checklist on a history form that asks whether the patient has ever had a disease (Example 4-3).

When trying to encourage the patient to open up and talk, ask **open-ended questions,** also referred to as *exploratory questions,* that allow the patient to formulate a response and elaborate if necessary. Questions that begin with *what*, *when,* or *how* or with phrases such as *tell me about*, *describe to me,* or *explain to me* are considered open ended because they allow you to bring forth information from patients without making them feel as though they are being cross-examined.

EXAMPLE 4-3

Open- versus Closed-Ended Questions

Open: What is the name of the physician referring you?

Closed: Were you referred by a physician?

Open: When did the doctor say you need to be seen?

Closed: Did the doctor say you need to be seen today?

Open: How do you want to take care of the bill?

Closed: Will you be paying for the bill?

EXAMPLE 4-4

Avoid "Why" Questions

No: Why are you calling?

Yes: What may I help you with today?

No: Why are you upset?

Yes: Please describe what has upset you.

No: Why don't you call back later?

Yes: Please call back this afternoon.

For example, "Please describe the type of pain you are having." It is a nonthreatening way to gather additional information.

Questions that begin with *why* should be avoided because they often sound judgmental or harsh and cause people to respond defensively. The patient may feel like he or she is being accused of something, and it may incite a negative response (Example 4-4).

Summarizing

Stating a brief summary of the information you have obtained helps give the patient a chance to clarify and correct misinformation. Use this review technique when given lots of detail or a confusing message. For instance, if the patient states that he has come in to get a flu shot, but he is sick with a cold, and he then elaborates on all of his symptoms, and then says that he also has an open sore that he is worried about on his foot, review what he has said in words, such as "I understand that you wanted to get a flu shot today, but since you have a cold you would like to be seen for the cold, and also have the doctor take a look at the open sore on your foot." Leave time for the patient to respond and correct any misinformation. Highlight main points and use this technique to transition to a new topic.

The Silent Pause

People are often uncomfortable with periods of silence during conversation, but they can be very beneficial. Controlled silence is a well-placed pause that can be used to get someone's attention, emphasize a message, reiterate or restate thoughts, add additional information, put events in sequence, state feelings, or take the conversation in a different direction. Do not allow silent pauses to be filled with chatter or let the conversation wander. Instead, use this time wisely to gather your thoughts and formulate additional questions. Remember the power of well-placed silence—it can be an effective exclamation mark or speak louder than a raised voice.

ELEMENTS THAT INFLUENCE AND INTERFERE WITH COMMUNICATION

A number of elements can affect, interfere with, or make communication more difficult. Consider the personality type and conversational style of the person you are communicating with. Realize that a person's emotions come from within and reflect mental states such as anger, anxiety, confusion, depression, fatigue, fear, nervousness, pain, sadness, and so forth that can interfere with communication. You may have to adapt your communication style to get your message across.

Try to stay neutral instead of agreeing or disagreeing with the patient's thoughts, ideas, or perceptions. By doing this, the patient cannot conclude that you think he or she is right or wrong and will understand that he or she is allowed to have personal opinions and conclusions. If you vocalize that you share the same opinion, patients may think that you agree with them, and therefore they are right. Also, if you share that you do not agree with them, they may perceive this as disapproval and then think of you as the opposition instead of someone who is trying to help them. By neither agreeing nor disagreeing, you prevent displaying a moralistic attitude that implies a particular judgment about the patient. Regardless of the communication difficulty, imagine the trip to the physician's office through the eyes of the patient and then take the necessary steps to improve that experience. Refer to Table 4-3 for a list of things to avoid when communicating.

Environmental Elements

Outside interference can also cause difficulty in communication. Noise, visual stimuli, and touch can be distractions and can cause your concentration to wander. Distractions can come from sounds within the room, such as the conversations of others, or sounds outside the building, like the gardener operating a leaf-blowing machine. It could also be someone sighing, giggling, or coughing; someone looking at a watch,

rolling his eyes, or closing his eyes; someone grabbing you, hugging you, or bumping into you; or being uncomfortable with people who are in close proximity. Temperature deviations (being too hot or too cold) can be disturbing and affect your ability to focus. Also, being preoccupied, uncomfortable because of a poor sitting arrangement, or embarrassed because you feel half exposed in a gown can all be barriers to the communication process.

Gender

Gender is probably one of the first things noticed about a person. Although generalizations about men and women should not be relied on, they should be considered. Men, for instance, often do not show their feelings and have a hard time admitting to disease and illness. Thus, they come to the physician less frequently and may not be open to admitting they have pain. Women, on the other hand, usually feel free to describe their illness and are often more in tune with their bodies. When it comes to describing intimate details about their health, however, both genders feel more comfortable with a member of the same sex. This wish should be honored if at all possible. If it cannot be honored, the issue should be discussed with the physician and the patient. Try to make the patient feel as comfortable as possible.

People declaring alternative lifestyles such as homosexuality, bisexuality, or transgender orientation should be allowed to voice their concerns with the physician and not be discriminated against. They especially need to feel safe and know that confidentiality is a mandatory requirement of all medical staff.

Age

Age is always a factor to consider when communicating. Infants, toddlers, little children, adolescents, teenagers, young adults, middle-aged persons, and older adults are all in different stages of development. Their age, life experiences, and the phase of life that they are going through affect their communication styles and abilities.

Children

When going to a physician's office, children will often base their opinions on their past experiences and what they have been told by their parents. These beliefs will vary greatly and affect the communication process.

TABLE 4-3 Things to Avoid When Communicating

Things to Avoid	Reasons
• Do not advise patients about their health care or other situation.	• This could be construed as practicing medicine without a license.
• Never belittle patients or the feelings they have.	• This reflects judgment on your part and minimizes their situation or the pain they are feeling. All feelings are justified and it should never be insinuated that they are not important.
• Do not challenge patients.	• This makes them feel as though they have to prove what they have said is true.
• Do not change the subject if you become uncomfortable with patients who are conveying their feelings.	• Instead, acknowledge their feelings. For instance, if a patient presents at the window and says, "I could hardly get up today I am so depressed," do not just ask them to sign in and have a seat. Instead, address them as best you can by saying something like "I'm sorry you are feeling so down; hopefully the doctor can help you with this."
• Do not take a defensive attitude.	• This may make patients feel as though they must defend themselves.
• Be careful about reassuring or giving approval.	• When you reassure patients, they may believe that there is no need for the anxiety or pain they are feeling; instead demonstrate empathy.
• Do not jump to conclusions.	• This happens when you have preconceived ideas or you have your mind made up and can lead to misunderstandings and miscommunication.
• Do not advise patients starting with such words as: a. **I want you to** drink less soda. b. **You have to** take your medications as prescribed. c. **You need to** get more exercise. d. **You shouldn't** eat so much fast food. e. **Why don't you** stop smoking; it's the worst thing you can do for your heath.	• These words come across as harsh demands; it is much better to start sentences with words such as: a. **You might consider** drinking less soda. b. **What we've noticed** is that patients who do not take their medications as prescribed experience increased health care issues and need to see the physician more frequently. c. **I encourage you to** get more exerciser. d. **You might** write down about how much fast food you consume in a week. e. **Research shows that** smoking is very harmful to your health.

A parent's reaction in a health care setting is often mimicked by children. If the parent is confident and trusting, the child will feel secure and open. If the parent is worried and fretful, the child will feel anxious. If a child associates the visit with being sick or getting a shot, he or she may become frightened and act out that fear in the physician's office. Do not dismiss these emotions; instead, recognize them and let them be expressed freely.

Always tailor your communication to the child's age and needs. Comprehension can vary greatly, and although a child may not understand what is said, he or she will likely respond to tone of voice, gestures, and facial expressions. Use such body language to calm the child's fears and make her feel at ease. A child needs to feel safe, so your goal should be to establish trust. Speak to the child directly and inform children of all ages, along with their parents, of what will happen during the appointment. This information and style of communicating will help correct erroneous preexisting ideas, clarify wandering thoughts of the unknown, and establish honesty. Procedure 4-2 will help facilitate communication with children.

PROCEDURE 4-2
Communicate with Children

OBJECTIVE: Practice techniques to help learn how to communicate effectively with children.

EQUIPMENT/SUPPLIES: An adult and a child (substitute role-play as needed).

DIRECTIONS: Follow these step-by-step directions to help facilitate communication with children. Job Skill 4-3 in the *Workbook* is presented to practice this skill.

1. Position yourself so that you can speak to children at eye level.

2. Speak with a soft, low-pitched voice.

3. Talk at a level they can understand and ask simple questions, rephrasing them when necessary until they are understood.

4. Allow the child to be involved—give him or her a clipboard and writing tool to use while the parent fills out the patient information form.

5. Offer a toy and use it or a puppet in a playful manner when asking questions. This can gain the child's attention and cooperation.

6. Recognize situations the child may be fearful of and allow each child to express fear and to cry.

7. Realize that a child may return to a lower developmental stage in order to receive comfort during an illness. For example, a child may revert to thumb sucking during a stressful event or start wetting the bed again because of fear.

PATIENT EDUCATION
Parent Pamphlets

Parents may not realize the anxieties a child may face when he or she is ill and must continually come to the physician's office or undergo frequent tests and procedures. The parents of a seriously ill child may not know how to deal with the situation. Written pamphlets are available to help them cope with a child's illness, understand the child's anxieties, and relate to the child's fears. Having pamphlets on display in the waiting room and offering them to parents will help educate them without judging their responses and actions.

Adolescents and Teenagers

Be receptive of all communication from adolescents and teenagers without being startled. If you express shock, they may assume you are judging them, which can close the channel of communication. Young people may request that their parents not come into the treatment room. Teenagers may be reluctant to divulge information or ask questions if someone else is present and should be given the opportunity to speak to the physician alone. Be sensitive to such requests and inform the physician so that he or she can assess the situation and decide if the parent should be included.

Older Adults

Senior patients have special needs, and older adults do not all communicate on the same level. Mental and physical changes such as impairment in memory or judgment may have resulted from illness, disease, or the aging process, and these changes may cause confusion or affect oral communication. Alzheimer's disease and senility are two common causes of impaired communication skills, although similar symptoms may be brought on by a head injury, depression, alcohol or drug abuse, and medication misuse. Always speak to older adults with respect, and expect them to comprehend on an adult level unless you have been advised differently. Do not speak down to them or patronize them. Recognize that they may need extra patience, assistance, and instruction or explanations. When senior patients are accompanied by a spouse, relative, or friend, always look directly at and speak to the patient, giving him or her a chance to respond and speak for himself or herself (Figure 4-8). If they are unresponsive, forgetful, or you are concerned about whether their recollection is accurate, ask the other adult if he or she has anything to add. Guidelines to follow when communicating with older adults are found in Procedure 4-3.

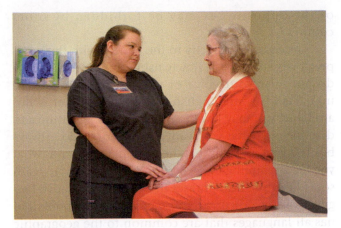

FIGURE 4-8 The medical assistant looks directly at the patient, communicating warmth, empathy, and concern

Economic Status

The medical assistant will interact with patients from different economic classes—both affluent and impoverished—which may lead to varied views regarding health care. The high cost of medicines, procedures, and hospitalizations continues to cause stress and worry among patients. Some individuals struggle to pay insurance premiums, deductibles, and copayments and for others their primary concerns may be the daily issues of survival. These factors should be considered when communicating with patients, and the health care professional should be aware of community assistance and government programs that they can refer patients to in such circumstances.

Wealthy patients and those in the upper middle class may not have to worry about financial problems. They are able to pay expensive premiums and use traditional fee-for-service options that offer more choices when selecting physicians and treatment alternatives. Thus, they are able to afford better insurance coverage. However, the economic status of patients, whether they are wealthy or poor, should not affect the way they are treated in the physician's office nor should it affect the way they are spoken to. All patients should be shown respect and common courtesy.

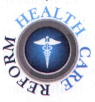

In the year 2011, community health centers received $11 billion in increased funding to provide medical care to patients who could not afford it. And, in the year 2014, uninsured individuals and small businesses were able to select a private health plan from a menu of choices offered through state-based insurance exchanges. Although the Health Care Reform bill constitutes the biggest expansion of federal health care in more than four decades, the Agency for Healthcare Research and Quality (AHRQ) found that high-quality health care varies according to patient income levels, the cities in which they live, and the states in which they reside.

PROCEDURE 4-3

Communicate with Older Adults

OBJECTIVE: Practice techniques to help learn how to communicate effectively with older adults.

EQUIPMENT/SUPPLIES: Medical assistant and older adult (substitute role-play as needed).

DIRECTIONS: Follow these step-by-step directions to help facilitate communication with older adults. Job Skill 4-4 in the *Workbook* is presented to practice this skill.

1. Avoid misconceptions and do not prejudge.
2. Speak clearly and slowly, offering simple explanations.
3. Form short sentences and ask brief questions.
4. Analyze communication, encouraging responses and feedback.
5. Rephrase statements or questions as necessary.
6. React calmly if the patient seems confused or forgetful.
7. Do not make excuses for patients or make up explanations as to why they seem confused.
8. Tell patients if you do not understand what they have said and ask them to repeat it.
9. Be gentle but honest and truthful in your communication, so you do not mislead patients or yourself.
10. Offer written instructions.

Language Barriers

As a health care professional, you will likely communicate with patients who do not speak English well enough to carry on a conversation. They may, however, understand or read English. Even patients who are usually proficient in English may feel more comfortable and revert to speaking their primary language during times of stress, such as illness or injury. First determine their level of fluency and, if necessary,* use a qualified health care interpreter who is professionally trained in translating medical terminology to layman's terms and who can communicate precisely in the patient's first language.

Whenever you have a non–English-speaking patient, an *interpreter* should be scheduled when the appointment is made to ensure that the patient will receive the best medical care. Workers' compensation provides professional interpreters, and physicians who treat Medicaid or State Children's Health Insurance Program (SCHIP) patients are required to create a plan for serving patients with limited English proficiency (LEP). The Department of Health and Human Services published guidelines that require physicians to consider four factors: (1) Number (or proportion) of patients with limited English proficiency, (2) frequency of encountering individuals with limited English proficiency, (3) importance of services provided, and (4) resources available. Staff members may be hired because they are bilingual, or telephone or video interpreting can be used, and patients may be referred to physicians with specific language capabilities. A member of the patient's family or a friend who speaks English may also be able to help; however, permission must be given by the patient, and it is important to make sure that both parties understand exactly what is being said. Some medical terms and phrases do not translate into other languages and difficulties arise when trying to communicate them accurately to a person who is not trained for this purpose.

Select an interpreter of the same sex because he or she will always be a part of personal discussions and will accompany the patient during the examination. Be aware that when discussing personal issues about the human body, interactions with members of the opposite sex may be forbidden by other cultures.

Always speak directly to the patient with the interpreter close by. Speak slowly using simple English and do not raise your voice or use slang. If the patient understands some English or if an interpreter is not available, you may have to improvise using gestures to demonstrate what you want the patient to do. Always be observant for signs that the patient understands what you are attempting to get across. You may want to learn some basic medical phrases in the patient's native language or use a dictionary or medical phrase book that has all languages that are common to the geographic region. Also, keep a notepad on hand to write down key words. Depending on the office's location, medical forms and patient information pamphlets in other languages should be made available. Bilingual classes, such as medical Spanish, are offered in many areas for health care professionals.

Cultural Differences

People move to the United States from all over the world and bring with them various cultural behaviors, traditions, and values that have been passed down through many generations. The United States was once called a melting pot because of its ethnic and cultural diversity, and the hope was that all of the diverse groups would blend together as a whole. The blending, however, does not mean ignoring heritage, and today more than ever, people are embracing their ethnic background and want to know more about where they came from. We have cultural differences that affect patterns of speech (accents), food preparation, beliefs, attitudes, and environments.

As a medical assistant you will interact with people from varied **ethnic** (racial) backgrounds and cultural origins who bring with them beliefs and values that may differ from your own; those beliefs and values are not superior or inferior. Keeping an open mind and understanding those differences can aid communication and thereby improve patient care. Be sensitive to the fact that an immigrant's health care needs may differ from native citizens' needs, as do their experiences and emotional makeup.

Variances within Cultures

The following list includes factors that the medical assistant should consider when shaping his or her communication with patients who have different cultural backgrounds.

---

*State guidelines vary and some states may mandate the use of professional interpreters for various federal or state-sponsored health plans (e.g., workers' compensation, Medicaid).

- Most Americans are familiar with, and believe in, Western medicine; however, other cultures practice Eastern medicine or holistic health, which has to do with treating the body, mind, and spirit. Some cultures believe in homeopathic treatment, folk remedies, medical rituals, or healing ceremonies. Others have superstitions that affect the way they look at disease, illness, and treatment.

- Personality trends vary among cultures. In some cultures, people tend to be forward or outgoing; in others, they are quiet and reserved.

- The philosophy on the use of medications and invasive tests or treatments may differ among cultures, as might views on pain and how people respond to it.

- Nonverbal signals, such as gestures and body language, may have different meanings from yours.

- Eye contact is very important in the American culture and indicates interest and involvement. In other cultures, such as Native American, Asian, and Latin, it may be considered disrespectful to look someone straight in the eyes. Trying to maintain eye contact with someone who is uncomfortable may be perceived as aggression and create a communication barrier.

- Although Americans may feel that touch is an important way to communicate the feeling of empathy, many adults do not like to be touched by people they do not know. A handshake is a sign of respect in some cultures, whereas touching is off-limits in others. Asian children's heads, for example, are considered sacred and should only be touched by a parent or elder in the family.

- Time may be viewed differently among people in general and especially among people from other cultures. For instance, in another culture, arriving 15 to 30 minutes after a scheduled appointment would be acceptable, but in the typical American medical office it would be deemed inconsiderate.

- Each person sees people and situations differently; this is referred to as perception. Cultural background, social upbringing, and religious beliefs influence perception as well as personal values, beliefs, and convictions. Latinos, for instance, value a warm, personal relationship with their health care provider, but they often also expect an authoritative manner and

professional dress from their physician. If the physician is dressed casually, trust may be harder to establish between the patient and the physician because casualness may be viewed as being carefree.

Since it is impossible to learn of all the variances in other cultures, the medical assistant should concentrate on whatever population the medical practice serves. If the health care worker practices active listening, exhibits empathy, is genuine, and treats patients in a professional manner with equal respect, misunderstandings caused by cross-cultural differences will be minimized. Trust will be established because patients' dignity will be preserved and their sense of self-worth maintained.

Stereotyping

Patients of different ages, cultures, genders, races, religions, lifestyles, and sexual orientation make up a medical practice, and their values may differ from yours. Judgments are often made when people are put into categories such as those mentioned above. Generalizations should not be made, and it should never be assumed that people from the same race or culture will respond in the same way. To **stereotype** is to hold an attitude that all people from the same ethnicity (or category) are the same; this should be avoided. Statements such as "Retired people always sleep in" and "Those people are lazy and don't work for a living" are types of negative stereotyping and demonstrate **prejudice**, a judgment that is formed prior to gathering all facts. Prejudice leads to **discrimination**, which means to treat an individual or group unfairly based on the category into which they fall. All patients should be viewed individually and treated equally. When you form a **bias**, your opinion is one sided and your judgment is negatively influenced.

Today's society holds biases that may include the belief that people who cannot afford health care should not receive the same level of care as people who can pay

---

✓ **COMPLIANCE**

Discrimination

Discrimination in the workplace because of race, color, national origin, religion, gender, age, handicap, or family status is illegal.

Civil Rights Act of 1964, Amended in 1972

for full services. The prejudices of our society should not affect the communication we have with patients or the type of health care we deliver. All patients should be treated impartially and all health care services provided equally. Guard against discrimination, avoid stereotyping, and do not jump to conclusions or make determinations about patients based on the differences mentioned.

Patients with Special Needs

Many patients seeking treatment in a health care setting have special needs. Being prepared to cope with those individual needs and disabilities is very important. When a person's understanding is limited or the senses are impaired, communication can be a challenge. People with physical and other types of disabilities can fall prey to discrimination: Eye contact can be avoided, staring can occur, rude remarks can be made, or an oversolicitous attitude can make the individual feel uncomfortable. Patients with disabilities prefer to be treated like other individuals. Never assume that a person with a disability needs help. Instead, ask the

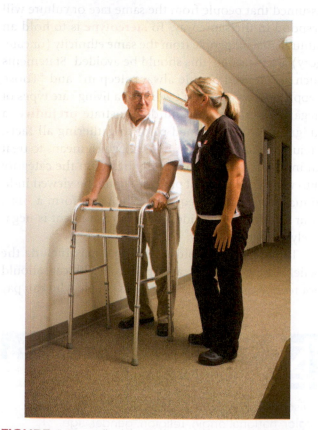

FIGURE 4-9 medical assistant asking a patient using a walker if he needs assistance

patient how you can be of help and follow his or her requests (Figure 4-9). Giving assistance without calling attention to a disability requires sensitivity and tact, and special consideration must be given in order to communicate effectively. The medical assistant can be empathetic toward a patient with special needs without offering gratuitous expressions of sympathy. The following sections offer guidance on communicating effectively with patients who have specific disabilities.

Hearing-Impaired Patients

There are many types of hearing impairments ranging from presbycusis, which is found in older patients who are hard of hearing, to congenital problems that can cause complete hearing loss at an early age. Exhibit diplomacy, patience, and tact when trying to communicate with patients who cannot hear what you are saying. If you have several hearing-impaired patients or are working for a large clinic, the use of an assistive listening device may be helpful. Guidelines to follow when communicating with hearing-impaired patients can be found in Procedure 4-4.

Visually Impaired Patients

When communicating with visually impaired patients, use verbal descriptions. Impaired eyesight may range from blurred vision to complete blindness and can include presbyopia, macular degeneration, cataracts, and glaucoma. If a patient loses his or her vision at an early age, other senses often take over. The patient may have more acute hearing, smell, and equilibrium, which give him or her the ability to quickly recognize sounds and voices and a sense of where he or she is after entering a foreign space. Patients who lose their sight later in life usually have a more difficult time adjusting. When communicating with a sight-impaired patient, follow the guidelines given in Procedure 4-5.

Speech-Impaired Patients

Speech impairments can be caused by medical conditions (e.g., traumatic brain injury, multiple sclerosis) or can result from congenital abnormalities. Stroke patients often have dysphasia or difficulty speaking. Usually they know exactly what they want to say, but may be unable to form the words they are trying to speak. Be patient and allow plenty of time to communicate without putting words in their mouths. A physical condition can leave a patient with dysphonia or voice

PROCEDURE 4-4

Communicate with Hearing-Impaired Patients

OBJECTIVE: Practice techniques to help learn how to communicate effectively with hearing-impaired patients.

EQUIPMENT/SUPPLIES: Medical assistant and hearing-impaired adult (substitute role-play as needed).

DIRECTIONS: Follow these step-by-step directions to help facilitate communication with hearing-impaired patients. Job Skill 4-6 in the *Workbook* is presented to practice this skill.

1. Select a quiet place to communicate and give the patient your complete attention.

2. Eliminate distractions or background noises such as traffic, running water, or office music that may disrupt the conversation or cause confusion.

3. Choose the best seating arrangement by determining whether the patient hears out of one ear better than the other, uses a hearing aid, or reads lips. Sit on the side of the person's good ear and reduce the distance between you and the patient. A hearing aid helps but does not restore normal hearing; optimal distance for a hearing aid's effectiveness is about 10 feet.

4. Face the patient in an area with good light so that he or she can see your facial expressions, but do not exaggerate them while speaking. Some patients may be able to lip read, so do not turn your head away from them, cover your mouth, or chew while talking.

5. Touch the patient lightly if necessary to gain his or her attention, or alert the patient by saying his or her name and then announcing the topic.

6. Speak in a natural tone, slowly, and distinctly, enunciating clearly and using a low-pitched voice; high-pitched sounds are often lost with auditory nerve damage. Do not over-pronounce, shout, or distort your speech.

7. If the patient speaks with an accent, select someone with a similar accent to speak with him or her. Trying to communicate with an accent that is different than the patient's can make communication more difficult.

8. Use short, simple sentences and repeat or rephrase any misunderstood statements.

9. Continue to speak directly to the patient if a sign language interpreter is present but wait for the message to be interpreted.

10. Use gestures as needed. Remember the importance of body language.

11. Write down words or phrases that you are having difficulty communicating using a spelling board or dry erase board.

12. Practice active listening techniques and obtain feedback by asking questions to verify understanding.

---

impairment. Also a lisp, stutter, or strong accent may cause a breakdown in communication. Procedure 4-6 offers suggestions for communicating with speech-impaired patients.

Impaired Level of Understanding

Individuals who are developmentally disabled, emotionally disturbed, have suffered acquired or traumatic brain injury, or are suffering from senility or Alzheimer's disease may have below-normal ability to think and reason. It is important to work closely with caregivers and to be aware of each patient's limitations. Offer assistance to each individual with dignity. Treat all such patients equally and give them the same respect and attention as other patients.

A patient's ability to communicate can be impaired by many types of diseases, brain injury, mental illnesses, mental retardation, or psychiatric disorders. Common problems that occur may include patients repeating themselves, not being able to communicate at all or at the appropriate level, sitting in silence, or having outbursts or using inappropriate language. Use the guidelines in Procedure 4-7 when communicating with patients who have an impaired level of understanding.

PROCEDURE 4-5

Communicate with Visually Impaired Patients

OBJECTIVE: Practice techniques to help learn how to communicate effectively with visually impaired patients.

EQUIPMENT/SUPPLIES: Medical assistant and visually impaired adult (substitute role-play as needed).

DIRECTIONS: Follow these step-by-step directions to help facilitate communication with visually impaired patients. Job Skill 4-7 in the *Workbook* is presented to practice this skill.

1. Approach the patient cheerfully and identify yourself by name when he or she enters the office.

2. Look directly at the patient and speak clearly in a normal tone and at a normal speed.

3. Inform the patient of others who are in the same room or area, for example, "Please have a seat in the waiting room, Mrs. Bartlett. There are a few other patients who are also waiting for Dr. Practon."

4. Let the patient know exactly what you will be doing. For example, "The medical assistant will be calling you shortly to take you to an exam room."

5. Ask the patient: "May I take your hand to show you the . . . counter, chair, doorframe, and so forth." This will help the patient become familiar with the surroundings.

6. Ask if the patient needs your assistance with filling out paperwork and comply with his or her wishes.

7. Escort the patient to the inner office or interview room by offering your arm or elbow (as directed by the patient) and helping to guide him or her. Look out for any obstacles that may be in the path. Provide verbal cues for turns, steps, and so forth, but do not steer the patient.

8. Inform the patient of the location, and tell him or her when you are leaving the room. Be sure to knock before reentering the room.

9. Explain the sounds of unusual noises or office machines that may be running nearby.

10. Use large-print material whenever possible or provide instructions on audiocassette.

PROCEDURE 4-6

Communicate with Speech-Impaired Patients

OBJECTIVE: Practice techniques to help learn how to communicate effectively with speech-impaired patients.

EQUIPMENT/SUPPLIES: Medical assistant and speech-impaired adult (substitute role-play as needed).

DIRECTIONS: Follow these step-step directions to help facilitate communication with speech-impaired patients. Job Skill 4-8 in the *Workbook* is presented to practice this skill.

1. Look directly at patients without making them feel self-conscious.

2. Allow patients time to think through what they are going to say and give them time to speak.

3. Do not speak for patients or rush the conversation; ask them to speak slowly.

4. Be sensitive to the circumstances and to the type of message being delivered.

5. Do not pretend to understand. Instead, say that you are having a little difficulty understanding, and ask them to repeat the statement.

6. Do not shout; people with speech difficulty are not hard of hearing.

7. Be courteous; rudeness is never acceptable.

8. Offer a notepad or message board if necessary.

PROCEDURE 4-7

Communicate with Patients Who Have an Impaired Level of Understanding

OBJECTIVE: Practice techniques to help learn how to communicate effectively with patients who have an impaired level of understanding.

EQUIPMENT/SUPPLIES: Medical assistant and adult with an impaired level of understanding (substitute role-play as needed).

DIRECTIONS: Follow these step-by-step directions to help facilitate communication with patients who have an impaired level of understanding. Job Skill 4-9 in the *Workbook* is presented to practice this skill.

1. Introduce yourself in a friendly manner.
2. Be professional and keep the conversation on a single subject and focused.
3. Speak slowly and in a calm manner.
4. Select simple words and short phrases using both verbal and nonverbal clues.
5. Use your tone of voice to express your concern; avoid letting impatience creep into your voice, because that implies the patient is slow to understand or is unintelligent. Do not raise your voice.
6. Repeat and rephrase the message you are trying to convey; it may be necessary to start over more than once.
7. Use demonstration when appropriate to reinforce the message.
8. Allow more time than usual because patients with impaired understanding may have short-term memory loss and need more explanation than is typical.
9. Reassure patients, and do not overload them with information.
10. Inform patients of what to expect prior to it happening.
11. Exhibit tolerance with patients who are withdrawn or mute; do not force answers.
12. Remind patients why they are at the physician's office and orient them to reality as appropriate.
13. Inform the supervisor or physician if you feel unsafe while trying to communicate.

Anxious Patients

Anxiety and anger impair communication. It is common for patients to be anxious when visiting a physician; this reaction is called the *white-coat syndrome.* When dealing with an anxious patient, realize that she may need help focusing and assume that she will not be able to remember all of the details of the conversation. Proceed at a slower pace and validate the patient's concern.

Severe anxiety may lead to an anxiety attack. Symptoms include increased heart rate (pulse rate), elevated blood pressure, diaphoresis (sweating), shaking or trembling, fast or uneven respirations, and hyperventilation. Patients may also complain of appetite changes, sleep disturbances, and being short tempered or irritable. If an anxiety attack occurs in the office, notify the physician and stay with the patient until the physician arrives. Try to calm anxious patients acknowledging that they are afraid and getting them to talk about their fears. Follow the guidelines listed in Procedure 4-8 when assisting anxious patients.

Angry Patients

Patients may enter the office angry or may become upset while in the office. The reason for the anger may be something completely unrelated to the office visit; this type of response is referred to as **displaced anger**. Or it may be caused by something that has occurred during waiting time or the visit. In either case, try to help the person identify the source and do not take it personally. Allow the patient to vent and do not let the patient's anger become contagious by responding with anger yourself. If the office has made an error, admit the mistake and apologize for it. Disarm anger by offering to help in any way you can. Do not argue—it will only add fuel to the fire. Instead, soften your response and avoid phrases that may ignite the situation (Example 4-5). If the person becomes loud, volatile, or threatening, take the patient aside or move to a private office. You may have to tell that person that he or she is acting inappropriately and that shouting will not be allowed because other patients are being disturbed.

PROCEDURE 4-8

Communicate with Anxious Patients

OBJECTIVE: Practice techniques to help learn how to communicate effectively with anxious patients.

EQUIPMENT/SUPPLIES: Medical assistant and anxious adult (substitute role-play as needed).

DIRECTIONS: Follow these step-by-step directions to help facilitate communication with anxious patients. Job Skill 4-10 in the *Workbook* is presented to practice this skill.

1. Recognize the signs of anxiety and acknowledge them.

2. Pinpoint possible sources of anxiety, such as fear of needles.

3. Make the patient as comfortable as possible and give him or her ample personal space.

4. Demonstrate a warm and caring attitude.

5. Speak with confidence, calmness, and empathy, asking the patient to describe what is causing his anxiety. Allow him or her to describe his or her feelings and thoughts.

6. Listen attentively without interruption, maintain eye contact, and have an open posture.

7. Accept the patient's thoughts and feelings; do not belittle them; demonstrate empathy.

8. Help the patient recognize the anxiety and cope with it by providing information and suggesting relaxation techniques such as visualization and deep breathing.

9. Inform the physician of the patient's concerns.

EXAMPLE 4-5

Soft Responses to Help Calm Patients

Responses That May Agitate	Soft Responses
"We cannot do that!"	"That's a difficult one, Mrs. Brown. Let's see what we can do."
"I don't know!"	"That's a good question, Mr. White. Let me check that out and get back to you."
"I'll be right back."	"Can you hold, Miss Gray, while I check on this? It may take me a couple of minutes."
"You'll have to …"	"Here is how we can help you with that, Mr. Gold.…"

Collect information and try to pinpoint the reason for the anger. Common reasons may include feelings of resentment due to an invasion of privacy, disappointment or frustration because of an illness or circumstances beyond their control, and financial problems. If patients cannot be accommodated in the appointment schedule and cannot see their physician

when they are sick and hurting, they may become frustrated. Oftentimes that frustration unravels into anger. Little things tend to agitate patients when they are feeling ill, and they may be angry about their own responses and lack of coping skills. Prolonged waiting times only aggravate these emotions. Emotional responses to physical situations are not uncommon, and otherwise calm patients might become distressed over confusing aspects of their illness or treatment. Follow the guidelines given in Procedure 4-9 when dealing with angry patients.

PROFESSIONAL COMMUNICATION

As a health care professional, you will communicate with patients; their family members and friends; other members of the health care team; your superiors, such as the office manager and physician; and other outside professionals, such as members of the hospital staff, pharmacies, and ancillary facilities. The following section will describe techniques and guidelines that can help you communicate professionally in an efficient, constructive, and productive manner.

PROCEDURE 4-9

Communicate with Angry Patients

OBJECTIVE: Practice techniques to help learn how to communicate effectively with angry patients.

EQUIPMENT/SUPPLIES: Medical assistant and angry adult (substitute role-play as needed).

DIRECTIONS: Follow these step-by-step directions to help facilitate communication with angry patients. Job Skill 4-11 in the *Workbook* is presented to practice this skill.

1. Recognize that the patient is angry. Most of the time this emotion is obvious, but some people may disguise it by seeming disinterested, ignoring your attempts to communicate, speaking in a monotone or unnatural voice, or avoiding eye contact.

2. Honor the patient's personal space, hold yourself with an open posture, maintain eye contact, and position yourself at the patient's eye level; do not stand over the patient.

3. Remain calm and show that you care about the patient's feelings by continuing to demonstrate genuineness, respect, and positive body language.

4. Focus on why the patient is there in order to uncover emotional, physical, and medical needs.

5. Listen attentively with an open mind and ask the patient to describe the cause of his or her anger and how it makes him or her feel. Let him or her vent openly. The patient has a right to his or her own feelings and perceptions; be empathetic.

6. Do not take a defensive attitude or try to talk the patient out of being angry by trying to rationalize the angry response.

7. Allow the patient time alone if he or she is so angry that it interferes with communication.

8. Determine a time frame to get back to the patient with an answer or solution.

9. Do not stay in the room with the patient if you feel threatened or are worried about the potential for violence. Leave the room and inform the physician or another staff member.

Patients and Their Family Members and Friends

In their research, psychologists have learned that the manner in which the medical staff interacts with a sick person can foster wellness or it can unintentionally aggravate a physical condition. They have also determined that preserving the patient's mental state is often more important than performing expert medical skills. The medical assistant should know how to create an atmosphere that will communicate a caring attitude toward the patient's feelings.

As a member of the health care team you, along with the physician, will be responsible for communicating details in order for patients to actively participate in their health care decisions. As an administrative medical assistant, you will gather information about the patient's demographics, insurance, and medical history, as well as organize referrals and tests, procedures, and follow-up examinations.

Family members and friends who accompany patients to the office can provide emotional support and offer another opportunity to understand and retain detailed instructions or specific information about the patient's illness and treatment plan. Acknowledge family members and friends who accompany patients to the office and communicate with them in the same way you do with patients (Figure 4-10).

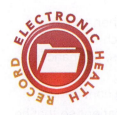

The dynamics of patient communication has changed with the implementation of the EHR. *Patient relationship-centered care (PRCC)* focuses on communication among patients, families, and physicians or other health care providers, which occurs moment-by-moment when encounters take place in and out of the examination room. There are few guidelines in how to optimize using the computer while building relationships; however, it has been determined that having good baseline communication

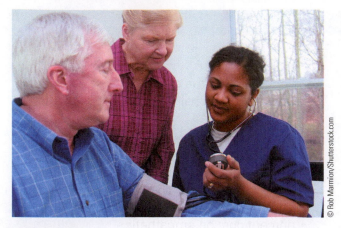

FIGURE 4-10 Communicate with family members and friends in the same way you communicate with patients

skills tends to integrate computing into relationships with patients.

Wherever an exchange is taking place with patients, being too focused on the EHR may cause missing important clues related to their diagnosis, treatment, and management. Each staff member must recognize that the EHR is not a neutral party, but instead often becomes a third-party participant in exchanges that take place. There is a need to be creative both in and out of the exam room to bridge this gap; for example, use the computer screen as a visual aid and share it with patients. By recognizing how you will use this tool to improve health care and communicate with patients, you will help fulfill the potential of the EHR in today's medical environment. Follow the guidelines in

PROCEDURE 4-10

Communicate with Patients and Their Family Members and Friends

OBJECTIVE: Practice techniques to help learn how to communicate effectively with patients and their families and friends.

EQUIPMENT/SUPPLIES: Medical assistant and another adult (substitute role-play as needed).

DIRECTIONS: Follow these step-by-step directions to help facilitate communication with patients and their families and friends. Job Skill 4-12 in the *Workbook is* presented to practice this skill.

1. Greet patients and their family members or friends with a warm smile and kindhearted words.

2. Introduce yourself and explain what you will be doing.

3. Use a genuine, friendly approach in all interactions whether verbal or nonverbal; respect the comfort zone.

4. Display a positive attitude when giving instructions or explaining such things as insurance delays, procedures, or financial statements.

5. Answer questions regarding confidentiality.

6. Focus on and speak to the patient so that he or she receives your undivided attention; instruct according to the patient's needs.

7. Listen carefully and allow time for questions.

8. Be aware how your personal appearance will affect the patient's response and demonstrate

confidence in the job you are doing so that the patient will know you are well trained and knowledgeable.

9. Be assertive and communicate succinctly and accurately, answer questions honestly, and admit when you do not know something. Tell the patient that you will find out the answers to his or her questions and follow through.

10. Keep the patient informed throughout the visit regardless of delays or interruptions.

11. Put the patient at ease by acknowledging any sources of anxiety or concern. Demonstrate sensitivity and empathy; do not minimize the patient's fears regardless of how trivial they may appear to you.

12. Obtain feedback to be sure that the message has been received correctly.

13. Reward the patient's compliance with the physician's treatment plan with praise. Health care professionals can offer support and guidance in things such as taking the correct medications, weight loss, smoking cessation, and so forth.

14. Do not let the EHR distract you from building a relationship with the patient; instead explain the positive aspects of having a computerized system and incorporate it into the visit, as necessary.

Procedure 4-10 when communicating with patients and their families and friends.

The Health Care Team

Communicating with coworkers can present some of the most difficult communication problems. Sometimes thoughtless comments are made or a *condescending attitude* (e.g., snobbish, patronizing) is displayed, which makes the other person feel inferior. Each person on a health care team is important and each job has value. Without all team members working together, a medical office would not run smoothly and the physician would not be able to treat all of the patients' needs successfully.

Communicate with each individual professionally, and do not talk down to anybody. Regardless of the job you are doing, always show respect and be caring and thoughtful in your actions and words while displaying empathy for the other person. Even a part-time file clerk

has an important job and is a vital part of the health care team. Offer words of appreciation to other members of the staff when you see that they are doing a good job.

Save lunchtime or breaks for discussion of non-work-related topics. An unprofessional atmosphere is created when whispers, excessive laughter, joking, and so forth are overheard by patients. The patient in the next room may be distressed, ill, or receiving bad news from the physician, and if office staff chatter can be overheard it would appear as though the staff does not care about their patients' needs.

Refer to the guidelines given in Procedure 4-11 to ensure positive communication between yourself and members of your health care team.

Office Manager

Your relationship with your supervisor differs from that of your coworkers. Your supervisor is typically

---

PROCEDURE 4-11
Communicate with the Health Care Team

OBJECTIVE: Practice techniques to help learn how to communicate effectively with coworkers and the health care team.

EQUIPMENT/SUPPLIES: Medical assistant and another adult (substitute role-play as needed).

DIRECTIONS: Follow these step-by-step directions to help facilitate communication with coworkers and the health care team. Job Skill 4-13 in the *Workbook is* presented to practice this skill.

1. Be polite and cheerful, using a friendly approach with each member of your office staff.
2. Include "please" and "thank you" in your everyday language.
3. Use correct names and titles when communicating and ask if you do not know the preference of other members of your health care team.
4. Use tact and diplomacy when attempting to resolve problems.
5. Speak calmly and respectfully and do not become angry or defensive.
6. Use proper channels of communication. Always try to work out problems on a

"one-to-one" basis prior to going to the office manager or other supervisor.
7. Do not judge your coworkers; instead practice empathy.
8. Have a positive attitude in all your work assignments.
9. Bring issues that bother you to the forefront; do not let them fester. Be assertive about your feelings and opinions and be open to discussing them.
10. Perform all your duties and responsibilities and cheerfully bear your share of the workload.
11. Offer to help a coworker when needed and do not refuse because the task is not in your job description.
12. Avoid gossip, arguments, and uncomplimentary statements about coworkers.
13. Do not complain; instead be a problem solver.
14. Maintain your work space in an organized and orderly fashion. Respect others' work spaces and property.
15. Treat coworkers as you would like to be treated.

your teacher, trainer, evaluator, and one who may discipline you if the need arises. Employees often have difficulty communicating with employers; however, employees who communicate well are invaluable to a medical practice, physicians, and supervisors. A good relationship will be one with mutual respect. Always be professional when communicating with a supervisor or manager. To establish an open and honest relationship, you will need to be able to receive critiques as well as constructive criticism. Show initiative and do not fall into the habit of saying "That is not in my job description." Be willing to try new things, pitch in when necessary, and act as a team member. Be willing to share your ideas. When presented and communicated correctly, they are typically welcomed and greatly appreciated.

Keep the office manager informed of problems that occur with patients, coworkers, office equipment, and so forth. Ask if you are unsure about a request, a task, or a medical term. If you do not understand something, do not try to muddle through because you are fearful of what someone will think. It is better to ask and verify the correct way to do something than to go blindly along and make mistakes. If you do not find out the correct way of doing a task the first time you are asked, then in the future you will face an even bigger problem when the office manager expects you to know how to do the task but you do not.

Periodically schedule time to communicate with your supervisor in a relaxed manner, telling him or her how you are doing, sharing concerns, and offering suggestions. Before beginning such a discussion, one should find the right time to approach and differentiate between an urgent and nonurgent problem. Consider the supervisor's needs and word your request accordingly by stating either "I need to speak to you at your earliest convenience," "I need to speak to you," or, in order to minimize interruptions, you could ask, "Do you have a minute?" "Is this a good time to talk?" or "Can I interrupt you for a moment?" If you cannot resolve a problem with a coworker or you need to report a situation that has occurred, be open, honest, and report the facts accurately.

Physician

Communicating with physicians in a professional manner is essential. Always address the physician as "doctor" using his or her last name unless told otherwise. Approach the physician between tasks and let him or her know what it is that you wish to discuss.

Ask if he or she would like to speak now or at a later time. Speak slowly, confidently, and use correct medical terminology.

Listen carefully when given instructions by the physician to relay to a patient. The physician depends on you to communicate information to patients in a professional, accurate, and timely manner. Doctors will also rely on you to receive messages, complaints, and other data that are being relayed from patients. Do not feel intimidated if you do not understand an order. Be honest and ask for the information to be repeated or say that you do not understand and ask for an explanation. Remember that learning continues to take place in the medical office, not just in the classroom.

Outside Health Care Professionals

Whether you are making referral appointments, retrieving laboratory results, or calling the answering service for messages, you will be communicating with outside professionals who are an extension of the health care team. Use the same level of professionalism with outside professionals as you do with other office staff. Remember that you are representing the physician and the medical practice each time you communicate; always promote the practice through positive public relations.

To help the office physician, the medical assistant may act as a *liaison*, communicating with a variety of hospital employees in numerous departments so that they can work together for the benefit of patients. A successful assistant will build a rapport with hospital personnel. The medical staff coordinator notifies the physician of required staff and committee meetings, requests updated copies of credentials and licenses for hospital files, records continuing education credits, and supervises all administrative duties of the physician at the hospital. The nursing staff reports the changing conditions of patients to the physician and receives telephone orders. You may also work with employees in the radiology, physiology, and laboratory departments to schedule tests and receive test results. It is important to understand each of the resources that outside departments and facilities provide.

Take the time to visit the hospital departments, local pharmacies, home health care agencies, and test facilities that you deal with on a regular basis. Introducing yourself to the staff who talks with you over the telephone will go a long way toward improving communications. Always be courteous, polite, respectful, and helpful but do not be afraid to stop and clarify information if you do not understand it.

For instance, if you are receiving laboratory results and the laboratory technician reads the results so fast that you cannot write them down, ask him or her to please slow down or repeat them so you can record them accurately. Likewise, if an outside physician speaks to you in a demeaning matter or too rapidly, do not be intimidated. Be courteous and ask him or her to repeat the message.

STOP AND THINK CASE SCENARIO
Feedback

SCENARIO: You are speaking with Mrs. Jacobson, who stopped by the office and said, "I am really not feeling well and I don't know what is wrong. I wonder if the pills the doctor gave me are making me sick. I feel queasy and can't seem to keep anything down, I'm really exhausted, and sometimes I feel light-headed like I'm going to faint. I am so tired of feeling this way! By the way, I also have a rash on my body. Do you think it's related? Could you please let the doctor know what is going on with me? I have to get home, and I'll be there if you need to get in touch with me."

CRITICAL THINKING: Determine which kind of feedback would be most appropriate to verify that you have heard the message correctly. Formulate a written response that could be given to the physician.

_____
_____
_____
_____
_____
_____
_____
_____
_____
_____
_____
_____
_____
_____

STOP AND THINK CASE SCENARIO
Communication Challenges

SCENARIO: You are speaking to Mrs. Stork, a long-time patient of Dr. Practon's. All of a sudden she breaks into tears and starts sobbing. You freeze and feel like walking away because you are not used to dealing with someone who is emotionally upset.

CRITICAL THINKING: Name at least three things you would avoid doing and state the right way to help someone who breaks down.

1. _____
_____
2. _____
_____
3. _____
_____

STATEMENT:
_____
_____
_____

STOP AND THINK CASE SCENARIO

Socioeconomic Fairness

SCENARIO: Mrs. Marra drives up in a Mercedes and comes in to talk about the blood test the physician has ordered for her. Your coworker is speaking with her and the patient demands that she call the insurance company to find out if the test is covered, what percentage they will pay, and whether any preauthorization is needed. Both you and your coworker know that it is a simple, inexpensive test and no preauthorization is required by the type of insurance plan she has. Your coworker communicates this to the patient, but she insists that the insurance company needs to be called to make sure. Your coworker agrees and then leaves the front desk mumbling about how much money Mrs. Marra has, how cheap she is, how demanding she is, saying, "Just because she has money she thinks she can boss everybody around, I'm not going to waste my time calling the insurance company," even though she told Mrs. Marra she would.

CRITICAL THINKING: How would you have handled the situation with Mrs. Marra?

_____
_____
_____
_____
_____
_____
_____
_____
_____
_____
_____
_____
_____
_____
_____
_____
_____
_____
_____
_____
_____
_____
_____
_____
_____

STOP AND THINK CASE SCENARIO
Positive versus Negative Attitude

SCENARIO: You arrive at the office early, in a good mood and ready to tackle the day. The lead receptionist, Sylvia, is there looking over the daily schedule and she starts complaining (like she does every day) and says, "Oh boy, Mrs. Yabarro is coming in today. What a pain she is. I hope she no-shows. And Mr. Harrington is coming back to see Dr. Practon this afternoon. I thought we got rid of him last week when he was here for 3 hours. What a day it's going to be! We have 30 patients scheduled and you know Dr. Practon will be late arriving from the hospital."

CRITICAL THINKING:

1. How has the receptionist's comments affected your mood?

_____

_____

_____

_____

2. How will you respond to the lead receptionist's comments?

_____

_____

_____

_____

3. What can you do to change this daily morning routine?

_____

_____

_____

_____

FOCUS ON CERTIFICATION*

CMA (AAMA) Content Summary
- Medical terminology
- Developmental/behavioral theories
- Human growth and development
- Adapting communication
- Verbal and nonverbal communication
- Listening skills
- Communication barriers
- Professional communication
- Patient interviewing techniques
- Evaluating effectiveness of communication

RMA (AMT) Content Summary
- Medical terminology
- Age-specific responses

- Professional conduct
- Communication methods
- Cultural and ethnic differences
- Prejudice
- Interpersonal relations
- Verbal/oral communication skills
- Active listening skills
- History-taking techniques
- Subjective and objective information

CMAS (AMT) Content Summary
- Medical terminology
- Human relation skills
- Professionalism
- Interview questions
- Oral communication

*This textbook and the accompanying Workbook meet the entry-level administrative and general competencies for the CMA outlined by the AAMA Examination Content Outline and Occupational Analysis and for the RMA and CMAS outlined by the AMT Competencies, Construction Parameters, and Examination Specifications (see Competency Grid in Appendix B.

REVIEW EXAM-STYLE QUESTIONS

1. Basic elements in the communication cycle include:
   a. sender, receiver
   b. sender, message, receiver
   c. sender, message, channel, receiver, feedback
   d. sender, message, channel, receiver, questions
   e. sender, message, verbal/nonverbal, receiver, feedback

2. Select the three primary ways messages are communicated in the order of importance.
   a. Spoken word, body language, tonality
   b. Body language, tonality, spoken word
   c. Tonality, body language, spoken word
   d. Spoken word, tonality, body language
   e. Body language, spoken word, tonality

3. If a patient makes up a reason to justify unacceptable actions or behavior in order to avoid something, the defense mechanism is known as:
   a. avoidance
   b. compensation
   c. displacement
   d. rationalization
   e. regression

4. In a health care setting, the comfort zone is approximately:
   a. 1 to 2 feet
   b. 2 to 3 feet
   c. 3 to 4 feet
   d. 4 to 5 feet
   e. 5 to 6 feet

5. When using nonverbal communication:
   a. the eyes, face, and hands can be used to communicate
   b. gestures are utilized
   c. it is referred to as body language
   d. touch can send signals
   e. all of the above are correct

6. Active listening involves:
   a. dwelling on or mulling over what the speaker has said
   b. giving the speaker your undivided attention
   c. verbal and nonverbal responses to a message
   d. focusing on yourself in addition to the speaker
   e. intuitive and immediate responses

7. Questioning, requesting examples, and paraphrasing a message are:
   a. ways to improve active listening
   b. types of nonverbal communication
   c. types of feedback
   d. not recommended when listening actively
   e. interpersonal skills

8. Which of the following is an example of negative stereotyping?
   a. All Italians are loud.
   b. I don't like Italian food.
   c. Italians should not be allowed in this medical office.
   d. I'm married to an Italian, therefore I know what they're like.
   e. I love all Italians.

9. Verbal descriptions are needed when communicating with:
   a. hearing-impaired patients
   b. patients with an impaired level of understanding
   c. visually impaired patients
   d. speech-impaired patients
   e. patients undergoing stressful situations

10. Some of the most difficult communication problems exist when communicating with a/an:
    a. physician
    b. office manager
    c. coworker
    d. patient
    e. outside health care professional

11. An example of objective information is a/an:
    a. lesion
    b. eye ache
    c. side pain
    d. odd taste
    e. upset stomach

12. An example of subjective information is a:
    a. blood pressure
    b. pulse rate
    c. temperature
    d. ringing in ear
    e. lesion

WORKBOOK ASSIGNMENT

To develop competency-based job skills, refer to the *Workbook* and complete the:
- Abbreviation and Spelling Review
- Review Questions

- Critical Thinking Exercises
- Job Skill activities, which are listed at the beginning of the chapter under *Performance Objectives in the Workbook*.

RESOURCES

Books

Effective Communication Practices for Healthcare Professionals, DVD, 1st edition
> Crosstown Production, 2011

Multicultural Manners: Essential Rules of Etiquette for the 21st Century
> Dresser, Norine
> Wiley Publications, New York, 2005

Racial and Ethnic Relations in America, 7th edition
> McLemore/Romo
> Addison-Wesley Publishers, 2004

Therapeutic Communications for Health Care, 3rd edition
> Tamparo/Lindh
> Cengage Learning, 2008
> Website: http://www.cengagebrain.com

Transcultural Communication in Health Care
> Luckmann, Joan
> Cengage Learning, 2000
> Website: http://www.cengagebrain.com

Dictionary

The Nonverbal Dictionary of Gestures, Signs & Body Language Cues
> Givens, Ph.D., David B.
> Spokane, WA, Center for Nonverbal Studies, 2002

Internet

2013 Yearbook of Immigration Statistics
> Office of Immigration Statistics
> Homeland Security

Find Articles
> Search: Key terms (e.g., multicultural patients, language barriers)

Migration Policy Institute
> Search: Migration information

Soft Skills
> Wikipedia—free encyclopedia
> Search: Soft skills

CHAPTER 5

RECEPTIONIST AND THE MEDICAL OFFICE ENVIRONMENT

LEARNING OBJECTIVES

After reading this chapter and learning step-by-step procedures to gain job skills,* you should be able to:

- Open the medical office, ready it for daily activities, and welcome patients in a cordial manner.
- Explain the "Red Flags Rule" and state how it deters medical identity theft.
- Register patients by obtaining vital information.
- Understand the purpose of the office privacy notice.
- Respond appropriately to patients who experience a delay in their appointment.
- Inspect and maintain confidentiality and orderliness in the reception area.
- Obtain community resources for patient referrals and education.
- State OSHA's role in regulating safety and health standards for the medical office.
- Identify ergonomic factors that affect the medical assistant's work environment.
- Describe steps to maintain office security.
- Discuss electrical and fire safety in a medical facility.
- List ways to prepare for environmental emergencies and other disasters.
- Assist in an office emergency.
- Perform necessary duties to close the medical office for the day.

PERFORMANCE OBJECTIVES (PROCEDURES) IN THIS TEXTBOOK

- Open the medical office (Procedure 5-1).
- Assist patients with in-office registration procedures (Procedure 5-2).
- Assist patients in preparing an application form for a disabled person placard (Procedure 5-3).
- Develop a list of community resources (Procedure 5-4).
- Develop a patient education plan for diseases or injuries related to the medical specialty (Procedure 5-5).
- Work at a computer station and comply with ergonomic standards (Procedure 5-6).
- Prevent and prepare for fires in the workplace (Procedure 5-7).
- Learn how and when to use a fire extinguisher (Procedure 5-8).

---

*This textbook *and the accompanying* Workbook *meet the educational components for entry-level administrative and general competencies outlined by CAAHEP and ABHES.*

- Develop an emergency disaster plan (Procedure 5-9).
- Close the medical office (Procedure 5-10).

PERFORMANCE OBJECTIVES (JOB SKILLS) IN THE WORKBOOK

- Prepare a patient registration form (Job Skill 5-1).
- Prepare an application form for a disabled person placard (Job Skill 5-2).
- Research community resources for patient referrals and patient education (Job Skill 5-3).
- Assess and use proper body mechanics (Job Skill 5-4).
- Evaluate the work or school environment and develop a safety plan (Job Skill 5-5).
- Take steps to prevent and prepare for fires in a health care setting (Job Skill 5-6).
- Demonstrate proper use of a fire extinguisher (Job Skill 5-7).
- Determine potential disaster hazards in your local community (Job Skill 5-8).
- Develop an emergency response template with an evacuation plan (Job Skill 5-9).

KEY TERMS

biohazard

community resources

disaster

ergonomics

face sheet

hazardous waste

infectious waste

Material Safety Data Sheets (MSDS)

medical identity theft

Occupational Safety and Health Administration (OSHA)

Pandemic emergency

patient instruction form

reception area

Red Flags Rule

registration form

registration kiosks

sharps containers

standard precautions

HEART OF THE HEALTH CARE PROFESSIONAL

Service

Old adage: "It takes months to get a new patient—and only seconds to lose one." As the first one who greets patients, the receptionist sets the tone of the office with a smile, helpful attitude, and caring approach. As the last person the patient talks to when leaving, the receptionist should seize all opportunities to leave a good impression while serving patients' needs.

OFFICE RECEPTIONIST

In past years, the front office assistant was expected to welcome patients in a friendly manner, obtain demographic information, answer the telephone, make appointments, and take messages.

The emerging role of the medical receptionist includes knowing and understanding a wide variety of laws and regulations; serving as a diplomat, a negotiator, a psychologist, and a director of public relations; answering an almost constantly ringing telephone; reviewing insurance cards and determining insurance types or managed care plans; confirming the practice's participation in plans and patients' eligibility and copayments; entering demographic data into the computer; explaining financial and medical procedures; posting a variety of transactions; and keeping up to date by reading monthly bulletins and newsletters. In other words, a person applying for a position as a receptionist in a medical office should be a professionally trained medical assistant who is flexible and prepared for a variety of duties.

First Impression

The medical receptionist plays an important role in how the physician's office is perceived and remembered. No matter how stressful the situation becomes,

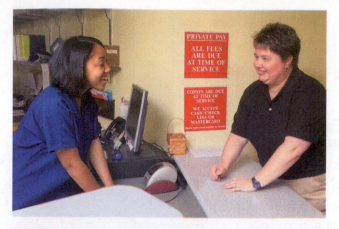

FIGURE 5-1 A friendly greeting with a smile from the medical assistant/receptionist sends a welcome message and is reassuring to most patients

first impressions always count and interruptions are a matter of daily routine. The receptionist must project a professional but empathetic and sympathetic attitude. A clean and orderly office with a friendly, well-groomed, attentive receptionist will help ease tension and make patients feel more comfortable. It is important for the assistant to be alert for cues to a patient's emotional state and to remember that most people arrive at the office ill, in pain, and anxious about their physical condition. Being attentive to the patient's needs can elicit a positive response from a patient awaiting an appointment, thereby aiding the physician at the initiation of medical treatment (Figure 5-1).

Multitasking

Multitasking involves rapidly shifting your focus from one task to another. This takes experience and becomes possible only when one of the tasks is so ingrained that it becomes automatic or second nature. Trying to perform several tasks simultaneously when not familiar with the tasks, as well as haste in trying to get them done quickly and being distracted or interrupted can cause mistakes.

Managing multiple tasks awaits the receptionist each day, and an organized approach is mandatory along with a calm demeanor. Priorities should be established, communicated, and adjusted as necessary; however, be careful about letting others change your priority list. If you are asked to do something for someone else, ask in what time frame it needs to be completed. That will allow you to determine where on your priority list the task should fit. If you are working on a task, let your coworkers and patients know the time frame you expect to complete it. Desk management systems can assist with multiple tasks and help you obtain organization skills if you are not experienced in managing your time. Although interruptions are constant, if patients are treated with respect, dignity, and kindness, they will in turn respect the receptionist's time and the job that he or she is doing.

OPENING THE MEDICAL OFFICE

Generally, the first and last duties of each day are to open and close the office just as you would any place of business. Refer to Procedure 5-1 for guidelines on opening the medical office.

Preparing Records

With electronic medical records, there will be no charts to pull for established patients. With a paper medical record system, returning patient charts typically have been retrieved from locked cabinets the evening before and put on the receptionist's desk (see Closing the Medical Office, later in this chapter). They were pulled in alphabetical order but are now arranged in the order in which patients will be seen, according to the office schedule.

Regardless of the type of system, each established patient's medical record needs to be viewed. If it is noted that consultation reports or test results have not been received, you now have ample time to check the incoming mail or call the appropriate facility to obtain an electronic copy or fax prior to the patient's arrival.

New patient records will be created or made up either at the time the appointment is made, when the registration and history forms are obtained, the evening before the appointment, or the morning of appointment (see Chapter 9, *Medical Records*).

Retrieving Messages

Call the answering service or retrieve messages from the answering machine and note all messages on appropriate forms. Deliver urgent messages to the physician and other messages to staff members as appropriate. Return telephone calls and take action on messages that pertain to the receptionist's duties. Chapter 6, *Telephone Procedures*, has information on telephone guidelines and message taking.

PROCEDURE 5-1

Open the Medical Office

OBJECTIVE: Open the office at the beginning of the day to promote efficient operation of the medical practice all through the day.

EQUIPMENT/SUPPLIES: A simulated office setting.

DIRECTIONS: Follow these step-by-step directions, which include rationales, and role-play the actions outlined to practice this procedure. Describe the action and rationale while performing each step.

1. Unlock the outside door and disarm the security system so that the alarm will not be triggered in error.
2. Turn on the office lights to ensure proper lighting throughout the day.
3. Check the room temperature for comfort in both front and back office and adjust thermostats, if necessary, or open windows for fresh air.
4. Turn on the sound system and office equipment; for example, computer, printer, photocopier, autoclave, diagnostic equipment, and so forth.
5. Check the fax machine for documents and distribute them as needed. Important data may be communicated via facsimile while the office is closed.
6. Unlock drawers, cabinets, and files that are usually unlocked during business hours and open those that require quick access.
7. Check the answering machine or call the answering service for messages. Turn off the answering machine during business hours. Record, relay, or respond to messages.
8. Check email messages; deliver or answer as necessary.
9. Unlock the door and check the **reception area** to make sure it is neat and clean. Vacuum, dust, and water plants when necessary to ensure a pleasant environment.
10. Straighten magazines, check for condition, and discard if old, torn, or damaged.
11. Check for possible safety hazards such as frayed electric wires, damaged furniture, or flooring that might cause a patient to fall. Report unsafe conditions to the office manager.
12. Check bathrooms to be sure they are adequately stocked and clean.
13. Restock daily office supplies (pens, pencils, note pads, paper clips).
14. Check the desk area to be sure it is tidy and uncluttered. Open the daysheet and fill in the date, if a manual bookkeeping system is used.
15. Check to see that all coworkers have arrived before transferring telephone calls.
16. Unlock the outside door to the reception area when the office is scheduled to open.

Greeting Patients

The appointment schedule is either printed from the computer system or copied from the appointment book the evening before or the morning of appointments. Before each patient arrives, the receptionist should note the name on the appointment schedule and watch for the patient's arrival in order to greet him or her by name, making sure to pronounce the name correctly. Ask if you are not sure how to pronounce the name and record the pronunciation of a particularly difficult name phonetically on the patient's chart. Take the time to update names in cases such as marriage or divorce. Customizing your welcoming remarks by adding the patient's name will prevent you from sounding like a broken record (Example 5-1).

EXAMPLE 5-1

Welcoming Remarks

- "Good morning, Mrs. Baker. Dr. Practon will be with you in a few minutes."
- "Hello, Mr. Cain. How is that new grandson of yours getting along?"
- "Nice to see you again, Mrs. Steinhouse."
- "How are you today, Mr. Atkins? Nancy, our clinical medical assistant, will be taking you back shortly."

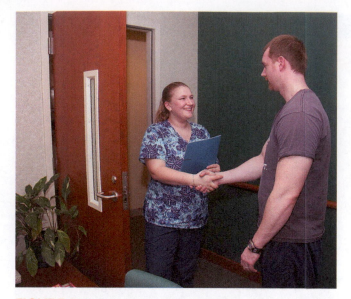

FIGURE 5-2 A medical assistant offering a warm greeting with a friendly handshake while making eye contact makes patients feel at ease

Using a personalized greeting, special comment, or expression with the right choice of words adds a personal touch that is cordial but not unprofessional. To accomplish this, place a self-adhesive note on the chart regarding something that is happening in the patient's life (e.g., wedding, trip, move), so the patient can be asked about it at the next visit—it is appreciated. For example, "You sure look rested. Did you have a great time in Hawaii, Mr. Warner?" A comforting touch or handshake (Figure 5-2) also conveys warmth and friendliness, as does noticing something unique about the patient and commenting on it. For example, "That's a beautiful scarf, Mrs. Anderson," "Is that your granddaughter Mr. Huang? She sure is adorable." By offering compliments, you add sincerity to your greeting and convey interest in the patient's life. Acknowledge those accompanying patients such as friends or family members. Get their names and offer them a handshake, as appropriate.

Calling out patients' names who are seated in the reception area is not a violation of the Health Insurance Portability and Accountability Act (HIPAA). However, sometimes you may need to select alternatives because names alone can reveal health information in highly specialized facilities. For example, having your name associated with a fertility clinic or oncology unit can reveal protected health information (PHI). Take precautions to protect health information at all times and in special situations assign each patient a number or pager instead of using names.

Addressing Patients

It should be standard practice to get to know patients' names and to learn how they prefer to be addressed. Greet patients using a professional but friendly tone. Address them with the correct title (e.g., Mr., Mrs., Ms., Miss) and use their last names unless they indicate to you that they would like to be called by a first name or nickname. If so, indicate the name of choice on the chart so that all medical personnel can use it. Children or young teenagers may be called by their given names. Do not refer to patients or staff by only their last names or by their medical conditions (e.g., "Smith is in the waiting room," "Sprained foot in Room 3," "Phone call for Practon on Line 1"). Even if only overheard by other staff members, it sounds degrading and can lead to bad habits. Never use terms that belittle the individual's dignity such as *darling*, *honey*, *sweetie*, and so forth. These terms may be offensive if used in a professional setting and are typically used in personal communication, such as with your family, loved ones, or close friends.

When speaking to someone in the reception area or talking on the telephone as patients arrive, the assistant should look up, nod, and smile to acknowledge their arrival. Later a more personal welcome can be extended. Although a patient may see the physician only a few times in the course of treatment, the medical assistant who establishes positive personal relations will build trust and confidence.

Patient Visit Log

Some medical offices still use a patient visit log attached to a clipboard and have patients sign in as they arrive. This reduces the chance of a waiting patient being overlooked; however, legally a sign-in sheet is a breach of confidentiality if it prompts patients to reveal "reason for visit." If they are there because of a sensitive medical condition, it would violate privacy rules to have it written on a sign-in sheet. The open display of patients' names seen that day to all who sign in or just want to take a look is also a violation of privacy.

Secure methods to protect confidentiality while logging patients' arrival times and processing patients' information are:

1. Obtain a confidential patient sign-in log that uses layered, perforated, prenumbered tickets printed on no-carbon-required (NCR) paper (Figure 5-3A). When the patient arrives, he or she prints arrival time, name, reason for visit, and the physician's name on the ticket. The ticket is then detached from the log, and either placed it in a box or given to the receptionist. The prenumbered sheet underneath is darkly obliterated, and when pulled apart the bottom sheet contains all the patients' data as recorded on sign-in (Figure 5-3B). This may be retained in a three-hole binder for future reference.

2. Purchase small preprinted, prenumbered adhesive labels (Figure 5-4A). Upon arrival, the patient can write appointment time, name, arrival time, and the physician's name. The receptionist removes the label and adheres it to the patient visit log, which is kept out of sight (Figure 5-4B). This may be retained in a three-hole binder for future reference.

COMPLIANCE

Patient Privacy

In 2003, federal laws made it mandatory to protect patient privacy. Methods of tracking patients' arrivals and obtaining necessary data while retaining confidentiality should be incorporated into all medical practices.

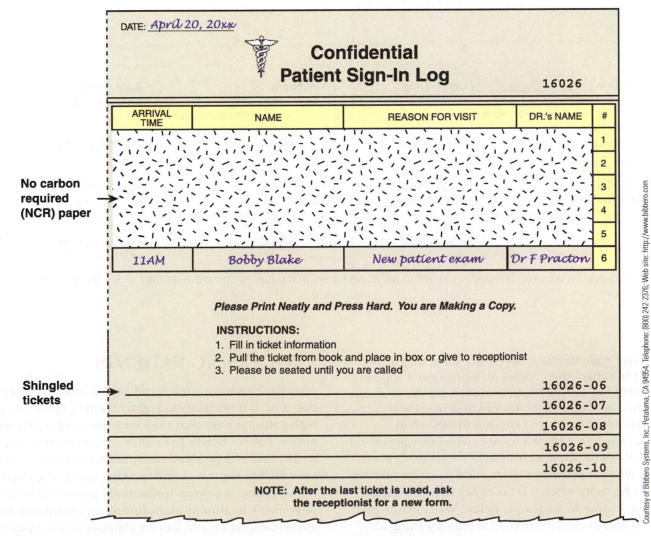

FIGURE 5-3A Confidential patient sign-in log with layered, perforated shingled tickets

FIGURE 5-3B Confidential patient sign-in log revealed under NCR paper

FIGURE 5-4A Small, preprinted, prenumbered adhesive labels that patients complete as they arrive for an office appointment

3. Have patients check in verbally when they arrive. Either check their names off a preprinted appointment log, noting the time of their arrival, or stamp their encounter form (or progress note) with a date/time stamp and attach it to their chart.

4. Assign each patient a number when they arrive and call out the number instead of the patient's name.

5. Give each patient an electronic device that vibrates or lights up when it is his or her turn to enter the back office to see the physician. Such devices are similar to ones distributed to guests waiting for tables in restaurants.

PROCESSING PATIENTS

After patients have arrived and signed in at the reception desk, it is necessary to register them or update their registration, verify that they have received a privacy notice, collect health insurance information (Chapter 18), and address all administrative issues before they are called to see the physician. After seeing the physician, patients are given instructions pertaining to the physician's treatment plan, future appointments are made (Chapter 7), and fees are collected or their health insurance is billed (Chapter 13).

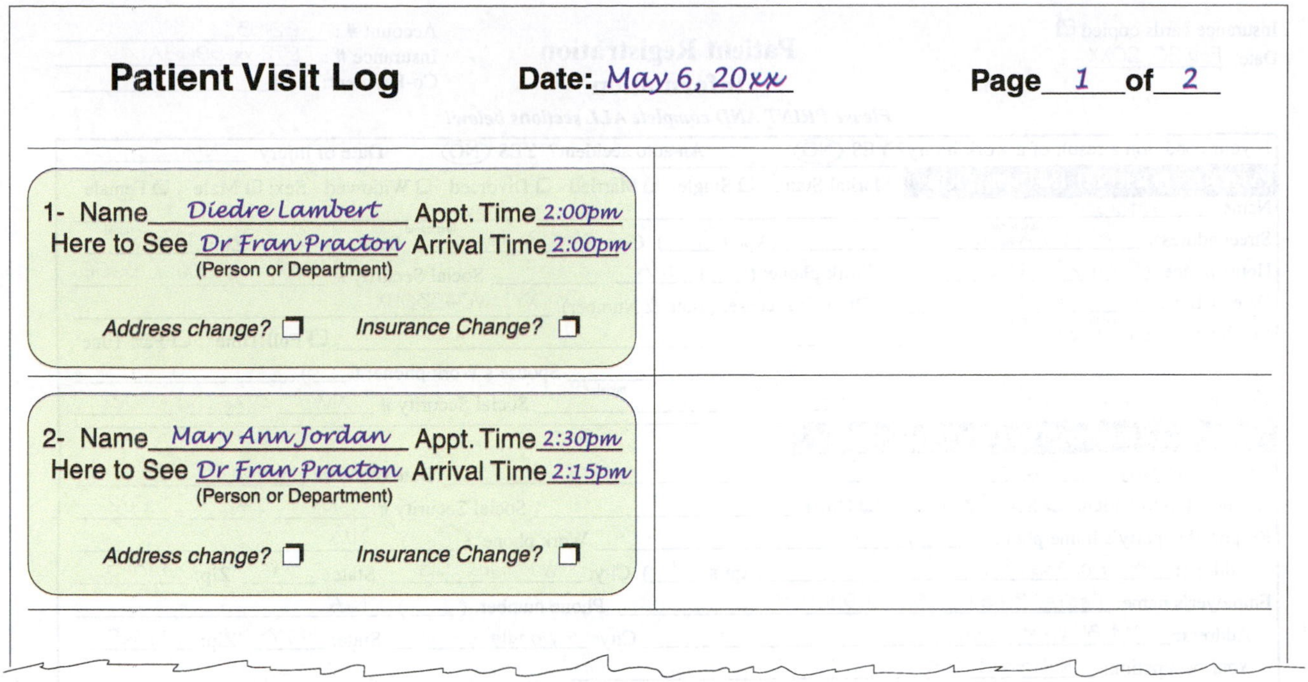
Patient Visit Log **Date:** May 6, 20xx **Page** 1 **of** 2

1- Name Diedre Lambert Appt. Time 2:00pm
Here to See Dr Fran Practon Arrival Time 2:00pm
(Person or Department)
Address change? ☐ *Insurance Change?* ☐

2- Name Mary Ann Jordan Appt. Time 2:30pm
Here to See Dr Fran Practon Arrival Time 2:15pm
(Person or Department)
Address change? ☐ *Insurance Change?* ☐

Courtesy of Bibbero Systems, Inc., Petaluma, CA 94954. Telephone: (800) 242-2376; Web site: http://www.bibbero.com

FIGURE 5-4B Adhesive labels placed on the patient visit log after completion by each patient

Patient Registration

At the patient's first office visit, a comprehensive but concise **registration form** (Figure 5-5) designed to record and index a patient's personal and financial data should be obtained. If the patient is to record the information at the first office visit, request that he or she arrives at least 20 minutes early so ample time is allowed to complete the form. Preprinted registration or information forms are commercially available or can be designed by office management and supplied by a printing company.

The receptionist should make sure that all necessary information is collected on the registration form. This information will be used in many ways and by a variety of office staff for treatment and billing purposes. If the information is inaccurate or incomplete, it will have an effect on the efficiency of the office staff to provide the best experience possible for the patient.

Some patients may refuse to divulge certain information on the form. In such instances, it is wise to adopt a pay-at-the-time-of-service office policy. If a patient expects insurance to pay for services and has not provided information, such as insurance policy number or birth date, the insurance company will probably deny payment. This should be explained to the patient in a concerned manner. It may not be something the patient has thought about or considered.

Red Flags Rule and Red Flags Program Clarification Act

Identity theft is the leading nonviolent crime in America and the medical practice setting is a place where personal information must be protected and secure; otherwise, it may be stolen. When someone uses another person's name or insurance information to falsely obtain medical services or products, such as durable medical equipment or prescription drugs, it is called **medical identity theft**. If someone steals a patient's identity, medical records can be altered and the patient's treatment compromised. Section 114 of the Fair and Accurate Credit Transactions Act (FACTA) addresses this issue in what is called the **Red Flags Rule**. Developed in 2008, the rule states that financial institutions and those who act as "creditors" need to have a written prevention and detection program for identity theft. Such a program would list reasonable policies and procedures to verify a patient's identity and target areas (red flags) where identity theft may occur.

The *Red Flag Program Clarification Act* of 2010 was subsequently passed which excludes most doctors, lawyers, and other professionals who do not receive full payment at the time services are rendered. Although the "Rule" no longer applies to doctor offices, medical identity theft is a real problem and a policy should be

Insurance cards copied ☑
Date: Feb 20, 20XX

Patient Registration Information

Please PRINT AND complete ALL sections below!

Account # : 62153
Insurance # : 572-xx-8966A
Co-Payment: $ N/A

Is your condition a result of a work injury? YES (NO)   An auto accident? YES (NO)   Date of injury: N/A

PATIENT'S PERSONAL INFORMATION   Marital Status ☐ Single ☑ Married ☐ Divorced ☐ Widowed   Sex: ☐ Male ☑ Female

Name: Peterson _____ Mayze _____ F.
      last name   first name   initial
Street address: 851 So. Adams   (Apt # 12) City: Woodland Hills   State: XY   Zip: 12345
Home phone: (555) 289-4413   Work phone: (___) N/A   Social Security # XXX - XX - 8966
Date of Birth: Aug. / 07 / 1936   Driver's License: (State & Number) XY V045369X
            month day   year
Employer / Name of School   Retired _____   ☐ Full Time ☐ Part Time
Spouse's Name: Peterson _____ Roy _____ ____   Spouse's Work phone: (___) _____
            last name   first name   initial
How do you wish to be addressed? Mrs. Peterson   Social Security # XXX - XX - 6022

PATIENT'S / RESPONSIBLE PARTY INFORMATION

Responsible party: Roy Peterson   Date of Birth: March 03, 1937
Relationship to Patient: ☐ Self ☑ Spouse ☐ Other _____   Social Security # XXX - XX - 6022
Responsible party's home phone: (555) 289-4413   Work phone: (___) N/A
   Address: 851 So. Adams   (Apt # 12) City: Woodland Hills   State: XY   Zip: 12345
Employer's name: Retired Pasadena School District   Phone number: (___) N/A
   Address: 44185 West Colorado Blvd.   City: Woodland Hills   State: XY   Zip: 12345
   Your occupation: Retired Teacher
Spouse's Employer's name: N/A   Spouse's Work phone: (___) _____
   Address: _____   City: _____   State: ____   Zip: ____

PATIENT'S INSURANCE INFORMATION   Please present insurance cards to receptionist.

PRIMARY insurance company's name: Medicare
Insurance address: P.O. Box 879   City: Los Angeles   State: CA   Zip: 12345
Name of insured: Mayze Peterson   Date of Birth: 8/7/36   Relationship to insured: ☑ Self ☐ Spouse ☐ Other ☐ Child
Insurance ID number: XXX-XX-8966A   Group number: N/A
SECONDARY insurance company's name: Blue Cross
Insurance address: P.O. Box 1022   City: Woodland Hills   State: XY   Zip: 12345
Name of insured: Mayze Peterson   Date of Birth: 8/7/36   Relationship to insured: ☑ Self ☐ Spouse ☐ Other ☐ Child
Insurance ID number: XXX-XX-8966   Group number: 00276A
Check if appropriate: ☑ Medigap policy ☐ Retiree coverage

PATIENT'S REFERRAL INFORMATION

Referred by: Glenda Marshall (Mrs. T.K.)   If referred by a friend, may we thank her or him? (YES) NO
Name(s) of other physician(s) who care for you: Patrick King, M.D.   (please circle one)

EMERGENCY CONTACT

Name of person not living with you: Kathryn Miller   Relationship: cousin
Address: 691 So. Brand Ave.   City: Woodland Hills   State: XY   Zip: 12345
Phone number (home): (555) 362-5711   Phone number (work): (____) N/A

Assignment of Benefits • Financial Agreement

I hereby give lifetime authorization for payment of insurance benefits to be made directly to Dr. G. Practon , and any assisting physicians, for services rendered. I understand that I am financially responsible for all charges whether or not they are covered by insurance. In the event of default, I agree to pay all costs of collection, and reasonable attorney's fees. I hereby authorize this healthcare provider to release all information necessary to secure the payment of benefits.
I further agree that a photocopy of this agreement shall be as valid as the original.
Date: Feb. 20, 20XX   Your Signature: Mayze Peterson
Method of Payment: ☐ Cash ☑ Check ☐ Credit Card

FORM # 58-8423 • BIBBERO SYSTEMS, INC. • PETALUMA, CA. • TO ORDER CALL TOLL FREE : 800-BIBBERO (800-242-2376) • FAX (800) 242-9330   (REV. 7/94)

FIGURE 5-5 Patient registration information form showing completion of personal and financial data obtained from the patient prior to or on her first visit to the office

developed to guard against it. Therefore, the following steps, which comply with the Red Flags Rule are listed as a guideline.

First, every new patient's identity needs to be verified. Copy all new patients' driver's licenses and compare them to other forms of identification. If the patient's photo ID does not show a current address, you may request a recent utility bill or other valid document. The license should be kept in the patient's file and the picture compared each time the patient comes in to see the physician. Do not use Social Security numbers as medical record identifiers and shred protected information when disposing of it. Employee training in fraud prevention should also occur, as needed.

The Federal Trade Commission (FTC) defines creditors as, "any business or organization that regularly provides goods or services first and allows customers to pay later." Health care providers who require payment at the time of service, accept credit cards, or bill and accept payment from an insurance carrier where the patient has no responsibility are not considered creditors. However, providers who offer payment plans, bill for services after they are provided, wait for insurance payment before billing patients for residual amounts, or offer specialized health care credit cards constitute creditor status. Red flags to look for include:

- Address inconsistencies when comparing identification documents
- Billing inconsistencies or services the patient did not receive
- Driver's license photograph that does not match the person in the office
- Clinically inaccurate medical records
- Missing insurance card, only an identification number is provided
- Patient's assertion that he or she is a victim of identity theft
- Post office box with no street address

If you suspect medical identity theft, contact the patient, secure the patient's medical record, close the patient's account, notify law enforcement, and have the patient file a complaint with the Federal Trade Commission and put a fraud alert on his or her credit report.

Preregistration

To ease and reduce in-office work, some offices mail, email, or fax the patient a registration form to complete in the comfort of his or her own home and a map giving directions so the patient can easily find the office.

COMPLIANCE
Medical Identity Theft

Although HIPAA addresses the protection and privacy of patient health information, the Red Flags Rule goes beyond this act, covering credit card and insurance claim information, tax identification numbers, and background checks for employees and service providers. To spot and prevent medical identity theft, one should monitor explanation of benefit forms, request and read credit reports, review a listing of yearly benefits paid to health care providers, and be attentive to security issues.

Ask the patient to bring the completed form in when he or she comes for the first visit.

Some offices may prefer to obtain new patient information by telephone. Be sure to verify you have the correct person; then the patient can be interviewed and data entered directly into the computer system. The assistant needs to review the data entered on the form while the patient is present to verify its accuracy and completeness.

Registration Kiosks—In large medical clinics, self-service **registration kiosks** may be found in the entrance or waiting room. Using computers in these stand-alone structures, patients can self-register, update demographic information, and process payments. Kiosks are an efficient way to increase patient flow and allow patients to control their health care experience.

Regardless of where the registration form is completed, all elements need to be addressed by either completing them or referencing "not applicable" (NA) in the blank area. Refer to the guidelines in Procedure 5-2 when assisting patients with in-office registration.

Registration Member Cards—Some medical practices have started issuing "premier member" cards to regular patients. The first time the patient is seen, you collect all of the patient's information and enter it into the computer system. A plastic member card is generated with the patient's own account number or personal code, which contains all patient information. Each time the patient calls for an appointment or is seen after that, the information is brought up on the computer screen and the patient is asked whether any changes should be made. If changes occur, new information can be

PROCEDURE 5-2

Assist Patients with In-Office Registration Procedures

OBJECTIVE: Obtain pertinent identifying information and properly register new and established patients.

EQUIPMENT/SUPPLIES: Patient registration/information form, clipboard, pen, patient information booklet, consent form, assignment of benefits form, appointment list, and photocopy machine.

DIRECTIONS: Follow these step-by-step directions, which include rationales, to learn this procedure. Job Skill 5-1 is presented in the *Workbook* to practice this skill.

1. Greet the patient and hand him or her a registration form on a clipboard with a pen. Ask the patient to complete the form, offering to assist as needed. Use of a clipboard allows the patient to sit comfortably and write independently on a hard surface.

2. Instruct the patient to answer all questions and complete all blank lines, indicating not applicable (NA) for areas that do not apply. This ensures that the patient has read all areas and addressed all questions on the form.

3. Give a patient information booklet outlining the policies of the medical practice unless it is office policy to mail a welcoming letter, map, booklet, and questionnaire before the first visit.

4. Ask for an insurance card and photocopy both sides or scan into the computer system.

5. Verify that the physician is covered by the health insurance contract.

6. Confirm patient eligibility and enrollment for insurance coverage or monthly capitation.

7. Ask for a prior authorization form if the patient is in a managed care plan and has been referred by another physician. An authorization to see the patient must be approved and received by the physician before the patient arrives for an appointment; otherwise, the physician would be denied payment for the service.

8. Collect and review the form for legibility, completeness, and accuracy. Ask the patient for information for any areas left blank. Correct information assists in billing and collections. The form should contain:

    a. Patient's full name (verify spelling and compare with insurance card and driver's license)

    b. Marital status

    c. Gender

    d. Home address (including street address if a post office box is listed) and email address

    e. Telephone, cell phone, and fax numbers—home and business (including extension number)

    f. Social Security number

    g. Birth date recorded as eight digits for computer processing (01-16-1945)

    h. Driver's license number

    i. Occupation with name and address of employer

    j. Spouse's or legal guardian's full name, work phone, and Social Security number

    k. Name and telephone number of person responsible for payment (guarantor)

    l. Insurance information; names, addresses, and telephone numbers—with policy and group numbers—of primary and secondary insurance (copy of insurance card may be placed in this area if all information is included)

    m. Name of person who referred patient and other physicians caring for patient

    n. Name of close friend or relative with daytime telephone number for emergency contact

9. Collect the copayment amount before the visit. This helps avoid sending bills for small amounts, thus reducing overhead costs.

10. Explain the patient's financial responsibility. Collection is made easier if the patient knows his or her financial obligation before receiving service.

(continues)

PROCEDURE 5-2 (continued)

11. Ask if there is any changed information if the patient is an established patient. Patients may not remember to let you know about changes in personal information, for example, new insurance, new married name, and so on.

12. Ask the patient to sign the consent form, assignment of benefits form, and responsibility for the account (guarantor) section of the form.

13. Insert a check mark on the appointment list indicating the patient has arrived for the appointment. This record must be retained as documentation for financial purposes.

14. Scan the patient registration form into the EMR or affix the form to the front inside cover of the patient's chart.

15. Place the history form and any other forms and reports into the patient's medical record or scan each item into the computer system.

16. Secure a multipurpose billing form (encounter form) on the patient's chart. The multipurpose billing form is explained in detail in Chapter 13, *Fees, Credit, and Collection*.

17. Ask the patient to be seated, and give an approximation of how long it will be before the examination. This keeps the patient informed and will reduce his or her anxiety.

18. Put the patient's medical record with the multipurpose billing form in the appropriate place to indicate to the physician or clinical medical assistant that the patient is in the reception room and ready to be seen.

---

downloaded to the card, and if not, the card can be swiped at any affiliate location to obtain information.

Registering Patients Under Managed Care Plans

As more patients enroll with managed care plans, the medical assistant is faced with increased information requirements to avoid insurance and billing problems. At or prior to the initial visit, one of the first questions the assistant should ask is: "Do you have your insurance card so that I can determine if the physician participates in the plan?" Identify the patient's particular plan and the name of the insurer. Then, scan or photocopy both sides of the insurance card. Additional important information includes the following:

- Authorization requirements for the patient to see the physician for a visit or for elective or major surgery
- Name and telephone number of the referring physician
- Patient's identification numbers for the plan (policy and group)
- Copayment? (Yes/No) Amount/percentage?
- Exclusions: lab, x-ray, waiting period, other
- Preventive health visit covered/authorized? (Yes/No)
- Well-baby/child visit covered/authorized? (Yes/No)
- Allergy treatments covered/authorized? (Yes/No) What is authorized?

- Vision/hearing examinations covered/authorized? (Yes/No)
- Plan telephone number/fax number, address, city, state, and zip code

For reference, an alphabetic listing of all plans to which the physician is a participant should be handy—perhaps on a grid or in the computer system. If the office does not belong to the prospective patient's plan, explain that the physician does not participate in that plan. If the physician does belong, more screening information may be necessary prior to scheduling the office visit.

Authorization for Visits—For the primary care physician who is a participant in a managed care plan, an authorization is not required for patient visits. A great number of plans require the patient to receive an authorization from the primary care physician to see a specialist or to receive outside services. If plans require authorizations, the assistant can remind patients to bring the authorization forms at the time of their scheduled visit. If test results are to be sent, transmitted, or faxed to the practice, the assistant in charge of scheduling may want to put a special note in the appointment log to confirm that the results have been received—preferably 1 or 2 days before the scheduled visit. Otherwise, the patient's appointment may have to be rescheduled pending necessary test results.

Registering Patients Coming from a Hospital

If you work for a surgeon, a new patient who the physician has already seen or performed emergency surgery on at the hospital may come to the office. Often the only information you get is the patient's name, diagnosis, and the procedure the surgeon performed. First, obtain the **face sheet** from the hospital admitting office or have the physician bring a copy from the patient's hospital record. If the hospital face sheet does not contain all the needed information, call the hospital ward unit coordinator or the insurance verifier in the admitting office. The patient's primary care physician can also be contacted regarding basic insurance information. If the doctor does not remember the patient's name, call the operating room desk at the hospital to identify the patient. Remember, HIPAA does not forbid sharing patient information for the purpose of treating the patient; however, if the hospital does not want to divulge the information the physician may need to call or take up the problem with the medical records supervisor.

Updating Information

When a patient returns, the original registration information is reviewed to make sure it is still accurate. This can be accomplished by printing the patient information and having the patient review it and make any changes in red ink. A patient information update form is also available for this purpose. Some offices use a confidential patient sign-in log that may be used to determine if there have been any changes (address, telephone number, insurance data) since a previous visit. Verifying patient information should be done at 3-month intervals for all patients who are not being treated for ongoing problems (Figure 5-6).

Medical History and Reports

A history form can be mailed with the new patient registration form, allowing the patient time to look up pertinent information and complete it accurately. To facilitate gathering medical information, ask new patients to request previous medical records from their former physician or to come in to sign an authorization to release information in advance of their appointment. The physician will then have time to review the past history, allowing a more relaxed initial interview. If laboratory or other test results are to be sent, transmitted, or faxed to the practice, the medical assistant will need to make sure that they are in the medical record prior to the patient's visit.

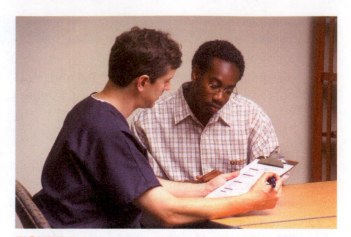

FIGURE 5-6 A medical assistant and patient are in a private area discussing the patient's completed registration/information form

Privacy Notice

After the patient is registered with the medical practice, a privacy notice should be presented to the patient and signed. HIPAA's privacy rule and practices were described in Chapter 3. The privacy notice needs to be posted in the reception room and on the practice's website where patients can easily find it. The medical assistant must be trained in presenting this notice to the patient (Example 5-2).

A privacy officer should be available to discuss the privacy rule with the patient if there are complex questions. A common question is, "Will you release information to my family members?" The answer would be, "The privacy notice addresses to whom your health information may be released." This is a good time to find out whether the patient would like to have a family member or friend listed in case of an emergency or unusual situation. Some computer software allows the date the patient received the privacy notice to be noted

---

EXAMPLE 5-2

Privacy Notice Distribution

Spoken to the patient when handing out the privacy notice: "Federal privacy law requires that we provide this notice to inform you how we will use your health information. It also outlines your rights regarding your own health information. Please sign this acknowledgement to indicate you have received a copy."

on the patient registration screen. This will help document the distribution process. If such software is not available, an area on the patient registration form could be designed to include a receipt statement with date, or a date stamp could be made with the information.

Waiting in Reception Area

After the patient has been registered and the privacy notice obtained, insurance information must be collected. The patient is then seated to wait for the medical assistant to escort him or her to the back office to see the physician. Waiting is expected but should be kept to a minimum. A study has shown that the average person can sit and wait for approximately 20 minutes before getting bored, fidgeting, worrying, or getting angry. Following are ways to ease the tension during long wait times:

- Post a sign in the waiting room that says, "Please approach the reception desk if you have waited more than 15 minutes."
- Keep patient expectations reasonable by including a statement in the waiting room, in the patient brochure, and on the medical practice website that states, "Our goal is to keep all appointments as scheduled, and we know your time is valuable. If a delay occurs we apologize and hope that you will understand that we are trying to accommodate all patients in the time frame allowed."
- Make patients aware of all delays and give options. If a situation occurs causing a delay and the 20-minute threshold is approaching, try to find out what is causing the delay and inform patients how long they can expect to wait before seeing the physician. Be honest! If the wait time is expected to run 30 or more minutes, ask the patient, "Would you like to reschedule, leave to do an errand and return in a half-hour, or continue to wait?" This common courtesy will go a long way toward smoothing patient relationships. Patients will appreciate having choices and being informed.
- In some locations, patients can become aware of wait times by accessing "MedWaittime" on the Internet via computer or mobile device. This site acts as a tool to help medical professionals and their patients communicate. If the office schedule is running late, the receptionist can enter "green, yellow, or red" to correspond to the wait situation and patients can view wait expectations up to 2 hours prior to their scheduled appointment. Physicians using this system can also communicate if

EXAMPLE 5-3

Patients Who Should Not Be Kept Waiting

Patients with:

- Contagious disease
- Continuous coughing
- High fever
- Nausea and vomiting
- Profuse bleeding
- Signs of rash (e.g., chicken pox, measles)
- Syncope (feeling dizzy or faint)
- Visible illness

they accept "walk-in" appointments, and patients can verify appointment times and insurance coverage. There is also an option to sign up for alerts via text or email, and patients can rank and choose participating facilities based on wait times.

Do not ignore patients by shutting the security window, avoiding eye contact, or acting as though you do not know how long they have waited or will have to wait—find out. If a patient becomes disruptive or irate because of a long wait time, escort him or her into an inner office and speak privately.

Example 5-3 lists patients with conditions that should not be kept waiting in the reception area.

Escorting Patients

Generally, patients will arrive and approach the reception desk, check in and fill out paperwork, and then have a seat in the reception area. It is usually the responsibility of the clinical medical assistant to call and direct patients into the treatment area of the physician's office; however, on occasion the administrative medical assistant may need to escort or direct a patient. If you see a patient fumbling with the front door, go assist by holding the door open. If you are working in a large clinic, patients will need to be directed to various departments. Good communication skills should be utilized to give clear directions.

The assistant can reduce the likelihood of a patient misplacing or losing a personal article such as a sweater or purse by suggesting that patients hold their belongings or leave them in a closet with a posted sign stating "Not Responsible for Personal Items." Not all visitors to the medical office will be patients and it may be necessary to screen visitors. Chief complaints need to be obtained from walk-in patients and a physician-endorsed problem list referred to, so proper triage can take place. The clinical medical assistant or physician may need to be advised if the receptionist is not able to determine the urgency of the patient's problem. Family members should be escorted to the location of their relative. Other physicians should be greeted pleasantly and ushered into the back office immediately. Visits from salespeople and pharmaceutical representatives may be handled by the assistant, postponed, or scheduled for another time if the physician is busy.

Patients with Special Needs

Processing a patient with special needs takes skill and forethought. Patients who are *physically impaired* with disabilities that alter their functions or appearance may require preliminary steps from the receptionist to ensure a pleasant atmosphere and an expedited visit. Consider the following when arranging for the arrival of older adult or functionally impaired patients:

- Give consideration when setting up the appointment to allow extra time, a special treatment room, and concern for transportation; reserve time for midday appointments.
- Reserve at-the-door parking.
- Watch for the arrival of the patient and promptly escort him or her into the office after asking whether assistance is needed. By posing this question a direct response is given, and the patient can describe how you can help; this attentiveness conveys a caring attitude.
- Become familiar with mobility devices such as canes, crutches, walkers, or wheelchairs (Figure 5-7). It may be necessary to prepare a place for a wheelchair in the waiting room, provide a footstool for a patient who arrives on crutches, or move furniture to ease navigation.
- Speak to a person with a disability at eye level, if possible, to ensure eye contact. There should be no awkwardness or hesitation when speaking to these patients.
- Verify in the patient's file that an appropriate contact is noted for emergencies.
- Enunciate clearly and speak slowly, especially if the office treats patients from different ethnic

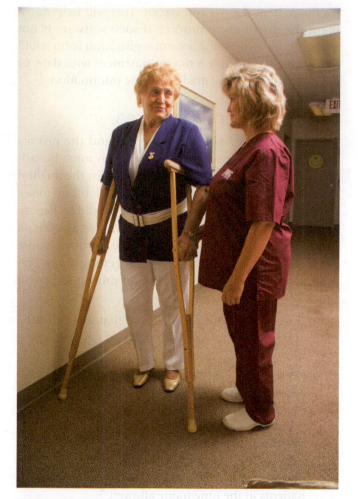

FIGURE 5-7 A medical assistant guiding a patient using crutches

backgrounds. Concentrate on the speaker and do not interrupt.

- Avoid terms that are offensive such as *crippled*, *deformed*, or *handicapped*. More acceptable terms are *people with functional needs*, *disabled*, and *impaired*.
- Provide help in filling out insurance forms in a well-lit area and provide privacy.
- Maintain a warm temperature in examination rooms.
- Keep carpet in good repair and attach handrails where needed, for example, entrance, stairs, by examination chair, and so on.
- Provide information sheets in large print (e.g., surgery aftercare).
- Provide information sheets on special subjects related to geriatric infirmities, such as arthritis and osteoporosis.

- Distribute emergency stickers with the physician's name and telephone number to be attached to the patient's telephone.
- Offer to complete a special parking permit if the patient has a temporary or permanent disability (refer to Procedure 5-3).
- Maintain a file with information on various senior citizen agencies that provide activities, transportation, and senior daycare.
- Provide maps for directions and a list of public transportation services, with schedules.
- Be alert to those patients who may not ask for assistance but have difficulty completing forms and may sign documents that they do not understand.

Disabled Driver Placard or License Plate Form

Form—A patient with physical disability who wishes to park in specially labeled spaces to reduce walking distance to a business or office may obtain a permit by getting a form provided by the Department of Motor Vehicles (Figure 5-8). Most state agencies provide standardized forms to individuals with legitimate physical problems. The physician may be required to provide a complete description of the illness or disability.

Instructing Patients

At the conclusion of the patient's visit, a **patient instruction form** completed by the physician with handwritten short statements will improve compliance by the patient, legally protect the physician because items are in writing (documented), reduce telephone calls, and cement the bond between the physician and patient (Figure 5-9). The form designed by the physician can be developed in a single-page format modified for the particular practice with the patient's identifying data (i.e., name, date of appointment, and diagnosis) and a checklist of topics that can include:

1. Tests
2. Medications
3. Precautions
4. Expectations
5. Activities to decrease or increase
6. Miscellaneous
7. Date of next appointment

When reviewing physician instructions with a patient, try to make the conversation as private as possible, so other patients cannot hear the exchange. The original form with the physician's signature would be scanned into a computer system or filed in the patient's medical record with a copy given to the patient.

PROCEDURE 5-3

Assist Patients in Preparing an Application Form for a Disabled Person Placard

OBJECTIVE: Assist the patient with a disability in completing a form for a parking placard or plate.

EQUIPMENT/SUPPLIES: Application/statement of facts for disabled person parking placard or plates form, clipboard, and pen or pencil.

DIRECTIONS: Follow these step-by-step directions, which include rationales, to learn this Procedure. Job Skill 5-2 is presented in the *Workbook* to practice this skill.

1. Obtain a form provided by the state for the patient with a physical disability who wishes to park in specially labeled parking spaces. As a courtesy, many medical practices may keep the forms on hand.

2. Hand the patient a pen with the form attached to a clipboard. Use of a clipboard allows the patient to sit comfortably and write on a hard surface.

3. Direct the patient to complete the applicant's section of the form (top area) and to sign and date in the appropriate area. Offer to assist in its completion. Areas may be highlighted for the patient.

4. Ask the patient to make out a check to the Department of Motor Vehicles for the necessary fee.

5. Review the filled-in form for legibility, completeness, and accuracy.

6. Complete the attending physician's statement (bottom portion) and obtain the physician's signature certifying that the patient is temporarily, moderately, or permanently disabled.

7. Make a photocopy of the form before sending it to the Department of Motor Vehicles in your state.

DMV
Nevada Department of Motor Vehicles

555 Wright Way
Carson City, NV 89711
Reno/Sparks/Carson City (775) 684-4DMV (4368)
Las Vegas area (702) 486-4DMV (4368)
Rural Nevada or Out of State (877) 368-7828
www.dmvnv.com

APPLICATION FOR DISABLED PERSONS LICENSE PLATES AND/OR PLACARDS
NRS 482.384

You may select either plates and one (1) placard, or two (2) placards.

☑ Disabled Plates *(permanent disability only)*   Disabled Placard(s) ☑ One ☐ Two

☐ Disabled Motorcycle Plates *(permanent disability only)*   Disabled Motorcycle Sticker ☐ One ☐ Other _____

First time applications for a Disabled Persons license plate or motorcycle sticker must be made in person.

In order to apply for disabled persons license plates or disabled motorcycle stickers(s) your name must appear on the vehicle registration certificate. If your vehicle is currently registered, you have the option of maintaining your current vehicle registration expiration date, or renewing for a full twelve (12) month period. Credit for any unused portion of your current registration is transferable to your disabled license plate registration. In applicable counties, if you are renewing for a full 12-month period, and your previous evidence of compliance with emissions standards was obtained more than 90 days ago, the vehicle must be re-inspected prior to registration. **You must have a permanent disability to qualify for Disabled Persons license plates** *(see description below).*

Please Print or Type

Applicants Name ___Connie_____Pauline_____Raymond_____ __10_/_14_/_20XX__
(Disabled Person)   First   Middle   Last   Date of Birth

Address ___10844 Koala Way, Las Vegas_____ _NV_ __12345__
              Address   City   State   Zip Code

County of Residence ___Clark___ Nevada DL or ID No. ___12345XXX___ Daytime Telephone No (_444_) _258-1229_

Signature of Applicant _____ Date _____

A LICENSED PHYSICIAN MUST COMPLETE THIS PORTION*

As a Physician for the above-named patient, I hereby certify that the applicant:

1. _____ Cannot walk two hundred feet without stopping to rest.

2. __✓___ Cannot walk without the use of a brace, cane, crutch, wheelchair, or other device or another person.

3. _____ Has a cardiac condition to the extent that functional limitations are classified as a Class III or Class IV according to standards adopted by the American Heart Association.

4. _____ Is restricted by a lung disease.

5. _____ Is severely limited in his/her ability to walk because of an arthritic, neurological, or orthopedic condition.

6. _____ Is visually handicapped.

7. _____ Uses portable oxygen.

I further certify that my patient's condition is a:

☐ **Temporary Disability** (6 months or less) Must indicate length of time not to exceed 6 months *beginning* _____
ending _____

☐ **Moderate Disability** (reversible but disabled longer than 6 months)
Must indicate length of time not to exceed 2 years *beginning* _____ *ending* _____

☑ **Permanent Disability** (irreversible, permanently disabled in his/her ability to walk, certification is valid indefinitely).

Please Print or Type

Physician's Name ___Jonathan Bojorquez, MD_____

Mailing Address ___56390 Broadway_____ _Las Vegas_ _NV_ __12345__
                        Address   City   State   Zip Code

Physicians License Number _N2402X_____ Telephone No (_444_) _967-4001_

Physicians Signature ___Jonathan Bojorquez, MD_____ Date ___2/12/XX___

* Physicians Assistant Certified (PA-C) or Advanced Practice Nurse (APN) are not authorized to complete this document.

SP27 (Rev 4/2007)

Courtesy of the Nevada Department of Motor Vehicles

FIGURE 5-8 Application/statement of facts for disabled person parking placard or plates completed by the patient and attending physician

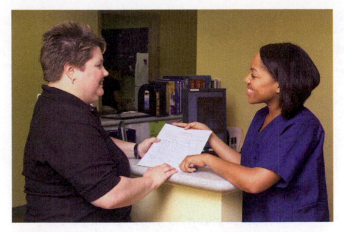

FIGURE 5-9 A medical assistant and patient reviewing a patient instruction form that was completed by the physician

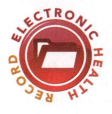

A patient instruction feature is often included in an electronic health record software program. Physician-approved instructions may be selected from a "drop-down list" within the computer program, or you may compose your own and type them directly into an open window. Record in the EHR when the instructions were provided to the patient; this may occur automatically when the instructions are generated.

Community Resources

National, state, county, city, and private agencies offer programs and resources about health maintenance, diet and nutrition, disease prevention, support groups, and various types of assistance that can be of value to patients. Local resources vary from city to city. Following are some examples of **community resources:**

- Alternatives to Violence
- Brain Injury Association
- Children's Speech and Reading Therapy
- Convalescent and Rehabilitation Care
- Disabled Resource Services
- Elder Care
- Food and Nutrition Information Center or Academy of Nutrition and Dietetics
- Hospice Care
- Meals on Wheels
- Support groups for various diseases (e.g., Alzheimer's Association, American Heart Association, American Diabetes Association, Multiple Sclerosis Society, and so forth)
- Twelve-step recovery groups (e.g., Alcoholics Anonymous, Anorexics and Bulimics Anonymous, Depressed Anonymous, Gamblers Anonymous, Narcotics Anonymous, Sex Addicts Anonymous, and so forth)
- Visiting Nurses

The list goes on and on. Patients may need referrals to various resource agencies, so it is wise to determine which agency contact information the physician would like you to have on hand. You may obtain this information by looking in the telephone directory or on the Internet. You may also want to contact a local social service agency or the local news press office as they may publish such a list. Refer to Procedure 5-4 for guidelines on developing a list of community resources.

RECEPTION AREA

The first area that people see when they enter a physician's office is the reception room. Create a welcoming area, a place where people will want to spend time when waiting for appointments. It should be well designed, meticulously maintained, and attractive.

Patients often spend more time in the reception room with the staff than in the examining room with the physician; for this reason, a clean appearance and an atmosphere of relaxation are desirable (Figure 5-10).

A counter with a window or shoulder-high shield assists to secure privacy and security. If the reception room is separated from the office by a sliding window, a

COMPLIANCE

Incidental Disclosures

Health care providers are permitted to talk with others even if there is a possibility of being overheard. This is referred to as an *incidental disclosure.* It is permissible to discuss a patient's condition or laboratory test results over the telephone, in a joint treatment area, or in a semi-private room with the patient, a provider, or a family member. When sharing protected health information (PHI) in these situations, use lowered voices or talk away from others. Exceptions include emergency situations, loud emergency rooms, or cases involving the hearing impaired.

PROCEDURE 5-4

Develop a List of Community Resources

OBJECTIVE: Create a current list of local resources related to patient health care needs.

EQUIPMENT/SUPPLIES: Telephone and telephone directory or computer with Internet connection and printer; paper and pen or pencil.

DIRECTIONS: Follow these step-by-step directions, which include rationales, to learn this procedure. Job Skill 5-3 is presented in the *Workbook* to practice this skill.

1. Determine what resources would be helpful to patients in your medical practice. This would vary depending on the physician's specialty, his or her personal preference, and the average age of patients; you may want to focus on specific areas.

2. After compiling a list, show it to the physician and verify which resource information he or she would like you to make available to patients.

3. Research agencies using:
   a. Telephone and phone directory
   b. Computer with Internet connection (see the *Resources* section at the end of this chapter)
   c. News press listing
   d. Local social service agency

4. Contact agencies to determine:
   a. Correct name or title
   b. Street address, city, and state
   c. Local telephone number
   d. Web page, email address, or other contact information
   e. Hours of operation
   f. Whether information pamphlets are available

5. Compile a list of resources in a computer database, either listing them alphabetically or grouping them into categories. This will depend on the length of the list and type of resources.

6. Ask how the physician would like the list made available to patients (e.g., posted on the bulletin board, compiled in printed form to hand out, used as a desk reference, or made into a PowerPoint presentation that plays on the TV screen in the waiting room).

7. Take on the role of patient navigator to help direct and facilitate patient referral of community resources.

8. Determine a method to follow up on referrals.

9. Verify the information on the list frequently to keep references current.

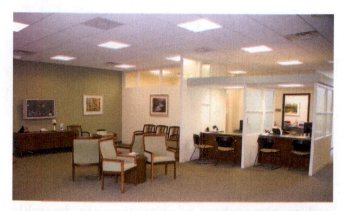

FIGURE 5-10 An inviting and pleasant reception area has seating arranged so that patients are comfortable sitting together or away from other patients

bell should be placed by it so that the medical assistant knows when a patient has arrived. The medical assistant should open and close the window quietly to reduce noise. Some patients react negatively to a closed window because they feel cut off from the staff—it seems to depersonalize the office.

Open reception rooms are acceptable according to HIPAA; however, be sure that patients cannot view computer screens or charts. Protected health information should never be overheard, so private discussions should not take place in waiting rooms or hallways. Portable room dividers may be utilized to add privacy, and privacy filters for computer screens may be used to safeguard documents.

COMPLIANCE
Computer Screen Saver

If the receptionist is frequently called away from the workstation, adjust the timing of the computer screen saver to protect open documents. Most screen savers can be set to come on after 1 to 60 minutes of inactivity. Select a setting by right clicking the mouse while on the desktop. Select "Properties," and then "Screen Saver." Choose how many minutes of time you would like to lapse before the screen saver is activated where it says "Wait ___ minutes."

COMPLIANCE
HIPAA Notice/Sign

A notice should be posted in the reception area explaining the office's HIPAA policy on confidentiality.

Features of the Reception Area

The reception area should include stable but comfortable chairs. Couches may be used, but they are less durable and are not as flexible for seating arrangements. The carpet should be of an industrial type that provides a cushion to walk on, reduces noise, and offers the feel of a comfortable living room. Window dressings should be simple and shades or blinds used to control lighting. The type of furniture, colors, and fabrics vary according to the taste of the physician or designer and create whatever atmosphere is desired. All items should be durable enough to handle large volumes of patient traffic and easy to maintain. A coatrack is a functional item often placed near the outside door where patients may put coats and umbrellas during inclement weather. Following are other features typically found in the reception area.

Business Cards

Business cards for all physicians and physician extenders (nurse practitioner, physician assistant) of the medical group should be available on the reception counter. Sometimes other office personnel (e.g., office manager, bookkeeper, medical insurance biller) also have business cards displayed for patients.

Signs

Signs in the reception area should be simple and direct. They should help people feel welcome as well as advise. A "No Smoking" sign could be displayed in a conspicuous place and a receptacle provided outside to extinguish cigarettes before entering the office.

Air, Temperature, and Lighting

Air should circulate freely in the waiting room. A door or window left ajar, a ceiling fan moving slowly, or air circulating through the air conditioning system can help avoid a stale smell. The temperature should be adjusted so that the thermostat registers between 68 and 72 degrees Fahrenheit and is comfortable to staff members. Be aware of outside temperatures and the way the office is facing (i.e., sunny exposure versus northern exposure), which can affect inside temperatures. Periodically check with patients to see that they are comfortable, and be aware that senior patients and babies may feel a draft or cold when others are comfortable. Lighting should be bright and cheerful to allow for easy reading of materials and viewing of surroundings.

Music

Music from a stereo system or CD player may help create a peaceful atmosphere but should be inoffensive, light, breezy, and quiet so as not to bother anyone—just loud enough to provide a soothing background and calm nerves. Light jazz, classical music, and soft rock are appropriate choices.

Plants and Decorative Items

Plants and terrariums can add decorative accents to the reception area and help create an inviting place for patients to wait. Be careful when adding fresh flowers; although they are beautiful, many flowers emit strong fragrances and can cause allergic reactions. Decorative items such as paintings, sculptures, mobiles, and aquariums provide a focus and add interest to the waiting area.

Reading Material

Reading material that reflects the interests of the patient population should be available in racks or on tables. Select a variety of recent issues of magazines that will appeal to both men and women, young and old, without being controversial or political in nature. Popular

PROCEDURE 5-5

Develop a Patient Education Plan for Diseases or Injuries Related to the Medical Specialty

OBJECTIVE: Formulate and carry out a plan to properly educate patients about treatment of diseases or injuries related to the specialty.

EQUIPMENT/SUPPLIES: Patient information booklet, information pamphlets from professional medical associations, office schedule of physicians and staff, paper, pen or pencil, and bulletin board.

DIRECTIONS: Follow these step-by-step directions, which include rationales, to learn how to develop a patient education plan.

1. Carefully assess the medical practice patients' needs for education.

2. Obtain patient educational devices, for example, information pamphlets from professional medical associations about

diseases and treatments, plastic anatomic models, and pamphlets explaining surgical procedures.

3. Devise methods to educate those patients with disabilities, for example, vision or hearing impaired, limitations of mobility, or language barriers (e.g., audiotapes).

4. Read information so you can be knowledgeable and answer questions.

5. Document information given to the patients in their medical record.

6. Place a suggestion box in the reception room with a short questionnaire requesting patient opinions about the quality of their care, office efficiency, and staff promptness and courtesy.

---

magazines may be brought in by staff or patients, but they should be in good condition with the address labels removed. Patient information pamphlets in the reception area can supply information about the medical practice and brochures can educate patients (see Procedures 5-4 and 5-5) about diseases and other topics such as pregnancy, child rearing, menopause, and so forth (Figure 5-11). See Chapter 19 on designing office brochures.

Food and Drink

Food and drinks may be made available, depending on the type of practice. A water cooler is always welcome and items such as coffee, tea, or even baked goods communicate to patients that they are welcome. Food, however, can easily soil carpet and furniture and should be discouraged in certain reception areas.

Television

Television programs playing constantly disrupt the quiet setting of the reception area and should be avoided; it sends the message that you expect patients to wait. Playing educational materials is acceptable, but the sound should be turned to a low volume so as not to disturb patients who are trying to read or are not interested in listening.

PATIENT EDUCATION

Disease Pamphlets

To enhance patient education, display health-oriented information pamphlets published by associations, such as the National Kidney Foundation, American Cancer Society, American Red Cross, American Lung Association, or American Health Association (see the *Resources* section at the end of the chapter for contact information). A bulletin board could also be used for this purpose. Patients could read information while waiting and would be encouraged to take the pamphlets home (Figure 5-11), some of which could include pictures of a physician examining children.

Bulletin Board

A bulletin board hung in the reception room can be filled with interesting items for patients to look at; for example, color pictures of the office staff with names and brief biographies. In an obstetrician's office, color pictures of new mothers and their infants would be appropriate. A colorful wall map to guide patients to

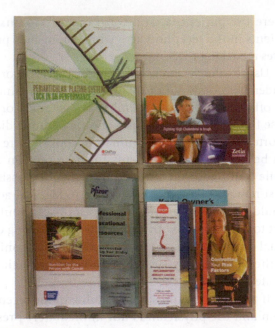

FIGURE 5-11 Brochures and handouts should be accessible and inviting to patients and office visitors

local laboratories and testing facilities would simplify directing patients to other sites.

In a multiphysician group, items tacked to the bulletin board might include new office schedules for physicians and staff, letters from patients, announcement cards, and newspaper clippings that have been date-stamped. It can be divided into sections for each physician so that reminders, articles, and notes for each one can be written or pinned on it. Check the bulletin board at least once a week to discard outdated material.

Children's Toys, Puzzles, and Books

Toys and puzzles help entertain children and are best placed in an activity center or corner of the room, so children do not disturb other patients while playing. Do not select noisy or active toys. Disinfect or sanitize items on a regular basis and be sure to avoid ones that are easily breakable and small toys or ones that can be pulled apart and swallowed. Cover all accessible light switch plates and place electric cords behind furniture, so they are not accessible to children. Select and view all items in the reception area with safety in mind and consider all ages when choosing books and playthings. Remember, the best feature of any waiting room is an immediate acknowledgment and friendly welcome when people arrive.

Maintaining the Reception Area

If a medical office is orderly and immaculately clean, patients will associate its cleanliness with good medical

practices. Many medical offices contract with private cleaning agencies or janitorial services to clean their facilities (see Chapter 19, *Office Managerial Responsibilities*) but regular light cleaning is usually left up to the office staff.

Divide housekeeping chores equitably among all office personnel so that no one person will feel imposed on, and the result will be an accident-free, sanitary office for both the patients and the staff.

Housekeeping Tasks

The medical assistant's housekeeping responsibilities begin where those of the cleaning service leave off. The medical assistant is assigned housekeeping duties to create a comfortable place for patients to wait, as opposed to cleaning the office. However, everything within reach should be polished and dusted by the assistants in an orderly process with items such as mirrors and medical equipment given special attention.

Avoid making patients feel as though someone is picking up after them when stepping into the reception room to straighten magazines, adjust lighting, empty wastebaskets, and arrange furniture. If the office closes for lunch, this would be a good time to freshen up the reception room.

Plants usually need to be watered weekly and fertilized occasionally. An assistant who does not have a green thumb might contact a plant service. Periodicals can be protected from theft and from becoming thumb-worn by placing them in vinyl covers or binders.

Additional housekeeping tasks might include emptying wastebaskets in the front and back office, sweeping the reception room quietly with a carpet sweeper if someone has dropped something, replenishing paper supplies, removing fingerprints from workstation divider windows, and tidying restrooms.

Most housekeeping tasks assigned to the administrative medical assistant are in the outer office, where, for instance, an uncluttered workstation with personal items out of sight should be the rule. To increase desktop space and secure personal items, each staff member may be assigned a drawer, locker, or cupboard that can be locked. Storing office paperwork in a desk drawer or file upon completion is recommended.

Unsightly or dangerous conditions, such as something spilled in any part of the medical facility or debris on the floor, should be attended to immediately by the first staff member to observe it, without regard to who is responsible.

Wear gloves for protection when doing any cleaning, and remove stains when first noticed. Blot the stain, apply cleaning solution, create friction while rubbing, and use cold water instead of hot to rinse the area. If infectious waste such as blood and urine (body fluids) or human waste, which can be dangerous to individuals and the environment, needs to be cleaned up in the reception area, use *universal precautions*, which means that you treat all as if it were infectious. You probably will not have to worry about hazardous waste, such as needles, scalpels, or slides with cultures contaminating the reception room; however, a patient may remove a wound dressing, which would necessitate using universal precautions and following hazardous waste guidelines. Hazardous waste kits may be purchased for such situations and the waste deposited in a biohazard container. Cleaning equipment and supplies are more economically priced if purchased from a wholesaler or discount supplier.

OFFICE SAFETY AND EMERGENCY PREPAREDNESS

We all want a safe and secure working environment, for practitioners, the patients, and ourselves. It is the responsibility of each employee in a medical office to learn about safety laws and regulations, office security, and fire prevention. It is also important to prepare for medical emergencies and disasters that may affect the medical practice and our community. This section covers these topics and helps provide a working knowledge so that you can comply with regulations and assist in these various areas.

Handling a Medical Emergency

The medical receptionist needs to maintain a flexible attitude to be able to adjust on a moment's notice to the unexpected. Reacting calmly in a situation that demands immediate attention includes following planned procedures and is especially important if the reception room is crowded with patients awaiting their own appointments.

Emergency protocols should be established and the administrative assistant may be the staff person to coordinate emergency efforts within an office. If an emergency arises in a treatment room, the clinical assistant would typically notify the receptionist who then calls an ambulance. This frees the clinical medical assistant to assist the physician with the patient until emergency personnel arrive. The receptionist could direct the ambulance to the back door of the office suite, lead emergency personnel to the area

where the patient is, and warn or oversee anxious patients in the reception area while emergency procedures are taking place.

Usually the person who has had an accident or who suddenly becomes seriously ill will be accompanied to the office by an anxious member of the family or by a close friend or neighbor. They should be immediately escorted into an inner examination room where they can be isolated from patients in the reception area. While waiting for the physician, the medical assistant must remain calm, yet show concern. Medical advice should not be given, and verbal responses should be kept to a minimum with conversation conveying emotional support. Relevant medial information confided by the patient may be related to the physician in private.

If a patient should stop breathing in the reception room and the physician is not immediately present, the medical assistant should be prepared to start cardiopulmonary resuscitation (CPR) until other help arrives. First aid training can also help the receptionist be prepared for office emergencies. The American Red Cross and the American Heart Association offer CPR and first aid classes in most local communities. All medical assistants should take these hands-on courses and become certified to a provider level. Continuing education and recertification need to be kept current.

For information about legal issues pertaining to emergency care of patients, see Chapter 3. For information about telephone calls from patients about emergencies, refer to Chapter 6.

Safety and Health Standards (OSHA Compliance)

Safety and health conditions in the medical office are regulated by the Occupational Safety and Health Act administered by the Department of Labor's Occupational Safety and Health Administration (OSHA). Employers must be knowledgeable about all job safety issues and health standards that apply to their work situation. They must be responsible for complying with the Occupational Safety and Health Act's "general duty" clause, Section 5(a)(1), which states that each employer "shall furnish . . . a place of employment which is free from recognized hazards that are causing or are likely to cause death or serious physical harm to his employees." Training to protect the medical staff from on-the-job health and safety hazards and to learn proper disposal of medically related hazardous materials is usually managed by the safety officer, who is often the office manager. This person is also responsible for developing a safety manual and compliance plan, performing inspections, keeping records, and correcting hazards. The safety manual should be located in a designated area, easily accessible to staff. Employees must comply with all rules and regulations, and employers who fail to meet the government standards established by OSHA are subject to fines of thousands of dollars. Offices may be checked for violations by an inspector who arrives unannounced or by advance appointment.

Medical Waste Management

The employer shall ensure the office is maintained in a clean and sanitary condition with a written schedule outlining cleaning and decontamination procedures that will include the following guidelines:

1. All equipment such as pails, bins, receptacles, and work surfaces must be cleaned and decontaminated with an appropriate disinfectant.
2. Any protective covering must be removed and replaced when contaminated.
3. Broken glassware shall not be picked up directly with the hands.
4. Contaminated needles, blades, and glass must be placed in **sharps containers** that are labeled and are closable, puncture-resistant, sturdy, and leakproof (Figure 5-12). They must be located in designated areas, easily accessible to employees, maintained upright during use, and closed immediately prior to moving, storage, or transport.
5. Any regulated waste such as liquid or semiliquid blood or infectious material must be contained and disposed of in a manner ensuring the protection of the employee.
6. Contaminated laundry must be handled as little as possible with a minimum of agitation and a color-coded label attached. It must be bagged or containerized at the location it was used and not sorted or rinsed. Employees handling contaminated laundry must wear gloves or other protective equipment.
7. Waste containers in treatment rooms should be out of reach of children.
8. Waste must be hauled by a registered hauler or an approved person and it must be properly identified.

Federal and state laws affect physicians who generate, store, haul, or treat biohazardous waste. Examples of medical waste include cultures; specimens; blood

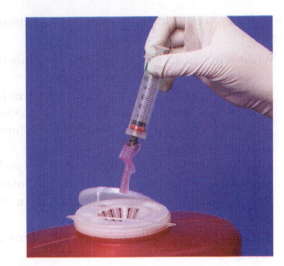

FIGURE 5-12 An approved puncture-proof sharps container is used to dispose of anything sharp such as needles with syringes attached, blades, and glass

products; sharps such as needles, blades, and glass; and items with rigid corners or edges. These waste items might be generated as a result of diagnosis, testing, treatment, and immunization. In some states, physicians are required to register as either a small- or a large-quantity generator. Usually, an accumulation of over 200 pounds of waste per month is considered to be a large generator. (Refer to Chapter 10 about disposal of controlled or uncontrolled substances.)

Waste may be treated on-site or at an approved medical waste treatment facility by incineration, by discharge into a public sewage system if it meets specific requirements, or by steam sterilization.

Some of the specific regulations regarding the medical office staff and outlined by OSHA will be summarized briefly; for more detailed fact sheets, booklets, and guidelines on bloodborne pathogens, contact the nearest state OSHA office or write to OSHA Publications Office, 200 Constitution Avenue, N.W., Room N3101, Washington, DC 20210.

Exposure Control Plan

An employer must have a written plan accessible to employees and updated and reviewed annually to eliminate or minimize employees' exposure to contaminated items.

Any new employee who will be exposed to bloodborne pathogens must receive formal training at the medical practice's expense during regular working hours; current employees who are assigned tasks that risk exposure must also receive training once a year in May.

A control plan would include occupational exposure such as:

- When skin, eye, or mucous membrane comes in contact with blood or infectious materials
- When pathogenic microorganisms are present in human blood that can cause disease in humans, such as hepatitis B virus (HBV) and human immunodeficiency virus (HIV)
- When there can be contact with body fluids such as saliva, semen, or vaginal secretions, or contact with unfixed tissue or organs from a living or dead human
- When accidental needle sticks occur in a clinical setting

Personal Protective Equipment (PPE)

Appropriate personal protective clothing shall be provided by the employer at no cost to the employee with assurance that the protective item is accessible to the employee. When gross contamination is anticipated, a lab coat or gown must be worn. Special protective clothing shall be cleaned, replaced, repaired, or disposed of at no cost to the employee. Gloves must be worn when there is anticipated contact with blood or infectious material or when the medical assistant has broken skin or a wound in the hand area. Gloves must comply with indicated standards, and surgical caps and shoe coverings shall be worn when contamination is anticipated and should be removed before the employee leaves the work area. Masks or eye protection equipment should be worn when droplets or splashes of blood or body fluids might be anticipated.

Immunizations

Hepatitis B is a potentially life-threatening pathogen that is transmitted through exposure to blood or other infectious body fluids and tissues. Employers must offer (free of charge) the hepatitis B virus (HBV) vaccine to all employees who are exposed to blood or other potentially infectious materials as part of their job duties. However, administrative medical assistants are not required to receive this injection.

At-Risk Employee Records

The employer must establish and maintain accurate records for each employee indicating those who are at risk to exposure by bloodborne pathogens or other infectious agents. The confidentiality of all records must be ensured and records must be maintained for the duration of employment plus 30 years. Training records are retained for 5 years and are not confidential; they must include

COMPLIANCE

OSHA and CDC

To comply with the Occupational Safety and Health Administration regulations, employers must display the Department of Labor poster informing employees of the protections of OSHA job safety and health protection guidelines in areas accessible to all employees.

In a medical practice, the employer must also post standard precautions developed by the Centers for Disease Control and Prevention (CDC), which are "minimum infection prevention practices that apply to all patient care, regardless of suspected or confirmed infections status of the patient, in any setting where healthcare is delivered." These include: (1) hand hygiene, (2) use of personal protective equipment, (3) safe injection practices, (4) safe handling of potentially contaminated equipment, and (5) respiratory hygiene/cough etiquette.

training session dates, summary of session, and the trainer's name with qualifications. Training records must be provided by the employer upon request from employees and any work-related injuries or illnesses must be documented on OSHA Form No. 200 and kept on file for 5 years for employee and compliance officer requests.

Ergonomics

Ergonomics is the science of fitting workplace conditions to the capabilities and natural movement of the human body. Working comfortably in a well-designed office without sitting or standing too long, overreaching, or using awkard postures can be achieved with furniture and equipment changes or occasionally redesigning a task. Workstations, treatment rooms, and other work sites in the medical office need to be assessed with ergonomics in mind. Employees need to be trained to comply with recommendations—the goal is optimal safety and productivity. Ergonomic products can be found in most office supply stores. Hand pads on telephones, adjustable standing desks, keyboards, mouse pads or trackballs, and special lighting are some common items that have been ergonomically designed. When the medical assistant works at a computer in one position hour after hour performing repetitive movements, injuries can occur (Figure 5-13). These problems are known as cumulative trauma disorders (CTDs) or

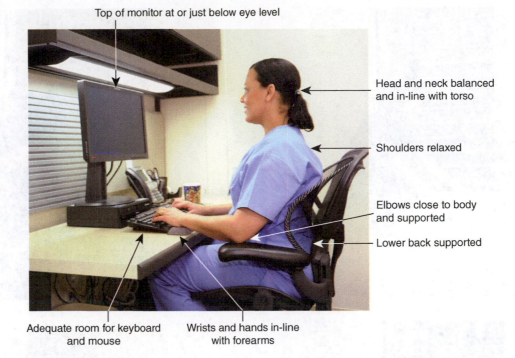

Top of monitor at or just below eye level

Head and neck balanced and in-line with torso

Shoulders relaxed

Elbows close to body and supported

Lower back supported

Adequate room for keyboard and mouse

Wrists and hands in-line with forearms

FIGURE 5-13 Ergonomic workstation illustrating proper computer-operator position to avoid injury and strain to the body

repetitive stress injuries (RSIs). It is important that the computer keyboard have wrist support (Figure 5-14). Other office tasks may require bending and carrying heavy objects. Figures 5-15 and 5-16 illustrate correct methods to execute these movements so that strain and injury to the body do not occur, as well as incorrect methods to avoid. Refer to Procedure 5-6 to learn how to work at a computer station according to ergonomic standards.

Office Security

Medical offices may be the target of theft because of the presence of expensive equipment and drugs. The administrative medical assistant can encourage the entire staff to be aware and take steps to prevent theft. Following are recommended steps to ensure security:

1. Encourage all staff members to keep valuables such as cellular telephones, purses, and cash locked in desk drawers or cabinets to alleviate temptation.
2. Minimize the number of prescription pads to one per doctor and securely lock away remaining pads.
3. Never leave the reception room unattended; leave one or two lights on in the reception area and hallways and close all blinds and curtains tightly at the end of the day.
4. Lock filing cabinets, cash boxes, and cupboards containing medical records, financial records, and controlled substances.

5. Make certain all unattended doors cannot be opened from the outside during the day.
6. Lock office doors and secure all windows if you are the last staff person leaving the office, even if the physician remains on the premises.
7. Leave the office with other staff members after dark.
8. Be alert for loiterers when leaving the office to make a bank deposit; vary times and patterns to avoid predictability.

Other security measures recommended by insurance carriers to keep the facility safe and well protected include using unbreakable mercury and metallic vapor lamps to keep the parking lot well lit; installing cylinder guards

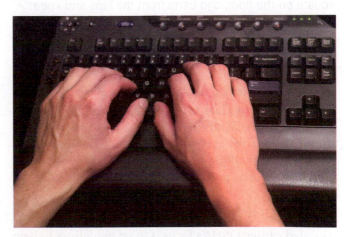

FIGURE 5-14 Keyboard with built-in wrist support

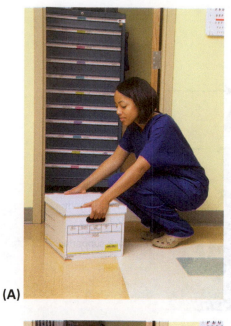

(A)

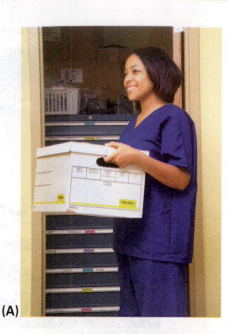

(A)

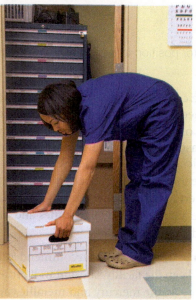

(B)

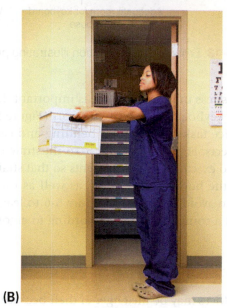

(B)

FIGURE 5-15 (A) Get close to the object, place feet square on the floor, and bend from the hips and knees. Use thigh muscles and lift gradually, keeping your spine straight. (B) Never bend from the waist

FIGURE 5-16 (A) When carrying heavy objects, divide the weight between your hands and hold them close to the body. (B) Never carry heavy objects away from your body

and deadbolts locks, digital coded burglar alarms, and burglar-resistant glass on windows; tracking keys that have been distributed; keeping outside shrubbery trimmed; advertising security measures with alarm company stickers; marking all equipment and computers with identifying marks; and not using a single master key.

Safe Working Environment

As stated earlier, OSHA's focus is to set guidelines to help create and maintain a safe working environment. It is,

however, up to the office management and all employees to implement safe working practices. Following are several areas to focus on when working toward this goal.

Slips, Trips, and Falls

Slipping, tripping, or falling in the workplace can be a common cause of major injury. Such accidents can occur when views are obstructed or where there is poor lighting. Slippery surfaces and wearing wrong footwear (e.g., open-toe or high-heel shoes) are two culprits that

PROCEDURE 5-6

Work at a Computer Station and Comply with Ergonomic Standards

OBJECTIVE: Avoid on-the-job injuries while using a computer by instituting ergonomic principles.

EQUIPMENT/SUPPLIES: Computer terminal with monitor, keyboard, wrist support, office chair, footrest, ergonomic mouse or trackball, and copyholder.

DIRECTIONS: Follow these step-by-step directions, which include rationales, to practice this procedure. This may be done at home or in the classroom.

1. Select an adjustable surface for the computer to sit on. This allows for change in height according to the person's size and will increase productivity.

2. Adjust a properly designed chair to the individual's height and build. This reduces fatigue and tension. Both seat depth and tilt, as well as lumbar support for the chair back, should be considered. Both feet should be flat on the floor. For a short person, a small footstool or telephone book to raise the feet will help avoid back problems.

3. Use a copyholder to place the document at eye level. This prevents fatigue, neck aches, backaches, and eyestrain.

4. Place the computer keyboard low, so the arms relax comfortably. Forearms should be parallel to the floor and wrists kept straight to prevent frozen shoulders and carpal tunnel syndrome. Installation of a hand and wrist support is also useful.

5. Place the computer monitor at or below eye level. It should be approximately 18 to 24 inches from the eyes; charts and written material should be 15 to 20 inches.

6. Turn down the brightness on LCD screens. This helps improve vision and reduce eyestrain. Periodically (i.e., every 10 minutes) focus the eyes on distant objects to eliminate eyestrain.

7. Take frequent breaks, stand up, and periodically do body and wrist stretches. This increases blood flow and decreases fatigue.

8. Apply ice, not heat, to painful areas during office breaks and after work. This prevents inflammation.

---

lead to mishaps. Beware of weather hazards, loose or unanchored rugs or mats, and spills causing wet or oily surfaces. Wrinkled carpet, uncovered cords, room clutter, low drawers left open, and uneven walking surfaces can all cause accidents.

To prevent these types of injuries, wear proper shoes and do not hurry or carry too much; overloading with bulk can be dangerous. Pay attention to where you are walking, especially if you must walk on a wet surface. Go slow and take small steps while keeping a hand free for balance. Use handrails on stairways and avoid bending when seated in a chair with wheels. Always turn on the lights before entering a room and open doors carefully. Keep cabinet drawers closed when not in use and inspect your work area to make sure extension cords or cables are not exposed. Check all rugs to see that they are secured to the floor. Nonskid adhesive strips should be installed on areas that are likely to be slippery. Keep clutter to a minimum, remove obstacles from walkways, and clean up spills immediately. Use a "Wet Floor" sign when needed. Wear long hair up (above the collar) so that it does not get tangled with

equipment or contaminate clean surface areas. Keep personal food items in the kitchen refrigerator, not with drugs or lab specimens.

Electrical Safety

Electricity is a source of possible danger if not used properly. Inspect electrical equipment before using and do not use if the item feels unusually warm to the touch, an unusual noise is heard when turning on, or a burning smell or smoke is noticed.

To prevent an electrical fire and keep from receiving an electrical burn or shock, follow these safety rules:

- *Plugs*—Do not use if the plug does not fit into the outlet or does not have a third grounding prong. Do not remove the third prong, pull on the cord to unplug, or force a plug into an outlet.
- *Cords*—Use approved extension cords for temporary situations only, never permanent. Do not run a cord under a carpet or use if the cord is frayed, cracked, or longer than 10 feet. Turn off equipment if a cord overheats.

- *Power strips and surge protectors*—Use cautiously and do not overload outlets. If the wall is warm to the touch, the outlet is discolored, a circuit breaker flips, a fuse blows, or you notice a burnt smell, call an electrician to have it inspected and request to have a dedicated circuit installed.
- *Light bulbs*—Use only the correct size and wattage for fixtures. Screw bulbs in securely.
- *Wall plates*—Check and replace outlets that are broken, are missing, or have loose-fitting plugs. Childproof all outlets in areas where children might be present.
- *Appliances and equipment*—Do not place appliances or equipment near water or areas that may become wet. Make sure all equipment is properly grounded, and use a ground fault circuit interrupter (GFCI) in such areas to protect against electrocution.
- *Space heaters*—Use space heaters only if absolutely necessary and keep them 3 feet from combustible materials (e.g., clothing, drapes, furniture, rugs). Do not use heaters with extension cords. Turn off and unplug when not in use.
- *Office kitchen*—Keep cooking area clean and clear of combustibles (e.g., food packaging, paper napkins, towels, potholders). Turn off the coffee maker when not in use and unplug it each night before leaving the office. Supervise food when in a microwave. If a fire occurs, keep the door closed and unplug the microwave, or keep the oven door closed and turn off the heat. Have an appropriate fire extinguisher in the area.
- *Special occasions*—Select flame-resistant, flame-retardant, or noncombustible items when decorating the office for holidays. Use UL Mark on light strings; never use candles. Inspect new and old electrical decorations and replace damaged lights while unplugged. Hang lights with proper clips or hooks; do not staple or nail. Do not overload extension cords. Turn off all electrical lights and decorations before leaving the office.
- *Electrical outage*—During an electrical outage, unplug all nonessential equipment to protect it from power surges. Keep a self-powered or battery flashlight (with extra batteries) in every room; do not use candles or the elevator.

Fire Prevention and Safety

According to the American Fire Safety Council, "Each year fires kill more Americans than all natural disasters combined." On an average day, "there are more than

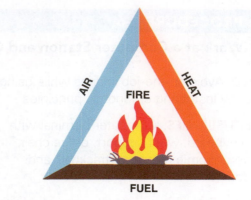

FIGURE 5-17 Fire requires all three sources

200 fires reported in the workplace in the United States." Air (oxygen), ignition (heat), and fuel are the three sources needed to start a fire.

Electrical equipment, hot surfaces, matches, machinery, open flames, smoking, and static electricity are common sources for ignition. Flammable gases (oxygen), liquids (adhesives, chemicals, paint), and solids (foam, packing material, paper, plastics, rubber, wood) are common sources of fuel. Oxygen is always present in the air as well as in oxygen canisters and oxidizing materials that can be found in many medical practices. In physician's offices, look for the following flammable substances and make sure they are stored safely: Acetone, Americlear (histology solvent), ethanol, methanol, isopropyl alcohol, peroxide, xylene, and any products containing the above such as Gram stain crystal violet, decolorizer, and safranin.

Material Safety Data Sheets (MSDS)

Material Safety Data Sheets (MSDS) should be kept on most chemicals and reagents in a medical facility. These sheets can be obtained from the manufacturer or medical supply company. OSHA's Hazard Communication Standard specifies the following information that must be included:

- Identification of chemical product
- Hazard(s) identification
- Composition/information on ingredients
- First-aid measures
- Firefighting measures
- Accidental release measures
- Handling and storage
- Exposure controls/personal protection
- Physical and chemical properties
- Stability and reactivity
- Toxicological information
- Ecological information

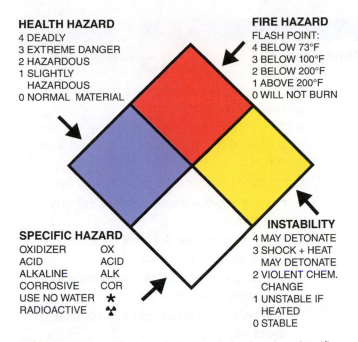

HEALTH HAZARD
4 DEADLY
3 EXTREME DANGER
2 HAZARDOUS
1 SLIGHTLY
  HAZARDOUS
0 NORMAL MATERIAL

FIRE HAZARD
FLASH POINT:
4 BELOW 73°F
3 BELOW 100°F
2 BELOW 200°F
1 ABOVE 200°F
0 WILL NOT BURN

SPECIFIC HAZARD
OXIDIZER   OX
ACID   ACID
ALKALINE   ALK
CORROSIVE   COR
USE NO WATER   ✱
RADIOACTIVE   ☢

INSTABILITY
4 MAY DETONATE
3 SHOCK + HEAT
  MAY DETONATE
2 VIOLENT CHEM.
  CHANGE
1 UNSTABLE IF
  HEATED
0 STABLE

FIGURE 5-18 Hazardous material labels showing classifications of health hazards (blue), fire hazards (red), specific hazards (white), and reactivity (yellow). Numbers (1–4) indicate the level of hazard, the higher the more dangerous.

- Disposal considerations
- Transport information
- Regulatory information
- Other information

MSDS have important information should a product be involved in an accident. They can be alphabetized and kept in a binder for quick reference. Individual sheets can also be placed in a sheet protector and stored near the chemical for emergency use.

Hazardous material labels showing classifications are used to mark products; the higher the number the more dangerous (Figure 5-18). Procedure 5-7 outlines steps to take to minimize the three sources needed to start fires and help prepare in the event of an office fire.

Fire Procedures and Evacuation

In the event of a fire, use the acronym RACER to guide your actions:

R = RESCUE Warn physicians and coworkers of fire and rescue patients and visitors in immediate danger, if safe to do so, while remaining calm. Assess the fire situation.

A = ALARM Activate the alarm by pulling the handle down sharply. Call for help and call 911 or the local fire department.

C = CONFINE Close all doors where fire is located and place wet blankets or towels at the bottom of doors; shut off oxygen valves and remove tanks from the fire area.

E = EXTINGUISH/EVACUATE Use a fire extinguisher to put out small fires. If unsuccessful, refer to the evacuation plan and assist where needed; do not use elevators.

R = RELOCATE Relocate patients from the area of fire to a safe place.

Until the fire department arrives, the person in charge should oversee and manage the emergency by doing the following:

- Send assistance to the fire area, if safe to do so.
- Assign employees to help relocate patients to an area farthest from fire and smoke.
- Evacuate rooms and clearly mark doors with the date and time rooms were cleared.
- Assign employees to clear hallways and exit routes.
- Send an employee outside to meet the fire department.
- Assign supervision of patients needing special attention.

Upon arrival of the fire department, the senior fire authority shall take charge. You may be required to provide critical information, such as location of chemicals and hazardous materials, floor plans, or information related to the cause of the fire.

If you have to evacuate the building because of a fire, get out fast, test doors before opening them, and close doors behind you. If doors are hot, DO NOT ENTER; use another route. Do not stop for anything and crawl low if smoke is present. Do not use an elevator; evacuate by stairs. If your clothes catch on fire, STOP, DROP, and ROLL. If you see someone else whose clothes have caught on fire, throw a blanket or towel over them and direct them to stop, drop, and roll. Once outside, stay outside. Leave the rescue of others in the building to the firefighters.

Fire Protection Systems and Equipment—Most large medical facilities have fire alarms, and all offices should have fire extinguishers. Manufacturer instructions need to be read and kept available for reference. The alarms and extinguishers should be strategically placed around the office; the local fire department can make recommendations. The equipment needs to be inspected, tested, and maintained on a regular basis; this may be performed by qualified staff or a certified/licensed third-party service provider. A log

PROCEDURE 5-7

Prevent and Prepare for Fires in the Workplace

OBJECTIVE: Learn ways to prevent and prepare for medical office fires.

EQUIPMENT/SUPPLIES: Medical office, home, or classroom (can simulate); paper and pen or pencil.

DIRECTIONS: Follow these step-by-step directions, which include rationales, to learn how to reduce the sources needed to start a fire and prepare for the likelihood of an office fire. *Workbook* Job Skill 5-6 is designed to practice this skill.

1. To reduce sources of ignition:
   a. Do not use open flames (e.g., Bunsen burners, candles).
   b. Extinguish any smoldering material (e.g., cigarettes).
   c. Implement a safe-smoking policy in designated areas.
   d. Properly use and maintain heat-producing equipment.
   e. Remove unnecessary sources of heat (e.g., space heaters).

2. To reduce sources of fuel:
   a. Correctly transport, store, and use flammable substances.
   b. Keep flammable substances to a minimum and store highly flammable substances in a fireproof cabinet.
   c. Discard waste materials regularly.
   d. Check furniture with foam upholstery and repair or replace when exposed.

3. To reduce sources of oxygen:
   a. Curb the use and storage of oxygen cylinders.
   b. Check to make sure oxygen canisters are not leaking.
   c. Do not store oxidizing agents near flammable materials or heat sources.

   d. Close doors and windows that are not needed for ventilation.
   e. Turn off ventilation systems that are not essential to the function of the medical office.

4. In the event of an office fire, prepare by:
   a. Posting the fire department telephone number.
   b. Becoming familiar with the location and operation of fire alarms.
   c. Learning the location and operation of all fire extinguishers.
   d. Testing smoke detectors and sprinkler systems.
   e. Developing a floor plan marking the location of fire alarms, fire extinguishers, smoke detectors, stairwells, and routes out of the office.
   f. Memorizing and posting evacuation routes.
   g. Determining evacuation procedures for at-risk patients (e.g., infants, children, pregnant women, persons with disabilities, and older adults).
   h. Ensuring good housekeeping practices (e.g., emptying trash regularly, ensuring exit routes are not blocked, and servicing fire extinguishers annually).
   i. Training employees and practicing fire drills on a random basis and at unexpected times, at least twice a year.
   j. Memorizing the path between your workstation and the nearest exit route, noting the number of doors, desks, workstations, and other objects in case smoke accumulates and you need to exit in the dark.
   k. Establishing a meeting place for all employees in the event of an evacuation.

needs to be maintained with documentation of training, inspections, testing, and maintenance that is available to the fire marshal upon request.

Fire Extinguishers—Fires are classified by type of burning material. Fire extinguishers are designed to put out specific types of fires, and either an alpha system (i.e., A, B, C, D) or picture labels are used to mark the extinguishers. Refer to Table 5-1 for the various types of fire extinguishers and their uses and Procedure 5-8 for guidelines on how to use an extinguisher.

TABLE 5-1 Fire Extinguisher Types and Uses

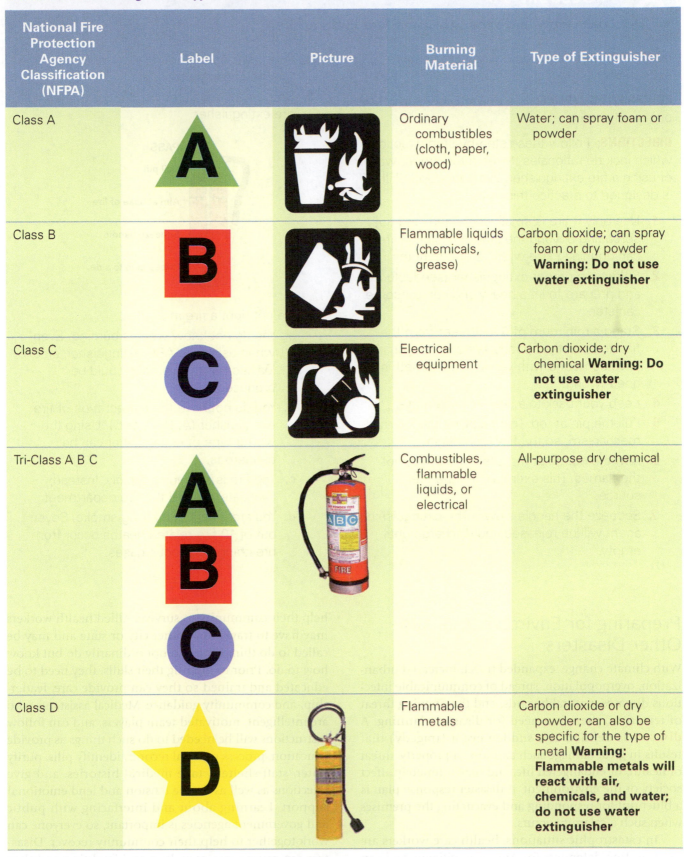

National Fire Protection Agency Classification (NFPA)	Label	Picture	Burning Material	Type of Extinguisher
Class A	A		Ordinary combustibles (cloth, paper, wood)	Water; can spray foam or powder
Class B	B		Flammable liquids (chemicals, grease)	Carbon dioxide; can spray foam or dry powder **Warning: Do not use water extinguisher**
Class C	C		Electrical equipment	Carbon dioxide; dry chemical **Warning: Do not use water extinguisher**
Tri-Class A B C	A B C		Combustibles, flammable liquids, or electrical	All-purpose dry chemical
Class D	D		Flammable metals	Carbon dioxide or dry powder; can also be specific for the type of metal **Warning: Flammable metals will react with air, chemicals, and water; do not use water extinguisher**

PROCEDURE 5-8

Learn How and When to Use a Fire Extinguisher

OBJECTIVE: Learn how and when to use a fire extinguisher.

EQUIPMENT/SUPPLIES: Fire extinguisher and office or school setting.

DIRECTIONS: Follow these step-by-step directions, which include rationales, to learn the proper way of using a fire extinguisher. *Workbook* Job Skill 5-7 is designed to practice this skill.

1. Use only if fire is small, contained, and not spreading beyond the starting point. A fire can double in size within 2 or 3 minutes.

2. Select the proper extinguisher (see Table 5-1) and prepare to lift a heavy and cumbersome canister.

3. Stand a minimum of 6 to 10 feet from the fire and use the "buddy system," so you have someone with you in case something goes wrong.

4. Keep your back to a clear escape route.

5. Pull the pin at top. This releases the locking mechanism, so the flow can begin.

6. Aim the nozzle at the base of the fire, not the flames. This extinguishes the fuel source.

7. Squeeze the handle slowly. The extinguishing agent will be released and discharge until empty.

8. Use a sweeping motion (back and forth) until the fire is completely out.

9. Remember the acronym PASS when using a fire extinguisher.

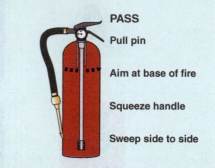

PASS

Pull pin

Aim at base of fire

Squeeze handle

Sweep side to side

10. Do not fight a fire if:

   a. You do not know what is burning. Even when using the ABC extinguisher, an exploa. sion or toxic smoke could be produced.

   b. You do not have the correct type of fire extinguisher (A, B, C, or D). Using the wrong type of extinguisher can be dangerous.

   c. The fire is spreading rapidly. Instead, evacuate and call the fire department.

   d. You are at risk of inhaling smoke. Seven out of 10 fire-related deaths occur from breathing poisonous gases.

Preparing for Environmental and Other Disasters

With climate change, expanded travel, increased urbanization, overpopulation, spread of communicable infectious diseases, natural hazards, and the ongoing threat of terrorism, there is a need for disaster planning. A **disaster** is defined as a sudden event (tragedy) that results in great damage such as a loss of property, threat of health, or endangered life, and may ultimately affect society or the environment. A disaster response plan is a blueprint for responding and evacuating the premises when such a calamity occurs.

In catastrophic situations, health care workers are the frontline defenders for American citizens and can help their community to survive. Allied health workers may have to travel to another city or state and may be called to do things they do not ordinarily do but know how to do. Prior to offering their skills, they need to be educated and trained so they can provide care, leadership, and community guidance. Medical assistants who are intelligent, motivated team players, and can follow instructions will be needed to do such things as provide education, process medical records, identify pills, purify water, staff shelters, take medical histories, and give injections as well as defuse tension and lend emotional support. Learning about and interfacing with public and government agencies is important, so everyone can work together to help their community recover. Disasters can cause mass casualties and fatalities, and they can strike our most vulnerable populations. During disasters, there will not be enough public safety and medical resources; therefore, health care facilities will be overwhelmed.

In a large-scale disaster, you may not be able to rely on technology. You may be called to do things the "old way." Therefore, it is essential to learn fundamental skills and techniques. The principles of triage need to be followed, which focuses on the entire population instead of individual citizens. The key priorities will be to prevent loss of life, "do the most good for the most people," work to alleviate harmful conditions, prevent or minimize property loss, and maintain services if at all possible.

Four core areas that the Federal Emergency Management Agency (FEMA) concentrates on are (1) mitigation/prevention, (2) preparedness, (3) response, and (4) recovery. Refer to Table 5-2 for a listing of potential

disasters. Procedure 5-9 gives guidelines for emergency disaster planning for each of these areas.

Pandemic Emergency

In a **pandemic emergency**, a new infectious virus appears that is capable of being transmitted from human to human (e.g., Ebola virus). The world population will have no or little immunity. Pandemic preparedness involves slowing the spread of the disease by focusing on nonpharmaceutical interventions such as social distancing, isolation or quarantine, and public health education. The World Health Organization (WHO) has a six-phase alarm system used to prepare for and implement during a pandemic emergency.

If a simulated environmental or other disaster event takes place in your community, you may want to volunteer to take part. By acting out real-life disaster

TABLE 5-2 Emergency Disasters and Potential Locations

Disaster	Potential Location
Airplane Accident	Airport or flight pattern
Bioterrorism	Large city
Civil Disturbance	Large city or one that has a large minority population
Earthquake	Structures at risk for collapse (Search FEMA Internet site: "Earthquake Risk by State and Territory")
Explosion	Near ammunition, chemicals, flammable material, natural gas, nuclear energy, or oil wells and rigs
Fire	Near forest or flammable site; potentially, all buildings have some risk
Flooding	Facility downstream from a dam or behind a dike; flooding is the most common hazard in the United States
Hazardous Materials	Near nuclear power plant, industrial facility, dumpsite, or storage area
Hurricane	Near the Gulf of Mexico or on the East Coast
Lightning or Extreme Heat	Areas susceptible to severe weather patterns causing power outage, utilities and phone disruption
Mud Slides	Hillsides or below hillside
Terrorism	Large city
Tornado	Susceptible areas such as the Midwest or South (Search FEMA Internet site: "Wind Zones in the United States" or "Tornado Alley Maps")
Tsunami (Tidal Wave)	On coast or near ocean water, less than 25 feet above sea level and 1 mile from shoreline
Windstorms or Heavy Rains	Areas with vulnerable weather patterns

PROCEDURE 5-9

Develop an Emergency Disaster Plan

OBJECTIVE: Evaluate possible disaster scenarios in your area and prepare for them by establishing a disaster plan.

EQUIPMENT/SUPPLIES: Medical office or school building, library or computer with Internet connection for research and printer; paper and pen or pencil.

DIRECTIONS: Follow these step-by-step directions, which include rationales, to learn how to cope with and respond during a disaster. Job Skill 5-9 is presented in the *Workbook* to practice this skill.

1. Involve all physicians and staff in emergency planning.

2. Determine goals of the emergency disaster plan (e.g., safe evacuation/treatment of staff and patients, quick restoration of business operations).

3. Delegate a responsible employee or student (facility charge person) to oversee emergency planning.

4. Designate teams of employees or students to conduct an analysis of potential hazards that could create a need for an emergency response in your area (see Table 5-2). This information may also be available through your local emergency preparedness agency.

5. Develop an Emergency Operations Plan (EOP) for all identified hazards. Tailor each plan to specific needs according to the hazard analysis. For example:

   • Earthquake safety: Fasten file cabinets and shelving to walls; secure pictures and strap water heater. Move to a safe place, according to the "Triangle of Life" or "Drop, Cover, and Hold On" survival plans.*

   • Floods: Move to higher ground; disconnect electrical equipment and utilities.

6. Review systems that may be lost (e.g., medical building or school damage, road and freeway closure, no electricity or water, satellite services interrupted, and so forth).

7. Assume appointment schedules, patient records, financial data, and other valuable documents may not be accessible, plus employee information and essential contacts such as creditors, insurance carriers, suppliers, utility companies, and so forth; determine how they can be duplicated or backed up and stored and retrieved from a remote location.

8. Develop an emergency kit that includes items to help the practice run smoothly if unable to return to the office (e.g., basic forms, prescription pads, lab request forms).

9. Identify services that will be most used in the emergency.

10. List "safe places" inside and outside the medical facility (e.g., under furniture, against walls, away from glass; away from trees, telephone lines, bridges, and overpasses).

11. Decide on an alternative site (e.g. school) or means of operating if the present site is compromised or destroyed.

12. Determine lines of communication (e.g., employee phone numbers, email addresses, and home addresses used to disseminate information about the disaster quickly).

13. Indicate the means of informing patients and staff of a new location or how the practice is recovering (e.g., staff telephone tree, practice website).

14. Prepare a script for the telephone answering machine to inform patients of why the practice has temporarily shut down, who they should call for medical emergencies, and other pertinent contact information.

15. Locate a facility or housing to be used if quarantine is necessary.

16. Establish procedures for closing of the medical office or campus if necessary.

---

*The "Triangle of Life" and "Drop, Cover, and Hold On" are both survival methodology used in earthquakes.

(continues)

PROCEDURE 5-9 (*continued*)

17. Develop an emergency response template including an evacuation plan to be used for various emergencies. Partial or full evacuation emergencies could include armed intruder, bomb threat, chemical spills, dam or levee failure, explosions, fire, gas leaks, industrial accidents, plane crash, terrorism, and other natural hazards.

    Include such things as:
    - Draw a diagram of the medical office with fire alarms and extinguishers, exits, and escape routes clearly marked.
    - Mark all office or school exits and keep doors unlocked during business hours.
    - Obtain emergency supplies such as blankets, bottled water, gloves, instant hot and cold packs, self-powered or battery-operated radio and flashlights, sturdy shoes, and so forth in addition to clinical supplies (e.g., bandage, splints) and common medications.

18. Identify the role of employees involved in evacuating patients and visitors and define expectations. For example:
    - Each physician's medical assistant will check his or her treatment rooms, shut the door when leaving, mark "empty" with the date and time on the door, and escort those patients to a predetermined safe place.
    - The medical insurance biller and accountant will help "at-risk patients" who may move slower and need special attention.
    - The receptionist will escort all patients from the waiting room to a predetermined safe place.

19. Establish a command post and chain of command.
20. Recognize criteria for calling an end to the emergency and reopening the medical office or campus.
21. Include emergency policies and procedures in the appropriate office manual and conduct training sessions.
22. Calculate how long your practice can survive financially and determine your insurance needs; research coverage for all possible disasters.
23. Coordinate your plan with neighboring businesses.
24. Identify relevant psychological and emotional issues that may be experienced by responders in emergency situations.
25. Investigate state agencies and list community resources that are involved with emergency disaster planning. Review their guidelines so that you can collaborate with disaster experts, for example:
    - American College Health Association
    - American Red Cross
    - Centers for Disease Control and Prevention
    - Department of Health and Human Services
    - Local law enforcement or fire service agencies
    - Medical Reserve Corps
    - State Health Care Department
    - State, county, or local emergency management agencies

situations, you can gain confidence and experience that will help you be prepared should a tragedy strike. The local, city, or county government office of emergency services, the local hospital, or a community college may design mock disaster drills or exercises to train staff and community members.

CLOSING THE MEDICAL OFFICE

In preparing to close the office, make sure all patients have left and follow the guidelines presented in Procedure 5-10.

PROCEDURE 5-10

Close the Medical Office

OBJECTIVE: Close and secure the office at the end of the day in an organized manner.

EQUIPMENT/SUPPLIES: A simulated office setting.

DIRECTIONS: Follow these step-by-step directions, which include rationales, to learn this procedure. You may role-play each step and describe the action and rationale.

1. Straighten the reception area and your desk, if there is time.

2. Organize your desk and restock items, as needed.

3. Print and photocopy a list of the patients to be seen with appointment time, or photocopy the appointment book page to distribute to physicians and staff the following day.

4. Pull charts if medical records are not kept in a computerized system and place in the order of scheduled appointments.

5. Date-stamp the hard-copy progress note and review the medical record to determine studies that were ordered; locate and file results.

6. Call the appropriate facility and make arrangements to have all missing information electronically transmitted or faxed.

7. Pull ledger cards, if financial information is not in the computer system, and place in order of patient appointments.

8. Leave the fax machine on and place in standby mode; make sure it is loaded with paper.

9. Log off computer and shutdown properly.

10. Turn off or unplug all other office equipment, including the coffee maker, to eliminate the chance of an electrical fire.

11. Put cash received in a safe, lock in a secure area, or deposit at the bank.

12. Place files in cabinets. Close and lock drawers, cabinets, and files including areas where drugs are stored.

13. Turn off the photocopy machine and fill with paper.

14. Turn on the answering machine or call the answering service letting them know when you will return and where and how the on-call physician can be reached in an emergency. Notify building security, if necessary.

15. Turn off lights, lock all doors, and activate the security system.

STOP AND THINK CASE SCENARIO

Privacy Protection

SCENARIO: You are sitting at the reception desk and there are two patients sitting in the adjoining waiting room. A new patient appears at her scheduled appointment time and begins asking you questions related to her medical condition.

CRITICAL THINKING: Determine three possible ways you could respond to her in order to protect her privacy without seeming rude or noncaring.

1. _____

_____

2. _____

_____

3. _____

_____

STOP AND THINK CASE SCENARIO

First Impression

SCENARIO: You are the patient and enter a medical office. You notice a faint smell of urine and approach the reception desk where the receptionist is talking on the telephone. She never looks up and you wait at the desk for a few minutes but finally give up and sit down. She keeps talking while chewing gum and you notice her blouse is low cut.

CRITICAL THINKING:

1. What is your first impression of the medical office and the receptionist?

_____

_____

2. How do you feel when the receptionist does not look up to acknowledge you?

_____

_____

3. If you were the receptionist, what would you have done in this situation?

_____

_____

STOP AND THINK CASE SCENARIO

HIPAA Violation versus Incidental Disclosure

SCENARIO A: A patient is waiting in the examination room and overhears the medical assistant speaking in the hallway telling the physician another patient's test results.

SCENARIO B: A waitress overhears the medical assistant telling a friend about a famous actress who visited the medical office today.

CRITICAL THINKING: In each scenario, distinguish the difference between "incidental disclosure" of protected health information and a HIPAA privacy-rule violation. State which it is and explain your reasoning.

A. _____

_____

_____

B. _____

_____

_____

STOP AND THINK CASE SCENARIO

Signs, Symbols, and Labels

SCENARIO: You are working in a medical office and have been introduced in this chapter to a number of signs, symbols, and labels having to do with fire and hazardous material.

CRITICAL THINKING: Consider all locations in and around the medical office and name other signs, symbols, and labels that might be found.

_____

_____

_____

FOCUS ON CERTIFICATION*

CMA (AAMA) Content Summary

- Medical terminology pertaining to the receptionist
- Professional communication and behavior
- Maintaining confidentiality
- Physical environment of the medical office
- Office maintenance (facility, furniture, and equipment)
- Patient information booklet

RMA (AMT) Content Summary

- Medical terminology pertaining to the receptionist
- Patient instruction
- Patient instruction regarding: health and wellness, nutrition, hygiene, treatment and medications,

pre- and postoperative care, body mechanics, personal and physical safety
- Patient brochures and informational materials
- Communicating, greeting, and receiving patients
- Basic emergency triage in coordinating patient arrivals
- Screening visitors and salespersons
- Patient demographic information
- Confidentiality during check-in procedures
- Preparing patient records
- Assisting patients into exam rooms

CMAS (AMT) Content Summary

- Receive and process patients and visitors
- Screening visitors and vendors
- Coordinating patient flow into examinations rooms

REVIEW EXAM-STYLE QUESTIONS

1. The emerging role of the administrative medical assistant serving as a receptionist includes:
   a. knowledge of operative procedures
   b. performing account collection calls at the front desk
   c. assisting the physician in the examination room
   d. serving as a diplomat, a negotiator, a psychologist, and a director of public relations
   e. managing the medical office

2. Two things that are important while performing multiple tasks are:
   a. energy and a desire to accomplish things fast
   b. organizational skills and a calm demeanor
   c. a dynamic personality and professional presentation
   d. a slow, deliberate manner with methodical tendencies
   e. the ability to always stop what you are doing and do whatever is asked of you by whoever asks it

3. After the medical office is opened, the answering machine should:
   a. be turned off during business hours after picking up messages
   b. be left on in case you get busy and cannot get to the telephone
   c. be left for the office manager to pick up all messages; they may be important
   d. be left for the physician to pick up all messages; they might be personal
   e. never be used; an answering service should be used instead

4. When greeting patients, the easiest way to customize requests or comments is to:
   a. ask the question, "How are you today?"
   b. start all conversations with, "Welcome to Dr. Practon's office."
   c. add the patient's name
   d. look straight into the patient's eyes
   e. think of a different phrase to say to each patient, so you never repeat the same phrase in the same day

---

*This textbook *and the accompanying* Workbook *meet the entry-level administrative and general competencies for the CMA outlined by the AAMA Examination Content Outline and Occupational Analysis and for the RMA and CMAS outlined by the AMT Competencies, Construction Parameters, and Examination Specifications (see Competency Grid in Appendix B).*

5. Select the correct statement regarding HIPAA's view of confidentiality in the reception area (waiting room).
   a. It would be nice if confidentiality could be kept in the reception area, but HIPAA understands that you have no control over that area in your office.
   b. HIPAA requires all offices to have a privacy screen or window separating the receptionist from patients in the waiting room.
   c. The one area HIPAA does not address is the reception area of a medical office.
   d. HIPAA forbids calling out of patients' names in the reception area.
   e. HIPAA is as important in the reception area as it is anywhere in the medical practice.

6. Select the correct statement regarding HIPAA's view of patient visit logs.
   a. All sign-in logs are forbidden according to HIPAA.
   b. HIPAA does not address regulations for sign-in logs in medical offices.
   c. Sign-in logs are permitted as long as patients are not prompted to reveal sensitive medical conditions by asking "reason for visit."
   d. Sign-in logs are no longer used in physicians' offices, so HIPAA does not address this issue.
   e. Physicians are being forced by HIPAA to obtain expensive alternatives to sign-in logs.

7. When registering patients who have not been seen in the medical office but who have been treated by your physician at a hospital facility, first obtain:
   a. the patient registration form from the hospital
   b. the history and physical report from the hospital
   c. as much information as possible from all other physicians who have been treating the patient
   d. the face sheet from the hospital admitting office
   e. the face sheet from the surgical unit

8. When appointment delays have occurred and patients are waiting in the reception area:
   a. post a sign that asks them to approach the front desk
   b. give them options so that they can make a decision to wait, return, or reschedule
   c. shut the security window so that you are not disturbed while conducting office business
   d. avoid eye contact because it will incite complaints
   e. both a and b

9. A patient instruction form will:
   a. improve patient compliance
   b. legally protect the physician
   c. reduce telephone calls
   d. cement the bond between the patient and physician
   e. all of the above are correct

10. The best feature of any waiting room is:
    a. cheerful décor
    b. an immediate acknowledgement and friendly welcome when people arrive
    c. stable but comfortable furniture arranged for flexible seating
    d. signs that are simple but direct patients
    e. features such as music, plants, decorative items, reading material, and so forth that give it a special touch

11. Housekeeping tasks in the medical office:
    a. include keeping the reception area neat and clean throughout the day
    b. are all left up to a professional cleaning service, which is usually hired by the office manager
    c. are all performed by the medical assistant acting as receptionist
    d. always include cleaning the office from top to bottom so that it is spotless
    e. are never done by the medical assistant

12. An office emergency:
    a. is always taken care of by the physician and should not involve the administrative medical assistant
    b. includes following planned procedures by the administrative medical assistant
    c. always dictates calling 911 for help
    d. is always handled by the clinical medical assistant
    e. should always involve evacuation of the waiting room by the receptionist

13. OSHA stands for:
    a. Occupational Safety and Health Administration
    b. Occupational Safety and Health Authorities
    c. Oversight Safeguards and Health Acts
    d. Operations Safety and Health Administration
    e. Operations Security and Health Authorities

14. Working at a computer in one position hour after hour performing the same movements over and over can cause injuries referred to as:
    a. repetitive trauma disorders
    b. cumulative stress injuries
    c. repetitive stress injuries
    d. ergonomic injuries
    e. movement disorders

15. Each year, what kills more Americans than all natural disasters combined?
    a. Fires
    b. Tornadoes
    c. Flooding
    d. Hurricanes
    e. Earthquakes

WORKBOOK ASSIGNMENT

To develop competency-based job skills, refer to the *Workbook* and complete the:
- Abbreviation and Spelling Review
- Review Questions

- Critical Thinking Exercises
- Job Skill activities, which are listed at the beginning of the chapter under *Performance Objectives in the Workbook.*

RESOURCES

Internet

Community Resources

Search: Community Resources, which enables you to sort through social service, health, and disability agencies in local areas.

Disaster Center Ranking of Tornado Risk by State

Search: Disaster Center—Tornado, to locate state rankings

Disaster Preparedness
- Use favorite search engine and key terms: Disaster, public health emergency, or mass casualty
- Disaster Kit: Go to FEMA website "ready.gov" for list of supplies

Earthquake Risk by State and Territory (FEMA)

Search: FEMA.gov—earthquake hazard

Federal Trade Commission Protecting America's Consumers
- Red Flags Rule
- Red Flags Clarification Act
- Identity Theft

Hurricane Preparedness

High Wind Risk Areas

Material Safety Data Sheets (MSDS)

United States Department of Labor (recommended format)

Serenity Found

Links for 12-step recovery resources

Journal

Disaster Medicine and Public Health Preparedness

American Medical Association

National Organizations

Alzheimer's Association

Enhance care and support

American Association of Retired Persons (AARP)

Membership benefits

American Cancer Society

Learn about cancer

American Diabetes Association

Risks, complications, and treatment

American Foundation for the Blind (AFB)

Programs and services

American Heart Association
- Mission
- Warning signs

American Lung Association

Lung disease

American Society on Aging (ASA)

Aging in America

Arthritis Foundation Information Line

Living with arthritis

Asthma & Allergy Foundation Hotline

Educational resources

Centers for Disease Control and Prevention

Diseases and conditions

Website: http://www.cdc.gov

Meals on Wheels Association of America (MOWAA)

About senior hunger

Search: Find a Local Program by ZIP code

Mental Health of America

Finding help and treatment information

National Association of Nutrition and Aging Services Programs (NANASP)

Resources and publications

National Center on Elder Abuse (NCEA)

Prevention and detection

National Clearinghouse on Alcohol & Drug Information (NCADI)

Materials, organizations, and agencies

Substance Abuse and Mental Health Services Administration (SAMHSA)

Topics and publications

National Council on the Aging

- Improve health
- Public policy

National Federation for the Blind

Publications and resources

National Institute on Deafness & Other Communication Disorders

A—Z index

National Kidney Foundation

Stages and treatment options

National Stroke Association

Prevention, signs and symptoms, recovery

CHAPTER 6

TELEPHONE PROCEDURES

LEARNING OBJECTIVES

After reading this chapter and learning step-by-step procedures to gain job skills,* you should be able to:

- Communicate effectively over the telephone.
- Be aware of telecommunication devices and operate a 12-button touch-tone telephone.
- State how a cellular telephone is useful in keeping the office in contact with the physician.
- Describe different types of telephone services that can be used in a medical office.
- Place and receive calls using proper telephone guidelines.
- Explain telephone screening and triage protocols.
- Respond appropriately to callers who have specific questions.
- Determine telephone reference aids used in a physician's office.

PERFORMANCE OBJECTIVES (PROCEDURES) IN THIS TEXTBOOK

- Prepare and leave a voice mail message (Procedure 6-1).
- Take messages from an answering service (Procedure 6-2).
- Answer incoming telephone calls (Procedure 6-3).
- Place outgoing telephone calls (Procedure 6-4).
- Screen telephone calls (Procedure 6-5).
- Identify and manage emergency calls (Procedure 6-6).
- Handle a complaint from an angry caller (Procedure 6-7).

PERFORMANCE OBJECTIVES (JOB SKILLS) IN THIS WORKBOOK

- Screen incoming telephone calls (Job Skill 6-1).
- Prepare telephone message forms (Job Skill 6-2).
- Document telephone messages and physician responses (Job Skill 6-3).
- Role-play emergency telephone scenario(s) (Job Skill 6-4).

---

* This textbook and the accompanying Workbook meet the educational components for entry-level administrative and general competencies outlined by CAAHEP and ABHES.

KEY TERMS

answering service

callbacks

cellular telephone

conference call

electronic messaging system

emergency care

protocols

screening

speakerphone

telecommunication

telephone routing decision grid

telephone log

telephone reference aid

time zones

triage

urgent care

voice mail

HEART OF THE HEALTH CARE PROFESSIONAL

Service

The telephone becomes a lifeline to a patient calling in distress. The medical assistant who handles telephone calls can assist in calming the patient and serves as the vital link between the patient and the physician.

PATIENT EDUCATION

General Office Policies

An effective medical assistant informs patients of general office policies such as office hours and direct extension numbers to conduct business. Patients should be encouraged to call the office during designated hours and given directions on where to call if an emergency arises.

COMMUNICATION BY TELEPHONE

The most important public relations responsibility of the medical assistant is to place, receive, and screen telephone calls for the physician in a friendly, efficient, and courteous manner. In fact, it has been said that telephone technique can mean the success or failure of a medical practice (Figure 6-1).

Good listening habits and the ability to interact verbally are two of the most important communication skills demanded of the administrative medical assistant.

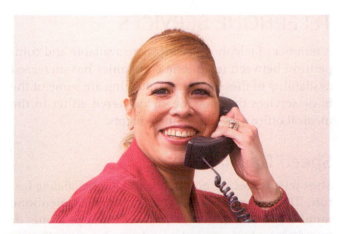

FIGURE 6-1 An administrative medical assistant pleasantly greeting the patient, with a smile in her voice, via the telephone

They become routine only with continued practice. Two exercises that can help develop them are role-playing and tape-recording a conversation and relistening to it to evaluate voice tone, inflection, and clarity. The assistant should cultivate a cheerful and calm voice, speaking as courteously over the telephone as in face-to-face conversation. The manner in which the assistant speaks will determine the caller's response. Listen carefully and take into account patients' limitations. Use the appropriate tone of voice—this will give the caller the assurance that his or her needs will be taken care of.

TELEPHONE EQUIPMENT

To telecommunicate is to transmit voice or data over a distance. The medical office assistant should periodically determine if the office is utilizing the most efficient and cost-effective **telecommunication** devices available. There is a continual need for this because telephones and services change frequently, with new equipment constantly being introduced. Telephone companies and electronic supply businesses will demonstrate and assess the telephone demands of the office. Choice of a telephone system depends on the number of telephone calls the office makes and receives daily, and the number of physicians and staff using the equipment. A multiphysician clinic in a city would need more telephone lines than a one-doctor office in a rural location.

Touch-Tone Telephone

The standard *12-button touch-tone telephone* is arranged with 10 buttons (digits 0–9) plus 2 special buttons, a star (*) and a pound (#), that activate automatic electronic features. As each button is pressed, a tone indicates the number has been sent to the central office equipment.

This type of telephone may also accommodate multiple lines and have additional buttons that may be pressed to place a call, hold a call, transfer a call, signal, or access other office extensions (Figure 6-2). A steady button light indicates a line is in use and a flashing light indicates a line is on hold.

Wireless Headset

A telephone accessory that reduces telephone fatigue and allows you to be more productive is the wireless headset. It allows mobility so you can work, walk, and talk with both hands free. Another benefit is eliminating the need to wedge a telephone receiver between your ear and shoulder, which may result in acute neck, shoulder, upper back, and arm pain.

Cellular Telephone

A **cellular telephone** is a wireless telephone that communicates through cell sites (antenna towers). The caller's and receiver's signals are automatically transferred from cell to cell as they travel. Mountainous or airport areas may cause signal interference. Cellular phone usage has become more popular and many households now have only cellular telephones and no landline phones.

Cellular phones can be used in vehicles and may be permanently installed or portable. Having hands-free operation (e.g., Bluetooth earset, headset, or

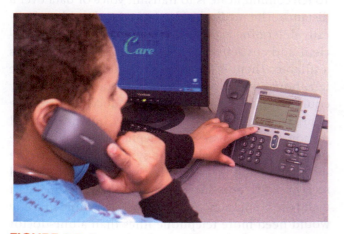

FIGURE 6-2 Example of a multiline telephone system

COMPLIANCE

Cellular Phone Security

Cellular signals are not secure, which means that other people may be able to listen to the conversations with a scanning radio. Therefore, staff and physicians should be very careful *not* to use patients' full names or reveal any confidential information when using a cellular telephone.

speakerphone) is a law in many states and should be used by physicians who take calls in the car.

Physicians have found cellular telephones to be the best tool for maintaining constant contact with their office staff and hospital personnel.

Vibration Mode Pager

The vibration mode on a cellular telephone is used when a ringing telephone would not be appropriate and when privacy is required. The medical assistant may need to contact a physician who is on hospital rounds or who is attending a luncheon business meeting; the caller merely dials the cell number and the phone carried by the doctor vibrates. A text message could also be sent via cellular telephone.

Confidentiality and privacy are better ensured when the vibration mode is used. When the phone vibrates, a physician can leave the current location quietly without interrupting others and conduct the conversation in a private location or use a nearby telephone to return the call.

TELEPHONE SERVICES

A number of telephone services are available and competition between telephone companies has increased availability of these services. Following are some of the basic services that may be encountered either in the medical office or while calling patients.

Speed Dialing

Most telephones are equipped with a *speed dialing* feature. This component electronically stores telephone numbers so that at the touch of a button or a one- or two-digit code, frequently used numbers are directly dialed. The medical assistant, with the physician's input, may determine the most commonly dialed numbers to program into the telephone memory. This listing can be retrieved from memory and displayed for quick access.

Redialing

An automatic *redialing* feature electronically stores the last telephone number dialed, which may be redialed by the push of a button. This redial feature may monitor a busy number for 30 minutes and alert you when the call may be put through.

Call Forwarding

A *call forwarding* feature allows all incoming calls to be automatically directed to another internal station, an outside telephone number, or to voice mail when no one is available to answer the telephone. This service may be turned on and off by dialing a sequence of numbers using activity keys.

Special call forwarding features may have the capacity to forward several (e.g., 12) preselected numbers within your service area to the telephone where you can be reached. All other calls ring as usual and may be routed to voice mail or an answering machine.

Caller ID

Caller ID reveals the name and telephone number of the caller in a display panel before the call is answered. If you need to return a call because you were disconnected or did not obtain the caller's number, or if an emergent patient cannot give you that information, then this feature is helpful. If your system does not have this feature, most local telephone companies provide automatic call return when you dial *69, which dials the last incoming telephone number whether it is answered or not.

Speakerphone

Most telephones have a **speakerphone**. This feature offers hands-free conversation without holding a receiver by using a built-in microphone and speaker. This feature is activated by pushing a button, and then the volume may be adjusted. Speakerphones have many advantages: (1) You can take notes, search for a record in a file, or handle patient charts with both hands while speaking on the phone; (2) you can continue working when placed on hold awaiting an answer; and (3) a group of people can talk using one telephone. However, it is not good policy to initially answer calls

COMPLIANCE

Speakerphone Confidentiality

Etiquette requires that the medical assistant ask whether the caller wishes the call to be on a speakerphone. Medical ethics requires confidentiality. The caller may not want to have the conversation overheard because it may be a private matter.

using the speaker because it infringes on the caller's privacy, often provides a weak connection, and changes the voice quality.

Automated Attendant

Some busy medical practices choose to use an automated answering system that allows all calls to be answered immediately, without busy signals or waiting on hold. The *auto-attendant*, which is voice activated, offers a menu of choices and routes calls to the appropriate person, such as the appointment scheduler, insurance biller, and so forth. Some patients have physical or sensory problems that make using auto-attendant difficult. The option of pressing "0" or saying "customer service" and reaching a live person should always be available.

An automated answering system can offer a menu in several languages. To get the most use out of an automated system, both staff and patients must accept it and use it properly. Following are suggestions for implementing such a system:

1. Advise patients in writing about the system and how it works.
2. Instruct patients clearly on how to select options.
3. Give callers the option to select "medical emergency" right after the medical practice is identified; otherwise, a medical malpractice claim could result.
4. Provide useful options such as "to schedule, change, or cancel an appointment . . .," "to speak to the billing office . . .," "to refill a prescription . . .," and so forth.
5. Allow the option of leaving a message for the physician, but do not provide the option of speaking directly to the physician. A staff person can take messages and relay them to the doctor.
6. Maintain a separate telephone line with an unlisted number for use by other physicians, the hospital staff, and physician personal calls.

Voice Mail

Voice mail is a type of answering system used to store and forward messages for someone who is unavailable. Access to the system may be either an automatic connect or involve entering a code on a touch-tone telephone. A recording tells the caller to dial the voice mail number and to speak after a beep. When the recipient dials into the system, the message is replayed. When the party is not in, always ask the caller whether he or she would like to be connected to voice mail. Voice mail can be an effective way to leave detailed and more complex messages. It allows the medical assistant or other staff members to pick up messages when not busy.

Make sure the voice mail setup has no more than four or five options for mailboxes. These options may be appointment scheduling, insurance and billing, clinical medical assistant, and prescription refills. Voice mail numbers may be printed on the monthly statement or given to frequent callers such as pharmacists, pharmaceutical representatives, relatives, or business callers. Another option might be to give frequent callers a phone number that bypasses the normal menu and puts callers speedily in contact with the mailbox they wish to reach, such as a special pharmacy line.

To reduce telephone traffic to the receptionist, consider voice mail as a backup for receiving messages. An example of a typical voice mail message, activated on the fourth ring, when the assistant is not able to answer the phone might be, "This is Dr. Practon's office. I'm sorry we are away from the desk. Please leave a message after the beep with your name and phone number and we will return your call shortly. Thank you." When a call comes in regarding a prescription refill, the message might be "This is the pharmacy line, which will be monitored at 9 a.m., 11 a.m., 1 p.m., and 3 p.m. If your call is urgent, call 654-7150 or, if an emergency, call 911. Please leave a message with your name, telephone number, the medication you wish to fill or refill, and your choice of pharmacy. Start your message after the beep. Thank you."

Voice Mail Guidelines

If the medical office records voice mail greetings for incoming calls, instructions must be clear to be effective. Review these suggestions before recording greetings:

- Keep the recorded instruction menu short and update the greeting regularly.
- Indicate who to call in the event of an emergency.
- Make certain the calling party can select zero to quickly reach an actual person.

- Ask an employee with a pleasant voice to record the outgoing message.
- Specify in the message when calls will be received and/or returned.
- If the system has an extension directory, be certain it can be verified with the caller before forwarding the call. Example: "You have reached the insurance department, extension 567. If this selection is correct, please press star." This will prevent the caller from being connected to the wrong person.
- For after-hours medically related calls, record a special night message that goes into effect at the close of the day and tells the caller what steps to take.

Leaving a Voice Mail Message

The medical assistant should also be aware of steps to take when preparing to leave a telephone message on a voice mail or answering machine. See Procedure 6-1 for instructions on preparing and leaving a voice mail message and Example 6-1 for a sample message.

Electronic Messaging

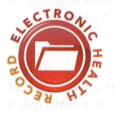

A *total practice management system* (*TPMS*) allows secure messages to be sent via the computer to members of the health care team. This computerized approach is replacing voice mail in many large offices and is referred to as an **electronic messaging system**. When used, the administrative medical assistant who answers the telephone, takes the incoming inquiry, inputs the message into the EHR system, and then sends it to the appropriate staff member (e.g., physician, office manager, clinical medical assistant, insurance biller). An electronic notification is sent to let the staff person know that a message has been received so that action can be taken. Assigning and managing tasks electronically, by using electronic messaging, affects workflow by increasing efficiency.

Answering Service

Most physicians contract with a telephone **answering service** to personalize and handle medical calls when the office is closed. Although some medical offices use an answering service during the lunch hour, use of a staggered lunch hour for staff is preferable. Unlike automatic answering, the answering service operator can execute the physician's telephone directions and be of assistance to patients.

COMPLIANCE

Telephone Voice Mail Confidentiality

The office staff should be aware of some major confidentiality concerns when using voice mail to convey messages. There are safe and unsafe ways to leave a message on a patient's home telephone. Following are some examples:

Specialists' Office: When leaving a message confirming an appointment with a specialist such as an oncologist or cardiologist, the identification of the type of procedure may reveal a lot about the patient and his or her medical problem. In this situation, say, "This is Erma from Dr. Practon's office. Please have Marjorie call me at (555) 486-9002."

Laboratory Test Results: When leaving a voice mail message about laboratory test results, the assistant might say, "(Patient's name) test results are in; please contact our office." This guarantees that someone other than the patient will not hear the actual test results, which the patient may not want divulged.

Highly Confidential Information: Caution needs to be taken when leaving a message for a patient to call the office regarding highly confidential information. To ensure the person being spoken to is the patient,

some practices assign each patient a personal identification code known only to the practice and patient. Then, to get any test results, the patient must first give his or her identification code. By following this protocol, there is a reasonable balance between the protection of confidentiality and meeting the patient's need to access personal information without having to make an office appointment.

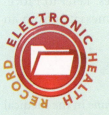

Electronic Transfer of Information: Patients may be requested to sign an authorization to allow the electronic transfer of information, acknowledging that the telephone might not be secure.

Prerecorded Information: Numerous software systems have been designed to maximize the use of the office telephone. One system provides individual test results and follow-up advice recorded by the physician for 24-hour accessibility. Confidentiality is ensured because each patient is assigned a special telephone number to reach the message.

PROCEDURE 6-1

Prepare and Leave a Voice Mail Message

OBJECTIVE: Leave a voice mail message.

EQUIPMENT/SUPPLIES: Telephone, message pad, and pen or pencil.

DIRECTIONS: Follow these step-by-step directions, which include rationales, to learn this procedure. Exercises are presented throughout the *Workbook* to enhance this skill for future practice.

1. Write down and plan the message before placing the call, assuming in advance that the caller cannot be reached.

2. Give your name, the name of the medical practice, and the date and time.

3. State your telephone number *twice* (slowly) because network noise may garble one of the numbers and the person receiving the call may not be able to return the call.

4. Speak clearly and slowly, sounding conversational rather than automatic.

5. Make the message brief and simple, avoiding details and humorous remarks. Never reveal any health information when leaving a voice message.

6. Specify a time when a telephone call may be returned.

EXAMPLE 6-1

Leaving a Voice Mail Message

"This is Jane from Dr. Practon's office and we are trying to contact Glen. If possible, please call our office at (555) 486-9002 (repeat number) today (give date). If Glen is unable to return the call today, please tell him that we called and would like him to return our call as soon as possible. Thank you."

The selection of a competent answering service is very important because charges of negligence can be made by patients against a physician if messages are not transmitted or are incorrectly conveyed. The Yellow Pages of the telephone directory list the names of answering services, and recommendations from other physicians can help determine a reliable service.

To verify that the service is relaying messages and doing the job satisfactorily, a physician might periodically call his or her own office number from another telephone. Since contract fees for a service are based on a predetermined number of calls per month, it is imperative that the medical assistant contacts the service promptly to avoid additional charges. Refer to Procedure 6-2 for instructions on taking messages from an answering service.

Answering Machine

The use of a telephone *answering machine* in the medical office is not recommended because an anxious caller needs personal contact. Usually a new patient will not leave a message. However, if the office uses a machine, the caller should be asked to include his or her name and home, work, and cellular telephone number along with the date and time of the call to verify that the return call has been made within a specific period. The use of an answering machine obligates a return call as soon as possible.

TELEPHONE POLICIES AND PROCEDURES

Training employees in, and advising patients of, telephone policies and procedures is part of the foundation of a medical office. Management consultants have determined that telephone calls to the medical office can be reduced by as much as 30% if patients understand the phone rules, particularly if the procedures have been outlined in an information booklet. To establish telephone policies and determine what information might be included in a patient information booklet, the following questions must be answered:

1. Who will answer telephone calls and who is the backup person?
2. What phrase will be used when answering the telephone to identify the medical practice and person answering?
3. How soon will the telephone be answered and what is the protocol for placing calls on hold?
4. What are the designated times for patients to call the office?
5. When will the physician and other personnel return calls?
6. What telephone number should patients call when the office is closed?
7. Who should patients call in a medical emergency?
8. What type of calls will the physician accept when in the office or when busy seeing patients?

PROCEDURE 6-2

Take Messages from an Answering Service

OBJECTIVES: Retrieve, record, and prioritize messages from an answering service.

EQUIPMENT/SUPPLIES: Telephone, message pad or telephone log, and pen or pencil.

DIRECTIONS: Follow these step-by-step directions, which include rationales, to learn this procedure.

1. Call the answering service and check for messages as soon as the office opens or reopens. Callers expect responses to messages as soon as a business opens.
2. Identify yourself and the practice and say you are calling to obtain messages.
3. Record the messages in the order given.
4. Write down complete information for each message on a message pad or telephone log (name of caller, business affiliation, date, time of call, reason for the call, and home, work, and/or cellular telephone number including area code), so action can be taken and/or return calls made.
5. Confirm the correct spelling of all names and repeat any information that you are unsure of for clarification.
6. Prioritize the messages and deal with urgent calls at once and then respond to or route the rest of the calls.
7. Pull medical records for clinical calls from patients and put the messages and charts in the proper location for staff or physician to respond to.

9. How will messages be taken?
10. What are the telephone extension numbers to call for business matters, such as questions about insurance, financial accounts, or authorizations?
11. What is the protocol the patient should follow to obtain laboratory test results?
12. What is the physician's policy for approving prescription refills by telephone?
13. Does the physician diagnose or give medical instructions by telephone—and if so, what is the fee charged?
14. How will calls be handled when the physician is out of the office or out of town?
15. Will patients be allowed to use the office telephone?

A number of medical practices are increasing their phone availability by answering phones ½ to 1 hour before the office opens, during the lunch hour, and ½ to 1 hour after closing time. This should be decided after analyzing patient calling patterns. Depending on the type of specialty, patients may be more likely to call early in the morning (e.g., OB-GYN, pediatrics, family practice), during the lunch hour (e.g., internal medicine), or late in the day. A telephone traffic study can be done by simply designing a sheet with spaces for each hour; a separate sheet should be made for each day. Check off times when calls are received. Heavy traffic days and hours are best determined when the study has been conducted for at least 6 weeks. The practice may experience seasonal peaks and a high volume of calls after billing statements are sent out.

Telephone Guidelines

Because appointment scheduling requires asking multiple questions, many practices have found that it is best to move the phone responsibilities and appointment scheduling away from the reception desk. Answering the telephone and placing outgoing calls are job skills a medical assistant must master. By practicing Procedures 6-3 and 6-4, you will develop expertise and competence in professional and efficient telephone communication.

PROCEDURE 6-3
Answer Incoming Telephone Calls

OBJECTIVES: Answer the telephone in a physician's office in a proficient manner, take action, and accurately record messages.

EQUIPMENT/SUPPLIES: Telephone, notepad, appointment schedule, and pen or pencil.

DIRECTIONS: Follow these step-by-step directions, which include rationales, to learn this procedure. Exercises are presented throughout the *Workbook* to enhance this skill.

1. Answer an incoming telephone call before the third ring. A telephone that cannot be answered quickly may indicate inadequate staffing or a low priority toward incoming calls. The caller may hang up if the call is not answered in a reasonable amount of time.
2. Smile when answering the telephone and use a friendly, low-pitched voice with the mouthpiece held about an inch from the lips. This procedure aids the caller in clearly hearing your message.

EXAMPLE 6-2

Answering the Telephone

Single Physician

a. "Good morning, Dr. Practon's office, Joan Miller speaking."
b. "Good afternoon, Dr. Practon's office. This is Joan Miller, may I help you?"

Multiphysician Office

a. "Good morning, doctor's office."
b. "Practon Medical Group."

3. Identify the office and yourself (Example 6-2). Most people do not hear the first couple of words, so use a few buffer words to help avoid questions about what office they have reached. By identifying yourself, you will make the patient feel more comfortable and will inform him or her of whom to ask for in future calls.

(continues)

PROCEDURE 6-3 (continued)

4. Listen attentively and obtain the identity of the caller with his or her home, work, and/or cell number. Do not answer questions from people who cannot be identified with certainty. Try not to use one-word responses as this indicates a lack of interest.

5. Repeat the caller's name during the conversation to show attentiveness and personalize the call.

6. Stay alert to what is being said, identify emergency calls, offer assistance, transfer calls when appropriate, and take a message when necessary. Repeat the message to the caller to confirm the facts are accurate and complete. This reduces errors.

7. Be pleasant and friendly, but not too familiar. Speak in a natural, conversational tone and manner. The caller should never feel the call is an intrusion, rushed, or unimportant.

8. Pause for emphasis, avoiding monotone delivery. Speak distinctly and be expressive, pronouncing words carefully.

9. Use the words "please" and "thank you" often.

10. Be prepared to repeat or spell words when unsure or speaking to an older adult patient.

11. Use proper *hold techniques* if a second call should come in on another line. Politely ask the first caller to hold one moment while the other ringing line is answered. Use a notepad to jot down the name and which line the caller is on. Never put an emergency call on hold, and periodically check all calls that are placed on hold to let the caller know you have not forgotten him or her.

12. After the second caller has been identified, prioritize the two callers—an emergency (first), long distance (second), or short message (third). Never leave the caller waiting on the telephone without an explanation or without identifying the caller, as it may be another physician or your employer/physician. Offer to call the patient back if a delay of more than 3 to 5 minutes is anticipated and complete all calls on hold in a timely manner.

13. Screen calls carefully referring to a telephone decision grid when necessary, and to protect a busy schedule; just say, "The doctor is unavailable."

14. Direct any call of a clinical nature to a clinical medical assistant who can obtain pertinent facts and either respond to the caller, relay the message, or route the call to the appropriate physician.

15. Avoid comments and discussions with others while the caller is on the line; this interrupts your focus and conveys a lack of interest.

16. End the telephone call in a pleasant manner by asking if there are any other questions and thanking the caller using his or her name. Concluding the call in this manner conveys professionalism and gives the caller a positive image of the office. Let the caller hang up before you disconnect and replace the receiver gently.

17. Follow through on messages, accurately document the information and action taken on the message form or in the medical record, and route it to the proper person or department. Do not put the message on the physician's desk if it is important and needs action or if the physician will not be in the office that day. Carry through with some predetermined action or follow-up procedure.

PROCEDURE 6-4

Place Outgoing Telephone Calls

OBJECTIVE: Place outgoing telephone calls in a physician's office in a proficient manner.

EQUIPMENT/SUPPLIES: Telephone, notepad, reference documents (test results and/or patient's medical record), and pen or pencil.

DIRECTIONS: Follow these step-by-step directions, which include rationales, to learn this procedure. Exercises are presented throughout the *Workbook* to enhance this skill.

1. Ask patients whether messages can be left at their residence or work and how to do so. Consider developing a form with a list of check-off possibilities, then have patients sign it and place it in their medical record so that their preferences may be followed.

2. Follow established callback routines at prescheduled times. The physician may choose certain times of the day to return calls to eliminate "telephone tag"; that is, calls being made and returned without the parties being able to reach each other. Calls to outside laboratories may be placed in the morning before the office gets busy with patients; calls regarding prescription refills or for appointment reminders may be made at slow times during the day or at the end of the day.

3. Plan the conversation and gather important papers (e.g., authorization, financial documents) and/or the patient's medical record for reference before placing the call.

4. Identify yourself and the office immediately when the party answers the telephone.

5. Identify party at other end.

6. Speak in a congenial but businesslike manner.

7. End each call in a friendly manner and let the other party hang up first.

Telephone Screening

The key to effective telephone control lies in formulating a plan for channeling and prioritizing calls, known as **screening**. Screening involves asking good questions and then following a standardized plan to route calls to the proper person. "Medical assistants are allowed to convey verbatim physician-approved information and directions without exercising independent professional judgment or making clinical assessments or evaluations."[*] The physician should indicate to the medical assistant his or her preference with regard to the transfer of calls. A **telephone routing decision grid** will guide the assistant as calls are screened and transferred (Table 6-1). Follow the steps in Procedure 6-5 to determine what action to take.

Telephone Triage

Triage literally means to sort things out. Telephone triage involves conducting an oral interview to access a patient's health status and to offer treatment or referral. Establishing a good triage system will free up physicians' time and optimize constructive time spent on patient calls by determining whether patients need to be seen today, tomorrow, at a later date, or treated at home. Three levels of triage have been established to ensure accurate decision making (Table 6-2). The risk factors of telephone triage should be identified, strategies established, triage levels understood, and telephone **protocols** (reference instructions) followed. "The general legal principle is that physicians are allowed to delegate screening, but not triage, to competent and knowledgeable medical assistants working under their direct supervision in outpatient settings."[*] All medical decisions are made by the physician, and only by following a strict protocol put in place by the physician would the medical assistant be legally able to make determinations. Always error on the side of caution and document the patient's statement, understanding, compliance, and action taken.

---

*Donald A. Balasa, JD, MBA, Executive Director, Legal Counsel for the American Association of Medical Assistants, CMA Today, Mar-Apr 2012.

TABLE 6-1 Telephone Routing Decision Grid

Type of Call and Referral

Acute Illness or Injury with STAT Referral to MD or NP:

- Bites: animal, human, snake
- Difficulty swallowing, choking
- Foreign object in eye
- Head injury, seizure
- Heat stroke or hypothermia
- High fever, vomiting
- Hospital registered nurse, regarding patient orders
- Hospital surgical unit, regarding patient in post-op
- Internal bleeding (bloody stools, shock)

- Physician's colleague (ask if you need to interrupt the physician)
- Severe pain
- STAT reports
- Sudden onset of critical symptoms (chest pain, breathing difficulty, severe burns)
- Uncontrolled bleeding
- Vehicle collisions (head trauma, neck or back injury)

Routine Calls with Return Call by MD or NP:

- Business calls (attorney, broker, CPA, medical society)
- Hospital surgical unit, regarding patient scheduled for surgery
- New patient, ill, wants to speak to physician
- Patient questions about nonurgent medication side effects

- Patient, under treatment, requests physician's response
- Personal calls from physician's family (ask if urgent)
- Pharmacy regarding new prescription (ask if patient is waiting)
- Requests for test results (positive)

Routine Calls with Referral to Clinical Personnel (RN, LPN, PA, or MA):

- Laboratory and test results
- Patient questions about treatment plan
- Patient or pharmacy regarding prescription refill
- Patient questions about medication

- Patient's family requesting medical information
- Progress reports from patients
- Requests for test results (negative)
- Schedule tests and procedures

Routine Calls with Action Taken by Administrative Medical Assistant:

- Appointments (new, established, cancel, change)
- Fees and billing questions
- Insurance company requesting patient information
- Managed care organization inquiry
- Medical practice questions

- Patient account information
- Pharmaceutical representative
- Referral from another physician's office
- Request for consultation
- Supply sales person

MD = medical doctor   NP = nurse practitioner   RN = registered nurse   LPN = licensed practical nurse   PA = physician's assistant   MA = medical assistant

PATIENT EDUCATION

Office Telephone Procedures

Patients should be given a booklet that outlines office telephone policies and procedures. Advise patients that telephone guidelines are included in this booklet and instruct them according to their level of understanding.

It should be noted that about two-thirds of all incoming calls deal with appointments, health insurance inquiries, financial matters, and requests for laboratory test results, most of which can be handled by the administrative medical assistant or transferred to a staff member.

Telephone Policies in Office Procedure Manual

In a physician's office, the telephone policy section of an office procedure manual should summarize directives and suggest scheduling guidelines to help the

PROCEDURE 6-5

Screen Telephone Calls

OBJECTIVE: Screen incoming telephone calls and route or process according to office policies.

EQUIPMENT/SUPPLIES: Telephone, notepad, reference documents (e.g., telephone decision grid), and pen or pencil.

DIRECTIONS: Follow these step-by-step directions, which include rationales, to learn how to screen telephone calls in a physician's office. Job Skill 6-1 is presented in the *Workbook* to practice this skill.

1. Gather identifying information; identify caller (name and age), relationship to patient, and health plan information.

2. Listen attentively and record what the caller tells you; use quotes, for example, "I have severe stomach pain."

3. Record patient statements regarding objective measures, such as what the patient sees, hears, or records (e.g., blood pressure, temperature, and so on).

4. Record your actions and the patient's compliance with the action plan.

5. If the call is transferred to a clinician, advise the patient of the extension and the name of the person you are transferring the call to along with the basic information.

6. Sign your name with credentials.

7. Document the conversation in the patient's medical record (see Chapter 9).

assistant determine whether and when to schedule an appointment. Any protocol involving assessment of symptoms should be developed and approved by the physician. The administrative medical assistant should be able to determine what action to take after asking three or four pertinent questions; however, if a determination cannot be made, the call should be transferred to a clinical staff member.

Following are suggestions for the telephone section of an office procedure manual:

1. Make the manual user friendly; arrange frequently seen medical conditions with symptoms on individual sheets in alphabetical order for quick reference.

2. Define each medical condition at the top of a sheet in a main heading.

3. Determine level of care and write separate paragraphs describing actions to take for each condition, listing emergencies first for an EMS (911) call, followed by situations when a patient should be seen immediately, seen within 4 hours, seen within 24 hours, and seen within 72 hours.

4. Have physician sign each protocol.

5. Assemble pages in a three-ring notebook for easy replacement or updating; encourage assistants to suggest additions and revisions at staff meetings.

Urgent and Emergent Telephone Calls

Two types of critical situations requiring medical care may arise, and it is important to distinguish the difference between them. The first is urgent care, also known as after-hours care. This involves an urgent situation requiring treatment of injuries or conditions that need prompt medical attention within 24 hours to prevent serious deterioration of a patient's health, but is not life threatening.

The second is emergency care and is a much more critical situation requiring immediate treatment to avoid putting a person's life in danger. Because time is an important element in handling any critical situation, help should be sought immediately.

It is absolutely essential that the medical assistant understand what to do should an emergency arise. In most urgent and emergent situations, the receptionist would not put the call on hold but would transfer the call to the physician, nurse practitioner, or clinical assistant. A note may be delivered to the physician in the treatment room, indicating the caller's name and the nature of the emergency while remaining on the line. Or the call could be transferred immediately to a clinical triage person who could determine the seriousness of the condition and direct the patient to the office or emergency room or advise him or her to call an ambulance immediately.

TABLE 6-2 Telephone Triage Levels and Risk Factors

Triage Level	Risk Factors
Level I: Low Risk Nonclinical (e.g., sore throat, diarrhea, cough)	• Patient problem documented by administrative medical assistant who is competent. • Policy in place for processing calls. • Physician makes decision based on documentation for a low-risk patient. • Nonclinical staff does not make independent decisions. • No triage protocol.
Level II: Urgent (e.g., severe high blood pressure, acute abdominal pain, worsening headache)	• Patient problem documented by trained clinical staff who questions patient regarding problem. • Information given to physician to review and make decision. • All communication documented, including patient's understanding and willingness to comply. • No triage protocol; well-defined triage policies and procedures in place.
Level III: Emergent (e.g., chest pain, loss of vision, suicidal)	• Patient problem documented by clinical staff (a licensed practitioner may be required in some states, e.g., NP, RN, LVN). • Communication skills and written protocol used to determine what instructions are given to patient. • All communication documented; physician to review at later time. • Well-defined written triage protocols in place.
All Triage Levels: (risk factors to consider)	• Cannot visually see patient when using a telephone. • Caller does not give accurate or complete information; it may be misleading. • Caller may not be honest or who they say they are. • Communication problems may exist but not be apparent. • Proper questions may not be asked. • Medical record not accessible to staff. • Documentation not complete. • Staff does not follow policies, procedures, and protocols or act within their scope of practice. • Physician is not consulted appropriately. • Patients get "lost" in system and/or no follow-up provided.
High-Risk Patients	• Those not seen but who make repeated calls. • Those anxious about their symptoms or a child's status. • The very old and very young (older adults, infants, toddlers). • Pregnant patient with concerns. • Self-care home problems. • Those with language barriers or communication problems.
All Triage Levels: Risk management considerations—staff to understand that they:	• Do not provide medical diagnoses. • Do not provide treatment advice. • Give general health information only; otherwise route to physician. • Are expected to know what to do when a situation does not follow exact written protocol. • State who they are (i.e., telephone screener, triage assistant). • Should not ignore or minimize routine complaints. • End all calls by advising patients to call back if symptoms worsen. • Put patients on hold only after determination is made that they do not have a medical emergency. • Understand the three triage categories. • Document all communication including patient's understanding.

When the physician is not in the office, an on-call physician may handle the emergency or contact may be made to the physician's cellular phone. When the physician is out of town and another doctor is covering in his or her absence, the assistant would notify the substitute physician.

It is recommended that all medical assistants attend a cardiopulmonary resuscitation (CPR) class as well as classes on emergency care offered by the American Red Cross or American Heart Association. Certain managed care contracts require that a person certified in CPR be on staff. Some medical problems that threaten life have been previously listed in Table 6-1.

Minor medical problems such as colds, flu, or sore throats are not legitimate medical emergencies unless the patient states that they are. The medical assistant is not the one to decide whether a case is an emergency; the patient usually makes the determination. Yet the assistant might have to stress the need for immediate medical attention in cases where the injured or sick person is unaware of the possible serious consequences. Refer to Procedure 6-6 for instructions on identifying and managing emergency calls.

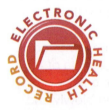

Responses to Typical Telephone Calls

A number of responses involve "pulling the patient's chart," so the medical record is available to refer to. In an office using electronic health records, the patient's EMR would be located using the patient's name or medical record number and brought up on the computer screen. The following are typical phone calls and appropriate responses.

Caller Who Fails to Identify Himself or Herself

Always screen incoming callers who request to speak to the physician. Be sure to obtain the name of the caller and the reason for the call (when appropriate). If the caller does not identify himself or herself, possible responses include those in Example 6-3.

Whether it is an incoming or outgoing call, steps should be taken to properly identify the party with whom you are speaking. Common questions include the patient's birth date or driver's license number. To ensure only authorized callers receive information, some practices assign code numbers or a password to the patient. The first or last three digits of the patient's account

number could be used for this purpose. The patient is then responsible for controlling the number/password and is informed that anyone calling with the number/password will be given information. In a suspicious situation where doubt occurs, ask for a callback number and verify it with the phone number(s) on record. In rare situations, you may need to ask for written authorization or ask the patient to fax the medical practice a document for a signature comparison.

Referral Inquiries

When patients call their physician for names of medical specialists, they should be given two or three names or be referred to the local county medical society for assistance. A referral list should be prepared by the physician and made available to the medical assistant for reference.

Insurance Queries

If a patient wants to talk to the physician about medical insurance, the assistant could give one of the responses in Example 6-4. When calling the insurance company for eligibility verification, the assistant needs to have a copy of both sides of the insurance card in order to know the

PROCEDURE 6-6

Identify and Manage Emergency Calls

OBJECTIVES: Determine whether a telephone call is an emergency and perform the action necessary to get help for the patient.

EQUIPMENT/SUPPLIES: Telephone triage response guide; telephone numbers of emergency rooms, poison control centers, and ambulance services; message pad or telephone log; pen or pencil.

DIRECTIONS: Follow these step-by-step directions, which include rationales, to learn this procedure. Several exercises are presented in the *Workbook* for practice.

1. Allow the caller/patient time to state the problem without interruption.

2. Identify whether the call is regarding an *urgent* or *emergent* situation to determine what action should be taken.

3. Maintain a calm, even, low-pitched tone of voice and take deep breaths; recognize that persons involved in an emergency medical situation may have physical and emotional responses.

4. Use the caller/patient's name when asking specific questions about the patient. This personalizes your conversation.

5. Ask whether the patient has experienced this same problem at a prior time.

6. Ask what is being done for the patient.

7. Obtain information accurately and as quickly as possible, such as:

   a. Caller/patient's name and location of patient with telephone number (home, work, cell) and address. Obtain this first in case the patient loses consciousness or the caller gets disconnected.

   b. Caller's relationship to the patient if the patient is not calling.

   c. Patient's age.

   d. Patient's symptoms fully explained.

   e. Description of the accident or injury.

   f. Explanation of the patient's current status.

   g. Details of any treatment administered.

8. Read back the information to verify and ensure that you have written it down accurately.

9. Interrupt or transfer the call immediately to the physician, clinical assistant, or nurse practitioner for advice. Never diagnose. If the physician is not in the office, follow established office guidelines for handling the emergency call, which may require one or more of the following:

   a. Transfer the call to the doctor on call, clinical assistant, or nurse practitioner. *Never put the caller on hold.*

   b. Have the caller remain on the line and dial 911 to obtain an ambulance for the patient. If the patient is the caller in a true emergency, he or she may become too ill (e.g., pass out) and not be capable of following through with a telephone call. Speak to the EMS dispatcher slowly and clearly. Give the name, exact location of the sick or injured person, and the telephone number.

   c. Instruct the patient to go to the nearest emergency room.

   d. Call the poison control center while the patient remains on the line or give the caller the telephone number of the poison control center.

   e. Contact the physician.

name and telephone number of the insurance carrier, the certificate and group number, and the effective date.

 Starting October 2013, over 8 million previously uninsured individuals applied and are now insured under private health plans through state insurance exchanges offered via the Affordable Care Act. You may receive telephone calls asking if your physician participates in a particular insurance plan. Keep up to date with the health plans your doctor contracts with so that you can readily answer incoming calls regarding plan questions. Refer to Chapter 18 for eligibility requirements for specific insurance types and additional information on this topic.

Prescription Calls

When a patient calls requesting a prescription refill, the assistant needs to know the name and telephone number of the pharmacy the patient patronizes, the name of the medication, dosage the patient is taking, the number of pills last prescribed, and the prescription number. Usually this information may be obtained from the patient or the medical record before the message slip is handed to the physician. In the event the doctor needs to talk to the patient about the renewal or wants the patient to schedule an appointment, the patient's home, work, and/or cellular telephone number should be recorded on the message slip (Figure 6-3). Often office policy instructs the patient to call the pharmacy directly. Refer to Chapter 10 for additional information on this topic.

Caller Who Will Not Terminate Conversation

A medical assistant's office time is precious and if a call turns into a long-winded conversation, it is wise to attempt to bring the call to a close by using one of the responses listed in Example 6-5.

EXAMPLE 6-5

Responses to Conclude a Call

a. "Excuse me, I must end this call to help other patients in the office. Could you please call back after 4:30 p.m. Mrs. Smith?"

b. "I'm sorry, Mr. Brown, but Dr. Practon needs me in the office now. Can I call you back?"

c. "I'm sorry, Mrs. Snyder, but I need to assist another patient now."

Angry Caller Concerned about a Bill or Delinquent Account

A call from an angry patient who is concerned about a bill or delinquent account may be avoided if billing practices have been thoroughly discussed at the time of the first office visit. The response to this call involves extreme patience and usually is the responsibility of the medical assistant—only in extreme situations would the physician be involved in collection matters. A suggested reply is shown in Example 6-6. See also Procedure 6-7.

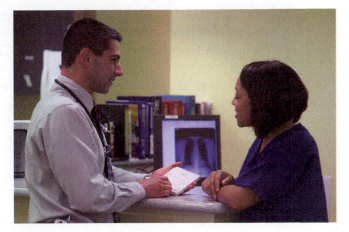

FIGURE 6-3 Prescription telephone messages that need immediate approval should be directed to the physician between seeing patients

---

EXAMPLE 6-6

Response Regarding a Delinquent Account

"Mrs. Black, I'm sorry you are upset about the amount owed on your statement. May I transfer your call to Roberta, who handles Dr. Practon's billing and helps patients make arrangements for settling their accounts?"

Inquiries from Outsiders about Patients

Do not divulge medical information about a patient without the patient's signed authorization; refer to the privacy notice. If it is a family member, the call may be transferred to the physician or you may give the response in Example 6-7.

EXAMPLE 6-7

Response to a Request to Divulge Medical Information

"I'm sorry, Mr. King, according to federal laws I'm not able to give you any information without a signed authorization for release by the patient."

When the Physician Is Not in the Office

If the call is for a physician who is not in the office, refer the caller to the doctor who is on call or ask the caller to leave a message. Some responses are listed in Example 6-8.

PROCEDURE 6-7

Handle a Complaint from an Angry Caller

OBJECTIVE: Respond to a complaint from an angry caller in a professional manner while expressing empathy and taking action to resolve the problem.

EQUIPMENT/SUPPLIES: Telephone, message pad, and pen or pencil.

DIRECTIONS: Follow these step-by-step directions, which include rationales, to learn this procedure.

1. Identify the person's anger and treat it seriously.

2. Slow down your rate of speech and lower your voice (pitch and volume). This practice soothes and calms the angry caller.

3. Remain calm and take time to listen carefully to the caller's complaint. This allows the caller to express the situation, release built-up feelings, and "get it off his or her chest" without forgetting something or having to repeat information.

4. Let the person have a chance to express anger without feeling rushed. Do not interrupt unless it is a medical emergency that must be taken care of immediately.

5. Use helpful phrases (see Example 6-16).

6. Do not monopolize the conversation—the angry person often can suggest the most appropriate solution to a problem if given a chance to verbalize it.

7. Change your physical position (stand up) to regain composure and take deep breaths when the irate caller is upsetting you. One cannot combat anger with anger.

8. Repeat the information to verify that you understand the problem or complaint. This procedure lets the caller know you are listening and fully understand the complaint.

9. Express your concern to help and then take action to resolve the problem or complaint.

10. Document the call and complaint on a notepad to be retained for future reference.

11. If you instruct the caller, ask him or her to repeat the instructions. People who are upset or stressed tend not to listen or comprehend parts of important conversations.

12. End the call in a cordial manner, stating what action you will take. Telephone etiquette states that the person who initiates the call should end the call.

13. Report complaint and/or angry callers to the physician or office manager and document the call and action taken in the medical record. This is important in the event of litigation by a patient or if the physician wishes to follow up with a telephone call to extend more personal service.

EXAMPLE 6-8

Response When Physician Is Not in Office

a. "Dr. Practon was delayed at the hospital, but I expect him shortly."

b. "Dr. Practon is not in the office, but I do expect him to call in soon. Would you care to leave a message?"

c. "Dr. Practon is not in the office. If this is an emergency or an urgent matter, Dr. Benson is on call."

When Another Physician Calls

If the call is from another physician, try to put the call through to the doctor or ask if the physician should be interrupted. Example 6-9 shows a possible response.

EXAMPLE 6-9

Response to a Physician

"Dr. Olivas, Dr. Practon is with a patient right now. Would you like me to interrupt him or have him call you back? If you will be discussing one of the doctor's patients, I would be happy to pull the record for Dr. Practon to refer to."

When the Physician Is Busy

If the call is from a patient requesting to speak to the physician and the physician is busy or behind schedule, obtain the home, work, and/or cellular telephone number so a return call can be made later in the day. Example 6-10 shows a possible response.

EXAMPLE 6-10

Response to Patients

"Mrs. Wells, Dr. Practon is with a patient now. However, I realize your call is important so please give me your telephone number and I'll have your medical record available for Dr. Practon to refer to. You can expect a return call after 4:00 p.m."

Verifying a Statement Made by the Caller

If you do not receive a clear message, always repeat or rephrase it back to the caller for verification. Use one of the suggested responses in Example 6-11.

EXAMPLE 6-11

Response to Verify a Statement

a. "Will you please repeat that?"

b. "I'm sorry, I didn't hear your name."

c. "Will you spell your name again, please?"

d. "Let me see if I understand what you are saying." Then repeat the statement or rephrase it, giving the patient an opportunity to verify it.

Obscene or Crank Call

If you receive an obscene or crank call, either hang up immediately or respond as shown in Example 6-12 if this happens frequently.

EXAMPLE 6-12

Response to an Obscene Call

"Are you there, operator? This is the call I asked you to trace—the party is on the line now."

Complaints

When handling complaints, the assistant needs to listen to the entire problem without interruption. This will allow the assistant to determine the best response, offer a solution, and then follow through on any actions promised (Example 6-13). As a general rule, the louder the caller talks, the softer the assistant should reply. A calm, quiet voice may calm the caller and make him or her listen more attentively to what is being said. If unable to meet the patient's request or needs, the assistant should explain the reason and suggest what can be done (refer to Procedure 6-7 presented earlier).

EXAMPLE 6-13

Response to a Complaint

"I'm sorry, no openings are available on Friday, Mr. Daventia, but I will call you if we have a cancelation."

Personal Calls

When personal calls from family or friends come in for you or a coworker, be specific and helpful, discreet, and truthful (Example 6-14). If the caller indicates it is an urgent matter and the person is busy, slip a note in front of them or interrupt politely.

EXAMPLE 6-14

Response to a Personal Call

"I'm sorry, Mr. Amberly, but Cindy (his wife) is assisting the physician in a treatment room right now. Can I give her a message as soon as she's through?"

Waiting on Hold

A patient who has made an incoming telephone call should not be left waiting on the line. Studies show that two-thirds of telephone callers say being put on hold makes them very angry.

If several lines are ringing and putting someone on hold is unavoidable, identify the caller, ask the person's permission to be put on hold, and do not leave the caller on hold for more than 30 seconds without speaking again, even if it is just to reassure him or her that you have not forgotten the call (Example 6-15). Be appreciative when you return,

PATIENT EDUCATION

Educational Telephone Messages

Play educational messages while telephone callers are on hold. Messages may include office hours, office policies, payment policies, or information on common illnesses that the medical specialist treats.

and if possible, explain briefly to the caller why you had to put him or her on hold. If the assistant must locate a medical chart, financial record, or other document, or the information cannot be quickly accessed on the computer, it is best to inform the patient and suggest a return call. It is acceptable for the assistant to suggest that the patient wait if it will be difficult to return his or her call and if the patient agrees. If it is foreseen that the wait may be more than 5 minutes, take the patient's name and number so the call may be returned.

Transferring Calls

When transferring telephone calls to another extension, give the caller the extension number and name of the person you are transferring the call to. Try to inform the coworker who will be receiving the call the reason for the call. If time allows, give as much information as possible so that the patient does not have to repeat himself or herself. Stay on the line and introduce the patient, if possible, and then release the call.

Example 6-16 offers helpful phrases to use when conversing with a patient over the telephone.

Callbacks

A designated time for routine **callbacks** that is printed in the information brochure reduces the number of incoming calls, since the patient will know when to expect a return call. Patients appreciate knowing their calls will be returned by the physician at an approximate time. Return calls might be made during the last half hour prior to lunch and at day's end when the answering service can pick up the incoming calls and transfer only the emergency calls to the physician.

RECEIVING TELEPHONE CALLS AND MESSAGES

To receive telephone calls from patients and to chart resultant data, the proper procedure is to write messages on callback slips, repositionable adhesive notes, a telephone log, or directly into an EMR. All patient telephone calls regarding treatment should be documented in writing and signed by the physician for transfer into the patient's medical record. Key elements include:

- Date and time of call
- Caller and patient's name with chart number

- Home, work, and/or cellular telephone numbers
- Reason for call; accurate but brief description
- Indicate if "urgent" and process immediately
- Pharmacy name and telephone number (if applicable)
- Action to be taken
- Name and/or initials of message taker

Telephone Message Slips

Numerous types of telephone record pads and booklets are designed for physician offices in many formats and may be purchased at stationery stores or through medical office supply companies. Message slips with no-carbon-required (NCR) paper are available in wire-bound books. One type of repositionable adhesive message slip with a response portion can be placed on the outside of the patient's chart. After the follow-up call has been made and noted, it may be removed from the front of the patient's folder and affixed to either the progress sheet or a telephone message carrier. Other types of message slips may be attached to the front of the patient's charts, then during free moments or at predetermined times, the physician can return calls. In a multiphysician office where telephone lines are often busy, transferring telephone-answering responsibilities to the answering service a few minutes before the noon hour and before the end of office hours (with the understanding that all emergency messages will be put through)

provides an uninterrupted time to follow through on telephone responses. Refer to Figures 6-4 and 6-5 for examples of two types of common message slips.

Telephone Logs

Use of a **telephone log** provides a duplicate copy as a permanent chronologic record; the original with repositionable adhesive may be placed in the patient's chart either on the progress sheet or in chronologic order attached to a telephone message carrier (Figure 6-6). This is known as "shingling." Logs are important for medicolegal reasons, as a reference when patients have unlisted numbers, or when it is necessary to contact a patient on short notice. If a daily log is maintained, the procedure is similar; obtain key elements as mentioned above, and then pull the chart and give both the message and the chart to the physician to prepare answers to questions or requests. Calls in the log that show no action has been taken can be flagged to prevent being overlooked or forgotten.

SPECIAL TELEPHONE CALLS

The majority of telephone calls are local calls; however, depending on the type of practice and location, other types of calls may also be common. The office manager should periodically have the telephone company monitor the practice's telephone traffic to verify the volume

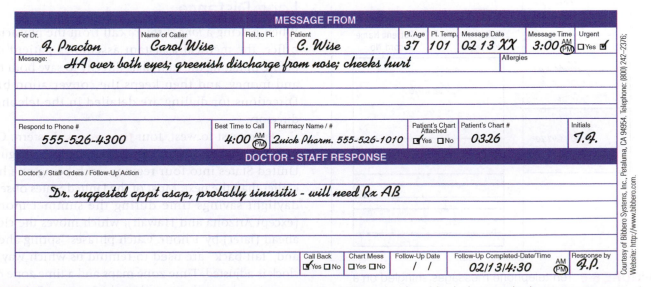

FIGURE 6-4 Repositionable adhesive telephone message slip designed to be shingled on a telephone message carrier sheet or affixed directly to the progress sheet

PATIENT'S NAME	*Robert Mayheu*		
ADDRESS *516 So. Palm Temecula*	INSURANCE	*Medicare*	
TEL. NO *555-423-1127* REFERRED BY ~	OCCUPATION *retired* AGE *66* SEX *M* S Ⓜ W D		

DATE	SUBSEQUENT VISITS AND FINDINGS
08/03/XX	*Office visit-Difficulty breathing + coughing, pain on*
	inhalation slight rales in LLL, Order CXR
	Advise ibuprofen 2 every 4 hours
	F. Practon, M.D.

PRIORITY ☐

PATIENT *Robert Mayheu* AGE *66*	
CALLER " "	
TELEPHONE *555-423-1127*	
PREFERRED TO	
CHART # *4163*	
CHART ATTACHED ☑ YES ☐ NO	
DATE *08/06/XX* TIME RECD BY *W.C.*	

Copyright 1976 Brochero Systems Inc
Printed in USA.

TELEPHONE RECORD ☎

MESSAGE
Pt. Robt Mayhew called to report
he's improving — wants results of X-ray

TEMP *98.6*   ALLERGIES *NKA*

RESPONSE
X-rays negative; continue ibuprofen
until pain is resolved. Call back prn.

PHYSICIAN INTIALS *C.K.*	DATE *08/06/XX*	TIME *4:00pm*	HANDLED BY *W.C.*

FIGURE 6-5 Chronologic telephone message record book slip. Duplicate copy remains in permanent record book and original with repositionable adhesive is filed in the patient's chart.

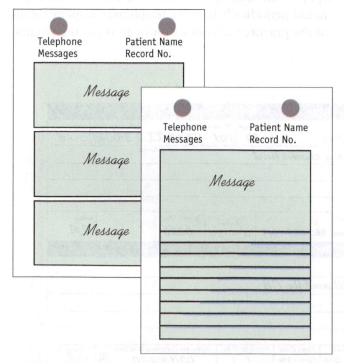

FIGURE 6-6 Ten telephone messages shingled on a message carrier and a full view of three messages affixed to the carrier

of calls, types of calls, and busy signals received. This will aid with decision making when a telephone service plan must be contracted.

Long Distance

When placing a *long-distance* call from the physician's office, the medical assistant assembles patient data before initiating the call, dials directly to save both time and money, and then keeps the conversation brief. Directions for dialing are detailed in the telephone directory.

From east to west, four **time zones**, Eastern, Central, Mountain, and Pacific divide the contiguous United States into four regions, each being one hour earlier than the next. Most of the United States observes daylight savings time during the summer months (except Arizona and Hawaii), which moves the clocks ahead (later) by 1 hour. Catch phrases "spring ahead" and "fall back" are used to remind us which way the clock is adjusted. Time zone maps and a time zone converter may be easily located on the Internet. Refer to the *Resources* section at the end of this chapter.

Some phone plans have discounted or free long distance and telephone records should be kept so that they may be checked against the telephone statement. Other offices block long-distance calls on all telephones except those of the physician and office manager. If "800" or "888" numbers are listed, they should be used instead of calling long distance.

Conference Calls

Occasionally, the physician may seek immediate consultation with specialists concerning treatment for a patient. The conference call, often referred to as *teleconferencing*, is an electronic means of permitting several physicians to consult with one another at the same time from different locations. Most telephones have this electronic capability and one party can arrange the conference call from his or her office. Another method of setting up a conference call is to have the operator connect all parties with the special conference operator, who will, in turn, manually connect them with one another. This type of call is expensive because each call is charged at the operator-handled rate.

International Communications

As *international telephone communication* grows more common, the more likely it becomes that you may speak to someone in another country. The International Communicator's Alphabet provides clarity and ease of understanding when satellite transmission is less than perfect. For example, when saying the name "Brent" you would say, "B as in Bravo, R as in Romeo, E as in Echo, N as in November, and T as in Tango." This alphabet is also standard in voice-input computer systems. Because numeric pronunciations differ internationally as well, recommended pronunciations include spelling the numbers as words. Refer to Table 6-3 to make communications clear when particular words are misunderstood.

TELEPHONE REFERENCE AIDS

A medical office may have many frequently used telephone numbers. To save time, place a comprehensive, alphabetized list of names and telephone numbers near the telephone for reference. Such a telephone reference aid or list might be on a sheet of paper protected with a clear, acetate cover, laminated, or placed under the corner of a glass-covered desk, on a wall near the telephone, or on the side of a filing cabinet—wherever it is handy to see. Alternatively, the list could be in a computer file and easily viewed and updated from time to time. The list could include unlisted numbers and the numbers of hospitals, emergency services, convalescent homes, physicians, staff members, local pharmacies, business machine

TABLE 6-3 International Communications Telephone Aid

International Communicator's Alphabet			International Numerical Pronunciations	
Alpha	**J**uliette	**S**ierra	Zero	0
Bravo	**K**ilo	**T**ango	Wun	1
Charlie	**L**ima (Leema)	**U**niform	Too	2
Delta	**M**ike	**V**ictor	Tree	3
Echo	**N**ovember	**W**hiskey	Foe-er	4
Foxtrot	**O**scar	**X**-ray	Fife	5
Golf	**P**apa	**Y**ankee	Six	6
Hotel	**Q**uebec	**Z**ulu	Seven	7
India	**R**omeo		Ate	8
			Niner	9

repair companies, and physicians designated to take over patient care when the physician is away from the office.

Callback List

Many practices are too large for the physician to have an index listing all patient telephone numbers. If the office is computerized and the physician has a computer station in his or her office, numbers can be accessed via the computerized database. A callback list consists of patients who the physician may wish to call on a regular basis—perhaps for no other reason than to give assurance. The physician who shows a personal interest by occasionally calling patients to inquire about their condition often contributes to their physical improvement. A patient might be on such a list because he or she:

1. Is trying a new medication
2. Has been unresponsive to a prescribed drug
3. Has missed an appointment, a patient usually calls when there is a good reason for missing an appointment; fear and apprehension may be involved when there is no call
4. Is depressed
5. Is experiencing a personal crisis that could affect his or her illness
6. Has seen a consulting physician
7. Has had outpatient surgery, in which case, an inquiry may be made on his or her condition
8. Is on the physician's "worry list," that is, has a condition that the physician is concerned about and wants to monitor closely

---

STOP AND THINK CASE SCENARIO

Respond to Personal Call from Friend

SCENARIO: Office policy states "Do not take personal telephone calls during business hours unless it is a family emergency." A friend who telephones you continually at the medical office calls to discuss an upcoming theater date. Tickets are going fast and the play will be sold out soon.

CRITICAL THINKING: How would you respond to your friend? Compose a personal response.

_____

_____

_____

_____

_____

_____

STOP AND THINK CASE SCENARIO

Evaluate Telephone Equipment

SCENARIO: You are the receptionist answering all incoming telephone calls. The office manager informs you that she will be looking at new telephone equipment and would like your input.

CRITICAL THINKING: What information would you gather to give to the office manager prior to purchasing new telephone equipment? Determine questions that should be answered in order to gather data.

_____

_____

_____

STOP AND THINK CASE SCENARIO
Compose Outgoing Voice Mail Message

SCENARIO: You are the receptionist for Practon Medical Group and the office manager has asked you to record the voice mail message for all incoming calls.

CRITICAL THINKING: Write a script for the message and be prepared to either read it or record it on a tape recorder to be played back to the class.

_____

_____

_____

_____

_____

STOP AND THINK CASE SCENARIO
Prioritize Incoming Telephone Calls

SCENARIO: You are the receptionist answering five incoming telephone lines; assume that 30 seconds after you answer one line the next line starts ringing.

CRITICAL THINKING: Read the scenario for each line and determine what action you will take, either to answer the caller's inquiry, place the call on hold, transfer the call, or tell the caller you will return the call. If the call is placed on hold, determine when you will return to the caller. If you decide to call back, determine the time frame in which you will place the call.

Line 1: A patient is calling for the results of his or her CT scan that was done last week.

_____

_____

Line 2: A surgical patient is calling to make a post-op appointment.

_____

_____

Line 3: A drug representative is calling to see if Dr. Fran Practon is in, and if not, he or she is asking when he or she can make an appointment to see the doctor.

_____

_____

Line 4: An angry patient is calling saying she has been disconnected twice by Dr. Gerald Practon's clinical medical assistant, who she has called to give a requested update on her sick husband.

_____

_____

Line 5: A new patient is calling with questions about the medical practice.

_____

_____

FOCUS ON CERTIFICATION*

CMA (AAMA) Content Summary

- Telephone modalities for incoming and outgoing data
- Prioritizing incoming and outgoing data
- Telephone techniques for incoming calls
- Telephone screening
- Maintaining confidentiality while on the telephone
- Gathering data over the telephone
- Multiple-line competency
- Transferring appropriate calls
- Identifying caller, office, and self
- Taking messages
- Ending telephone calls
- Monitoring special calls (problem calls/emergency calls)

RMA (AMT) Content Summary

- Employ appropriate telephone etiquette
- Perform appropriate telephone techniques
- Instruct patient via telephone
- Inform patients of test results per physician instruction
- Employ active listening skills

CMAS (AMT) Content Summary

- Address and process incoming telephone calls from outside providers, pharmacies, and vendors
- Employ appropriate telephone etiquette when screening patient calls and addressing office business
- Recognize and employ proper protocols for telephone emergencies

REVIEW EXAM-STYLE QUESTIONS

1. To telecommunicate is to:
   a. use a teletypewriter to communicate data
   b. use a computer to communicate data
   c. use the Internet to communicate data
   d. transmit voice or data over a distance
   e. use the telephone to communicate voice

2. Most medical offices will be using a:
   a. cellular telephone
   b. pager
   c. 12-button touch-tone telephone
   d. voice-activated telephone
   e. video phone

3. A telephone service that is a type of answering system used to store and forward messages is:
   a. voice mail
   b. automated attendant
   c. call forwarding
   d. speakerphone
   e. caller ID

4. A speakerphone in the medical office:
   a. should only be used by the physician
   b. should be used only after asking permission from the caller
   c. cannot have the volume adjusted
   d. cannot be used while being placed on hold
   e. cannot be used by more than one person at a time

5. An answering service is preferable to an answering machine because:
   a. answering machines are expensive
   b. you do not have to play back messages
   c. you do not have to listen to patient complaints
   d. they will not break down
   e. they offer personalized handling of medical calls

6. How many levels of triage are there?
   a. 1
   b. 2
   c. 3
   d. 4
   e. 5

---

*This textbook and accompanying Workbook meet the entry-level administrative and general competencies for the CMA outlined by the AAMA Examination Content Outline and Occupational Analysis and for the RMA and CMAS outlined by the AMT Competencies, Construction Parameters, and Examination Specifications (see Competency Grid in Appendix B).

7. Which level of triage represents a "low-risk" problem?
   a. Level I
   b. Level II
   c. Level III
   d. Level IV
   e. Level V

8. When screening a telephone call, it is important to:
   a. ask good questions
   b. gather information
   c. listen and record what the caller tells you
   d. sign your name with credentials
   e. all of the above

9. Some medical problems that threaten life are:
   a. sunburn or skin rash
   b. colds, flu, or sore throats
   c. breathing difficulty, head trauma, and bites
   d. constipation, nosebleeds, and indigestion
   e. headaches, eye aches, and earaches

10. A caller who fails to identify himself or herself but insists on speaking to the physician should be:
    a. disconnected
    b. told to call back
    c. put through to the physician
    d. advised of office policy stating you have to announce each caller to the physician
    e. put through to the office manager

11. When you have a caller who will not terminate the call, it is proper to:
    a. allow him or her to continue; hanging up would be rude
    b. advise him or her that you must terminate the call to tend to other work
    c. listen until he or she stops talking
    d. hang up on him or her
    e. put him or her on hold indefinitely

12. Regarding putting patients on hold, standard practice should be to:
    a. say, "just a minute," and place them on hold
    b. say, "I'm putting you on hold"
    c. say, "I'll be right back"
    d. try not to put patients on hold but if you must, ask their permission first
    e. place them on hold as necessary

WORKBOOK ASSIGNMENT

To develop competency-based job skills, refer to the *Workbook* and complete the:
- Abbreviation and Spelling Review
- Review Questions

- Critical Thinking Exercises
- Job Skill activities, which are listed at the beginning of the chapter under *Performance Objectives in the Workbook*.

RESOURCES

Books

Adult Telephone Protocols, 3rd edition
Thompson MD, FACEP, *David* A.
American Academy of Pediatrics, *2012*

Pediatric Telephone Protocols: Office Version, 14th edition
Schmitt MD, FAAP, Barton D.
American Academy of Pediatrics, 2012

Tele-Nurse: Telephone Triage Protocols
Lafferty/Baird
Delmar Cengage Learning, 2001
Website: http://www.cengagebrain.com

Internet

Time Zones
Search: Time zone maps and time zone calculator

CHAPTER 7

APPOINTMENTS

LEARNING OBJECTIVES

After reading this chapter and learning step-by-step procedures to gain job skills,* you should be able to:

- Discuss various ways an appointment template and matrix can be used.
- Describe how electronic appointments are made via computer.
- List considerations when selecting an appointment book.
- Explain various flow techniques for scheduling appointments.
- State methods of handling various types of problem appointments diplomatically.
- Determine procedures when scheduling convalescent home and house call appointments.
- Identify the requirements for setting up diagnostic tests and therapeutic appointments.
- Choose an appointment card appropriate for the medical practice.
- Explore various appointment reminder systems.

PERFORMANCE OBJECTIVES (PROCEDURES) IN THIS TEXTBOOK

- Prepare an appointment matrix (Procedure 7-1).
- Execute appointment procedures (Procedure 7-2).
- Schedule appointments in a paper-based system (Procedure 7-3).
- Schedule electronic appointments (Procedure 7-4).
- Reorganize patients in an emergency situation (Procedure 7-5).
- Schedule surgery, complete form, and notify the patient (Procedure 7-6).
- Schedule an outpatient diagnostic test (Procedure 7-7).

PERFORMANCE OBJECTIVES (JOB SKILLS) IN THIS WORKBOOK

- Set up appointment matrix (Job Skill 7-1).
- Schedule appointments (Job Skill 7-2).
- Prepare an appointment reference sheet (Job Skill 7-3).
- Complete appointment cards (Job Skill 7-4).
- Abstract information and complete a hospital/surgery scheduling form (Job Skill 7-5).
- Transfer surgery scheduling information to a form letter (Job Skill 7-6).
- Complete requisition forms to schedule outpatient diagnostic tests (Job Skill 7-7).

This textbook and the accompanying Workbook meet the educational components for entry-level administrative and general competencies outlined by CAAHEP and ABHES.

KEY TERMS

appointment and patient care
   abbreviations

appointment block

appointment book

appointment cards

appointment schedule

automated appointment reminder
   system

clustering

computer program

established patient

fixed interval

matrix

modified wave

new patient

no-show

open access

software

stream

template

true wave

HEART OF THE HEALTH CARE PROFESSIONAL

Service

The ultimate art of appointment making is accomplished when the physician's schedule is blended with patients' needs and convenience. Taking these three items into consideration, multiple times in a day, is a challenge. Accomplishing this task is gratifying because the office runs smoothly, you satisfy your employer, and you serve the patients' needs.

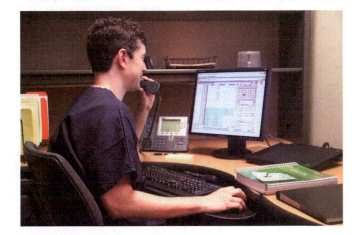

FIGURE 7-1 Medical assistant making an appointment for a patient using computer software

APPOINTMENT SCHEDULE TEMPLATE

In the era of two-career families, children involved in countless activities, and primary care physicians being asked to see more patients in fewer hours, a well-planned **appointment schedule** is essential.

A variety of schedule types will be introduced in this chapter, but a basic schedule consists of a list designating chronological times for patients to meet with the physician and receive medical services.

One of the most important and challenging responsibilities assigned to the medical assistant is coordinating appointments according to fixed time intervals and taking into account patient needs while maintaining a smooth schedule for patients and others who visit the physician (Figure 7-1). This task is made easier if the physician prepares a list of routine services and procedures with an estimate of the time needed for each type of visit. A **template**, which serves as a guide for scheduling various types of appointments, could be created to:

- Indicate each doctor's preferred time frames
- Cut down on decision making

- Allow faster access for new patients
- Provide for urgent and emergent situations
- Decrease patient waiting times

The template is preformatted with a certain number of slots for various types of appointments per hour. For example, one physician may choose to see established patients every 10 minutes with open periods for two new patients in the morning and three in the afternoon. An **established patient** is one who has received professional health care services within the past 3 years from the physician or another physician of the same specialty who belongs to the same group practice. The patient's history would be somewhat familiar to the physician, thus requiring less time. A **new patient** is one who has *not* received any professional services from the physician or another physician of the same specialty who belongs to the same group practice within the past 3 years. Although the new patient may have been seen before by the physician and a history may be on file, if more than 3 years have passed, the physician will need a longer appointment to review the patient's history and get up to date on the patient's current problems.

Selected times could be set aside for routine procedures (e.g., sigmoidoscopies on Tuesdays and Thursdays from 8:00 a.m. to 9:00 a.m.). A list of typical ailments could also be composed by the physician with time intervals needed to treat each problem. The medical assistant can then refer to this template when scheduling patient appointments.

SCHEDULING SYSTEMS

Scheduling systems can be either computerized or manual, and there are a variety of innovative scheduling techniques available. The following questions should be considered when determining what type of system will satisfy office and patient needs:

1. Will the system fit in with the unique demands of the specialty?
2. Will the system offer flexibility?
3. Will the system complement the physician's style and choice of time segments for examining patients and performing procedures?

To determine a scheduling system that not only satisfies patient needs but is also flexible, the staff,

including the physician, should periodically review patient flow by analyzing the schedule for a specific length of time—at least 6 weeks—and then adjust the times for required office procedures to better utilize the physician's time and to provide a smoother patient flow. First, the optimum number of patients that can be seen per day and half day should be determined. This decision is made by the physician. Second, determinations need to be made about how many emergencies or walk-in patients typically occur. Also, carefully consider whether the practice experiences higher volumes on certain days of the week or during certain seasons (e.g., ski season for an orthopedic surgeon). Tracking the schedule for a period of 6 to 12 weeks can help determine these factors and aid in the choice of a scheduling system (Figure 7-2).

 The Affordable Care Act requires all insurance policies to cover a broad range of benefits including preventive medicine services such as screening for breast and colon cancer, cholesterol, depression, diabetes, and substance abuse. Appointment time slots for such services need to be determined and made available for patients.

Appointment Schedule Tracking Grid

Week	Monday	Tuesday	Wednesday	Thursday	Friday	Saturday 1/2 Day
1 (work-ins)	40 ✓✓✓✓✓✓✓	32 ✓✓✓✓✓	31 ✓✓✓	29 ✓✓✓✓	45 ✓✓✓✓✓✓✓	23 ✓✓✓✓✓
2 (work-ins)	36 ✓✓✓✓✓✓✓✓	31 ✓✓✓✓	37 ✓✓✓✓	32 ✓✓	39 ✓✓✓✓✓✓✓	20 ✓✓✓✓✓✓
3 (work-ins)	42 ✓✓✓✓✓✓✓	30 ✓✓✓	29 ✓✓✓✓✓	30 ✓✓✓	42 ✓✓✓✓✓✓	19 ✓✓✓✓
4 (work-ins)	38 ✓✓✓✓✓✓	29 ✓✓✓✓	30 ✓✓✓✓	27 ✓✓✓✓✓	46 ✓✓✓✓✓	25 ✓✓✓✓✓✓✓✓✓✓
5 (work-ins)	33 ✓✓✓✓	33 ✓✓✓✓✓	30 ✓✓✓✓	30 ✓✓✓✓	37 ✓✓✓✓✓	22 ✓✓✓✓✓✓✓✓
6 (work-ins)	39 ✓✓✓✓✓✓✓	35 ✓✓✓	38 ✓✓✓	30 ✓✓✓✓	35 ✓✓✓✓	24 ✓✓✓✓✓✓
Average Daily Appts.	38	31.66	32.5	29.66	40.66	23.83
Work-ins (✓)	High: 8 Low: 4 Avg: 6.5	High: 5 Low: 3 Avg: 4	High: 5 Low: 3 Avg: 3.16	High: 5 Low: 2 Avg: 3.66	High: 7 Low: 4 Avg: 5.5	High: 10 Low: 4 Avg: 6.5
Walk-ins	✓✓				✓	✓✓✓
Emergencies		✓			✓✓	
Cancellations			✓	✓✓		✓
No-shows	✓✓	✓				

FIGURE 7-2 Appointment schedule tracking sheet for a six-week period showing the number of total appointments in one day. Included in the total number are number of appointments that have been worked into the schedule each day (indicated by an "✓") along with the number of walk-ins, emergencies, cancelations, and no-shows

Computerized Appointments

The majority of offices schedule appointments using a computer software program, which is often included in a *total practice management system (TPMS)*. Software is defined as instruction that directs the computer or word processor to perform tasks; it is also referred to as a computer program. Software programs can be developed for a particular type of practice, or a generic program may be purchased. The ideal appointment system will have software that performs key functions according to the unique requirements of a particular practice. The computer system supplier or vendor will assist in installation, training, and support. A good vendor will be available for questions and will assist in using the system to its full potential.

Electronic appointment scheduling may be included with medical billing software and used by a single practitioner; however, it is most useful in clinics or large medical facilities because the system can handle numerous doctors and be accessed from a number of different locations. The computer software program can be used to manage all appointments, free times, days off, and search for available openings in the schedule. For instance, if a patient can come in only on Thursdays at 2:00 p.m., you can insert that criteria and search for the next available time that meets the patient's needs. Such systems can also be used to coordinate and schedule specific treatment rooms and equipment.

An appointment matrix can be set up so that the system can block segments of time when the physician is out of the office and reserve segments of time for specific patient types, services, or procedures. This is referred to as an appointment block. For example, if a consultation requires 45 minutes, the appointment scheduler would search for a 45-minute block and offer that time slot. You can view schedules for multiple providers and practice locations on the same screen and can also keep a list of patients who have requested to be notified if an earlier appointment becomes available.

If the physician wishes to be reminded of personal or professional appointments and to have regularly occurring events scheduled in the appointment calendar, time for all these should be blocked off. If the physician wants personal reminders kept off the appointment calendar but wants to be reminded of such things as outside appointments and scheduled meetings, these may be noted on a monthly desk calendar. Calendars with large squares provide room for physician and office staff reminder notations.

The appointment software can record a patient's appointment on the computer's scheduling calendar, in the patient's electronic medical record (EMR), and in an electronic tickler file, so the medical assistant can send a reminder notice or telephone the patient before the appointment. If a patient calls to find out when the appointment is scheduled, the system can search by name or account number to find the time and date. From the electronic appointment schedule, a daily list of appointments can be printed for each physician (Figure 7-3).

Appointment Book

Choosing an appointment book consisting of lined pages used to schedule and record times set aside for patients to see health care practitioners for procedures or services involves decisions about (1) size, (2) available desktop area, (3) style requirements (taking into consideration how far in advance the appointments are to be made), (4) number of physicians in the group, and (5) medical specialty.

In a group practice, one medical assistant may schedule all the physicians' appointments on a large, multiple-column sheet, often color-coded with a different color for each day of the week and with a physician's name heading each column (Figure 7-4). If standardized columns contain too much or too little space devoted to particular items, self-designed, custom-made appointment sheets may be printed for a three-ring binder at reasonable cost.

Patient Flow Techniques

The goal of the administrative medical assistant serving as a receptionist is to stay on schedule because if the appointment system fails, he or she must deal with irate patients and frustrated physicians. The choice of scheduling methods depends on the size and specialty of the practice, the number of physicians in the practice, and the doctors' preferences, so consider these factors and the goal of maintaining smooth patient flow with a minimum of waiting time as you evaluate the following scheduling systems.

Stream Schedule

Most doctors' offices use stream or fixed interval scheduling (Figure 7-5), which gives each patient a specific appointment time. Patients seen for the first time are usually assigned 45- to 60-minute appointments, whereas follow-up examinations are scheduled every

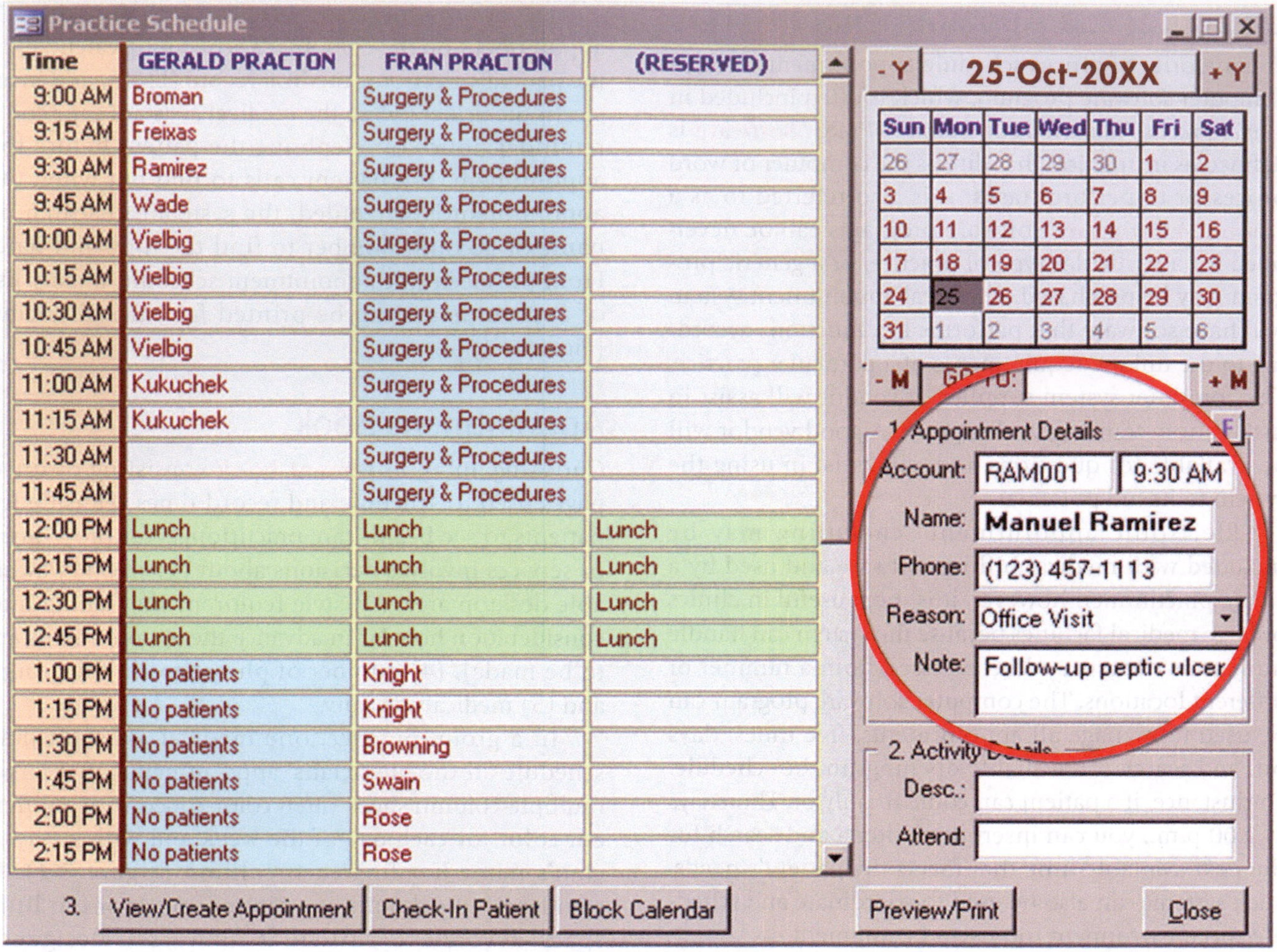

FIGURE 7-3 Patient appointment screen showing appointments for October 25, 20XX, for two providers. Note appointment details (displayed by single-clicking on a patient name) and patients with more than one (15 minute) time slot, indicating blocked time for longer appointments

10, 15, or 20 minutes. The time allotment will vary depending on the physicians' specialty and the circumstances.

Specialty and consulting practices also use this technique because it allows the physician time to prepare for each office visit with the knowledge that the day will begin and end on schedule if patients adhere to their assigned times. The disadvantage is that there can be little deviation from the schedule for late arrivals, emergencies, walk-ins, or patients who need more or less time than scheduled.

Clustered Appointments

Clustering is a plan that sets aside blocks of time for similar patient problems, especially when it is known that several patients will require the same services. Physicians have determined that this system speeds up each

case. Using this method, all patients with diabetes might be scheduled in the early morning and all patients with hypertension in the afternoon. Family practice physicians may have sports physicals or preschool checkups at the beginning of the school year. Arranging blocks of time to be used exclusively for similar services allows the staff to anticipate what is required to provide these services in the most efficient manner.

Single Book

Single booking or *time-specific* is a scheduling technique used when an appointment may take a great amount of time. Specialty and consulting practices such as psychiatry and physical or occupational therapy use this method because patients are seen for consultations, counseling, patient education, or types of therapy. Appointments may be for 45 to 50 minutes of each hour.

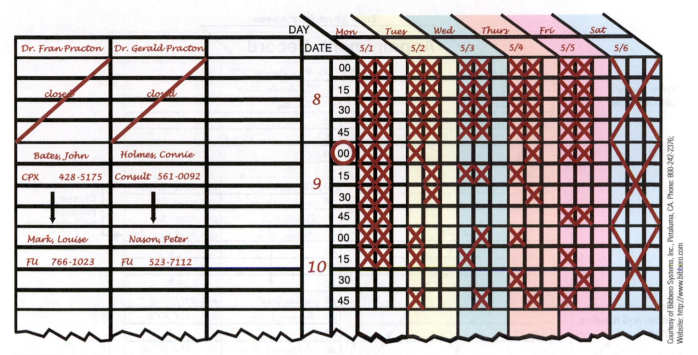

FIGURE 7-4 Two physician appointment sheets for one week showing part of Monday's schedule and indicating (with Xs) appointments already blocked or booked for the rest of the week

Double Book

Double booking is a scheduling technique that allows two or more patients to have an appointment for a particular time, depending on the proper combination of patient complaints; for example, checking a strep throat and changing a dressing take a brief time. This system is used to work in emergencies and book in an already full schedule but involves risking the goodwill of patients if they must always wait to see the doctor.

True Wave

True wave scheduling is a flexible appointment system that attempts to keep patient flow moving smoothly from one hour to the next (Figure 7-6A). When utilizing a true wave system, all patients are told their appointments are on the hour and each is seen in the order they arrive. If one patient is late, there should be another waiting to be seen. It presumes there will be some no-show patients, some walk-in patients, and some late arrivals; the expectation is that visits will average out during the hour. The number of patients to be seen in an hour depends upon the physician's specialty, which can be determined by finding the average amount of time used for each appointment and then dividing that number into 1 hour. In other words, if the average visit is 15 minutes, four patients could be seen in

1 hour. This schedule prevents a waste of the physician's productive time. The disadvantages are that patients may wait for longer time periods and may talk to each other and discover their appointments were scheduled at the same time.

Modified Wave

In **modified wave** scheduling, patients are scheduled at the first half of each hour with single 10-minute appointments; no appointments are scheduled the second half of the hour allowing for work-ins (Figure 7-6B). Another example of modified wave is to schedule more than one patient at specific intervals throughout the hour, but the same number is seen during each hour. So if five patients can be seen in 1 hour, two are scheduled at the hour, two at 20 minutes past the hour, and one 20 minutes prior to the next hour. With staggered appointments, the patients do not have to wait unreasonable lengths of time.

This system was developed as a compromise to minimize patient waiting and to maximize use of physicians' office hours to keep the patient flow smooth. The number of patients seen is affected by the number of examination rooms available. This system works best if there is no overscheduling and if it is used consistently by both the physician and the staff.

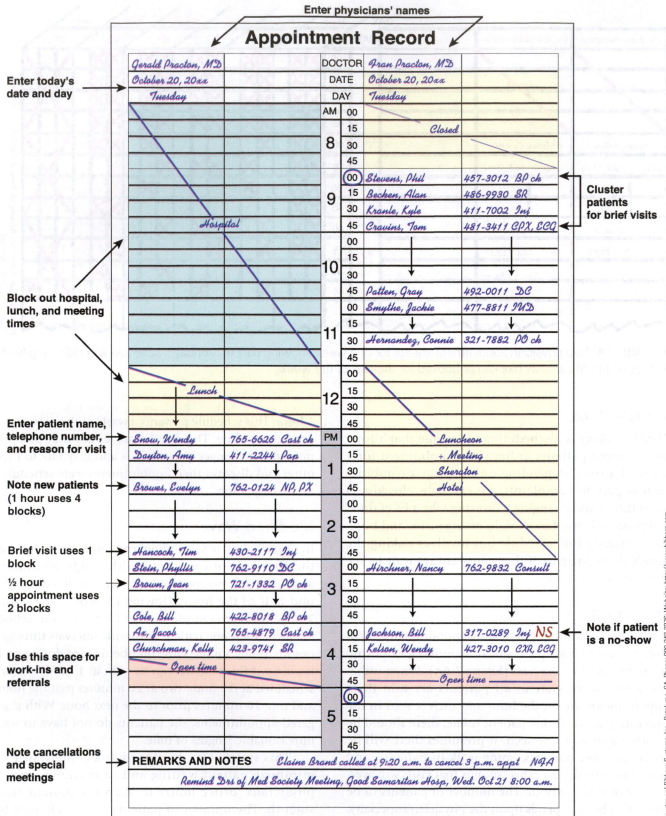

Enter physicians' names

Appointment Record

		DOCTOR	Fran Practon, MD	
Gerald Practon, MD		DOCTOR	Fran Practon, MD	
October 20, 20xx		DATE	October 20, 20xx	
Tuesday		DAY	Tuesday	

Enter today's date and day →

Block out hospital, lunch, and meeting times →

AM	00		
	15	Closed	
8	30		
	45		
	00	Stevens, Phil	457-3012 BP ch
9	15	Bechen, Alan	486-9930 SR
	30	Kranle, Kyle	411-7002 Inj
	45	Cravins, Tom	481-3411 CPX, ECG
	00		↓
	15		
10	30		
	45	Patten, Gray	492-0011 DC
	00	Smythe, Jackie	477-8811 IUD
	15		↓
11	30	Hernandez, Connie	321-7882 PO ch
	45		
	00		
	15	Luncheon	
12	30	+ Meeting	
	45	Sheraton	
PM	00	Snow, Wendy 765-6626 Cast ch	Hotel
	15	Dayton, Amy 411-2244 Pap	
1	30		
	45	Browes, Evelyn 762-0124 NP, PX	
	00		
2	15		
	30		
	45	Hancock, Tim 430-2117 Inj	
	00	Stein, Phyllis 762-9110 DC	Hirchner, Nancy 762-9832 Consult
3	15	Brown, Jean 721-1332 PO ch	↓
	30		
	45	Cole, Bill 422-8018 BP ch	↓
	00	Ax, Jacob 765-4879 Cast ch	Jackson, Bill 317-0289 Inj **NS**
4	15	Churchman, Kelly 423-9741 SR	Kelson, Wendy 427-3010 CXR, ECG
	30	Open time	↓
	45		Open time
5	00		
	15		
	30		
	45		

Cluster patients for brief visits →

Hospital

Lunch

Enter patient name, telephone number, and reason for visit →

Note new patients (1 hour uses 4 blocks) →

Brief visit uses 1 block →

½ hour appointment uses 2 blocks →

Use this space for work-ins and referrals →

Note if patient is a no-show →

Note cancellations and special meetings →

REMARKS AND NOTES Elaine Brand called at 9:20 a.m. to cancel 3 p.m. appt NA

Remind Drs of Med Society Meeting, Good Samaritan Hosp, Wed. Oct 21 8:00 a.m.

Courtesy of Bibbero Systems, Inc., Petaluma, CA. Phone: 800-242-2376; Website: http://www.bibbero.com

FIGURE 7-5 Appointment sheet for two physicians illustrating blocked time periods, appointments, no-show, canceled appointment, and special notations

A. True Wave

Dr. Fran Practon				Wednesday, May 10, 20XX
Time	Patient	Phone	Reason for visit	Comments
9:00	Cathy Villa	488-0987	CHF F/U	
	Shirley Nass	985-9800	BP ✔	
	Robert Crest	480-9870	well-baby ✔	
	Mary Chin	481-9675	Pap/pelvic	
10:00	Paul Nye	988-4551	post-op visit	
	Cindy White	488-6322	cast change	
	Paul Vega	988-1200	diabetes ✔	

B. Modified Wave

Dr. Fran Practon				Wednesday, May 10, 20XX
Time	Patient	Phone	Reason for visit	Comments
9:00	Cathy Villa	488-0987	annual Px	
9:10	Shirley Nass	985-9800	BP ✔	
9:20	Robert Crest	480-9870	well-baby ✔	
9:30	Mary Chin	481-9675	Pap/pelvic	
9:40				
9:50				
10:00	Paul Nye	988-4551	post-op visit	
10:10	Cindy White	488-6322	cast change	
10:20	Paul Vega	988-1200	diabetes ✔	

FIGURE 7-6 (A) Example of true wave scheduling (B) Example of modified wave scheduling appointment page

Open Access

Open access, also called *same day scheduling, same day access,* or *advanced access,* allows most patients to obtain appointments the same day they call. In order to make this system work, the backlog of current patients must be cleared. After the schedule is freed, open access will lead to a regular flow of patients and visitors who simply call and come in the same day. Many practices, including large clinics such as the Mayo Clinic in Rochester, Minnesota, have adopted open access scheduling.

Modified Open Access

A *modified open access* schedule is a patient-centered model which focuses on established patients who support the practice—therefore, there is a limit on new patient bookings. An "open access" time limit is set, usually around 11:00 a.m. so that established patients can have priority access up until that time and are encouraged to make same-day appointments. After 11:00 a.m., the remaining two-thirds of the day is left open and new and established patients are scheduled giving each equal access. The time can be adjusted to provide for trends in the practice and patient care demands. Established patients cannot schedule beyond 7 days and at no point are new patients offered appointments beyond that day. As the schedule opens up, however, callbacks are often made to accommodate new patients.

Open Hours

Open hours allows patients to walk in anytime within a specified time frame; they sign in with the receptionist and are seen in order of their arrival. Medical laboratories and x-ray facilities often use this scheduling procedure.

Triage

If the medical assistant is working overtime because of problems in scheduling or because many of the emergency appointments turn out to be false alarms, consideration might be given to more creative appointment scheduling and screening procedures. An example would be a system based on *triage*, as described in

Chapter 6. Appointment scheduling triage sorts out those patients who need to be seen quickly from those who can wait. By establishing appropriate criteria and obtaining relevant information, triage can be used by the staff to improve patient scheduling and to increase the certainty that real emergencies, based on the physician's determination, will receive prompt attention. Flexible appointment systems based on triage are the *true wave*, the *modified wave*, and the *clustering* or *appointment blocking* system.

Appointment and Patient Care Abbreviations

Standard **appointment and patient care abbreviations** should be used to save space and enable all staff members to understand what is noted. When training new employees, a list of acceptable abbreviations should be accessible for quick reference. Refer to Table 7-1 for a list of standard abbreviations used in this *textbook* and *Workbook*. The table may also be located in Appendix B of the *Workbook*.

TABLE 7-1 Appointment and Patient Care Abbreviations

Abbreviation	Definition
a	allergy; abortion
AB	antibiotic
abd, abdom	abdominal, abdomen
abt	about
Acc, acc	accommodation
acid	accident
adm	admit; admission; admitted
adv	advice
aet.	at the age of
AgNO$_3$	silver nitrate
AIDS	acquired immune deficiency syndrome
alb	albumin
ALL	allergy
a.m., AM	before noon
AMA	American Medical Association
an ck	annual check
an PX	annual physical examination
ant	anterior
ante	before
A & P	auscultation and percussion

Abbreviation	Definition
AP	anterior posterior; anteroposterior; antepartum care
AP & L	anteroposterior and lateral
approx.	approximate
apt	apartment
ASA	acetylsalicylic acid (Aspirin)
asap, ASAP	as soon as possible
ASCVD	arteriosclerotic cardiovascular disease
ASHD	arteriosclerotic heart disease
asst	assistant
auto	automobile
ba	barium
BI	biopsy
BM	bowel movement
BMR	basal metabolic rate
BP, B/P	blood pressure
BP ck, BP	blood pressure check
breast ck	breast check
Brev	Brevital (drug)

(continues)

TABLE 7-1 Appointment and Patient Care Abbreviations (*continued*)

Abbreviation	Definition	Abbreviation	Definition
BS	blood sugar	diag.	diagnosis, diagnostic
BUN	blood urea nitrogen	diam.	diameter
Bx, BX	biopsy	diff.	differential
C	cervical; centigrade; Celsius	dilat	dilate
C & S	culture and sensitivity	disch.	discharged
Ca, CA	cancer, carcinoma	DNA	does not apply
canc, cncl	cancel, canceled	DNKA	did not keep appointment
cast ck	cast check	DNS	did not show
Cauc	Caucasian	DOB	date of birth
CBC	complete blood count	dr, drsg	dressing
CC	chief complaint	DSHA	does she have appointment
CDC	calculated date of confinement	DTaP*	diphtheria, tetanus, and pertussis (vaccine)
chem.	chemistry	Dx, Dg, dx	diagnosis
CHF	congestive heart failure	E	emergency
chr	chronic	ECG	electrocardiogram; electrocardiograph
ck	check		
CI	color index	ED	emergency department
cm	centimeter	EDC	estimated date of confinement; due date for baby
CNS	central nervous system		
CO, C/O	complains of	EEG	electroencephalogram; electroencephalograph
CO₂, CO2	carbon dioxide		
comp	comprehensive	EENT	Eye, ear, nose, and throat
compl	complete	EKG	electrocardiogram; electrocardiograph
con, CON, Cons, Consult	consultation		
		EMG	electromyogram, electromyelogram
Cont.	continue	epith.	epithelial
COPD	chronic obstructive pulmonary disease	ER	emergency room
		ESR	erythrocyte sedimentation rate
CPE, CPX	complete physical examination	est.	established; estimated
C section, C/S	cesarean section	etiol.	etiology
CT	computerized tomography	EU	etiology unknown
CV	cardiovascular	Ex, exam.	examination
CVA	costovertebral angle; cardiovascular accident; cerebrovascular accident	exc.	excision
		ext	external
		F	Fahrenheit; French (catheter)
CXR	chest x-ray	FH	family history
Cysto, cysto	cystoscopy	FHS	fetal heart sounds
D & C	dilatation and curettage	flu syn	influenza syndrome
dc	discontinue	fluor	fluoroscopy
DC	discharge, dressing change	ft	foot; feet
del	delivery	FU, F/U	follow-up (visit)
Dg, dg, Dx, dx	diagnosis		

*Abbreviations approved by local Joint Commission as the preferred abbreviation.

(*continues*)

TABLE 7-1 Appointment and Patient Care Abbreviations (continued)

Abbreviation	Definition	Abbreviation	Definition
FUO	fever of unknown/undetermined origin	i.e.	that is
FX, Fx	fracture	IM	intramuscular
G	gravida (number of pregnancies)	imp., IMP	impression
g, gm	gram	inc	include
GA	gastric analysis	inf, INF	infection, infected
GB	gallbladder	inflam., INFL	inflammation
GC	gonorrhea	init	initial
GGE	generalized glandular enlargement	inj., INJ	injection
GI	gastrointestinal	int, INT	internal
GTT	glucose tolerance test	intermed	intermediate
GU	genitourinary	interpret	interpretation
Gyn, GYN	gynecology	IPPB	intermittent positive pressure breathing
H	hospital call	IQ	intelligence quotient
HA	headache	IUD	intrauterine device
HBP	high blood pressure	IV, I.V.	intravenous
HC	house call; hospital call; hospital consultation	IVP	intravenous pyelogram
HCD	house call, day	JVD	jugulovenous distention
HCl	hydrochloric acid	K35	kollmann (dilator)
HCN	house call, night	KUB	kidneys, ureters, bladder
hct	hematocrit	L	left; laboratory; living children; liter
HCVD	hypertensive cardiovascular disease	lab, LAB	laboratory
HEENT	head, eyes, ears, nose, and throat	lac	laceration
hgb, Hb	hemoglobin	LBP	low back pain
hist	history	L&A, l/a	light and accommodation
H₂O, H2O	water	L&W	living and well
hosp	hospital	lat, LAT	lateral
H&P	history and physical	lb(s)	pound(s)
HPI	history of present illness	LLL	left lower lobe
hr, hrs	hour, hours	LLQ	left lower quadrant
HS	hospital surgery	LMP	last menstrual period
Ht, ht	height	lt., LT	left
HV	hospital visit	ltd.	limited
HX	history	LUQ	left upper quadrant
HX PX	history and physical examination	M	medication; married
I	injection	MA	mental age
I&D	incision and drainage	med., MED	medicine
IC	initial consultation	mg	milligram(s)
		MH	marital history
		ml	milliliter(s)
		mm	millimeter(s)

(continues)

TABLE 7-1 Appointment and Patient Care Abbreviations (*continued*)

Abbreviation	Definition	Abbreviation	Definition
MM	mucous membrane	PC	present complaint; pregnancy confirmation
MMR	measles, mumps, rubella (vaccine)	PD	permanent disability
mo	month(s)	PE	physical examination
MRI	magnetic resonance imaging	perf.	performed
N	negative	PERRLA, PERLA	pupils equal, round, react to light and to accommodation
NA, N/A	not applicable	PFT	pulmonary function test
NaCl	sodium chloride	pH	hydrogen ion concentration
NAD	no appreciable disease	PH	past history
neg.	negative	Ph ex	physical examination
New OB	new obstetric patient	phys.	physical
NFA	no future appointment	PI	present illness
NP, N/P, (N)	new patient	PID	pelvic inflammatory disease
NPN	nonprotein nitrogen	p.m., PM	after noon
N/S, NS	no-show	PMH	past medical history
NTRA	no telephone requests for antibiotics	PND	postnasal drip
N&V	nausea and vomiting	PO	postoperative check, phone order
NYD	not yet diagnosed	P Op, Post-op	postoperative check
O₂, O2	oxygen	pos.	positive
OB	obstetrical patient, obstetrics; prenatal care	post.	posterior
OC	office call	postop	postoperative
occ	occasional	PP	postpartum care
ofc	office	Pre-op, preop	preoperative (office visit)
OH	occupational history	prep	prepare, prepared
OP, op.	operation, operative, outpatient	PRN, p.r.n.	as necessary
OPD	outpatient department	procto	proctoscopic (rectal) examination
OR	operating room	prog	prognosis
orig.	original	P&S	permanent and stationary
OT	occupational therapy	PSP	phenolsulfonphthalein
OTC	over the counter	Pt, pt	patient
OV	office visit	PT	physical therapy
P	pulse; preterm parity or deliveries before term	PTR	patient to return
PA	posterior anterior, posteroanterior	PX	physical examination
P&A	percussion and auscultation	R	right; residence call; report
PAP, Pap	Papanicolaou (test/smear)	RBC, rbc	red blood cell
Para I	woman having borne one child (Para II, two children, and so on)	Re:, re:	regarding
		rec	recommend
		re ch	recheck
		re-exam, reex	reexamination
PBI	protein-bound iodine	REF, ref	referral

(*continues*)

TABLE 7-1 Appointment and Patient Care Abbreviations (*continued*)

Abbreviation	Definition	Abbreviation	Definition
reg.	regular	Tb, tbc, TB	tuberculosis
ret, retn	return	TD	temporary disability
rev	review	temp.	temperature
Rh-	Rhesus negative (blood)	TIA	transient ischemic attack
RHD	rheumatic heart disease	TMs	tympanic membranes
RLQ	right lower quadrant	TPR	temperature, pulse, respiration
RO, R/O	rule out	Tr.	treatment
ROS	review of systems	TTD	total temporary disability
rt., R	right	TURB	transurethral resection of bladder
RT	respiratory therapy	TURP	transurethral resection of prostate
RTC	return to clinic		
RTO	return to office	TX, Tx	treatment
RUQ	right upper quadrant	U	unit
RV	return visit	Ua, U/A	urinalysis
Rx, RX, ℞	prescription; any medication or treatment ordered	UCHD	usual childhood diseases
S	surgery	UCR	usual, customary, and reasonable
SD	state disability	UGI	upper gastrointestinal
SE	special examination	UPJ	ureteropelvic junction or joint
sed rate	sedimentation rate	UR, ur	urine
sep.	separated	URI	upper respiratory infection
SH	social history	UTI	urinary tract infection
SIG, sigmoido	sigmoidoscopy	vac	vaccine
SLR	straight leg raising	VD	venereal disease
slt	slight	VDRL	Venereal Disease Research Laboratory (test for syphilis)
Smr, sm.	smear		
S, M, W, D	single, married, widowed, divorced	W	work; white
SOB	shortness of breath	WBC, wbc	white blood cell or count; well baby care
sp gr	specific gravity	WF	white female
SubQ*	subcutaneous	WI, W/I	walk-in, work-in
SR	suture removal; sedimentation rate	wk	week; work
STAT, stat.	immediately	wks	weeks
STD	sexually transmitted disease	WM, W/M	white male
strab	strabismus	WNL	within normal limits
surg.	surgery	WR	Wassermann reaction (syphilis test)
Sx.	symptoms		
T	temperature; term parity or deliveries at term	WT, Wt, wt	weight
		x, X	x-ray(s); multiplied by
T&A	tonsillectomy and adenoidectomy	XR	x-ray(s)
		yr	year

*Abbreviations approved by local Joint Commission as the preferred abbreviation.

(*continues*)

TABLE 7-1 Appointment and Patient Care Abbreviations (*continued*)

Abbreviation	Definition
Symbols	
*	birth
$\overline{c}$, /c, w/	with
$\overline{P}$	after
$\overline{s}$, /s, w/o	without
$\overline{c}$ c, $\overline{c}$/c	with correction (eyeglasses)
$\overline{s}$ c, $\overline{s}$/c	without correction (eyeglasses)
+	positive

Abbreviation	Definition
–, $\overline{o}$	negative
±	negative or positive, indefinite
Ⓛ	left
Ⓜ	murmur
Ⓡ	right
♂	male
♀	female
μ	micron

SCHEDULING APPOINTMENTS

Five goals to aim for when scheduling appointments include:

1. Filling all available time slots
2. Reducing appointment handling, that is rescheduling
3. Decreasing no-show rates
4. Enhancing providers' schedule and flexibility
5. Increasing patient satisfaction

Five things to consider regarding patients satisfaction include the patient's:

1. Ability to get an appointment when needed
2. Convenience regarding the appointment time
3. Being seen by their own provider
4. Respectful treatment by office personnel
5. Receiving regular reminder notices, as appropriate

Refer to Procedure 7-1 for instructions on preparing an appointment matrix. Procedure 7-2 offers step-by-step directions to execute appointment procedures. Refer to Procedure 7-3 for instructions on scheduling paper-based appointments and Procedure 7-4 for scheduling electronic appointments.

Managing Appointments

Physicians and their assistants often forget that a medical appointment may be just one event in a patient's or a parent's busy day. The available opening in the physician's schedule may conflict with school, work, or a family crisis. Therefore, the medical assistant should maintain a flexible attitude toward scheduling appointments and try to give some consideration to patients' busy schedules and personal priorities. Late

PROCEDURE 7-1

Prepare an Appointment Matrix

OBJECTIVE: Set up, block out, and enter information in an appointment schedule for a: (A) paper system, and (B) computer system in accordance with an established format or template called a *matrix*.

EQUIPMENT/SUPPLIES: Office policy for office hours and physician's schedule. **(A) Paper System:** Page from appointment book, calendar, and pen or pencil. **(B) Computer System:** Computer with electronic scheduling software.

DIRECTIONS: Follow these step-by-step directions, which include rationales, to learn this procedure. Job Skill 7-1 in the *Workbook* is presented to practice this skill in a paper-based system.

(A) PAPER SYSTEM

1. Enter the physician's name, date, and day of the week in ink at the top of each appointment page.
2. Note the time the office opens and closes by circling the hour (see Figures 7-4 and 7-5).
3. Block out the hours when patients are not scheduled by inserting a diagonal line through these time slots with a notation indicating the reason. At least 3 months of appointment sheets should be blocked out to avoid having to reschedule patients.

(continues)

PROCEDURE 7-1 (continued)

(B) COMPUTER SYSTEM

4. Turn on the computer, open the scheduling program, and select "Appointment Schedule" from the Main Menu.

5. Click on the scheduling calendar and select a date. Note: Arrows or plus and minus signs (e.g., +M and –M and +Y and –Y) typically appear at the top of the calendar to move forward or backward to another month and/or year.

6. Select "Block Calendar," and click on the time slot you would like to block.

7. Click "Yes" to create a new calendar block.

8. Follow the prompts in the "Description" field and enter the reason for the block and how you would like it applied (e.g., to all Mondays, to all days of the week, etc.).

BOTH SYSTEMS:

9. First, block all lunch periods and holidays.

10. Next, block other ongoing physician responsibilities, for example, staff meetings, hospital rounds, and so on.

11. Note and block off any special luncheons, meetings, conventions, vacations, and so forth for the upcoming months.

12. Indicate time reserved for unscheduled patients (i.e., write "open" by time slots). This will allow some open time in the morning or afternoon for patients with urgent needs, emergencies, referred patients, and walk-ins, or to let the physician and staff catch up and return calls.

13. Verify to be sure that all time blocks are complete before returning the appointment book to the scheduling desk or clicking "save" in the computer program and returning to the Main Menu.

PROCEDURE 7-2

Execute Appointment Procedures

OBJECTIVE: Gather information to execute appointment procedures in accordance with office policy and in preparation to make appointments in a paper-based system (Procedure 7-3), or in an electronic computerized system (Procedure 7-4).

EQUIPMENT/SUPPLIES: Office policy for office hours, physician's schedule, description of patient visits to be scheduled, list of standard abbreviations (Table 7-1), and appointment page or computer with electronic scheduling system that has the matrix determined, that is, appointment times blocked off according to the physician's schedule.

DIRECTIONS: Follow these step-by-step directions, which include rationales, to learn this procedure. Job Skill 7-2 is presented in the *Workbook* to practice this skill.

1. Write legibly and erase neatly when needed, or enter data accurately in a computer system. All staff who view the appointment schedule should be able to quickly read and locate information.

2. Determine whether the patient is new or established, which physician the patient will

be seeing, and the nature of the visit (chief complaint). This information sets the stage for determining the appointment time, length, and availability. Consult office policy to determine the length of time necessary for each patient's appointment (see *Workbook*, Appendix A).

3. Discuss with the physician and patient any special appointment needs when making a follow-up appointment such as specific appointment times, procedures, and use of medical equipment.

4. Use abbreviations shown in Table 7-1. Standard abbreviations save space and can be understood by all staff members.

5. Record the appointment in the appointment book following step-by-step instructions in Procedure 7-3, or in a computer system following step-by-step instructions in Procedure 7-4.

6. Complete an appointment card to give to the patient; cards may be printed from a computer system. This eliminates errors between the recorded appointment and what is documented on the card.

PROCEDURE 7-3

Schedule Appointments in a Paper-Based System

OBJECTIVE: Schedule appointments in a paper-based appointment system in accordance with office policy.

EQUIPMENT/SUPPLIES: Page from appointment book with matrix set up, calendar, and pencil.

DIRECTIONS: Follow these step-by-step directions, which include rationales, to learn this procedure. Job skill 7-2 is presented in the *Workbook* to practice this skill.

1. Search the appointment book for a mutually agreeable date and time. Allowing for the patient's agenda is as important as considering the office schedule.

2. Write the patient's last name in pencil, followed by the first name, telephone number (home, work, or cell), and reason for the visit, known as the *chief complaint*. Listing the patient's last name first makes locating an appointment easier. The telephone number assists in appointment confirmation, thus eliminating the need to view the medical record. Patient's names may be written over in ink at

the end of the day to create a permanent record, or a copy of the page may be made.

3. Indicate appointment length clearly, using vertical arrows (↓).

4. Indicate patients requiring special preparations (preps) using a red pen or other mark, such as an asterisk (*), to ensure a call can be made to verify that correct procedures have been followed prior to arrival.

5. Reschedule all canceled appointments and indicate those not rescheduled at the bottom of the appointment sheet or on a separate list. Then, record the cancelation in the patient's medical record with the current date, reason, and your signature. Follow up according to office protocol.

6. Indicate on the appointment sheet when the patient is a no-show by writing N/S or NS in the margin with a colored pen. Then record the no-show in the patient's medical record with the current date and your signature. Follow up according to office protocol.

PROCEDURE 7-4

Schedule Electronic Appointments

OBJECTIVE: Schedule electronic appointments in a computerized system in accordance with office policy.

EQUIPMENT/SUPPLIES: Computer with electronic scheduling program.

DIRECTIONS: Follow these step-by-step directions, which include rationales, to learn this procedure.

1. Open the computer-scheduling program from the Main Menu.

2. Select the scheduling calendar and the physician the patient will be seeing.

3. Use the scheduling calendar and click on the month, day, and year desired. Note: Use the plus (+) and minus (−) signs on the top of the calendar to move forward or

backward to the next or previous month; you may select the "search" option to find the next available appointment for the timeframe required.

4. Select a time slot with the correct timeframe for the type of appointment you will be scheduling and click on it to create an appointment. Depending on the type of scheduling software program you are using, you may double click to create an appointment or select "create appointment" from available options.

5. Select the patient's name to be scheduled, and click "add" or "add new patient." If a new patient has not been registered in the computer system, you will have to complete

(continues)

PROCEDURE 7-4 *(continued)*

the registration process, save it, and then return to the appointment scheduler.

6. Indicate the length of the appointment if you are not already using a template that has established timeframes.

7. Insert the patient's telephone number and then indicate the reason for the visit (chief complaint); a "note" field may be used for

this purpose or a "reason list" may appear in a drop-down menu.

8. View to verify that the data input is correct and then click "save."

9. When complete, view the Appointment Schedule to make sure all the information is entered and then close the window and return to Main Menu.

---

afternoon appointments may be set aside for patients who work during the day, or the needs of working patients may have to be satisfied by an occasional evening, early morning, noon appointment, or a Saturday morning office visit. Midday appointments may be reserved for the older adults. Toddlers and preschoolers are generally less fussy if seen early in the day, and it is best to schedule after-school hours for children's office visits. An occasional adjustment in the schedule may have to be made for a child who must be picked up at school, a college student home for the weekend, or an office worker whose only time to see the physician is during the lunch hour.

Patients who need blood work done while fasting should be scheduled early in the day. New patients, who generally require more time, might also be scheduled early so that they can be seen as close to their scheduled times as possible; this creates a good first impression. New patients who have not completed their paperwork should be brought in at least 30 minutes before their appointment time.

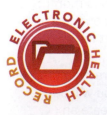 Electronic scheduling systems offer the availability to have patient portals in various locations where patients can schedule their own appointments and quickly fill out forms using templates. Medical applications (apps) are also becoming available for mobile devices such as smartphones and tablets that can be used to make appointments, complete questionnaires, access medical records, and allow providers to securely message patients.

Do not schedule long or time-consuming patients in the last appointment hour of the day, and speak to the physician about when he or she wants a talkative patient to be brought in. Offering patients a brief form (Figure 7-7) may help talkative patients to curtail their discussion and focus on the reason for the visit; it also helps prompt forgetful patients.

SCHEDULING TIPS AND TYPES OF APPOINTMENTS

To plan for unexpected patients and interruptions in scheduling, it is wise for the medical assistant to allow two 15- or 30-minute free periods during the day to fix a delayed schedule, perhaps just before the lunch hour and in midafternoon. It is also wise to schedule lightly during the first hour of the day, leaving heavier scheduling, if necessary, for hours later in the afternoon.

Bringing patients in before the actual morning start time is a good idea as long as the physician is ready to see the patient at the scheduled time. This allows time for the clinical medical assistant to take vital signs, and the patient has time to disrobe and be ready for the physician. It is not good practice or realistic to process patients into multiple treatment rooms prior to the doctor's arrival; this will put the schedule immediately behind. Do not schedule according to the number of rooms available; instead schedule according to the number of health care practitioners who can see patients.

Long waiting times are equated with poor service and patient dissatisfaction. Extended waits may also leave a negative impression about the quality of health care delivered. It is noted that more patients complain about waiting times than about high fees, and according to the American Journal of Public Health, "Waiting times of 30 minutes or longer sharply reduced the likelihood that men would visit a doctor again."

In certain specialties, a letter can be sent to all patients that informs them that because of the nature of the practice, appointment times are approximate and an attempt will be made to contact the patient if a delay of more than 20 minutes is expected. Noting each patient's arrival time and noting the time the patient is escorted to the treatment room help to monitor the appointment schedule. There are many types of appointments that a medical assistant manages during each day and these will be described subsequently.

Patient/Physician Form

Patient Name: _____ Date: _____

To help maximize your visit, please fill out this form and present it to your physician in the treatment room. Thank you for your cooperation.

1. List the main reason for today's visit: _____
_____

2. If you have been in an accident, please list when, where, and how it occurred. _____
_____

3. List any other problems or concerns that you would like to speak to the physician about: _____
_____

4. If you need any of the following, please indicate with check marks and additional details as needed.

_____ Prescription renewal
If "yes" please list the medication, dosage, and how you are taking it.
_____

_____ Forms
List type _____

_____ Excuse from work or school

_____ Other
Please explain _____

FIGURE 7-7 A brief form the patient fills out before seeing the physician to help outline the reason for the visit

Follow-Up Appointments

Usually a patient's need for a follow-up appointment will be decided by the physician and the patient at the close of a visit. If the patient is to return, the appointment should be made at the reception desk, with the date and time made mutually clear. While the patient is determining the best time for the appointment, the assistant can guide him or her to a convenient time slot to hasten the decision. It is not advisable to schedule a patient appointment too far in advance because calendar events may not be known and the appointment may be forgotten.

The importance of writing down all appointments the moment they are made, whether by telephone or in person, cannot be overemphasized; the physician's presence in the office is often determined solely by the appointments scheduled. If an appointment is made and the assistant fails to record it, embarrassing problems can result. If possible, schedule appointments one after the other to prevent gaps in the physician's time while awaiting the next patient. When a patient is to have a series of office visits, try to schedule them at the same time and day of the week to help establish them in the patient's mind.

Unscheduled Patient and Nonpatient Appointments

Occasionally, a patient may walk in to see the doctor without a scheduled appointment. Check office policy regarding such situations. In order for an appointment determination to be made, it is advisable to obtain the most precise assessment of the patient's medical problem and ask the physician whether you should work the patient into the day's schedule, send the patient to the emergency room, or make an appointment for another day.

Unscheduled visits at peak office hours by sales representatives or pharmaceutical representatives can result in wasted time for both the office staff and the sales representatives. The assistant may want to block off one or two quiet periods in the middle of the week, perhaps around the noon hour, for this type of business call. Then the salesperson will have time for a brief talk about products, and no patient care time will be lost.

Emergency Situations

When a genuine emergency situation occurs, playing havoc with a carefully planned day, the medical assistant should assess the problem and then take one or more of the following actions:

- Refer the patient to a hospital emergency facility.
- Suggest the patient come to the office immediately.
- Schedule the patient for one of the appointment periods left open for urgent or emergent problems.
- Work the patient into the schedule and flag the appointment with a colored pen or notation in the computer.

Patients with scheduled appointments that are interrupted by an emergency should be handled in one of the ways mentioned in Procedure 7-5.

Referral Appointments

Because physicians depend upon patient *referrals* from other doctors, it is important that these patients be given appointments as soon as possible. If the referring physician calls the doctor directly, the appointment requirements may be assessed at that time.

Depending on the specialty, it may be appropriate to allow a block of time for referral appointments, which often require priority. In the managed care setting, primary care physicians refer patients to specialists when necessary.

COMPLIANCE

Continuity of Care

Generally, it is not necessary to obtain a signed authorization for release of medical information from a patient who is being referred to another physician for the same condition. If the patient agrees to the referral, continuity of care applies and medical records regarding that specific condition may be forwarded.

If the physician refers many patients to other physicians, ask those physicians for their business or appointment cards. This provides the patient with the new physician's name and address and expedites the referral. Referral appointments may be flagged, so the medical assistant can follow up with the referring physician to find out whether the patient kept the appointment or was a no-show.

Habitually Late Patients

When a patient is habitually late for appointments, schedule him or her either 15 minutes before the real appointment time or at the end of the day. This can prevent the patient's tardiness from disrupting the day's schedule. A coded notation could be written on

---

PROCEDURE 7-5

Reorganize Patients in an Emergency Situation

OBJECTIVE: Reorganize patients in an emergency situation.

EQUIPMENT/SUPPLIES: Section of the office procedure manual regarding emergencies, appointment book, telephone, and pen or pencil.

DIRECTIONS: Follow these step-by-step directions, which include rationales, to learn this procedure.

1. Candidly explain to patients awaiting appointments that an emergency has interrupted the day's schedule.

2. Give patients an option to (a) reschedule their appointments, (b) run an errand and return, (c) use the telephone if they need to alert a family member or babysitter of the delay, or (d) remain and wait.

3. If possible, notify patients by telephone about the delay, politely explaining and apologizing for the inconvenience; offer the previously mentioned options.

4. If a scheduled patient arrives before he or she can be reached, apologize and explain the situation, offering the previously mentioned options.

5. Be aware that stress can result for staff members and waiting patients when emergency situations arise. By maintaining a calm demeanor, patients will assume that the emergency is being handled correctly and will gain confidence in the actions of staff members.

the patient record as a reminder if the problem continues.

No-Show Patients

Every practice needs to establish and enforce a policy for dealing with no-show appointments. For example, the patient who misses a first appointment might be called at the end of the day to suggest rescheduling the visit; after a second missed appointment, an immediate call might be made to find out the reason and to remind the patient that a third no-show would result in dismissal by the physician; after a third appointment is missed, a certified letter should be sent to release the patient.

Each time an appointment is missed, the assistant should note the occurrence in the patient's medical record along with the action taken, as further explained in Chapter 9. No-shows may also be highlighted on the appointment sheet, indicated by NS or N/S with a colored pen, or noted in a computer system.

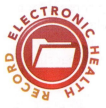

Canceled Appointments

When using an electronic scheduling system, enter the Appointment Schedule, select the physician's calendar and date, and then clink on the time slot where the patient is scheduled. Depending on the software, you can either double-click on the time slot you want canceled or click "cancel." Scheduling software programs usually track canceled appointments so that another record is not necessary.

In a paper-based system, if a patient cancels an appointment and does not set up an alternative time, the name should be listed on a cancelation sheet for tracking purposes or remain on the appointment page with a line drawn through it and a notation in the margin to indicate a cancelation was requested by the patient. At the end of the day, the date, time, and reason for the cancelation or missed appointment are then written in the patient's medical record. If the physician thinks the missed appointment will jeopardize the patient's physical condition, the assistant or physician should telephone the patient to suggest making another appointment.

When a patient reschedules, the medical assistant should cross out the original appointment before writing in the new appointment to reduce the chance of scheduling the appointment twice.

COMPLIANCE

Accurate Appointment Book

An accurate appointment book serves as a permanent record of all appointments and can be used for documentation in medicolegal cases. Omission of information about a canceled appointment can have serious legal consequences.

If the patient does not reschedule, the canceled appointment should be noted in the appointment schedule and the patient's medical record. A certified letter with return receipt requested may also be sent with a copy retained in the medical record.

Some offices charge for failure to keep an appointment. To institute this policy, the patient must be notified in advance. However, few physicians actually collect because of the poor public relations that may result.

Managed Care Appointments

One of the important factors managed care organizations (MCOs) use as a measure of the provider's quality of care is how well appointment scheduling is organized and facilitated. This requires maximum cooperation between the front and back office staff. Services must be scheduled correctly according to a specified time frame so that quality of care will not suffer. Poor appointment scheduling may provide an excuse for an MCO to closely monitor a practice's patient relations and medical outcomes. This in turn may lead to increased paperwork, reduced reimbursements, or being dropped from the MCO's network of physicians at the end of the contract period.

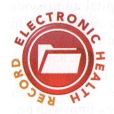

Internet Appointments

As more people use the Internet on a daily basis and more medical practices use Web-based software, more offices are communicating with patients online. Cloud-based software now includes electronic health record (EHR) management as well as electronic claims processing, e-prescribing, customized reporting, collection management, storing documents, and scheduling appointments. Patients can access the schedule via their cell phone and like the convenience of making their own appointments.

Tele-Appointments

In some rural areas after the initial appointment, telephone appointments (tele-appointments) can be arranged in a medical practice if no formal office visit is required. Patients are given designated times when they may call and talk to the physician. The physician must document the information in each patient's medical record. A nominal charge may be made for this service and billed to the insurance company using appropriate *Current Procedural Terminology (CPT)* codes. Refer to Chapter 2 for telemedicine services.

Scheduling Surgery

The physician will determine the surgical procedure, specify an assistant surgeon, indicate the amount of time required, and specify the hospital preference before the assistant makes any arrangements. Then, a surgical scheduling form—often distinctive in color to make it stand out—may be used. This form may be designed by the staff for the physician with sections to be completed by the physician, patient, and scheduler. The form will help coordinate all details involving outside facilities, prevent scheduling problems, and ensure adherence to insurance requirements. The purpose of this form is to make certain that all sequential tasks are completed.

Referring to Figure 7-8, Section 1 concerns the medical procedure and would be completed by the physician before surgery; Section 2 would be completed by the patient in the presence of the staff so that items could be explained and insurance information reviewed; Section 3 would be completed by the office staff as each step is performed with dates documented and with the name of the person who did the scheduling indicated.

After the surgery has been scheduled with the surgery department and with the hospital admissions office, the medical assistant posts the arrangements in the appointment schedule indicating date, time, patient's name, procedure, name of hospital, and assistant surgeon. Telephone calls are made to assisting or referring physicians for confirmation. After thorough verbal instructions are given, a letter or a form with pertinent information may be sent to the patient and distributed to each person involved; one copy should be filed with the patient's medical record (Figure 7-9). Refer to Procedure 7-6 for step-by-step directions for scheduling surgery and completing the surgical scheduling form.

PATIENT EDUCATION

Inform Patients of Surgical Procedures

The physician and the medical assistant often share the responsibilities of informing the patient about a surgical procedure including what to expect before, during, and after surgery. The physician usually explains the details about the procedure, why it is needed, how it will correct the problem, how long it will take, and so forth. The medical assistant may be the one asking the patient to sign the surgical consent form, explaining when to go for preoperative testing, directing the patient to the hospital admissions office, explaining postoperative care (dietary restrictions or activity levels), and advising when a postoperative appointment should be made.

The medical assistant witnesses the correct signature on the form and is not actually witnessing the consent. This is an important issue in the event the patient claims he or she did not understand or was not fully informed when verifying consent for a procedure. Special care should be taken to show awareness of the patient's concerns, answer all questions, and provide a telephone number should additional questions arise.

The written responsibilities of the medical assistant conclude after all items on the form have been addressed. However, the assistant may want to relieve patient anxiety by telling the patient what to expect upon arrival at the hospital.

Preoperative and Postoperative Appointments

The medical assistant usually sets up the preoperative appointment the week of surgery and makes appointments for laboratory tests and x-rays. He or she should exercise careful judgment in scheduling a sick person for numerous tests in sequence because too many appointments in one day may be tiring. The assistant must also have knowledge of the patient's insurance requirements that dictate in-network facilities and may require preauthorization. The postoperative appointment is typically scheduled at the time surgery arrangements are made. The time interval after surgery would be specified by the surgeon and would depend on the type of procedure.

HOSPITAL/SURGERY SCHEDULING FORM

Section 1   **Completed by physician**

1. ___✓___   Patient's name __*Alice Ruth Buckely*__
2. ___✓___   Procedure __*incision and drainage deep neck abscess*__
3. ___✓___   Emergency: Urgent _____   Elective ___✓___
4. ___✓___   Diagnosis: 1. __*Right neck abscess*__
                2. _____
5. ___✓___   Hospital/Facility name __*College Hospital*__   Surgeon __*Daniel Marks, MD*__
6. ___✓___   Inpatient ___✓___   Outpatient _____   Day Surgery _____
7. ___✓___   Surgical assistant required?   Yes ___✓___   No _____
          Who preferred? __*Ralph Curtis, MD*__
8. ___✓___   Anesthesia required?   Yes ___✓___   No _____
          Who preferred? __*William Able, MD*__
9. ___✓___   Referring physician __*Mary Tsongas, MD*__

Section 2   **Completed by patient**

10. ___✓___   Age of patient __*54*__ Date of birth __*1-15-XX*__ Smoker _____ Nonsmoker ___✓___
11. ___✓___   Room accommodations: Private _____   Semi-private ___✓___
12. ___✓___   Telephone numbers: Home (__*555*__) __*486-1135*__   Work (_____) __*N/A*__
13. ___✓___   Insurance Company __*Acme Insurance Co.*__ Policy Number __*XXX-XX-9532*__
          Secondary Insurance __*None*__   Policy Number _____
14. ___✓___   Second surgical opinion needed for insurance?   Yes ___✓___   No _____
15. ___✓___   Name of nearest relative __*Charles Buckely*__
          Address __*49267 West Cota Drive*__   Phone number __*555-486-1135*__
16. ___✓___   Admitted to this facility previous?   Yes _____   No ___✓___
          Date _____ Type of procedure _____
17. ___✓___   Patient has had preadmission testing of CBC ___✓___, EKG _____, Chest x-ray _____
          within __*1*__ weeks.
18. ___✓___   Admission and procedures reported to patient on   Date: __*October 3, 20XX*__
19. ___✓___   Preadmission and operation instructions given to me?   Yes ___✓___   No _____
20. ___✓___   Insurance and financial arrangements discussed with me?   Yes ___✓___   No _____

Section 3   **Completed by medical assistant**

21. ___✓___   Operation room reserved for surgery on this date __*Oct. 10*__ and time __*8:30 a.m.*__
          Name of hospital employee that scheduled surgery __*Betty Chapman*__
22. ___✓___   Name of surgical assistant scheduled and called __*Ralph Curtis, MD*__
23. ___✓___   Name of anesthesiologist scheduled and called __*William Able, MD*__
24. ___✓___   Reported to referring physician's office and talked to __*Ruth Raines, CMA(AAMA) 10/1*__
25. ___✓___   Hospital/Facility admission confirmed/preadmission test scheduled   __*10/8/20XX*__
26. ___✓___   Preauthorizations/second opinions obtained
          Authorization/precertification # __*1001-62-40*__   Date provided __*10/2/20XX*__
          Who provided number? __*Acme Insurance/James Brown*__
27. ___✓___   Admitting date and surgical procedure entered in appointment book   __*10/2*__
28. ___✓___   Arrangements confirmed with patient   __*10/2*__
29. ___✓___   History and physical report ready
          Name of office employee that scheduled surgery __*Marcia Lopez, MA*__ Date __*10/2/20XX*__

FIGURE 7-8 Example of a completed hospital surgery scheduling form

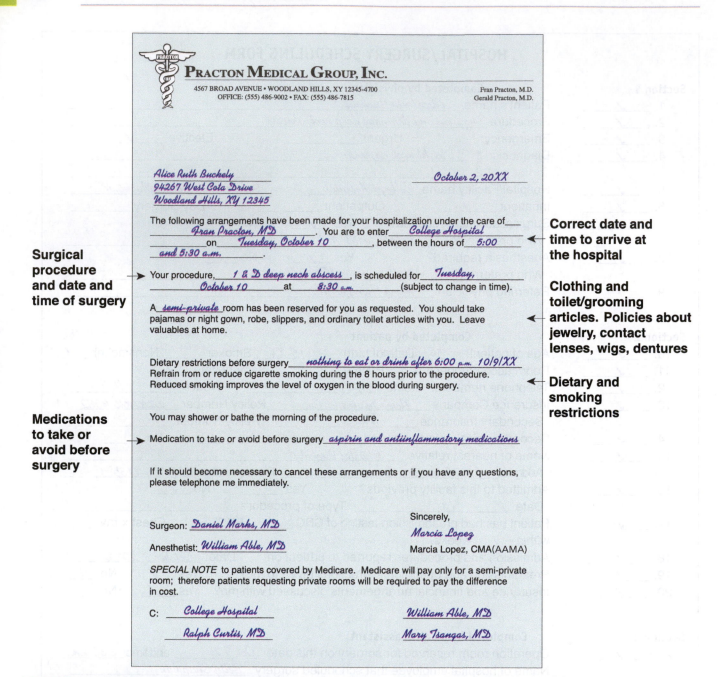

Surgical procedure and date and time of surgery

Medications to take or avoid before surgery

Correct date and time to arrive at the hospital

Clothing and toilet/grooming articles. Policies about jewelry, contact lenses, wigs, dentures

Dietary and smoking restrictions

FIGURE 7-9 Example of a completed form letter illustrating important information related to a patient's schedule surgery

PROCEDURE 7-6

Schedule Surgery, Complete Form, and Notify the Patient

OBJECTIVE: Schedule surgery and complete a hospital/surgical scheduling form and notify the patient.

EQUIPMENT/SUPPLIES: Patient's chart, hospital/surgery scheduling form, surgical scheduling guidelines, calendar, telephone, letterhead, envelope, and pen.

DIRECTIONS: Follow these step-by-step directions, which include rationales, to learn this procedure. Job Skill 7-5 in the *Workbook* is presented to practice this skill.

1. Obtain detailed information from the physician and patient for Section 1 of the hospital/surgery scheduling form.

(continues)

PROCEDURE 7-6 *(continued)*

2. Show awareness of the patient's concerns regarding the procedure and explain that you are going to be scheduling the procedure and making all the arrangements.

3. Obtain detailed information from the patient for Section 2.

4. Telephone the surgical scheduling unit at the hospital to reserve the operating room, naming the surgeon, assistant surgeon, the time (hour and length), procedure, preferred date, and patient's name, address, telephone number, date of birth, age, gender, and insurance/authorization information.

5. Call the hospital admissions office to give information and arrange for the patient to be admitted on the day of surgery; verify the time to arrive.

6. Arrange for preadmission testing (e.g., laboratory or radiology).

7. Complete Section 3 of the hospital/surgery scheduling form.

8. Post the surgical arrangements in the appointment schedule blocking the appropriate time segments and indicating date, time, patient's name, procedure, name of hospital, and assistant surgeon.

9. Telephone assisting or referring physicians for confirmation of scheduled surgery.

10. Compose a document or letter for the patient with pertinent instructions about the scheduled surgery and send a copy to each person involved, retaining a copy for the patient's medical record (Figure 7-9).

11. Schedule the preoperative and postoperative appointments.

12. Telephone one business day before surgery to remind the patient of his or her arrival time.

Diagnostic Testing and Therapeutic Appointments

The type of medical specialty will determine the type of diagnostic tests that are typically scheduled. Some examples are laboratory tests (blood chemistry, microbiology, pathology, cultures), radiology (x-ray, MRI, CT), physiology (ECG, treadmill, echocardiogram), and nuclear medicine (bone scan, IVP, thyroid uptake).

Examples of therapeutic appointments include physical therapy, occupational therapy, speech therapy, and nutritional counseling.

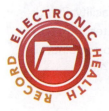

Laboratory tests and diagnostic images can be ordered electronically and test results sent directly to the health care provider's office; some EHRs link results directly to patients' EMR. Electronic prompts can be setup to remind health care providers of a test or procedure that is due. Procedure 7-7 gives step-by-step directions for scheduling outpatient diagnostic tests.

Hospital Visits

Postoperative visits for surgical patients and hospital visits for acutely ill patients are made by the physician at least once and sometimes twice daily. The physician may also make daily visits to patients in intensive care units, the newborn nursery, and other specialized hospital units. Because patient records generally do not leave the office and to facilitate recordkeeping during hospital rounds, the physician may choose to carry a mobile device (e.g., android device, smartphone, iPad) or a notepad on which the name of each patient to be seen is listed. An example of a card filled in for outside visits is shown in Figure 7-10.

A small handheld computerized portable device has the ability to connect to the Internet and serves as a personal information manager with an electronic visual display and entries made via a virtual keyboard; some recognize handwritten notes. It can capture, store, and manipulate a variety of information and be used for simple organizational tasks, e-prescribing, ordering and checking laboratory tests, keying progress notes, and reading captured data. The doctor can log hospital visits and charges at the time the patient is seen and this information can later be transferred to the patient's financial records by attaching the device to a computer. Such devices can handle encryption, so data downloaded from hospitals are safe. A clock and calendar is also included that has scheduling notification which can be used by physicians managing their own outside appointments.

PROCEDURE 7-7
Schedule an Outpatient Diagnostic Test

OBJECTIVE: Schedule an outpatient diagnostic test ordered by the physician within a certain time frame. Confirm a mutually agreeable date with the patient and give test instructions and location of test site.

EQUIPMENT/SUPPLIES: Physician's written or oral order for diagnostic test; patient's medical record; test scheduling and preparation guidelines; name, address, and telephone number of diagnostic test facility; calendar; telephone; and pen.

DIRECTIONS: Follow these step-by-step directions, which include rationales, to learn this procedure.

1. Obtain detailed information from the physician for the diagnostic test to be performed and determine the time frame for results. If it is urgent, schedule the test immediately and request STAT results. This affects the date of the return appointment.

2. Find out from the patient a mutually agreeable date and time for the test.

3. Telephone the insurance carrier to determine if preauthorization is needed and, if so, obtain it.

4. Telephone the diagnostic facility and schedule the test needed.

5. Obtain a date and time and give the patient's name, age, address, telephone number, and insurance information.

6. Notify the facility if the test results are urgently needed.

7. Obtain any special instructions for the patient, for example, dietary restrictions, fluid intake, or medications to avoid.

8. Notify the patient of the arrangements for the test, including the name, address, and telephone number of the facility and the date and time to report for the test. Ask the patient to repeat the instructions to verify he or she has a clear understanding of the requirements for the test.

9. Ask the patient if he or she has any concerns regarding the test that is to be performed.

10. Prepare the requisition slip and arrange for the patient to pick it up or fax/transmit it to the facility.

11. Insert documentation in the patient's medical record indicating the current date, the name of the facility, name of the test, date and time the test is scheduled, and any special instructions. Indicate the patient's understanding of the test and affiliated appointments (Example 7-1).

12. Make a posttest appointment for the patient.

13. If the results are to be conveyed to the patient over the telephone, put a reminder in the tickler file or computer system so that appropriate follow-up can be made.

EXAMPLE 7–1

Chart Documentation for Diagnostic Test

5/15/XX   Scheduled MRI, College Hospital, 5/17/XX, 3:30 p.m.; no pacemaker, implants, claustrophobia. RTO 5/27/XX 10:00 a.m. Adv. pt. via phone and sent requisition slip elec. to facility. Pt indicated understanding of test procedures and need for a follow-up appointment. *Lani Bardsdale, CMA (AAMA)*

Hospitalist

A trend that has evolved to reduce hospital costs and shorten hospital stays is the *hospitalist*. These physicians take over when a patient is admitted to the hospital and provide inpatient care in place of primary care physicians (PCPs). They oversee tests and results, monitor changes in the patient's condition, consult with families, and discharge patients back to their regular doctor. Usually they are internists or family practitioners or have completed residency training. Most hospitalists are employed by managed care organizations, large clinics, or hospitals, but others are

MONTH: JUNE 20XX

Patient Name	KEVIN BLAKE	Admission Date	6/1/20XX	Physician	GERALD PRACTON MD
Account No.	1784-96	Discharge Date	6/4/20XX	Patient Referred By:	
Birthdate	MARCH 28, 1958	Hospital	COLLEGE HOSPITAL	Diagnosis	HERNIATED INTERVERTEBRAL DISC

Circle Correct Code	1	2	3	4	5	6	7	8	9	10	11	12	13	14	15	16	17	18	19	20	21	22	23	24	25	26	27	28	29	30	31
HOSPITAL ADMIT																															
99221 (99222) 99223	X																														
HOSPITAL VISITS																															
(99231) 99232 99233		X	X																												
HOSPITAL DISCHARGE																															
(99238) 99239				X																											
HOSPITAL CONSULT																															
99251 99252 99253 99254 99255																															
EMERGENCY ROOM VISIT																															
99281 99828 99283 99284 99285																															
NURSING FACILITY ADMIT																															
99304 99305 99306																															
NURSING FACILITY VISITS																															
99307 99308 99309 99310																															

FIGURE 7-10 Hospital tracking form carried by the physician to the facility for daily recordkeeping. Patient admitted 6/1/XX, seen 6/2 & 3/XX, and discharged 6/4/XX. Form is given to the medical insurance biller after the patient is discharged or at end of month for posting charges

COMPLIANCE

Electronic Mobile Device Security

Any electronic mobile device used for business should have access controls and employ encryption. Passwords must be used on all mobile devices containing protected health information and should be different from other office computer network passwords, be a minimum of six characters, and incorporate letters and numbers. A mobile device should never be left unattended. Electronic mobile devices, whether employee- or physician-owned, may be subject to audits like any other office electronic device depending on their usage for the medical practice.

independent physicians who have agreements with PCPs and are paid for their work by insurance companies. Hospitalists do not substitute for specialists, such as surgeons or obstetricians.

Convalescent Hospital Visits

Convalescent hospital or nursing home calls are made on a monthly basis and more frequently if a patient becomes unstable. With the input of the physician, blocks of time are set aside for these outside calls, usually after hospital rounds in the morning or after office hours before the physician returns home at the end of the day. Tracking systems similar to those described for hospital visits may be used to record convalescent hospital visits (see Figure 7-10).

House Call Visits

Fewer house calls are made today because most physicians do not have the time. However, they do occur on occasion especially in oncology and internal medicine. A portable device, similar to those used for hospital visits, or a list is prepared in advance indicating each patient's name, address, and telephone number (home, work, cell). As the physician makes each call, he or she records the pertinent information about the visit. It is the medical assistant's responsibility to record financial charges for each visit to individual patient accounts in the computer system or on the patient's ledger card and daysheet.

APPOINTMENT REMINDER SYSTEMS

Experience has shown that custom-printed **appointment cards** simultaneously completed as the appointment is made are by far the best means of avoiding misunderstandings about future office visits and help prevent errors (Figure 7-11).

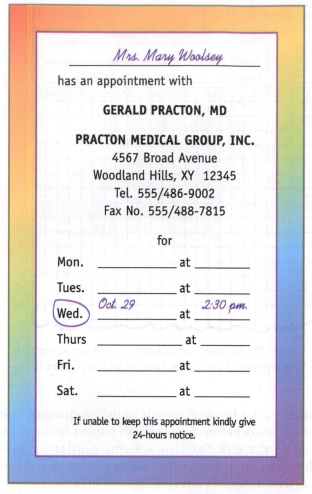

Mrs. Mary Woolsey

has an appointment with

GERALD PRACTON, MD

PRACTON MEDICAL GROUP, INC.
4567 Broad Avenue
Woodland Hills, XY 12345
Tel. 555/486-9002
Fax No. 555/488-7815

for

Mon.	_____	at	_____
Tues.	_____	at	_____
(Wed.)	_Oct. 29_	at	_2:30 pm._
Thurs	_____	at	_____
Fri.	_____	at	_____
Sat.	_____	at	_____

If unable to keep this appointment kindly give
24-hours notice.

FIGURE 7-11 Example of a completed appointment card

There are many types of successful recall systems and each depend on the medical assistant's ability to utilize the system and fine-tune it to meet the specific needs of the medical practice; it may be necessary to use several systems. A system can be as simple as placing a colored dot on patient charts, and then pulling charts at specified intervals. Or, a reminder card may be addressed as the patient is leaving the office and placed in a monthly tickler file; at the appropriate time, the card is mailed. Refer to Chapter 8, Procedure 8-3 for step-by-step directions to set up a tickler reminder file.

Confirmation telephone calls made by the medical assistant to patients scheduled to be seen within 1 or 2 days virtually eliminate failed appointments. Dental offices usually confirm all appointments because many are made months in advance; medical facilities typically confirm only new patient, longer appointments, or appointments for in-office procedures. Early morning or late afternoon is usually the best time to reach people at home to remind them of their appointments. Many daytime confirmation calls get "no-answers";

COMPLIANCE

Confidential Reminder Notices

For confidentiality purposes, a reminder card should be mailed in an envelope; _never use a postcard_ (Figure 7-12). Information for the reminder card may be obtained from a patient's encounter form, from dictation about the patient's visit, or from recall data entered into the computer software program.

therefore, it might be worth having an assistant make calls in the early evening hours. A flex schedule could accommodate this need. Even if it requires extra pay for the work, the expense will be more than made up if only one long appointment is saved.

Decreasing the missed appointment rate can be expected to improve continuity of care and free up appointment times, so others can be served more expediently. Always indicate when the appointment is confirmed in the appointment record and the follow-up procedure in the patient's medical record.

Automated Reminder Systems

An **automated appointment reminder system** retrieves appointment data from the computer's scheduling system and supports integrated phone, email, text, and mobile app messaging that allows the office to communicate with patients the way they prefer (Figure 7-13). The software can be programmed to determine the dates that follow-up appointments are due or past due and then print or activate various types of computer-generated reminder messages. Computerized phone messages state the appointment time and instruct patients to call the office and cancel their appointment if necessary. Messages can be placed in several languages. If there is no answer, the program can be setup to call the patient back up to five times. Such programs allow you to select which patients to call, which messages to use, and the preferred call date and time.

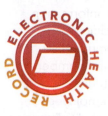

APPOINTMENT REFERENCE SHEET

At the end of the previous day or before the first patients arrive each day, the medical assistant prepares a schedule of patients to be seen by the physician. It can be

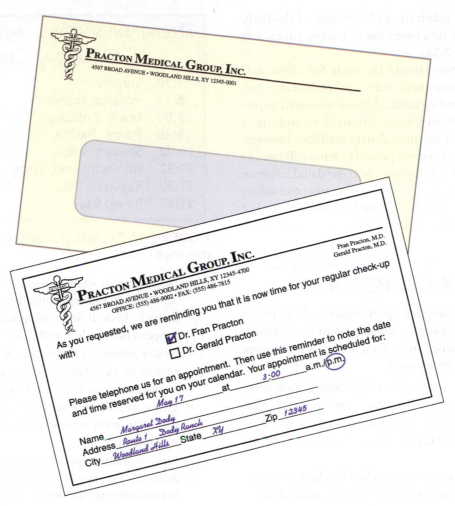

FIGURE 7-12 Recall reminder card to be mailed with address showing through a window envelope

---

Electronic Mail (E-mail) Message

Subj: **Appointment Reminder**
Date: April 19, 20XX
From: Front Desk Staff <office@practonmedicalgroup.com>
To: Mary Avery <mavery@smartmail.com>

This email is to remind you of the following appointment:

When: Thursday, April 20, 20XX
Where: Practon Medical Group—Woodland Hills
Address: 4567 Broad Street (Map)
Phone: (555) 486-9002

In the event you wish to make changes to your appointment, please call Practon Medical Group during normal business hours.

NOTE: THE INFORMATION CONTAINED IN THIS E-MAIL TRANSMISSION IS INTENDED TO BE SENT ONLY TO THE STATED RECIPIENT OF THE TRANSMISSION. IF THE READER OF THIS MESSAGE IS NOT THE INTENDED RECIPIENT OR THE INTENDED RECIPIENT'S AGENT, YOU ARE HEREBY NOTIFIED THAT WE DO NOT INTEND TO WAIVE ANY PRIVILEGE THAT MIGHT ORDINARILY ATTACH TO THIS COMMUNICATION AND THAT ANY DISSEMINATION, DISTRIBUTION, OR COPYING OF THE INFORMATION CONTAINED IN THIS E-MAIL IS THEREFORE PROHIBITED. YOU ARE FURTHER ASKED TO NOTIFY US OF ANY SUCH ERROR IN TRANSMISSION AS SOON AS POSSIBLE AND TO RETURN THE E- MAIL TO US. THANK YOU FOR YOUR COOPERATION.

FIGURE 7-13 E-mail message reminding a patient about an upcoming appointment, with confidentiality statement

either a computer printout, a photocopy of the daily appointment sheet, or a typed list of names, times, and procedures (Figure 7-14).

Additional copies should be made for office staff members. The reference sheet enables the physician to preview the day and recall established patients in order to prepare for each patient's visit. Medical records in a computerized system are immediately available; however, if using a paper-based system, patients' charts will need to be pulled from the file and placed near the dated reference sheet sequenced in the order of the appointment schedule. As patients arrive, names may be checked off or the time of their arrival stamped or noted in the computer system.

GUIDELINES TO AVOID AUDITS AND IMPROVE SCHEDULING

It has been determined that appointment scheduling is one of the most important parts of patient care. Following is a summary, which includes a few ways to improve scheduling and avoid an audit:

- Make sure the telephone receptionist knows how much time to allow for appointments based upon the physician's determinations and guidelines.
- Block off several urgent and emergent slots during the day.
- Notify the supervisor immediately when an urgent appointment cannot be given to an established patient on the same day.

APPOINTMENT SCHEDULE, FRAN PRACTON, M.D.

Tuesday, July 7, 20XX

Time	Patient	Procedure
7:30	Surgery	College Hosp.
8:15	Hospital rounds	College Hosp.
9:00	Lewis, Anthony	Annual phys.
9:45	Frame, Martha	MMR
10:00	Stewart, Adele	Heart eval.
10:30	Womochiewski, Leroy	NP; CPX
11:30	Ragland, Bill	BP check
11:45	Rowe, Ray	Chest pain

FIGURE 7-14 Example of a daily appointment reference sheet

- Note the time each patient is actually seen using 15 minutes as the maximum waiting time; after a 2-week check, if the waiting time is longer, bring scheduling into line with back-office reality.
- Notify patients if the physician is running 20 minutes or more behind schedule and offer the option to reschedule or continue to wait.
- Utilize physician extenders to provide routine care. This gives waiting patients another immediate option.
- Limit primary care office visits to the national average of six per hour, until it has been determined whether the work pace should be increased or decreased.

STOP AND THINK CASE SCENARIO

Handle a Patient with an Unverified Appointment

SCENARIO: Mr. Frederickson shows up at the office Monday morning on May 10 at 10:00 a.m. stating he has an appointment with Dr. Gerald Practon. Dr. Practon is overbooked and very busy all day. You search the appointment schedule and locate an appointment for the patient on the next day, Tuesday, May 11, at 10:00 a.m. When you advise Mr. Frederickson that the appointment was made for Tuesday, he becomes very agitated. He did not bring his appointment card with him but is adamant, stating, "It says Monday, May 10."

CRITICAL THINKING: Options are to (1) stand firm because the appointment is documented, (2) work the patient in as soon as possible, (3) work the patient in later in the morning, or (4) ask the patient to come back in the afternoon and you will work him in. Decide which option you would take and elaborate on how you would word your response; give a rationale for your choice

_____
_____
_____
_____
_____
_____
_____
_____
_____

STOP AND THINK CASE SCENARIO

Determine a Routine, Urgent, or Emergency Appointment

SCENARIO: Dr. Fran Practon's Friday schedule is full and Mrs. Charlene Pratt, an established patient, calls at 1:00 p.m. requesting to be seen that day for a migraine headache she has had for 1 week.

CRITICAL THINKING: Following are four possible ways to respond in this situation. First, determine if this is an emergency, urgent, or routine appointment. Next, select one of the possible choices. Third, compose a response and comment on various factors used in your critical thinking and decision-making process. And last, comment on why you did not select the other choices.

a. Send her to the emergency room.

_____

_____

_____

_____

b. Have her see Dr. Gerald Practon, who has an opening that afternoon.

_____

_____

_____

_____

c. Have her come into the office and wait to see Dr. Fran Practon.

_____

_____

_____

_____

d. Make an appointment for her first thing on Monday morning with Dr. Fran Practon.

_____

_____

_____

_____

_____

STOP AND THINK CASE SCENARIO

Explain Office Policy for Urgent and Emergent Appointments

SCENARIO: In Scenario 2, Mrs. Pratt indicates that she does not want to see a male doctor and decides to wait to see Dr. Fran Practon; she is worked into the schedule at 2:00 p.m. Mr. Belgum, who has an appointment at 2:00 p.m., is sitting in the waiting room and gets upset because Mrs. Pratt is taken back to see the physician before he is.

CRITICAL THINKING: What would you say to Mr. Belgum?

_____
_____
_____
_____
_____
_____
_____
_____
_____

STOP AND THINK CASE SCENARIO

Reasons Physicians Refuse to Accept and Treat Patients

SCENARIO A: Mei Yuen-Chung called the doctor's office to make a new patient appointment; she was refused an appointment.

SCENARIO B: Nathaniel Conner, an established patient was dismissed from the physician's practice.

CRITICAL THINKING: In each scenario, consider reasons that the physician would not want to accept and/or treat the patient and list reasons that might be appropriate to refuse treatment.

A. _____
_____
_____
_____
_____
_____

B. _____
_____
_____
_____
_____

*This textbook and the accompanying Workbook meet the entry-level administrative and general competencies for the CMA outlined by the AAMA Examination Content Outline and Occupational Analysis and for the RMA and CMAS outlined by the AMT Competencies, Construction Parameters, and Examination Specifications (see Competency Grid in Appendix B).

FOCUS ON CERTIFICATION*

CMA (AAMA) Content Summary

- Utilizing appointment schedules/types
- Appointment guidelines
- Appointment protocol
- Physician referrals
- Appointment cancelations/no-shows
- Scheduling outside services
- Appointment reminders/recalls

RMA (AMT) Content Summary

- Employ appointment scheduling systems
- Employ proper procedures for cancelations and missed appointments

- Understand referral process
- Understand and manage patient recall system
- Schedule nonoffice appointments

CMAS (AMT) Content Summary

- Schedule and monitor patient and visitor appointments
- Address cancelations and missed appointments
- Prepare information for referrals
- Arrange hospital admissions and surgery, and schedule patients for outpatient diagnostic tests

REVIEW EXAM-STYLE QUESTIONS

1. A template:
   a. serves as a guide for scheduling various types of appointments
   b. indicates each doctor's preferred time frames
   c. cuts down on decision making
   d. is preformatted with a certain number of slots for various types of appointments
   e. all of the above

2. A new patient is one who has:
   a. never been seen by the physician
   b. never been seen by the physician or a member of the medical practice
   c. never been seen by the physician or a member of the same specialty of the group practice
   d. not been seen by the physician or a member of the same specialty of the group practice for 3 years
   e. not been seen by the physician or a member of the same specialty of the group practice for 5 years

3. Indicating time-slots on the appointment schedule for lunch hours, hospital rounds, regular meetings, and so forth is referred to as a/an:
   a. block
   b. hold
   c. reservation
   d. entry
   e. flag

4. To evaluate a scheduling system, periodically review patient flow by analyzing the schedule for a minimum of:
   a. 2 weeks
   b. 4 weeks
   c. 6 weeks
   d. 8 weeks
   e. 10 weeks

5. Scheduling patients in the first half of each hour with single 10-minute appointments and no scheduled appointments the second half of the hour is called:
   a. true wave scheduling
   b. modified wave scheduling
   c. stream scheduling
   d. clustered appointments
   e. open access

6. Open access is also called:
   a. single booking
   b. double booking
   c. same-day scheduling
   d. open hours
   e. triage

7. A tickler file may be used:
   a. as a template for appointment scheduling
   b. to file incoming test results
   c. to file incoming documents
   d. to place reminder cards
   e. to look up telephone numbers

8. Select what action to take when a genuine emergency situation occurs.
   a. Refer the patient to a hospital emergency room
   b. Suggest the patient come to the office immediately
   c. Schedule the patient for one of the appointment slots left open for such problems
   d. Work the patient into the schedule
   e. All of the above

9. All referral appointments should be:
   a. referred to the physician
   b. referred to the doctor on call
   c. scheduled as soon as possible
   d. treated as typical new patient or established appointments
   e. handled by the office manager

10. An appointment reference sheet:
    a. can be used by all staff members
    b. is for the physician only
    c. is made for the receptionist
    d. should be kept as a permanent record
    e. is not used in computerized offices

11. Hospital visits are typically made by the physician:
    a. once a day
    b. once, and sometimes twice a day
    c. every other day
    d. as needed
    e. whenever the physician has time

12. A patient who is in a convalescent or nursing home is visited by the physician:
    a. every time the patient makes a request to see the doctor
    b. each week
    c. each month
    d. every time the nursing staff calls to report on the patient's condition
    e. whenever the physician feels there is a need

WORKBOOK ASSIGNMENT

To develop competency-based job skills, refer to the *Workbook* and complete the:
- Abbreviation and Spelling Review
- Review Questions
- Critical Thinking Exercises

Job Skill activities, which are listed at the beginning of the chapter under *Performance Objectives in the Workbook*.

RESOURCES

Appointment Scheduling

American Academy of Family Physicians

Search key term: open access scheduling

View software selections and Internet services for medical office appointment scheduling. Use one of the search engines, for example www.google.com.
- Google
- Lycos
- Web Crawler
- Yahoo

Search key phrases:
- improve patient flow
- office productivity
- physician appointment scheduling
- reducing patient wait times

RECORDS MANAGEMENT

CHAPTER 8

FILING PROCEDURES

LEARNING OBJECTIVES

After reading this chapter and learning step-by-step procedures to gain job skills,* you should be able to:

- Create and file electronic documents.
- Discuss security measures used in an electronic health record storage system.
- Summarize electronic confidentiality guidelines.
- Maintain computerized reports.
- State the differences between electronic, alphabetical, subject, indirect, chronological, and tickler filing systems.
- Memorize and apply ARMA filing rules.
- Select equipment and supplies to set up a filing system.
- Develop a charge-out system and conduct a search for a lost record.
- Determine the retention period for temporary and permanent records.
- Understand various methods used in record storage.
- Compare methods to transfer and dispose of records including confidential materials.

PERFORMANCE OBJECTIVES (PROCEDURES) IN THIS TEXTBOOK

- Set up an email filing system (Procedure 8-1).
- File using a subject filing system (Procedure 8-2).
- Organize a tickler file (Procedure 8-3).
- Determine filing units and indexing order to alphabetically file a patient's medical record (Procedure 8-4).
- Label and color-code patient charts (Procedure 8-5).
- Prepare, sort, and file documents in patient records (Procedure 8-6).
- Locate a misfiled medical record file folder (Procedure 8-7).

---

*This textbook *and the accompanying* Workbook *meet the educational components for entry-level administrative and general competencies outlined by CAAHEP and ABHES.*

PERFORMANCE OBJECTIVES (JOB SKILLS) IN THE WORKBOOK

- Determine filing units (Job Skill 8-1).
- Index and file names alphabetically (Job Skill 8-2).
- File patient and business names alphabetically (Job Skill 8-3).
- Index names on file folder labels and arrange file cards in alphabetical order (Job Skill 8-4).
- Color-code file cards (Job Skill 8-5).

KEY TERMS

alphabetical filing	download	open-shelf files
Association of Records Managers and Administrators (ARMA International)	downtime	outguide
	electronic files	password
	encryption	purge
backup	file folder	recycle
binder file folder	file guide	scores
caption	file label	subject filing
charge-out system	file tab	surname
commercial filing system	given name	tickler file
cut	indexing units	virus
databases	lateral file	
diagnostic file	numerical filing	

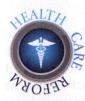

HEART OF THE HEALTH CARE PROFESSIONAL

Service

Patients appreciate a medical assistant who can expedite their care by performing behind-the-scenes tasks. Having information at your fingertips and being able to locate documents quickly are of great service to patients.

COMMERCIAL FILING SYSTEMS

There is an abundant variety of recorded information in physician practices, and the administrative medical assistant needs to protect and file it in an accurate and expedient manner. The information can be paper documents such as progress notes, hardcopy reports, handwritten memos, or messages; electronic documents such as medical records, medical claims, financial records, databases, or emails; or graphic images such as x-rays, CT scans, or MRIs. Because medical records constitute the collective memory of a physician's practice, a filing system should be easy to understand and also meet the office needs for security, expansion, and retrieval. Regardless of the system chosen, general rules should be written so that all staff members follow the same guidelines. Compliance by all employees is mandatory or the system will not work.

Properly managing files containing protected health information (PHI) while ensuring HIPAA compliance are two important implementations the administrative medical assistant can take part in to ensure the health care provider can obtain monetary incentives provided under the Health Care Reform Act. Incentives are also obtained by demonstrating meaningful use when adopting electronic medical records and recording demographic information for more than 50% of patients seen as well as other requirements.

Office management considerations when choosing a filing system are (1) number of active records, (2) number of inactive records, (3) frequency of record retrieval, (4) amount of filing and/or equipment space, (5) convenience of file or computer terminal locations, (6) cost of the system, and (7) overall size of the medical practice to be compliant with electronic health record (EHR) mandates. Medical offices may purchase some form of patented **commercial filing system** (alphabetical and/or numerical), which uses folders and guides manufactured for professional office use, or a *total practice management system (TPMS)*, which includes electronic medical records and the capability to transmit and receive electronic files in and outside of the medical office. Following, an electronic filing system is discussed.

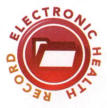

ELECTRONIC FILING SYSTEMS

Electronic medical records (EMR) are legal documents and information should be scanned, entered, and retrieved with care by using at least two identifiers, such as the patient's name, medical record number, or date of birth. Various **electronic files** or **databases** are used to store a collection of information electronically, either on the hard drive of the computer system or on the Internet, if using a "cloud-based" system. At the end of each month, the data may be downloaded onto two media storage devices—one kept in the office for reference and one stored off-site for backup safety. The data may consist of files pertaining to patient demographics, diagnoses, procedures, diseases, surgeries, drugs, financial records, or other categories used to monitor information.

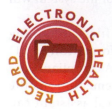

Creating Electronic Documents

Computerized medical practices use a scanning machine to scan and index documents that are collected via the paper route, such as patient registration forms, history forms, authorization documents, and insurance cards. The information is digitized, sorted, and filed according to the design of the software program or the medical practices' preference.

Original documents may be shredded, so little office space is needed for storage.

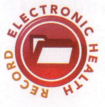

Electronic Security

A patient's medical information must always be kept confidential; therefore, it is important to maintain security of the computer system. This is the responsibility of the medical practice and every employee. Access to the system can become threatened if medical assistants are not aware of basic security measures. HIPAA's Security Rule addresses physical safeguards, such as facility access and control along with workstation device and security. Technical safeguards are also addressed, such as audit controls, integrity controls, and transmission security. A covered entity, such as a medical practice must adopt reasonable and appropriate policies and procedures to comply with the provisions of the Security Rule.

A secure form of retaining confidentiality is a software program that stores files in coded form. This process is known as **encryption**, which makes the data look like gibberish to unauthorized users.

In addition, using security codes or passwords to enter the computer system assures that unauthorized users will not gain access. When an individual leaves a place of employment, his or her password or means of access needs to be changed.

COMPLIANCE
Security Codes

There are several options for controlling access to data. Those most frequently used are identification (ID) numbers and electronic passwords, also called *security codes*. A **password** can be a word or phrase, but it should contain a sequence of letters and numbers so it remains private and cannot be guessed by others to gain access (see Example 8-1). Badges, cards, and keys may also be used to access individual terminals. Biometric access controls unique to each individual may consist of fingerprints, eye patterns, or voice prints. As discussed in Chapter 3, there are statements that clearly outline the consequences of violating confidentiality rules and regulations.

Another safeguard is to classify employees and limit access to specific computer functions. To guard against theft and embezzlement, an employer should consider whether employees need simple inquiry functions versus data entry and update functions. Many computer programs are designed to record the dates and times files are altered. With a log-on feature, any employee who alters a file can be identified. Only responsible employees should be given the task of deleting and updating information.

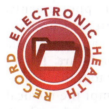

Maintaining Computerized Reports

Computer files can grow tremendously and then become unmanageable when the medical assistant tries to find a letter or report, especially when the patient is not registered with the office and reports or medical records are received in preparation for a scheduled visit. Computerized file management systems are available to assist in arranging electronic files. Using such a system not only helps with quick retrieval but also saves space on the computer hard drive.

Maintaining Email Files

The medical office may get electronic mail from vendors, patients, government agencies, and other outside sources. Email files need to be managed the same way paper files are managed so that information can be easily retrieved. It is important to sort email regularly so that you can determine what is important, label it, and file it so that it is easily found. Procedure 8-1 lists steps for setting up an email filing system.

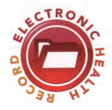

Backing Up Computer Files

Electronic files should be backed up periodically and always at the end of the day. A full **backup** is an exact copy of the entire hard drive that is stored on a digital versatile (Video) disc (DVD), compact disc read-only memory (CD-ROM), flash drive, or an external hard drive. Frequency of backups will depend on the amount of information being input. If the amount is large, then it is wise to back up (save data) often during data entry. It is possible to establish an automated backup system, in which the computer itself regularly initiates the backup process. Some software programs display a screen prompt that asks, "Do you want to backup now" before the program is closed.

Information may be lost because of a power spike, computer breakdown, or a **virus,** which is a hidden program that enters the computer by an outside source and can destroy data or memory and cause the system to crash. To prevent a virus from infecting the computer and to prevent outsiders from viewing computer data,

---

PROCEDURE 8-1
Set Up an Email Filing System

OBJECTIVE: Prepare an email file designed for filing email messages.

EQUIPMENT/SUPPLIES: Computer, Internet access, and email account.

DIRECTIONS: Follow these step-by-step directions, which include rationales, to learn this procedure.

1. Separate and delete junk mail immediately upon receiving it. If you want to keep mail temporarily, it may be left after reading it; most email systems will automatically delete read mail in 7 to 14 days.

2. Sort through business-related emails to determine which ones need to be printed for action, filed in office files (e.g., patient charts), and stored electronically.

3. Create a filing system for important email items. Determine email file folder names that will allow you to find them easily and quickly when you need them. For example, folders could be named "Contracts," "Supply Companies," "Maintenance," and so forth.

4. Save and insert emails in appropriate folders.

5. Purge mail in folders periodically to eliminate old information.

use a firewall or security-oriented router. Software can also be installed to display a message when infected media are inserted. The antiviral program should be updated periodically with the latest version.

When the computer is not functioning properly, this is referred to as **downtime**. A power *surge suppressor*, preferably with backup capability, will prevent computer and data file damage.

About once a week have the computer compare the original records with the backup. This verification can take 20% to 30% longer than an ordinary backup, but if a comparison is not made, there is no way to ensure information has been backed up properly. Another good practice is to select one backup per month to keep indefinitely. Then if something should happen to the computer, it is possible to restore data from an earlier point in time and update from that point. Always retain the three most recent backups. Delete the older version and use the storage device for the newer version. It is important to store backup copies away from the office because of fire, flood, and theft.

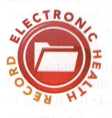

Electronic Confidentiality Guidelines

To comply with confidentiality requirements and avoid problems with computer files, follow these guidelines:

1. Never leave any storage media (e.g., flash drive, DVD) unguarded on desks or anywhere else in sight.
2. Always log off of the computer terminal before you leave your workstation.
3. Never write down log-on sequences, passwords, or any other codes that regulate personal access to a system; change your password periodically. If you must write down your password, hide the paper and scramble what is written (Example 8-1).
4. Never **download** (transfer data) public domain software, files from electronic bulletin boards, or other communications systems, because a virus can get into the office system.
5. Never bring in portable storage devices (e.g., DVDs) from outside your office.
6. Always back up files regularly to save data that might get lost through a breach of security.
7. Respect other employees' computer files the same way you do those kept in a desk file drawer. If you use another employee's computer, do not move or alter files or change the screen format.

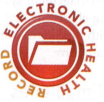

Electronic Tickler File

A **tickler file**, also called a *suspense* or *follow-up* file, is used in medical offices so that the staff can remind patients of preset appointments, follow up on patients who have missed or canceled appointments, and note tests patients may need scheduled in the future. Tickler files are a type of time management tool that can be set up in computer systems to prompt the medical assistant to take action at specific times, such as check on an expected referral letter or laboratory report due by a specified date, order a depleted inventory item, or follow up on an unpaid insurance claim. These files may also be used to remind the physician of personal appointments, subscription renewal dates, income tax payments, and meeting dates.

Most medical office computer systems include some type of electronic tickler file. Some options include:

1. Built-in reminders that can be selected and set automatically for such things as patients' monthly blood pressure checks or annual physical exams.
2. Drop-down calendars that allow reminder notes to be placed in certain dates, then pop up and appear on that date as a reminder.
3. Links to the patient's progress notes, where reminders can be recorded and later present as a reminder.

PAPER-BASED FILING SYSTEM

Paper-based filing systems have been around for years, and although electronic medical records are becoming the norm, most offices have some sort of paper files, so it is important to understand how a paper-based filing system is organized.

Alphabetical Filing System

The simplest and most popular filing method is by alphabetical name sequence, because it is easy to understand and does not require a cross-reference index. Also, if an alphabetical entry is especially confusing, the telephone book, which is a classic example of alphabetical name filing, provides an excellent reference.

Alphabetical Color-Coding

Management consultants recommend color-coded alphabetical filing that consists of colored tabs for each letter of the alphabet. Depending on the size of the practice, tabs are selected for the first, second, and sometimes third letters in the patient's last name and secured to the edge of the file folder for easy reference. Any misfiled record would break the color pattern and stand out, for example, when filing the name "Franklin," the letter **F** could be red and the **R** would be color-coded green. You would quickly locate the "**FR**" section in the file cabinet and file the chart using the remaining letters of the patient's surname alphabetically. An example of an open-shelf file folder using this type of color coding is shown in Figure 8-1.

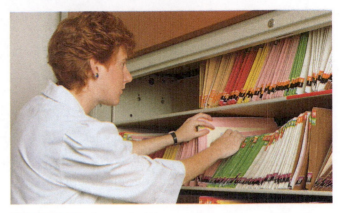

FIGURE 8-2 Open shelf lateral file cabinets with colored charts

Alphabetical color-coding of medical file folders has the advantage of reducing misfiles, speeding retrieval, and making office filing more efficient. The labels are readable from front and back for open-shelf file cabinets (Figure 8-2). In addition to using color-coded alpha labels, various colors may also be used to distinguish medical charts.

Subject Filing System

Subject filing is an alphabetical arrangement of records filed by topic or grouped under a main theme. These themes are assigned titles that become signposts to direct you to the right file.

Business papers other than those dealing with patients are usually stored in a separate cabinet or desk drawer and filed in alphabetical order by subject. Miscellaneous communication dealing with matters other than patient treatment may be filed under "Correspondence."

If the physician does research, lectures, or writes for periodicals, the assistant may be in charge of organizing materials in a **diagnostic file**. The main heading in this type of subject file might be the name of the disease. Then after the main heading, patient cards can be alphabetized with name, diagnosis, treatment, prognosis, and additional information outlined.

If the physician keeps medical articles for future reference, the physician can determine and note a subject heading for each article or highlight the title of an article in the table of contents that is of special interest. The assistant will then remove the article and assign a main heading and secondary heading for a subject file. Both main subject and secondary subject headings may be referenced (see Example 8-2). If the article is on an

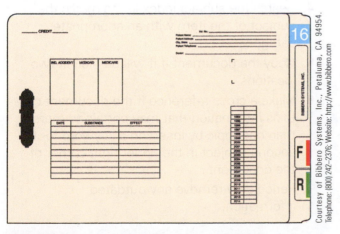

FIGURE 8-1 Preprinted lateral file folder with color-coded alphabetical designation for first two letters of the last name and year tab

EXAMPLE 8–2

Subject Headings for Medical Articles

a) **Article title:** *Advance Clues to Heart Attacks*

   Main subject heading: *Heart Attacks*

      Secondary subject heading: *Advance Clues*

b) **Article title:** *Living with Multiple Sclerosis*

   Main subject heading: *Multiple Sclerosis*

      Secondary subject heading: *Activities of Daily Living (MS)*

c) **Article title:** *The Menopausal Woman and Breast Cancer*

   Main subject heading: *Breast Cancer*

      Secondary subject heading: *Menopause*

obscure topic, it is helpful to give it a fairly general heading. Since no two subject files are the same, the medical assistant handling the business matters of the practice usually determines the captions for the guides and folders. Examples of documents include employee information, financial documents, insurance policies, and taxes. Then subcategories are created under each category, for example, taxes (federal and state).

Physicians can also insert current articles directly into a patient's chart, so a discussion of the latest treatment option can be held when the patient returns. Maintaining a patient database by disease, symptom, medication, or device (e.g., pacemaker) will make locating patients for this purpose easier. Refer to Procedure 8-2 for instructions on how to use a subject filing system.

Indirect Filing System

If privacy and convenience of expansion are important considerations, an indirect filing system may be preferable. An indirect filing system, also referred to as a **numerical filing** or *unit numbering* system, is used primarily to handle rapidly growing files in hospitals, clinics, and large medical practices. It is termed an "indirect" system because an auxiliary cross-reference index is used to determine a patient's assigned number before locating the file. A *numerical file register* with consecutive numbers is usually maintained to determine the last assigned number. After a number has been assigned, it is either keyed into a computer filing program or typed with the patient's name on a small index card and filed alphabetically by last name. A cross-reference file provides rapid access to patient numbers; however, a disadvantage is the time the extra step takes (i.e., locating the number to find the file).

PROCEDURE 8-2

File Using a Subject Filing System

OBJECTIVE: Demonstrate filing of documents using a subject filing system.

EQUIPMENT/SUPPLIES: Documents to be filed by subject, subject index list, highlighter pen, and pencil.

DIRECTIONS: Follow these step-by-step directions, which include rationales, to learn this procedure.

1. Read the document to find the main subject.

2. Highlight or underline the keyword that best describes the subject of the document.

3. Write the subject header in the upper right corner if it does not appear in the document.

4. Search the subject index list to match the subject of the item with an appropriate category.

5. Copy the document if it will be filed in two locations.

6. Make a cross-reference if the document contains information that may pertain to more than one topic by inserting a keyword for the second subject in the upper right corner of the document.

7. Periodically remove any outdated information.

The following methods of filing by consecutive numerical sequence result in more even distribution of active and inactive records. The *middle-digit numbering sequence* arranges records by six-digit numbers. The *terminal-digit* and *triple-digit* systems use numbers to designate shelves or drawers to find charts, and all digits are color-coded. Hospital record numbers, x-ray numbers, and telephone numbers are often used as a basis for arranging records by the last digits (Example 8-3).

Chronological Files

In a *chronological* filing system, numbers are used based on dates. Files, or sections within a file, are listed by year, month, and day with the most recent files in the front of the file drawer or the most recent documents in the front of the folder. In a physician's office, chronological filing is one method used to file documents within a chart so that the latest visit, laboratory test, x-ray, hospitalization, and so forth are at the beginning

of each section of the file (see Chapter 9 for more information).

Tickler Card Filing System

Even when the medical office is using a computer system, there may be a need for a tickler card filing system. Refer to Figure 8-3 for an illustration of a tickler file and Figures 8-4, 8-5, and 8-6 for various types of cards used for reminders. See instructions in Procedure 8-3 to organize a tickler card file.

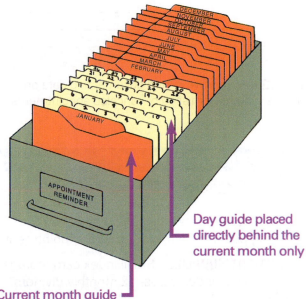

Day guide placed directly behind the current month only

Current month guide placed at the front of the tickler file

FIGURE 8-3 Tickler card file used as an appointment reminder system

---

EXAMPLE 8–3

Indirect Numerical Color-Coded Filing

Middle-Digit Numbering Sequence

To retrieve Mrs. Doe's case, number 294597, begin with the last number sequence and locate 97, then look for the middle number sequence 45, and finally look for the first number sequence 29.

Record No. 294597 = 974529

Terminal-Digit System

To obtain Mr. Benton Thomas's patient record, number 516204, begin with the last number and go to Section 4, which appears as 00000<u>4</u> (sections 0 to 9). Then, look at the next two preceding digits and go to Row 20, which appears as 000<u>20</u>4 (rows 00 to 99). Next, look at the preceding two digits and go to Shelf 16, which appears as 0<u>16</u>204 (order 00 to 99). And last, look at the final number to find Chart 5, which appears as <u>5</u>16204 (order 0 to 9).

Record No. 516204 = 4 (section) 20 (row) 16 (shelf) 5 (chart)

PRACTON MEDICAL GROUP, INC.
4567 Broad Avenue
Woodland Hills, XY 12345
Tel. 555/486-9002

As you requested, we are reminding you that it is time for your six-month checkup with *Dr. Fran Practon*

Please phone today for an appointment. Then use the space below to note the date and time reserved for you.

Tuesday   *March 12*   *3:00 p.m.*
DAY   DATE   TIME

FIGURE 8-4 Preprinted tickler card used as appointment reminder

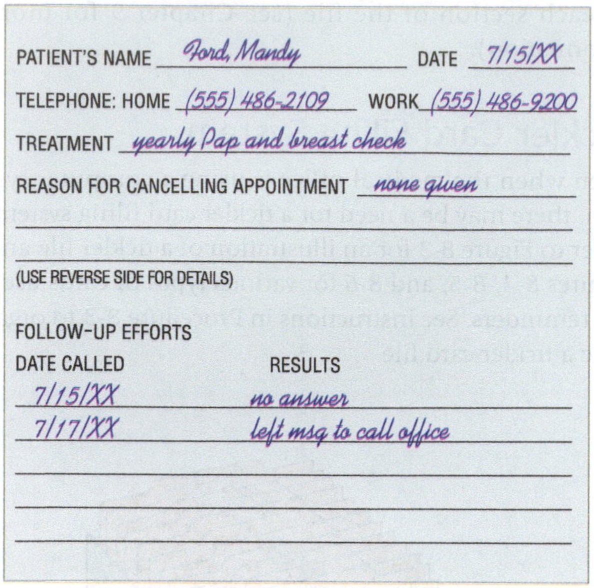

PATIENT'S NAME *Ford, Mandy* DATE *7/15/XX*

TELEPHONE: HOME *(555) 486-2109* WORK *(555) 486-9200*

TREATMENT *yearly Pap and breast check*

REASON FOR CANCELLING APPOINTMENT *none given*

(USE REVERSE SIDE FOR DETAILS)

FOLLOW-UP EFFORTS

DATE CALLED	RESULTS
7/15/XX	*no answer*
7/17/XX	*left msg to call office*

FIGURE 8-5 Follow-up card documenting data on patients who have missed or canceled appointments

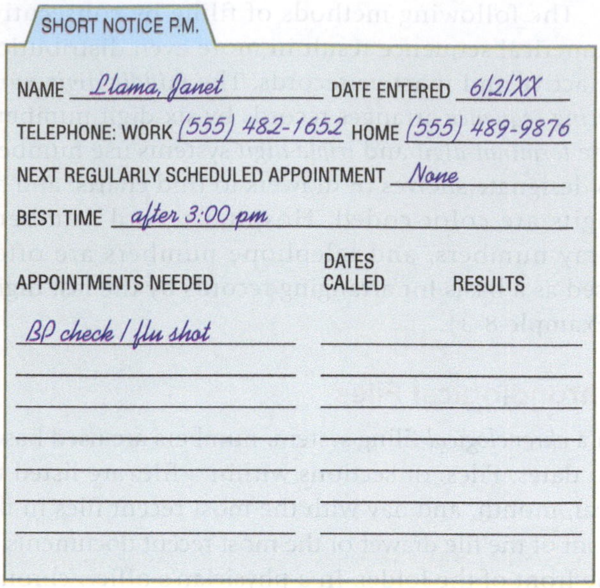

SHORT NOTICE P.M.

NAME *Llama, Janet* DATE ENTERED *6/2/XX*

TELEPHONE: WORK *(555) 482-1652* HOME *(555) 489-9876*

NEXT REGULARLY SCHEDULED APPOINTMENT *None*

BEST TIME *after 3:00 pm*

APPOINTMENTS NEEDED	DATES CALLED	RESULTS
BP check / flu shot		

FIGURE 8-6 Tickler card used as a reference to call patients on short notice for fill-in appointments

PROCEDURE 8-3

Organize a Tickler File

OBJECTIVE: Prepare a tickler file designed for recalling patients by mail for future appointments.

EQUIPMENT/SUPPLIES: Small index card storage box, 3" by 5" index cards, 12 monthly dividers, and pen.

DIRECTIONS: Follow these step-by-step directions, which include rationales, to learn this procedure.

1. Type or write the names and addresses of patients on cards; patients can self-address preprinted reminder cards when leaving the office. These will be mailed to patients as reminders of upcoming appointments.
2. Insert the month and year of the recall appointment on each card.
3. File each card behind the month preceding the patient's recall appointment. Allow enough time for mailing and response.
4. Check the tickler file at least once or twice a month and send out recall notices. This should be done enough in advance so that patients can call and reserve times during the appropriate month for their future appointments.

Short-Notice Reminder File

In a short-notice reminder system, a file is divided into time categories appropriate to the practice, such as *urgent, anytime, a.m.*, and *p.m.* When making appointments, patients are asked if they are interested in coming on short notice or anytime there is an opening. This information is placed on a card and filed in the appropriate category (Figure 8-6). Then when there is a cancelation, the assistant can refer to the short-notice reminder file to select one of these people as a substitute.

ALPHABETICAL FILING RULES

In 1986, the **Association of Records Managers and Administrators (ARMA International)** developed rules for alphabetizing that are the basis for most **alphabetical filing** systems in use today.

To standardize filing procedures and ensure consistency, simplified general rules considered appropriate for the medical office will be summarized with examples from *Alphabetic Filing Rules* published by the ARMA International Standards Program.

General Guidelines

Names are divided into sections called *units* (last name, first name, middle name). The alphabetical process starts by comparing the last name—first unit—letter by letter. If only a last name is known, this single unit is filed before a last name with a first initial. A last name with only an initial is filed before a last name with a first name beginning with the same initial; this rule is often stated as "file nothing before something."

As patterns for naming offspring have changed, moving away from the traditional use of the male's last name (surname), rules must be adopted to reflect these trends. Example 8-4 shows alternative sources of surnames.

EXAMPLE 8–4

Sources of Surnames

Using the example of the mother's name, **Mary Dearfield**, and the father's name, **Richard Lange**, study the following options:

a. Some parents give one child the mother's maiden name (surname) and the next child the father's name, for example, Jerry Dearfield and April Lange.

b. Others choose to give their children a hyphenated version of the last two names, for example, Jerry Dearfield-Lange.

c. Others develop a hybrid surname linking parts of the parents' two names to form a new surname, for example, Jerry DeLange.

When filing a confusing surname (last name), or when it is difficult to distinguish a last name from a first name, it is advised to setup a cross-reference file (Example 8-5).

EXAMPLE 8–5

Cross-Referencing

When filing a foreign surname, such as *Huang Lon*, use the last name as the first filing unit and then cross-reference.

Primary File:	Lon, Huang
X-Reference File:	Huang, Lon (**See** Lon, Huang)

Rule 1: Individual Names

Names of patients are assigned **indexing units** and alphabetized by comparing the first unit in each name, letter by letter, in this order: **surname** (last name), first indexing unit; **given name** (first name), second indexing unit; and middle name (if any), third indexing unit (see Example 8-6). Second units are considered only when the first units are the same, third units are considered only when the first and second units are the same, and so on. Any additional names are filed as successive units. If only initials are listed, for example, E. J. Hoover, the first initial is considered a complete unit and filed before names with additional letters.

EXAMPLE 8–6

Filing Individual Names

Name	Unit 1	Unit 2	Unit 3	Names Appearing in File Order
Thomas Andrew Johnson	Johnson	Thomas	Andrew	JONG, NEUYEN
T. K. Johnson	Johnson	T	K	JOHNSTONE, THOMAS
Thomas Johnstone	Johnstone	Thomas		JOHNSON, THOMAS ANDREW
Neuyen Jong	Jong	Neuyen		JOHNSON, T.K.

Rule 2: Prefixes

Last names with prefixes are called *surname particles* (e.g., "D," "de," "Del," "Des," "Mac," "Mc," "Saint," "St.," "Van") and are filed like other surnames as one indexing unit whether the prefix is followed by a space or not (see Example 8-7). The prefix is considered part of the surname. When filing "Saint" and "St.," they either may be filed exactly as spelled or "St." may be spelled out, depending on office preference, but remember, both "St." and "Saint" are handled as a prefix to the last name.

EXAMPLE 8–7

Filing Names with Prefixes

Name	Unit 1	Unit 2	Unit 3	Names Appearing in File Order
Marilyn McFadden	McFadden	Marilyn		vonDYKE, ROBERT
John MacArthur	MacArthur	John		ST. JAMES, MARCIA
Harvey Schmidt S	Schmidt	Harvey		SCHMIDT, HARVEY
Robert vonDyke	vonDyke	Robert		McFADDEN, MARILYN
Marcia St. James	St. James	Marcia		MacARTHUR, JOHN

Rule 3: Hyphenated Names

All hyphenated names—whether first names, middle names, or surnames—are considered to be one indexing unit. For example, when a husband and wife combine their surnames with a hyphen, ignore the hyphen and file the two names as one unit. Surnames on folder labels may be typed without a hyphen, a space, or any punctuation marks. Hyphenated words in a business name, however, are indexed as separate units. Example 8-8 shows how to file hyphenated names.

EXAMPLE 8–8

Filing Hyphenated Names

Name	Unit 1	Unit 2	Unit 3	Names Appearing in File Order
Leslie Newton-Ross	NewtonRoss	Leslie		NEWTONDAVIS, ANNAMARIE
Loretta Jane Newtonberg	Newtonberg	Loretta	Jane	NEWTONROSS, LESLIE
Anna-Marie Newton-Davis	NewtonDavis	AnnaMarie		NEWTONJOHN, ARTHUR
Arthur Newton-John	NewtonJohn	Arthur		NEWTONBERG, LORETTA JANE

Business Names

Smyth-Barnes Cosmetics				SMYTH-BARNES COSMETICS
Churchill-Clayton Pharmacy				CHURCHILL-CLAYTON PHARMACY

Rule 4: Abbreviated Names and Nicknames

Abbreviations of personal names (i.e., first names) are indexed as they are written (see Example 8-9). Shortened names or nicknames, such as Al or Kate, are alphabetized as written if they are true names or if the true names are not known.

EXAMPLE 8–9

Filing Abbreviated Names

Name	Unit 1	Unit 2	Unit 3	Names Appearing in File Order
Virgil Robt. DeKalb	DeKalb	Virgil	Robt (Robert)	DeKALB, VIRGIL ROBT
Jas. Charles Baker	Baker	Jas (James)	Charles	BAKER, JAS CHARLES
Charles L. Baker	Baker	Charles	L	BAKER, CHARLES L

Rule 5: Titles and Degrees

Titles, degrees, and seniority terms following the name are not units and are *disregarded in the indexing unless they are needed to distinguish identical names*. Alphabetic suffixes (e.g., Jr. or Sr.) are filed before Roman numerals (I, II, III). Both alphabetic abbreviations, such as "Jr.," and numerical suffixes, such as "II" and "III," are filed before alphabetical suffixes such as "Prof.," "Dr.," or "PhD."

A man with a name identical to his father's is called "Jr." as long as his father is alive; when his father is dead, he may drop the "Jr." A male is a "III" when his father is a "Jr." A male named after his grandfather, uncle, or cousin is a "II." These terms may be enclosed in parentheses and placed at the end of the name on file labels.

Exception: When a name consists of a title and a given and/or middle name, such as Reverend Brown or Sister Mary Margaret, the name is not transposed and the title is the first indexing unit. Example 8-10 shows how to file names with titles and degrees.

EXAMPLE 8–10

Filing Names with Titles and Degrees

Name	Unit 1	Unit 2	Unit 3	Unit 4	Names Appearing in File Order
Dr. Robt. Crespi, Jr.	Crespi	Robt.	(Jr)	(Dr)	REVEREND BLAKE
Reverend Blake	Reverend	Blake			ESPINOZA, ROBT. A (PROF.)
Prof. Robert A. Espinoza	Esinoza	Robert	A	(Prof.)	CRESPI, ROBERT (JR) (DR)
Samuel T. Blake, III	Blake	Samuel	T	(III)	BLAKE, SAMUEL T (III)

Rule 6: Married Women

Typically, the surname is the only part of her husband's name a woman assumes when she marries. Her legal name, however, could be anyone of the following: (1) her own first and middle names together with her husband's surname, (2) her own first name and maiden surname together with her husband's surname, or (3) her first (given) name and her own (maiden) surname (see Example 8-11). The title "Mrs." is not typically used on file folder labels anymore but may be considered part of the third unit and placed in parentheses; adding the husband's first and middle names or initials is optional, typed to the side or below the woman's legal name.

EXAMPLE 8–11

Filing Names of Married Women

Name	Unit 1	Unit 2	Unit 3	Names Appearing in File Order
(1) Mrs. Callie Justine White (Karl W.)	White	Callie	Justine	WHITE, CALLIE JUSTINE
(2) Mrs. Callie Campbell White	White	Callie	Campbell	WHITE, CALLIE CAMPBELL
(3) Mrs. Callie Campbell	Campbell	Callie	(Mrs.)	CAMPBELL, CALLIE (MRS.)

Rule 7: Hospitals, Medical Facilities, and Businesses

The names of hospitals, pharmacies, and other business facilities are indexed in the same order as written on the letterhead unless the firm name includes the complete name of a person, in which case the surname would be followed by the given name or initials. Some offices follow an *optional* rule that does not transpose the full name in a business. Thus, in Example 8-12, Wm. Ingram's Pharmacy would be the last name in the group.

Numbers are indexed as though written out and are filed as one unit. Compass directional terms are usually considered separate units. Prepositions, conjunctions, and articles are not units except when "a," "an," "and," "the" are the first words, in which case they become the last filing unit.

EXAMPLE 8-12

Filing Names of Hospitals, Medical Facilities, and Businesses

Name	Unit 1	Unit 2	Unit 3	Unit 4	Names Appearing in File Order
The Good Samaritan Hospital	Good	Samaritan	Hospital	The	WM INGRAM'S PHARMACY
Wm. Ingram's Pharmacy	Wm	Ingram's	Pharmacy		TWENTYFIFTH ST AMBULANCE
25th St. Ambulance	Twenty-fifth	St	Ambulance		GOOD SAMARITAN HOSPITAL THE

Rule 8: Addresses When Names Are Identical

When patients have identical names, alert each patient to that fact and suggest that both remind the staff at each office visit to prevent confusion about records. If two names are identical and the physician or hospital sees patients from more than one city or state, the address may be used to make the filing decision. Index by name first, then state, city, street, and finally by number from the lowest to the highest number (see Example 8-13). Geographic names such as Las Vegas are treated as two separate indexing units.

Refer to Procedure 8-4 when alphabetically filing a patient's medical record.

EXAMPLE 8-13

Filing Addresses When Names Are Identical

Name	Unit 1	Unit 2	Unit 3	Unit 4	Unit 5	Unit 6
John Almonzo, 120 Adams, Rye, New Hampshire	Almonzo	John	New	Hampshire	Rye	Adams (120)
John Almonzo, Portage, New York	Almonzo	John	New	York	Portage	
John Almonzo, 450 Adams, Rye, New Hampshire	Almonzo	John	New	Hampshire	Rye	Adams (450)

Names Appearing in File Order

ALMONZO, JOHN NEW YORK PORTAGE

ALMONZO, JOHN NEW HAMPSHIRE RYE ADAMS 450

ALMONZO, JOHN NEW HAMPSHIRE RYE ADAMS 120

PROCEDURE 8-4

Determine Filing Units and Indexing Order to Alphabetically File a Patient's Medical Record

OBJECTIVE: Determine each filing unit given a surname, given (first) name, and middle name to alphabetically file patients' medical records.

EQUIPMENT/SUPPLIES: Patients' medical records with names on labels and pen or pencil.

DIRECTIONS: Follow these step-by-step directions, which include rationales, to learn this procedure. Job Skills 8–1 and 8–2 are presented in the *Workbook* to practice this skill.

1. Obtain the patient's surname (last name), considered unit 1. Filing records in alphabetical order creates efficiency in filing and retrieving charts. Look carefully at each letter of the name when placing it in the file.

2. Study each filing rule to see which one applies to the surname you are trying to file.

3. Consider the second unit, the given (first) name, only when the first unit is the same as the other names in the file.

4. Study, letter by letter, the patient's given (first) name, which becomes unit 2.

5. Consider the third unit, the middle name or middle initial, only when the first and second units are the same.

6. Study, letter by letter, the middle name or middle initial (if any); this is unit 3 in the sequence of filing. Remember "file nothing before something," so an alike name without middle initials or names would be filed first.

7. Find the proper location on the shelf or in the file drawer.

8. Use your hand to make space between the existing records and place the file in the proper location.

9. If refiling a file folder where an outguide exists, pull the outguide halfway out, insert the file folder in front of the outguide, and remove the outguide. Outguides must be removed each time you refile a record that has been borrowed

FILING EQUIPMENT

Filing equipment consists of the storage units used to keep files. Size (floor space used), accessibility (ease of use), durability, security, and appearance are all considered when selecting filing equipment.

Lateral Files

The most popular file cabinets used for storing patient medical records are the upright shelf files referred to as **lateral files**. They typically have sliding doors that open upward and recede into the top of the shelf, which resembles a bookcase. An **open-shelf file** unit with seven 36-inch shelves will hold approximately 1000 records (Figure 8-7). File cabinets are available in colors to harmonize with office décor.

Open-shelf or lateral files are popular in medical offices because they require less floor space than conventional steel drawer cabinets. There is no drawer opening and closing to cause cabinets to tilt, record access is quicker, and misfiling is reduced, especially if

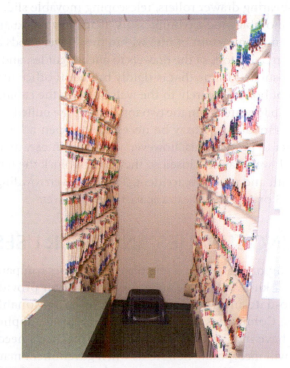

FIGURE 8-7 Charts in an open-shelf cabinet file

folders are color-coded. Doors that can be pulled out and down can provide security with locks.

Lateral shelves can be located on a wall or double as a room divider near the medical assistant's desk, and they can be found in modular-stationary or rollout models. It is important to secure these types of files to the walls to prevent tipping during any earth movements. File dividers keep materials upright, and visible file folders are stored perpendicularly with tabs and color-coded labels extending beyond the side of each folder to clearly show the patient's name.

Full-Suspension Drawer Files

The traditional upright steel cabinet with three to five drawers is still popular for the storage of business records in a medical office (e.g., payroll records, insurance explanation of benefit documents).

Desirable features in cabinets with drawers are ball-bearing drawer rollers, telescoping movable slides, steel movable blocks (compressors) that allow for expansion and contraction of files within the drawers, rods at the top or bottom of the drawers to anchor guides, and a fire-insulated frame that is rigidly braced. If office files are not bolted securely to the wall or floor, the cabinet may tip forward when the two top drawers are pulled out simultaneously. It may be necessary to open a lower drawer to prevent this; however, when not in use, try to keep lower drawers closed so they do not block the traffic path and cause an accident. To avoid overcrowding, leave 3 or 4 inches of extra space in each drawer.

FILING SUPPLIES AND THEIR USES

It is important to find a reliable office supply company with a knowledgeable salesperson who can provide up-to-date information and supplies at reasonable costs. Companies that specialize in medical supplies will have items specific to a medical practice's needs and will incorporate new items when government mandates become law (e.g., HIPAA-regulated consent forms,

latest CMS-1500 claim form). Following are general supply items found in a medical practice.

File Guides

File guides are pressboard, manila, metal, or plastic dividers that sit slightly higher than the file folders in order to be more visible on the shelf or in the drawer. They provide support for folders and serve as signposts to direct the eyes to labeled sections. Along the top of the best quality guides is a reinforced metal tab in which labels may be inserted so that the guides can be reused. Less sturdy guides with plastic-coated tabs are also available. Typically, one divider is used for 25 folders, allowing 4 to 6 inches of empty space for working. In a lateral filing system, alpha-guide labels can be placed in the extreme left position or staggered throughout the files. As the number of folders increases, two-letter (color-coded) secondary guides may be added to serve as additional signposts (Example 8-14).

Guides for shelf files are side-tabbed and as a rule are not staggered (Figure 8-8). A sturdy metal hook projects

EXAMPLE 8–14

Two-Letter Secondary Guides

Primary Guide

B

Secondary Guides

Be

Bi

Bo

Br

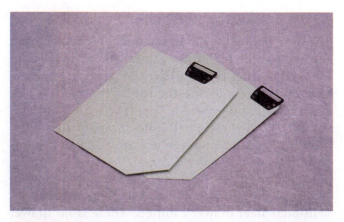

FIGURE 8-8 Guides used to separate file folders into subsections

from the back of each guide to keep it attached to the cabinet, so it will not work forward. Guides for file drawers have tabs on the top and are equipped with a projection at the bottom center with a metal-reinforced hole in the middle. A metal guide rod attached horizontally to the bottom of a file drawer is placed through these holes to secure the guides in place within each drawer.

File Folders

Letter-size **file folders** (8 ½″ by 11″) are designed to hold information to be stored in open-shelf cabinets or file drawers. Ordinary kraft or manila folders in 11-point stock are suitable for average medical practices. The choice of weight ranges from 8-point, which is very light, to 24-point, which is extra heavy, and will depend on the extent of handling. If folders are to be handled often, sturdier file folders should be purchased because redoing folders is not only time consuming but also expensive.

The assistant can be creative in designing preprinted chart covers, so important information can be recorded on both the inside and outside (Figure 8-9). Commercially printed folders are economically sensible when a practice initiates a great number of new patient records per day or per week.

Information available on the outside of chart covers might include the patient's allergies, drug reactions, nicknames or titles, for example, a patient with a Ph.D. who prefers to be addressed as "doctor." If protected health information is listed on the front of the file folder (e.g., diabetic), careful attention should be given to turning the chart cover when left unattended.

The inside of the chart cover might include coded notations or pressure-sensitive colored labels alerting the staff of a patient's failure to pay a bill, legal problems, or specific medical problems.

The back half of a standard folder extends about one-half inch beyond the front to form a protruding tab. Creases at the bottom of folders, called **scores**, permit expansion of file folders.

Binder File Folders

Binder file folders are designed with clamps or file fasteners to secure papers inside, preventing lost items. Disadvantages of binder folders include the tendency of the files to bulge where the clamps are located and the time it takes to insert documents in the folder and remove them for photocopying or when filing new paperwork.

Information is placed in folders with correspondence headings visible and with most recently dated papers at the front (Figure 8-10). Special medical reports may be filed according to type of report; that is, all ECG results together, all urinalysis reports together, and so forth. It is best for a medical assistant to set aside a specific time each day to transfer and file patient data.

Stapled and Shingled Documents

Because paper clips slip off or attach to neighboring papers, stapling continuation sheets or related items diagonally in the upper left corner is preferable.

A telephone message or small laboratory test report may be stapled, taped, or glued to a standard-size sheet of paper so that it will not be misplaced or overlooked. It may also be *shingled* as described in Chapter 6 (Figure 6-6). This method is not preferred, because data are covered and it is time consuming to take documents apart before photocopying a medical record.

When it is time to dispose of the contents of a folder, the assistant should remove labels and save the folder for reuse by placing a new label directly on top of the old one or by replacing a removable label. Old folders may be used for inactive storage because they will not be reviewed often.

Color-Coding File Folders

When several physicians are associated but maintain separate practices, patient folders may be color-coded to distinguish each physician's patients (Figure 8-11). An inexpensive way to convert ordinary manila folders to color is to purchase colored tape, colored dots, or preglued colored tabs to affix directly to the folder tabs.

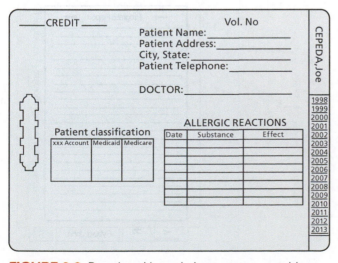

FIGURE 8-9 Preprinted lateral chart cover—outside view

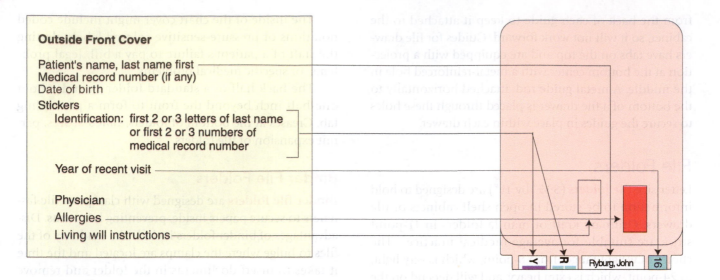

Outside Front Cover

Patient's name, last name first
Medical record number (if any)
Date of birth
Stickers
    Identification: first 2 or 3 letters of last name
                     or first 2 or 3 numbers of
                     medical record number

    Year of recent visit

    Physician
    Allergies
    Living will instructions

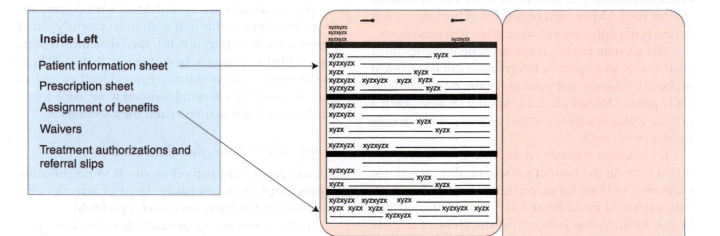

Inside Left

Patient information sheet

Prescription sheet

Assignment of benefits

Waivers

Treatment authorizations and
referral slips

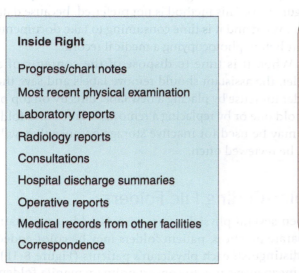

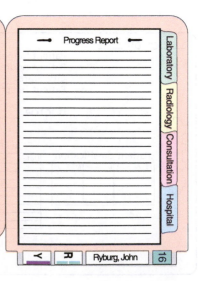

Inside Right

Progress/chart notes

Most recent physical examination

Laboratory reports

Radiology reports

Consultations

Hospital discharge summaries

Operative reports

Medical records from other facilities

Correspondence

FIGURE 8-10 Patient's medical record and its contents

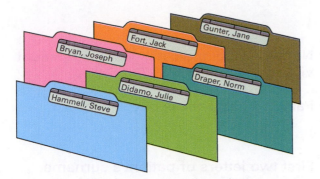

FIGURE 8-11 Colored file folders for physicians in same office maintaining separate practices

Miscellaneous Colored Labels

Other kinds of labels are also useful, such as those indicating restrictions for private health information (Figure 8-12).

A small wraparound self-stick label printed with the last digit of each year can be attached to the edge of the folder to indicate the most recent year of service. This can be covered with a new sticker each year after the patient has seen the physician. Folders with old dates that need to be purged from the active files can be seen easily.

A fluorescent sticker placed on the front of the chart alerts the physician to a patient's drug allergies. Dots indicating type of insurance coverage assists the physician when prescribing medication according to specific insurance formularies and when sending patients to in-network facilities. It also speeds the completion of insurance claims

(Figure 8-13). For example, all Medicare folders are put in one pile and completed at one time. For heavy usage, file labels can be covered with Mylar overlays.

File Tabs

File tabs are staggered projections in varying widths above or on the sides of the body of a file folder or guide, also used as signposts to direct the eye to a specific label. The width of the tab, called the **cut,** is usually expressed as a fraction. *One-half cut* means that the tab takes up one-half of the back flat of the folder, while a *one-third cut,* which is the most popular, allows for three tabs of equal length to fit across the top of a standard folder. A *full tab,* often with a reinforced edge, extends the length of the back of the folder and may be used to attach color-coded labels. Straight-cut folder tabs with rounded corners stay in the best condition (Figure 8-14). To be visible, folder tabs used in open-shelf files extend beyond the right side of the back leaf. Names arranged vertically on these side tabs are not as easily read as numbers.

File Labels

File labels are small stickers usually covered with acetate or a protective overlay to keep them from wearing. After a **caption,** which is a name or number used as a heading to locate a file, has been typed on a label, it is affixed to the tab of a folder. A small space is left between the top of the label and the top of the folder,

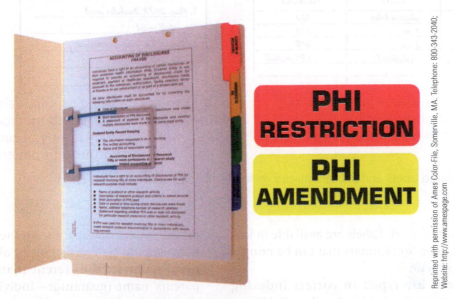

Reprinted with permission of Ames Color-File, Somerville, MA. Telephone: 800-343-2040; Website: http://www.amespage.com

FIGURE 8-12 HIPAA divider sets are used in patient files to quickly identify records with protected health information (PHI); fluorescent labels are placed on the cover of the folder to alert office staff of PHI

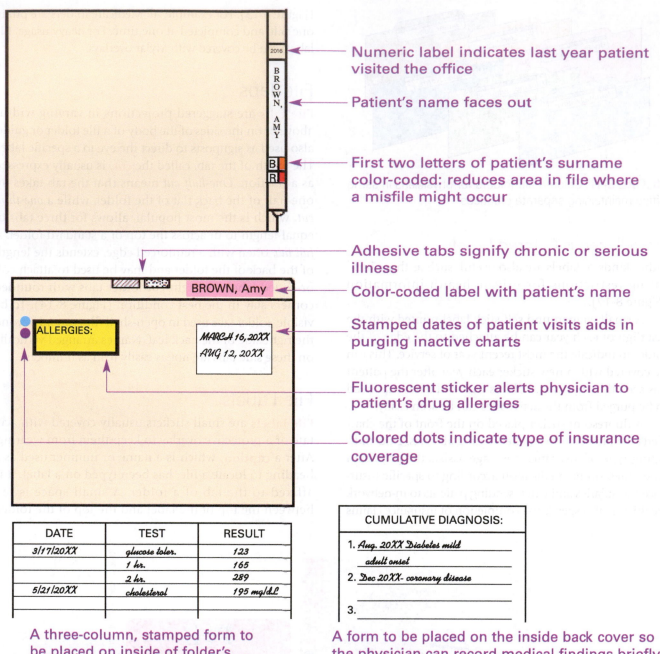

Numeric label indicates last year patient visited the office

Patient's name faces out

First two letters of patient's surname color-coded: reduces area in file where a misfile might occur

Adhesive tabs signify chronic or serious illness

Color-coded label with patient's name

Stamped dates of patient visits aids in purging inactive charts

Fluorescent sticker alerts physician to patient's drug allergies

Colored dots indicate type of insurance coverage

DATE	TEST	RESULT
3/17/20XX	glucose toler.	123
	1 hr.	165
	2 hr.	289
5/21/20XX	cholesterol	195 mg/dL

A three-column, stamped form to be placed on inside of folder's front cover to identify lab work

CUMULATIVE DIAGNOSIS:

1. Aug. 20XX Diabetes mild
   adult onset
2. Dec 20XX- coronary disease

3. _____

A form to be placed on the inside back cover so the physician can record medical findings briefly in the order in which they occur; saves time by not having to go through patient's records

FIGURE 8-13 Colored labels and stickers placed on the front and inside covers of chart

so the label will not peel off. Labels are available in various styles, colors, sizes and formats that can be printed from a computer system.

Name captions are typed in correct indexing arrangement (last name first) either in all capital letters or in a combination of uppercase and lowercase letters, as shown in Figure 8-15. The patient's name should start two or three spaces from the left edge of the label on the second line space from the top edge, and placement should be consistent on all labels. When children's names are different than their parents', the parents' name (guarantor—individual responsible for the bill) should be cross-referenced on the chart, as this will help locate the account for billing. Refer to Procedure 8-5 for instructions on labeling and color-coding patient charts.

PROCEDURE 8-5

Label and Color-Code Patient Charts

OBJECTIVE: Label and color-code patient charts using a specified color-coding system to quickly file and locate charts.

EQUIPMENT/SUPPLIES: Patient charts, color-coding system guidelines, file folders, and colored name labels.

DIRECTIONS: Follow these step-by-step directions, which include rationales, to learn this procedure. Job Skill 8-5 is presented in the *Workbook* to practice this skill.

1. Assemble patient charts.
2. Arrange each name in indexing order so that charts can be color-coded in sequence.

3. Begin with the first patient and note the first and second letters of the patient's surname (last name) and select alphabetical labels of the correct color.
4. Type in indexing order the patient's last name, first name, and middle initial and adhere the label to the file folder tab.
5. Repeat steps 3 and 4 until all charts are labeled and color-coded.
6. Look through the group of file folders to be sure the order and color of the file folders are correct and that all charts are of the same color within each letter of the alphabet grouped together.

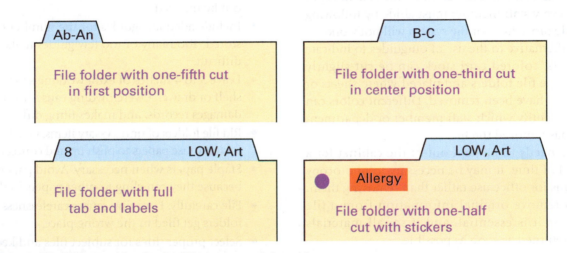

Ab-An — File folder with one-fifth cut in first position

B-C — File folder with one-third cut in center position

8 · LOW, Art — File folder with full tab and labels

LOW, Art · Allergy — File folder with one-half cut with stickers

FIGURE 8-14 File folders with tabs in different cuts and positions

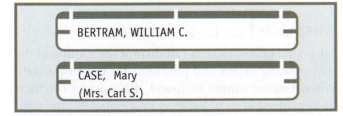

BERTRAM, WILLIAM C.

CASE, Mary
(Mrs. Carl S.)

FIGURE 8-15 Typed file folder labels

CHARGE-OUT AND CONTROL SYSTEMS

To track charts when removing from files, a **charge-out system** is used to indicate when and by whom a record has been removed. One person should

supervise the system and all members of the staff who remove records, charts, or folders should be admonished to return them promptly. A team effort should be made to avoid misplacement. Patients have the right to expect that their medical records will be safeguarded from unauthorized use or disclosure and that the filing system adopted by the office will ensure accurate retrieval.

Outguide

An **outguide**, which replaces a file folder that has been removed until the folder has been returned, is required if control of patient records is to be maintained. It is usually made of heavy pressboard with a tab labeled "OUT." Some are designed with lines to record the patient's name, medical record number, date taken out and returned, who removed the record, and why the record was removed or location it was taken to. Others are designed with pockets in which a written requisition form can be inserted. The form is made out by the borrower and should be filled out completely and consist of an original and a copy. One can be filed in the outguide folder and one attached to the medical record. It cannot be overemphasized that once an outguide system is put into place, every staff member must abide by following the outguide procedures or the system will not work.

As an alternative to the use of outguides to indicate pulled charts, colored card stock can be cut slightly larger than the file folders and placed where sheets or whole folders have been removed. Different colors can be used to identify which staff member or department employee has removed the file.

If a file needs to be kept out of the cabinet for a long period of time, it may be necessary to photocopy needed items for office use rather than removing them. Try not to remove original information from a file folder unless it is essential, and if so, all materials should be returned as soon as possible.

Outfolder

An *outfolder* serves the same purpose as an outguide except that it provides a place to store incoming items (e.g., laboratory reports) until the regular folder is returned. Charge-out information may be written on the front of the folder, which is often printed with ruled lines.

FILING DOCUMENTS IN PATIENT RECORDS

In Chapter 9, you will learn about the various elements comprising a medical record, such as:

- Patient information sheet
- Medical history questionnaire

- Progress and chart notes
- Electrocardiogram reports
- Laboratory (log) reports
- Radiological reports
- Prescription log
- Medical reports (history and physical, consultation, operative reports, discharge summaries)

Each of these documents must be placed within every patient's file folder in an organized manner so that data can be accessed quickly. Procedure 8-6 will take you through the steps of getting documents ready for filing in a patient's medical record in a paper-based system.

Misfiling

To avoid the misfiling of information, study the following guidelines and common causes of misfiling:

- Type patient names legibly using a standardized form. Changes in the typed format of headings can be misread.
- Include adequate guides for the number of files stored. Too many or too few guides make filing difficult.
- Leave 3 to 4 inches of extra working space per shelf or drawer. Overcrowding causes misfiling, damages records, and makes filing difficult.
- Rid file folders of unnecessary items. Overloaded folders cause papers to push up and conceal file tabs.
- Staple papers when necessary. Avoid paper clips because they can cling to other papers in the file.
- File carefully. Hurrying causes carelessness and folders get filed in the wrong place.
- Select proper titles for subject files and keep headings simple. Failing to properly designate the subject or name results in lost files.

Misplaced or Lost Records

Misplaced or lost records can disrupt the routine of the day, creating delays and problems for the entire staff. When a record cannot be found, the assistant conducts an organized search. Refer to Procedure 8-7 for step-by-step instructions on locating a patient's lost record.

RECORD RETENTION AND STORAGE

There are both federal and state laws that pertain to the requirements for keeping records; however, in some cases a law cannot be found for the retention of a

PROCEDURE 8-6

Prepare, Sort, and File Documents in Patient Records

OBJECTIVE: Prepare, sort, and file documents in patient records.

EQUIPMENT/SUPPLIES: Documents (letters, medical reports, diagnostic test reports), file sorter, tape, stapler, and pen or pencil.

DIRECTIONS: Follow these directions, which include rationales, to learn this procedure.

1. Separate and group documents to be filed in patient medical records, financial records, business files, and so forth.

2. *Patient Files:* Examine documents that are to be filed in patients' medical records, making sure they have been date stamped and initialed by the physician. All reports must be viewed by the doctor and released before filing.

3. *Business Files:* Index and code documents to be filed by subject. *Indexing* is deciding on the caption; *coding* is marking the caption on the material to be filed, usually by underlining or by writing a word in the upper right corner. Both steps can be performed simultaneously. Captions chosen and marked might be letterhead name, signature name, reference name, or the name of the person or institution to whom the letter is addressed. Coding may be unnecessary when files are supervised by one person who will be familiar with correspondents and able to quickly scan for the caption.

4. Photocopy and cross-reference data when it applies to more than one patient or subject.

5. Sort documents in filing sequence; documents are arranged in either alphabetical or numerical order. A desk sorter with a series of dividers using alphabetical or numerical classifications facilitates this step before the documents are placed in file folders. It is efficient to file in order since one patient may have several reports to be filed (Figure 8-16).

6. *File Documents:* Items are placed in the appropriate file folder and under the appropriate file division (e.g., laboratory) face up, top edge to the left, with the most recent item placed to the front.

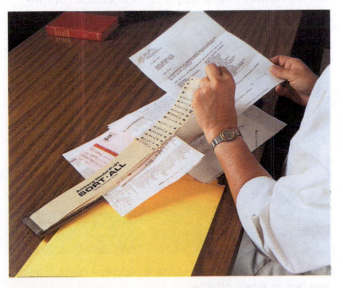

FIGURE 8-16 Medical assistant using a desk sorter to alphabetize reports to make filing easier

particular type of record. All records should be retained for at least the number of years included in the statute of limitations and if federal laws and state laws do not agree, always keep the record for the longer period stated. Most states have statutes requiring medical or hospital records to be kept anywhere from 7 to 25 years. Because records chiefly contain information on patient care, the records may be of value to patients in later years or even to their offspring. It is, therefore, the policy of most physicians to retain paper medical records indefinitely.

Record Retention Schedule

Setting up a records retention schedule will ensure that records are kept according to law but not retained unnecessarily. A retention schedule is a list of record

PROCEDURE 8-7

Locate a Misfiled Patient Medical Record File Folder

OBJECTIVE: Search for a misfiled patient medical record.

EQUIPMENT/SUPPLIES: File cabinet (shelves or drawers).

DIRECTIONS: Follow these step-by-step directions, which include rationales, to learn this procedure.

1. Check in the spaces in front of and behind where the patient's file folder should be located.

2. Check above and below the shelves where the record should be kept, or in the bottom of the drawer.

3. Look for the first two colors of the patient's last name among other records if using a color-coded system. The color, if misfiled, should stand out.

4. Look under the patient's first name, instead of the last; sometimes, it is difficult to distinguish between first and last names or the file folder could be set up incorrectly.

5. Search through the entire section of the first letter of the patient's last name.

6. Determine other ways the patient's name could have been spelled, as well as misspelled, transposed, and so forth.

7. Look for similar names; names that sound the same but are spelled with a different vowel.

8. Explore different areas of the office; that is, look in desk trays or in-baskets, on top of and beneath folders, and among the charts of other patients seen the same day; a variety of employees may need to use the file.

9. As a last resort, if the record remains missing after a thorough search, set up another file folder or sheet, flag it for identification, and label it with the word "Duplicate" and the patient's name.

---

types and the length of time each record should be kept. Steps to take when preparing a policy for retention are:

1. Sort records according to type (e.g., patient inactive records, payroll records, appointment sheets).

2. Refer to the schedule for retention and determine how long to keep each type of record.

3. Obtain the physician's approval.

4. Implement the schedule by moving records from active to inactive files, packing storage boxes to move off-site, or processing for destruction.

5. Use 15" by 12" by 10" storage boxes, which will hold both letter and legal papers and are easier to lift than larger cartons (Figure 8-17).

6. Leave records in standardized manila folders; if binders or hanging files are used, remove items before sending them to storage.

7. Place all similar records in one container with the same destruction date.

8. Clearly label the storage box with the type of records and the "from" and "to" dates of the materials enclosed or the last date (by year) the patient was seen.

9. Compile an inventory list of contents for future reference (e.g., payroll 20XX).

10. Conduct random inspections to ensure compliance with the schedule.

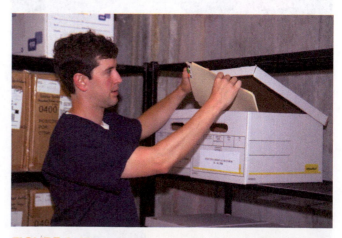

FIGURE 8-17 Medical assistant placing a chart in a storage box to retain off-site

Financial and Legal Records

Vital papers such as financial reports and legal documents are considered permanent records and are kept indefinitely in a secure file (see Table 8-1). A loose-leaf notebook can hold a record of the physician's personal inventory; changes and additions may be made simply by adding and deleting pages.

Active and Inactive Patient Files

Medical charts should be **purged** (removed) at predetermined intervals to increase shelf space and eliminate looking through inactive records when trying to file. It is often difficult for the medical assistant to determine when to transfer patient files from active to inactive status without having to read all the details on each chart. This problem can be solved by date-stamping visits on the front of each folder or by attaching colored tabs to indicate the last year of treatment (as previously shown in Figure 8-13).

In a typical medical office, patient files are purged and moved from active to inactive status every 3 to 5 years. However, the assistant should review all files at least once a year to remove useless data, making it easier to find things and reducing bulk. This task may be worked into the regular filing routine.

Typically, the charts of a surgeon would be kept in the active file for a shorter period of time than those of a pediatrician or family practitioner, whose patient care is more likely to continue over years. Physicians located near military bases or resort areas see many transient patients, whose records would be purged frequently.

Proof materials, such as x-rays, laboratory reports, and pathology specimens, should be kept indefinitely. If a patient is a minor, records should be retained until the patient reaches the age of majority, that is, 18 to 21 years, plus the time allowed in that state for a lawsuit to be instituted for injuries the patient sustained as a minor. In most states, that period is 1 to 4 years beyond the age of majority. Everything pertaining to a patient who has had a negative attitude toward his or her care should be retained.

Calendars, appointment books, and telephone logs should also be filed and stored. Cases involving radiologic injury, such as leukemia, may be considered under the statute after the injury is discovered, and this can occur 20 to 30 years after radiation exposure. Before purging records, the medical assistant should refer to the office records retention schedule. Refer to Table 8-1 for suggested guidelines. The physician should have the final say on the length of time that files should be kept active, depending on the type of medical specialty.

COMPLIANCE

Authorization to Release Information Form

The medical assistant should retain requests made by patients to transfer or release medical information to other parties (e.g., other physicians, insurance companies). These documents become part of the permanent medical record.

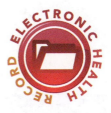

Electronic Storage

The advantage of computerized medical records is that they can be downloaded from the computer to other media (e.g., flash drive, external hard drive, DVD) for storage. The transfer of such records is accomplished quickly and the media can be stored in a fireproof safe or off-site for safe keeping.

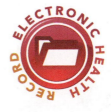

Online Record Storage

Online personal health record (PHR) services are emerging where patients can import records from various health providers to be stored online and create their own personal health profile. Some online sites offer free access and storage of electronic medical records which are used by large employers; others are targeted to health care providers.

COMPLIANCE

HIPAA and CMS Retention Requirements

The HIPAA Administration Simplification Rule requires "a covered entity, such as a physician billing Medicare, to retain required documentation for 6 years from the date of its creation or the date when it last was in effect, whichever is later."

The Center for Medicare and Medicaid services requires Medicare managed care program providers to retain records for 10 years.

TABLE 8-1 Records Retention Schedule

Temporary Record	Recommended Retention Period (Years)	Temporary Record	Recommended Retention Period (Years)
Accounts receivable (computerized or ledger cards)	7	Duplicate bank deposit slips	1
Appointment sheets	3	Employee time cards/sheets and schedules	5
Balance sheets	5	Employment applications	4
Bank deposits and statements (reconciliations)	2	Expense reports	7
		Financial statements	5
Cash receipt records	6	Insurance policies (canceled or expired)	3
Contracts and leases (expired)	7		
Contracts with employees	6	Inventory records	7
Copies of estimated tax forms	6	Invoice and billing records	6
Correspondence, general	5	Payroll records	7
Deceased patients' medical records	5	Petty cash vouchers	3
		Postal and meter records	1
Depreciation schedules	3		

Permanent Record (Retained Indefinitely)	
Accounts payable ledgers	Equipment records
Audits	Inactive patient medical records purged from active files
Balance sheets	Income tax returns and documents
Bills of sale for important purchases	Insurance policies and records
Canceled checks and check registers	Journals
Capital asset records	Legal correspondence
Cashbooks	Media tapes or storage devices
Certified financial statements	Patients' medical records including x-ray films
Charts of accounts	Professional liability insurance policies
Credit history	Property appraisals
Deeds, mortgages, contracts, leases, and property titles/records	Telephone records

Website privacy policies differ and according to the U.S. Department of Health and Human Services, protection laws created by HIPAA that govern the health care industry do not apply to personal health record storage services. Therefore, it is extremely important to investigate security and confidentiality measures if you are going to use such a service.

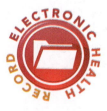

Document Imaging

Paper-based medical and financial records can be converted into electronic documents using document-managing software. Records are scanned into the computer system, digitized, and stored on the hard drive or transferred to one of the previously mentioned media for storage.

Archived electronic documents may then be retrieved using electronic search capabilities, saving time and space. Advanced programs have the capability of sorting similar documents and organizing them by date, check number, and so forth. The type of scanning equipment would determine how fast this process could be done, but the money saved on medical record storage might be worth the effort and expense.

Prior to the use of computers, images were taken of documents and reduced on film using micrograph technology by hospitals, clinics, and insurance companies.

Microfiche technology, or a *microfilming* photographic process was often used and older medical records may still be found which have been stored on this type of media.

DESTROYING DOCUMENTS

Some large medical facilities may contract with outside vendors to destroy medical documents while others may use small paper shredders that attach to waste baskets and shred two to five sheets at a time or stand-alone machines that shred up to 27 sheets simultaneously.

Purging Computer Files

Records are increasingly being stored electronically, that is, on computer hard drives, flash drives, microfilm, optical disks, and various types of backup media. Disposal methods may include degaussing (wiping out information using a magnet) and zeroization (which involves writing binary code zeros over the data). Refer to Table 8-2 for methods of recycling and destroying various types of media.

Dated electronic documents hamper retrieval, increase supply costs, and use up valuable storage space, so whenever computers are used, data need to be purged frequently. One way to assist purging of electronically stored files is to print a list of document types and indicate the retention time (e.g., 3 days, 6 months, 1 year).

COMPLIANCE

Deleting Confidential Files

The HIPAA Privacy Rule requires appropriate administrative, technical, and physical safeguards to protect the privacy of health information through the disposal process. Deleting confidential files may not be sufficient to prevent unauthorized disclosure of information. The impression that the information, once deleted, has been removed from the system and is inaccessible to others may not always be true. Measures to prevent unauthorized disclosure of information are as follows:

1. Encrypt confidential files.
2. Use utility software to specifically overwrite files that have been deleted.
3. Physically destroy disks that are being discarded.
4. Monitor the printer while printing, and destroy "bad" copies of confidential printouts.
5. Carefully control, or do not permit, utility software designed to read and restore deleted files.

TABLE 8-2 Methods of Recycling and Disposing of Protected Health Information

Type of Media	Method of Recycling and Destruction
Audiotape	Record over original tape to recycle Shred tape or crush cassette to destroy
Computer CDs, DVDs, or flash drives	Overwrite all data to recycle Crush or magnetically erase and incinerate to destroy
Labels for PHI created on media devices	Remove and shred or incinerate to destroy
Laser disk	Overwrite rewriteable disks to recycle Crush rewriteable and write-it-once disks to destroy
Magnetic media	Reformat and overwrite tape to recycle Magnetically erase, shred, and incinerate to destroy
Microfilm/Microfiche	Crush or shred to destroy
Videotape	Record over original content to recycle Crush or shred tape and cassette to destroy

Any one of the following types of files is probably an unnecessary file that can be targeted for deletion:

1. A file that has been superseded by another file.
2. A backup or temporary file created by an application program.
3. An older version of a software program if the newer version is on the hard drive.
4. An infrequently used file that should have been transferred to another media.

Whatever the method, it is essential that all information be completely eradicated.

Recycling and the Green Team

Concerns about our environment have motivated medical offices to "go green." A *green team* should be selected from concerned employees who would be willing to evaluate all aspects of the office then suggest improvements. Water conservation, energy efficiency, and purchasing environmentally preferable products are common areas to review. On the top of the list would be an office-recycling center placed in a prominent location. A three-level recycling system would target disposal of regular waste, paper waste, and biohazard waste. The adoption of green policies should focus on changing the behavior and attitudes of all workers so that compliance is achieved.

Medical assistants can show concern for the environment by volunteering for a *green team* or by supervising a waste paper **recycle** plan that is neat, efficient, and orderly. A small box placed near the photocopy machine will provide storage for unclear photocopies that can be used for scrap paper as long as they are not of a confidential nature (e.g., medical records).

Most breaches of confidentiality related to paper recycling occur before the paper ever leaves the medical office. Use of closed containers with slots with one person assigned to empty them can solve the problem. Under most recycling programs, envelopes, gummed labels, rubber bands, cellophane, plastic report covers, and photographic paper are not recyclable. Check with your community's waste disposal program to obtain a list of acceptable recyclable products in your area.

STOP AND THINK CASE SCENARIO
Locate a Missing Record

SCENARIO: Kathryn Holcomb's medical record cannot be located in the file cabinet and the patient is coming in this afternoon for a postoperative recheck with Dr. Fran Practon.

CRITICAL THINKING: You have methodically checked the file cabinet. What staff members might have the file and for what purpose?

a. _____

b _____

c. _____

d. _____

e. _____

f. _____

g. _____

What procedures can be used to prevent missing records?

_____

_____

_____

STOP AND THINK CASE SCENARIO

Determine Document Types and Filing Systems

SCENARIO: Dr. Fran Practon arrived at the office this morning and handed you the following documents to be filed: (a) list of email addresses, (b) last month's bank statement, (c) recipe for apple crisp, (d) list of personal books for reading, (e) laboratory test results on patient Mary Higgins, (f) MRI results on patient Clark Brenneman, (g) phone message on patient Linda Downey, and (h) recall notice for patient Sandra Inez.

CRITICAL THINKING: Decide (1) what type of documents these are (electronic, financial, medical, or personal), (2) how these documents should be filed (alphabetical, chronological, by subject), and (3) where these documents should be filed (medical record, personal file, tickler file). Suggest and note file names.

Example: Transcribed chart note for patient Cindy Hopkins
1. patient's medical record
2. file chronologically
3. in progress notes

a. Email addresses
1. _____
2. _____
3. _____

b. Bank statement
1. _____
2. _____
3. _____

c. Recipes
1. _____
2. _____
3. _____

d. Books (personal)
1. _____
2. _____
3. _____

e. Laboratory report
1. _____
2. _____
3. _____

f. MRI report
1. _____
2. _____
3. _____

g. Telephone message
1. _____
2. _____
3. _____

h. Recall notice
1. _____
2. _____
3. _____

FOCUS ON CERTIFICATION*

CMA (AAMA) Content Summary

- Needs, purposes, and terminology of filing systems
- Alphabetic, numeric, and subject filing
- Color-code, tickler, electronic data processing, and cross-reference files
- Storing, protecting, and transferring files
- Retaining and purging files (statute of limitations)
- Scanning equipment

RMA (AMT) Content Summary

- Prepare patient record (by filing information)
- Manage patient medical record system
- File patient and physician communication in chart
- File materials according to proper system (chronological, alphabetical, subject)
- Protect, store, and maintain medical records according to proper conventions and HIPAA privacy regulations

CMAS (AMT) Content Summary

- Manage documents and patient charts using paper methods
- File records alphabetically, numerically, by subject, and by color
- Employ indexing rules
- Arrange contents of patient charts in appropriate order
- Document and file laboratory results and patient communication in charts
- Store, protect, retain, and destroy records appropriately
- Perform daily chart management
- Observe and maintain confidentiality of records, charts, and test results

REVIEW EXAM-STYLE QUESTIONS

1. Information to be filed may be in the form of:
   a. paper documents
   b. electronic documents
   c. graphic images
   d. manila file folders
   e. a, b, and c are all correct

2. When selecting a filing system, determine two things to consider.
   a. Should be difficult to understand so files cannot be tampered with
   b. Security and expansion
   c. Appearance and mobility

   d. Lightweight and attractive
   e. Sturdy and long lasting

3. A total practice management system (TPMS) is a/an:
   a. patented commercial filing system
   b. alphabetical or numerical filing system
   c. electronic filing system designed to transmit within the medical office
   d. electronic filing system designed to transmit within and outside of the medical office
   e. professional filing system using folders and guides

---

* *This* textbook *and the accompanying* Workbook *meet the entry-level administrative and general competencies for the CMA outlined by the AAMA Examination Content Outline and Occupational Analysis and for the RMA and CMAS outlined by the AMT Competencies, Construction Parameters, and Examination Specifications (see Competency Grid in Appendix B).*

4. An electronic database may consist of files pertaining to:
   a. patient demographics
   b. drugs
   c. procedures
   d. diagnoses
   e. all of the above

5. When scanning, entering, or retrieving patient information from an electronic filing system, you should:
   a. verify the patient by his or her date of birth
   b. verify the patient by his or her driver's license
   c. verify the patient by his or her medical record number
   d. verify the patient by at least two identifiers
   e. verify the patient by three identifiers

6. A password, used as a security code to safeguard entrance to a computerized system should:
   a. always start with a capital letter
   b. consist of a phrase
   c. consist of a series of numbers
   d. be a sequence of letters and numbers
   e. both a and b

7. A tickler file system is also called a/an:
   a. alphabetical filing system
   b. chronological filing system
   c. suspense file
   d. inactive filing system
   e. short-notice reminder file

8. For patient medical records, the most common filing system is:
   a. indirect
   b. numerical
   c. alphabetical
   d. subject
   e. tickler

9. A subject filing system is usually used for:
   a. patient medical records
   b. hospitals, large medical practices, and clinics
   c. reminder notices
   d. business records
   e. electronic records

10. In an indirect filing system, you begin to look for a file by:
    a. going to the cross-reference index
    b. looking for the number 0
    c. looking for the patient's last name in the file cabinet
    d. looking at the middle digit
    e. looking at the terminal digit

11. A chronological filing system:
    a. is out of date and not frequently used
    b. uses numbers to identify and locate patient records
    c. is frequently used to file documents within a chart
    d. is based on the alphabet
    e. is only used for business files

12. Which organization developed the rules for alphabetical filing that are still used today?
    a. AHIMA
    b. ARMA
    c. HIPAA
    d. AAMA
    e. AMA

13. The most popular file cabinets used for storing patient medical records are:
    a. lateral or open shelf files
    b. drawer files
    c. vertical files
    d. automated files
    e. telescoping files

14. The "cut" of a file folder describes the:
    a. thickness of the folder
    b. type of edge the folder has (rough, smooth)
    c. number and position of tabs
    d. number of folders in a box
    e. manufacturer

15. A records retention schedule is a:
    a. list of active records
    b. list of inactive records
    c. list of active and inactive records
    d. list of record types and the length of time each should be kept
    e. list of destruction methods used for old records

WORKBOOK ASSIGNMENT

To develop competency-based job skills, refer to the *Workbook* and complete the:

- Abbreviation and Spelling Review
- Review Questions

- Critical Thinking Exercises
- Job Skill activities, which are listed at the beginning of the chapter under *Performance Objectives in the Workbook*.

RESOURCES

Books

Medical Filing, 2nd edition
Claeys, Therese
Cengage Learning, 1997
Website: http://www.cengagebrain.com

Internet

American Health Information Management Association
Search: Articles and federal regulations regarding record management

Association of Records Managers and Administrators (ARMA International)
Search: Archives, compliance, federal rules, record management, and organization of records

Bibbero Systems, Inc.
Filing equipment and medical office products
Website: http://www.bibbero.com

Keywords for Internet Searches

- Electronic health record
- Electronic medical record
- Filing rules
- Filing systems
- Go green
- Health record systems
- Medical record filing
- Medical record retention
- Medical record storage
- Recycling
- Tickler files

CHAPTER 9

MEDICAL RECORDS

LEARNING OBJECTIVES

After reading this chapter and learning step-by-step procedures to gain job skills,* you should be able to:

- List reasons for maintaining medical records.
- Compare the benefits of an electronic medical record (EMR) and a paper-based medical record.
- Outline "meaningful use" objectives.
- Describe the operation of an electronic health record (EHR) practice management system.
- Name three basic types of medical record organization systems.
- State the functions of a flow sheet.
- Explain several ways information can be entered into a medical record.
- Determine who is qualified to provide computerized provider order entry (CPOE) into an electronic medical record system.
- Cite various titles the physician may have in the treatment of patients.
- Summarize the differences between a manual, an electronic, and a digital signature.
- Itemize contents of a patient's medical record file.
- Discuss two types of documentation formats.
- Understand the contents of a history and physical examination report.
- Define an internal and external audit of medical records.

PERFORMANCE OBJECTIVES (PROCEDURES) IN THIS TEXTBOOK

- Prepare and compile a medical record for a new patient (Procedure 9-1).
- Follow documentation guidelines to record information in a medical record (Procedure 9-2).
- Correct a medical record (Procedure 9-3).
- Abstract data from a medical record (Procedure 9-4).

*This textbook and the accompanying Workbook meet the educational components for entry-level administrative and general competencies outlined by CAAHEP and ABHES.

PERFORMANCE OBJECTIVES (JOB SKILLS) IN THE WORKBOOK

- Prepare a patient record and insert progress notes (Job Skill 9-1).
- Prepare a patient record and format chart notes (Job Skill 9-2).
- Correct a medical record (Job Skill 9-3).
- Abstract from a medical record (Job Skill 9-4).
- Prepare a history and physical (H & P) report (Job Skill 9-5).
- Record test results on a flow sheet (Job Skill 9-6).

KEY TERMS

abstract	electronic health record (EHR) practice management system	problem-oriented medical record (POMR)
attending physician		
audit	electronic medical record (EMR)	prognosis
case history	flow sheet	progress report
CHEDDAR	health information management (HIM)	referring physician
cloaning		sign
computerized provider order entry (CPOE)	laboratory report	SOAP
	meaningful use	source-oriented record (SOR)
consulting physician	medical record	symptom
diagnosis	medical report	treating or performing physician
electronic health record (EHR)	ordering physician	x-ray report

HEART OF THE HEALTH CARE PROFESSIONAL

Service

Although a medical record is the property of those who create it, the patient owns the information within. Consider the medical record as a diary put in your care, and have a high regard for it. By respecting patients' privacy and keeping personal information confidential, you will be serving all patients.

PATIENTS' MEDICAL RECORDS

A patient's **medical record** is a recording of information that documents facts and events during the administration of patient care—it contains sensitive, personal information and tells a story starting with the patient's medical history and includes all medical complaints as well as the care received. The legal task force of the American Health Information Management Association (AHIMA) defines the legal health record (LHR) as "the documentation of healthcare services provided to an individual, in any aspect of healthcare delivery by a healthcare provider organization." The principal reasons for maintaining medical records are:

1. To aid in the diagnosis and treatment of a patient
2. To provide a basis for evaluating the adequacy and appropriateness of care
3. To communicate between the physician and other members of the health care team and ensure continuity of care
4. To verify that services were medically necessary
5. To provide clinical data for research and education
6. To substantiate procedure and diagnostic code selections to process insurance claims for appropriate reimbursement
7. To comply with federal and state laws
8. To provide legal protection and defend the physician in the event of a lawsuit

Patient records are also used in completing various reports required by law, such as reports on communicable

PROCEDURE 9-1

Prepare and Compile a Medical Record for a New Patient

OBJECTIVE: Prepare and compile a medical record for a new patient.

EQUIPMENT/SUPPLIES: File folder, patient information form, file folder label, labels for special information (current year, allergies, insurance information), computer, forms (flow sheet, progress notes, laboratory reports, and so forth), two-hole punch, and pen.

DIRECTIONS: Follow these step-by-step directions, which include rationales, to learn this procedure. Job Skills 9-1 and 9-2 are presented in the *Workbook* to practice this skill for a paper-based system.

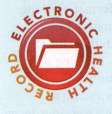

ELECTRONIC MEDICAL RECORD (EMR):

Preparation of a new patient electronic medical record (EMR) happens at the point of registration, as discussed in Chapter 5, *Receptionist and the Medial Office Environment.*

1. As new patient information is input into the computer system, a medical record number and electronic chart are created.

2. As progress notes, test results, and other documents accumulate, everything is electronically filed and arranged according to the software program or the medical practice's preference.

PAPER-BASED MEDICAL RECORD:

3. Select a file folder, either lateral or vertical.

4. Key or type a label for the patient's file folder with the last name followed by the first name and middle initial; charts are filed by last name.

5. Adhere the label to the tabbed edge of the file folder, which may be located at the right, left, or middle top portion of the folder—or on the side.

6. Select colored tabs for the first two letters of the patient's last name if a color-coded filing system is used. In larger offices, additional labeling may be required. This label must be visible when the patient's record is in the filing cabinet or drawer and assists in filing and locating lost charts.

7. Add a current year label, either to the end or top tab of the file folder for a new patient. To update an established patient's record, add a year label the first time the patient comes in for an appointment for the current year. This helps when purging inactive files (see Chapter 8).

8. Adhere an allergy label and indicate all allergies; if there are *no known allergies*, write the abbreviation NKA. Allergy labels alert all staff members and help avoid adverse reactions.

9. Adhere an insurance label indicating the type of plan. Labels identify patients who are in specific insurance plans or categories (e.g., Medicare, HMO).

10. Insert blank forms used by the medical practice into the patient's file folder. Label each sheet with the patient's name or record number. This helps identify each page of the record.

11. Punch holes in the sheets, if necessary, and affix them to the folder. This will secure pages and help position information that may otherwise fall out.

---

diseases, child abuse, gunshot wounds, stabbings from criminal actions, diseases and illnesses of newborns and infants, and injury or illness that occurs in the workplace. A medical record must be prepared for all new patients who will be seen in the medical practice (Procedure 9-1). Various parts of the medical record will be examined in this chapter, as well as electronic recordkeeping; medical record filing systems were discussed in Chapter 8.

MEDICAL RECORD SYSTEMS

With the onset of documentation guidelines and the increase of medical record audits, it is important that a proper medical record system be used. It assists with accessing patients' conditions, provides others with critical information, furnishes statistical information, protects against liability suits, and is a key to quality care.

Medical record information is available through data retrieval systems that provide computer readouts so that traditional patient charts can be updated constantly.

Paper-Based Medical Record System

Paper-based medical records still exist; however, they are inefficient, easy to misplace and misfile, and costly to manage, move, and store. Many people feel secure with a hard copy of information in hand, so while converting to an electronic system some practices maintain *hybrid records* (i.e., using electronic recordkeeping but having some portion of the record on paper). Paper records are time consuming to maintain and more vulnerable to a variety of security threats such as tampering, theft, and loss. There is also no easy way to search for clinical data in a paper-based system.

Health Care Reform

In 2009, President Barack Obama signed the American Reinvestment and Recovery Act (ARRA—stimulus act), which included the Health Information Technology for Economic and Clinical Health (HITECH) Act. The president stated, "The current, paper-based medical records system that relies on patients' memory and reporting of their medical history is prone to error, time-consuming, costly, and wasteful. With rigorous privacy standards in place to protect sensitive medical records, we will embark on an effort to computerize all Americans' health records in five years (by 2014). This effort will help prevent medical errors, improve health care quality, and is a necessary step in starting to modernize the American health care system and reduce health care costs."

Meaningful Use

The term **meaningful use** means that electronic health record technology be used in a meaningful manner to

COMPLIANCE

Electronic Recordkeeping Mandates

One provision in Title II of HIPAA directs federal government programs to adopt national electronic standards for automated transfer of certain health care data among health care payers, plans, and providers.

support efficient, quality, and coordinated patient care. Each eligible provider who demonstrate that certified EHR technology is used for the purposes of electronic exchange of health information, electronic prescribing, and submission of information on clinical quality measures is given an incentive bonus. The EHR incentive program final rule defines the payments that are available from both the Medicare and Medicaid programs for non–hospital-based eligible providers (EPs), also referred to as eligible professionals. EHR technology must be used for 80% of patients.

The following three stages have a set of objectives that are to be met in order for the health care provider to receive the incentive payment. As an example, Table 9-1 lists core- and menu-set objectives that must be met for Stage 2.

- **Stage 1 (2011–2013)*:** Set the criteria for capturing patient data in a standardized format, tracking clinical conditions, and coordinating care by sharing health information with the patient or other health care professionals. In doing so, the provider received an incentive bonus—up to $43,720 for Medicare providers and up to $63,750 for Medicaid providers. Over time, incentive payments decrease. Successful reporting must be completed before moving to Stage 2.

- **State 2 (2014–2015):** Stage 1 objectives expanded— requires better health information exchange between providers, increases e-prescribing, incorporates laboratory test results, promotes patient engagement by giving patients secure online access to their health information, and uses secure electronic messaging to communicate with patients on relevant health issues (see Table 9-1). Again, Stage 2 must be successfully completed before moving on to Stage 3.

- **Stage 3 (2016–2017):** Rule is not finalized but draft recommendations include continuing to expand meaningful use objectives and improve efficiency, quality, and safety leading to improved health care outcomes; include diagnostic imaging and increase the threshold for medication and laboratory orders. Over time, physicians who were eligible but did not implement EHR in a meaningful way are penalized through payment adjustments.

---

*Forty-eight percent of all health care practices meet basic guidelines for meaningful use of certified EHR technology under Stage 1 of the Medicare and Medicaid EHR Incentive Programs. *Modern Healthcare*, January 20, 2014.

TABLE 9-1 Stage 2 Core-Set and Menu-Set Electronic Objectives for Eligible Providers*

Core-Set Objectives: Report on all 17	Menu-Set Objectives: Report 3 of 6
1. Perform computerized provider order entry (CPOE) for medication, laboratory, and radiology orders	1. Submit electronic syndromic surveillance data to public health agencies
2. Generate and transmit electronic prescriptions	2. Record electronic notes in patient records
3. Record demographic information	3. Have imaging results accessible through Certified Electronic Health Record Technology (CEHRT)
4. Record and note changes in vital signs	4. Record patient family health status
5. Record smoking status for patient 13 years and older	5. Identify and report cancer cases to a state cancer registry
6. Use clinical decision support to improve performance on high-priority health conditions	6. Identify and report specific cases to a specialized register; other than cancer
7. Provide patients the ability to view online, download, and transmit their health information	
8. Provide clinical summaries for patients for each office visit	
9. Protect electronic health information	
10. Incorporate clinical lab test results into EHRs	
11. Generate lists of patients by specific conditions to use for quality improvement, reduction of disparities, research, or outreach	
12. Use clinically relevant information to identify patients who should receive reminders for preventive and follow-up care	
13. Use certified EHR technology to identify patient-specific education resources	
14. Perform medication reconciliation	
15. Provide summary of care record	
16. Submit electronic data to immunization registries	
17. Use secure electronic messaging to communicate with patients on relevant health information	

*Eligible *Medicare providers* are non–hospital-based licensed doctors of medicine/osteopathy, doctors of dental surgery/medicine, doctors of pediatric medicine, doctors of optometry, and chiropractors. Eligible *Medicaid providers* are non–hospital-based licensed doctors of medicine, osteopathy, dental surgery/medicine, podiatry, and optometry; chiropractors; nurses; nurse practitioners; certified nurse-midwives; dentists; and physician assistants in federally qualified health centers or rural health clinics that are led by a physician's assistant.

To go a step further, the use of *patient-generated health data (PGHD)* is now being incorporated into many practice management systems. PGHD includes the patient's health history, symptoms, treatment history, lifestyle choices, and ongoing biometric data, such as blood glucose or blood pressure readings, or other health-related data created, recorded, and gathered to assist the patients with their health concerns. Patients may gather supplemental data and record changes in their health condition using smartphones, tablets, and online patient portals.

Concerns about using PGHD are the ability to store the data and monitor the status of the information as reviewed by the physician, or not reviewed.

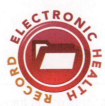

Converting Paper Records to Electronic Records

To digitize medical records is to convert paper documents to electronic images using a scanner. Some health care enterprises process more than 2500 different types of documents. The most common are patient history and physical evaluations, consultations, prescriptions, reports (laboratory, EKGs, radiology), insurance claims, and billing statements. Advanced scanners can handle taped strips from fetal monitors or electrocardiography machines, envelopes, self-adhesive notes, and other odd-sized items without misfeeding or errors while reading the material.

If you are responsible for managing the conversion of a paper record to an EMR, it is important to consult with a **health information management (HIM)** professional to develop a plan, write a proposal, and select a vendor. A HIM professional collects, integrates, analyzes, and codes health care data. Goals should be clarified and the physician needs to lead the effort. Visit other offices, network with managers who have gone through the conversion process, and attend vendor demonstrations. Verify the references of all potential vendors prior to making a selection, obtaining a commitment, and negotiating a contract. A successful conversion is tied to having an open mind, ample education, and on-site training. Refer to Figure 9-1 for an example of a letter sent from a clinic to inform patients of the transition to an electronic medical record system.

WOODLAND HILLS CLINIC

2300 Main Street • Woodland Hills, XY 12345
Telephone (555) 486-2300

January 1, 2016

Ms. Stephanie Moes
2369 Palomar Avenue
Woodland Hills, XY 12345

Dear Stephanie:

Woodland Hills Clinic is improving the way we manage your health care information so we can continue to deliver the highest quality service to all of our patients.

We are launching a new electronic health record system that will provide complete electronic documentation of the care you receive at Woodland Hills Clinic. It will create a single and continuously updated electronic chart for each patient, which means records will be complete and accessible by your health care providers from anywhere at any time.

This will strengthen the collaboration of our entire team by orchestrating the activities of our physicians, nurse practitioners, nurses, medical assistants, and administrators in our 18-plus departments and 15 locations.

This transition from paper charts to electronic health records is a big project that requires technical changes across all of our facilities. When you come in for your next appointment, things may be a little different. We have outfitted our exam rooms with computers and we encourage you to read the enclosed brochure which details the many ways you will benefit from this electronic approach. This is an exciting step forward and one of our most ambitious projects in our 50-year history.

Thank you for your patience as we move into 2016 and continue to improve the exceptional care you have come to expect from Woodland Hills Clinic.

Sincerely,

Richard Rennell

Richard Rennell, MD
CEO and President

FIGURE 9-1 Sample letter informing patients of the transition to an electronic health record system

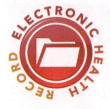

Electronic Health Record Practice Management System

For years now, medical offices have had practice management systems that consist of computer software programs for appointment scheduling and financial records. Many years later, offices started using **electronic medical records (EMR)**, which are digital versions of patients' paper charts. The EMRs were used within the medical practice or in an **electronic health record (EHR)** system that had the capability to capture and store data in electronic form but information could only be shared within one medical practice or organization. Soon after, *electronic health record practice management systems* were developed, often called an *interoperable system* that provides the capability of sharing data outside the medical practice, with other providers involved in the patient's care including other EHR systems found in hospitals, nursing homes, laboratories, and radiology departments; also referred to as a *total practice management system* (TPMS).

When a medical practice adopts an **electronic health record (EHR) practice management system**, everything goes electronic and a database is maintained in the computer that consists of a master patient list with demographics and account numbers, practice physicians and health care practitioners in the area and their identifiers, and insurance carrier information. As previously discussed, the patient data file is first created when a new patient is seen. The patient's history and physical; problem, allergy, and medication lists; outside test results; and diagnosis and prognosis would be included in the data repository and added to each time the patient is seen or when any action is taken or a report or communication received.

In an EHR practice management system, every examination room can be set up with a computer terminal, or more often a laptop is brought into the room. Some physicians are concerned about patients viewing monitors or feel the computer might be a distraction. They prefer to use computers outside the exam room (in the hallway or at the physician's desk) so that they can maintain eye contact and use a hands-on approach; it is a matter of personal style and some doctors use a combination of both. Also, various electronic mobile devices are used to input, store, and transfer data. A *digital pen*, much like a regular ballpoint pen, equipped with a small camera can be used and is especially accurate when marking check-off boxes on a template. It picks up ink from the page, and the mark is uploaded as a single image into the computer system. Although not as accurate, it can also be used for handwriting. While the physician writes, the pen records its own position and movement. After the user is done writing, the digital pen is docked in a cradle attached to a computer's USB port, where the data are uploaded. A copy of the handwritten page is then produced in electronic form.

EHR management systems are continuing to improve, and upcoming technology enables the physician to make "mouse calls" to patients over the Internet for a fee. They offer fast, secure, and centralized access to health care data that can be viewed electronically through in-office terminals and in satellite offices, patient portals, homes, and other outside locations such as the emergency room or intensive care unit by using protected passwords. In some hospital settings, wireless networks are now in place where a wireless computer on a cart can be moved from room to room allowing nurses to view and input patient data (e.g., vital signs) directly into the electronic system.

Laboratory results may come directly from outside laboratories and automatically populate various fields in the patient's electronic record. Hospital radiology and operative reports as well as discharge summaries may be received directly and filed electronically. Prescriptions may be routed to pharmacies through a process called *e-prescribing*. Legal documents and other correspondence would be stored, and a special medical/surgical note area may be available to document phone calls and messages. Virtually, all components of a medical practice are integrated into an EHR practice management system.

Some benefits of an EHR system include the ability to:

- Have information readily available
- Search and track patient histories, clinical data, prescription drugs, consultations, and a variety of data
- Detect inconsistencies in diagnoses
- Monitor quality assurance standards
- Share information, quickly and smoothly
- Deliver prompt reports
- Achieve timely billing and reimbursement
- Decrease errors and miscommunications

- Increase legibility by reducing handwritten notes
- Alert the physician when prescribing a drug to which the patient is allergic
- Warn the physician of drug interactions or a diagnosis that contradicts the use of a drug
- Reduce or eliminate transcription costs
- Save time with centralized chart management, thus eliminating filing and file storage expenses
- Provide electronic faxing
- Create customized reminder notices
- Streamline and facilitate the documentation process

Other functions of an EHR practice management system are listed throughout this *textbook*, such as generating customized patient information, authorization, or encounter forms (Chapters 3, 5, 13); utilizing portals (e.g., kiosks) so that patients can communicate with the office (Chapters 2, 5); going online to verify insurance eligibility (Chapter 18); scheduling e-appointments (Chapter 7); and generating requisition forms and specific written instructions for patients (Chapter 8).

In subsequent chapters, the following will be discussed: E-prescribing of drugs (Chapter 10), data processing for written correspondence (Chapter 11), charge capture for bookkeeping purposes (Chapter 15), auto-coding for procedures and diagnoses (Chapters 16, 17), electronic processing of health insurance claims (Chapter 18), and electronic financial management (Chapter 20). This chapter will focus on EMRs. Refer to Example 9-1 for some of the most common features used in an EHR system and doctor responses to experienced benefits.

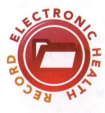

Electronic Health Record Software

There are many types of EHR software packages; however, the key to successful operations is the ability to be compatible and communicate with other software programs outside of the medical facility. Formatting standards for data content, as well as standards guidelines for sending and receiving data is critical. Patient privacy and security are two other considerations, so it is best to communicate all of your office's needs prior to making your selection and make sure you can store, send, and receive information outside of your network.

Common Features in an EHR System*

- Viewing drug lab results (80%)
- Ordering electronic prescriptions (74%)
- Recording clinical notes (67%)
- Generating patient lists by demographic criteria (34%)
- Generating quality metrics (31%)
- Providing electronic copies of health information to patients (14%)

National Survey of Doctors Reporting on Benefits**

- Sending electronic prescriptions saves time (82%)
- More efficient functioning of the medical practice (79%)
- Receives lab results faster (75%)
- Data confidentiality enhanced (70%)
- Electronic features an asset when recruiting physicians (68%)

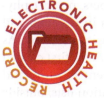

Using An Electronic Medical Record

When a user enters an EMR, which is the equivalent of a patient chart, a drop-down menu or tool bar often occurs which makes navigating through the medical record easier (Example 9-2). Tabs, similar to those used in a paper-based system, can assist when going to various sections of the medical record and data can be entered into specific areas.

In an EMR chart, the health care provider can document clinical findings in a free-text narrative by keying information directly into the computer or by dictating a report and having it transcribed and electronically fed into the record. Various types of dictation software are available, and "pick lists" on

---

Annals of Internal Medicine study; 1820 primary care physicians surveyed from 2011 to 2012.
**National survey of doctors conducted by HealthIT.

EXAMPLE 9-2

Menu Bar

- Appts
- Doctors
- Consults
- EKGs
- H & P
- Lab Tests
- Meds
- Notes
- Progress Notes
- Radiology
- Results
- Scans
- Other

templates can also generate narratives. The physician can choose the typical language for normal findings already stored in the software or mark an insertion point for edited remarks and later dictate that section of the report. The report is then released to be finalized by the medical transcriptionist, who reviews and edits it for accuracy of grammar and spelling, enters any information that has been dictated, and returns the report to the physician for final review and signature.

The practitioner can also use templates with specific data fields associated with various history and examination requirements. Several different templates are available, and the vendor may be able to design customized templates to suit the needs of the medical practice and the physician. Templates, however, may not be designed for a specific problem or visit type, nor should they be made to meet specific reimbursement criteria. Example 9-3 shows a series of typical questions designed to find more information about the patient's chief complaint, which is "fever." This would appear in a pop-up screen after entering the reason for the patient's visit.

One screen may contain ongoing data about a patient, including allergies and past history of complaints. There may be a history and physical screen with two different templates. The type of visit often "drives" the templates, for example, one may be for a well-child preventative visit and one may be for an ill-child visit. When the examination has been completed, the software program may prompt the physician through a series of templates and screens to assist in the assignment of procedural codes.

When the diagnosis has been determined, a diagnostic screen appears. There are usually several diagnostic codes listed—those that were previously assigned

and those relating to the current problem. The physician selects the appropriate ones according to the description. With this data input, it is then possible for the system to generate either an electronic claim for transmission or a paper claim for mailing depending on how the insurance utility was set up.

Electronic records should be considered a new tool designed to improve the work of a medical practice. For most paper chart elements, there is an electronic equivalent and they are constantly evolving as a means to provide better care and meet the ever-changing documentation requirements.

Although the benefits seem to outweigh the problems, EMR systems are not perfect. There is a learning curve and some physicians are not computer savvy or do not have the time or desire to implement a completely new way of doing things.

EXAMPLE 9–3

Computer Template Questions

Chief Complaint: Fever

The questions appearing in a pop-up screen might ask, "How long has the patient had a fever?" "What is the highest temperature reading?" "What other symptoms (chills, sweats, nausea, vomiting, rash, headache, pain) accompany the fever?"

COMPLIANCE

Electronic Data and System Security

It is imperative that an EMR system provides security for both data and the system.

- *Data security* offers protection from improper disclosure or unauthorized or unintended alteration of information.
- *System security* incorporates safeguards to protect the system and its resources and data from defined threats.

You can customize the security features of an EHR system by deciding who has access and setting rules for password complexity. An audit trail is provided, which locates suspicious patterns of access.

Certain treatment rooms may have dead spots that drop the signal from a wireless network, making electronic documentation in the exam room impossible. Disruption of the Internet connection may occur, such as when a fiber-optic cable is severed. And, an electrical outage can prove disastrous because no records can be accessed.

Medical Record Access

As stated in Chapter 3, both the Privacy Act and the Health Insurance Portability and Accountability Act established laws that permit patient access to their medical records. If such a request is made for the patient's personal use, it is wise for the physician or medical assistant to sit down with the patient and explain medical abbreviations, medical terminologies, sensitive diagnoses, and answer any questions prior to the patient leaving with the medical record.

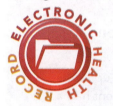

With an EHR system, all providers who take part in the patient's care for a particular problem have instant access to the medical record pertaining to that health issue. For instance, if the patient is in the hospital, the provider can access the patient's medical record from the hospital room, nurse's station, and office cubical as well as the laboratory, pharmacy, and medical records department. During a medical emergency or when an on-call physician sees another doctor's patient, it is imperative for the medical record to be available.

Electronic Medical Record Backup

Numerous backups are required because an EHR vendor cannot guarantee that a patient record can be retrieved for the entire statute of limitations time frame.

An hourly or daily backup system to a CD, DVD, or flash drive should be instituted and a full backup using an external hard drive, dedicated server, or online backup system are all possible choices. Whatever method is used, an alternative power source is needed because an EMR system cannot function without electricity and is at risk if a temporary blackout occurs or a natural disaster causes the electrical circuits to be down for several days or weeks.

*Professional Data Systems.

EMRs are now being used in litigation, and the federal court system has implemented rules for discovery of electronically stored information. Unlike a paper record, an electronic record system can capture the time that an entry was made, when the record was accessed, who looked at it, and if it was altered. In litigation, security practices may be called into question in an attempt to cast doubt on the validity of the record. The medical practice's adherence to applicable standards and security laws (e.g., HIPAA) may also be called into question. Steps should be taken to ensure that the electronic system provides mechanisms that establish the trustworthiness of the record during legal proceedings.

Medical Record Organization Systems

The medical record should be arranged in a way that will reduce the likelihood of critical information being overlooked. Three basic types of medical record organization systems used by most physicians' offices are:

- Problem-oriented medical record
- Source-oriented record
- Integrated record

Problem-Oriented Record System

During the 1960s, Dr. Lawrence Weed developed a **problem-oriented medical record (POMR)** system. The system has been modified for use by individual disciplines, including the medical profession (Figures 9-2 and 9-3).

The example in Figure 9-2 illustrates a form that includes identification data and lists in tabular form all of the patient's permanent and temporary problems, each one numbered and dated. The patient's continuing and temporary medications are cross-referenced (by number) to the problem for which they were prescribed, along with dosage information and the start and stop dates of the medication.

Some data are hard to track in narrative progress notes; on the other hand, flow sheets, charts, or graphs allow the physician to quickly find information and perform comparative evaluations. They provide an organized method of documentation that leads to quicker diagnosis and treatment and better patient care. These, however, do not replace documentation in the progress notes in the

medical record. The example in Figure 9-3 indicates allergies and the patient's blood type and illustrates several **flow sheets** in the bottom portion of the form that allow the physician to quickly find information.

One flow sheet lists consultations, the specialty and name of the physician, and the date the appointments occurred. The type of problem is cross-referenced by number to the problem list shown in Figure 9-2. Another flow sheet lists immunizations and the dates they were received. A third one lists hospitalizations, the year they occurred, and the reason for the admission. There are also flow sheets for Pap tests, mammograms, and prostate-specific antigen (PSA) tests along with a tracking form for blood pressures.

In addition to the types of flow sheets mentioned, they are commonly used to record blood sugar levels for patients with diabetes; prothrombin levels for patients taking blood-thinning agents (e.g., Coumadin); weight for obstetric, obese, or undernourished patients; as well as medication refill information. They can be developed for any type of continuous problem, for example, cardiovascular cases (see Example 9-4).

Using a POMR system helps the physician retrieve information quickly, have an ongoing review of the patient's health status, plan for medical care, and handle large patient workloads. There is less reliance on the physician's memory, so errors are reduced and the patient receives more efficient, continuous care. The disadvantage of using this format in a paper-based system is the time it takes to develop the problem list and to do the necessary repetitious recording.

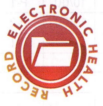

Using a computerized system, the POMR approach is frequently found and referred to as a *Problem Oriented Medical Information System (POMIS)*. The computer is able to populate various flow sheets automatically, saving input time and making retrieval fast and easy. Some EHR systems have the capability of bringing the patient's established problem list to each visit. This can be used as long as the provider is treating each one of the established problems on that date of service and the documentation supports the diagnosis billed for.

Source-Oriented Record System

The **source-oriented record (SOR)** system is the most common paper-based management system. Documents are arranged according to sections, for example, history and physical section, progress notes, laboratory, radiology, surgical operations, and so forth. Some SOR systems

PATIENT RECORD—COMPREHENSIVE FLOW SHEET (page 1)

Name: Morani   Betty   A.   **Account No.:** 00621

Address: 4040 Third St.   New Hill   XY   00421   **Telephone:** (555) 897-6543

Date of Birth: 6/20/45   **Sex:** F **Status:** M   **Social Security No.:** XXX-XX-3333

Employer: Retired   **Occupation:** Hair stylist

Next of Kin: John Morani   **Relationship:** H   **Telephone:** (555) 897-0060 work

Address: Same

Insurance: Medicare   **Policy No.:** XXX-XX-3333A   **Group:**

Address: ABC Insurance Company Fiscal Intermediary   **Telephone:** (555) 499-0101

Date	PERMANENT PROBLEMS	Problem Number	Date	TEMPORARY PROBLEMS	Problem Number
10/08	Hypertension—essential	P-1	1/09	L. Retinopathy	T-1
10/08	Diabetes mellitus—type II	P-2	3/13	Conjunctivitis	T-2
4/10	Atherosclerosis with cerebral	P-3	7/16	UTI	T-3
	vascular insufficiency		11/16	Otitis media	T-4
4/10	Hearing loss	P-4			
1/12	Left bundle branch block	P-5			
1/12	Bilateral grade II retinopathy	P-6			

Date Start	CONTINUING MEDICATIONS	Date Stop	Problem Number	Date Start	TEMPORARY MEDICATIONS	Date Stop	Problem Number
10/08	Sinoserp 1 mg b.i.d.	10/00	P-1	3/13	Tetracycline 250 mg	10d	T-2
10/08	Orinase 0.5 gm daily	10/00	P-2	7/16	Amoxil 250 mg	10d	T-3
10/10	Hydrodiuril 50 mg am		P-1	11/16	Amoxil 250 mg	7d	T-4

FIGURE 9-2 Comprehensive flow sheet (page 1) used for problem-oriented medical record printed on or attached to inside front cover listing permanent and temporary medical problems and continuing/temporary medications

PATIENT RECORD—COMPREHENSIVE FLOW SHEET (page 2)

Name: Morani, Betty A.   **Allergies:** Codeine

Acct No. 00621   Sulfa

Date of Birth: 6/20/45   **Blood Type:** A+

Physician: Fran Practon MD   **Health Care Directive.:** Yes

Date	CONSULTATIONS	Problem Number	✔	IMMUNIZATIONS	Dates			INFLUENZA Date
1/09	Ophth. – Dr. Metz	T-1		**Haemophilus (b)**				10/08
4/10	ENT – Dr. O'Farrell	P-4		**Hepatitis A**				9/09
1/12	Ophth. — Dr. Metz	P-6		**Hepatitis B**				9/10
			✔	**Inactivated Polio**	'51	'52		11/11
			✔	**MMR**	had			10/12
				Pneumococcal				9/13
			✔	**Small Pox**	'53			10/15
			✔	**Varicella**	had			9/16

Date	HOSPITALIZATIONS	Problem Number	✔					
			✔	**TB**	'52	'98		
1950	T&A		✔	**DPaT**	'46	'59	'80	
1978	TAH							

Date	PAP TEST	Date	MAMMOGRAM	Date	PSA
10/08	Class I	10/08	Normal		
1/09	Class I	4/10	R Microcalcification		
4/10	Class I	1/12	R Microcalcification		
1/12	Class I	7/14	Normal		
3/13	Class I	11/16	Normal		
7/14	Class I				
11/16	Class I				

DATE	10/08	1/09	4/10	1/12	3/13	7/14	11/16			
BP	140/88	150/90	160/86	128/78	130/84	190/90	160/80			
DATE										
BP										

FIGURE 9-3 Comprehensive flow sheet (page 2) used for problem-oriented medical record printed on or attached to inside front cover listing various data for tracking purposes

use color laminated tab dividers for each section, which make locating information quick and easy. The information in each section is sequenced in chronological order, with the most recent on top. Sequencing of the sections varies from practice to practice. The disadvantage of the SOR system is the lack of an overall picture of the patient's health or problem because documentation related to these issues is filed in different sections of the record.

Integrated Record System

The *integrated record* system files all documents in chronological order without regard to their source.

EXAMPLE 9-4

Cardiovascular Flow Sheet

Patient's Name: Clare McDonald		Acct No. 486-932		Physician: F. Practon, MD	
Normal Values ABC Lab	135–199	30–85	<130	L=<3.7 M=>3.7 H=>4.7	35–180
Date	Cholesterol	HDL	LDL	Cardiac Risk Ratio	Triglycerides
1/18/2010	204	59	116	3.5	145
2/3/2011	232	61	160	3.80	57
2/17/2012	245	55	142	4.5	242
10/9/2013	256	62	178	4.1	80
2/16/2014	277	59	181	4.7	186
5/4/2015	266	50	186	5.3 Start Zocar 40 mg/d	149
9/14/2016	187	70	102	2.7	99

Trying to compare information from the same source—for example, laboratory test results—is difficult because they are scattered throughout the record.

RECORDKEEPING

With the appearance of computers and communication equipment, there are a variety of ways to keep records and record data. Following are four basic ways information can be entered into the medical record:

- *Physician hand-enters data*—Entries in the patient's record are handwritten. Physicians have been held liable when medication has been given to a patient in error as a result of handwritten notes that were incorrectly read. All hand-written entries must be legible.
- *Physician dictates*—Many physicians dictate their notes or comments. Dictation terminals may be available at the physician's desk, in the treatment room, or at office workstations. Portable equipment may be used by the physician when off-site. The transcriptionist listens to voice-recorded data and keys the information using a computer. The record or report is then reviewed and signed by the physician.
- *Physician keys data*—Data are entered via a remote device or terminal that is available in every examination room where the physician can key in information about the patient's visit. This information can be printed in the form of a progress note or medical report.

- *Medical assistant or scribe enters data*—A checklist, form, or template is used with common problems and procedures specific to the medical practice. The assistant fills in blanks, completes phrases and sentences, or keys in dictated text as the physician narrates findings and recommendations. Medical assistants acting as scribes should be meticulous and document what the doctor says and not insert their own impressions; scribes should take no clinical role in patient visits. The advantage of this system is that the physician can focus his or her full attention on the patient and the medical record is completed before the physician leaves the examination room. The scribe must include (1) who performed the service with title, (2) who recorded the service, with qualifications, and (3) signature and date for both (see Example 9-5). The physician can review the input before leaving the room or at a later time (Figure 9-4).

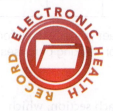

Order Entry

In 2012, the Centers for Medicare and Medicaid services (CMS) established the criteria for **computerized provider order entry (CPOE)** into an EHR system for the CMS Incentive Programs. "Meaningful use" medical record auditors have the authority to determine whether entry of medication, laboratory, and radiology orders has been made by licensed health care professionals or credentialed medical assistants.

Documentation by Scribe

(1) State, who performed the service with title: "I, Gerald Practon, MD, personally performed the services described in this documentation as scribed by Lynda Winter in my presence, and it is both accurate and complete."

(2) State, who performed the service with qualifications: "I, Linda Winter, CMA (AAMA), am scribing for, and in the presence of Dr. Gerald Practon."

(3) Signature and date for both the physician and scribe: "Physician's Signature: *Gerald Practon, MD*, Date: 10/14/20XX; Scribe's Signature: *Linda Winter, CMA (AAMA)*, Date: 10/14/20XX."

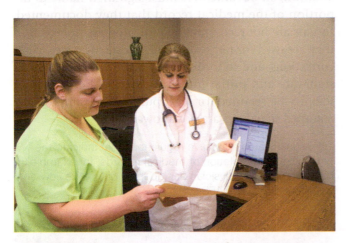

FIGURE 9-4 A medical assistant is shown clarifying information with the physician about a patient's condition before recording it in the medical record

Medical assistants carrying the American Association of Medical Assistants (AAMA) CMA certification meet this requirement; however, since the only individuals eligible for this certification examination are those who have graduated from a postsecondary medical assisting program accredited by either CAAHEP or ABHES, in 2014 AAMA established an *Assessment-Based Recognition (ABR) program* in order entry for electronic health records (EHRs). Individuals who pass this assessment-based certification program meet the "credentialed medical assistant" requirement for CPOE. The program assesses knowledge and experience and the candidate has to complete five AAMA continuing education courses covering key elements of electronic order entry.

Recordkeepers

In each medical practice, an individual should be named as the recordkeeper. In a small practice, this may be a duty of the administrative medical assistant. In a large medical practice, one person is usually in charge of all medical records. The larger the practice, the more duties the medical recordkeeper has. He or she may be in charge of overseeing the medical record system and all file clerks, documentation requirements, coding, internal audits, processing authorization requests for records, and obtaining patient records from other facilities. As mentioned in Chapter 3, this person would need to comply with all regulations regarding the use and transfer of private health information, including answering subpoenas.

Office policies vary, but records are usually sent to other physicians with no charge when the need has to do with continuation of care or transfer of care. When records are requested from patients for their personal use or for reasons that do not involve treatment (e.g., life insurance application), the physician's office usually charges for the copying and release of records (e.g., 25 cents per page up to $25 for the entire record). Most offices notify insurance companies of the charge when signed requests are received and only release the records after the fee has been obtained. This saves billing insurance companies for miscellaneous fees and trying to collect small amounts of money.

Documenters

All individuals who provide health care services may be known as *documenters* because they chronologically

COMPLIANCE

HIPAA Rule on Copying Records

The amount that health care organizations can charge for providing patients with copies of their medical information is limited by HIPAA to a "reasonable, cost-based fee," and HIPAA narrowly defines what costs can be included. The rule is not nearly as strict for release of information (ROI) requests and charges from outside entities, which vary state by state and can run as high as $1.18 per page plus retrieval and handling fees. Patients requesting copies of their records should do so in writing. Typically, the doctor's office has 5 days to produce the record allowing time to process the request and retrieve charts that may have been sent to an outside storage facility.

record facts and observations about the patient and the patient's health.

The receptionist may record canceled or no-show appointments and messages, the insurance specialist may record authorization requests or alerts for patients who have been sent to a collection agency, and the clinical medical assistant may record vital signs, scheduled tests, and other clinical data—each taking the role of a documenter. A *Clinical Documentation Improvement Specialist (CDIS)* may be utilized to help the provider strengthen the overall patient record. A CDIS reviews clinical data to verify that it is accurate, complete, legible, and done in a timely manner.

There are instances when the physician's title may change, depending on the specialty and services rendered. Because this can be a confusing issue and because it is important when submitting insurance claims, clarification of these various roles is detailed here.

- **Attending physician** refers to the medical staff member who is legally responsible for the care and treatment given to a patient.
- **Consulting physician** is a provider whose opinion or advice regarding evaluation or management of a specific problem is requested by another physician.
- **Ordering physician** is the individual directing the selection, preparation, or administration of tests, medication, or treatment.
- **Referring physician** is a provider who sends the patient for testing or treatment. It may also be the

provider who transfers the management of a patient to another physician.

- **Treating** or **performing physician** is the provider who renders a service to a patient.

Regardless of who the documenter is, entries need to be made in a timely manner*—at the time of service or shortly thereafter. If clarification or additional information is needed, it is acceptable to delay the entry for a reasonable length of time (i.e., 24 to 48 hours). It is never reasonable to expect a provider to recall details of an examination several weeks after the encounter took place. Entries should never be made in advance.

Authentication of Documents

Each document must be authenticated by signature, which attests to the content of the entry and its accuracy. The treating or attending physician must sign each progress note as well as all test results and reports. In addition, all documenters must sign their name to the portion of the medical record that they documented. Initials are not recommended for progress notes, but if they are used for test results, telephone messages, chart corrections, and so forth, it is recommended that a staff signature and initial log which establishes signature identity be retained for legal purposes (Example 9-6). Stamped signatures are not allowed.

---

*Individual states may have regulations that indicate the timeliness of completion of medical records, for example, in Pennsylvania, the physician has up to 10 days to review and sign the record (§ 18.158.d.4).

EXAMPLE 9-6

Signature/Initial Log for Office Staff

Date	Name	Position	Credential	Signature	Initials
January 3, 20XX	Gerald Practon	General Practitioner	MD = medical doctor	*Gerald Practon MD*	GP
January 3, 20XX	Fran Practon	Family Practice Physician	MD = medical doctor	Fran Practon MD	FP
January 5, 20XX	Suzanne Davenport	Office Manager	CMA (AAMA) = certified medical assistant (American Association of Medical Assistants)	*SD Suzanne Davenport CMA (AAMA)*	SD
January 6, 20XX	Andrea Roddick	Administrative Medical Assistant	CMAS = certified medical administrative specialist	*Andrea Roddick CMAS*	AR
January 6, 20XX	Sondra Kovitz	Clinical Medical Assistant	RMA = registered medical assistant	Sondra Kovitz RMA	SK
January 6, 20XX	Beatrice Federrer	Medical Insurance Biller	CPC = certified professional coder	*Beatrice Federrer CPC*	BF

Medicare Signature Requirements*

Medicare contractors have reported that "one of the most common errors is missing or illegible physician signature." When a Medicare audit is performed and documentation is not accepted due to an illegible signature, a signature log or attestation statement to support the identity of the illegible signature may be submitted. If the original record contains a printed signature below the illegible signature, this may be accepted.

Manual Signatures

Handwritten or typed entries made during the continuing care of the patient should be signed by the treating or attending physician. For a chart to be admissible as evidence in court, the physician who dictated or wrote the entries must attest that the entries were true and correct at the time of writing. A physician's signature after the typed notes indicates this fact. If the physician is away from the office after dictating a document and the correspondence is urgent, there are two choices:

1. The assistant can sign the physician's name with his or her own initials after it.
2. A photocopy of the record (letter) may be sent, stating that the physician will sign and forward the original upon his or her return.

Electronic Signatures

Documents generated via computer may contain signatures created in several different ways. A pen and electronic signature pad, similar to those found in retail stores, may be used. Electronic signatures or digital signatures are more common. An *electronic signature* refers to a method of authenticating documents by the insertion of a facsimile of a person's actual handwritten signature or typed name that is affixed electronically at the end of a document. Because it can be altered, deleted, or forged by anyone with access privileges, an electronic signature creates obvious problems.

A *digital signature* is secure because it cannot be forged or altered without detection, and if the content of the signed document is altered, the signature is invalidated. To authenticate portions of the medical record using a digital signature, an individual with computer access uses an identification encryption system such as a series of letters or numbers (alphanumeric computer key entries), an electronic writing, or a biometric system, such as voice print, handprint, or fingerprint transmissions; and facial, iris, or retinal scans. See Example 9-7 for an illustration of a chart note using an electronic signature and view the following list of acceptable electronic signature formats:

- Authenticated by Gerald M. Practon, MD
- Authorized by Fran T. Practon, MD
- Chart accepted by Gerald M. Practon, MD
- Closed by Fran T. Practon, MD
- Confirmed by Gerald M. Practon, MD
- Digital signature: Fran T. Practon, MD
- Digitalized signature: Gerald M. Practon, MD— handwritten and scanned into the computer
- Electronically approved by Fran T. Practon, MD
- Electronically signed by Gerald M. Practon, MD
- Finalized by Fran T. Practon, MD
- Released by Gerald M. Practon, MD
- Reviewed by Fran T. Practon, MD

EXAMPLE 9–7

Electronic Signature

Patient: Marlo Lewis   MR No: 1007
DOB: 12/14/1939

Informed Consent for Radical Nephrectomy: Detailed informed consent was given to the patient regarding radical nephrectomy. The risks and benefits of surgery were discussed in detail. Both open and laparoscopic approaches were discussed in detail. The risks of both surgeries include bleeding, infection, need for transfusion, damage to surrounding tissue, need for further treatment including surgery, chemotherapy, radiation, myocardial infarction, pulmonary embolism, and even death. The risks of anesthesia were detailed as well. No guarantees were made or implied. Time was allowed, and all questions were answered. She understands these risks and accepts them.

Electronically signed by CEDRIC EMMERSON MD 6/3/2016 17:59:58

---

*As of May 2011, CMS has agreed to rescind the rule requiring a physician's signature on Medicare laboratory requisitions.

- Signed: Gerald M. Practon, MD
- Signed before import by Fran T. Practon, MD
- Signed by Gerald M. Practon, MD
- This is an electronically verified report by Fran T. Practon, MD
- Verified by Gerald M. Practon, MD

DOCUMENTATION GUIDELINES

Documentation is a communication tool that should paint a clear picture of what was found, what was done, and why. An on-call or consulting physician should be able to look at another physician's documentation and determine his or her thought process in arriving at the diagnosis and treatment recommendation.

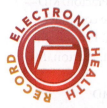

Electronic medical records follow the same documentation requirements as a paper-based system. All documentation must contain sufficient, accurate information to:

1. Support the diagnoses
2. Justify the treatment or procedures performed
3. State the course of care

4. Identify test results
5. Promote continuity of care

Complete, but not extraneous documentation is the goal. The medical assistant is often the one to document the following:

- Email messages
- Faxed communications
- Informed consents
- Patient education sessions
- Patient instructions
- Patient's failure to keep an appointment
- Patient's noncompliance; failure to follow the physician's advice
- Prescription refills and medication samples
- Telephone conversations

A variety of documentation formats are accepted by insurance companies as long as the information is discernible. Some data may be obtained using a questionnaire, check-off list, or template. If forms are used, they need to be initialed by the physician and all positive findings expanded upon. They do not take the place of narrative documentation in the medical record.

Procedure 9-2 takes you through step-by-step documentation guidelines that should be adhered to in maintaining each patient's medical record. If a medical assistant is aware of documentation deficiencies, it is

---

PROCEDURE 9-2

Follow Documentation Guidelines to Record Information in a Medical Record

OBJECTIVE: Follow documentation guidelines to record information in a medical record and verify that the record is accurate and complete.

EQUIPMENT/SUPPLIES: Medical record and patient data; computer or word processor and pen.

DIRECTIONS: Read the step-by-step directions, which include rationales, to locate the type of entry to be documented, then follow the directions pertaining to the type of chart note entry you will be performing. Documentation entries typically done by the medical assistant are indicated with an asterisk (*). Job Skills 9-1, 9-2, and 9-5 as well as the scenarios in Critical Thinking Exercise No. 2 are presented in the *Workbook* to practice this skill.

1. *Record the patient's name and date (month, day, and year) for each entry.

2. Include the patient's past medical history (serious illnesses, accidents, and operations).

3. Document smoking habits and history of alcohol or substance abuse.

4. State the patient's ethnicity and language spoken.

5. *List all allergies and history of adverse reactions.

6. List each patient encounter in complete form, legibly, accurately, and in chronological order.

7. *Enter all documentation in a timely fashion; state information objectively and be specific, including:
   - *Reason for the encounter (chief complaint)
   - Relevant history, physical examination findings, and prior diagnostic test results

(continues)

PROCEDURE 9-2 (continued)

- Assessment, clinical impression, or diagnosis
- Plan of action including necessary follow-up care
- *Date and legible identity of the observer

8. Document the patient's progress, response to and changes in treatment, and revision of diagnosis.

9. *Record all immunizations or injections given to the patient.

10. Identify appropriate health risk factors.

11. Present the rationale for ordering diagnostic and other ancillary services; if not stated, the documented rationale should be easily inferred.

12. List the reasons for deviations from standard treatment.

13. *Use standard, approved abbreviations.

14. *Prominently display the patient's problem list, and document significant illnesses and medical conditions so the list is kept current.

15. Have past and present diagnoses accessible to the treating or consulting physician.

16. *Document all telephone conversations with or regarding the patient.

17. Support procedure and diagnostic codes reported on the health insurance claim form or billing statement with documentation in the medical record.

18. *File the results of laboratory, x-ray, electro-cardiogram (ECG), and other tests with the most recent report on top, or scan into the EHR.

19. *Photocopy prescriptions written for the patient if not prescribed electronically.

20. *List the names of the staff members who assisted in any procedure.

21. *Document any sample drugs that are given to the patient and the patient's agreement to accept the samples.

22. *Indicate patient education and instructions.

23. *Read through written entries to verify that everything is legible.

24. *Verify that each entry is signed or initialed by the author and include professional credentials.

25. *Make all corrections using standard technique.

---

his or her responsibility to bring them to the physician's attention in a tactful manner.

Medicare Documentation Guidelines

In November 1994, the American Medical Association (AMA) and the Centers for Medicare and Medicaid Services (CMS) developed documentation guidelines for the Medicare program. They are referred to as the 1995 guidelines. Subsequently newer guidelines were developed in 1997. These policies affect reimbursement for procedure codes used for evaluation and management services and are routinely used by government programs and private carriers.

Physicians may use either the 1995 or 1997 guidelines; there is no formal requirement. Medicare and other claims processors and auditors may use them when reviewing documentation to determine that the reported services were actually rendered and that the level of service was provided.

PATIENT EDUCATION

Document Patient Education

Whenever an opportunity presents itself, or when the physician asks you to educate a patient, find a quiet area so that you can speak confidentially. Let the patient know what you would like to inform him or her about. The educational session may consist of verbal communication such as going over an instruction sheet, a handout of reading material, or possibly a demonstration such as showing how to go to a website address for information that the physician would like the patient to view. Be sure to get feedback, so you know that the patient understands any instructions given and allow time for questions. Document each educational session with details about what was communicated or given to the patient. And, do not forget to follow up, if necessary.

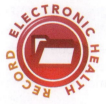

Electronic medical records have applications that allow the use of templates and "smart phrases"; however, Medicare states that "each note must stand alone" and therefore frowns upon entries that are worded exactly alike or similar to previous entries. Providers must use caution when applying electronic "templated" language. For example, when using an EMR, the program automatically brings up the history of present illness from the previous office visit so all the provider has to do is make changes based on the current illness. If the physician forgets to review the previous information, a "cloned" record is created. **Cloaning** is the use of imported text in the medical record and results in documentation that is worded exactly the same or similar to previous entries or encounters; also referred to as "cut-and-paste" documentation. Medicare says that documentation in the EMR should mirror that of a handwritten note. Each note should be unique and specific to the patient and his or her situation at the time of the encounter.

When significant aberrant reporting patterns are detected by Medicare or other insurance carriers, then a review is conducted. Because these federal guidelines affect reimbursement, many medical practices have begun using these documentation policies for Medicare patients as well as those under private or managed care plans.

Documentation Terminology

Accurate words or phrases are of utmost importance when documenting a patient encounter and determining what charges to bill or verifying services that have been billed. Often a physician will list a normal situation or negative result by either dictating or writing "noncontributory" or "within normal limits (WNL)." Such phrases *cannot* be used when referring to an affected body area or to determine a diagnostic code assignment. These terms should not be used if the

COMPLIANCE
Documenting Medical Necessity

Government programs and private insurance carriers have an obligation to those enrolled to ensure that services paid for have been provided and were medically necessary. Documentation must support the level of service and each procedure.

EXAMPLE 9–8
Documentation Terminology

A statement such as "All extremities are within normal limits" does not indicate how many extremities or which extremities were examined. Documentation must indicate which limb was examined and the reason for examination. For example, "The left lower extremity was examined for skin rash, and no abnormalities were found."

---

patient was not questioned or no examination was performed on the body part (Example 9-8).

Likewise the term *negative* as in "chest x-ray, negative" does not indicate what service the physician provided. Instead, state details such as "PA and lateral chest films were reviewed and no abnormalities were seen."

When describing the status of a condition, that is, acute or chronic, the word *acute* refers to a condition with a sudden onset that runs a short but relatively severe course. The word *chronic* means a condition persisting over a long period of time. However, the word *persistent* or *intermittent* may be preferred for certain ailments. For example, "chronic asthma" is listed in the diagnostic codebook as "mild intermittent asthma" or "mild, moderate, or severe persistent asthma."

Documentation guidelines say, "describe the condition," so if the physician states "controlled hypertension" or "controlled diabetes," this is stating a fact that describes the state of the hypertension or diabetes and the reason for the visit (chief complaint). In addition, the patient should be questioned about blood sugar level results or diet, and the physician should document the response; then a finding has been identified supporting the state of the chronic condition.

Acronyms, Abbreviations, and Symbols

Acronyms, abbreviations, and symbols appear in handwritten chart notes because physicians need to document quickly and eliminate long words. In many instances, it would be difficult for a layperson to interpret a medical record because of the physician's shorthand. The medical assistant needs to be familiar with all the acronyms, abbreviations, and symbols used by the physician and use standard ones that are commonly understood by the general medical community. Do not invent an abbreviation. Each medical office should develop a list of standard abbreviations applicable to the specialty.* To assist in this task, each local hospital has its own list of abbreviations acceptable in its facility that might be available to staff physicians on request for medical office use.

Official American Hospital Association policy states that "abbreviations should be totally eliminated from the more vital sections of the record, such as final diagnosis, operative notes, discharge summaries, and descriptions of special procedures." Many physicians are, however, unaware of this policy, and the final diagnosis may yet appear with abbreviations on the patient's record.

The current trend is to omit periods with specialized abbreviations, acronyms, and metric abbreviations as well as physicians' academic degrees (e.g., MD). Latin abbreviations are typed in lowercase letters with periods (e.g., b.i.d., a.m.), and many of these are pharmaceutical abbreviations (see Chapter 10). The patient care abbreviations are listed in Chapter 7, Table 7-1. The medical assistant can use a medical dictionary to look up abbreviations not included in this table.

Illustrations

Illustrations may be used by the physician to document an area of the body where a problem occurs. They may also depict a finding, symptom, or procedure and may help educate the patient or verify a completed service. Some EHR software programs have templates with illustrations that the physician can use to record such things as where the patient's pain is located. Illustrations may also be purchased or hand-drawn and labeled by the doctor, then scanned into an EMR or filed in the patient's chart. Illustrations that are used for some aspect of a patient encounter become part of the medical record and must be legible, dated, and signed. Include the patient's name and date of birth on the drawing.

Digital Images

Some physicians (e.g., plastic surgeons, oral surgeons) may take photographs of the patient that become part of the medical record. These may be digital images that are imported into a document using word processing software while transcribing medical reports. Images may also consist of scans of various body organs or radiographic x-rays. If EMRs are used, the image can be

attached so that other physicians can view it. A graphic may help the physician determine what corrective measures to take and also makes it easier for patients to understand their condition or disease because it is visual and gives more comprehensive detailed documentation. If photographs are part of the medical record, be sure to label them with the patient's name, date of birth, and date taken; the right or left side should also be indicated, as appropriate. Remember that if a patient's digital image is requested for publication, the authorization form must contain wording that indicates the digital image is to be used in this manner.

Measurements

Measurements that pertain to lacerations, lesions, burns, nerve and skin grafts, neoplasms, tattoos, cysts, injection material, and so forth commonly appear in patients' medical records and operative reports. Most of the time, the metric system (e.g., centimeters) is used when measuring skin lacerations and lesions. Avoid using terms such as small, medium, or large. Documentation should consist of the location and site, the size, the number of lesions treated, the method of destruction, and any extenuating circumstances. Reimbursement is affected by the size or area documented and subsequently reported on insurance claims.

CORRECTING A MEDICAL RECORD

To alleviate confusion and prevent medicolegal problems, it is important to know how to correct a medical record. Never erase or use correction fluid on handwritten or typed entries and do not obscure or put self-adhesive typing strips over an original entry to correct later. When the physician discovers an error, such as a progress note that has been inserted into the wrong record or is missing, it must be added as an addendum.

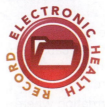 EHR systems need to have EMR correction capabilities, so providers can make amendments, track corrections, and identify that an original entry has been changed. Refer to Procedure 9-3 for instructions on making a simple or long correction, adding an addendum, and performing corrections in an EMR. For further information on making corrections in business correspondence, see Chapter 11.

---

*The Joint Commission states, "Any reasonable approach to standardizing abbreviations, acronyms, and symbols is acceptable," and lists "standardized abbreviations developed by the individual organization" as an example.

Michael Otani

February 22, 20xx	The patient is a Japanese-American male, age 32, who came in complaining of rectal discomfort, rectal bleed ing, and severe itching. PE revealed multiple soft ~~external~~ *internal* hemorrhoids.
DIAGNOSIS:	Multiple internal hemorrhoids. *36 fp*
TX:	Rx Americaine Suppositories #24 i a.m. & p.m. and after each bowel movement and 1 oz Americaine ointment appl. sm amt a.m. and p.m. Pt. to return in 2 weeks for a re– examination

Corr. 2/24/XX fp

Fran Practon, MD
Fran Practon, MD

mtf

FIGURE 9-5 Medical record chart note with examples of corrections made by physician Fran Practon (FP) on the day she read and signed entries

---

PROCEDURE 9-3

Correct a Medical Record

OBJECTIVE: Insert a correction entry in a medical record using standard procedures.

EQUIPMENT/SUPPLIES: Patient's medical record, reference documents for making correction (transcribed notes, telephone notes, physician's comments, correspondence), and pen or computer.

DIRECTIONS: Follow these step-by-step directions, which include rationales, to learn this procedure. Job Skill 9-3 is presented in the *Workbook* for practice.

SIMPLE CORRECTION

1. Draw a line neatly through the incorrect entry. It should remain readable because you do not want to suggest any altering or obliteration of a medical record.
2. Write or type the correct information where there is adequate space, either above or below the line being corrected.
3. Write "Corr.," the date, and your initials in the margin of the page.

LONG CORRECTION

1. If there is no room for the correction above or below the error, the correction must be made after the original entry.
2. Enter the current date and corrected data stating, "Correction to medical record on (give date)."
3. Enter the correction.
4. Initial and sign at the end of the notation.

CORRECTION WITH ADDENDUM OR ATTACHED DOCUMENT

1. If an addendum or attached document is necessary to correct the error or omission and there have been office visits after the error is found, date the entry with the current date and refer to the date of the entry being corrected (e.g., "9/6/20XX: Addendum to entry on 8/10/20XX").

(continues)

PROCEDURE 9-3 (continued)

2. Note in the original record where to find the addendum or attached document (e.g., "See addendum after entry on 10/24/20XX").

3. Initial and sign at the end of the addendum.

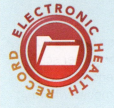

ELECTRONIC CORRECTION

1. Maintain the original entry in the computerized electronic file. Never delete or key over an original entry to correct data unless it is in the process of being entered.

2. Always verify all entries prior to clicking "save." If an error is immediately noted, highlight, underline, or score-through the section in error using editing features

found under "tools" (track changes or edit).

3. If the entry has been "saved," in the computer system, it cannot be altered. To edit the record so that a correction or an addendum can be made, most software programs offer an "edit" feature. A warning sign may occur stating that you cannot edit the record, but offering steps to take to make a change or add an addendum.

4. Follow the steps offered in the software program and correct the error or add the addendum, noting the date of the entry being corrected; the software program will automatically record the date and time of the new entry and the user's name when the save feature is activated.

CONTENTS OF A MEDICAL RECORD

Patient records consist of a variety of documents that are outlined in the following section.

Patient Information Form

As explained in Chapter 5 and shown in Figure 5-5, the patient registration form is used to obtain demographic and insurance information. It is primarily a business record but also helps acquaint the physician with a patient's personal data and becomes part of the medical record. It may be scanned into an EHR system.

Patient Medical History

The medical history is the starting point of the medical record and should be detailed and complete with no blanks left on the patient history form. If interviewing the patient, use open-ended questions and reflective listening. Document patient statements while repeating back to the patient what he or she has said. The physician will determine what entries will be made on the history and physical report.

The levels of evaluation and management (E/M) services, which will be discussed in more detail in Chapter 16, *Procedure Coding*, are based on four types of history: Problem focused (PF), expanded problem focused (EPF), detailed (D), and comprehensive (C).

E/M services is a phrase used for various types of office visits when referring to documentation and appropriate procedure codes selected from the *Current Procedural Terminology* codebook. See Tables 16-3 and 16-4 in Chapter 16.

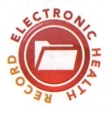

In an EHR system, a history section specific to a specialty (e.g., urologic history) will be included. Then, anything that pertains to the urologic history may be listed (e.g., cystoscopy or prostate ultrasound; diabetes, thus explaining the symptom of frequent urination). Each **case history** includes some or all of the following elements as seen in Figures 9-6A and 9-6B.

Chief Complaint (CC)

The chief complaint (CC) is a concise statement, usually in the patient's own words, describing the **symptom**, problem, condition, or other factor that is the reason for the encounter. This is usually *subjective* information describing any indication of the disease or disorder that is perceived or experienced by the patient. If more than one, list them in the order of importance. *The CC is required for all levels of history.*

Complaints can also be *objective* if a patient complains of something that can be seen, felt, heard, or measured (e.g., a rash or a bump). Objective evidence or an observable physical phenomenon that is typically associated with a given condition is referred to as a **sign**.

Larson, Vivian P.
February 12, 20XX

80-02-48

HISTORY

CHIEF COMPLAINT:

Pain and restricted motion of the right arm; cut on the head—patient has a headache and feeling dizzy and nausiated.

HISTORY OF PRESENT ILLNESS:

This 65-year-old Caucasian female was walking on the street when she slipped on some loose gravel and fell, landing on her right arm and striking her head against the curb. She sustained a laceration of her scalp and an injury to her right shoulder. She went home to change her clothes and started experiencing dizziness and blurred vision. She then went to the University Hospital Emergency Room by automobile where an x-ray of her right arm revealed a fracture involving the greater tuberosity of the humerus and a CAT-Scan of her head revealed a subdural hematoma.

PAST FAMILY AND SOCIAL HISTORY:

Past History: The patient states that her general health has always been good except that in recent years she has suffered from spastic colitis. She had a flare-up of this condition about six months ago. Operations: T & A at age 13. Total abdominal hysterectomy in 1956. Allergies: No known allergies.

Social History: She smokes cigarettes occasionally and drinks alcohol socially only.

Family History: Her father died at age 72 of a cerebrovascular accident. Her mother died at age 74 of a myocardial infarction. Three brothers, all deceased, two with cancer (age 67 and 71), and one with heart disease (age 60). Two sisters, alive and well, one has heart problems. No family history of tuberculosis or diabetes.

REVIEW OF SYSTEMS:

GENERAL: No fever, no chills, no night sweats, or weight loss.
HEENT: Blurred vision, headache, and head pain. No earaches, deafness, sore throats, hoarseness, or difficulty in swallowing.
CV/R: No chest pains, tachycardia, or ankle edema. No shortness of breath, chronic cough, or wheezing.
GI: Appetite good, slight nausea, no vomiting, diarrhea, constipation, or melena.
GU: No dysuria, hematuria or pyuria.
GYN: No spotting since her hysterectomy.
CNS: Dizziness reported. No fainting or seizures.

PHYSICAL EXAMINATION

GENERAL

This patient is a well-nourished, well-developed, 65-year-old Caucasian female who is awake, alert, and experiencing head pain, headache, dizziness, blurred vision, and slight nausea. She also is experiencing pain in her right shoulder when she attempts to move her right arm. Height 5'8". Weight: 155 lb. Blood pressure: 170/90. Temperature: 99°. Pulse: 100. Respirations: 20.

HEENT:

The pupils are dilated, equal, and react slowly. Extraocular movements are normal. Nasopharynx is clear. Upper and lower dentures. Ears are clear. There is a laceration measuring 2.3 cm on occipital region of scalp.

FIGURE 9-6A The first page of a medical history depicting various history components in full block report style

Larson, Vivian P.
February 12, 20XX
Page 2

NECK:

Supple with a full range of painless motion. Thyroid is not enlarged. No lymphadenopathy and no venous engorgement.

CHEST:

Symmetrical with normal expansion. Breasts: No atrophy and no masses. Lungs: Clear to auscultation. Heart: Normal sinus rhythm, no murmurs, and no enlargement.

ABDOMEN:

Soft, nontender and somewhat obese. Liver, kidneys, and spleen are not palpable.

GENITALIA:

Normal external female.

RECTAL:

Deferred.

NEUROLOGICAL:

No motor deficits. Dizziness experienced without relation to head movement. Patient is oriented to person, place, and time. Slight drowsiness occurring.

MUSCULOSKELETAL:

There is a small bruise over the anterior aspect of the left knee. The hips, knees, and ankle joints are otherwise normal. Good peripheral pulses. The right upper arm is moderately swollen and discolored. There are no other gross deformities. The patient has considerable pain with any attempt at either active or passive movement of the right shoulder.

DIAGNOSIS:

1. Laceration—occipital region of scalp measuring 2.3 cm.
2. Subdural hematoma.
3. Relatively undisplaced fracture proximal right humerus (greater tuberosity).
4. Hypertension.

TREATMENT PLAN:

Suture scalp wound. Fracture treatment (without manipulation) with right arm placed in a long arm fiberglass cast. Admit patient to hospital observation unit directly from Emergency Department. Place patient under head trauma precaution and monitor blood pressure every hour.

Gerald Practon, MD
Gerald Practon, MD
mtf
D: 2-12-XX

T: 2-13-XX

80-02-41

FIGURE 9-6B The second page of a medical history and results of a physical examination prepared in full block report style

History of Present Illness (HPI)

The chief complaint is followed by a detailed account of how the patient was injured or when he or she first noticed the illness, called history of present illness (HPI). The HPI is a chronological description of the development of the patient's present illness from the first sign or symptom or from the previous encounter to the present. It includes the following elements: location, quality, severity, duration, timing, context, modifying factors, and associated signs and symptoms (Example 9–9). Members of the medical staff cannot collect this information; the billing provider must perform the HPI. If the patient has been treated by another physician for the same or a similar problem, this will be discussed, along with the possible diagnosis and treatment prescribed.

Past, Family, and Social History (PFSH)

Either the physician, medical assistant, or patient may complete the Past Family and Social History questionnaire, check-off list, or template but the provider must note his or her review of the information. A PFSH may be used from a previous encounter; however, the physician must list the date of the earlier visit and review all elements of the previous encounter listing any changes or elements not reviewed. The PFSH consists of a review of the following areas:

Past History (PH)—The past history is a personal history, including usual childhood diseases (UCHD), previous illnesses, physical defects, operations, accidents or injuries, treatments, immunizations, and medications including drugs the patient has taken recently or is currently taking.

Allergies should also be listed including any reactions the patient may have to drugs, food, or the environment. In a paper record, allergies should be underlined in red in the medical record and placed on the front of the chart, boldly visible. Some medical practices list allergies at the top of each page in the patient's progress notes, and most electronic software programs have "alerts" that prompt the recording of allergies that must be addressed before proceeding to another area in the medical record. Because new allergies may appear as individuals age, questions should be asked to verify allergies each time a patient is seen for an appointment.

Family History (FH)—The family history is a review of medical events in the patient's family (i.e., blood relative), including diseases that may be hereditary or

EXAMPLE 9–9

Elements of History of Present Illness

If a patient has chest pain, the physician may describe (1) the location of the pain (e.g., midsternal), (2) the quality of the pain (e.g., dull, sharp, stabbing), (3) the severity of the pain to further define the magnitude of the problem usually using a scale of 1 to 10, (4) the duration of the pain (when the symptom first occurred), (5) the timing or relationship to a specific place or time of day, (6) the context or when the pain occurs, (7) all remedies and interventions that have been tried to resolve the pain (modifying factors), and (8) any associated signs and symptoms (other problems that contribute to the pain).

place the patient at risk. Notations are made regarding whether the mother and father are living and well (M & F, l & w), ages at death, cause of death, and similar information for siblings and grandparents. The place and circumstances of the patient's birth (e.g., adoption) might also be noteworthy.

Social History (SH)—The social history is an age-appropriate review of past and current activities and occupational history (OH), habits, diet (e.g., caffeine use), marital history (MH), exercise, recreational interests, and alcohol, drug, or tobacco use. Sexual activity and numbers of sexual partners are also noted.

Review of Systems (ROS)

A review of systems (ROS), or systemic review (SR), is an inventory of systems that begins at the top of the body and continues down through each body system as questions are asked about current and previous medical problems (Figure 9–6A). The ROS should not be confused with the examination of body systems, which will follow.

As with the PFSH, either the physician, medical assistant, or patient may use a check-off sheet for the ROS but the provider must note his or her review of the information. Also, a ROS from a previous encounter may be used as long as the provider notes the date of the earlier ROS, reviews all elements of the previous encounter, and notes any changes or elements not

TABLE 9-2 List of Body Systems for Review with Abbreviations

Body System	Abbreviation
Constitutional symptoms	
Eyes, nose, throat	ENT
Cardiovascular	CV
Respiratory	R
Gastrointestinal	GI
Genitourinary	GU
Musculoskeletal	MS
Integumentary (skin and breast)	
Neurological	CNS
Psychiatric	psychiat
Endocrine	Endo
Hematologic/lymphatic	HEM/Lymph
Allergic/immunologic	AL

reviewed. To transcribe this information, the medical assistant must be able to recognize the body part and divide the information as it is dictated. Table 9-2 contains a list of body systems to be reviewed with common abbreviations. Go to student resources at www.cengagebrain.com for a comprehensive list of body systems with descriptions.

Physical Examination

The physical examination (PE or PX) is objective (O) in nature; that is, it consists of findings the physician can discover by examination or through tests (Figures 9-6A and 9-6B). The thoroughness of the examination and the determination of what body systems will be covered depend on the patient's illness or injury and on the specialty of the physician. The physician dictates the entire physical examination for the patient's medical record expanding upon irregular findings. Diagrams showing different parts of the anatomy may also be used by the physician to make notes and draw arrows to various organs as mentioned

previously under *Illustrations*. Go to student resources at www.cengagebrain.com for descriptions of physical examinations of various body parts and systems with examples.

If the patient is going to be admitted to the hospital and has had a physical examination 1 week before admission, the Joint Commission permits a copy of the PE to become part of the hospital record instead of a new history and physical (H & P) on the date of admission. If the patient has had any new development or changes between the examination date and the admission date, then these are noted in the hospital record when the patient is admitted.

During the PE, the physician goes through four basic procedures:

1. *Inspection*, or observation, of the patient's physical characteristics and body parts
2. *Palpation*, or touching and feeling, of various parts and organs of the body
3. *Percussion*, or striking, of parts of the body with short, sharp blows, during which attention is fixed on the resistance of the tissues under the fingers and on the sound elicited to determine tissue size, density, and location
4. *Auscultation*, or listening, to sounds of the internal parts of the body with the aid of a stethoscope

In addition, the physician can perform *mensuration*, that is, measuring various parameters of the body, and *manipulation*, that is, moving muscles and bones to access mobility or as a form of treatment.

Levels of Examination, Body Areas, and Organ Systems

The levels of evaluation and management (E/M) services are based on four types of examination that are defined as follows:

- *Problem focused (PF)*—A limited examination of the affected body area or organ
- *Expanded problem focused (EPF)*—A limited examination of the affected body area or organ system and other symptomatic or related body areas or organ systems
- *Detailed (D)*—An extended detailed examination of the affected body area or organ system and other symptomatic or related body areas or organ systems

- *Comprehensive (C)*—A general multisystem examination or complete examination of a single organ system and other symptomatic or related body areas or organ systems

The extent of the examination and what is documented depends on clinical judgment and the nature of the presenting problem(s). They range from limited examinations of single body areas or complete single organ system examinations to general multisystem examinations.

Table 9-3 lists the body areas and organ systems that are recognized for purposes of examination. See Chapter 17 for more information.

Complexity of Medical Decision Making

Medical decision making is the thought process that the physician goes through. It refers to the complexity of establishing a diagnosis and selecting a management option. The levels of E/M services recognize four types of medical decision making:

- Straightforward (SF)
- Low complexity (LC)
- Moderate complexity (MC)
- High complexity (HC)

The following three elements are considered to qualify for a level of decision making:

Management Options

The number of diagnoses or management options is based on the number and types of problems addressed during the visit, the complexity of establishing a diagnosis, and the management decisions made by the doctor.

Amount and Complexity of Data

The amount and complexity of data to be reviewed is based on the amount and complexity of diagnostic testing ordered or reviewed. A decision to obtain and review old medical records or to obtain history from sources other than the patient increases the amount and complexity of data to be reviewed.

Risk

The risk of significant complications, morbidity, comorbidities, or mortality levels is based on (1) significant complications, (2) other conditions associated with the presenting problem(s) (morbidity), (3) underlying diseases or other conditions present at the time of the visit (comorbidity), (4) the risk of death associated with the problem (mortality), (5) the diagnostic procedure(s), and (6) the possible management options (treatment rendered—surgery, therapy, drug management, procedures, and supplies).

Diagnosis

The **diagnosis** is an impression, an assessment, or a final conclusion of the nature of the disease or illness

TABLE 9-3 List of Body Areas and Organ Systems for Purposes of Examination

Body Areas	Organ Systems
Head, including the face	Constitutional (vital signs, general appearance)
Neck	Eyes
Chest, including the breasts and axillae	Ears, nose, mouth, and throat
Abdomen	Respiratory
Genitalia, groin, buttocks	Cardiovascular
Back, including the spine	Gastrointestinal
Each extremity	Genitourinary
	Lymphatic
	Musculoskeletal
	Skin
	Neurological
	Psychiatric

based on history, physical examination findings, and, sometimes, diagnostic tests such as x-rays, laboratory tests, or electrocardiogram (ECG).

Treatment

This is a recommended plan or treatment for the diagnosis. It might include admission to the hospital, physical therapy, additional tests, medication, diet and exercise recommendations, and scheduling a future appointment.

Prognosis

Prognosis is a probable outcome of the disease or injury and the prospect of recovery. It includes an estimate of partial or total disability in an accident or industrial case.

Progress Notes

After the initial visit, the history and physical examination are recorded in the chart as seen in Figure 9-6, and each subsequent patient visit is documented with

progress notes chronologically entered in the medical record as seen in Figures 9-5 and 9-7.

Progress notes document a patient's clinical status, compare past to current condition, review particulars of the case, communicate findings, and detail a treatment plan. These notes may be requested to be seen by attorneys, other physicians, and insurance companies, and may be used as evidence during litigation; therefore, documentation should be descriptive, legible, neat, accurate, complete, and include the following technical elements:

- Date of service
- Patient's name on each page
- Signature with credentials

Both the plan for and the importance of follow-up need to be communicated to the patient, as well as the level of seriousness of the patient's condition. Document the patient's understanding of the treatment plan and remember the progress note needs to "stand alone."

Self-Adhesive Paper-Based Chart Notes

Some companies manufacture pressure-sensitive paper in single sheets or as continuous sheets that are perforated at various intervals. A series of chart notes for different patients can be typed on the paper, then the notes are placed on the physician's desk for signature. Finally, each note can be carefully separated at perforations or cut apart. The backing is peeled off and each note is secured in the next available blank space of the patient's progress sheet, so information previously entered is not obliterated. If the note is continued to another page, write the patient's name and date of service at the top, indicating "continued."

> **COMPLIANCE**
>
> **Initial Plan of Care**
>
> Medicare reports problematic trends in the lack of documentation for the *initial plan of care*, especially for physical therapists. Each health care provider seeing the patient needs to clearly state what the plan and recommendations are for the patient's care.

Goldberg, Arlene   No. 0697

1-7-XX   Wt: 169 lbs   BP: 136/72

1-7-XX   CC: Malaise, anorexia, epigastric pressure with sensation of fullness, nausea, headache, vertigo, and vomiting.

PE: Abdomen tender and rigid; esophagitis with pain and dysphagia; and severe epigastric pain.

Dx: Acute gastritis.

Plan: Discontinue alcohol, IM inj Prochlorperazine, 10 mg.

Gave Rx for 20 Meperidine, 50 mg, q4h, orally. Pt is told of the importance of follow-up and indicates an understanding of the seriousness of her condition. Retn 4 days.

Gerald Practon, MD

Gerald Practon, MD

mtf

FIGURE 9-7 Typed progress note signed by the physician

Patient Name						Date of Birth: 6 / 16 / 45	Chart# 1209

Patient Name _Morani_ _Betty_ _A_
LAST · FIRST · MIDDLE

Prob. No. or Letter	DATE	**S** Subjective	**O** Objective	**A** Assess	**P** Plans	Page 2

#1 12/8/xx Pt returns for scheduled visit following neg. work up
for primary causes of recently diagnosed hypertension.
No new symptoms since last visit of 11/10/xx. Pt relieved
that all tests were neg. & is very anxious to start therapy
for control.

BP 150/105 RA & LA sitting. Recheck of heart
& lungs normal.

Pt's essential hypertension asymptomatic.
Prescribed Esidrix 25 mg Tabs #14.
Take 1 after breakfast & dinner.
Retn 1 wk. Follow low sodium & high
potassium diet. Given diet slip #3 MS.
Discussed side effects. If dizziness or
lightheadedness occur on standing,
reduce Esidrix to i after dinner.
Pt. advised alcohol & barbituates
may worsen side effects.

Gerald Practon, MD

Courtesy of Bibbero Systems, Inc., Petaluma, CA 94954. Telephone: (800) 242–2376; Web site: http://www.bibbero.com

FIGURE 9-8 Progress note from a problem-oriented medical record with an example of the SOAP format

Take care when dividing the notes for placement because brief notes can easily be placed on the wrong patient's chart. Using self-adhesive chart notes eliminates the time-consuming work of obtaining each medical record and locating the proper page to type in the information. If a chart is dropped and the pages scatter, the medical assistant should be able to pick up each piece of paper and put the chart back together, after identifying the patient and date of service, by page.

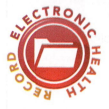

Electronic Progress Notes

In electronic record management, progress notes may be dictated or transcribed directly into the computer system and signed electronically. Care must be taken to make sure that the note is entered into the correct patient's EMR.

Documentation Format

Patient progress notes can become voluminous and an organized system to dictate and record enables the physician and staff to locate certain sections quickly and find information. The following methods are used by physicians because they are consistent and complete. They have enjoyed some popularity because they were developed from acronyms that can be remembered easily.

SOAP Format—The SOAP format is illustrated in Figure 9-8, showing a POMR that is divided into four sections. The acronym is derived from the following:

S: *Subjective*—statements about how the patient feels and symptoms experienced. This would include comments by the patient about the history of present illness, responses to review of systems, and statements about the past, the family, and social history.

O: *Objective*—data from laboratory reports, x-rays, other diagnostic tests, and physical findings on examination by the physician. All objective data are seen (inspection and observation), heard (auscultation), felt (palpation), or measured as in diagnostic testing.

A: *Assessment*—analysis of the subjective and objective portions of the chart note used to attain a diagnosis.

P: *Plan*—therapeutic treatment plan and instructions to the patient by the physician. This includes further testing, medications, return visit, and outlook or prognosis of the case.

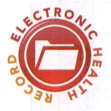

In some software programs, an EMR may be designed to utilize a SOAP format. The first window to appear would be for the "subjective" documentation. After data are entered and "saved," the program would automatically take the user to the next window for the "objective" data, and so forth.

CHEDDAR Format—This format breaks down in further detail each element of the patient encounter. The **CHEDDAR** acronym is derived from the following:

C: *Chief complaint* stated by the patient as the main reason for seeing the doctor. This is usually a subjective statement.

H: *History of the present illness*, including social history and physical symptoms as well as contributing factors.

E: *Examination* by the physician.

D: *Details* of problems and complaints.

D: *Drugs and dosages* of the current medications the patient is taking.

A: *Assessment* of the diagnostic process and the impression (diagnosis) made by the physician.

R: *Return visit information or referral* to a specialist for additional tests.

Medical Reports

A **medical report** is a permanent, legal document in either letter or report format that formally states the elements performed and the results of an examination and recommended treatment. Following are some common types of medical reports:

- **Consultation Report:** Report describing either a consultation with diagnosis and recommendations, or a consultation and treatment provided sent to the referring physician. A consulting physician is one who has expert knowledge and experience in a specialized area. Contents typically include elements of an H & P directed at the patient's problem in the consulting physician's specialty area. Any diagnostic tests ordered—with results, medications recommended or initiated, treatment provided, and follow-up arrangements are included.

- **Operative Report:** Report detailing a surgical procedure performed in a hospital or an outpatient surgical center. Included are the names of the primary and assistant surgeon, preoperative and postoperative diagnosis, full description of the procedure including the approach and any intraoperative complications, finding of the procedure, specimens removed, estimated blood loss, and the date and time recorded.

- **Hospital Discharge Summary:** This report lists the reason for the admission, significant findings, treatment and procedures provided, patient's discharge condition, and a final diagnosis along with follow-up instructions including discharge medications, activity level recommendations, dietary restrictions, therapy, and who the patient is to follow up with. The summary must be filed in the patient's medical record within 48 to 72 hours of discharge from a hospital setting.

Outside Tests

Often, patients are sent to outside testing facilities to have diagnostic tests performed. Following are some of the more typical tests that are scheduled by the medical assistant and procedures for processing test results.

Laboratory Reports

Laboratory tests may be performed in the physician's office laboratory (POL), by an outside freestanding lab, or by a hospital laboratory, which sends or transmits test results to the physician's office. In the report, normal value ranges are typically indicated, and abnormal values can be easily identified (Figure 9-9). The medical assistant should never interpret a **laboratory report**.

Laboratory Report

PATIENT: PETER, JAMES B.

REFERRED BY: 51829   9909

AGE/SEX 78 / M   COLLECTED 01/23/16
SPECIMEN NO. X1006401   RECEIVED 01/23/16 1:40PM
PANEL   REPORTED 05/22/16 12:55PM

TEST	RESULT	HI LO	AGE/SEX SPECIFIC EXPECTED VALUES			VERY LOW	LO	RESULT DISPLAY EXPECTED	HI	VERY HI
GOLD 3										
CHEMISTRY										
GLUCOSE	318	H	85.	–	125.	MG/DL					X
BUN	51	H	8.	–	22.	MG/DL					X
CREATININE	6.4	H	0.7	–	1.5	MG/DL					X
BUN/CREAT	8		7.0	–	37.0				X		
URIC ACID	7.9	H	2.8	–	6.6	MG/DL				X	
CALCIUM	12.3	H	8.5	–	10.5	MG/DL					X
PHOSPHORUS	7.3	H	2.0	–	4.5	MG/DL					X
SODIUM	128	L	135.	–	150.	MEQ/L		X			
POTASSIUM	6.1	H	3.5	–	5.5	MEQ/L				X	
CHLORIDE	121	H	95.	–	110.	MEQ/L					X
CO2	20		20.	–	34.	MEQ/L			X		
TOT PROTEIN	5.2	L	6.0	–	8.5	GM/DL	X				
ALBUMIN	3.4	L	3.6	–	5.4	GM/DL			X		
GLOBULIN	1.8		1.5	–	3.7	GM/DL			X		
A/G	1.9		1.1	–	2.3				X		
IRON	265	H	40.	–	200.	MCG/DL				X	
GGTP	95	H	5.	–	40.	U/L					X
SGPT(ALT)	134	H	0.	–	45.	U/L					X
SGOT(AST)	178	H	0.	–	41.	U/L					X
LDH	408	H	90.	–	270.	U/L					X
ALK PHOS	422	H	119.	–	309.	U/L				X	
TOTAL BILI	5.1	H	0.1	–	1.2	MG/DL					X
CHOLESTEROL	156		140.	–	200.	MG/DL			X		
TRIGLYCERIDE	163		30.	–	250.	MG/DL			X		
TOTAL LIPIDS	596		400.	–	1000.	MG/DL			X		
HDL CHOLEST	55		> OR = 36			MG/DL					
CHOL/HDL	2.84		1/2 AVG. RISK = 3.3								
			AVERAGE RISK = 4.4								
			2X AVG. RISK = 7.1								
			3X AVG. RISK = 11.0								
CBC										
WBC	10.0		3.5	–	11.0	TH/CMM				X	
RBC	5.00		3.5	–	5.5	M/CMM			X		
HGB	17.0	H	11.7	–	15.7	GM/DL				X	
HCT	40.0		35.	–	47.	%			X		
MCV	87		80.	–	107.	MICRNS			X		
MCH	34.0		26.	–	34.	PG				X	
MCHC	33.0		28.	–	36.	%			X		
PLATELET CNT	375		140.	–	440.	TH/CMM				X	
DIFFERENTIAL										
NEUTROPHIL	75		42.0	–	75.0	%				X	
LYMPHS	25		16.0	–	52.0	%			X		

*** FINAL REPORT ***

FIGURE 9-9 Example of a laboratory report showing the names of each test and an indication of whether the results are low, in the expected normal range, or high

Radiology Reports

Some physicians take x-rays in their offices and store the x-ray films in a separate file using a numerical system because of their size. Other physicians send their patients to a radiology group or hospital radiology department to have films taken by a radiographer and interpreted by a radiologist; these are kept by the facility. An **x-ray report** indicates the number and type of views taken (e.g., lateral, panoramic), quality of the study, description of the anatomy, observations or findings, and an impression or conclusion, which are sent to the physician ordering the study to be included in the patient's medical record. If the physician takes the films and dictates the findings, the results may be included in the patient's initial history and physical examination report, included in a progress note, or dictated in a letter form. When using an EMR system, radiology images and reports can be received electronically.

Besides x-ray reports, radiology reports may consist of computed tomography (CT) scans, fluoroscopy studies, interventional radiology procedures, magnetic resonance imaging (MRI), nuclear imaging, mammography, and ultrasound reports.

Electrocardiograms

Some offices perform electrocardiograms (ECGs or EKGs) on patients while others refer patients to the physiology department of a local hospital to have the study done. An EKG is a recording of the electrical activity of the heart through the entire cardiac cycle. It calculates the heart rate and rhythm, measures the voltage of each wave, and notes any abnormalities. Modern EKG machines produce computer-generated reports immediately. In a paper-based system, a hard copy of the ECG and written interpretation is placed in the patient's record. There are ECG machines that interface with EHR software allowing results to be imported directly into the patient's EMR.

Other reports generated by the physiology department are cardiac stress tests, 2-D echocardiograms, Holter monitors, and vascular studies.

Test Results

When patients or their specimens are sent to an outside testing facility, it is important to be sure that the test has been done, the report has been received, the physician has read it, and the proper response has been made. Test results may be mailed, faxed, phoned, or sent electronically to the physician's office. All test results need to be reviewed and initialed by the physician who indicates any action to be taken. The physician may telephone the patient if there are abnormal results or have the medical assistant call to set up a follow-up appointment.

For a paper-based system, maintaining a log in a notebook or desk calendar, or using a preprinted form is quick and easy—more importantly, it is imperative if trying to identify which patient's results are pending. Refer to Figures 9-10 and 9-11 for examples of office test-tracking devices. Enter each report that is received and identify if a report is missing. Hard copy test results are typically filed within a specific section of the medical record labeled for this purpose, for example, all laboratory tests are filed under "Lab" and all electrocardiogram results are filed under "EKG."

Outside Test Log

Date Ordered	Patient Name	Test Ordered	Facility Name	Date of Test	Date Report Rec'd	Test Results to Patient (Date & Initial)
1/6/XX	Kim Chang	CBC c̄ Sed Rate	ABC Lab	1/7/XX	1/9/XX	✓
1/6/XX	Bruce Johnson	UGI	College Hosp.	1/4/XX	1/17/XX	
1/7/XX	Joe Felipe	3 hr GTT	College Hosp.	1/8/XX	1/11/XX	✓
1/8/XX	Lori Carr	Serum Beta HCG Quan	ABC Lab	1/10/XX		

ORDER #74-9052   BIBBERO SYSTEMS, INC., PETALUMA, CA   TO REORDER CALL TOLL FREE (800) BIBBERO (800/242-2376) OR FAX (800) 242-9330

FIGURE 9-10 Example of entries made in a test log showing when tests have been ordered and reports received

June	22
Maria DiPetro	treadmill– College Hosp
Cecilia Chung	protime– ABC Lab

FIGURE 9-11 Example of entries made on the page of a flip calendar used as a tickler file to track tests

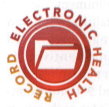

When using an EMR system, an alert may signal the physician to check the patient's "in box" where the pending test results can be reviewed, signed off, or assigned to a staff member so that a telephone call or follow-up appointment can be made. The completed test report is then imported directly into the patient's medical record. Some systems highlight (in red) all abnormal values, record the results next to the last results for easy comparison, and produce a graph to show how values fluctuate.

Miscellaneous Documents

If a patient has a durable power of attorney for health care or a living will and/or wishes to donate organs at the time of death, this information should be flagged in the patient's EMR or noted on the face sheet or chart cover.

The patient's account or ledger, which contains financial information, is also considered part of the record but is not filed with the medical record; it is maintained in a separate file.

There are many types of other documents that may be filed in a medical record. Some common documents are consent forms, correspondence, emails, and fax transmissions. It is the medical assistant's responsibility to assist the physician in keeping medical records current and accurate.

ABSTRACTING FROM MEDICAL RECORDS

An **abstract** of data is required to complete reports, forms, and insurance claims. During this process, information is extracted from various places in the medical record and used to answer questions, code procedures, fill in blanks on forms, or compose a *medical summary*. The summary should include such information as the patient's name, address, birth date, height, weight, marital history, social history, objective findings on physical examination, laboratory results, x-ray findings, diagnosis, anticipated further treatment, and prognosis.

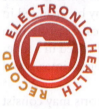

For industrial or work-related injuries or illnesses, initial medical reports and subsequent **progress reports** are submitted until the patient has fully recovered, or until the condition is declared permanent and stationary.

Some EHR systems have a "chart abstraction" feature, which can ease locating information and compiling a summary report. Refer to Procedure 9-4 for step-by-step instruction when abstracting data from a medical record.

AUDIT OF MEDICAL RECORDS

To perform an **audit** of medical records is to periodically examine or review a group of patient records. The purpose of an audit is to verify that good recordkeeping is in place, that documentation is valid for the level of service provided and billed, that proper medical care is being provided, and that only authorized users are accessing or making entries to medical records. An audit compliance plan gives providers written details of what is expected and/or permitted for documentation and billing purposes.

Internal Review

When an audit is done by the medical office staff, this process is called an *internal review*, and records may be picked at random. There are two types of internal reviews: the *prospective review*, which is done before billing is submitted, and the *retrospective review*, which is done after billing insurance carriers. Worksheets may be used, which separate the components of the medical

PROCEDURE 9-4

Abstract Data from a Medical Record

OBJECTIVE: Abstract data from a medical record.

EQUIPMENT/SUPPLIES: Patient's medical record, form to insert abstracted data, and pen or pencil.

DIRECTIONS: Follow these step-by-step directions, which include rationales, to learn this procedure. Job Skill 9-4 is presented in the *Workbook* for practice.

1. Read and review all parts of the patient's medical record that relates to the data being sought in order to become familiar with all aspects of the case.

2. Answer the following questions to see if you understand all aspects of this patient's medical record.
   a. Does the patient's past history show anything of consequence?
   b. Does this patient have any drug or food allergies?
   c. Did this patient have surgery, and, if so, what was performed?
   d. What is the patient's diagnosis?
   e. Was any medication prescribed?
   f. Was any laboratory work performed or ordered?
   g. Were any x-rays performed or ordered?
   h. What is the etiology (cause) of this disease, injury, or illness?
   i. What is the prognosis for this patient's case?

3. Define all abbreviations listed in the patient's history and physical examination and the progress notes.

4. What documents helped you find the answers to these questions?

record to check off various items and to simplify and expedite the process.

Following are some of the important and most error-prone areas when reviewing documents during the process of performing an internal review:

1. Confirm that patient names or identification numbers are listed on each page of documentation for the dates of service reviewed.

2. Make sure dates are recorded for all entries and that dates of service match dates listed on insurance claims.

3. Look to see if all medical record entries are signed or initialed by the attending physician.

4. Identify prominent notations of allergies and adverse reactions so that patients are not prescribed medications that will cause an allergic reaction.

5. Substantiate that evaluation and management procedure codes conform correctly to either 1995 or 1997 documentation guidelines.

6. Check for documentation of a request from a third party when a consultation is billed.

7. Determine if all handwritten entries are legible to an outside reviewer.

8. Establish that proper authorization forms for release of records are in place and signed by the patient.

9. Cross-check *CPT* codes representing procedures and services for accuracy, and make sure medical necessity is documented.

10. Verify that documented diagnoses are consistent with current *ICD-10-CM* diagnostic codes on insurance claims and that they match correct dates of service.

External Audit

Government programs, managed care organizations, and private insurance carriers that have a contract with a physician have the right to do an *external audit* of medical records. This usually occurs as the result of unusual billing patterns by a medical practice and after insurance claims have been submitted and paid. During the external audit, medical records may be selected by the insurance carrier and various elements are categorized and awarded points according to the extent of the documentation. For example, the history would be one category. Other categories would include the extent of the physical examination, complexity of medical decision making, time, and so forth. No points are given when elements are missing. This system shows where documentation deficiencies occur and whether billed diagnostic and procedure codes are substantiated. Investigators may question the patient, review the medical documentation and financial records, and interview the staff and all physicians who participated in the care of the patients' cases being audited. If improper coding patterns are discovered, the physician may have to refund monies or may be penalized.

One type of external audit that Medicare performs is a "Recovery Audit Contractor" (RAC) review, which includes:

- Review of medical records for medical necessity and compliance with Medicare payment rules
- Automated claims review for such things as duplicate payment
- Review areas of concern identified by CMS or the Office of Inspector General (OIG)

For future reference, Table 9-4 lists where to look in this *textbook* to find various types of documents in a medical record.

TABLE 9-4 Examples of Documents Found in a Medical Record

Title	Chapter	Figure/example number	Page number
Treatment authorization request		Figure 2-3	36
Patient information/registration form	5	Figure 5-5	144
Telephone message slips	6	Figures 6-4, 6-5, and 6-6	197, 198
Flow sheets	9 and 10	Figures 9-2 and 9-3; Example 9-4	280, 281, 282
		Figure 10-7	330
Soap chart note	9	Figure 9-8	298
Correction to chart note	9	Figure 9-5	290
Medical history	9	Figures 9-6A and 9-6B	292, 293
Physical examination	9	Figure 9-6B	293
Chart note example	9	Figures 9-5, 9-7	290, 297
Laboratory report	9	Figure 9-9	300
Advance Beneficiary Notice	18	Figure 18-16	590
Insurance cards	18	Figures 18-1, 18-2, 18-3, 18-5, and 18-10	562, 565, 567, 577
Doctor's First Report for workers' compensation	18	Figure 18-11	580

STOP AND THINK CASE SCENARIO

Physician Roles and Titles

SCENARIO: Kay Lenzer has been under the care of Dr. Practon for her annual physical examinations. She falls at home, suffering a compound fracture of her left tibia. Dr. Practon determines that the fracture requires treatment by a specialist and sends her to Dr. Skeleton, an orthopedic surgeon who orders x-rays and performs surgery to stabilize the fracture. During the recovery phase, Ms. Lenzer develops a peculiar skin rash and Dr. Skeleton sends her to a dermatologist, Dr. Cutis, for an opinion about the skin ailment.

CRITICAL THINKING: What roles do the following physicians play and what are their correct titles? Remember, a physician can take on more than one role.

Dr. Practon:

_____

_____

Dr. Skeleton:

_____

_____

Dr. Cutis:

_____

_____

STOP AND THINK CASE SCENARIO

Chart Documentation

SCENARIO: You are the administrative medical assistant and have the certification of CMA (AAMA). It is Friday, October 16, 20XX, at 2:00 p.m. and an established patient, Mrs. Beverly Brooks, stops by the office and wants to see Dr. Fran Practon. Neither doctor is in the office this afternoon and the patient complains that they are never there when she needs them. She refuses to tell you what is wrong or to see the doctor on call, go to an urgent care center, or go to the hospital emergency room; she just says she is not feeling well. She leaves upset and does not schedule an appointment or answer questions as to when she will be home to receive a telephone call.

CRITICAL THINKING: Write a narrative chart note describing the interaction that will serve both as a message and as documentation for the medical record.

_____

_____

_____

_____

_____

_____

_____

_____

_____

_____

_____

_____

_____

_____

_____

_____

FOCUS ON CERTIFICATION*

CMA (AAMA) Content Summary

- Documentation and reporting
- Medical records
- Medical record ownership
- Formats (chart notes)
- Records management
- Paper and electronic records
- Organization of patient records
- Problem- and source-oriented records
- Collecting information
- Making corrections
- Components of a patient history
- Equipment operation (computer)
- Storage devices
- Computer applications (word processing, database, security/passwords, patient data)

RMA (AMT) Content Summary

- Understand and utilize proper documentation
- Prepare patient record
- Records and chart management
- Record diagnostic test results in patient chart
- Problem-oriented medical records
- Identify and employ proper documentation procedures
- Adhere to standard charting guidelines
- Identify and understand application of basic software and operating systems

- Recognize software application for patient record maintenance
- Encryption, passwords, access restrictions, and activity logs
- Obtain patient history employing appropriate terminology and abbreviations
- Differentiate between subjective and objective information
- Understand and employ SOAP and POMR charting systems

CMAS (AMT) Content Summary

- Demonstrate knowledge and manage patient medical records
- Manage documents and patient charts using paper methods
- Manage documents and patient charts using computerized methods
- Arrange contents of charts in proper order
- Document and file laboratory results and patient communication in charts
- Perform corrects and additions to charts
- Transfer files
- Perform daily chart management
- Prepare charts for external review and audits
- Observe and maintain confidentiality of records, charts, and test results

REVIEW EXAM-STYLE QUESTIONS

1. One advantage of a paper-based medical record system is:
   a. management costs are reasonable
   b. they are easy to move
   c. they are easy to store
   d. people feel secure with a piece of hard copy information in hand
   e. they are less vulnerable to security threats

2. Select the correct definition for "meaningful use."
   a. Providers "mean to" and treat patients according to quality of care standards.
   b. EHR technology is used in a meaningful manner.
   c. Physicians "use" medical recordkeeping technology in a "meaningful" way.

   d. Medical offices follow "meaningful use" rules for security of their computer systems.
   e. Practice management organizations mandate "meaningful use" rules for office security.

3. Select the sentence that best describes an EHR practice management system.
   a. A digital version of patients' paper charts.
   b. An EMR system that shares electronic information within the practice setting.
   c. An interoperable system that shares data outside the medical practice.
   d. A database that is accessible electronically.
   e. Both a and b

---

* This textbook *and the accompanying* Workbook *meet the entry-level administrative and general competencies for the CMA outlined by the AAMA Examination Content Outline and Occupational Analysis and for the RMA and CMAS outlined by the AMT Competencies Construction Parameters, and Examination Specifications (see Competency Grid in Appendix B).*

4. A flow sheet:
   a. takes the place of listing data in the medical record
   b. can be used instead of dictating such things as lab results, blood pressure, and immunizations
   c. can be used to help view continuous problems and comparative values
   d. is one of the three basic medical record organizational systems
   e. is no longer allowed according to HIPAA

5. Documents are arranged according to sections in the:
   a. flow sheet
   b. POMR system
   c. SOR system
   d. integrated record system
   e. SOAP format

6. In a patient medical record, data can be:
   a. hand-entered by the physician
   b. dictated by the physician
   c. keyed into the system by the physician
   d. entered by the medical assistant
   e. all of the above

7. Documenters of the medical record:
   a. should be only physicians in the medical practice
   b. are all individuals who provide health care services
   c. need to be licensed health care providers
   d. have to be the attending or ordering physician
   e. all of the above

8. The provider who renders service to the patient in an office setting is referred to as the:
   a. attending physician
   b. consulting physician
   c. ordering physician
   d. referring physician
   e. treating physician

9. Medicare documentation guidelines state that:
   a. the 1997 guidelines replace the 1995 guidelines
   b. outpatient physicians should use the newer 1997 guidelines
   c. outpatient physicians should use the 1995 guidelines
   d. outpatient physicians can use either the 1995 or the 1997 guidelines
   e. both a and b

10. The difference between an electronic signature and a digital signature is:
    a. the digital signature is a facsimile of a person's actual handwriting, and an electronic signature is a series of letters or numbers that cannot be altered
    b. the digital signature is a series of letters or numbers that cannot be altered, and an electronic signature is a facsimile of a person's actual handwriting
    c. the electronic signature is affixed electronically to the end of the document, and the digital signature is a facsimile of a person's actual handwriting
    d. the digital signature is secure and cannot be forged, and the electronic signature uses an encryption system to make it secure
    e. the electronic system uses such things as a voice print, handprint, or fingerprint, and the digital system uses a biometric system

11. When an error in a paper-based medical record is discovered, the first step is to:
    a. draw a single line through the incorrect entry
    b. use white correction fluid to obscure the incorrect entry
    c. use correction tape to obliterate the incorrect entry
    d. draw a heavy line through the incorrect entry
    e. erase the incorrect entry

12. An example of subjective information would be a/an:
    a. laboratory test
    b. EKG reading
    c. blood pressure reading
    d. temperature
    e. patient's expression of the pain level

13. The HPI is:
    a. the patient's family history: all illnesses, diseases, and a list of deceased relatives
    b. the chief complaint; reason for the visit
    c. a chronological description of the development of the patient's present illness
    d. a review of all body systems from top to bottom
    e. the patient's social history including smoking, alcohol consumption, and sexual practices

14. During a comprehensive physical examination, the physician examines:
    a. the body area mentioned in the chief complaint first
    b. the body starting at the feet and working toward the head
    c. all areas that do not look normal first
    d. the body starting at the head and working toward the feet
    e. the body starting in the core (chest and stomach) first, then works toward the extremities and head

15. The complexity of medical decision making is dependent on which three items?
    a. The level of (1) personal, (2) family, and (3) social history.
    b. The (1) number of diagnoses and management options, (2) amount and complexity of data to be reviewed, and (3) risk of complications, morbidity, and comorbidities or mortality.
    c. The (1) diagnoses, (2) treatment, and (3) prognosis

    d. The (1) review of systems, (2) body areas examined, and (3) organ systems examined.
    e. The level of (1) history, (2) physical examination, and (3) number of diagnoses.

16. The acronym "SOAP" stands for:
    a. Subjective, Operative, Action, Plan
    b. Sensible, Operational, Analogy, Plan
    c. Subjective, Objective, Assessment, Plan
    d. Subjective, Objective, Appraisal, Program
    e. Secure, Object, Aim, Purpose

17. A type of internal review where medical staff look at medical records to verify that good recordkeeping is in place and that documentation is valid before billing is submitted is called a/an:
    a. self-audit
    b. retrospective review
    c. external review
    d. external audit
    e. prospective review

WORKBOOK ASSIGNMENT

To develop competency-based job skills, refer to the *Workbook* and complete the:
- Abbreviation and Spelling Review
- Review Questions

- Critical Thinking Exercises
- Job Skill activities, which are listed at the beginning of the chapter under *Performance Objectives* in the Workbook.

RESOURCES

Books

Electronic Health Records: A Practical Guide for Professional Organizations, 5th edition
  Amatayakul, Margaret
  AHIMA Press, 2012

Electronic Health Records: Transforming Your Medical Practice, 2nd edition
  Amatayakul, Margaret
  Medical Group Management Association, 2010

Ethical Best Practices: Resource Guide for Healthcare Documentation Specialists
  Association for Healthcare Documentation Integrity (AHDI), 2010

The Paperless Medical Office: Using Optum PM and Physician EMR, 1st edition
  Ferrari/Heller
  Cengage Learning, 2015
  Website: http://www.cengagebrain.com

Today's Health Information Management: An Integrated Approach, 2nd edition
  McWay, Dana
  Cengage Learning, 2014
  Website: http://www.cengagebrain.com

The Total Practice Management Workbook: Using 3-Medsys Educational Edition
  Brasin/Favreau

Cengage Learning, 2010

Website: http://www.cengagebrain.com

Using the Electronic Health Record in Health Care Provider Practice, 2nd edition

Maki/Petterson

Cengage Learning, 2014

Website: http://www.cengagebrain.com

Internet

Agency for Health Research and Quality

U.S. Department of Health and Human Services

Evaluates EHR technology

American College of Physicians

Articles: Electronic systems, e-prescribing, running a practice

Health Information Technology

American Health Information Management Association (AHIMA)

Search: Electronic medical records, health records

ARMA International

Leading authority on managing records and information

Search: EHR, EMR

Center for Health IT

American Academy of Family Physicians

Tools for accessing and implementing electronic medical record software

Centers for Medicare and Medicaid Services

Electronic Health Records Overview and Incentive Programs

Certification Commission for Health Information Technology (CCHIT)

Certification standards and process

Electronic Medical Records

Search: Free EMR software (e.g., PracticeFusion)

Institute of Medicine

Article: Key Capabilities of an Electronic Health Record System

Washington DC: National Academies Press, 2003

Medical Group Management Association (MGMA)

EHR Systems

Office of the Inspector General (OIG) and Federal Bureau of Investigation

OIG national fraud hotline

Magazine

ADVANCE for Health Information Professionals

Information on medical records, medical recordkeeping, medical transcription, and diagnostic and procedure coding (published biweekly—free subscription).

10

DRUG AND PRESCRIPTION RECORDS

LEARNING OBJECTIVES

After reading this chapter and learning step-by-step procedures to gain job skills,* you should be able to:

- Compare the five schedules of controlled substances.
- Understand when and how to renew a physician's narcotic license.
- Explain the three types of drug names.
- Name the components of a prescription.
- Discuss how e-scripts are used and state the benefits of using an electronic prescription program.
- Define terms and abbreviations pertaining to drugs.
- Know the requirements of "order entry" of drugs into a computerized system.
- Document telephone calls regarding prescriptions in the medical record.
- State the prevention measures used to track prescription refills and avoid prescription errors.
- Describe the methods used to store, control, and dispose of drugs.

PERFORMANCE OBJECTIVES (PROCEDURES) IN THIS TEXTBOOK

- Use a drug reference book to spell and locate drug information (Procedure 10-1).
- Read and interpret a written prescription (Procedure 10-2).
- Record medication in a patient's medical record and on a medication log (Procedure 10-3).

PERFORMANCE OBJECTIVES (JOB SKILLS) IN THIS WORKBOOK

- Spell drug names (Job Skill 10-1).
- Determine the correct spelling of drug names (Job Skill 10-2).
- Use a drug reference book to locate information (Job Skill 10-3).
- Translate prescriptions (Job Skill 10-4).
- Record prescription refills in medical records (Job Skill 10-5).
- Write a prescription (Job Skill 10-6).
- Interpret a medication log (Job Skill 10-7).
- Record on a medication schedule (Job Skill 10-8).

---

*This textbook and the accompanying Workbook meet the educational components for entry-level administrative and general competencies outlined by CAAHEP and ABHES.

KEY TERMS

brand name	generic name	prescriptions
chemical name	inscription	shelf life
Drug Enforcement Administration (DEA)	pharmaceutical	signature
	pharmaceutical representative	subscription
e-prescribing	pharmacist	superscription
Food and Drug Administration (FDA)	*Physicians' Desk Reference (PDR)*	transcription

HEART OF THE HEALTH CARE PROFESSIONAL

Service

When patients are prescribed medications, they need to take them regularly. And as medications run out, patients rely on the medical assistant to handle the prescription renewal in an expedient manner. The administrative medical assistant is often the one at the front desk who serves as the bridge between the patient and the physician as he or she receives telephone calls and answers questions about medications. The knowledge received in this chapter will help fulfill this important responsibility efficiently and will serve the patient in ways you may never fully realize.

INTRODUCTION

Prescription drug use has steadily increased in the United States for the past decade and in 2013 it was reported, "Nearly 70% of Americans are on at least one prescription drug, and more than half take two.*" The U.S. Department of Health and Human Services reports that for the years 2007–2008, 76% of adults 60 years of age or older used two or more prescription drugs and 37% used five or more.** Safe use and distribution of these products is a health concern that affects all health care workers as well as consumers. Accurate medication records and prescription processing is necessary to prevent misuse and adverse drug events "that occur in 15% or more of older patients presenting to offices, hospitals, and extended care facilities.***"

*Mayo Clinic, Olmsted Medical Center, Rochester, MN. Newsnetwork.mayoclinic.org, June 29, 2013.
**U.S. Department of Health and Human Services, Centers for Disease Control and Prevention, National Center for Health Statistics Data Brief, No. 42, September 2010.
***American Family Physicians article, 2013 March 1;87(5):331–336.

HISTORY OF DRUG LAWS

Federal drug laws are designed to ensure the safety of drugs while minimizing the availability and diminishing the opportunity for abuse of controlled substances; a prescription drug may or may not be considered a "controlled substance." State laws vary from state to state; as a rule, a state can add restrictions to federal laws, but almost never reverse or reduce them. Pharmacies and doctors must conform to all applicable laws within their jurisdiction.

The Harrison Narcotic Act

The United States became increasingly involved in world affairs after the Spanish-American War and the State Department called for an international conference dedicated to address the opium problem and the eradication of worldwide drug traffic.

The State Department's efforts were headed by Dr. Hamilton Wright, who enlisted the help of Representative Francis Burton Harrison to introduce legislation to control the prescription, sale, and possession of drugs such as cocaine, heroin, morphine, and opium within the United States. In June 1914, the passing of the Harrison Narcotic Act heralded the beginning of a long history of narcotic control legislation. The act called for all doctors, pharmacists, and vendors to register and submit paperwork for all drug transactions, but it was also used to shut down legitimate medical practices as well as dope clinics that were in violation.

The Volstead Act

In 1919, Congress passed the *National Prohibition Act*. Authored by Andrew Volstead, it was also known as the Volstead Act. The law prohibited the manufacture, transportation, and sale of beverages containing more than 0.5% alcohol. This act did not address pharmaceutical substances, but it was a precursor of regulations that were to come.

The Marijuana Tax Act

During the 1930s, there was disagreement among the medical profession as to the dangers of marijuana. The pharmaceutical manufacturers managed to keep cannabis out of the Harrison Act, so marijuana was legal. The Treasury Department's Prohibition Unit hired Harry J. Anslinger, the first federal commissioner of narcotics, to be in charge of improving the effectiveness and enforcement of the Volstead Act, which made alcohol illegal. At this time, many civil organizations and local law enforcement officials began to pressure the federal government to outlaw marijuana. Hearings were held by Congress to consider the evidence for federal-level prohibition and the Marijuana Tax Act was passed in 1937, which required a transfer tax for all who sold marijuana.

Medical Marijuana

As evidence was brought forth that marijuana has some clinical use in the treatment of several conditions, such as decreasing nausea in patients undergoing chemotherapy, decreasing intraocular pressure in patients with glaucoma, and improving appetite in patients with AIDS-induced anorexia, the *California Compassionate Use Act of 1996* was passed in that state to ensure that people who are seriously ill have the right to obtain and use marijuana for medical purposes. Each state has the option of passing such laws and as of this printing, 25 states and the District of Columbia have legalized medical marijuana.

Legalized Recreational Marijuana

At present, the states of Alaska, Colorado, Oregon, and Washington have legalized recreational marijuana and several other states have ballet initiatives pending. Problems with regulation have occurred where the drug was legalized and a distribution system implemented without regulations, so lawmakers are looking closely at the states that have legalized marijuana for recreational use prior to pushing forward legislation. It must be noted that federal laws have not approved legalizing marijuana for medical or recreational use and can override state laws that are in place.

The Food, Drug, and Cosmetic Act

The Food, Drug, and Cosmetic Act of 1938 was aimed at controlling cosmetics and medical devices and required the first labeling of drugs with adequate directions for safe use. It also mandated premarket approval from the Food and Drug Administration (FDA) for all new drugs.

In 1951, the Durham-Humphrey amendment to the Food, Drug, and Cosmetic Act changed over-the-counter (OTC) availability for the most effective therapeutic agents and mandated prescription status.

Today, the FDA is under the jurisdiction of the U.S. Department of Health and Human Services and has the responsibility to patients as consumers to enforce all drug legislation, thereby protecting the public and keeping them informed of the potential dangers of drugs. It also determines which drugs are prescribed and which can be distributed over the counter. It ensures that drugs are safe before it permits them to be marketed and guarantees the identity, strength, and quality of drugs shipped in interstate commerce. As a result, the drugs used in the United States are standardized. Information on new drugs is gathered and published periodically by the FDA.

The Drug Enforcement Administration

With the social changes and political upheavals of the 1960s, intolerance of drug use changed. Debates increased about the decriminalization and legalization of drug use, and President Nixon launched a vigorous campaign to sway the public against these forces, calling for a "War on Drugs." The Drug Enforcement Administration (DEA) was established as well as the *National Institute for Drug Abuse*.

The DEA, which is part of the U.S. Department of Justice, regulates the manufacturing and dispensing of dangerous and potentially abused drugs.

The Controlled Substances Act

The *Comprehensive Drug Abuse and Control Act*, which replaced the Harrison Narcotic Act, the Food, Drug, and Cosmetic Act, and the Durham-Humphrey laws, is commonly referred to as the Controlled Substances Act (CSA) of 1970 (Title II). It is a federal law that requires the pharmaceutical industry to maintain physical security and strict recordkeeping for certain types of drugs in order to limit and control access to drugs that intoxicate or can make a person "high," such as hallucinogens, narcotics, stimulants, and some depressants. Other drugs of abuse such as anabolic steroids used by athletes to increase muscle mass are also controlled through this act. This act allows for finer control of drugs by using five categories to classify drugs according to the danger they present and apply restrictions to the highest categories. Most states have passed laws that mirror the Controlled Substances Act; however, state schedules may vary from federal schedules.

Schedule of Controlled Substances

Controlled drugs, which include both narcotics and certain nonnarcotics, are divided into five schedules on the basis of their potential for abuse, accepted medical use, and safety. Substances found in Schedule I have a high potential for abuse, no accredited medical use, and a lack of accepted safety. The potential for abuse decreases for drugs found in Schedules II to V; therefore, control varies depending on the schedule in which the drug is placed, as seen in Table 10-1.

All controlled substance labels and packaging must clearly show the drug's assigned schedule (Figure 10-1). This is written to the right of the drug name.

To prevent unauthorized use of controlled substances, the nine-digit (alphanumeric) number the DEA issues must appear on all the physician's narcotics prescription blanks, purchase orders, and any other documents of transfer for Schedules III, IV, and V substances. It must be noted that some drugs in Schedule V do not require a prescription in some states. Schedule II substances must be ordered with a federal triplicate order form (DEA-222). In some states, when ordering Schedule II substances from out-of-state companies, a copy of the purchase agreement (not the federal triplicate order form) must be sent within 24 hours of placing the order to the office of the state attorney general.

Physician Narcotic License

If a physician administers, prescribes, or dispenses drugs listed in the Controlled Substances Act, he or she must be registered with the DEA. Physicians are required to register every 3 years if prescribing only and every year when dispensing. In some states, a physician with offices in more than one DEA region must also contact the district or regional branches and register at each. If drugs are administered and dispensed only at a main office, then registration at the DEA regional branch near the principal office is sufficient.

A note on a calendar will signal the assistant to remind the physician to renew the narcotic license prior to his or her date of birth. If the physician is late in renewing, there is a 3-month grace period after a registration expires during which controlled substances can be prescribed. The physician must keep a record of all drugs dispensed under the act for 2 years.

Dispensing and Recordkeeping

Some doctors dispense medication including controlled substances from their offices. Controlled substances must be kept separate and secure, under lock and key, with limited access of clinical personnel. Inventory must be taken every 2 years and include the following:

- Date and time of inventory
- Provider's name, address, and DEA registration number
- Signature of person who took inventory

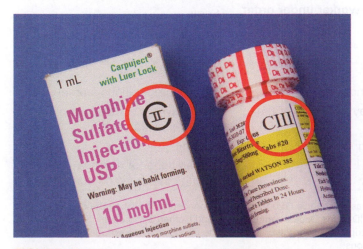

FIGURE 10-1 Two examples of controlled substance labels. The large "C" stands for "controlled substance." The Roman numerals (II and III) indicate the assigned schedule number.

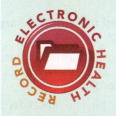

COMPLIANCE

Electronic Prescriptions for Controlled Substances

In 2013, regulations were passed for practitioners to issue electronic prescriptions for controlled substances in Schedules II through V. Pharmacists may accept, annotate, dispense, and electronically archive such prescriptions. In December 2014, the DEA approved a certification process for electronic prescriptions developed by the Electronic Healthcare Network Accreditation Commission. EHR software companies and pharmacy systems have been working together to take additional security and technology steps to comply with the DEA's final rule. As of March 27, 2015, it became mandatory for practitioners to issue electronic prescriptions for controlled and noncontrolled substances.

TABLE 10-1 **Five Schedules of Controlled Substances**

Schedule	Use and Abuse	Examples of Substances
I	• High abuse potential • Limited medical use; with special permission, these drugs can be used for research • Use leads to severe dependence • Must be ordered on a DEA form only by certain qualified medical researchers	Heroin LSD Marijuana* Mescaline Peyote
II	• High abuse potential • Limited medical use in the United States • Severe psychic and/or physical dependence • DEA order form for Rx (triplicate) handwritten by physician • No refills by telephone • Rx must be filled within a specific time period (6 months in CA, 7 days in some states) • In emergency, physician may telephone or fax Rx, but written Rx must go to pharmacy within a specific time period (e.g., 72 hours in CA) • Records retained in a separate file	Amphetamine Cocaine Codeine Demerol Fentanyl Methadone Methamphetamine (injectable liquid) Morphine Opium Percocet
III	• Lower abuse potential than in Schedules I and II • Moderate to low physical dependence; high psychological dependence • May contain limited quantities of substances from Schedules I and II • Written or verbal telephone order by physician only • Refillable up to five times in 6 months	Anabolic steroids Barbiturates (short acting) Codeine combinations (e.g., Tylenol w/codeine, Fiorinal w/codeine) Hydrocodone combinations
IV	• Lower abuse potential than in Schedule III • Limited physical or psychological dependence • **Rx may be written by health care worker but signed by physician**** • **Rx may be phoned in by health care worker under order of the physician**** • Refillable up to five times in 6 months	Ativan Librium Meprobamate Phenobarbital Serax Valium Xanax
V	• Lowest abuse potential • Limited physical or psychological dependence • State laws vary—may require Rx or may be sold over the counter • Purchaser must be 18 years old and sign Exempt Narcotic Registration Form with the pharmacist in some states	Antibiotics (some) Cardiac preparations (some) Cough syrups containing codeine and similar narcotics Lomotil Preparations for diarrhea (e.g., paregoric mixture)

*The federal government is reviewing the classification of marijuana as a Schedule I drug. Any recommendation to change the classification will need to be approved by the National Institute of Drug Abuse (NIDA), the Department of Health and Human Services (HHS), and the DEA.
**In some states, medical assistants are allowed to handwrite prescriptions under the direction of the physician. Drug schedule requirements vary by state; check your state's requirements for regional regulations.

All records, including inventory for Schedule I and II substances, must also be kept separate and maintained for 2 years. Records for Schedule III, IV, and V substances must be kept separate or made readily available for DEA inspection upon request.

The Omnibus Budget Reconciliation Act (OBRA)

In 1990 Congress enacted the Omnibus Budget Reconciliation Act (OBRA), which included provisions that directly affect Medicaid pharmacy programs and providers. Effective since 1993, pharmacies have been responsible for the following:

- *Prospective Drug Utilization Review (ProDUR)*— Requires evaluation of drug therapy problems, therapeutic duplication, drug–disease contraindications, multiple drug interactions (including OTC drugs), incorrect drug dosage, duration of drug treatment, drug–allergy interactions, and evidence of clinical misuse and abuse.
- *Patient Counseling Standards*—Governs patient counseling, which involves the pharmacist offering to discuss the unique drug therapy regimen of each Medicaid recipient when filling prescriptions.
- *Maintenance of Patient Records*—Requires pharmacy providers to obtain, record, and maintain basic patient information such as name, address, telephone number, age, gender, history, disease states, known allergies, drug reactions, and a comprehensive list of medications.
- *Drug Use Review Board*—Requires that state Medicaid programs maintain a board; individual states may require the board to be comprised of specific types of professionals.

Because of this federal mandate directed at Medicaid patients, pharmacies across the nation have begun to include similar provisions for non-Medicaid patients as well.

DRUG NAMES

When communicating with patients, completing medical reports, or inputting information in patients' charts, the assistant needs to understand that drugs have more than one name:

- Brand name
- Chemical name
- Generic name

EXAMPLE 10–1

A Drug's Three Types of Names

Brand Name	Chemical Name	Generic Name
Tylenol®	N-acetyl-para-aminophenol	acetaminophen

In addition to understanding these categories, the assistant must be able to spell drug names correctly and locate specific information under each category in reference books or databases (Example 10-1).

Chemical Name

The **chemical name** indicates the chemical content of the drug compound. It is usually very long and the drug is not commonly referred to by that name.

Brand Name

The **brand name** indicates ownership by a manufacturer and serves as a trademark that is protected from competition for a specific length of time. A superscript ® to the right of the name indicates that the trademark has been registered with the U.S. Patent and Trademark Office. A superscript ™ to the right of the name indicates it is being used as a trademark but is not officially registered.

Brand names are chosen to be easier to spell and pronounce than chemical names. They are used for marketing purposes and may also suggest a characteristic of the drug. Patients often remember the brand name, even when taking a generic form. Drugs with brand names begin with a capital letter when written, with a few exceptions, such as pHisoHex. Most hyphenated brand names have capital letters after the hyphens such as Ser-Ap-Es or Cytosar-U. There are also names, such as NegGram, that contain no hyphen but nonetheless have a capital letter in the middle of the word. Some drug names, such as penicillin, may appear either capitalized or not; however, specific types of penicillin, such as Penicillin V, are capitalized.

Generic Name

When a patent expires from the pharmaceutical company that originally developed and manufactured a drug, the drug may then be manufactured by other pharmaceutical companies. At that time, the drug may be given a **generic name** that is slightly different for each manufacturer. Manufacturers who market the compound may promote the product under either its generic name or a branded generic *trade name*. Since 1961, generic drug names in America have been assigned by the United States Adopted Name (USAN) Council. The council consists of one member from each of the following organizations: (1) American Medical Association, (2) United States Pharmacopeial Convention, (3) American Pharmacists Association, (4) Food and Drug Administration, and (5) a member at large. When typed or written, a generic drug name is not capitalized, unless the generic name is identical to the brand name.

Patients are often confused about generic drugs and may think that because the price is greatly reduced that the generic drug is a different drug than the brand name. Federal law mandates that the generic drug be manufactured according to the same chemical formula and be "bioequivalent" to the original product. The generic version may appear different in size, shape, and color, and the "fillers" (powders and liquids in which the chemicals are suspended) may also differ.

Other drugs may be evaluated by the FDA and released as over-the-counter (OTC) drugs at a lower strength, while remaining in prescription form at a higher strength (e.g., ibuprofen/Motrin). This may cause confusion for the patient, so the medical assistant needs to have current reference books and keep up to date with the latest drug releases.

Legislation in some states allows patients to request generic drugs if the prescription does not specify a particular brand. In other states, pharmacists can substitute generic for brand name drugs if they get the patient's and the physician's permission. Generic drugs are almost always less expensive; therefore, it is likely that more patients will request generic drugs. Note that not all drugs have generic equivalents.

Generic drugs are used on all drug formularies developed by insurance companies. By utilizing generic formularies when possible, the overall costs of health care can be reduced. A *drug formulary* is a listing of a wide range of drugs that have been preapproved by a third-party organization. If the physician is associated with a health organization utilizing a drug formulary and prescribes these preapproved drug products, the patient can usually buy the medication with a reduced copayment. If the physician does not follow the formulary, or feels that a medication that is needed is not included on the formulary, the cost to the patient is usually much higher. Most drug formularies have an "exception clause," so the provider can appeal if medical necessity warrants the patient taking a brand name

---

PATIENT EDUCATION
Medication Assistance Programs

Many pharmaceutical companies offer free medicine for low-income patients and Medicare patients who are disabled. Check with pharmaceutical representatives to obtain information or see *Resources* at the end of this chapter to locate the Directory of Prescription Drug Patient Assistance Programs on the Internet. Patients may also use the Internet as an economic way to purchase medications. Encourage patients to use only sites certified by the Verified Internet Pharmacy Practice Site (VIPPS) that comply with federal regulations and address safety concerns.

---

instead of the generic. A current list of the top 200 brand and generic drugs may be found on the Internet (see the *Resources* section at end of this chapter).

DRUG REFERENCES

It was determined in the mid-1800s that there was very little uniformity in the strength of drugs. The *United States Pharmacopeia (USP)* was published around this time to provide drug standards for identification, to indicate the purity of drugs, and to ensure uniformity of strength.

The American Pharmaceutical Association sponsors another book entitled *National Formulary (NF)*, which contains formulas for drug mixtures. Drugs selected for this reference book are chosen on the basis of therapeutic value.

Physicians' Desk Reference

A useful reference book, which some physicians have in their libraries, is the **Physicians' Desk Reference (PDR)**, published annually with supplements provided during the year by PDR Network (Figure 10-2). This reference book, which provides essential prescription information on major **pharmaceutical** products, is invaluable to the physician and medical assistant. However, it lists only those drugs that the pharmaceutical companies pay to have listed; therefore, not all drugs are included. It is now available as a free download (mobilePDR) to MDs, DOs, NPs, and PAs practicing medicine in the United States as well as U.S. medical students and residents.

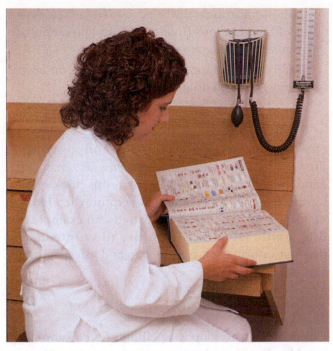

FIGURE 10-2 The medical assistant is using the *Physicians' Desk Reference* to obtain information about a drug

The *PDR* is divided into sections that may vary in color designation and titles among the different editions, but typically include those seen in Table 10-2.

The product identification guide can be particularly helpful to the medical assistant. For example, a patient who regularly takes Coumadin has called for the results of her weekly INR blood test. The physician has changed the dosage from 3 mg to 2 mg. The patient has been on a variety of dosages and she indicates that she has leftover pills. The patient asks what color the new dosage is in order to determine whether she already has that pill on hand. The assistant can refer to this guide to identify the medication and ensure that the instructions given to the patient will be correct (Figure 10-3). Enhanced pill identification displays may also be accessed via the Internet, using a computer or handheld device (see *Resources* section at the end of this chapter).

Other Drug Reference Books

Many drug reference books that are smaller than the *PDR* and that were originally developed for nurses may be useful to the medical assistant. Such drug handbooks provide an alphabetized index of drugs by generic and brand names. A modified description of the following information is usually included:

1. How supplied (e.g., capsules, tablets, solutions)
2. Mechanism of action (pharmacokinetics)
3. Route, indication, and dosage

TABLE 10-2 Physicians' Desk Reference (PDR) Sections and Uses

Section	Name of Section	Color	Use
Section 1	Manufacturers' Index	White	Lists drug manufacturers in alphabetical order with address and phone number; used to contact drug companies
Section 2	Brand and Generic Name Index	Pink	Product listing by brand and generic name with cross-reference table and page numbers where complete drug descriptions are found; most commonly used section to locate drugs and spell drug names
Section 3	Product Category Index	Blue	Drugs categorically listed by type of agent (e.g., antibiotics, anti-inflammatory); helpful if you have difficulty understanding the name of the drug but know the category
Section 4	Product Identification Guide	Light gray	Full color reproductions of the actual size and color of tablets, capsules, bottles, tubes, and packages; used to identify pills
Section 5	Product Information	White	Largest section that lists over 2500 drugs and products alphabetized by manufacturer and then by product name within each manufacturer's list; used to find complete drug information
Section 6	Dietary Supplements	White	Alphabetical list of dietary supplements by manufacturer; used to locate herbal preparations and nutritional supplements

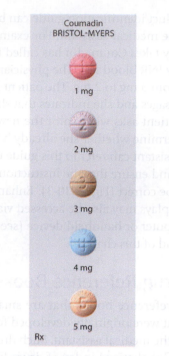

Coumadin
BRISTOL-MYERS

1 mg

2 mg

3 mg

4 mg

5 mg

Rx

FIGURE 10-3 Sample from a drug reference guide of Coumadin® medication (brand name), showing the various strengths the pill comes in and the color and shape of each pill.

4. Adverse reaction
5. Contraindications (interactions and precautions)
6. Nursing considerations

Refer to Procedure 10-1 for instructions on how to locate drugs using a drug reference book.

Over-the-Counter Drugs

One popular reference book for nonprescription drugs is the *Physicians' Desk Reference for Nonprescription Drugs*. Although much smaller, this book is similar in design to the *PDR* and is helpful when looking up OTC drugs. Figure 10-4 illustrates an example of a drug bottle label that identifies the contents and product information for the safe and effective use of an OTC drug.

Word Books

Excellent tools to help in spelling of medications are word books of brand and generic drug names. They are inexpensive, compact, and provide a simple arrangement for locating terms quickly because the words are listed alphabetically and detailed drug information is

---

2 3

PROCEDURE 10-1

Use a Drug Reference Book to Spell and Locate Drug Information

OBJECTIVE: Obtain the correct spelling of a drug name or search for drug information by using a drug reference book.

EQUIPMENT/SUPPLIES: *Physicians' Desk Reference* (*PDR*) or other drug handbook and pen or pencil.

DIRECTIONS: Follow these step-by-step directions, which include rationales, to learn this procedure. Job Skills 10-1, 10-2, and 10-3 are presented in the *Workbook* to practice this skill.

1. Using a **drug reference book**, such as the *Delmar Healthcare Drug Hand book*, go to the Index in the back of the book and look up the generic name (bold face) or brand name of the drug.

2. Note the page number and locate it within the largest section of the book. You may also use the book like a dictionary and look up the drug using the alpha letters found at the top or side of the pages as a guide.

3. Each drug listed may have some of the following subtitles: available forms,

indications/uses, dosages, action (how the drug acts on the body), adverse reactions, interactions, contraindications, side effects, laboratory test considerations, overdose management, drug interactions, how supplied, and nursing implications.

4. Using a **PDR**, find the name of the drug in the *Brand* and *Generic Index* section; note the page number listed.

5. Locate the page number in the *Product Information* section.

6. Locate the drug name and view a replica of the product information guide; like those included with the medication.

7. **Spelling:** If the physician writes or dictates an unfamiliar drug name, the assistant can use the *Brand* and *Generic Name* section of the *PDR* to determine the proper spelling and capitalization. Write each letter using uppercase (capitals) and lowercase letters for the drug name when spelling it out.

not included. Some books, by use of color or symbol, show whether a word represents the generic or brand name and what type of drug it is (narcotic, laxative, diet aid, hormone, and so forth). The Internet can also be used to help spell drug names (see *Resources* section at the end of this chapter).

UNDERSTANDING PRESCRIPTIONS

Multiskilled allied health professionals may be involved with preparing and reading prescriptions, explaining to patients the components of a prescription, and authorizing refills for medications that are Schedule IV or V controlled substances; refer to individual state laws regarding this. The medical assistant may draft prescriptions for the overseeing physician, but it is not legal to authorize, approve, or sign prescriptions on behalf of the physician. The prescription cannot be called in,

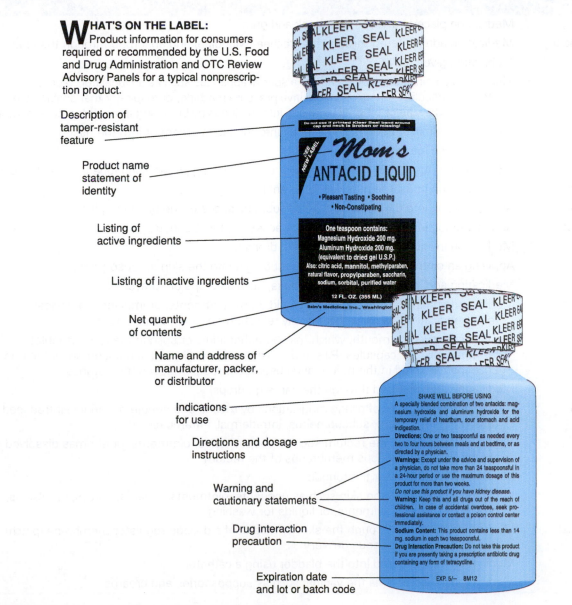

WHAT'S ON THE LABEL:
Product information for consumers required or recommended by the U.S. Food and Drug Administration and OTC Review Advisory Panels for a typical nonprescription product.

Description of tamper-resistant feature

Product name statement of identity

Listing of active ingredients

Listing of inactive ingredients

Net quantity of contents

Name and address of manufacturer, packer, or distributor

Indications for use

Directions and dosage instructions

Warning and cautionary statements

Drug interaction precaution

Expiration date and lot or batch code

Mom's ANTACID LIQUID
• Pleasant Tasting • Soothing • Non-Constipating

One teaspoon contains:
Magnesium Hydroxide 200 mg.
Aluminum Hydroxide 200 mg.
(equivalent to dried gel U.S.P.)
Also: citric acid, mannitol, methylparaben, natural flavor, propylparaben, saccharin, sodium, sorbital, purified water
12 FL. OZ. (355 ML)
Balm's Medicines Inc., Washington

SHAKE WELL BEFORE USING
A specially blended combination of two antacids: magnesium hydroxide and aluminum hydroxide for the temporary relief of heartburn, sour stomach and acid indigestion.
Directions: One or two teaspoonful as needed every two to four hours between meals and at bedtime, or as directed by a physician.
Warnings: Except under the advice and supervision of a physician, do not take more than 24 teaspoonful in a 24-hour period or use the maximum dosage of this product for more than two weeks.
Do not use this product if you have kidney disease.
Warning: Keep this and all drugs out of the reach of children. In case of accidental overdose, seek professional assistance or contact a poison control center immediately.
Sodium Content: This product contains less than 14 mg. sodium in each two teaspoonful.
Drug Interaction Precaution: Do not take this product if you are presently taking a prescription antibiotic drug containing any form of tetracycline.
EXP. 5/--   8M12

FIGURE 10-4 Components of an over-the-counter drug label

faxed, or transmitted electronically until the physician has reviewed, approved, and executed the order.

To understand a medical prescription, the medical assistant must be knowledgeable about the various routes used to administer medication, know prescription abbreviations, and be familiar with common errors found when writing or reading prescriptions.

Routes of Administration

Medication may be administered in various ways depending on how fast the drug is to be absorbed into the body. Also, convenience of administration is a factor. See Table 10-3 for an overview of different ways medication can be given.

Components of a Prescription

A prescription is an order to prepare medications written by a physician, directed to a pharmacist. The *Board of Pharmacy* in each state oversees the licensing of pharmacists, regulates the licensing of pharmacy technicians, and sets state law requirements and online operating guidelines.

All **prescriptions** follow a specific format, the components of which are shown in Figure 10-5. Each is pre-printed with the physician's name, address, telephone

TABLE 10-3 Drug Routes

Drug Route of Distribution	Method of Administration
Buccal	Medication placed between the cheek and gum
Endotracheal	Medication administered through the trachea (windpipe) and absorbed through the lung
Enteral	Medication given orally
Inhalation	Medication administration by means of a special apparatus such as an inhalator, vaporizer, atomizer, nebulizer, intermittent positive pressure machine, or respirator that enables the patient to draw air or other substances into the lungs by breathing through the nose or mouth
Injection	Medication administration either directly into the bloodstream or into the tissues
Intra-articular	Administration into a joint
Intradermal	Administration just beneath the outer layer of the skin (e.g., allergy and tuberculosis skin testing)
Intramuscular	Administration into large muscles (e.g., antibiotic injections)
Intrathecal	Administration into the subarachnoid or subdural space of the brain or spinal cord
Intravenous	Administration into a vein for immediate access to the bloodstream
Instillation	Medication in liquid form administered in drops
Inunction	Applying an ointment with friction (i.e., rubbing it into the skin for absorption)
Nasal	Medication administered through the nose, such as drops or sprays
Ophthalmic	Medication administered to the eye. Liquid drops, ointments, or implantable devices (e.g., medication disc) that continually release medication can be used
Oral	Medications given by mouth, which may be either liquid or solid in the form of tablets, lozenges, pills, or capsules. Pills and capsules are swallowed and absorbed by the body. Lozenges are held in the mouth and absorbed through mucous membranes
Otic	Medication administered through the ear (e.g., drops)
Parenteral	Describing all methods of giving medications by means of a needle or cannula introduced through the skin (e.g., subcutaneous, intradermal, intramuscular)
Rectal	Medications given via the rectum such as suppositories, ointments, or enemas dissolved and absorbed by the mucous membranes of the rectum
Sublingual	Medication placed under the tongue
Topical	Substances applied to the skin such as unguents, ointments, creams, sprays, emulsions, powders, plasters, liniments, or liquids for washing
Transdermal	Medication delivered through the skin by means of a dosage-regulator membrane (patch); also known as transcutaneous delivery
Urethral	Medication administered into the bladder using a catheter
Vaginal	Medications absorbed via the vagina, such as suppositories and creams

number, and often the DEA narcotic number, National Provider Identification (NPI) number, and state license number at the top. All prescriptions written for narcotics must contain the DEA number. Prescription pads for controlled substances may also contain the statement, "Prescription is void if the number of drugs prescribed is not noted." A space is provided for the patient's name, date of birth, address, and date to be completed by the physician. In the remaining space, the physician writes the four standard components of the prescription:

1. *Superscription*—The first element of a prescription, represented by the familiar symbol "Rx," which is Latin for "recipe" or "take" is usually imprinted on the prescription pad.
2. *Inscription*—The generic or brand name of the drug or medication, the quantity of ingredients, and the dosage amount and/or dose strength (DS for double strength). The amount of active drug in each capsule, tablet, or suppository is usually given in milligrams. The strength of creams, ointments, and topical liquid medicines is usually given as a percentage. The strength of oral liquid medications is given as milligrams per milliliter.
3. *Subscription*—Directions to the pharmacist on the total quantity of the drug to be given for the prescription and the form of the medication (e.g., capsules, tablets).
4. *Signature* or *transcription*—Instructions to the patient, which are included on the label, so the patient will know how to take or apply the

medication. The instructions may be written in Latin abbreviations, which the pharmacist must translate. Sometimes written instructions are supplemented with verbal directions to the patient; for example, whether to take the medication around the clock or during waking hours only.

The physician's signature is required in ink or indelible pencil. At the bottom of the prescription is a space where the physician can indicate how many more times the prescription may be filled (e.g., "Repeat ___ times" or "Rep. 0-1-2-3 PRN").

Prescription forms may have a line with a check box that states, "Do not substitute," referring to the substitution of a generic drug for the specified brand name drug. In some states, the physician must not only check the box or statement but also initial or sign in that area to signify no substitution. Some physicians either handwrite or have a section on their prescription forms that states "Dispense as written" or "Brand medically necessary." Other prescriptions may include the statement "Generic drugs are permissible."

State Prescription Regulations

Certain states have mandates over and above those required by federal law. Some states have replaced triplicate prescription forms with tamper-resistant security forms that have special features. Other states have special prescription form requirements for state Medicaid prescriptions, state-approved prescription paper printers, or prescription pads that can only be purchased

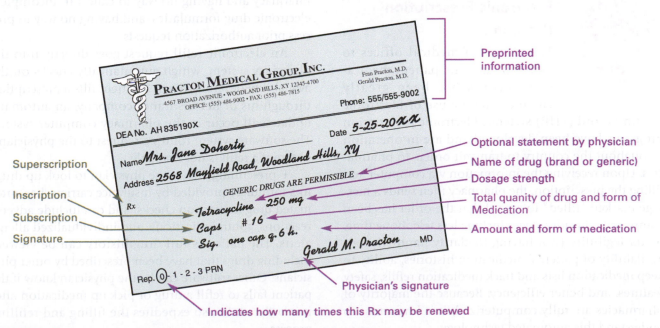

FIGURE 10-5 A completed prescription with components identified

directly from the state. Some of the security features for states that have special requirements include:

- Colored background—which is harder to copy
- Resistant paper—resists erasures and alterations
- Copy alerts—the word "VOID" appears when photocopied
- Tracking devices—identification and batch numbers
- Thermocratic ink—the reverse side reveals the word "SAFE" when rubbed

Check laws within your state to see if special forms or requirements are necessary.

Authorizing Prescriptions

When the physician prescribes medication, the order may be written by the physician or medical assistant, faxed or transmitted electronically to the pharmacy, or verbally given to the medical assistant or pharmacist. Because the prescription is a legal document, many physicians prefer to write out all orders themselves. If the writing is illegible, it is the pharmacist's responsibility to telephone the physician to make certain of the drug ordered. Table 10-1 outlines which schedule of drugs may be written by a health care worker and signed by the physician.

In some states, physicians must call pharmacies themselves with new prescriptions or to authorize refills for controlled substances; pharmacists may not be able to accept orders from office personnel.

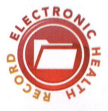

Electronic Prescription Programs

The ability of medical offices to maintain accurate patient medication records has been greatly enhanced by the use of Electronic Health Record (EHR) systems. Electronic prescription programs have been developed and are in operation throughout the country to transmit orders to pharmacies. Upon receiving the information via computer and filling the prescription, the pharmacy then sends a message marked "filled" to record that the order has been completed. The advantages include less telephone time, better legibility (not having to clarify handwriting), availability of patients' medication histories, ability to keep medication lists and track medication refills, safety features, and better efficiency. Because the majority of pharmacies are fully computerized, it is important to understand this automated technology.

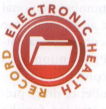

E-Prescribing—Electronic prescribing uses computerized software to create and authorize prescriptions. The two-way electronic communication between physicians and pharmacies includes filling new prescriptions, refill authorizations, changes in requests, canceled prescriptions, and verification of filled prescriptions. E-scripts can also be received via pharmacies by email or fax. Handwritten faxes should never be used for medication orders because of potential problems interpreting the physician's handwriting as well as the inherent difficulty of reading faxes.

Typically, a laptop or handheld device is used and prescriptions are created and entered into a software application during patient examinations. The software then electronically transmits the request to a pharmacy.

Although e-prescribing is supposed to eliminate drug errors, many software programs include a drop-down menu for drug product selection and it is very easy to select and click on the wrong drug. Also, standard or default prescription directions are included in many e-script programs, which must be overridden if they do not match how the prescriber wishes to order the medication. It is *extremely* important that the entire order be reviewed before transmitting the request to the pharmacy. Other complaints about e-prescribing include accidently sending a prescription to the wrong pharmacy and having no way to cancel it, incomplete electronic drug formularies, and having no way to process prior authorization requests.

An electronic refill request goes directly into the pharmacy system, which automatically checks on the availability of refills. When a patient fills a prescription through his or her insurance company, an automatic update will occur in the pharmacy computer system. The software system routes a request to the physician's system if a refill is not available.

E-prescribing allows the physician to look up drugs in a formulary provided by insurance carriers, has automated drug interaction checks, and can include adverse reactions, contraindications, and individualized allergy alerts. The patient's full drug history can be viewed, including drugs that have been prescribed by other physicians. Other software can let the physician know if the patient fails to refill a drug or pick up medication after it is ordered. It also expedites the filling and refilling process.

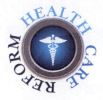

Electronic prescriptions or *e-prescribing* incentive programs for Medicare and Medicaid patients started in 2009 and ended in 2013. E-scripts are expected to save taxpayers millions of dollars because they make it easy for physicians to look at drug formularies and drug prices, and to see if a generic drug is available so a lower cost medication may be selected. Millions of injuries caused by drug-related errors are also expected to be reduced because there will be no more illegible handwritten prescriptions.

Preprinted and Duplicate Prescriptions

When writing prescriptions by hand, some physicians have found it efficient to use preprinted prescriptions for certain drugs; however, too many prescriptions in this format can result in wasted time sorting through the pads to find the right one.

Federal law does not require that a physician keep a copy of a patient's prescription, but it is a good idea in the event a physician is questioned about a prescribed medication. Prescription pads that have carbonless (NCR) paper can be obtained, allowing for a duplicate copy to be retained for the patient's medical record.

Prescription Abbreviations

All medical assistants should know prescription terms and abbreviations because they will use them when communicating with patients and pharmacy staff, when taking dictation, and for understanding instructions on the administration of medications. Table 10-4 in this text also appears in Appendix B of the *Workbook* and includes a list of common prescription abbreviations and symbols. The Latin abbreviations are a kind of shorthand that speeds writing or taking messages and relaying them to the physician.

Common Errors and Dangerous Abbreviations to Avoid

Because handwriting is sometimes difficult to decipher and poor penmanship is common, errors can occur when reading and filling a prescription.

The Joint Commission (TJC) publishes standards that must be met by all hospital facilities. To make sure that standard protocols are in place and followed, TJC surveys hospital facilities and issues sanctions in the areas of noncompliance. As of this date, TJC has not issued a comprehensive list of approved abbreviations for Health Information Management (HIM) departments; however, they did publish National Patient Safety Goals, which state, "Standardize the abbreviations, acronyms, and symbols used throughout the organization, including a list of abbreviations, acronyms, and symbols not to use."

The Joint Commission has published its own list of prohibited abbreviations that may not be used in patient charts, written orders, or notes. Although physician outpatient practices are not bound by TJC standards, physicians must comply in inpatient settings and it makes sense to follow these recommendations to avoid abbreviations that are easily misunderstood on medical records. Read through Table 10-4 to view recommended abbreviations and note the abbreviations in red, which are recommended to write out. Read Table 10-5 to view examples of some abbreviations to avoid in order to prevent misreading and misinterpreting prescriptions. The Institute for Safe Medical Practices (ISMP) is another organization that publishes a list of error-prone abbreviations which may be viewed online; see the *Resources* section at the end of this chapter.

Since many of these abbreviations have been long used by members of the health care community, a list of approved abbreviations needs to be in place. Also, a list of abbreviations to avoid needs to be printed for office use and staff members need to be educated regarding the dangers of their use.

Medication Documentation Errors—To avoid errors when documenting multiple medication names and dosages in a patient medical record, it is advisable to write them in list form instead of paragraph form. Lists are easier to read and locate data without error (see Example 10-2).

PRESCRIPTION DRUGS AND THE ROLE OF THE MEDICAL ASSISTANT

The administrative medical assistant's responsibility with regard to drugs and prescriptions is to assist the physician by being knowledgeable about federal and state statutes on medications, to field medication calls and help patients, and to record drug information. It is beyond the scope of the medical assistant's training to give advice about drugs or prescribe medication. This also includes administering or dispensing prescription or OTC medications, herbs, and drug samples unless under the direct order and supervision of a physician. Refer to Procedure 10-2 for instructions on interpreting a written prescription.

TABLE 10-4 Common Prescription Abbreviations* and Symbols

Abbreviations	Definitions	Abbreviations	Definitions
a	before	o.m.	every morning
aa	of each	o.n.	every night
a.c.	before meals	OTC	over-the-counter (drugs)
ad lib.	as much as needed	oz	ounce
a.m. or AM	morning, before noon	p	after
ante	before	p.c.	after meals
aq.	aqueous/water	p.o., or PO	by mouth (per os)
b.i.d.	two times a day	p.r.	per rectum
caps	capsule	p.r.n. or PRN	whenever necessary
c̄	with	**q	every
**cc, cc	with meals	**q.a.m.	every morning, every day before noon
comp. or comp	compound	**q.h.	every hour
d	day	**q.h.s.	every night, at bedtime
**DC or D/C	discontinue, discharge	q.i.d.	four times a day (not at night)
dos.	doses	**q.n.	every night
DS	double strength	**q.p.m.	every night
DSD	double starting dose	**q.2 h.	every two hours
elix.	elixir	**q.3 h.	every three hours
emul.	emulsion	**q.4 h.	every four hours
et	and	rep, REP	let it be repeated; Latin repeto
ext.	extract	Rx	take (recipe), prescription
garg.	gargle	s̄	without
gm or g	gram	sat.	saturated
gr	grain	SC, subc, subcut, subq, SQ	subcutaneous
gt.	drop	Sig.	write on label; give directions on prescription
gtt.	drops		
h	hour	SL	sublingual, under tongue
**h.s.	before bedtime (hour of sleep)	sol.	solution
ID	intradermal	SR	sustained release
IM	intramuscular	**ss	one-half
**inj.	injection; to be injected	stat or STAT	immediately
IV or I.V.	intravenous	syr.	syrup
kg	kilogram	tab.	tablet
liq	liquid	t.i.d.	three times a day
M or m.	mix	top	topically
mcg	microgram	Tr. or tinct.	tincture
mg or mgm	milligram	Tsp, tsp	teaspoon
ml or mL	milliliter (use instead of "cc" for cubic centimeter)	vag.	vagina, vaginally
		X or x	times (X10d/times ten days)
N.E. or ne	negative	i, ii, iii, iv, viii, etc.	1, 2, 3, 4, 8, etc.
noct.	night	5", 10", 15"	5, 10, 15 minutes, etc.
NPO or n.p.o.	nothing by mouth	5°, 10°, 15°, or 5', 10', 15', etc.	5 hours, 10 hours, 15 hours, etc.
O₂	oxygen		
**o.d.	once a day, every day	ʒ or dr.	dram (drachm)
o.h.	every hour	℥ or oz.	Ounce
oint	ointment		

*Many of these abbreviations are derived from Latin; they are usually typed in lowercase and with periods. Periods are especially important when an abbreviation does not have periods and would spell a word; for example, b.i.d. without periods spells the word bid.

**Recommendation: Write out this term or use alternative wording, so an abbreviation error does not occur.

TABLE 10-5 Common Errors and Dangerous Abbreviations to Avoid

When Penmanship Is Poor, This . . .	. . . Can be Misread as This . . .	. . . So Write This Instead or Use This Guideline
1.0 mg	10 mg	"1 mg" Do not use terminal zeros for doses expressed in whole numbers
.3 mg	3 mg	"0.3 mg" Always use zero before a decimal when the dose is less than a whole unit
10000	100000	Insert comma (10,000)
6 units regular insulin/ 20 units NPH insulin	120 units of NPH	Never use a slash
**AD (right ear)	AD (*atrium dextrum* 5 right atrium)	"right ear"
**AS (left ear)	AS (aortic sac)	"left ear"
**AU (each ear)	AU (*ad usum*) according to custom	"each or both ears"
BT (bedtime)	BID (twice daily)	"bedtime"
*cc	U (units)	"ml" or "mL"
D/C	discharge or discontinue	"discharge" or "discontinue"
*DPT	demerol-phenergan-thorazine or diphtheria-pertussis-tetanus	Completely spell out drug names
Every 3–4 hours	every ¾ hours	"every 3 to 4 hours"
HCl	KCl	Completely spell out drug names (hydrochloric)
HCT	hydrocortisone or hydrochlorothiazide	Completely spell out drug names
**IU	IU (International unit)	"unit" or "international unit"
*MgSO₄, *MSO₄, MS	magnesium sulfate or morphine	Spell out term
o.d. or **OD (every day)	OD "right eye" (oculus dexter)	"daily" or "right eye"
OU (each eye)	OU (outer upper)	"each eye"
per os	**OS (left eye)	"po," "by mouth," or "left eye"
q.d. or *QD	q.i.d. (four times a day)	"daily" or "every day"
qn	qh (every hour)	"nightly"
qhs	every hour	"nightly"
q6PM	every 6 hours	"6 p.m. nightly"
q.o.d. or *QOD	q.d. (daily) or q.i.d. (four times daily)	"every other day"
*SC, *sc, *sq	SL (sublingual)	"subcut" or "subcutaneously"
sub q	every	"subcut" or "subcutaneously"
TIW or tiw	three times a day	"three times weekly"
*U or *u	zero (0), 6, cc, or a four (4), causing a 10-fold overdose or greater (e.g., 4U seen as "40" or 4u seen as "44")	"unit"
*ug or mg	microgram	"mcg"
x3d	three doses	"for three days"

*Abbreviations prohibited by The Joint Commission.
**Abbreviations listed as "error-prone" by the Institute for Safe Medication Practices (ISMP).

EXAMPLE 10–2

Medication Formatting For Medical Records

Paragraph Form:
The patient is on Premarin 0.625 mg daily, Calcium 500 mg b.i.d., Zocor 40 mg at bedtime, Verapamil 180 mg SR q.a.m., Ambien 5 mg at bedtime, and Lasix 20 mg daily.

Suggested List Form:
MEDICATIONS:

Premarin 0.625 mg daily

Calcium 500 mg b.i.d.

Zocor 40 mg at bedtime

Verapamil 180 mg SR q.a.m.

Ambien 5 mg at bedtime

Lasix 20 mg daily

Medication Aides/Assistants

There is a growing need for capable health care personnel who are able to distribute medications in hospitals, assisted living homes, correctional institutions, skilled nursing facilities, and similar settings, so a number of states have created a category of medication aides or assistants. Typically, state laws require the completion of a short training course, and applicants may be required to pass a test.

A variety of titles exist for this new category of health care worker, such as certified medication technician, certified residential care medication aide, medication aide credentialed, medication assistive person, qualified medication aide, registered medication aide, trained medication aide, and so forth. "As long medical assistants work under direct physician supervision, they do not have to become medication aides/assistants in order to be delegated by the physician(s) the administration of medication (including intramuscular, subcutaneous, and intradermal injections, which includes vaccines/immunizations)."* The delegation of duties is determined by each state's medical practice act.

Order Entry Rule

As discussed in Chapter 9, only licensed health care professionals, medical assistants carrying the American Association of Medical Assistants (AAMA) CMA certification, and those who have passed the Assessment-Based Recognition (ABR) program offered by the AAMA meet the requirements for "order entry" for CMS incentive

---

PROCEDURE 10-2

2/3

Read and Interpret a Written Prescription

OBJECTIVE: Read and accurately interpret a written prescription.

EQUIPMENT/SUPPLIES: Patient's prescription, abbreviations (Table 10-3), and pen or pencil.

DIRECTIONS: Follow these step-by-step directions, which include rationales, to learn this procedure. Job Skill 10-4 is presented in the *Workbook* to practice this skill.

1. Read the patient's name on the prescription to verify spelling, accuracy, and legibility.
2. Read the patient's address to check that it has been inserted.
3. Confirm the date written on the prescription.
4. Review the inscription (brand or generic drug name).
5. Confirm that the drug dosage strength is listed and correct.
6. Look at the subscription (form of the medication—capsules, tablets) and the quantity (number or amount) of the drug prescribed for legibility.
7. Read the signature or transcription—directions to the patient on how to take or apply the medication and what time(s) to take or apply it. Translate the Latin into common English.
8. Validate that the renewal or refill times are indicated and note the number allowed.
9. Check the prescription for the physician's signature and indicate who prescribed the medication.

---

*Balasa, Donald A. (2010). Medical assistants do not need to become medication aides/assistants, *CMA Today*, 43(6), 6.

programs and are permitted to enter medication orders into the computerized provider order entry (CPOE) system.

Pharmaceutical Representative

Pharmaceutical representatives or "detail reps" may schedule an appointment to visit the physician and leave drug samples and literature. Detail reps are often allowed into the back office to view medication samples to determine the need for additional samples prior to writing the order for the physician to sign. In some clinics, representatives must sign in at the front desk. Others do not allow representatives to meet with the doctors during office hours. Instead, they create a drop box for pamphlets; however, if samples are left, the physician, nurse practitioner, or physician's assistant must sign for them. In lieu of having drug samples on hand, some medical practices establish a voucher system. Vouchers are distributed to patients, which are then given to the pharmacist for free medication.

Drug Classifications

If sample medications are kept in the office, the medical assistant must make sure that they have not expired and are organized so that all physicians can easily find them to give to patients. They can be located quickly if they are organized alphabetically or grouped by type or classification of substance in drawers, bins, or on shelves. The choice and number of identifying labels depend on the medical specialty and the supply of medications kept on hand. Go to student resources at www.cengagebrain.com for a list of drug classifications and their functions.

> ☑ **COMPLIANCE**
> ### Anti-Kickback Statutes
>
> According to an anti-kickback statute, physicians commit a felony if they knowingly and willfully offer, solicit, pay, or receive payment in exchange for drug referrals payable under Medicare, Medical Assistance, or other government health programs. Payment can be in the form of money, vacations, tickets to sporting events, and so on. Violations are punishable by fines, imprisonment, or exclusion from the Medicare program.

Medication Instructions

Pharmacists are encouraged by the FDA to provide printed instructions with every new prescription.

Some physicians ask their medical assistants to instruct patients about drug dosages and drug schedules. Such instructions supplement physician orders and do not replace directions given to patients by pharmacists. Past studies indicate that poor interpersonal communication is the cause of multiple medication errors. Be alert to discern whether the patient understands the directions given. Elderly patients may have difficulty hearing and seeing and may be reluctant to admit that they have not heard the instructions or are confused and do not comprehend.

Patients forget approximately 50% to 75% of what they have been told after leaving the office. Personal instructions will help prevent confusion when several medications are to be taken at various times and if drug names are similar. When patients confuse medications with names that sound alike, such as Lanoxin (for heart failure) and Levoxyl (for hypothyroidism), ask the patient to verify the drug by bringing it in, taking it to the pharmacy, or using the product identification section in the *Physicians' Desk Reference* (see previous section).

According to the Food and Drug Administration (FDA), among older adults, 17% of all hospitalizations are caused by side effects of prescription drugs. This is six times more than for the general population. And, according to a *New York Times* article (11/23/11), "Four medications or medication groups (none of which were labeled 'high risk')—used alone or together—were responsible for two-thirds of emergency hospitalizations among older Americans . . . which accounted for 33 percent of emergency hospital visits." Errors may also be made when a prescription is written, filled, or taken at home.

Drug Dispensing Containers

Various drug dispensing containers are sold at pharmacies or provided by pharmaceutical representatives to aid patients in separating their medications according to the days of the week and times of day they need to take them. If a friend or family member assists the patient in preparing and administering the medication, that person should be included when instructions are given. Medicine spoons and cups should be clearly marked; tableware and drinking glasses vary in capacity and do not provide accurate measurement.

PATIENT EDUCATION

Prescription Drug Instructions

When instructing patients about proper guidelines for taking prescription medication,* include the following:

1. Speak directly to the patient and ask him or her to repeat the directions to be sure that he or she clearly understands them.

2. Write the name of the medication, manufacturer (if generic), dosage, and directions for the patient.

3. Advise the patient to take the medication exactly as prescribed, at the right times, and in the correct amounts.

4. Instruct the patient about special precautions when taking certain medications. For example, Coumadin is a blood-thinning agent, so blood samples must be tested regularly to avoid blood clots or blood loss.

5. Tell the patient to inform the physician if any new symptoms or adverse effects develop when taking the drug.

6. Instruct the patient to take the medication for the prescribed duration of time, even if he or she begins to feel improvement. If the patient has been prescribed antibiotics, instruct the patient to:

   a) Always finish the complete prescription, even if symptoms subside and the patient is feeling better.

   b) Call and inform the doctor's office if, for any reason, the patient stops using the medication.

   c) Report all symptoms immediately if any adverse reactions occur.

7. Ask the patient to tell the physician if he or she decides not to take the medication.

8. Inform the patient not to take other medications, such as over-the-counter drugs, without first asking the physician.

9. Warn the patient not to take any medications that are prescribed for someone else and not to share their medication with anyone else, not even family members.

10. Inform patients of warning instruction labels, such as "refrigerate," "shake well," "do not take dairy products," or "store in a dark, cool place."

11. Instruct the patient to discard unused portions of prescription medications and medications that have expired dates.

12. Caution patients about taking medications that could cause sleepiness, interfere with concentration, or affect the ability to drive or operate machinery.

13. Inform patients not to mix old prescription medications with a new bottle of the medication; pills may not look the same and cause confusion and there is no way of tracking the expiration date of the older drugs.

*Instructing patients about taking prescription medication should be done only at the direction of the physician.

COMPLIANCE

Vaccine Information Statements (VIS)

The Centers for Disease Control and Prevention produces Vaccine Information Statements (VISs) that explain the benefits and risks of a vaccine. Federal law requires that these information sheets be handed out to vaccine recipients, their parents, or their legal representatives whenever certain vaccinations are given.

Medication Schedule Card

Medical practices participating in the Medicare and Medicaid Electronic Health Records Incentive Program provide patients at the end of their office visit with a clinical summary of care and a medication list in order to satisfy "meaningful use" requirements. This list can be printed on a wallet-sized card for easy access.

Some practices have developed patient medication schedule cards (Figure 10-6) to help patients keep track of their medicines. These cards are also useful if the patient has an emergency or sees a specialist and the primary care physician does not have an opportunity to supply medical records.

PRACTON MEDICAL GROUP, INC.
4567 Broad Avenue
Woodland Hills, XY 12345-4700
Tel. 555/486-9002

Patient's name:

Gloria V. Smith

Please bring this card with you for each appointment.

Your primary physician is:

Gerald Practon, MD

With so many potent medicines available today, the possibility of undesirable effects of single drugs, or adverse interactions of multiple drugs, is always present. If there is any question of side effects of drugs, or their potential toxicity, feel free to call and discuss this with your physician.

It is vital that you, and all health care professionals involved in your care, know exactly the names and dosages of ALL medicines you are currently taking. Please keep this card with you and show it to your doctor or dentist, during office visits, and to your pharmacist when prescriptions and/or over-the-counter preparations are purchased.

MEDICATION SCHEDULE

Name of Medication	Strength	Times to be Taken Each Day						
		AM		Noon		PM		Bed
Lasix	*40 mg*	*1*		*1*		*1*		
Sonata	*5 mg*							*1*

If you have any questions or problems with medications, please call (555) 486-9002

FIGURE 10-6 Example of a medication schedule card given to a patient with some medications recorded

Medication Log

Some offices use a drug flow sheet or medication log for all medications the patient takes, including drugs prescribed by the attending as well as other physicians. This is useful for patients on multiple medications and shows, at a quick glance, the usage habits of a patient or whether a drug might be contraindicated (Figure 10-7). It includes patient name, date of birth, date prescribed, name of medication, dosage, amount prescribed, directions, whether the medication is taken regularly or as needed, telephone or written order, name of the pharmacy, and the physician's initials indicating approval. This type of flow sheet can also be produced by electronic software programs and easily checked to see the frequency of drug refills; however, they should never replace the physician's initial documentation in the medical record.

Medication Refills

Each medical office may have different protocols for prescription refills. Often a separate pharmacy line is designated and the medical assistant must obtain the

MEDICATION LOG

PATIENT NAME: FOLEY , Mary Beth   **DATE OF BIRTH:** 9-30-52

ALLERGIES: KNA

DATE	MEDICATIONS	DOSE	#	INSTRUCTIONS (SIG)	PRN REG	TEL WRIT	PHARMACY	DR. SIG.
8/5/XX	Amitriptyline	100 mg	90	i p.o. bedtime	R	T	ABC Pharm	GP
9/23/XX	Glucotrol	10 mg	30	i p.o. a.c./a.m.	R	T	ABC Pharm	GP
9/23/XX	Verapamil SR	240 mg	30	i p.o. q. a.m.	R	T	ABC Pharm	GP
10/7/XX	Glucotrol	10 mg	90	i p.o. a.c./a.m.	R	W	mail order pharmacy	GP
10/7/XX	Tetracycline	250 mg	30	i p.o. a.c./a.m. yellow sputum	P	T	ABC Pharm	GP
10/16/XX	Verapamil SR	240 mg	90	i p.o. q. a.m.	R	W	mail order pharmacy	GP
10/28/XX	Amitriptyline	100 mg	90	i p.o. bedtime	R	T	ABC Pharm	GP

FIGURE 10-7 Medication log, also called drug flow sheet, showing recorded medications

following information from the patient before a refill can be processed:

1. Name and telephone number of the patient in case the physician needs to talk with the patient before prescribing the medication or renewing the prescription
2. Name and spelling of the medication
3. Dosage strength (e.g., milligrams)
4. Number of tablets or capsules in the prescription
5. Prescription number
6. Name and telephone/fax number on email address of the pharmacy. If the prescription approval is faxed or electronically transmitted, the form may list the birth date, Social Security number, medical insurance number, and the patient's telephone number.
7. How many refills remain on the prescription

Pull or view the patient's medical record and verify that you have the correct record by looking at least two patient identifiers, such as the patient's name and date of birth. Check on the date of the patient's last visit, when the last prescription was filled, and when the patient is due to return to the office. Prescription regulations for Schedule II controlled substances vary from state to state. In 2010, the DEA announced regulations on e-prescribing controlled substances that require using two of the following types of authentications: a biometric identifier (fingerprint or iris scan), a password or challenge question, or a hard device separate from the computer from which the practitioner gains access to the e-prescribing system.

If the physician does not use e-prescribing for controlled substances, the prescription must be handed directly to the patient or in some states may be prescribed by the physician over the telephone (or faxed) as long as the DEA number is given and a follow-up written prescription is sent immediately to the pharmacy. In such cases, the assistant might advise the patient by saying, "I'm sorry, Mr. Wayne, but that drug cannot be prescribed over the telephone. Could you please come into the office to pick up the prescription this afternoon?"

To eliminate the possibility of errors when telephoning in a prescription, ask the pharmacist to read back each prescription. If unsure of the pronunciation, spell the name of the medication. If the medical assistant handles the medication refills, advise the

Prescription Callback Protocols

a. Pharmacy callbacks are made after 4:00 p.m.

b. Pharmacy callbacks are made twice a day.

c. Refill requests will be faxed or electronically transmitted at the end of the day.

pharmacist of the office protocol regarding pharmacy callbacks and instruct patients about office procedures (Example 10-3). Individual office policies vary, but the following are a few common protocols. If the patient is taking an ongoing medication:

- Instruct the patient to call the office two working days in advance to request a refill.
- Instruct the patient to call the pharmacy where the prescription was originally filled two working days in advance to request a refill. The pharmacy will then call or transmit a request to the office to get an approval and have time to refill the medication.
- For a mail-order pharmacy, initially give the patient two written prescriptions, one for a 14-day supply and one for a 3-month supply. Instruct the patient to fill the 14-day prescription locally and begin taking the medication. The patient should then send the other prescription to the mail-order pharmacy. When the patient receives the mail-order prescription, any medication left from the first order should be put aside

PATIENT EDUCATION

Prescription Refill Protocols

Advise patients about office policies for prescription refills. Instruct patients to bring in their medications in the original bottles every time they see the physician or when they are admitted to the hospital. Encourage patients to call with questions regarding their medications.

to use as a backup if the mail order is delayed or if the patient forgets to allow for enough delivery time. The patient should begin taking the mail-order medication and mark the calendar to allow for a 2-week turnaround processing time for future refills.

Charting Prescriptions

The medical assistant must see that all prescription orders and refills are promptly committed to writing and documented in patients' medical records. The items to record are the date of refill approval, name of the medication, dosage strength, and number of tablets or capsules.

Adding the telephone number of a patient's **pharmacist** to the medical record is also a good idea, because it provides the assistant with a ready reference for telephoning a prescription refill. See Example 10-4 and Procedure 10-3 for an illustration and instructions when documenting a prescription refill.

EXAMPLE 10–4

Record of Prescription Refill in a Patient's Chart

Scenario A: On January 12, 20XX, Marjean Hope called at 10:15 in the morning to request a refill of her Lorazepam prescription, 30 tablets at a strength of 0.5 mg. The medical assistant looked at her medical record, which showed that her last refill was a month ago and that she was scheduled to see the doctor in 1 week. Approval for a refill was transmitted to ABC Pharmacy.

Chart note entry for Marjean Hope: January 12, 20XX—E-script refill Lorazepam 0.5 mg, #30 tabs, ABC Pharmacy. Medical assistant's name and credentials.

Scenario B: Patient Mindy Jones called on July 7, 20XX, asking for a written prescription for Diovan HCT tabs for her mail-order pharmacy (WellCheck). She said the strength is 160/12.5 and she takes one a day. Dr. Gerald Practon always gives her 90 pills with three refills. The chart was pulled and Dr. Practon verified the request and wrote the prescription.

Chart note entry for Mindy Jones: July 7, 20XX—Written refill for Diovan HCT tabs 160/12.5, #90 1 tablet each day, X3 refills (WellCheck Pharmacy). Medical assistant's name and credentials.

PROCEDURE 10-3

2
3

Record Medication in a Patient's Medical Record and on a Medication Log

OBJECTIVE: Record medication in a patient's medical record and on a medication sheet.

EQUIPMENT/SUPPLIES: Patient's electronic medical record or chart with progress sheet, medication log sheet, and pen.

DIRECTIONS: Follow these step-by-step directions to learn this procedure. The rationale for each step is to comply with CMS documentation guidelines as referred to in Chapter 9. Job Skills 10-5 and 10-8 are presented in the *Workbook* to practice this skill.

1. Write the date of the chart entry
2. State if it is a new prescription or a refill.
3. Insert the name of the medication.
4. Include the dosage.
5. List the amount given.
6. Write the directions.
7. Sign or initial the chart entry with your professional title.
8. Write the date of the prescription on the medication log.
9. List the name of the medication, dose, amount, instructions or directions (signature) to the patient, and whether taken regularly or as needed.
10. Indicate the telephone or written order and name of the pharmacy.
11. Sign or initial the log entry.

Drug Abuse Prevention Measures

Physicians may be approached by people who exhibit varying extremes of drug-seeking behavior. The medical assistant must be able to recognize those patients who might be drug misusers or abusers. One indication might be an unfamiliar patient's statement that a controlled substance being requested was previously prescribed by another physician. Another hint might be an unfamiliar patient's statement that he or she is the patient of another physician for whom the physician occasionally covers and that the patient wishes to have a prescription for a controlled substance renewed. In such situations, the assistant should ask the patient for the name of his or her regular physician and attempt to verify the story. A patient's hesitancy in answering or avoiding questions can also indicate a problem.

Good documentation in the medical record is the best way of tracking a patient's drug use habits. The medical record should always be consulted, not only to verify that the medication was prescribed, but also to check the correct dosage and amount (number of pills) prescribed. This will help verify if the patient has been taking the medication correctly and whether it is the proper time frame for a refill. Drug flow sheets and electronic records are useful for such tracking purposes, and sometimes pharmacies can be helpful in alerting the office staff if a patient has prescriptions from more than one physician for the same medication.

Protecting Prescription Pads

A prime target of drug abusers is the prescription pad. Some medical practices use computer-generated prescriptions. To discourage anyone from photocopying these prescription sheets, special paper is used, which, if copied, shows the word "copy" or "void" in bold relief on the photocopy. The assistant can protect the prescription pads in the office by:

1. Storing unused prescription pads in a safe place, preferably under lock and key, so they cannot be easily stolen
2. Minimizing the number of pads in use at one time; if the physician can carry a pad in his or her pocket where it is easily accessible at all times, pads in use could be limited to one
3. Not leaving prescription pads in unattended office areas, in examining rooms, or in the physician's car
4. Having prescription blanks numbered consecutively so that if one is missing, it will be noticed quickly
5. Asking the physician to avoid signing prescription blanks in advance
6. Making sure the physician writes and signs prescription orders in ink or indelible pencil to prevent alterations
7. Making sure the physician indicates "no refills" if the prescription does not have a place to check for "zero" refills
8. Checking to make sure the amount of medication prescribed is written out or in Roman numerals, as

well as expressed in an Arabic numeral, thus preventing changes; for example, "30 (thirty or XXX) tablets" cannot be changed to "80 tablets"

9. Not permitting prescription blanks to be used as memo pads for notes; drug abusers can erase notes and use the blanks to obtain drugs

10. Obtaining tamper-proof prescription pads that are printed in colored ink or tinted so that copying, erasures, or white correction ink is easily detected

Prescription blanks for nonrestricted medications could have a printed statement centered across the prescription that reads, "Rx not valid for narcotics, barbiturates, or amphetamines" or "not valid for Schedules II and III drugs"; the placement is important, so the message cannot be cut off. The DEA number can also be omitted and written when the prescription is filled.

If a pad is missing, it might be wise to clip the left or right lower corner of the remaining pads, and then notify local pharmacists to reject any whole sheets. Some communities have set up a telephone network for stolen prescription blanks, in which one pharmacist calls two pharmacists, those two each call two, and so forth until the entire community knows about the problem in a short time.

Drug Side Effects and Adverse Reactions

The Centers for Disease Control and Prevention reported that "74.4 percent of all outpatient visits to physicians result in prescriptions*." The assistant must be aware that medication taken in the correct dosage may produce side effects. Also, food, beverages, and other drugs taken in conjunction with prescribed medication may produce adverse reactions. The patient should be asked every time medication is prescribed if he or she has any medication allergies, because an individual may have developed one since the last time seen. Legally, the assistant is not permitted to tell the patient to stop the medication; this falls under medical care. In case a patient should take an overdose of medication, the telephone numbers of the nearest fire department and poison control center should be kept close at hand in the physician's office.

Information about a patient's previous adverse side effects from drugs should always be recorded in a prominent place near the front of the medical record. Brightly colored "ALERT TAGS" (Figure 10-8) may be used on the front cover of the patient's chart to bring this information to the attention of anyone handling the record.

*National Hospital Ambulatory Medical Care Survey: 2010.

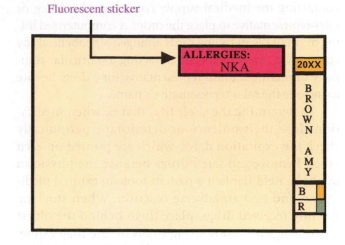

FIGURE 10-8 Fluorescent sticker on a file folder alerts the physician to a patient's drug allergies

If the patient does not have any allergies to medications, the abbreviation NKA (no known allergies) should be inserted, indicating that the patient has been questioned regarding allergic reactions. Be sure to ask the physician if a patient should be questioned regarding food allergies and "natural" medication or herbs.

CONTROL AND STORAGE OF DRUGS

The medical assistant can help the physician avoid potential liability by setting up a systematic plan for the management and storage of drugs. The clinical assistant who handles the medications daily is usually delegated the task of keeping an inventory—evaluating needs and recording the names of drugs that are running low. The administrative assistant may be the one to follow through by

---

PATIENT EDUCATION

Prescription Side Effects

When a patient is taking a prescribed or OTC drug, instruct him or her to call the office when experiencing one or more of the following complaints: *dizziness, drowsiness, nausea, vomiting, rash, respiratory trouble, sleeplessness, headache, blurred vision, hemorrhaging, constipation, decreased appetite, or weight loss.* The medical assistant, should then bring the situation to the physician's immediate attention.

contacting the medical supply company, pharmacy, or sales representative to place the order. A computerized listing or small file of calling cards arranged alphabetically by company name will speed contacting a particular company or pharmaceutical representative for a drug. Be sure to include the sales representative's name.

To determine the shelf life, that is, when medications lose their potency or deteriorate, periodically check the expiration dates, which are printed on each label. Remove outdated drugs because the physician might be held liable if a patient took an expired medication and had an adverse reaction. When stocking recently received drugs, place them behind the oldest dated drugs to ensure using drugs before they expire. Certain drugs must be refrigerated; others are kept in dark, dry cabinets. Be sure to follow specific storage instructions.

Drug Waste Disposal

Drugs should be discarded immediately when expired or if labels are detached or become illegible. Never throw medications where unauthorized people might have access to them. Types of wastes that might be encountered by medical office personnel are referred to as hazardous, medical, and universal wastes.

Hazardous wastes are solid, liquid, or gas wastes that can cause death, illness, or injury to people or destruction of the environment if improperly treated, stored, transported, or discarded. Substances are considered hazardous wastes if they are ignitable (capable of burning or causing a fire), corrosive (able to corrode steel or harm organisms because of acidic properties), reactive (able to explode or produce toxic cyanide or sulfide gas), or toxic (containing substances that are poisonous). Mixtures, residues, or materials containing hazardous wastes are also considered hazardous. Examples of hazardous wastes that might be found in a medical office are copier toner, fluorescent bulbs, batteries, pesticides, spilled chemicals, toilet bowl cleaners, mercury, x-ray film, nitrates, hydrogen peroxide, sulfuric acid, compressed gas cylinders like oxygen and spray cans, UV germicidal lamps, and cloths used to clean solvent spills.

Medical waste, also called biomedical waste, is any solid waste generated in the diagnosis, treatment, or immunization of human beings or animals, in research pertaining thereto, or in the production or testing of biologicals. Medical waste includes, but is not limited to, soiled or blood-soaked bandages, discarded surgical gloves, discarded surgical instruments, needles used to draw blood and give injections,

cultures, swabs used to inoculate cultures, removed body organs (tonsils, appendixes, limbs), and lancets.

Universal wastes are lower risk hazardous wastes that are generated by a wide variety of people rather than by the industrial businesses that primarily generate other hazardous wastes.

Disposal of Uncontrolled Substances

Drugs should not be discarded in trash bins or flushed down the toilet—even in small quantities—because trace amounts of chemicals (drug residue) can enter the environment and harm drinking water and the soil.

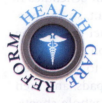

In 2011, the *Pharmaceutical Stewardship Act* was presented to Congress, which was designed to have pharmaceutical producers take responsibility for establishing comprehensive drug take-back programs available to consumers in every state. A number of states have engaged in pilot take-back programs; however, as of this date, no state has imposed mandatory take-back obligations on manufacturers. Check to see if any programs have been implemented in your state; some programs provide mail-back envelopes. For medical offices, the following options are available.

Expired drugs may be discarded with the hazardous or medical waste depending on county, state, or federal laws; the strictest law prevails. Check with the local pharmacy, hospital, or state agency to see if there is a hazardous waste collection program that can aid in the disposal of unwanted medications in your area.

Incineration may be another option and there are companies licensed to dispose of and incinerate drugs. If state laws permit, it may be possible to use the local hospital's incinerator. There are also several organizations that recycle drugs, for example, they give prescription drugs to HIV patients in the United States and in other countries.

Disposal of Controlled Substances

If controlled substances are kept in the medical office, recordkeeping, inventory, security, and correct disposal methods are all important responsibilities of the medical assistant.

In 2010, the *Secure and Responsible Drug Disposal Act* was signed to allow easy disposal of controlled substances by consumers and to help limit drug diversion. Proposed options include take-back events, mail-back programs, and collection receptacle locations. Implementation of these regulations allow for voluntary administration of authorized manufacturers, distributors, reverse distributors, narcotic treatment programs, hospital, clinics, and retail pharmacies.

Most states have return processors (reverse distributors) that pick up controlled substances for disposal. An unofficial list of reverse distributors may be obtained through the DEA. In some situations, drugs may be shipped to a disposal site and the medical assistant may obtain DEA Form 41, Inventory of Drugs Surrendered, from the nearest DEA office. Complete the form and have the physician sign it to verify its accuracy. Call the nearest DEA office for instructions prior to using this method because not all offices have facilities for storing and destroying controlled substances. To ship the drugs, use registered mail. Drugs may also be personally delivered to an Environmental Protection Agency (EPA)-approved incinerator; notify the DEA 14 days in advance. Two responsible individuals from the medical practice must accompany the controlled substances and actually witness their being rendered irretrievable. After they are destroyed, the DEA (or whoever destroyed them) should supply a receipt. File the receipt in a safe place.

Regardless of the procedure followed, all federal, state, and local requirements for the handling of controlled substances and for waste disposal must be followed.

STOP AND THINK CASE SCENARIO
Determine Correct Medication

SCENARIO: An established patient, Charlie Gutierrez, is seen for an evaluation of a red rash-like dermatitis on both feet. Dr. Practon hands the patient a written prescription. As the patient is leaving the office, Mr. Gutierrez hands you the prescription and asks you what it says. In reading it, the handwritten name of the medication looks like either Lamictal or Lamisil.

CRITICAL THINKING:

1. What would you do to determine the correct medication?

_____

_____

_____

_____

2. What are some preventive measures to help avoid cases of mistaken drug identity?

_____

_____

_____

_____

STOP AND THINK CASE SCENARIO
Determine Food and Drug Allergies

SCENARIO: An established patient, Sonja Tucker, is seen for an evaluation of severe back and side pain. It is suspected she may be passing a kidney stone, so Dr. Practon orders an intravenous pyelogram, which will require radiographic contrast material. You notice an alert tag on her medical record that states she is allergic to shellfish.

CRITICAL THINKING: Consider which process is necessary to determine the following:

1. What else might the patient also be allergic to?

_____

_____

2. What should you say to Dr. Practon in this situation?

_____

_____

3. Are there additional questions you might ask the patient?

_____

_____

FOCUS ON CERTIFICATION*

CMA (AAMA) Content Summary

- Documentation reporting
- Food and Drug Administration
- Drug Enforcement Administration (DEA)
- Disposal of biohazardous material
- Classes of drugs
- Drug action/uses
- Side effects/adverse reactions
- Substance abuse
- Prescription safekeeping
- Medication recordkeeping
- Control substance guidelines
- Immunizations
- Commonly used medications

RMA (AMT) Content Summary

- Determine terminology association with pharmacology
- Identify and define common prescription abbreviations

- Identify and define drug schedules and legal prescription requirements
- Understand procedures for completing prescriptions
- Identify and perform proper documentation of medication transactions
- Identify Drug Enforcement Administration (DEA) regulations for ordering, dispensing, prescribing, storing, and documenting regulated drugs
- Identify commonly used drugs
- Identify and describe routes of administration for parenteral, rectal, topical, vaginal, sublingual, oral, inhalation, and instillation drugs
- Demonstrate ability to use drug references (*PDR*)

CMAS (AMT) Content Summary

- Understand basic pharmacological concepts and terminology
- Chart patient information

REVIEW EXAM-STYLE QUESTIONS

1. The drug law that called for registration of all doctors, pharmacists, and vendors to submit paperwork for all drug transactions is the:
   a. Harrison Narcotic Act
   b. Volstead Act
   c. Food, Drug, and Cosmetic Act
   d. Controlled Substances Act
   e. Compassionate Use Act

2. The first federal commissioner of narcotics was:
   a. Reverend Charles Brent
   b. Hamilton Wright
   c. Francis Burton Harrison
   d. Andrew Volstead
   e. Harry J. Anslinger

3. The drug law that mandates drugs be put into five different schedules according to their potential for abuse is the:

   a. Harrison Narcotic Act
   b. Volstead Act
   c. Food, Drug, and Cosmetic Act
   d. Controlled Substances Act
   e. Compassionate Use Act

4. The following procedure(s) is typically followed when prescribing Schedule II narcotics:
   a. The physician writes an order for the narcotic on a triplicate prescription form.
   b. The physician writes an order for the narcotic on a regular prescription form.
   c. The physician telephones in the order for the narcotic prescription.
   d. The physician writes the prescription on a "narcotics only" prescription form.
   e. All of the above are correct.

---

* This textbook *and accompanying* Workbook *meet the entry-level administrative and general competencies for the CMA outlined by the AAMA Examination Content Outline and Occupational Analysis, and for the RMA and CMAS outlined by the AMT Competencies, Construction Parameters, and Examination Specifications (see Competency Grids in Appendix B).*

5. Less expensive drugs manufactured with the same chemical formula as the original drug whose patent has expired are called:
   a. brand name drugs
   b. generic drugs
   c. chemical duplicates
   d. pharmaceutical substitutes
   e. Class B drugs

6. A useful prescription drug reference book that most physicians have in their libraries is the:
   a. *United States Pharmacopeia*
   b. *National Formulary*
   c. *Physicians' Desk Reference*
   d. *Physicians' Desk Reference for Nonprescription Drugs*
   e. word book

7. The administration route for medication placed under the tongue would be called:
   a. sublingual
   b. otic
   c. buccal
   d. transdermal
   e. oral

8. The component of a prescription labeled "signature" is:
   a. the recipe
   b. where the name of the drug or medication goes
   c. where the instructions to the patient are written
   d. where the physician signs his or her name
   e. the directions to the pharmacist

9. When "e-prescribing" a drug:
   a. colored prescription pads are used
   b. tamper-proof prescription pads are used
   c. resistant paper is used
   d. thermocratic ink is used
   e. prescriptions are entered into software applications and transmitted electronically

10. The abbreviation "q.i.d." means:
    a. four times a day
    b. three times a day
    c. two times a day
    d. morning, noon, and nighttime
    e. every afternoon

11. A pharmaceutical representative is also called a:
    a. salesperson
    b. sales representative
    c. pharmacist
    d. detail rep or person
    e. medical representative

12. What device can be used when a patient has difficulty remembering when to take medications?
    a. medication schedule card
    b. drug dispensing container
    c. medication alert bracelet
    d. drug flow sheet
    e. both a and b

13. To educate a patient about possible drug side effects, advise the patient to:
    a. stop taking the medication if a side effect is suspected
    b. throw away the medication if a side effect occurs
    c. call the office if one of the typical symptoms occurs (e.g., dizziness, nausea, headache)
    d. go directly to the emergency room
    e. wait until the next office visit and advise the physician

14. Which of the following statements is correct?
    a. All Schedule I drugs should be kept under lock and key.
    b. All Schedule I and II drugs should be kept under lock and key.
    c. All Schedule I, II, and III drugs should be kept under lock and key.
    d. All Schedule I, II, III, and IV drugs should be kept under lock and key.
    e. All Schedule I, II, III, IV, and V drugs should be kept under lock and key.

15. Uncontrolled substances may be discarded by:
    a. throwing them in a waste receptacle
    b. flushing them down the toilet
    c. discarding them with hazardous medical waste
    d. contacting a reverse distributor for pick up
    e. shipping them to the DEA

WORKBOOK ASSIGNMENT

To develop competency-based job skills, refer to the *Workbook* and complete the:

- Abbreviation and Spelling Review
- Review Questions
- Critical Thinking Exercises

- Job Skill activities, which are listed at the beginning of the chapter under *Performance Objectives in the Workbook*.

RESOURCES

Books

2013 Delmar's Nurse's Drug Handbook™, 22nd edition
Spratto/Woods (published annually)
Cengage Delmar Learning
Website: http://www.cengagebrain.com

Physicians' Desk Reference (published annually)
PDR Network (hardcover or free download)

Physicians' Desk Reference for Nonprescription Drugs (published annually)
PDR Network

Internet

To obtain information on drugs, including newly approved drugs and developments in drug therapy, the following websites may be useful:

Be Med Wise®
Information on nonprescription products with quiz

Dictionaries
- MediLexicon
Abbreviations, drug search
- Merriam-Webster Dictionary
Thesaurus, medical dictionary, encyclopedia
- The Free Dictionary
Words that "start with ___" or "end with___"

Directory of Prescription Drug Patient Assistance Programs
Patient Assistance Programs

Drug Disposal Sites
- **Environmental Protection Agency**
Pharmaceuticals and Personal Care Products
Click on: How do I properly dispose of unwanted pharmaceuticals
- **Federal Drug Association (FDA)**
Guidelines for drug disposal
- **National Community Pharmacists Association**

Click on: Dispose my meds

Drug Enforcement Administration
Drug facts, scheduling, and prevention

Drugs A-Z List
Spell drug names

Drugs.com™
Pill identifier by size and shape

Food and Drug Administration
Click on "Drugs," then "Healthcare Professional Resources"
A–Z subject index for drug-specific information

Institute for Safe Medication Practices
Medication safety tools list
Error-prone abbreviations, symbols, and dose designations
High-alert medications

Look-Alike/Sound-Alike Drugs
List of confused drug names

MedWatch
U.S. Food and Drug Administration
FDA safety information and adverse event reporting program

The Medical Letter
Critical appraisals of new drugs, comparative reviews of older drugs

National Council on Patient Information and Education (NCPIE)
Drug education for safe usage

Top 200 Drug List in the U.S.A.
Administration routes
Alpha list by number of prescriptions dispensed
Practice tests

Vaccine Information Sheets (VISs)
Informational handouts on vaccines

White House Drug Policies
Office of National Drug Control Policy

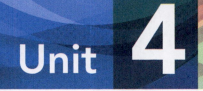

Unit 4

WRITTEN COMMUNICATION

CHAPTER 11

WRITTEN CORRESPONDENCE

LEARNING OBJECTIVES

After reading this chapter and learning step-by-step procedures to gain job skills,* you should be able to:

- Name office equipment and supplies used in written correspondence.
- State various functions word processing software can perform in an electronic health record system.
- Describe different letter formats and punctuation styles.
- List the parts of a letter.
- Assemble reference materials that aid in writing effective letters.
- Understand common writing rules.
- Outline the characteristics of a letter and discuss different types of letters.
- Identify types of memos and describe proper format.
- Demonstrate proper editing and proofreading techniques.
- Explain various ways to perform transcription tasks.
- Operate a photocopy machine and state solutions to common copier problems.

PERFORMANCE OBJECTIVES (PROCEDURES) IN THIS TEXTBOOK

- Compose, format, key, proofread, and print business correspondence (Procedure 11-1).
- Proofread a business document (Procedure 11-2).
- Transcribe a dictated document (Procedure 11-3).
- Prepare documents for photocopying (Procedure 11-4).

PERFORMANCE OBJECTIVES (JOB SKILLS) IN THE WORKBOOK

- Spell medical words (Job Skill 11-1).
- Key a letter of withdrawal (Job Skill 11-2).
- Edit written communication (Job Skill 11-3).

---

*This textbook and the accompanying Workbook meet the educational components for entry-level administrative and general competencies outlined by CAAHEP and ABHES.

- Compose and key a letter for a failed appointment (Job Skill 11-4).
- Compose and key a letter for an initial visit (Job Skill 11-5).
- Compose and key a letter to another physician (Job Skill 11-6).
- Compose and key a letter requesting payment (Job Skill 11-7).
- Key two interoffice memorandums (Job Skill 11-8).
- Abstract information from a medical record; compose and key a letter (Job Skill 11-9).
- Key a two-page letter (Job Skill 11-10).

KEY TERMS

edit	mail merge	proofreading
form letter	mixed punctuation	simplified letter style
full block letter style	modified block format	thesaurus
interoffice memorandum	open punctuation	transcriptionist
justification	photocopy	word processing
letter template	photocopy machine	word processing log

HEART OF THE HEALTH CARE PROFESSIONAL

Service

Communicating in written form is a special talent, and written words said "just right" can set the mood to induce positive action. Patients appreciate a goodwill message, short note, or comment directed personally. Developing written communication skills will help you serve patients' needs.

WRITTEN COMMUNICATION

Letter writing was the primary mode of personal and business communication before the onset of newspapers, telegrams, telephones, fax, email, and text messaging. At that time, many people maintained diaries, journals, and personal letter records. Today, because of convenience, much correspondence is communicated electronically; however, there are times when only professionally typed correspondence on business letterhead can convey the desired message and tone. If letters of an official or a legal nature (e.g., letter of withdrawal) must be sent by fax or email, the original should always be prepared on letterhead with original signatures and also sent via mail.

Clerical responsibilities assigned to the medical assistant involve composing and keying routine letters and memos, transcribing medical data, providing clinical summaries for each patient office visit, duplicating directives, generating financial reports, and sending patient statements.

Professionally written and accurately keyed office communications are indications of an orderly, well-run professional office. Handling medical communications requires composing written materials that clearly transmit the physician's ideas and office policy. It also requires expertise in operating computer equipment.

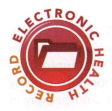

The Electronic Health Record and Word Processing Software

Word processing is an automated communication system that uses computer memory with specific software installed to create a variety of word documents. Refer to Figure 11-1 for an illustration of some word processing software features, such as margin controls, centering text, indentations, and boldface. Word processing systems have increased productivity and lowered office costs.

Data are stored on the hard drive, which can be duplicated and transferred to other data-storing media,

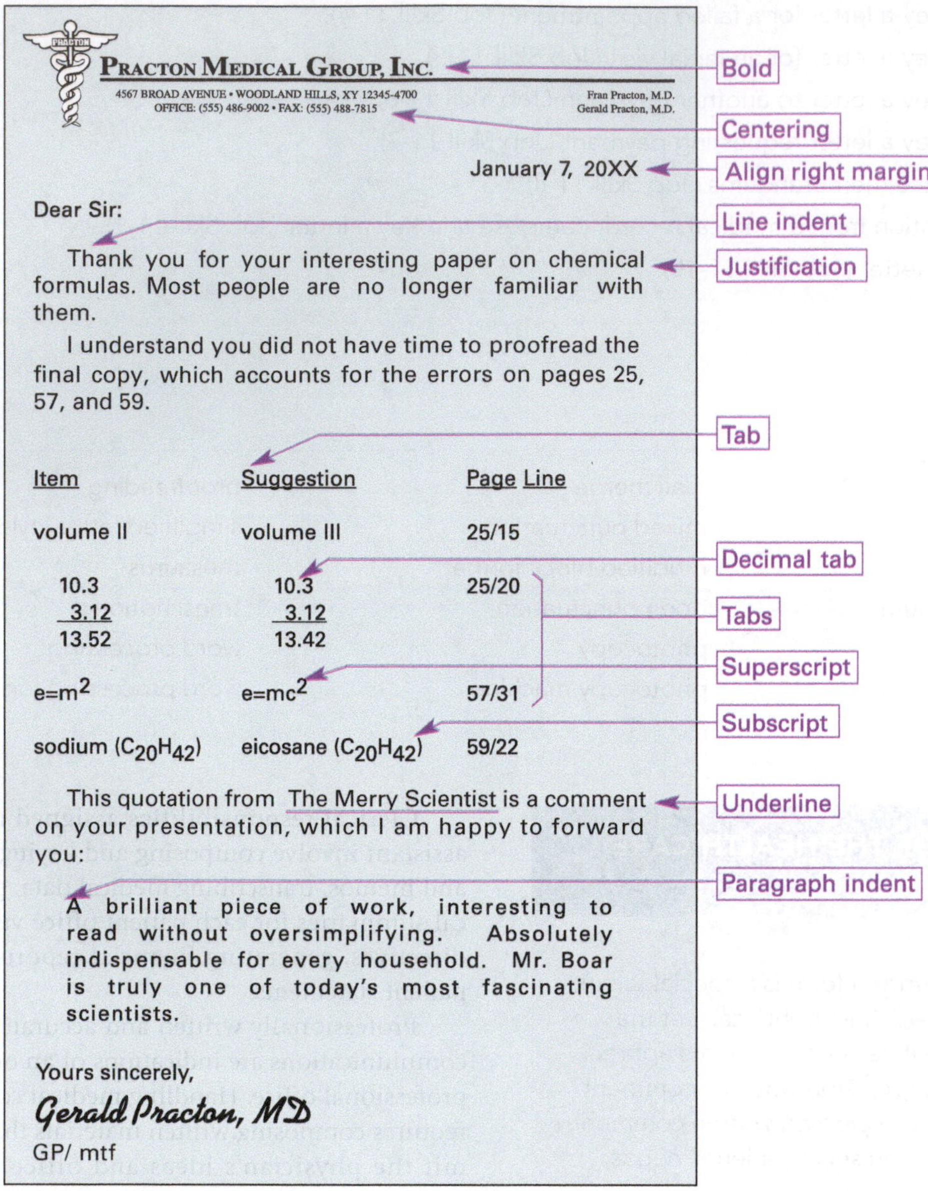

The following labels point to features in the letter:
- Bold
- Centering
- Align right margin flush
- Line indent
- Justification
- Tab
- Decimal tab
- Tabs
- Superscript
- Subscript
- Underline
- Paragraph indent

Letter content:

PRACTON MEDICAL GROUP, INC.
4567 BROAD AVENUE • WOODLAND HILLS, XY 12345-4700
OFFICE: (555) 486-9002 • FAX: (555) 488-7815

Fran Practon, M.D.
Gerald Practon, M.D.

January 7, 20XX

Dear Sir:

Thank you for your interesting paper on chemical formulas. Most people are no longer familiar with them.

I understand you did not have time to proofread the final copy, which accounts for the errors on pages 25, 57, and 59.

Item	Suggestion	Page Line
volume II	volume III	25/15
10.3	10.3	25/20
3.12	3.12	
13.52	13.42	
$e = m^2$	$e = mc^2$	57/31
sodium ($C_{20}H_{42}$)	eicosane ($C_{20}H_{42}$)	59/22

This quotation from The Merry Scientist is a comment on your presentation, which I am happy to forward you:

A brilliant piece of work, interesting to read without oversimplifying. Absolutely indispensable for every household. Mr. Boar is truly one of today's most fascinating scientists.

Yours sincerely,

Gerald Practon, MD

GP/ mtf

FIGURE 11-1 Some features of word processing software

such as CDs, DVDs, jump drives, or flash drives. In an EHR system, communication is often kept separate in the EMR portion of the software. A "Communication" menu tab often appears with a drop-down list naming the different types of communication. Another way of tracking various types of communication is to use a word processing log. The log can be kept in a separate computer file or in the EHR system labeled "Templates" or "Form Letters" with the names of specific types of letters (e.g., F. Practon Collection Letters). The menu tab or log needs to be updated each time items are deleted or added. Various types of letter formats may also be printed and kept in a three-ring notebook.

Computer Equipment and Supplies Used for Written Correspondence

Technological advances have moved medical offices into the electronic age. Forms that used to require the use of typewriters may now be scanned into the computer system to be filled in and manipulated using word processing software. Electronic letters may be created using templates, signed electronically, and printed in hard copy or sent via email or fax. The electronic letter must be able to include different types of communication in a variety of formats.

Letters should be printed on 20- or 24-pound bond paper that has a crisp surface and is receptive to both ink and printed copy. Plain or printed bond paper is used for continuation sheets (i.e., the second, third, or additional pages of a letter). Both large (No. 10) and small (No. 6 ¾) envelopes are used for business correspondence and patient statements.

LETTER STANDARDS, STYLES, AND COMPONENTS

An attractive, perfectly typed letter effectively conveys its message; a sloppy, carelessly keyed letter does not. Margins on all four sides should be as equal as possible, with spacing adjustments made between various components of the letter. Material placed too high or too low upsets the symmetry of the page and causes an imbalance. Mailability standards for a keyed communication require a perfect letter with balanced margins (Figure 11-2) and without grammatical or keyed errors. An unmailable letter is one that has any of the following:

1. Misspelled word
2. Keyed error or a poorly corrected error
3. Unbalanced margins; any of the four
4. Special lines omitted, such as a date line or a signature line
5. City name abbreviated, such as LA for Los Angeles or NY for New York City

Study the words listed in Table 11-1, which are some of the most commonly misspelled words in medical office correspondence.

Letter Styles

The most common letter styles are (1) **full block letter style**, which has all lines aligned at the left margin and adapts best to computerized preparation, as shown in Figure 11-3; (2) **modified block format**, which has the date and closing lines beginning at the center of the page, as shown in Figure 11-4 (note: this figure also labels the parts of a letter); and (3) impersonal **simplified letter style**, which eliminates both the salutation and the complimentary close and includes a subject

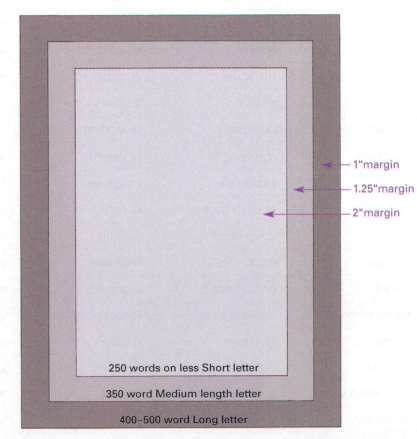

1"margin
1.25"margin
2"margin

250 words on less Short letter

350 word Medium length letter

400–500 word Long letter

FIGURE 11-2 Reduced version of a visual guide used for letter placement. Word processing margins set to 1 inch (dark gray) for long letters, 1.25 inches (medium gray) for medium letters, and 2 inches (light gray) for short letters.

TABLE 11-1 **Words Commonly Misspelled in Medical Office Correspondence**

A–C	C–I	I–P	P–R	R-W
abnormally	consensus	inadvertently	particular	reiterated
abrupt	convalescent	incision	penicillin	repetition
abscess	cough	indispensable	permissible	reviewed
absorbent	cycle	infectious	perseverance	rheumatism
acceptable	deficiency	inflammation	persistent	rhythm
accessible	definitely	inoculate	personal	schedule
accidentally	delinquent	insomnia	personnel	seizure
accommodation	demise	interfered	perspiration	senility
acknowledgment	described	intermittent	pharmaceutical	separate
acuity	diagnosis (sing.)	interpret	pharmacy	severity
administration	diagnoses (plur.)	irritated	physician	significance
admissible	diaphragm	jeopardize	precaution	specialist
admittance	diarrhea	judgment	precede	successful
affect (influence)	disappointed	labeling	prescription	sufficient
alcohol	disease(s)	laboratory	prevalent	superintendent
analysis	effect (result) (noun)	liquefy	principal (chief)	supersede
analyze	eligible	markedly	principle (rule)	surgeon
appointment	evidence	muscle	probably	susceptible
bandage	exertion	necessary	procedure	suture
behavior	existence	ninety	profession	symptom
beneficial	experience	noticeable	prognosis	technique
benefited	explanation	nourishment	pursue	temperature
brochure	facility	observation	quantity	thorough
cancel	fracture	occasionally	receiving	transferred
canceled*	height	occurrence	recognize	unconscious
capsule	hemorrhage	occurring	recommend	urinalysis
carcinoma	hygiene	omission	recovery	vaccine
cartilage	illegible	omitted	recurrence	visible
comparative	immediately	opportunity	referral	vitamin
conscious	immunity	paralyzed	referring	weight

*The past tense, "canceled" and "cancelled" are both considered correct.

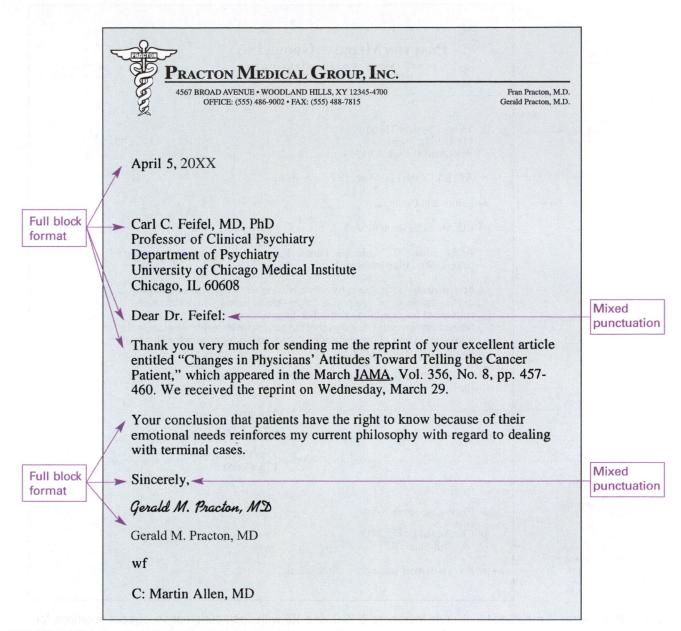

Full block format

Mixed punctuation

Full block format

Mixed punctuation

PRACTON MEDICAL GROUP, INC.

4567 BROAD AVENUE • WOODLAND HILLS, XY 12345-4700
OFFICE: (555) 486-9002 • FAX: (555) 488-7815

Fran Practon, M.D.
Gerald Practon, M.D.

April 5, 20XX

Carl C. Feifel, MD, PhD
Professor of Clinical Psychiatry
Department of Psychiatry
University of Chicago Medical Institute
Chicago, IL 60608

Dear Dr. Feifel:

Thank you very much for sending me the reprint of your excellent article entitled "Changes in Physicians' Attitudes Toward Telling the Cancer Patient," which appeared in the March JAMA, Vol. 356, No. 8, pp. 457-460. We received the reprint on Wednesday, March 29.

Your conclusion that patients have the right to know because of their emotional needs reinforces my current philosophy with regard to dealing with terminal cases.

Sincerely,

Gerald M. Practon, MD

Gerald M. Practon, MD

wf

C: Martin Allen, MD

FIGURE 11-3 Letter in full block style with mixed punctuation

line typed in all capital letters placed a triple line space after the inside address. In the simplified format, reference initials and notations are keyed in lowercase, two lines below the signature line, as in other styles. The simplified style is rarely used by physicians, because it is too impersonal. It is used in situations in which form letters are sent in the corporate setting. The physician's preference determines the letter style used in a particular office.

Letter Punctuation Styles

Letters have two types of punctuation styles—open punctuation and mixed punctuation. **Open**

punctuation is a style in which no punctuation mark is used after the salutation or complimentary close, as shown in Figure 11-4. **Mixed punctuation** is a style in which a colon or a comma is used after the salutation and complimentary close, as shown in Figure 11-3.

Margins

Right and left margins may be changed according to whether a letter is short or long. Most of the time the default (preset) feature of the word processing program is used to keep side margins of letters consistent in dimension. This default is usually set at 1 or 1.25 inches

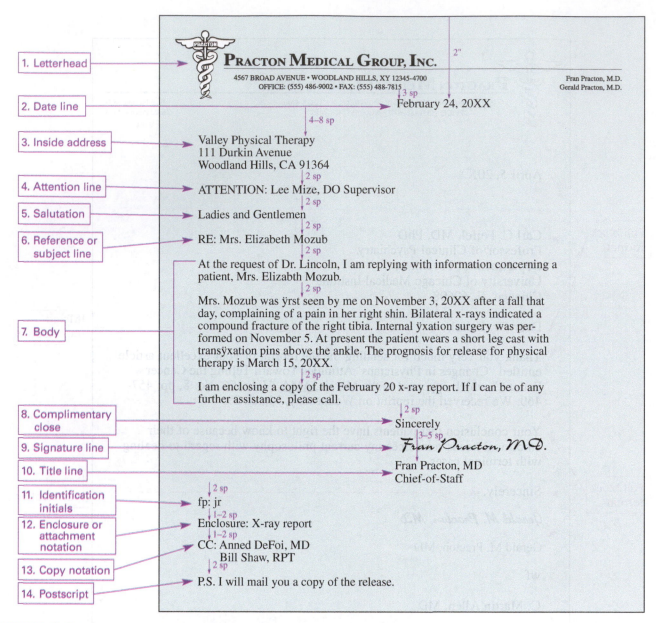

FIGURE 11-4 Letter in modified block style (numbers 2, 8, 9, and 10) with open punctuation, special notations for various parts of a letter, and spacing requirements

and is ideal for long- or medium-length letters. Side margins for short letters might be increased in width and set at 2 inches (Figure 11-2).

Defaults are also in place for top and bottom margins, usually set at 1 inch but they may be adjusted according to the letter size and side margins. If there is a second page to the letter, the bottom margin of the first page can be increased up to 2 inches (12 lines) so that lines can be better spaced on the additional page.

Word processing programs also have alignment options (Figure 11-5) that include a **justification** feature that automatically justifies both margins while

keying, if desired. *Justify* means to space words on each line of text so that the ends of the lines are flush at the right and left margins.

Parts of a Letter

Refer to the following letter parts in Figure 11-4.

Letterhead (1)

Letterhead lines are designed in an attractive format and are positioned in the upper 2 inches of a sheet of bond paper. They may include a specially designed

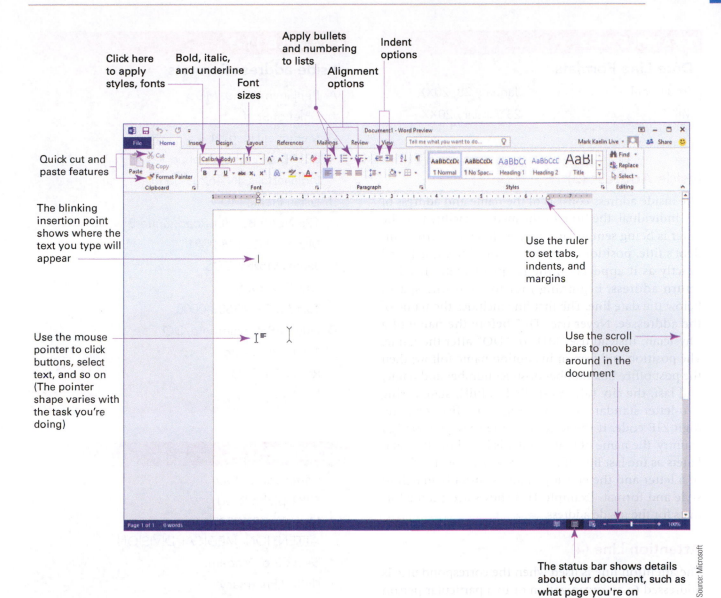

Click here to apply styles, fonts

Bold, italic, and underline

Font sizes

Apply bullets and numbering to lists

Alignment options

Indent options

Quick cut and paste features

The blinking insertion point shows where the text you type will appear

Use the mouse pointer to click buttons, select text, and so on (The pointer shape varies with the task you're doing)

Use the ruler to set tabs, indents, and margins

Use the scroll bars to move around in the document

The status bar shows details about your document, such as what page you're on

Source: Microsoft

FIGURE 11-5 Computer screen showing format features of a word processing program. The blinking insertion point shows where the left margin is set.

practice logo and generally contain the medical practice name, physician's name and title, address, telephone number, fax number, and possibly email address (Example 11-1). The return address on the envelope may match the letterhead format in miniature.

Date Line (2)

The date line is keyed 13 or 14 line spaces from the top of the paper or 3 spaces below the letterhead, depending somewhat on the size and position of the letterhead. Do not abbreviate the month or show the date in numbers only (e.g., 1/28/XX). Example 11-2 shows acceptable date line formats.

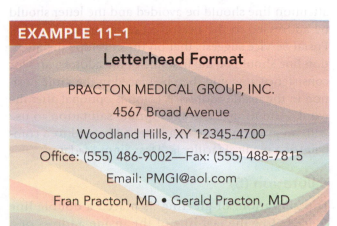

EXAMPLE 11–1

Letterhead Format

PRACTON MEDICAL GROUP, INC.

4567 Broad Avenue

Woodland Hills, XY 12345-4700

Office: (555) 486-9002—Fax: (555) 488-7815

Email: PMGI@aol.com

Fran Practon, MD • Gerald Practon, MD

<table>
<tr><td colspan="2">**EXAMPLE 11–2**</td></tr>
<tr><td colspan="2">**Date Line Formats**</td></tr>
<tr><td>Traditional</td><td>January 28, 20XX</td></tr>
<tr><td>Military</td><td>28 January 20XX</td></tr>
</table>

Inside Address (3)

The inside address consists of the name and address of the individual, the firm, or the medical facility that the letter is being sent to, and may include the correspondent's title, position, department, or office. It is keyed exactly as it appears on the recipient's letterhead or return address, beginning four to eight line spaces below the date line. The first line includes the name of the addressee. Never use "Dr." before the name of a physician; instead use "MD" or "DO" after the name. The position and firm or institution name follow; then the post office box number or street number and name; and last, the city (always spelled in full), state (using two-letter standard abbreviations), and five- or nine-digit ZIP code. If the letter is being sent to a foreign country, the name of that country is keyed in all capital letters as the last line of the address. The inside address of a letter and the envelope address usually match in style and format. Example 11-3 shows acceptable formats for the inside address.

Attention Line (4)

The attention line is used when the correspondence is addressed to an organization or to a particular person within the organization (Example 11-4). It usually precedes the salutation, starting at the left margin and a double line space below the last line of the inside address. Unless it is absolutely necessary, the use of the attention line should be avoided and the letter should be addressed to the person(s) receiving it. The U.S. Postal Service suggests that on the envelope the attention line should be the first line of the address, and for consistency, it would then be placed in the same position in the inside address. A colon is optional after the word "Attention." The appropriate salutation to use with an attention line in a letter addressed to a company or a medical facility is "Dear Sir or Madam."

Salutation (5)

The salutation, or greeting, is placed a double line space below the last line of the inside address or a

EXAMPLE 11–3

Inside address Formats

A. Benjamin Wong, MD
   Chief of Staff
   Memorial Hospital
   2211 East Eighth Avenue
   Indianapolis, IN 46205-0000

B. Lillian Frank, MD
   126 North Bender Road, Suite B
   Miami, FL 33136-2021

C. James Mozby, DDS
   P.O. Box 2338
   Toledo, OH 43503-0000

D. Guy DePetridiantonio, DO
   14017 Via Vento
   Rome 4LI 7523
   ITALY

EXAMPLE 11–4

A. Carter Laboratory
   198 Upjohn Road
   Mission, KS 66202-0000
   ATTENTION: MEDICAL DIVISION
   Dear Sir or Madam:

B. United Pharmacy
   198260 Main Street
   Somerset, NJ 40001-0000
   Attn: Ann Talbot
   Dear Ms. Talbot:

C. Attention: Art West, MD, and
   Jean Coe, MD
   One North 14th Street
   Las Vegas, NV 89102-0000
   Dear Drs. West and Coe:

double line space below the attention line. It typically begins with "Dear" and reflects the name of the person to whom the letter is addressed. In *open punctuation*, there is no punctuation after the salutation.

EXAMPLE 11–5

Salutations

A. **Open Punctuation**

Dear Dr. McGuirer

Dear Doctors

B. **Mixed Punctuation**

Dear Dr. Ames and Dr. Rulfo:

(when addressing two physicians)

Dear Drs. Ames and Rulfo:

Dear Sir or Madam:

(when gender is unknown)

To Whom It May Concern:

(when recipient is unknown)

Dear Ms. Troy:

(when marital status is unknown or when
Ms. was used on letter received)

EXAMPLE 11–6

Reference or Subject Lines

A. **Block Style**

Dear Dr. McMurtry:

RE: Faith Upton

B. **Modified Block Style**

Dear Miss Allison:

Refer to: Policy No. 5682

Dear Dr. Arthur:

SUBJECT: AMA Meeting

ABC Laboratory

2340 Main Street

Any City, XY 50201-6912

Dear Madam or Sir:

Re: Nancy Smith, Office Manager

In *mixed punctuation*, the salutation is followed by a colon (Example 11-5). "Ms." is used when a woman's title is not known or as a substitute for "Miss" or "Mrs." The best clue is what the letter writer uses to identify herself. "Dear Sir or Madam" is used when it is not known whether the addressee is a man or a woman.

Reference or Subject Line (6)

The reference or subject line draws the reader's attention to a subject or, in medical correspondence, to a patient's name or account number. It is customarily positioned a double line space after the salutation. In block style, it is always positioned at the left margin.

In modified block style, it may be centered or, for special emphasis, aligned with the left edge of the date line. Another placement variation is to type the subject line between the last line of the inside address and the salutation, in the same style and position as the attention line. An attention line and a subject line can be keyed in the same style if both appear in a letter (Example 11-6).

Body (7)

The body is the main part of the letter and contains the message to be conveyed to the recipient; it should begin two lines below the salutation or two lines after the reference or subject line if there is one. In block style, all paragraphs begin at the left margin. Paragraphs are single-spaced internally, with double-spacing separating the paragraphs. Extremely short letters can be double-spaced with indented paragraphs.

Complimentary Close (8)

At the end of a letter, one to three complimentary words are typed a double line space below the last line of the body of the letter, indicating that the sender has concluded the message; only the first letter is capitalized (Example 11-7). The closing line is followed by a comma if a colon has been used after the salutation in keeping with the *mixed punctuation* format; in *open punctuation*, no punctuation follows the closing.

Signature Line (9)

The signature line includes the first and last names of the person responsible for writing the letter and his or her credential (e.g., MD). It is keyed three to five line spaces

EXAMPLE 11–7

Complimentary Close Phrases

A. **Mixed Punctuation**

Sincerely,

B. **Open Punctuation**

Cordially

EXAMPLE 11–8

Signature Lines

A. *John D. Carter, MD*
   John D. Carter, MD
   Chief of Surgery

B. *Kim Hall*
   Kim Hall, CMT

C. *Roberta Avila, MD*
   Roberta Avila, MD, PhD
   Director, Medical Research

D. *Bryon Avery*
   Bryon Avery

E. *Sally Hartman-Fox*
   Sally Hartman-Fox, CMA-A (AAMA)
   Office Manager

F. *Marsha Cole*
   Marsha Cole
   Secretary to Dr. Blake

below the complimentary close to allow space for the handwritten signature. The space may be reduced or increased to improve letter placement. The signature line uses complete names rather than initials, so the reader can determine the title to use in response. Example 11-8 shows variations in signature lines.

Title Line (10)

A business or professional title associated with the person who has written the letter is keyed on the line below the signature line or immediately after the signature and preceded by a comma. Title lines are highlighted in Example 11-9.

Identification Initials (11)

Identification or reference initials to distinguish the writer and the person who has keyed the letter are

EXAMPLE 11–9

Title Lines

A. Marilyn Smythe, DDS
   Chairman, Dental Department

B. Robert Belasco, MD, Administrator

EXAMPLE 11–10

Dictator (Writer) and Typist's Reference Initials

A. Dg   (typist)
B. ABJ   (typist)
C. RBCJr:lm   (dictator and typist)
D. MF:CFP   (dictator and typist)
E. KL/me   (dictator and typist)

inserted a double line space below the signature or title lines (Example 11-10). If both the writer's initials and the initials of the person who keyed the letter appear, include a colon or slash in between. The trend is to omit the dictator's initials if the name has been keyed in the signature block or if it appears in the letterhead. (The assistant should be careful to avoid humorous or confusing three-letter combinations.)

The fact that a letter is dictated or written by someone other than the person who signs it is indicated by the writer's name or initials followed by the typist's initials (rather than the signer's and the typist's). Example 11-11 shows two ways to identify the person who wrote the letter.

Enclosure or Attachment Notation (12)

The enclosure notation is a courtesy to the correspondent to affirm that separate material is enclosed with the letter. The word "enclosure" or an abbreviation is keyed either a single or double line space below the identification initials. It is appropriate to list the enclosures or particular attachments when several items are included. When an enclosure is large or bulky, it may be

EXAMPLE 11–11

Writer's Identification Initials and Typist's Reference Initials

A. *James B. Moore, MD*
   James B. Moore, MD
   MHJ:bt

B. *Mary T. Washington, MD*
   Mary T. Washington, MD
   ATMcGuire/lw

EXAMPLE 11–12

Enclosure or Attachment Notations

A. Attachments (2)

B. Enclosures 2

C. Enc.

D. 2 encls.

E. 1 Enclosure

F. Enclosures: Pathology report
                     Operation schedule

G. Check enclosed

H. Enclosure—Software

I. Enclosure sent separately

---

best to indicate that the enclosure will be sent separately (see Example 11-12).

Copy Notations (13)

When several copies have been mailed to people other than the person whose name appears on the inside address, a copy notation is keyed at the bottom of the letter a single or double line space below the enclosure notation. "Copy," "CC," or "C" indicates that courtesy copies have been mailed or made for distribution to the named people; names or initials are given in alphabetical order (see Example 11-13). Never key a copy notation without a name following it.

The notation "bcc," "bc," or "BCC" is used for *blind copies*, when the writer sends a copy of the correspondence to a third party without the knowledge of the person receiving the original letter. For blind copies, do not make a copy notation on the original, but make a "bcc" notation on the file copy with the name of the recipient following it.

EXAMPLE 11–13

Copy Notations

A. c: Al Moore

B. bc: Carol Yu, MD

C. Copies to Dr. Alcott
          Dr. Sowell

D. BCC: Hal Ames

E. cc: James More, MD
          Carolyn Shaw, RPT

EXAMPLE 11–14

Postscripts

A. **Example of an Afterthought:**

   P.S. I spoke to the hospital electrician who said that nine plugs will be adequate.

B. **Example of Reiteration:**

   P.S. Don't forget the Thursday AMA meeting!

Postscript (14)

A postscript is an afterthought or a statement repeated (reiterated) for emphasis (Example 11-14). It is keyed a double line space below the last keyed line and may be preceded by "P.S.," if desired.

COMPOSING LETTERS

A medical assistant who can independently compose letters for the physician possesses a skill that is an asset to the practice. Letters written over the assistant's signature will deal with patient appointments, insurance, and routine business matters.

Letters written by the assistant for the physician's signature will usually concern medical matters, for example, abstraction of medical data from patients' charts in reply to requests for information. Such letters should emulate as much as possible the physician's usual degree of formality and professional style.

Reference Material

Useful references for letter writing include an English grammar reference book for punctuation and correct use of grammar, a medical dictionary for spelling and definitions, a secretarial manual for style and format, and a thesaurus. A **thesaurus** ("treasury" in Greek) is an alphabetical listing of synonyms and antonyms used to find alternative words to express the same or opposite ideas. It is a useful tool for preventing words in letters from sounding repetitious. These reference materials are available in printed form, as part of word processing software programs, and via the Internet (see the *Resources* section at the end of this chapter). A computerized reference file of well-written sample phrases, paragraphs, or letters can be assembled to save time and effort when similar letters are being prepared.

Outline and Tone

Before beginning to outline the content of a letter, the assistant should try to visualize the person receiving the correspondence and anticipate what the recipient needs or wants to know. Picture the reader and ask, "What would I say if the person was on the telephone or across the desk?" Proceed to write the letter as though talking with the recipient, using conversational language when writing to a familiar person. More reserved language may be used when writing to an unknown recipient.

The trend when writing business letters is to use a personalized approach. Eliminate the use of formal words or artificially worded phrases, and keep the number of words to a minimum, which increases clearness and avoids the possibility of overwhelming the reader. Simplicity, clarity, and conciseness are basic standards for every medical communication.

Use gender-neutral terms instead of "he/she" or "him/her" to avoid offending the recipient. Careful proofreading prevents the embarrassment of discovering an error in the letter's text or a misspelling of the recipient's name after the original letter has left the office. Medical correspondence deals primarily with routine matters, and letters of two or three paragraphs cover most subjects.

Introduction, Body, and Closing

The first paragraph of a letter (i.e., introduction) should be positive in tone and deal immediately with the subject matter in a friendly and courteous manner. It should include a personal comment and an expression of interest in the patient or his or her health problem. Thoughts are presented in logical order in the body of the letter with sentences averaging no more than 20 words. A concise and courteous closing statement includes some reference to an action to be taken by the recipient. Thanks are expressed if a service has been rendered or a response expected; otherwise, the assistant waits until the request has been fulfilled before following up with an acknowledgment. All correspondence should be answered promptly—within 24 hours if possible. If there is a delay, the letter, when it is written, should include a tactful explanation.

Characteristics of a Letter

A well-written letter has the following characteristics:

1. It creates a favorable impression by arousing the reader's interest with the first sentence.
2. It appeals to the reader's point of view and avoids the use of the pronoun "I."
3. It is correct in every grammatical detail.
4. It is courteous, friendly, and sincere—promoting goodwill.
5. It is accurate, clear, concise, and complete.
6. It flows smoothly from paragraph to paragraph and concludes by telling the reader how to respond.
7. It avoids jargon and stilted phrases such as "please be advised," "as per," "under separate cover," and "attached hereto." It also avoids sexism by deleting the role use of "he" or "she."
8. It concludes on a positive note, emphasizing a pleasant closing thought.

Common Writing Rules

There are many basic rules to follow when writing. Table 11-2 lists common punctuation and Table 11-3 lists some of the common writing rules, each with examples.

TABLE 11-2 Common Punctuation

Punctuation	Definition	Example
Apostrophe (')	Used to create possessive forms and denote omission of letters.	It is Dale's cell phone. Please don't (do not) do that.
Colon (:)	Used to introduce a series of items, to follow formal salutations, and to separate the hours from minutes indicating time.	The following employees will be going to the convention: Mary Adams, Margaret Kinsley, and Lynda St. George.
Comma (,)	Used to separate words or phrases in a series of three or more (the final comma before the "and" is optional). Also used to separate long introductory clauses or to connect independent clauses joined by "and," "but," "for," "nor," "so," and "yet."	She ran to the phone, answered it, and asked the patient to please call back tomorrow when the office was open.

(continues)

TABLE 11-2 Common Punctuation (*continued*)

Punctuation	Definition	Example
Diagonal (/)	Used in abbreviations, dates, fractions, and to indicate two or more options.	c/o, 2015/2016, 1/3, he/she
Ellipsis (. . .)	Used when quoting material and you want to omit some words. Also used to indicate a pause in the flow of a sentence.	"No matter who you are . . . when you're dealing with Alzheimer's . . . as the disease unfolds, you don't know what to expect."
Exclamation point (!)	Use at the end of an emphatic declaration, interjection, or command.	You have all been asked to please turn off the air conditioner at the end of the day!
Hyphen (-)	Used when writing numbers, to create compound words, and when adding certain prefixes.	Twenty-two, on-the-go, ex-husband
Parentheses ( )	Used to include material that you want to de-emphasize. Also used to enclose a number that is spelled out in a sentence.	The Centers for Medicare and Medicaid Services (formerly the Health Care Financing Administration) is offering a seminar on medical coding.
Period (.)	Used at end of an indirect question, at the end of a sentence, following a command, and following some abbreviations.	Dr. Practon asked when Mrs. Fields would be coming in again.
Question mark (?)	Use at the end of a direct question.	Is Dr. Practon going to be coming to the seminar?
Quotation marks (" ")	Used to set off spoken dialogue. Also used with some titles and words that are used in a special way (typically, commas and periods go inside quotation marks).	Dr. Practon said, "Do not be late for the seminar."

TABLE 11-3 Common Writing Rules

Topic	Rule	Example
Capitalization	*Capitalize:* • Addresses: Street, city, and state names • Compass points when used to indicate geographical parts of a country (not when used as part of proper names) • Days of the week, months, or holidays	• 123 Echo Lane, Hill Country, Nebraska • Eastern United States, Northern Canada (southern Illinois, eastern Texas) • Monday, February 14, 2011 Valentine's Day
	• Family indications when personally addressing an individual (not when used as a positive pronoun) • First word of every sentence, whether complete or not • Geographical terms when preceding or following names	• I am glad to see you Mother. • Hello, Mrs. Olivares. • Pacific <u>Ocean</u> Happy <u>Canyon</u> <u>Lake</u> Mead <u>Mount</u> Olives Palm <u>Desert</u> Niagara <u>Falls</u>

(*continues*)

TABLE 11-3 **Common Writing Rules** (*continued*)

Topic	Rule	Example

	• Government departments
	• Military names
	• Names of organizations
	• Names of people (proper names)
	• Political, racial, or religious designations
		• Federal Bureau of Investigation
		• U.S. Army, Marine Corps, Royal Air Force
		• Practon Medical Group, Inc.
		• Frances A. Witherberry
		• Democrat, Republican
		  German, Irish, Jewish
		  Catholic, Protestant

	• Sums of money written out • Titles: Academic and religious	• Three Thousand Fifty Dollars • <u>Doctor</u> Richard Reed <u>Professor</u> Darrell Larkin <u>Bishop</u> Mary Beth Stinson <u>Reverend</u> Walter A. Field

	• Titles: Books, newspapers, or magazines	• Administrative Medical Assisting
		  Wall Street Journal
		  Family Circle

	• Titles: Documents and reports	• U.S. Constitution American Cancer Society Annual Report
Numbers	• Spell out single-digit whole numbers • Use numerals for numbers greater than nine • Spell out simple fractions	• Please send <u>four</u> or <u>five</u> copies. • Please send <u>10</u> or <u>12</u> copies. • one-half, two-thirds

	• Spell out times of day when "o'clock" is being used; use numerals when exact times are emphasized
	• Spell out large numbers
	• Use commas when numbers have more than five digits
	• Use *noon* and *midnight* instead of a.m. and p.m.
	• Use numerals when writing laboratory results
	• Use numerals for mixed fractions (unless it is the first word in a sentence)
	• Write out a number if it begins a sentence
		• Your appointment is at four o'clock on March 23.
		  Please arrive at 8:30 a.m.
		
		• Please send one thousand syringes.
		• $1000
		  $52,000
		• Do not have anything to eat or drink after 12 *midnight*.
		• Your cholesterol was 162 mg/dl
		
		• Please pay 5½ percent interest.
		
		• Thirty local physicians will be attending the convention.

Plurals	• Medical terms ending in "a"
	  Keep the "a" and add "e"
	• Medical terms ending in "is"
	  Drop the "is" and add "es"
	• Medical terms ending in "oma"
	  Drop the "oma" and add "omata"
	• Medical terms ending in "um"
	  Drop the "um" and add "a"
	• Medical terms ending in "us"
	  Drop the "us" and add "i"
	• For most English words Add "s"
	
	• Words ending in "s," "ch," or "sh" (also x, z)
	  Add "es"
	• Words ending in "y" preceded by a consonant
	  Drop the "y" and add "ies"
	• Words ending in "y" preceded by a vowel
	  Add "s"
		• Singular: vertebra
		  Plural: vertebrae
		• Singular: diagnosis
		  Plural: diagnoses
		• Singular: fibroma
		  Plural: fibromata
		• Singular: bacterium
		  Plural: bacteria
		• Singular: bronchus
		  Plural: bronchi
		• Singular: pill, house
		  Plural: pills, houses
		• Singular: gas, church, brush
		  Plural: gases, churches, brushes
		• Singular: extremity
		  Plural: extremities
		
		• Singular: key
		  Plural: keys

(*continues*)

TABLE 11-3 Common Writing Rules (*continued*)

Topic	Rule	Example
Possessives	• Singular nouns that end in "s" Add an apostrophe and an "s" • Singular nouns that do not end in "s" Add an apostrophe and an "s" • Plural nouns that end in "s" Add an apostrophe • Plural nouns that do not end in "s" Add an apostrophe and an "s"	• Mrs. Jones's physician is Dr. Fran Practon. • The child's throat is red. • The seminar was three days' duration. • The children's play area needs cleaning.
Word Division	• Divide according to pronunciation • Divide after a prefix • Divide before "ing" • Divide hyphenated compound words at the hyphen • Divide compound words between the two words from which they derive • Divide the root word from the suffix • Divide between consonants	• carcinoma car-cin-oma • electrocardiogram electro-cardiogram • walking walk-ing • hysterosalpingo-oophorectomy • cardiomyopathy cardio-myopathy • cardiology cardio-logy • inject in-ject

Types of Letters

Basic types of letters used in medical offices include multipage letters, form letters, and interoffice memorandums. Refer to Procedure 11-1 for step-by-step instructions to compose, format, key, proofread, and print business correspondence.

Multipage Letter

When more than one page is needed for written correspondence, a simplified heading is placed at the top of each continuation sheet, using a horizontal or vertical format (see Example 11-21). Continuation pages are keyed on plain bond paper or preprinted second sheets.

The heading for all continuation sheets begins on line seven, which leaves a 1-inch top margin. The letter is continued on the third line space after the heading. It is best to conclude a paragraph at the bottom of each page, but if this is not possible, carry at least two lines of a paragraph to the continuation sheet. Never use a second page to key only the complimentary close. There must be at least a 1-inch bottom margin.

Always look at the document in print preview before printing. Check to be sure that the page-two markings appear where they were intended. If transcribing a document that will be printed at another site with no opportunity for you to review the final printout, be sure someone verifies the printer setup and checks the document.

PROCEDURE 11-1

2 3

Compose, Format, Key, Proofread, and Print Business Correspondence

OBJECTIVE: Compose, format, key, proofread, and print business correspondence following guidelines of commonly used business-letter style.

EQUIPMENT/SUPPLIES: Computer and printer, letterhead paper, envelope, attachments (if necessary), thesaurus, English dictionary, medical dictionary, and pen or pencil.

DIRECTIONS: Follow these step-by-step directions, which include rationales, to learn this procedure. Job Skills 11-4, 11-5, 11-6, 11-7, 11-9, and 11-10 are presented in the *Workbook* to practice this skill.

1. Assemble materials, determine the recipient's address, and decide on the letter style or format (modified or full block style).

(*continues*)

PROCEDURE 11-1 (*continued*)

2. Prepare an outline and/or draft of the letter, noting important points or topics to be included in a logical sequence.

3. Turn on the computer and select the word processing program (e.g., Microsoft Word).

4. Open a blank document or a letter template to be used. A template includes each component of a letter and allows you to create a new document with less keystrokes.

5. Using the "Format" and "Page Setup" functions, select the font size and type, desired spacing, document margins, paper size, and layout.

6. Create and key the *letterhead*.

7. Key the *date line* beginning at least three lines below the letterhead, making sure it is in the proper location for the chosen style.

8. Double-space down and insert the *inside address,* making sure it is in the proper location for the chosen style. Select a style to insert an *attention line* if necessary.

9. Double-space and key the *salutation,* using either open or mixed punctuation. A business letter is more formal than personal correspondence, so the salutation should include a title and the person's last name.

10. Double-space and enter the *reference line* ("Re:" or "Subject:") in the location for the chosen letter style. This helps the recipient identify the contents of the letter before thoroughly reading it.

11. Double-space and key the *body* (content) of the letter in single-space, making sure the paragraph style is proper for the format chosen. Double-space between paragraphs. Save your work to the computer hard drive every 15 minutes.

12. Proofread the letter on the computer screen for composition and make additions, deletions, or adjustments as needed.

13. Proofread for typographical, spelling, grammatical, and mechanical errors. Use the word processing software program's spell-check feature and any reference books to check for correct spelling, meaning, or usage.

14. Key the *second-page heading* on line 7 (name, page number, and date) in vertical or horizontal format if a second page is necessary (see Example 11-21).

15. Key a *complimentary close,* making sure it is in the proper location for the chosen style.

16. Go down four spaces and key the *sender's name and title* or credentials as printed on the letterhead. This makes it easier for the recipient to identify the sender.

17. Double-space and insert the sender and typist's *reference initials* in lowercase letters, separating the two sets of initials with a colon or slash.

18. Single- or double-space to insert *copy* ("CC"), *enclosure* ("Enclosure" or "Enc"), or *attachment* notations.

19. Double-space to insert a *postscript* ("P.S."), if necessary.

20. Save the file before printing a hard copy, and proofread the letter again. Make corrections, if necessary.

21. Print the final copy to be sent and proofread.

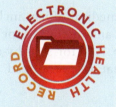

22. If the letter is composed using EHR software, have the physician review it and sign it electronically, then transmit a copy to the patient via email (if proper authorization forms have been signed), and send a copy to the patient's EMR.

23. If using a paper-based system, photocopy the letter to be retained in the patient's chart so that if questions arise, a copy of the letter can be referred to.

24. Save the file to the hard drive and to an electronic storage device for future reference.

25. Prepare an envelope, using the format for optical scanning. If sending the correspondence registered or certified, be sure to place special mailing instructions on the envelope.

26. Clip any attachments to the letter and give to the physician for review and signature.

Sample Letters

Sample letters for common situations are presented in Examples 11-15 through 11-20. See Chapter 3 for a letter of withdrawal from a case (Figure 3-11), a letter to a patient who fails to keep an appointment (Figure 3-12), and a letter to confirm discharge by a patient (Figure 3-13). See Chapter 13 for examples of collection letters.

Form Letters

Form letters, also known as *repetitive letters*, are often used when the physician communicates repetitious

---

EXAMPLE 11–15

Outlining Office Visit Fees

Dear Mrs. Chai:

In response to your request for information on fees charged for office visits, Dr. Practon has asked me to send you a range of the customary charges. Fees vary according to the level of history, medical examination, and decision-making process performed by the physician. They are:

Office visit, new patient from $33.25 to $132.28

Office visit, established patient from $16.07 to $96.00

If you have any questions, do not hesitate to call our office for additional information.

EXAMPLE 11–16

Canceling an Appointment

Dear Miss Wooley:

Dr. Fran Practon has asked me to cancel all of her scheduled appointments for the week of Monday, July 3, through Friday, July 7, because of a family emergency. Therefore, I have canceled your appointment for Wednesday, July 5, at 2:00 p.m. I have been unsuccessful in my attempts to reach you by telephone, so would you please contact this office as soon as possible to schedule another appointment. Dr. Practon regrets any inconvenience this change may have caused you.

EXAMPLE 11–17

Response to a Referral

Dear Dr. Ames:

Thank you for referring your patient, Mrs. Phyllis Green, for consultation. She was examined by me today, and there were no significant symptoms of pulmonary disease. Her episodic asthma seems to be exercise related and should improve with a continuous exercise program.

Her chest x-ray was normal, as were the results of the CBC, BUN, and spirometry. She has a short ejection systolic murmur that does not vary with maneuvers.

My recommendation is that Mrs. Green continue the medication and diet you recommended and that she enroll in a daily supervised exercise program. Please do not hesitate to contact me if you have further questions regarding my findings.

EXAMPLE 11–18

Transferring Care to Another Physician

Dear Dr. Bailey:

This letter confirms my April 7 telephone referral of Marjorie Lowe, transferring her to your care.

Mrs. Lowe has been my patient for five years and has experienced increased complaints of coughing and shortness of breath. I am referring Mrs. Lowe to you after a routine office exam and pulmonary function test indicated the possibility of emphysema. I appreciate your receiving Mrs. Lowe as a new patient for this condition, and I will continue to care for her other medical problems.

Her address and telephone number are 12135 Arbor Circle, Kearney, Nebraska 68845, Tel. 555/236-4068.

---

information, such as notifying the health department of an individual who has contracted a contagious disease or notifying the Department of Motor Vehicles that an individual has developed epilepsy.

Additionally, form letters are mailed to patients who fail to keep appointments, who do not follow the medical advice given to them, or who need to be advised, with written documentation, of the physician's withdrawal from a case. Contents for some of these are shown in Chapter 3. The assistant must always be aware of the legal implications for the physician inherent in writing any such letter and never diagnose or make any unethical statements about a patient's illness or the prognosis for recovery.

Letters that provide instructions and details of an upcoming hospital stay, which appeal a denied health insurance claim, or which deal with routine collections, are also typical instances in which form letters might be used. To save time and to reflect the physician's personality in writing form letters, templates of model form letters should be kept. These can be stored on CDs, DVDs, or a jump/flash drive. Such letters can be merged with address, salutation, and date

---

EXAMPLE 11–19

Letter About a Delinquent Account

Dear Miss Norton:

Two months ago on June 14, you visited our office for a complete physical examination. We have received no payment in response to our billing statements.

We would like to hear from you concerning the $250 balance. Please contact this office as soon as possible so we can set up a satisfactory payment plan. Your cooperation in this matter is appreciated.

EXAMPLE 11–20

Request for Information

Dear Sir or Madam:

In your Spring catalog on page 85, you advertised a designer-styled, steel stool with an adjustable seat. Dr. Davis would like to place an order; however, he first would like to know what type of padding is used in the construction of the seat and whether the stool is available with a washable cover.

Your prompt reply to this inquiry is appreciated.

EXAMPLE 11–21

Multipage Letter Headings

A. Leonard J. Warren, MD (2) May 1, 20XX
   (addressee)

B. RE: Lorraine Gonzaga (patient)
   Page 2
   November 19, 20XX

---

information. This is called **mail merge**. Top-quality form letters can be prepared in a few minutes, and most computer software programs (e.g., Microsoft Word, Pages) have various letter and memo templates that can be used.

Interoffice Memorandums

Interoffice memorandums (memos) are used by offices, clinics, and hospitals to facilitate the exchange of ideas among individuals and departments within the organization in situations when informal written communication is appropriate. The message, which is casual in tone, should communicate instructions or other messages in a concise, impersonal manner, so the reader can easily absorb the information.

Types of memos include the (1) *informative*, which provides facts with explanations; (2) *directive*, which gives brief instructions; and (3) *administrative*, which states policy or judgment on a specific topic.

A template of a memo format with appropriate guide words used as headings and followed by a colon may be saved and kept in the computer (Figure 11-6). Some memos are printed on letterhead, but usually the title "Interoffice Memo" or simply "Memo" is sufficient

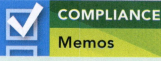

COMPLIANCE
Memos

Confidential matters should never be written in memos, because those messages are circulated throughout the office and may be part of permanent or temporary records.

typed either in a vertical or horizontal format (Example 11-22).

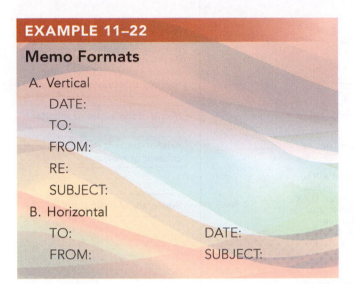

EXAMPLE 11–22

Memo Formats

A. Vertical

DATE:

TO:

FROM:

RE:

SUBJECT:

B. Horizontal

TO: DATE:

FROM: SUBJECT:

The vertical style is popular, easier to set up, and more appropriate when the subject line is lengthy. In the horizontal format, the two headings TO and FROM are double-spaced flush with the left margin; the DATE and SUBJECT (or RE:) lines would be placed to the right of the center of the page.

Margins are set at the point where the preprinted guide words begin or at a point two or three spaces after the longest guide word in the left column of the printed headings. Typist's initials, enclosures, and copy notations are single- or double-spaced at the conclusion of the message, just as in any letter. Keying the writer's initials is not required, but may be included according to office policy.

A keyed signature line is typically not used, nor does the author or dictator sign the memo. However, if the writer of the memo prefers to end the memo with a handwritten signature, then key the writer's name or initials on the fourth line below the last line of the message. If the writer inserts handwritten initials at the end of the memo or next to the typed name in the heading, as in Figure 11-6, omit the signature line altogether. Even if the memo is not signed, it should always be submitted to the author for approval before being distributed.

When a hardcopy memo is to be read by several persons , the names are listed either in alphabetical order or in order of seniority, with each person initialing his or her name after reading the information. If the memo continues to an additional page or pages, begin 1 inch from the top of the continuation page and key in headings: name of addressee, date, and page number. Triple-space and continue with the body of the memo.

When electronic mail is used to send memos, it is only necessary to insert the names of the recipients with their email addresses and the word "MEMO" in the subject line because the date and recipient's name will appear as a regular part of the email heading.

CORRECTIONS IN BUSINESS CORRESPONDENCE

Corrections occur in business correspondence in spelling, word division, spacing, punctuation, capitalization, grammar, use of figures and symbols, and data input (typographical errors). While keying data, it is common to transpose and alter the sequence of letters and numbers, which changes the spelling of a word or the numerical order. When some type of correction, alteration, or refinement is necessary, these changes are referred to as **edits**. Any editing done to letters or medical records should not change the content or meaning of the physician's dictation. If questions arise, ask the physician prior to making changes.

Text-Editing Features

Computer word processing software has special text-editing features, which include:

- Directional keys, which move the cursor up, down, left, and right
- Function keys, which perform tabulation, delete, and search operations
- Tool features, which flag misspelled words and misused phrases during the keying or scanning of a document; also provide word corrections and synonyms
- Edit features, which search for a page number or a word or phrase in the text and allow optional replacement

MEMO

DATE:	September 1, 20XX
TO:	Karen Avila Roberta Klein
FROM:	Fran Practon, MD *F.P.*
SUBJECT:	Certiÿciation Seminar for Administrative Medial Assistants

Dr. Lane Jackson of the Hollywood Children's Hospital will be the moderator and guest speaker at a symposium to be held on September 27, 20XX, at Los Robles Hospital in Thousand Oaks. The meeting will focus on medical terminology and emergency treatment as they relate to children. I recommend that you make every effort to attend as Dr. Jackson is a noted authority in pediatrics.

Additional information:

1. $25 registration fee (paid by Practon Medical Group) needs to be mailed to Los Robles Hospital on or before September 10.
2. Continuing education units will be awarded those persons who attend.
3. A buffet luncheon is included in the registration fee.

jf

Annotations:
- Date the message originated
- Alphabetical list of all names of persons or departments for routing; titles not necessary
- Name of the writer or dictator
- Brief statement describing content of memo
- Summary of main points

FIGURE 11-6 Preprinted headings on an interoffice memo to medical office personnel

- Print features, which prints multiple copies of documents and can merge letters with a list of names and addresses
- Format functions, which direct the:
  - Placement of information in the document such as indentation, centering, and right and left margin justification
  - Alignment of multiple columns
  - Use of boldface, italics, and underline
  - Removal and addition of words and sections with a cut-and-paste feature
  - Insertion and removal of punctuation
  - Hyphenation of words that go beyond the right margin

Automatic format features may also indicate a certain style, setup, or format. Inadvertent use of the above-mentioned features may result in a printout containing an incorrect format or an inappropriate word, phrase, or entire paragraph, so proofreading is always necessary. Word processing software also has the capability to convert partial words to complete words; however, when this occurs, the word should always be checked for correctness.

Proofreading

Proofreading may be done on-screen and also on hard copy after printing. Careful **proofreading** and correcting of all copy prevents the embarrassment of errors in information presented to patients and associates. Proofreading on-screen is more difficult than scanning the printed page because errors can be easily overlooked. Errors that are not corrected might seriously affect a medical case or research information, so take extra care to find and correct errors when they appear on-screen. Reread final hardcopy documents because in the process of making corrections using computer software, words may be lost, phrases may be duplicated, new paragraphs may be inserted, or old paragraphs may not be deleted.

Spelling and Grammar Check

Spell check, grammar check, and medical dictionary software programs are available, or may be packaged with a word processing program. Specialized software programs may be purchased for medical terms, pharmacology words, laboratory terminology, and so forth, which allow for medical words to be added so that the dictionary may be personalized to a medical specialty. Many of these programs use a marker system (i.e., highlight or wavy line) to point to problem words. Corrections can be made as the document is being keyed or after it is finished, using the search and replace function.

Some grammar checkers allow a choice of six types of writing styles: general, business, technical, fiction, informal, and custom. This gives the operator a tremendous amount of flexibility, so such a program is very useful. It is not perfect, however; you need to know basic grammar to make decisions about proper usage of words. Never rely on spell or grammar check programs to correct the overall document; stop if doubts occur about words and phrases and look them up. Researching these later is *not* a good idea, because they may not be picked up during the spell check and thus be overlooked or forgotten. Software that checks spelling offers tips for improvement, but the corrective action is still the proofreader's responsibility. Remember that the spell-check feature does not check for correct *use* of a word, and sometimes the spell-check feature may indicate that words or sentences are wrong when they are actually correct. Therefore, do not accept suggested corrections without question. Other times, a document may be run through spell check and no errors are found. However, when manually proofing, you may find a typographical error (e.g., *do* instead of *to*). Refer to the *Resources* section at the end of this chapter for online spelling and grammar help via the Internet.

Cut-and-Paste Features

Cut-and-paste features allow the operator to remove words or sections of text and rearrange by putting the removed (cut) item in another place. When using this editing feature, it is easy to make mistakes while inserting or rearranging words or paragraphs. Particular care must be taken whenever these procedures are performed.

Print Preview

When you are proofreading on the computer screen, the display can be deceptive as to how the format of a document may appear when printed. Most software programs offer a "print preview," allowing the proofreader to view the document on the screen as it will appear when printed. Always view the document using "print preview." Proofread work on-screen and train your eyes to spot the smallest of errors. Then print out and proofread the document again to see if anything slipped by unnoticed. This skill will improve with experience. Refer to Procedure 11-2 for instructions on proofreading a document.

ENVELOPE ENCLOSURES

A letter's first impression is made by the envelope in which it is enclosed; much the same way that the first impression of a book is determined by its cover. The envelope should always have a professional appearance and follow accepted business style. See Chapter 12 for envelope guidelines.

When a letter goes to the physician to be signed, it is paper-clipped under the flap of the envelope so the physician sees both together (Figure 11-7). The envelope size depends on the type of communication and the number of enclosures. Attachments are stapled to the back of the letter. When the letter has been signed and is ready to mail, it is folded and inserted into the envelope so that it will be in reading position when it is removed.

Folding Enclosures

To fold a letter for a large (No. 10) envelope, place the letter flat on the desk in reading position. First fold from the bottom to a point a little less than one-third of the page and crease. Next, fold downward from the top to within one-half inch of the first fold and crease. The last crease is inserted into the envelope first so that the top of the letter is at the top of the envelope (Figure 11-8).

PROCEDURE 11-2

Proofread a Business Document

OBJECTIVE: Proofread a business document on-screen and in hard copy to correct spelling, typographical, mechanical, grammar, and other errors.

EQUIPMENT/SUPPLIES: Computer, document with errors (on-screen and hard copy), and pen or pencil.

DIRECTIONS: Follow these step-by-step directions, which include rationales. Several job skills are presented in the *Workbook* for practice after keying a letter.

1. Proofread the document as you key in data using the word processing software program. You might turn off the automatic spell check to force yourself to read the completed document carefully and look for spelling errors and use of wrong or incomplete words.

2. Slowly read the material aloud, if you can, to keep from skimming over material too quickly. Increasing the size of the font to " 14 point" may make it easier to spot errors; however, be sure to reduce the font to the proper size and check the format before printing and sending. You may also increase (zoom) the size of the document to "200%" for easy viewing.

3. Check for typographical and mechanical errors. Then, review the document for style, spelling, grammar, and meaning. If you find one error, look carefully nearby for others.

4. Check punctuation. Watch for doubled periods, missing parts of paired punctuation such as parentheses and quotation marks, missing commas, missing semicolons, and so forth.

5. Check capitalization for beginning of sentences and proper use for drug names, names of places, and medical specialty abbreviations. Watch to make sure that the "auto-format feature" does not capitalize all words at the beginning of new lines.

6. Read titles and first lines carefully. Check that titles in headers match those in the text.

7. Check consistency of headings and subheadings (same font, size, alignment, capitalization).

8. Check numbered and alphabetically ordered lists for correct sequence. Look for repeated, missing, or out-of-order numbers or letters.

9. Use the spell-check feature only for obvious errors since it cannot select words out of context (e.g., *injection* for *infection*, *palpation* for *palpitation*) or correctly spelled homonyms (e.g., *their* for *there*, *callus* for *callous*).

10. Load a medical dictionary or update the dictionary in the software program to include terms or acronyms unique to the medical practice's specialty.

11. Review a revised (cut and paste) document carefully before and after revisions. Words can be omitted or rekeyed, a new paragraph inserted without deleting the old, or a paragraph moved without deleting it at its original position. This can be verified with the search and find feature.

12. Reread the on-screen copy that comes immediately before and after revisions.

13. Read it a second time, word for word, letter by letter, watching for errors in spelling, punctuation, and grammar and for accuracy of facts.

14. Print a hard copy of the document using one of the following recommendations:

    a. Use a plastic ruler to remain on the correct line and proofread the hard copy.

    b. Read each line backward, a word at a time for long, complicated documents. This method will help you catch spelling and other errors that sometimes get overlooked during the conventional reading.

    c. Divide the document into convenient viewing sections for proofreading, that is, paragraph by paragraph or 10 to 12 lines at a time.

    d. Look at the copy upside down to check spacing, placement, appearance, and format.

15. Always strive for a perfect first printing of the final copy and do not send a document with errors.

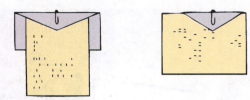

FIGURE 11-7 Two examples of paper-clipping a letter for signature to the underside flap of an envelope

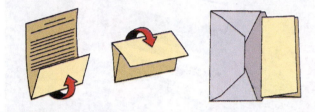

FIGURE 11-8 Folding a letter for insertion into a large (No. 10) envelope

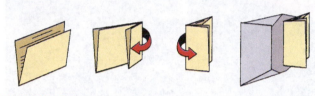

FIGURE 11-9 Folding a letter for insertion into a small (No. 6¾) envelope

For a small (No. 6¾) envelope, the letter is placed flat on the desk in reading position. First, fold from the bottom up to within one-half inch of the top and crease. Next, fold from the right a third of the way over to the left and crease; then fold from the left over to about one-half inch of the previous crease on the right. The last creased edge is inserted into the envelope first (Figure 11-9).

MEDICAL TRANSCRIPTION

A physician's transcription needs vary according to medical specialty, size of practice, amount of consultation work, involvement in medical and community affairs, and whether the office has an electronic health record or paper-based system. Documentation can be recorded using a dictation-transcription machine, mobile device, computerized template, or speech recognition system.

The medical assistant usually records the patient's chief complaint, vital signs, and medications in the patient's chart or inputs this information directly

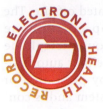

into the EMR. The review of systems' information may include a check-off sheet filed directly in the paper-based system or scanned into the EMR. The history may be taken in a similar way or the physician may interview the patient to obtain this information.

The physician may use a mobile electronic device, a template set up for specific types of examinations, or a speech recognition system to record the physical examination and any other portions of the record. If a digital recording system is used, a medical transcriptionist will listen to the recording and type the data for hard copy or directly into the EMR.

The medical **transcriptionist** (MT) or *medical language specialist (MLS)* may be a certified medical assistant (CMA [AAMA]), registered medical assistant (RMA), certified medical transcriptionist (CMT), or other health care professional. MTs may work in the physician's office, in a health care facility, or at home.

A service can also be contracted to do the transcription off-site; this is referred to as *outsourcing.* Outsourcing companies may be located in another city, state, or country. Regardless of the location, the Internet can be used to send and receive documents, expediting the turnaround time. Cost containment is the main reason medical practices outsource this type of work. Some cost-saving measures are lower wages, freeing work areas in the office for other uses, reducing employee benefits and not having to accommodate vacation schedules, and having workers focused on transcription around the clock—7 days a week.

Regardless of where the work is done, a transcriptionist should have an educational background in medical terminology and basic skills of business English, vocabulary, grammar, spelling, punctuation, and capitalization. These skills become paramount when an EMR system is used, because the transcriptionist is acting as an editor. A superior transcriptionist can transcribe 10,000 characters an hour, but this degree of proficiency comes only after much practice, and each organization has its own standards. Accuracy is more important than speed. With practice, the transcriptionist can learn to listen to a new group of words while still keying a previous group. Typically, a new transcriptionist is allowed a 3- to 6-month period to increase production to the expected level.

Large medical groups and hospitals may find it economically advantageous to combine high-volume transcription and typing tasks in a data input or word processing center, which may be located off-site. The physician dictates into a desktop microphone attached to a portable unit, or through telephone lines to the center. The dictation is either automatically recorded to be transcribed by personnel or received into a voice recognition system and is converted to text, which appears on-screen. Editing and corrections in a voice recognition system are keyed directly. Material can be printed as hard copy, and the information is saved in memory.

Transcription Procedures and Equipment

If the administrative medical assistant's position requires transcription, it is important to understand the equipment and methods of operating the system skillfully (Figure 11-10). Before using any transcription equipment, the assistant can read the basic operating instructions in the manual, discuss procedures with a coworker who has used the machine, or call the sales representative for a demonstration. Transcription systems range from the small portable dictation unit hand-carried by the busy physician, to combination dictation and transcription desktop models that use standard micro- or minicassettes. The physician dictates into the machine, which records the message on the *media*. The assistant then activates the media by using a foot pedal or by hand and listens to the dictated information through a headset or earpiece, while simultaneously keying data on medical report forms or letterhead paper, or directly into the EMR. Most machine dictation is transcribed using word processing software. All machines are equipped with a backspacing mechanism and can fast-forward to the next report. It is possible to select forward or reverse to listen to the prerecorded material. Tone, volume, and speed can be adjusted to each person's keying capabilities.

Sometimes the medical assistant is asked to transcribe from handwritten copy or edit a document. If handwritten copy is difficult to read, all the typist can do is try to figure out what the writer has in mind. Sometimes a word can be deciphered if the typist understands the context of the sentence. It may also help to look elsewhere for comparable letters; chances are that difficult areas can be figured out. However, if there are still problems, do not guess. Ask the writer (dictator) to clarify confusing words, and never change any wording without informing him or her.

When the assistant cannot make sense of a word or a phrase, he or she should leave a blank space and write

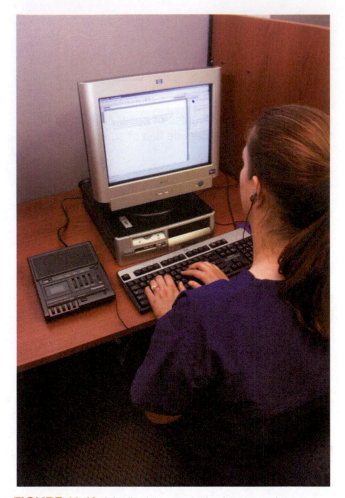

FIGURE 11-10 Medical transcriptionist operating a dictation-transcription machine, keying in data via computer

the physician a note indicating the page number and the line of the missing or indistinct information. This is known as "flagging" and can also be easily indicated by using repositionable adhesive tape flags or tabs.

Every physician has a unique dictation style, with which the transcriptionist becomes familiar. Most physicians prefer to dictate patient information into the machine at the end of the day or at quiet periods during office hours when the medical assistant may be working on other projects. At the convenience of the assistant, material may be transcribed later. Refer to Procedure 11-3 for instructions on transcribing a dictated document.

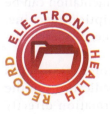

Templates

As stated previously, a *template* in an EMR is a predesigned format, used as a starting point to input documentation so it does not have to be recreated every time. The software company can customize it for the physician or medical specialty. Typically, it has a sequence of basic headings for content to help with creation of a document. The writer uses the template as a guide for the report elements that are needed. A template is often used for electronically captured information. In a computer system, it is a keystroke saver and speeds generating a document.

Speech Recognition

Some physicians use speech or *voice recognition* software to generate documents. While the dictator speaks into a microphone, the dialogue appears on the

✓ COMPLIANCE
Transcription Confidentiality

Quality assurance, security, and confidentiality measures need to be taken into consideration because the HIPAA does not prevail outside the United States. The HIPAA privacy rule does not prohibit the use of tapes for dictation, nor outsourcing of transcription. However, it requires that specific language addressing confidentiality be inserted in contracts with business associates (outside vendors).

PROCEDURE 11-3

Transcribe a Dictated Document

OBJECTIVE: Transcribe a dictated letter or report without errors into hard copy using a computer.

EQUIPMENT/SUPPLIES: Letterhead stationery, transcription equipment (headset, earphones, foot control, media containing dictation), English and medical dictionaries, drug book, computer, and printer.

DIRECTIONS: Follow these step-by-step directions, which include rationales, to learn this procedure.

1. Gather all necessary information and materials at the desk, including reference books.
2. Make sure the headset, earphones (or amplifier), and foot control are attached to the unit and comfortably positioned.
3. Verify that the unit is plugged in, turned on, and operating properly.
4. Insert the medium. Priority (STAT) reports are transcribed immediately. Then the oldest dictation is transcribed and the most recent dictation is keyed last.
5. Scan electronically to estimate the length of the report or letter, and listen for special instructions or comments before beginning to transcribe.
6. Adjust the volume, tone, and speed controls.
7. Set the margins and tabulator stops.
8. Select the paper and note how many copies are required.
9. Finally, begin transcribing after activating the recording; listen and remember a phrase, stop the voice, key the material, and repeat the process. Try to avoid rewinding and listening to

the same material twice. Listen for pauses to indicate punctuation or the end of a sentence.

10. Look up the meaning of English and medical homonyms to end confusion and help you decide how to spell them, such as *mucus* (noun) or *mucous* (adjective), *ileum* or *ilium*. Homonyms sound the same but have different meanings.
11. Proofread the document on-screen for content; typographical, spelling, grammar, style, and mechanical errors; and overall appearance.
12. Save the file to the hard drive before printing a hard copy, and proofread the document again. Make corrections, if necessary.
13. Transmit one finished copy to the recipient and one copy to the patient's EMR or other electronic file. If using a paper-based system, print two copies, one to be sent and one to be retained in the files. If questions arise, a copy of the document can be referred to.
14. Save the file to the hard drive and to a CD-ROM, DVD, or jump/flash drive to be stored for future reference.
15. Prepare an envelope using the format for optical scanning (presented in Chapter 12). If sending the correspondence by registered or certified mail, be sure to insert these special instructions on the envelope.
16. Clip any attachments to the document, and give to the physician for review and signature.
17. Turn off the transcription equipment.

computer monitor. The dictator is able to verbally order the record to be electronically signed when it is completed. The document is instantly available as hard copy or can become part of the patient's EMR. However, all speech engines must be initially trained and the dictator must practice speaking into the machine so that his or her voice, style, syntax (way in which words are put together), and vocabulary allow the software to work at its optimum. Dictation must be distinct, clear, and unhurried. It may be time consuming because physicians are used to dictating rapidly.

If punctuation, paragraphing, and capitalization are not vocalized, the *speech recognition technician (SRT)* must carefully edit the document at a later time. On-screen editing may also include inserting figures as numbers instead of as words.

PHOTOCOPYING PROCEDURES

The term **photocopy** means any process using light or photography to reproduce multiple copies of original (graphic) material, also known as reprographics. Medical offices are experiencing the need to make more copies of patient records, medical reports, correspondence, insurance claim forms, bills, memos, and other documents. A computer can send electronic medical records or print multiple copies, and the fax machine may also have reproduction capabilities; however, the most popular machine to reproduce documents is the photocopier.

When high-quality copies are needed quickly in limited quantities, the **photocopy machine** is one of the most important pieces of equipment in the medical office. Documents can be reproduced on ordinary paper stock, specially coated paper, copying paper, letterhead, preprinted forms, and colored stock. The copies resemble the original, the equipment is easy to operate, and paper and toner are the only supplies necessary. Some models can reduce or enlarge copy size, collate, and staple multiple documents. Although the cost of making one copy is small, employees should be discouraged from duplicating items unnecessarily.

Both sides of an insurance card can be copied using the same piece of paper and running it through a second time. Caution should be taken because certain copyrighted material cannot be legally copied without permission.

Multifunction Devices

A multifunction device (MFD) is linked to a computer system and provides a printer, scanner, copier, and often a fax in a single unit. It comes in small sizes, just larger than a printer, which saves desktop space, and in large sizes that offer all the functions of a deluxe photocopy machine.

Photocopy Machine

In most offices, the copier is a busy machine (Figure 11-11). Always place the machine away from file cabinets or walls to prevent overheating. Keep the area surrounding the machine neat and clean, and recycle used photocopy paper. Schedule lengthy copy projects for times when the machine is least busy. Study the operating manual for specific instructions and place it in a prominent place for reference.

To make a photocopy, the original material is either fed into the machine or placed facedown on the platen glass. After machine adjustments are

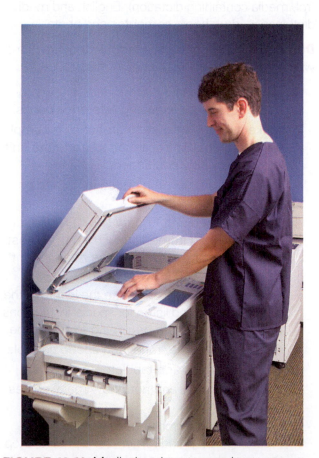

FIGURE 11-11 Medical assistant preparing to copy a medical document on a photocopy machine

PROCEDURE 11-4

Prepare Documents for Photocopying

OBJECTIVE: Prepare documents with multiple pages for photocopying.

EQUIPMENT/SUPPLIES: Photocopy machine, paper, equipment instruction book, document(s) to be photocopied, stapler with staples, and staple remover.

DIRECTIONS: Follow these step-by-step directions, which include rationales, to practice this procedure.

1. Warm up the photocopy machine if it has been turned off.
2. Assemble all pages of the document.
3. Check the original to see it is free of smudges and stains before making a copy.
4. Remove paper clips and staples, and assemble documents to be copied before taking them to the copier. Staples or paper clips may damage the photocopy equipment.
5. Copy only the portion of the medical record that is requested and that the patient has authorized. If the document is from a patient's medical record, verify that there is a signed authorization to release the information.
6. Use correction tape when lines, smudges, or phrases of a master copy need to be corrected. To avoid photocopy "lines" appearing where the tape is attached to the master, paint edges of tape with correction fluid or place adhesive tape over the correction tape.
7. Place the original(s) in the machine according to the instructions for the photocopy equipment. If single-sheet copying, place each page facedown on the glass. If the machine accepts the entire document, load the pages (facedown or faceup) into the feeder according to directions.
8. Select the correct format for size (e.g., letter or legal size paper, size of copy) and set the machine for the number of copies desired. Make at least one file copy of all documents.
9. Press the settings, so copies will be collated, stapled, or both, if the equipment has these features.
10. Regulate for light or dark copy if the machine does not automatically adjust for this. Careful preparation will save time and money by preventing running the job again.
11. Always make copies with the copier lid closed, because the drum picks up toner to cover the entire glass opening. An open lid wastes toner and may lead to more service calls, and intense light can be a health hazard.
12. Press the "start" or "print" button.
13. Arrange the document pages in the correct sequence, and staple if the equipment does not have the stapling feature.
14. Verify the number of document pages. If the patient or an attorney has requested copies, then submit the number of pages to the person responsible for billing.
15. Avoid lengthy exposure to sunlight or room light, which may damage the developing roller, if toner cartridges are used.
16. Notify the office manager if copy paper and supplies are at the reorder point.
17. Be sure to take all originals and photocopies from the trays before the next person copies a document.
18. Refill paper trays, unless another person has signed this duty.
19. Make sure the copier is turned off at the end of the day.

made according to size, darkness, and quantity, copies may be produced in seconds from paper stored in cassettes. The "print" button is pressed to activate the copy machine. Refer to Procedure 11-4 for instructions when preparing documents for photocopying.

Common Photocopy Machine Problems

To keep the photocopy machine running smoothly and free of paper jams, it should be cleaned and maintained regularly (Figures 11-12 and 11-13). Table 11-4 offers suggestions for troubleshooting some of the most common photocopy machine problems.

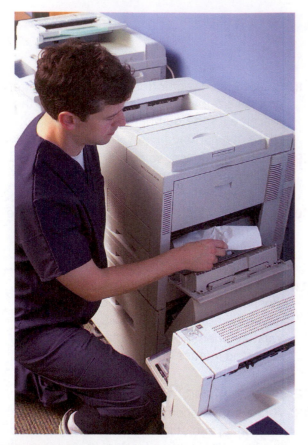

FIGURE 11-12 Medical assistant opening a copy machine to remove a paper jam

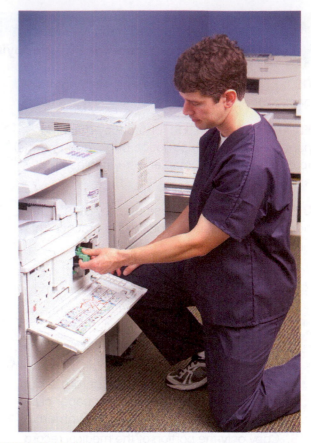

FIGURE 11-13 Medical assistant opening a copy machine to remove or install an ink cartridge

TABLE 11-4 Copier Problems with Possible Causes and Solutions

Difficulty	Possible Cause	Solution
Feeding problems	Letterhead or heavy-stock paper may cause static buildup	Substitute lighter-weight paper (20 lb is standard)
Misfeeding	Uneven edges or curl; may be caused by mixing weights of paper in the same tray or cassette	Open another ream of paper or turn the existing paper over; fan to allow air to circulate between sheets
Jamming in the bins or sheets sticking together	Excessive curl of paper; moisture or low humidity may be the cause	Turn the paper over; check storage conditions; ask maintenance or supplier to check static eliminator
Wrinkling	High moisture due to damp storage, or paper has remained in copy machine too long	Check storage conditions; substitute another ream of copy paper
Smoking or making strange noise	Cause unknown	Turn machine off immediately; contact person in charge of maintenance
Light or unreadable copy	Ink cartridge low	Check ink cartridge and replace when low

STOP AND THINK CASE SCENARIO
Edit a Thank-You Letter for Final Copy

SCENARIO: Dr. Fran Practon gives you a rough draft of a letter that she wants you to put into final copy to send to the patient, Jason Chieu. It reads as follows:

Dear Mr. Chieu, I wanted to express my thank-you due to the fact that you referred your friend, Cherry Hotta, to our medical practice. I recognize that this referral indicates that I provided good medical care for you and your family. I'm grateful for both your confidence and consideration. My staff and I are committed to deliver the same quality care that you have come to expect from me. Again thanks for your kindness in referring your friend to me. Sincerely,

CRITICAL THINKING: What should you do? Respond to each choice and list the changes you would make if you selected response 1, 2, or 3.

1. Rewrite it to give it a conversational tone.

2. Rewrite it to make it more concise and clear.

3. Rewrite it to give it a formal tone.

4. Send it as written.

_____

_____

_____

_____

_____

_____

_____

_____

_____

_____

_____

_____

_____

STOP AND THINK CASE SCENARIO
Edit a Transcribed Medical Report

SCENARIO: Dr. Gerald Practon dictated a medical report on Charlotte Greenwich, who came in with a right inguinal hernia. You transcribed the report, but certain sections are unclear and you have had to leave several blanks.

CRITICAL THINKING: What should you do? Respond to each choice stating whether you would or would not proceed in that manner and give the reasons behind your decision.

1. Look at the patient's medical record and try to obtain the data to insert.

_____

_____

2. Look at a medical record of another patient who had the same complaints and try to fill in the data by reading through that chart.

_____

_____

3. Mark the hard copy of the medical report with notes to the physician asking for clarification.

_____

_____

4. Other (please state).

_____

_____

STOP AND THINK CASE SCENARIO

Select the Correct Homonyms in a Medical Report

SCENARIO: Dr. Fran Practon dictated a medical report, and some sentences contained homonyms. You want to put it into final copy. A section reads as follows:

Mrs. Frye has completed one (coarse, course) of radiation therapy after her mastectomy. There was (mucous, mucus) draining from the site of treatment. She complained that the prescribed medication for her nausea had the (effect, affect) of making her drowsy. She cannot (bare, bear) to be lethargic.

CRITICAL THINKING: Look at each set of homonyms and decide how you would determine the correct word, then circle it. Respond to each of the following choices expressing why you would or would not proceed in the manner stated.

1. Look in the patient's medical record for any notes to decide which word is more appropriate.

_____

2. Look up each of the words in the medical dictionary and decide from the meaning which one suits the context of the sentence.

_____

3. Flag the section of the report and ask Dr. Practon which words are the correct ones.

_____

FOCUS ON CERTIFICATION*

CMA (AAMA) Content Summary

- Medical terminology
- Spelling
- Data entry
- Reports
- Documents
- Correspondence
- Letters
- Memos
- Messages
- Fundamental writing skills
- Sentence structure
- Grammar
- Punctuation
- Keyboard fundamentals
- Formats (letters, memos, reports)
- Proofreading
- Making corrections from rough draft
- Computer storage devices
- Word processing applications
- Report generation

RMA (AMT) Content Summary

- Medical terminology (word definitions, spelling)
- Apply proper written communication to instruct patients
- Understand and correctly apply terminology associated with secretarial duties
- Compose correspondence employing acceptable business format
- Employ effective written communication skills adhering to ethics and laws of confidentiality
- Transcription and dictation

CMAS (AMT) Content Summary

- Medical terminology
- Employ effective written communication
- Format business documents and correspondence appropriately
- Possess fundamental knowledge of word processing

---

*This textbook and the accompanying Workbook meet the entry-level administrative and general competencies for the CMA outlined by the AAMA Examination Content Outline and Occupational Analysis and for the RMA and CMAS outlined by the AMT Competencies, Construction Parameters, and Examination Specifications (see Competency Grid in Appendix B).

1. Computer software is programmed to permanently store data on the hard drive, which can be duplicated and transferred to other data-storing media such as:
   a. DVDs
   b. jump drives
   c. CDs
   d. flash drives
   e. all of the above are correct

2. Select the correctly spelled word.
   a. Indespensable
   b. Indispinsable
   c. Indispinseble
   d. Indispensable
   e. Indespinsable

3. What determines the letter style used in a physician's office?
   a. Equipment used
   b. Physician's preference
   c. Type of letter being sent
   d. Office manager's preference
   e. Personal choice of staff member

4. When a colon or comma is used after the complimentary close, it is referred to as:
   a. full punctuation
   b. open punctuation
   c. mixed punctuation
   d. internal punctuation
   e. closed punctuation

5. To *justify* means to:
   a. start all lines flush with the left margin
   b. space words so that the ends of lines are flush at the right and left margins
   c. align text flush with the right margin
   d. center text
   e. indent when starting a new paragraph

6. The date line is typically placed:
   a. one double space below the letterhead
   b. one space below the letterhead
   c. two spaces below the letterhead
   d. three spaces below the letterhead
   e. four spaces below the letterhead

7. Select the correct statement regarding the *salutation*.
   a. There is no punctuation after the salutation in *open punctuation*.
   b. There is a colon following the salutation in *open punctuation*.
   c. "Ms." is never used in the salutation.
   d. When a woman's title is not known, the salutation should read: "To whom this may concern."
   e. When it is not known whether the addressee is a man or woman, the salutation should read: "To whom this may concern."

8. Select the correct statement regarding the *body* of a letter.
   a. All paragraphs are single-spaced within the body of a letter.
   b. All paragraphs are double-spaced within the body of a letter.
   c. Paragraphs are typically single-spaced within the body of a letter with double spacing used for extremely short letters.
   d. The body of a letter begins four lines below the salutation
   e. The body of a letter begins four lines below the reference or subject line.

9. In the *complimentary close*:
   a. only the first letter of the first word is capitalized
   b. one to three complimentary words are used and each is capitalized
   c. one to three complimentary words are typed four line spaces below the body of the letter
   d. the closing line is followed by a comma in *open punctuation*
   e. no punctuation follows the closing in *mixed punctuation*

10. When the writer of a letter sends a copy to a third party without the knowledge of the person receiving the original letter, it is referred to as a:
    a. hidden copy
    b. back copy
    c. concealed copy
    d. blind copy
    e. secret copy

11. A thesaurus lists:
    a. synonyms
    b. antonyms
    c. definitions
    d. synonyms and antonyms
    e. all of the above

12. Basic standards for every medical communication include:
    a. simplicity, clarity, and conciseness
    b. detailed descriptions
    c. medical terminology
    d. elaborate language
    e. all of the above are correct

13. Ideas that are informally exchanged among individuals and departments within an organization or business are written on:
    a. form letters
    b. formal letters
    c. multipage letters
    d. repetitive letters
    e. interoffice memorandums

14. When moving sections of text in a letter using word processing software, the following text-editing feature should be used:
    a. format feature
    b. directional keys
    c. cut-and-paste feature
    d. spell check
    e. search feature

15. The job of a medical transcriptionist:
    a. is no longer needed with modern technology
    b. varies according to the use of EMRs, paper-based systems, and type of data entry
    c. is only found in large medical practices and hospitals
    d. is not needed with the use of templates
    e. is not needed with speech recognition software

WORKBOOK ASSIGNMENT

To develop competency-based job skills, refer to the *Workbook* and complete the:
- Abbreviation and Spelling Review
- Review Questions

- Critical Thinking Exercises
- Job Skill activities, which are listed at the beginning of the chapter under *Performance Objectives in the Workbook.*

RESOURCES

Books

The AMA Handbook of Business Letters, **4th edition**
    Seglin/Coleman
    AMACOM, 2012
At a Glance: Writing Sentences and Beyond, **6th edition**
    Brandon/Brandon
    Cengage Learning, 2015
    Website: http://www.cengagebrain.com
Basic Keyboarding for the Medical Office Assistant, **3rd edition**
    Moss, Edna Jean
    Cengage Learning, 2004
    Website: http://www.cengagebrain.com

Basic Grammar and Usage, **8th edition**
    Choy/Goldbart Clark
    Cengage Learning, 2011
    Website: http://www.cengagebrain.com
Building Better Grammar, **1st edition**
    Hogan, Gina
    Cengage Learning, 2013
    Website: http://www.cengagebrain.com
Get Writing: Sentence and Paragraphs, **3rd edition**
    Connelly, Mark
    Cengage Learning, 2014
    Website: http://www.cengagebrain.com

Grammar and Usage, Naturally, 1st edition
> Barkley/Sandoval
> Cengage Learning, 2015
> Website: http://www.cengagebrain.com

Grammar and Writing Skills for the Health Professional, 3rd edition
> Oberg, Doreen Villemaire & Villemaire, Lorraine
> Cengage Learning, 2018
> Website: http://www.cengagebrain.com

Write Right: A Desktop Digest of Punctuation, Grammar, and Style
> Venolia, Jan
> Ten Speed Press, 2001

Internet

Association for Healthcare Documentation Integrity (AHDI)
> Search: Professional Practices for Writing Tools and Guidelines

Big Dog Grammar
> Study parts of speech

The Blue Book of Grammar and Punctuation
> Grammar and Punctuation Rules

Common Errors in English Usage
> Go to: List of Errors

MedicineNet, Inc.
> Med Terms Dictionaries

Merriam-Webster Dictionary
> Dictionary, Thesaurus, Medical Dictionary, Spanish Dictionary, Encyclopedia Britannica, Word Games

MT Desk
> Grammar, Style, Usage

CHAPTER 12

PROCESSING MAIL AND ELECTRONIC CORRESPONDENCE

LEARNING OBJECTIVES

After reading this chapter and learning step-by-step procedures to gain job skills,* you should be able to:

- Select appropriate mail equipment and stationery supplies.
- Describe various options for purchasing postage and postal supplies.
- Explain how incoming mail is handled and sorted.
- State the characteristics of suspicious mail.
- Define methods for annotating incoming mail.
- Coordinate distribution of mail when the physician is gone.
- Determine the most economical classification for various mailings.
- Choose the safest service for mailing valuable items and important papers.
- Demonstrate the envelope address format that follows preferred U.S. Postal Service regulations.
- Discuss electronic mail etiquette, format, usage, and security.
- Summarize the advantages of an electronic communication system for a medical practice.
- Cite etiquette, guidelines, and operating procedures for fax transmissions.

PERFORMANCE OBJECTIVES (PROCEDURES) IN THIS TEXTBOOK

- Operate a postage meter machine (Procedure 12-1).
- Follow safety guidelines when handling large volumes of mail and suspicious mail pieces (Procedure 12-2).
- Open, sort, and annotate mail (Procedure 12-3).
- Prepare outgoing mail (Procedure 12-4).
- Complete Certified Mail and Return Receipt U.S. Postal Service forms (Procedure 12-5).
- Address a business envelope using U.S. Postal Service regulations (Procedure 12-6).
- Manage office mail (Procedure 12-7).
- Compose an email message (Procedure 12-8).
- Prepare a fax cover sheet and send a fax (Procedure 12-9).

This textbook and the accompanying Workbook meet the educational components for entry-level administrative and general competencies outlined by CAAHEP and ABHES.

PERFORMANCE OBJECTIVES (JOB SKILLS) IN THE WORKBOOK

- Process incoming mail (Job Skill 12-1).
- Annotate mail (Job Skill 12-2).
- Classify outgoing mail (Job Skill 12-3).
- Address small envelopes for OCR scanning (Job Skill 12-4).
- Complete a mail-order form for postal supplies (Job Skill 12-5).
- Compose a letter and prepare an envelope for Certified Mail (Job Skill 12-6).
- Key and fold an original letter; address a small envelope for Certified Mail, Return Receipt requested (Job Skill 12-7).
- Key and fold an original letter; address a large envelope for Certified Mail, Return Receipt requested (Job Skill 12-8).
- Prepare a cover sheet for fax transmission (Job Skill 12-9).

KEY TERMS

annotate	enclosure (enc)	Registered Mail
bar code sorter (BCS)	facsimile (fax) communication	service endorsements
Certified Mail	Federal Express (FedEx)	United Parcel Service (UPS)
DHL Worldwide Express	mail classifications	United States Postal Service (USPS)
domestic mail	optical character recognition (OCR)	zone improvement plan (ZIP + 4)
electronic mail (email)		

HEART OF THE HEALTH CARE PROFESSIONAL

Service

Processing mail is a "behind the scenes" job and not thought of as very important. However, when not done efficiently and in a timely manner, the entire office can grind to a stop and a variety of responsibilities that address patients' needs may not be met.

UNITED STATES POSTAL SERVICE

The volume of incoming and outgoing mail in the physician's practice is a major factor in determining mail procedures—each office may process mail differently. The medical assistant's goal is to take appropriate steps to sort and distribute incoming mail and to choose the service that speeds the delivery of outgoing mail at minimum cost. With the advent of the Internet, sending first-class letters and other documents using standard mail delivery (*snail mail*) has diminished. Sending documents by fax and electronic mail (email) has increased because of the ease and speed of sending and receiving a communication as well as the reduced cost.

The **United States Postal Service (USPS)** has one of the largest mail handling systems in the world and is used by the majority of citizens in the United States to deliver both domestic and international mail. To obtain quick and up-to-date information on regulations and take advantage of many online services, access the USPS website (see the *Resources* section at the end of this chapter). There you can obtain **domestic mail** (United States and its territories) and international mail postage rates, locate ZIP codes, register a change of address, find abbreviations for city names that exceed 13 characters, calculate postage according to the weight and size of the item, purchase stamps, print postage onto envelopes or labels (see "Click and Ship"), obtain forms and shipping supplies, create cards, locate a post office, track and confirm delivery, and obtain information about various shipping services. The USPS toll-free 800 number is also very helpful.

ZIP Codes

A nine-digit **zone improvement plan (ZIP + 4)** code on the envelope expedites sorting and delivery because mail can be processed by computerized equipment. Use of the ZIP code system decreases the potential for human error, reduces the possibility of misdelivery, and leads to better control of postal costs. The four-digit add-on number identifies a specific delivery segment such as a city block, floor of a building, department within a company, or group of post office boxes. A hyphen appears after the five-digit ZIP code and before the four-digit add-on code. If the ZIP + 4 code is known, it should be used.

Automated mail equipment reads the nine-digit code on first-class letters and cards using **optical character recognition (OCR)**. Then the **bar code sorter (BCS)** imprints a bar code on the lower right corner of the envelope. Local ZIP codes can usually be found in telephone directories in addition to on the USPS website.

SUPPLIES AND EQUIPMENT

In a small-volume mail operation, some or all of the following supplies will be useful: letter opener, postal scale, postage machine, postage meter, stapler, rubber stamps, labels, adhesive tape, stickers, and postage stamps. Check at your local post office to see what shipping supplies are free, for example, Priority Mail and Express Mail boxes, envelopes, and labels.

Postal Scale

The postal scale, used to determine the weight of mail, is available in spring, beam, pendulum, and electronic models. If the office has a pediatric scale, it can be used as a postal scale.

Postage Meter

Postage meters are used to print prepaid postage directly on envelopes or onto a meter tape that is affixed to large envelopes or packages. The imprint, or meter stamp, serves as postage payment, postmark, and cancelation mark. Because metered mail does not have to be canceled at the post office, mail handling is expedited. Envelopes that contain bulky items can be weighed, then run through the meter prior to inserting the contents, or a postage meter tape (label) can be affixed to the envelope. Write "Hand Stamp" in large letters on bulky envelopes under or to the left of the stamp.

Postage meters cannot be purchased, but they can be rented and fees are based on the amount of usage. The medical assistant should keep a daily record of postage costs to make sure the office is not being overcharged for minimum usage.

There are stand-alone meters and ones that operate within a *postage machine* (Figure 12-1). A postage machine may be purchased or leased. An automated machine can stuff, feed, and seal envelopes as they pass through the meter. Models vary in design, from lightweight, stand-alone, hand-operated machines to sophisticated machines with a computer-controlled meter that can weigh mail items while processing. When leasing a mail machine, most manufacturers will bundle the meter rental into the lease payment.

All postage meters are refilled electronically; some use an analog telephone line but most use a computer network. Postage meter manufacturers offer several ways to pay for the postage including the use of credit or debit cards, pay in advance, or post-in advance and pay when mailings are sent.

After the model has been selected from a list of manufacturers authorized by the USPS, an application for a postage meter license is submitted to the post office where the metered mail is to be deposited. The manufacturer typically does this; there are no fees. For bulk mailing and automated mailing, you must fill out a USPS form and pay an annual fee. All metered mail must be deposited at the post office where the permit was issued. Bulk mail drop-offs are recommended early in the day, early in the week, and early in the month. It is illegal to possess a postage meter without paying for meter rental. Refer to Procedure 12-1 for instructions on operating a postage meter machine.

Stamp Services

There are several ways to order postage without having to make a special trip to the post office. Ordering by mail, over the telephone, and via the Internet are three common ways.

Stamps by Mail

Stamps by Mail can be purchased by filling out Form 3227-A provided by the U.S. Postal Service and mailing it to the local post office. After indicating on the form the items needed and the cost, a check or money order for the total amount is inserted in a self-addressed attached envelope. Within 5 business days, the stamps are mailed to the medical office at no extra charge. Any

PROCEDURE 12-1

Operate a Postage Meter Machine

OBJECTIVE: Set up a postage meter and apply postage to an envelope or package for mailing, according to U.S. Postal Service guidelines.

EQUIPMENT/SUPPLIES: Postage meter, addressed envelope or package, and manual or electronic postal scale.

DIRECTIONS: Although postage meters differ in size and function, the following step-by-step directions, which include rationales, are basic to learning this procedure.

1. Rent or lease a postage meter from one of the USPS-approved manufacturers.

2. Contact the meter company and set up an account to pay for postage, so the meter can be activated.

3. Find the location where the meter registers the date. The date will change automatically but the correct date must be verified. USPS guidelines state that the day an envelope or package is mailed must be the date that appears on the postage label, or postage may be forfeited.

4. Verify that contents and enclosures are included in the envelope or package.

5. Weigh the item on a scale (unless the postage machine does this automatically) to determine if it is over 1 ounce.

6. Seal the envelope or package (unless the machine seals it).

7. Key in the amount of postage on the meter (unless done automatically) and press the *Enter* button. Proofread the amount as necessary. If postage is deficient, the article will be returned by the USPS.

8. Process the mail and packages:

   a. *ENVELOPES*—Apply postage to the envelope by holding it flat with the right side up, so the address can be read. Locate where to slide the envelope through near the bottom of the machine. Place the envelope to the left side and push toward the right. Make certain the postage is printed in the upper right corner of the envelope.

   b. *PACKAGES*—Weigh the package to determine postage. Create a postage label and affix to the package in the upper right corner.

9. Check the postmarked label to see if it is legible and to verify the printed date and the amount.

10. Reset the meter to zero when all mail has been metered.

11. Save all unused and spoiled postage-metered tapes and envelopes and apply for a refund within the year. Request a refund (up to 90% of postage value) if an error is made by the meter (poor ink or incorrect postage amount), and do not imprint further postage until the problem has been corrected.

12. Reorder postage prior to it running out, depending on how the account was set up.

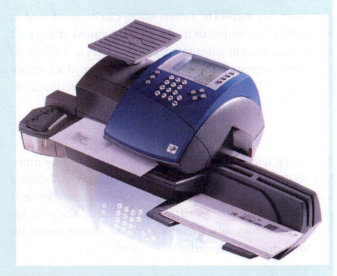

FIGURE 12-1 Optimail™ 30 Digital Postage System (Courtesy of FP Mailing Solutions, Addison, IL; website: http://www.fp-usa.com)

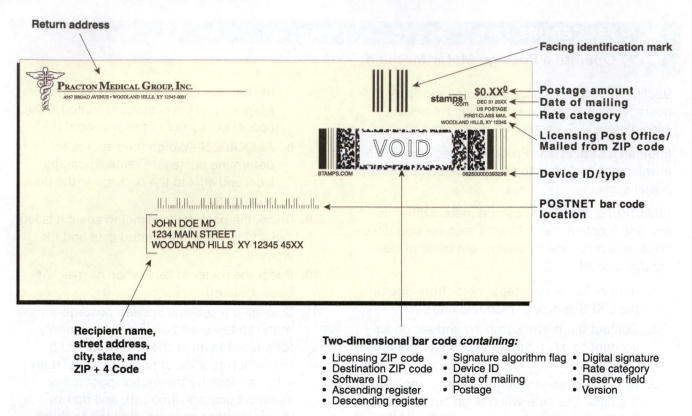

FIGURE 12-2 Example of an information-based indicia (IBI) bar-coded envelope shown addressed, printed, and electronically stamped using online postage

order totaling $200 or more is returned by Certified Mail and a signature is required upon delivery.

Forever Stamp—The *Forever stamp* can be purchased in a booklet (20 stamps) or in a roll (100 stamps) at any post office, online, or at automated postal centers and ATMs. As the name suggests, it can be used forever to mail a 1-ounce letter, regardless of when the stamp was purchased; its value will always remain that of a first-class stamp.

Stamps by Telephone

Stamps by Telephone involves a call to the toll-free number (800-STAMP-24) anytime 24 hours a day, 7 days a week. Stamps are delivered within 5 business days and may be charged to an office credit card. There is no minimum order, but there is a service charge based on the total price of the order.

Online Postage

Exact postage can be purchased and printed from a personal computer (PC) by using the U.S. Postal Service Online Store, or from an online software company that is approved by the U.S. Postal Service. Using these services, customers are able to purchase postage and print a two-dimensional bar code that is digitally encoded

and contains various information about the mail piece, such as mail processing and security-related data elements (Figure 12-2). It also allows the mail to be tracked. Two types of services offer PC postage: Offline postage hardware and online postage software (see *Resources* section at the end of this chapter).

HANDLING INCOMING MAIL

Incoming mail should be opened and processed expediently while keeping confidentiality and security in mind.

Mail Security

It is vital to know how to handle suspicious incoming mail safely, especially since the increase of terrorist activity in the United States. Suspicious characteristics are any mail that is:

- Unexpected or from someone you do not know
- Addressed to someone no longer at your address
- Postmarked with a city that does not match the return address
- Handwritten or poorly typed with no return address or bearing one that you cannot confirm is legitimate

- Showing misspelled common words
- Incorrectly titled
- Oddly sealed or excessively taped-over areas on the mailed piece
- Stamped with excessive postage
- Excessive in weight
- Marked with restrictive endorsements ("Personal" or "Confidential")
- Exhibiting signs of leakage of liquid (residue of a white, brown, or sandy-brown powdery substance on the exterior, oily stains, or discolorations)
- Lopsided or lumpy, containing an unknown item
- Having protruding wires or aluminum foil
- Visually distracting or contains ticking sounds

The USPS caution and commonsense guidelines for those handling a large volume of mail and suspicious mail pieces are outlined in Procedure 12-2.

Opening Mail

Each medical practice needs to have established procedures for opening the physician's incoming mail and the medical assistant should set aside a regular time each day to open the mail as soon as possible after delivery (Figure 12-3). Typically, the assistant handles the mail that deals with statements, payments, insurance, invoices, laboratory test reports, samples, and magazines for the reception room.

PROCEDURE 12-2

Follow Safety Guidelines When Handling Large Volumes of Mail and Suspicious Mail Pieces

OBJECTIVE: Follow safety guidelines when handling and opening large volumes of mail and when coming across mail pieces that are suspicious.

EQUIPMENT/SUPPLIES: Large volumes of incoming mail and suspicious signs of mail tampering.

DIRECTIONS: Follow these step-by-step directions when opening large volumes of mail or handling suspicious pieces of mail.

1. Wash your hands thoroughly with soap and water before and after handling any suspicious piece of mail.
2. Put on disposable latex gloves if you have open cuts or skin lesions on your hands.
3. Do not eat or drink around mail.
4. Do not handle a letter or package that you suspect is contaminated.
5. Stay calm. Do not panic. Do not open, empty, shake, bump, or sniff the contents of any suspicious envelope or package.

IF A SUSPICIOUS PIECE OF MAIL IS OPENED, FOLLOW THESE GUIDELINES:

1. Isolate the specific area of the workplace so that no one disturbs the item, and put the suspicious mail item into a plastic bag or other container.

2. Leave the room and close the door.
3. Keep others away from the area.
4. Wash your hands with warm water and soap for at least 1 minute. Have anyone who has touched the envelope or package do the same.
5. Do not allow anyone who might have touched the envelope to leave. List all people in the room and give the list to the local public health authorities or law enforcement officials.
6. Do not clean up spilled powder. Cover with plastic, paper, or a trashcan and leave the room.
7. Remove contaminated clothing, place in a plastic bag, and give it to emergency responders. Shower with soap and water. Do not use bleach or disinfectant on your skin.
8. Turn off fans and ventilation units if there is a question of room contamination by aerosolization. Leave the area immediately, close the door, seal off the area, and shut down the air-handling system in the building.
9. Notify your supervisor and local law enforcement authorities immediately.

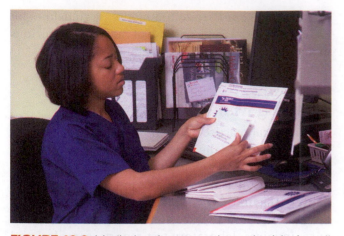

FIGURE 12-3 Medical assistant opening a physician's mail

Items needed when opening the mail include a hand or portable automatic letter opener, a stapler, paper clips, transparent tape, a date stamp, and an ink pad (stored upside down to allow the ink to soak into the top).

When correspondence requests patient data or requires background information, the physician will be able to view the electronic medical record (EMR) from multiple locations; however, if a paper-based system is used, the patient's chart should be pulled and placed with the letter on the physician's desk. If a letter refers to previous correspondence, gather the needed information and fasten it to the back of the letter, perhaps with "See attached" written in the margin. After the medical assistant has opened all the mail, it is then stacked and distributed according to distribution guidelines listed in Table 12-1.

Annotating Mail

The physician may request that you **annotate** all business correspondence. This means to read the correspondence and either underline or highlight important words and phrases or make explanatory notes in the margins, so action can be taken. Annotating should be done sparingly because it loses its value if it is overdone. When there is doubt about underlining a word or phrase, it is best not to do so. The assistant should approach each letter looking for the answers to who, what, why, when, and where. Colored pencils/pens will differentiate notes written by the assistant from those written by the physician, and different colors may be used to distinguish general information from items that require particular attention. In, out, and hold baskets on the physician's desk will keep both incoming and outgoing correspondence organized and prevent loss.

Handling Mail When the Physician Is Away

Before the physician leaves the office for an extended time, the assistant should discuss procedures for handling the mail in his or her absence. Some questions to pose might be:

TABLE 12-1 Typical Daily Mail in a Physician's Office and Its Distribution

Mail	Distributed to...
Faxes, certified or registered letters, express and priority mail, telegrams and mailgrams	Physician
Personal letters, email, and letters from other professionals	Physician/office manager
Checks from patients, insurance forms, invoices, letters about accounts	Medical assistant/bookkeeper/insurance specialist
Letters soliciting contributions	Medical assistant who annotates/office manager
Radiology and laboratory reports; other test results	Medical assistant who routes reports to the physician via EMR or chart
Announcements of meetings, medical society bulletins, professional materials	Physician/office manager
Journal reprints, medical journals, newspapers	Physician/office manager
Magazines for the office	Medical assistant/receptionist
Advertisements, catalogs, and equipment and supplies information	Office manager/medical assistant
Drug samples	Medical assistant who stores in cabinet

1. Should all *personal mail* be forwarded unopened, can it be opened at the office and a photocopy forwarded, or should it be held?
2. May the assistant decide which mail to forward after opening it?
3. Should any correspondence be answered?
4. Does the physician want all correspondence held until his or her return?
5. Should the assistant prioritize the mail into various piles with the most important on top (see Procedure 12-3)?

If the medical assistant is instructed to forward personal correspondence at different times to different addresses listed on the travel itinerary, numbering the envelopes consecutively will permit the physician to determine if all communications have been received. Items not forwarded could remain in a separate folder or they might be sorted into a four-pocket folder set up with sections headed:

- Correspondence Requiring Immediate Action
- Correspondence to Be Read
- Correspondence Awaiting the Physician's Signature
- Miscellaneous Items

Trays could be labeled:

- Urgent
- Not So Urgent
- Junk Mail
- Acknowledged Items (including business and personal mail)

If a communication arrives that requires an immediate response from the physician, the assistant should write a note to the correspondent or send an email to explain that the physician will reply promptly on his or her return.

When the entire office closes for vacation, arrangements must be made with the post office to hold the mail or forward it to a specific address.

PROCEDURE 12-3

②③

Open, Sort, and Annotate Mail

OBJECTIVE: Open, sort, annotate, and process incoming mail using a standard procedure.

EQUIPMENT/SUPPLIES: Letter opener, date and time stamp, ink pad, stapler, paper clips, transparent tape, and adhesive notes.

DIRECTIONS: Follow these step-by-step directions, which include rationales, to learn this procedure. Job Skills 12-1 and 12-2 are presented in the *Workbook* to practice this skill.

1. Tap the lower edges of a stack of envelopes on the desk to settle the contents, so no item will be accidentally cut as the envelope is opened. Any item cut by mistake should be immediately mended with tape.

2. Check the address on each letter or package to verify it has been delivered to the correct location.

3. Set aside all letters marked "Personal" or "Confidential," unless you have permission to open them. If opened by mistake, the letter should be resealed with transparent tape, labeled "Opened by mistake," and initialed, then placed with other personal mail on the physician's desk.

4. Arrange all envelopes with the flaps facing the same direction and slip the opener under the flap, and with one stroke, cut the edge open.

5. Open all envelopes.

6. Remove and flatten the contents of each envelope, and then hold the emptied envelope up to the light to make certain nothing remains inside.

7. Stamp bank checks and money orders with a restrictive endorsement, "For Deposit Only" and attach each envelope to every check and route to the bookkeeper or insurance clerk. When the check is scanned and the payment is posted, the patient's return address on the check or envelope can be compared with the patient account and verified.

8. Scan or attach all envelopes to the back of letters that do not have complete return addresses or lack a signature to identify a sender.

9. Verify all **enclosure (enc)** notations on each letter with the actual enclosures. If the enclosure is missing, write "No enclosure" opposite the notation at the bottom of the

(continues)

letter and contact the sender. Scan enclosures or clip single small enclosures to the front of the letter and large attachments to the back. Protect x-ray films and photographs by placing a small piece of paper over the material before attaching a paper clip.

10. Check the date of the letter with the postmark. If a delay is shown, scan or keep the envelope because this may be needed for reference in legal matters or cases of collection. If dates correspond, discard the envelope.

11. Date stamp and time stamp, if required, each piece of correspondence in the upper right corner. The date may have legal significance in fixing responsibility for any delay in delivery or response.

12. Sort and prioritize mail in the following order:
    - *FIRST ORDER*—Items sent by overnight delivery, Registered Mail, Certified Mail, special delivery, fax, or email.
    - *SECOND ORDER*—Personal or confidential mail.

- *THIRD ORDER*—First-class mail, airmail, express mail, and priority mail. Separate according to payments received, insurance forms, reports, and other correspondence.
- *FOURTH ORDER*—Packages (e.g., drug samples). Check contents to be sure that nothing is missing or broken.
- *FIFTH ORDER*—Magazines, medical journals, and newspapers. If journals have accumulated while the physician is gone, photocopy the table of contents for the physician to scan and review on his or her return.
- *SIXTH ORDER*—Advertisements, catalogs, equipment and supply information, and junk mail (unsolicited or inapplicable advertisements). Several sheets of advertising that arrive in one envelope should be stapled together, unless you have received instructions to discard.

13. Annotate letters by underlining or highlighting important words and phrases, and make notations on the front or back of the correspondence that requires action.

HANDLING OUTGOING MAIL

The medical assistant has numerous responsibilities when processing outgoing mail for the office. To choose the least expensive and most efficient system for mailing items, a knowledge of mail classifications and the steps to take before mailing documents is necessary.

Mail Classifications

Mail is classified by size, contents, weight, frequency of mailings, destination, and speed of delivery. *Shape-based pricing* was introduced in 2007 and you can now obtain a lower rate by changing the shape of a piece of mail. Types of mail classifications have changed over the years and obsolete but familiar titles have been included in parentheses to increase understanding. Procedure 12-4 offers instructions for preparing outgoing mail.

First Class

First-class mail includes letters, cards, flats, bills, statements of account, small parcels, and all matter sealed or otherwise closed to inspection. It is the fastest and most economic service because mail goes by air when air service is available without an added fee and it includes forwarding and return services. All sealed matter, up to and including 13 ounces in weight, fall into this category as well as post cards. *2nd Ounce Free* is now available for commercial mailers using first-class mail to enclose promotional and advertising materials.

Following are minimum and maximum requirements for standard types of first-class mail:

- *Postcard*:
  5 × 3½ inches—minimum length and height
  6 × 4¼ inches—maximum length and height
- *Letter*:
  5 × 3½ inches—minimum length and height
  11½ × 6⅛ inches—maximum length and height
  maximum weight: 3.5 oz
- *Large envelope*:
  15 × 12 × 3/4 inches—maximum dimensions
  maximum weight: 13 oz package (box, thick envelope, or tube)

PROCEDURE 12-4

Prepare Outgoing Mail

OBJECTIVE: Prepare outgoing mail for delivery.

EQUIPMENT/SUPPLIES: Manual or electronic postal scale, postage meter or PC stamps, envelope or package for mailing.

DIRECTIONS: Follow these step-by-step directions, which include rationales, to learn this procedure. Job Skill 12-3 is presented in the *Workbook* to practice this skill.

1. Sort all pieces of mail according to postal class for processing; bundled mail is processed faster.
2. Weigh the item to be mailed using a manual or electronic postal scale.
3. Compute the amount of postage needed to ensure fast delivery service.

4. Affix the correct postage to the item for mailing. Delivery is expedited by using online postage and postmarked labels applied by postal meters machines because this type of postage does not have to be canceled or postmarked at the post office.
5. *Optional*: Obtain a "Letter-Size Mail Dimensional Standards Template" from the post office. It has guides for maximum and minimum mailable dimensions of ¼-inch thickness or less and is an efficient way to measure outgoing mail accurately and quickly.
6. Place the mail in the office's designated outgoing mail area or take the mail to the post office. Establishing a central location for outgoing mail ensures quick pickup and delivery.

First-class mail to Mexico and Canada requires more postage than first-class mail sent within the United States.

Priority Mail

Priority mail is the designation for first-class mail that weighs more than 13 ounces, up to and including 70 pounds. The cost is based on distance and weight if over 1 pound. It is the fastest way to get heavier mail to its destination within 1 to 3 days. Using the free USPS priority mail envelopes, boxes, and tubes ensures first-class handling. Priority mail is also available in zone-based pricing and in flat-rate boxes and envelopes.

Priority Mail Flat-Rate Boxes/Envelopes—To ship using a flat rate, you select the size of box or envelope that fits your packaging needs, then purchase it for a flat rate. Anything that fits into the box or envelope, weighing less than 70 pounds, is mailed for the flat rate and the package reaches its destination within 2 to 3 days. Tracking is available and insurance is free up to $50. Following are the sizes of various flat-rate boxes and envelopes:

- *Large box*—12 × 12 × 5½ inches
- *Medium box*—13⅝ × 11⅞ × 3⅜ or 11 × 8½ × 5½ inches
- *Small box*—8⅝ × 5⅜ × 1⅝ inches

- *Legal envelope*—15 × 9½ inches
- *Padded envelope*—12½ × 9½ inches
- *Envelopes*—12½ × 9½ or 10 × 7 or 10 × 5 inches

Priority Mail Express

Priority mail express is the fastest and most reliable delivery service offered by the USPS. It includes tracking and insurance up to $100. Overnight service with date- and time-specific delivery (by noon or 3:00 p.m.) is available with a money-back guarantee. Delivery is made 7 days a week including holidays. The charge is based on weight, and the item must be 70 pounds or less. The local post office furnishes a network directory of cities served by express mail as well as labels and various sizes of envelopes and boxes.

Periodicals (Second Class)

Periodicals, formerly called *second-class mail*, include newspapers and periodicals that must be regularly issued at least four times a year, at which time the rate for mailing is computed. This class of mail is forwarded.

Media Mail (Third Class)

Media mail, formerly called *third-class mail* and sometimes referred to as *book rate*, is a special classification for mailing books, sound recordings, videotapes, and computer media (such as CDs and DVDs) that weigh at least 16 ounces and not more than 70 pounds. The endorsement, "Media Mail," must be written under the postage. Typically, media mail is not forwarded unless it contains a special endorsement.

Standard Post (Parcel Post/Fourth Class)

Standard post, formerly known as *parcel post* or *fourth-class mail*, includes thick envelopes, tubes, and packages containing gifts and merchandise weighing up to 70 pounds and mailed within the continental United States. The combined length and girth must not exceed 130 inches. Postage depends on the weight, shape, and destination. All standard post mail is forwarded; tracing and delivery confirmation is included at no extra charge.

Packages weighing more than a pound should be mailed in person at the post office. All packages should be sealed with glass-reinforced waterproof strapping (not masking tape) and address labels readable from a distance of 30 inches.

Bound Printed Matter (Special Fourth Class)

Bound printed matter, formerly called *special fourth-class mail*, is paid by permit imprint only and is applied to promotional material (advertising), directories, or educational material. No personal correspondence is allowed. Discounts are available for a minimum of 300 pieces.

Mixed Class

Mixed class, or *combination mailing*, may be used when a letter must be sent with a parcel. If it is sent parcel post, first-class postage is required on the letter, which either may be attached to the outside of the package or placed inside. When x-rays are mailed with a letter by a medical office, this classification is often used.

International Mail

There are many delivery options for *international mail*, each offering specific features, including volume mailing services. Delivery time and cost vary.

Special Services

The USPS offers *special services* to track mail, provide proof of mailing, and ensure delivery. The level of tracking and desired security will determine which service to use.

Registered Mail

Registered Mail is used when sending money and valuable or irreplaceable documents or packages. Items are placed under tight security from the point of mailing to the point of delivery. You can register first-class or priority mail, but a trip to the post office is required to complete the forms, which include proof of mailing and delivery (date and time). Insurance coverage based on the declared value of the item (up to $25,000) can be added. Extra services, such as Delivery Confirmation, Signature Confirmation, Collect on Delivery, Return Receipt, and Restricted Delivery can be combined with Registered Mail.

Certificate of Mailing

A *certificate of mailing* is a form that provides proof of mailing on a specific date (e.g., tax forms). The form is returned to the assistant to keep on file. Because the post office does not keep a record of the mailing, this certificate costs less than Certified Mail.

Certified Mail

Certified Mail is used when it is necessary to prove that a piece of mail has been mailed and delivered at a certain time and date. This type of mail service is used often by medical offices for collection purposes and for important letters (e.g., notification of practice relocation or closure, or dismissal of a patient). The sender is provided with a receipt of mailing and delivery can be verified online using the unique article number on the form. The receiver must sign a receipt of delivery when it arrives and this remains on file at the receiver's post office for 2 years. A copy of the signature record (*Return Receipt*) may be requested prior to or after delivery for an additional fee.

Certified Mail forms list detailed benefits on the back and may be kept in the office to eliminate special trips to the post office (Figure 12-4).

Delivery Confirmation

For a small additional fee, a *Return Receipt* can be requested for evidence of delivery for several classes of mail including Registered and Certified Mail. An electronic copy (or postcard) of the addressee's signature provides the date and time of delivery or attempted delivery (Figures 12-5A and 12-5B). *USPS Tracking* is also available, which provides end-to-end tracking including confirmation. First, determine what level of delivery confirmation is needed, then ask at your local

FIGURE 12-4 Front of a completed Certified Mail Receipt, U.S. Postal Service Form 3800 (Courtesy of U.S. Postal Service)

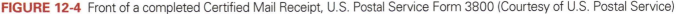

post office which service would accomplish your request. Refer to Procedure 12-5 for instructions on completing a USPS Certified Mail and Return Receipt form.

Restricted Delivery

Restricted delivery is available for Certified Mail, insured mail (over $200), or Registered Mail and ensures that only a specified person will receive a piece of mail. The signature of the person who signed for the item, along with the date and time of delivery or attempted delivery, is included.

Other Delivery Services

Many private carriers compete with the U.S. Postal Service to provide shipment of letters and packages. Some of the most popular are **United Parcel Service (UPS)**, **Federal Express (FedEx)**, and **DHL Worldwide Express** (formerly Airborne Express). The USPS may contract with an outside service for the transportation and delivery of mail, such as the alliance they have with FedEx for delivering Global Express Guaranteed (GXG) mail items.

Most delivery services offer next-day service, second-day service, and regular shipping service. Delivery times and costs vary according to the weight and size of the package and the distance involved. Rate calculations can be performed via the Internet and compared with various carriers. All shipping packages (envelopes and various size boxes) are free and can be ordered using each company's toll-free telephone number and delivered directly to the office.

The assistant may want to be familiar with the range of services and delivery schedules provided by mail carriers and to be aware of special packaging and labeling requirements. Free "Package Pickup" for Express and Priority Mail is available through the USPS and arrangements can be made with other carriers to have letters and packages picked up at the medical office. The Yellow Pages of the telephone directory provides names of other private shipping and courier companies listed with toll-free numbers under "Shipping Services."

ADDRESSING ENVELOPES FOR COMPUTERIZED MAIL

Two popular envelope sizes are used in the medical office:

- Personal size (number 6¾) 6½″ × 3⅝″
- Business size (number 10) 9½″ × 4⅛″

The upper left corner of the envelope is reserved for the name and address of the sender. If not preprinted, this is placed on line three about 1/2 inch from the left edge of the envelope.

The name and address of the person who is to receive the communication should be keyed as they appear in the inside address and should be placed

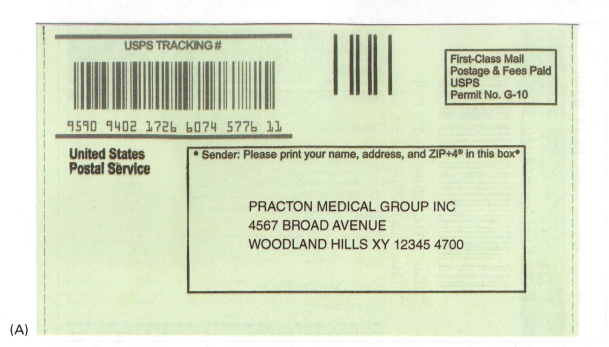

(A)

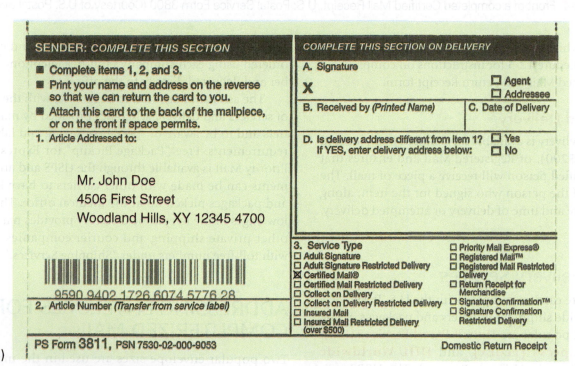

(B)

FIGURE 12-5 (A) Front of Domestic Return Receipt, U.S. Postal Service Form 3811, addressed with sender's information. (B) Back of receipt addressed with recipient's information and indicating unique article tracking number and type of service (Certified Mail). (Courtesy of U.S. Postal Service)

within the reading zone determined by the U.S. Postal Service for OCR electronic scanning.

Optical character recognition (OCR) is a fully computerized system that processes the mail by reading the complete address at a speed of 36,000 pieces an hour or 10 pieces every second. Specific typing and addressing standards must be adhered to when preparing an envelope for OCR processing. At the bottom right-hand corner of the envelope is a space reserved as a bar-code read area. After the OCR scanner has read the printed mailing address, it prints a bar code of minute vertical lines representing the nine-digit ZIP code in the

PROCEDURE 12-5

2
3

Complete Certified Mail and Return Receipt U.S. Postal Service Forms

OBJECTIVE: Complete a Certified Mail Receipt and Return Receipt delivery confirmation to accompany a letter.

EQUIPMENT/SUPPLIES: U.S. Postal Service Certified Mail Receipt (PS Form 3800), Domestic Return Receipt (PS Form 3811), and pen.

DIRECTIONS: Follow these step-by-step directions, which include rationales, to learn this procedure. Job Skills 12-6, 12-8, and 12-9 are presented in the *Workbook* to practice this skill.

1. *CERTIFIED MAIL RECEIPT FORM*—Handwrite and print legibly the addressee's name, street address, city, state, and ZIP + 4 code in the bottom right corner of the form. When processing this at the U.S. post office, the mail clerk will tear off and adhere part of the

receipt with the receipt number to the mail piece.

2. *RETURN RECEIPT FORM*—Handwrite and print legibly the sender's name, street address, city, state, and ZIP + 4 code on the front side of the form.

3. *BLOCK 1*—Handwrite and print legibly the addressee's name, street address, city, state, and ZIP + 4 code in the bottom left corner of the reverse side of the form.

4. *BLOCK 2*—Handwrite and print legibly the 20-digit number obtained from the front side of the form.

5. *BLOCK 3*—Insert a check mark indicating the appropriate service type (Certified Mail).

6. Attach this card to the back of the mail piece, or on the front if space permits.

---

bar-code read area (see Example 12-1). This reserved area must remain free of extraneous markings, such as printing and colored borders. Although the U.S. Postal Service accepts any color combination of ink and paper, black printing on white paper is the easiest to read.

Word processing software programs include a feature that addresses envelopes in the OCR format and inserts the bar code. These programs also have mail merge capabilities, so an address book can be accessed and names and addresses can be easily inserted into a set of similar documents, such as letters informing patients of a new office address or an upcoming immunization clinic.

All major U.S. cities employ computerized mail processing; therefore, medical assistants should adopt the required envelope format (Figure 12-6). The electronic "reader" scans the envelopes' zone area. In processing mail for delivery, both postal employees and sorting equipment ignore everything but the address in the line immediately above the city name. The last line

must always contain the city, state, and ZIP code. Nothing may be typed below the last line of the address because the computer will consider it an error and redirect the envelope for hand processing.

Envelope Guidelines

Guidelines in Procedure 12-6 are used to address business mail according to U.S. Postal Service OCR processing requirements.

COMPLIANCE

Address Errors

Average number of mail pieces processed by the USPS:

- 22 million mail pieces processed each hour
- 366,000 mail pieces processed each minute
- 6,100 mail pieces processed each second

*Approximately 25% of all mail pieces have something wrong with the address, for example:

- Missing apartment number
- Wrong ZIP code

*USPS 2012 statistics

EXAMPLE 12-1

Bar Code

PROCEDURE 12-6

Address a Business Envelope Using U.S. Postal Service Regulations

OBJECTIVE: Address business envelopes according to U.S. Postal Service regulations for accurate and timely delivery.

EQUIPMENT/SUPPLIES: Computer and printer with envelope tray.

DIRECTIONS: Follow these step-by-step directions, which include rationales, to learn this procedure. Job Skills 12-4, 12-6, 12-8, and 12-9 are presented in the *Workbook* to practice this skill.

1. Refer to Figure 12-6 for visual guidance in preparing envelopes.

2. Select the envelope format using a computer word processing program, usually found under "tools."

3. Key the sender's name, street address, city, state, and ZIP + 4 code in upper- and lower-case letters in the upper left corner of the envelope. If the letter needs to be returned to the sender for additional postage or address correction, a return address will ensure prompt return.

4. Start to the left of the center and at least 2 inches from the top of the envelope and key the receiver's mailing address using:
   a. Block format
   b. Left, uniform margin
   c. Single-spacing
   d. At least 10-point type
   e. All capital letters with no characters touching (preferred format)

f. No punctuation (except hyphen in ZIP + 4 code)

g. Four to six lines maximum

5. Leave a minimum of one space between the city name and the two-character state abbreviation and the ZIP + 4 code (see Table 12-2).

6. Use standardized address abbreviations (see Table 12-3 at end of chapter).

7. Use standardized state abbreviations (see Table 12-4 at end of chapter).

8. If a city name in an address exceeds 13 digits, refer to the "Address Abbreviation" section of the *National ZIP Code Directory*, published annually by the U.S. Postal Service, to find the accepted abbreviation. The computer is programmed to read only those cities listed in the directory.

9. Key any notation for special services as noted in Figure 12-6.

10. Key an attention line (when one is necessary) on the second line of the mailing address (see Example 12-2).

11. Mail destined for a foreign country must have that country's full name, typed in capital letters on the last line of the address.

12. Proofread the envelope or mailing label and make corrections before printing. Accurate address information and placement of data will ensure fast and correct delivery to the recipient.

Large Manila Envelopes

When addressing large manila envelopes, place the address to the right edge of the mail piece. If centered, the scanning equipment will no longer read it. Never use tape to seal a letter or manila envelope.

Two Delivery Addresses

When mail that has two delivery addresses, for example, a post office box (POB) number and street address, the mail is delivered to the address that appears directly above the city–state–ZIP code line (Example 12-3). If the two addresses have different ZIP codes, the ZIP must be the one that serves the address of actual delivery.

To speed mail delivery in this situation, always address the correspondence to the POB number. Recipients can pick up mail addressed to a POB as early as 8 or 9 a.m., whereas mail addressed to a street address may not be delivered until that afternoon. Also, when a medical office moves to a new location, the process of forwarding mail to a new street address can delay its

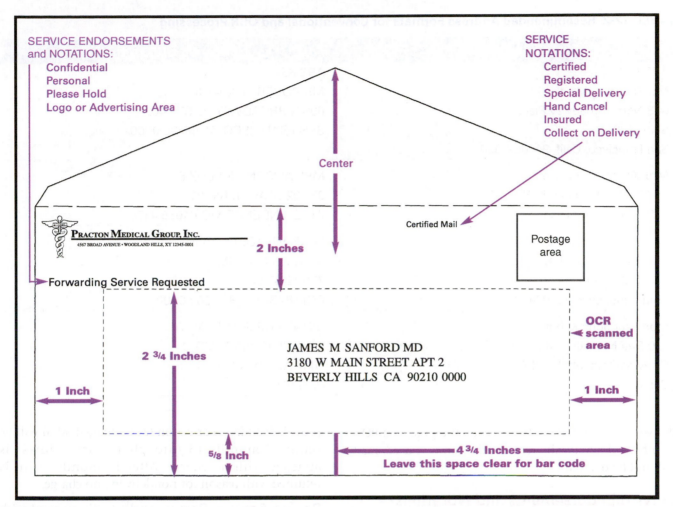

FIGURE 12-6 Completed number 10 business envelope (9½ inches by 4⅛ inches) using the OCR format for placement of recipient's address, sender's return address, and special service endorsements. Envelope is not shown to scale.

EXAMPLE 12-2

Envelope Address Attention Line

PRACTON MEDICAL GROUP INC

ATTN FRAN PRACTON MD

4567 BROAD AVENUE

WOODLAND HILLS XY 12345 4700

or

PRACTON MEDICAL GROUP INC

ATTN FRAN PRACTON MD

4567 BROAD AVENUE

WOODLAND HILLS XY

12345 4700

EXAMPLE 12-3

Two Addresses

MIDWAY PHARMACY

2221 W MAPLE STREET

PO BOX 54 *[mail would be delivered here]*

NEW YORK NY 10017 0000

MIDWAY PHARMACY

PO BOX 54

2221 W MAPLE STREET *[mail would be delivered here]*

NEW YORK NY 10017 0000

TABLE 12-2 Recommended Address Formats for Conventional and OCR Processing

Conventional	Preferred OCR Format
ARS 654 Mr. Robert L. Major 608 North Broadway Place Suite 402 San Francisco, Calif. 91400-0000	ARS 654 MR ROBERT L MAJOR 608 N BROADWAY PL STE 402 SAN FRANCISCO CA 94100 0000
Mrs. Alison McKenzie 35-102 West Avenue K, Rm. 21 Independence, Missouri 64055-4178	MRS ALISON MCKENZIE 35 102 W AVE K RM 21 INDEPENDENCE MO 64055 4178
Lane Memorial Clinic Attention: Dr. C. M. Kim 770 12th Street E Columbus, Ohio 43202-0000	LANE MEMORIAL CLINIC ATTN DR C M KIM 770 12 ST E COLUMBUS OH 43202 0000
Monsieur John Kaput 120 Rue Nepean, Apt 8 Ottawa (Ontario) K2P 0B6 Canada	MONSIEUR JOHN KAPUT 120 RUE NEPEAN APT 8 OTTAWA ON K2P 0B6 CANADA

delivery for 1 or 2 days. If, however, the practice's POB number, which usually remains the same, is used, mail will not be delayed.

Service Endorsements and Notations

Service endorsements are used to request a new address and to provide the USPS with instructions on how to handle undeliverable mail (see examples in Figure 12-6). The endorsement must appear in 8-point type or larger and should stand out clearly with a ¼-inch clear space on all sides. It cannot interfere with the return address or the mailing address that appears within the OCR-read area. Endorsements may appear in one of the following areas:

- Below the return address—line 9, flush with the left edge of the return address
- Below the postage area—clear of all stamp markings
- To the left of the postage area—clear of all stamp markings
- Above the delivery address—not interfering with the OCR-read area

A medical practice may request one of the following endorsement types:

Address Service Requested—Mail is forwarded for 12 months at no charge and notice of new address provided; address correction fee is charged. Mail will be returned months 13 through 18; new address is attached with no charge. After 18 months, mail is returned with reason for nondelivery; no charge.

Return Service Requested—Mail returned with new address and reason for nondelivery; no charge. To remail, new postage needs to be applied, so it is best to prepare a new envelope.

Change Service Requested—Mail disposed of and a separate notice of new address or reason for nondelivery provided; address correction fee charged.

Forward Service Requested—Mail forwarded to new address for 12 months at no charge; this is the same with no endorsement appearing. Between 13 and 18 months, the mail piece is returned with new address; may be minimal charge. After 18 months or if undeliverable, mail is returned with reason; no charge.

Other notations, such as *confidential*, typically appear below the return address and *special service notations* such as *certified* typically appear to the left or below the stamp, but cannot interfere with the OCR-scanned area for the address (Figure 12-6). When the office is notified of a new address, be sure to update the patient's personal information in the computer database.

Window Envelopes

Window envelopes are often used for mailing patient statements and are popular because their use eliminates the need to prepare an envelope. They also reduce the possibility of a letter being placed in the wrong envelope. Correspondence with address inserts for window envelopes must follow post office specifications. That is, they must be on white or very light-colored paper of a size that matches the opening to allow a clear view of the entire address. One-eight inch of clear space must be visible between the address and all edges of the window; the only information that may show through the window is the name, address, and any key number used by the sender. If any part of the address is hidden, the OCR will reject the envelope.

When folding a letter for a window envelope, the letter is placed flat on the desk in the reading position. First, fold from the bottom third up, and then fold the top third *backward*. The last crease goes in the envelope first, with the envelope window-side up (Figure 12-7). Be sure to check the placement of the address when using a window envelope.

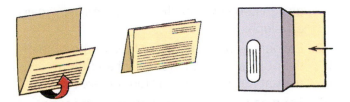

FIGURE 12-7 Folding a letter for insertion into a window envelope

Sealing and Stamping Envelopes

If hand sealing several envelopes at one time, hold 8 or 10 in your left hand (if right-handed) with flaps on the left edge facing up. Grab the top one by the flap and bring the flap under the next one until all flaps are open. Then, fan out several with address side down and use a damp sponge to wet the glue and seal the envelopes shut.

When stamping, tear about 8 or 10 stamps from a roll and fan-fold them so that they separate easily. Fan envelops, address side up and attach a stamp to the top envelope, and then proceed to the next.

A *sealer* on a mail machine may also be used to moisten and seal multiple envelopes prior to the meter printing postage directly on envelopes or labels.

Mail Tracking

When mailing important items, it is best to use a type of mail classification that offers mail tracking. Always

keep the receipt, which shows the tracking number until the mail-piece has arrived. If the mail item has not arrived within a specified time period, you can trace it by going online or calling the delivery service.

MANAGING OFFICE MAIL

Tight control of office mail procedures will expedite collections, save postage expense, and leave the staff time for other duties. Letters and packages that need to be rushed should be taken directly to the post office (Figure 12-8).

The medical assistant may want to use one of the many automated mailing stations and information centers that provide shipping information and help determine the type of service desired. The USPS website provides the information needed to mail everything from a letter to a 70-pound package. A "decision tree" is available; you choose the type of mail, size, and weight, and then indicate how many pieces you have and whether you want it sorted, and it will automatically give you the best option for mailing. Postage and labels for special services are dispensed and receipts are provided. Refer to Procedure 12-7 for guidelines on managing office mail.

ELECTRONIC MAIL

Electronic mail (email) is a type of mail service that electronically sends, receives, stores, and forwards messages in digital form over telecommunication lines. Electronic communication is often preferred because it can reduce telephone calls, eliminate phone tag, save

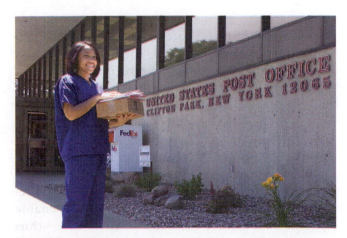

FIGURE 12-8 Medical assistant taking mail and packages to a U.S. post office

PROCEDURE 12-7

Manage Office Mail

OBJECTIVE: Follow U.S. Postal Service guidelines to ensure that all mail is expedited in a safe and expedient manner.

EQUIPMENT/SUPPLIES: Mailing supplies and mail; pen.

DIRECTIONS: Follow these step-by-step directions, which include rationales, to learn this procedure.

1. Check each outgoing letter for a written signature and for enclosures before sealing the envelope.

2. Avoid surcharges by keeping envelopes and cards within size limitations because nonstandard mail costs more.

3. Use window envelopes only if an address has four or fewer lines.

4. Indicate the proper mailing class to avoid being charged at the first-class rate.

5. Use a service endorsement on the outside of envelopes that instructs the post office to forward mail to a new address. This procedure ensures that patients will receive their bills with minimum delay.

6. Print the bar code on the envelope if the office has a computer or mail machine.

7. Use lightweight paper when sending international mail because rates are measured in 1/2-ounce increments.

8. Purchase a postage scale and keep it accurately adjusted or keep a supply of Stamps by Mail forms on hand to save a trip to the post office if mail is not metered.

9. Prepare computer media for mailing by placing them in cardboard or heavy plastic before inserting them into a box or padded envelope.

10. If staples or paper clips must be used, fold the material so the fasteners are on the inner part of the documents. Write "Non-Automation Compatible Mail," "Do Not Run on Automation Equipment," "Please Hand Stamp," "Do Not Bend," or "Media Enclosed" prominently on the envelope if the envelope is thick or contains media, x-rays, or delicate objects.

11. Include APO (Army/Air Force Post Office) or FPO (Fleet Post Office) initials followed by a designated city and ZIP code on military mail envelopes.

12. Encourage patients to pay fees at the time of their office visit or personally hand them their statement with a return envelope.

13. Send several health insurance claim forms to the same carrier in one large manila envelope.

time, is flexible, increase accessibility to information, and encourage a rapid response. The sender can leave a message in the electronic mail box of a distant computer, a handheld device, or a smartphone where it can be retrieved by the receiver at a convenient time. If a response is required, it can be returned using the same system. Physicians can easily access email from home, the office, a hospital, and distant locations. Errors are reduced through the elimination of verbal and handwritten data. Email can improve time management, create self-documenting medical records, and enable patients to be more involved in their care—thus improve patient satisfaction and enrich the provider-patient relationship.

Email Usage

Physicians have found multiple uses for email, and many medical practices have an active email address. Uses in a medical practice include:

- *Prescription requests and refills*—Whether using an EMR or a paper-based system, pharmacy requests can be expedited via email.

- *Test results*—Laboratory, radiology, and various test reports may be emailed to the requesting physician to review. After interpreting the results and determining what action needs to be taken, the reports would be automatically transferred to the patient's EMR or filed in the patient's chart.

The physician may email the normal findings with any comments to the patient's private email address; abnormal findings would warrant a telephone call to the patient.

- *Transfer of patient records*—If medical records are stored electronically in the physician's computer system, selected portions of the EMR or the entire record can be emailed to a consulting physician. In return, the consulting physician can email comments about the patient to the referring physician. This communication can be transferred to the patient's EMR or printed as a hardcopy and filed in the patient's chart.

- *Insurance processing*—Email has multiple uses for the insurance department. It may be used to verify the patient's eligibility; substantiate the deductible amount and status; obtain authorization for a referral, service, or procedure; follow up on outstanding claims; and appeal denied or downcoded claims.

- *Appointment scheduling*—Patients may request appointments online by entering dates and times they prefer. A return email message confirms the appointment.

- *Health news and information*—Notices can be sent regarding new health information or screening tests (e.g., blood pressure checks, cholesterol tests). Links to websites that offer patient education can be provided via email.

- *In-office communication*—Email is able to facilitate faster, more efficient business communications with colleagues and among coworkers who do not need an immediate response, unlike verbal messages, which may be forgotten. When computers are in a network, electronic mail can be transmitted to other areas of a medical facility and substitute for a hard copy interoffice memo. Large medical facilities may have an *intranet,* that is, an in-house website for employees that provides a network to disseminate information internally and cannot be accessed by the general public. In-office electronic messaging using a total practice management system is another way of communicating with coworkers (see Chapter 6).

Subscription Services

When subscribing to an online computer information service via the Internet (e.g., America Online, Google Mail, Yahoo) or by using a local service (cable or telephone company), it is possible to communicate with

PATIENT EDUCATION

Email

Email communication to patients can consist of data about the medical practice and the staff, for example, office hours, satellite locations, and announcements, such as when flu vaccines have arrived and are available or times for walk-in blood pressure checks. Patients need to be informed when a medical practice uses email and what they can use it for.

COMPLIANCE

Email Consent

Health care providers may not use or disclose protected health information without a valid authorization. The patient must sign an email consent form to communicate electronically. In the form, the patient should acknowledge that he or she understands the risks of emailing information (Figure 12-9).

any other person who has an email address around the world. Millions of people subscribe to these services to network information with each other.

Transmitting and Receiving Email

To use email, the computer needs to have access to a modem or router that is serviced by a long-distance telephone carrier or cable company for transmission of information across its lines. When sending a message, an online service is accessed by designating the mailbox code of the recipient and then keying in the message

COMPLIANCE

Data Transmission Security

Data transmission security must be ensured. The Health Insurance Portability and Accountability Act (HIPAA) requires the use of password protection, encryption, and authentication in transmission of patient information on an open network to ensure confidentiality.

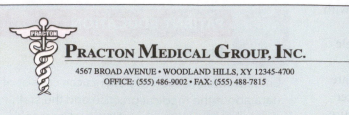

PRACTON MEDICAL GROUP, INC.

4567 BROAD AVENUE • WOODLAND HILLS, XY 12345-4700
OFFICE: (555) 486-9002 • FAX: (555) 488-7815

Fran Practon, M.D.
Gerald Practon, M.D.

CONDITIONS FOR THE USE OF EMAIL

Provider will use reasonable means to protect the security and confidentiality of electronic mail (e-mail) information sent and received. Provider cannot guarantee the security and confidentiality of e-mail communication, and will not be liable for improper disclosure of confidential information that is not caused by provider's intentional misconduct. Therefore, patients must consent to the use of e-mail for patient information. Consent to the use of e-mail includes agreement with the following conditions:

1. All e-mail messages to or from the patient concerning diagnosis or treatment will be printed and made part of the patient's medical record. Because they are a part of the medical record, other individuals authorized to access the medical record, such as staff and billing personnel, will have access to those e-mail messages.
2. Provider will not forward e-mail messages to independent third parties without the patient's prior written consent, except as authorized or required by law.
3. Provider cannot guarantee that any particular e-mail message will be read and responded to within any particular period of time. The patient shall not use e-mail for medical emergencies or other time-sensitive matters.
4. It is the patient's responsibility to follow up and/or schedule an appointment if warranted.

ACKNOWLEDGMENT AND AGREEMENT

I acknowledge that I have read and fully understand the risks associated with the communication of e-mail between the provider and me, and consent to the conditions outlined herein. I agree to the instructions outlined herein and any other instructions that the provider may impose to communicate with patients by e-mail. Any questions I may have had were answered.

_____   _____

Patient's Signature   Date

_____

Patient name:

_____

Patient address:

_____

Patient e-mail address:

FIGURE 12-9 E-mail consent form that can be adapted to a medical practice (see Example 12-4). When opening unsolicited or unknown email, there is a risk of exposing the computer system to viruses, so it is important to follow office guidelines in this regard.

When receiving a message, the user accesses an email service on the computer and enters the password for the appropriate "mailbox." Any message stored can be brought up on a screen and saved or printed. In some electronic mail systems, the message will be deleted after a period of time.

EXAMPLE 12-4

Electronic Mail (Email) Address

Dbrown@aol.com

Dbrown	Individual user (David Brown)
@	at
aol	site (America Online, an online service provider)
com	type of site (commercial business)

Email Etiquette

It is important to use proper email etiquette to retain good rapport with recipients and avoid legal problems. Court cases regarding issues of privacy and ownership in electronic communication systems indicate that email is company property. Make business email businesslike and do not write personal emails on company time. Do not send messages of a sensitive nature, such as a termination notice or a legal issue, via email. Email messages may not be confidential and should not contain any data that could prove embarrassing to the sender, the business, or other people. Compose the email, then reread it with this in mind.

Users need to be careful about expressing emotion in a message. Choose words carefully and eliminate humor, sarcasm, and anger. These can be misinterpreted easily because the receiver cannot see a grin or hear a chuckle. If you get emotional after receiving an email message, write a reply and put it aside until the next day. Emotional responses to messages should not be made immediately. Before sending the message, reread and rewrite it to make it sound less harsh. Do not write anything racially or sexually offensive. Assume messages are forever. Misdirected messages should not be ignored but followed through to the intended recipient.

Email Format

An email business communication should follow the format of the memorandum, as discussed in Chapter 11 and illustrated in Figure 11–6. Anything more formal should justify using a letter format, which can be attached to the email, sent instantly by fax, or sent via snail mail. Use a font that is clean-cut and professional looking, such as Times New Roman, 12 point, black, and minimize the use of color and design (see Figure 7-13).

Use a brief, meaningful, and specific subject line, such as "Request for a Meeting" or "Insurance Announcement" instead of one that is long or vague in nature. If there is a date or location involved, include this in the subject line.

Salutations may be formal; however, because the sender, recipient, and subject are identified in the heading, they may be informal and require no more than a name or an initial and a dash (see Example 12-5).

The message communicated in the body of the letter needs to be brief and to the point. *Pronouns may be omitted* if the interpretation is not lost in the reading of the message (see Example 12-6).

Left justify the message because this makes it easier to read and use correct grammar, word usage, and spelling along with standard capitalization and punctuation rules. Do not write in all capital letters; this is referred

---

EXAMPLE 12-5

Email Salutations

Dear Mrs. Smith: (formal)

Hi Joe, (informal)

Greetings or Good morning/afternoon (informal)

EXAMPLE 12-6

Email Grammar

A. Received lab report so please call for the results. (no pronouns)

We received *your* lab report so please call *us* for the results.

B. Sent x-ray films to Dr. Stevens on March 18. (no pronouns)

I sent *your* x-ray films to Dr. Stevens on March 18.

to as "shouting." The way you produce an email message reflects your professionalism and the importance of the message.

Do not use "emoticons," such as smiley faces ☺ and frowns ☹ in business email. Use these only in personal communications with people you know well. Use only well-known acronyms and abbreviations. Limit messages to a maximum of two screens.

If responding to a long email message, print out the letter and refer to it to ensure all items have been addressed accurately. Do not paraphrase from the message, but use quotes for the exact words when necessary. Create several paragraphs instead of one long body of text. Use numbered lists, when appropriate, to increase comprehension and speed reading. Be careful, however, when using formatting features such as bullets, underline, italics, and boldface because they may not transmit correctly.

Tell the recipient what you want him or her to do and when you want action taken. Indicate to the recipient if you want a confirmation upon receipt of your email. Proofread your email before sending it and always check your spelling.

A complementary close may be formal or informal (see Example 12-7). It is often acceptable to merely type your name.

Most email programs are able to append signature lines automatically to the end of each message you send. A standard may be required by the medical practice for employees' signature lines, such as employee's name, business address, and telephone number. A maximum of six lines is recommended (see Example 12-8).

Answering Email

Most email programs automatically save and include the text that you are answering. After going back and forth a few times, this history can get unwieldy, so use judgment regarding when to start a new email. Update the subject line when you receive or send a reply. Otherwise, the receiver may think that he or she has read the message and may accidentally delete it.

EXAMPLE 12-7

Email Complimentary Closings

Very truly yours, (formal)

Sincerely, (formal)

Thank you, (informal)

Call me if you have questions, (informal)

EXAMPLE 12-8

Email Signature Lines

A. (Ms.) Charlotte Evans
Insurance Billing Specialist
Practon Medical Group, Inc.
4567 Broad Avenue
Woodland Hills, XY 12345-4700
Phone: (555) 486-9002

B. Maria Valdez, Office Manager
Fran T. Practon, MD and Gerald M. Practon, MD
Telephone: (555) 486-9002

Use the "reply all" function with discretion. If four people received the message and you select "reply all," then all four people will receive your reply. Instead reply to the original sender unless the situation requires a "response to everyone."

Forwarding Email

Beware when forwarding a message and never forward chain letters. To protect against viruses, the message may be copied and pasted in a new email message. Clean it up if the message has been forwarded several times. Erase all the "forwarded from" information and anything else that is irrelevant. By doing this, your recipient will not have to scroll through screens of routing information to find the one paragraph to read.

Email Attachments

Limit the use of attachments, and if sending one refer to it in the body of the email. Attachments are useful for sending large, formatted documents but not as a substitute for the regular text of an email. Send attachments using a common format (e.g., Word doc., pdf., rtf.) to make sure the person you are sending an attachment to can open it. Do not open attachments from someone you do not know because they may contain a virus that could infect your computer.

Basic Guidelines for Using Email

Office policies should be instituted to regulate email use for personal correspondence and employees need to understand these policies regarding when telephone calls or face-to-face communication is preferred. There should also be an employer's policy on inspection of messages. Following are some basic email policy guidelines:

- Use strong encryption and password protection.
- Have the patient sign an informed email consent form. If a patient refuses, do not send or accept email from him or her.
- Do not provide any patient identifiers or personal health information in the body or subject field.
- Identify office staff who have permission to read and receive office email.
- Indicate appropriate times in the medial practice to send and receive messages.
- Print email if it contains important information or if there is need for a paper record. Append it to the patient's EMR when necessary.
- Save all emails that contain PHI.
- Set up and use distribution lists that include names to which you can legally send email messages.
- Set up a retention policy, that is, time limits or retaining and deleting messages to ensure appropriate messages are kept.
- Create an automatic reply function if you plan to be away from the office for an extended period of time. By letting people know when you will return, the sender will not be waiting for an immediate response.

Managing Email

An email management system should be developed so that you do not get overwhelmed with email communication. Following are management protocols that can be applied:

- Check and empty your email box regularly at designated times during the workday so that you will not miss time-sensitive messages or let email build up. Some email software will make an audio sound (beep) when email arrives; that is, if the software is up and running and the speakers are turned on.
- Limit how often you check your email inbox so that it does not interrupt your work focus.
- Be prepared to act on messages when opening them; this eliminates the need to open and read messages multiple times. If you cannot give an immediate response, let the sender know you will reply within a specified time, for example, within 24 hours.

- Organize your mailbox into several categories or folders where messages can be stored.
- Create a "miscellaneous" email folder for messages that do not fit into basic folders.
- Make a "temporary" email folder for messages that do not need to be kept permanently.
- Include a prompt when closing or deleting all email messages that says, "Do you want to make this a part of the health care business record?" This allows one last time to decide if the mail should be kept or deleted.
- Set up and use distribution lists that include names to which you can legally send email messages.
- Set time limits for retaining and deleting messages; a retention policy will alleviate confusion and help ensure appropriate messages are kept.
- Save all email responses that contain PHI.
- Refer to Procedure 12-8 for instructions on composing an email message.

Email Policies and Security

Use a secure messaging service that allows the sending and receiving of encrypted messages. When using such a service, messages are picked up and delivered through the Internet or the medical practice's website, which is linked to the vendor's Web server. The server is protected by a firewall. A secure messaging service also allows the physician to limit staff access to specific categories of messages, restrict forwarding messages to standard email systems, and permit patient communication for only those patients who have signed an informed consent and authorization document.

Post an informed email consent document outlining office policies and security capabilities and an authorization to use email forms on the medical practice's website. Statements about who has access to patient emails, where patient emails go after they are read and printed, expected response times, various ways patients can use email, and what topics are appropriate for email usage should be included. It should be noted that there is a significant risk that electronic messages may be misdirected or intercepted by unintended parties, so it is not possible to guarantee the confidentiality of messages sent via the Internet. If strict guidelines are not established, patients may attempt to use email for urgent needs, resulting in potential harm to themselves and liability for the physician.

Each workstation should have a password to ensure that unauthorized people cannot access patient information. Patients' email addresses must not be used for

PROCEDURE 12-8

Compose an Email Message

OBJECTIVE: Compose and prepare email messages for transmission via the Internet.

EQUIPMENT/SUPPLIES: Computer with Internet connection.

DIRECTIONS: Follow these step-by-step directions, which include rationales, to learn this procedure.

1. Use Times New Roman font, 12 or 14 point, black ink.
2. Insert the recipient's email address.
3. Insert a descriptive subject line.
4. Insert a salutation.
5. Compose a single-spaced, left-justified message in the body of the letter.
6. Append closing signature line(s) at the end of the message.
7. Proof message and check for spelling errors.
8. Click "Send" and wait for an on-screen message to indicate the mail has been sent.
9. Mail that has been returned as undeliverable will appear in your mailbox. If mail is returned, verify the address and read carefully the reason for nondelivery.

☑ COMPLIANCE

Email Privacy and Security

Email between patients and physicians involves protected health information (PHI) in electronic form, and HIPAA protects all patient information. Therefore, even though HIPAA does not directly address email in any of its standards, both the privacy and security rules apply.

marketing purposes and written consent must be obtained before sending patient-identifiable information to a third party, even another physician.

Review federal and state laws relating to email and Internet use (e.g., copyright laws) as well as laws that affect the use of email for transmitting confidential patient health information. Laws may vary from state to state; for instance, communicating with patients whose residence is outside of the state where the physician is located, unless the physician is licensed to practice medicine in that state, may be prohibited.

FACSIMILE COMMUNICATION

Facsimile (fax) communication, more commonly called *fax transmission*, is an important communications tool for sending and receiving printed copies of information because the transmission is instant, reliable,

and inexpensive. It prevents errors because it is an exact copy of the original document, whether it is typewritten, handwritten, or a graphic illustration.

To use fax transmission, each office needs a fax machine or a computer with fax capabilities, a printer, and a telephone line or cable connection. Although faxes are typically used less frequently than email in today's business world, when used properly they can add a useful dimension when forms or documents need to be sent quickly.

To determine whether a document should be faxed, decide whether a telephone call would be more appropriate, particularly if only a short reply is required. Physicians use fax machines to resubmit unpaid insurance claims, obtain preauthorization for services or procedures, and send medical documents such as laboratory, pathology, x-ray, and biopsy reports (Figure 12-10).

Fax Etiquette

It is inappropriate to send some documents by fax. Do not fax letters of appreciation, apology, or condolence or messages containing negative information, such as news of impending layoffs. Do not send insulting or sloppy messages or chain letters. Avoid sending a fax and asking the recipient to make and distribute copies. Do not send advertisements for wide distribution, and avoid using the fax machine for sending messages of a personal nature.

Cover Sheet

A cover sheet is mandatory to ensure protection and verify reception. It may consist of either a separate small

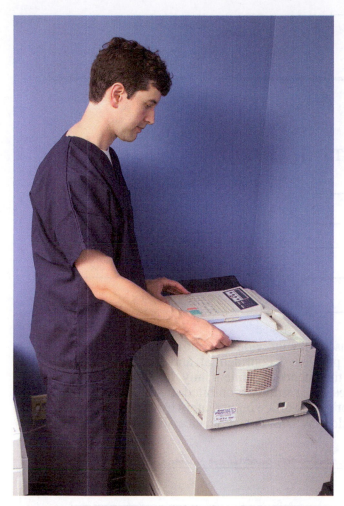

FIGURE 12-10 Medical assistant faxing a document

half-sheet or a full-sheet page, a small self-adhesive form attached to the top of the first page, or a stamp on page 1. The transmittal sheet or form may be handwritten or typed (Figure 12-11).

Fax Machine Features

Special features offered on fax machines are:

- Automatic document feeder (ADF); eliminates hand feeding of originals and saves time.
- Coded mailboxes; keep fax messages confidential.
- Automatic page cutting and collating for incoming documents.
- Store-and-forward (broadcasting) features; used to schedule specific times for transmission, resulting in reduced telephone costs, automatic image reduction, activity reporting, voice request, delayed transmission, memory, remote control, and polling.

Transmit faxes only to and from machines located in secure or restricted access areas to protect the patient's confidentiality.

Fax Operating Guidelines

When a document is placed in the fax machine, it is scanned and the text is converted to electronic impulses that are transmitted over telephone lines. The impulses are then converted back to text by the receiving fax machine. The medical assistant should be aware of certain general operating procedures when using a fax machine:

- Plug fax equipment into a special fax power surge suppressor, preferably one with an uninterruptible power supply (UPS), to prevent damage.
- Study the owner's manual for explicit information on the machine's care and use.
- Designate one or two staff members to monitor the fax machine.
- Keep the machine clean to avoid poorly reproduced copies.
- Write fax numbers in red and telephone numbers in black for easy identification.
- Avoid using pencil, correction fluid, or tape on documents; remove staples and paper clips to prevent damage to the machine.
- Wait for the signal that indicates receiving transmission has ended before trying to remove any document from the machine.
- Press the stop button to interrupt transmittal of a document; do not pull the paper out by hand.
- Try to transmit at times of the day when telephone rates are least expensive.
- Never leave the machine until the transmission is complete to ensure that the complete document went through.
- Place the machine away from direct sunlight or heat of any kind to avoid damage to documents.
- Turn the machine off when paper is replaced; failure to do so may cause incorrect sensor readings.
- Avoid sending documents that contain dark areas because they reproduce poorly. Lighten documents using photocopy machine settings prior to transmission.
- Reduce clerical time by maintaining a list of frequently used fax telephone numbers or program them into the fax machine.

PRACTON MEDICAL GROUP, INC.

4567 BROAD AVENUE • WOODLAND HILLS, XY 12345-4700
OFFICE: (555) 486-9002 • FAX: (555) 488-7815

Fran Practon, M.D.
Gerald Practon, M.D.

FAX TRANSMITTAL SHEET

To: _College Hospital_   Date _April 5, 20XX_

Fax Number: _555-487-6790_   Time _10:30 a.m._

Telephone No. _487-6789_

From: _Gerald Practon, MD_   Telephone No. _555-486-9002_

Number of pages (including this one): _1_ Fax No. _555-488-7815_

Note: This transmittal is intended only for the use of the individual or entity to which it is
addressed, and may contain information that is privileged, confidential, and exempt from
disclosure under applicable law. If you are not the intended recipient, any dissemination,
distribution, or photocopying of this communication is strictly prohibited. If you have
received this communication in error, please notify this office immediately by telephone and
return the original FAX to us at the address below by U.S. Postal Service. Thank you.

Remarks: _Please send immediately the lab and x-ray reports on patient, Irene Snell._

If you cannot read this FAX or if pages are missing, please contact:
PRACTON MEDICAL GROUP, INC.

INSTRUCTIONS TO THE AUTHORIZED RECEIVER: PLEASE COMPLETE THIS STATEMENT OF RECEIPT AND RETURN TO SENDER VIA THE ABOVE FAX NUMBER.

I, _Mary Smith_ , verify that I have received _1_
                                                (no. of pages including cover sheet)

from _Gerald Practon, MD_
      (sending facility's name)

FIGURE 12-11 Example of a completed fax cover sheet for medical document transmission

- Send legal-sized documents only if the target fax machine can handle them.
- Keep fax transmissions short, not more than 10 pages, if possible.
- Telephone the recipient and ask when it is a good time to transmit a lengthy fax (20 pages or more). A message may be lost if the recipient's machine runs out of paper, toner, or both.
- If a thermal fax is used, photocopy all documents received and scan or file them, destroying the original.

Faxing Confidential Records

When handling faxed records, the assistant should be aware of specific legal and confidential requirements. They are:

1. Fax health information only when it is absolutely necessary to save time critical to the patient's welfare, not for convenience.
2. Do not fax personal documents, psychiatric records except for emergency requests, or records containing information on sexually transmitted diseases, drug or alcohol treatment, or HIV/AIDS status.
3. Never fax a patient's financial data. In court, faxing medical information can be justified on the basis of medical necessity, but faxing financial information cannot be justified.
4. Fax only to machines located in physician offices, nursing stations, or other secure areas. Do not fax to machines in mail rooms, office lobbies, or other open areas unless someone is standing by to receive the fax or it is secured with passwords.
5. Before faxing medical records, remember that issues of patient confidentiality, physician liability, invasion of privacy, and potential breach of the patient-physician privileged relationship are serious concerns.
6. Edit your release of records authorization form and obtain patients' signatures to allow for fax transmission of confidential medial information.
7. Send and ask other senders to fax records by reference number (e.g., medical record number) rather than by patient name.
8. For confidential information, verify the telephone number and make arrangements with the recipient for a scheduled time of transmission or send it to a coded mailbox; otherwise, do not fax it. Coded mailboxes require the sender to punch in a code indicating the individual to whom the fax is addressed and the receiver to then punch in his or her own code to activate the printer. Place a telephone call to the recipient about 15 minutes after faxing patient records to verify receipt. Or request that the authorized receiver sign and return an attached receipt form at the bottom of the cover sheet on receipt of the faxed information.
9. Prepare a properly completed transmittal sheet with each transmission including a statement similar to that in Example 12-9.
10. If a fax document gets misdirected, note the incident along with the misdialed number in the patient's medical record.
11. Keep a fax report of all transmissions, indicating the date, time, and destination telephone number.
12. Monitor incoming faxes frequently to maintain confidentiality.

Legal Document Requirements

The Federal Rules of Evidence (Rule 803) of the Uniform Rules of Evidence (URE) apply to duplication of documents. More than half of the states have adopted rules based on the URE, which states, "a duplicate is admissible to the same extent as an original unless (1) a genuine question is raised as to the authenticity or continuing effectiveness of the original, or (2) in the circumstances it would be unfair to admit the duplicate in lieu of the original."

A number of states have adopted the Uniform Photographic Copies of Business and Public Records Act.

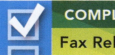

COMPLIANCE

When to Use a Fax

The American Health Information Management Association (AHIMA) recommends that fax machines not be used for *routine* transmission of patient information and should be used only when (1) hand or mail delivery will not meet the needs of immediate patient care, or (2) a third party requires it for ongoing certification of payment for a hospitalized patient.

COMPLIANCE

Fax Release of Information Form

For Medicare patients, wording on the release of information form must meet government requirements for confidentiality.

EXAMPLE 12-9

Facsimile Confidentiality Statement

Unauthorized interception of this telephonic communication could be a violation of federal or state laws. The documents attached to this transmittal contain confidential information. They belong to the sender and are legally privileged. The information contained here is intended for use only by the authorized receiver named above. It cannot be redisclosed or used by any other party. If the assistant is not the authorized receiver, he or she will be notified that any disclosure, copying distribution, or taking any action on the information contained here is prohibited. If the assistant has received this document in error, notify the sender immediately by telephone or arrange for the return of the original documents to sender or to receive instructions for their destruction.

This authorizes the admissibility of reproductions in legal cases that are made in the regular course of business without need to account for the original.

The Bureau of Policy Development of the Centers for Medicare and Medicaid Services (CMS) stated in June 1990 that the use of a fax machine to transmit physicians' orders to health care facilities is permissible. When a fax is used, it is not necessary for the prescribing practitioner to countersign the order at a later date. However, a legible copy of the physician's order must be retained as long as the medical record is retained. Some hospitals may not accept faxed physician orders, or they may limit transmission during certain times and require verifications of signature. The assistant should check with local hospitals or clinics about their fax policies.

Consult an attorney in your state to make sure documents (e.g., contracts, proposals, outlines, charts, graphs, plans, artwork composites, or photographs) requiring signatures are legal if faxed.

Refer to Procedure 12-9 for instructions on filling out a fax cover sheet and transmitting a facsimile.

PROCEDURE 12-9

Prepare a Fax Cover Sheet and Send a Fax

OBJECTIVE: Prepare a cover sheet and send information quickly and accurately by fax.

EQUIPMENT/SUPPLIES: Document to send, fax machine, and telephone line or cable connection.

DIRECTIONS: Follow these step-by-step directions, which include rationales, to learn this procedure. Job Skill 12-7 is presented in the *Workbook* to practice this skill.

1. Prepare a cover sheet for the document to be faxed, referring specifically to what is being sent and containing the:
   * Date
   * Time fax was sent
   * Name of recipient
   * Fax number of recipient
   * Telephone number of recipient
   * Name of sender
   * Telephone number of sender (in case of a transmittal problem; e.g., lost page or dropped line)
   * Statement that it is personal, privileged, and confidential medical information

   intended for the named recipient only (see Figure 12-11)
   * Total number of pages, including the cover sheet

2. Place the document face down in the fax machine to align it for transmission.

3. Dial the fax number of the recipient. Preprogram all commonly used fax numbers to prevent misdialing errors. If the fax machine has a digital display that shows the fax number dialed, verify it for accuracy.

4. Press start when you hear the fax tone.

5. Transmit the entire document, front and back, to be signed and not only the page to be signed, so the receiver has full disclosure of the agreement.

6. After the document has processed through the fax machine, press the button requesting a receipt if the machine does not automatically generate a report.

7. Remove the documents from the machine. If necessary, call the recipient to be sure the fax was received.

TABLE 12-3 Common Address Abbreviations

Address	Abbreviation	Address	Abbreviation	Address	Abbreviation
Alley	ALY	Harbor	HBR	Room	RM
Annex	ANX	Heights	HTS	Route	RT
Apartment	APT	Hill	HL	Row	ROW
Arcade	ARC	Hospital	HOSP	Run	RUN
Association	ASSN	Institute	INST	Rural	R
Avenue	AVE	Island	IS	Shoal	SHL
Bayou	BYU	Isle	ISLE	Shore	SH
Beach	BCH	Junction	JCT	Southeast	SE
Bend	BND	Lake	LK	Southwest	SW
Bluff	BLF	Lakes	LKS	Spring	SPG
Bottom	BTM	Lane	LN	Square	SQ
Boulevard	BLVD	Mall	MALL	Station	STA
Branch	BR	Manager	MGR	Street	ST
Bridge	BRG	Manor	MNR	Suite	STE
Brook	BRK	Mount	MT	Summit	SMT
Burg	BG	Mountain	MTN	Terrace	TER
Bypass	BYP	North	N	Track	TRAK
Camp	CP	Northeast	NE	Trail	TRL
Canyon	CYN	Northwest	NW	Tunnel	TUNL
Cape	CPE	Orchard	ORCH	Turnpike	TPKE
Causeway	CSWY	Palms	PLMS	Union	UN
Center	CTR	Park	PK	Valley	VLY
Circle	CIR	Parkway	PKWY	Viaduct	VIA
Cliffs	CLFS	Place	PL	View	VW
Club	CLB	Plaza	PLZ	Village	VLG
Court	CT	Point	PT	Ville	VL
Drive	DR	Port	PRT	Vista	VIS
East	E	Prairie	PR	Walk	WALK
Estates	ESTS	Ranch	RNCH	Way	WAY
Expressway	EXPY	Rapids	RPDS	Wells	WLS
Extension	EXT	Ridge	RDG	West	W
Freeway	FWY	River	RIV		
Grove	GRV	Road	RD		

TABLE 12-4 Two-Letter State Abbreviations for the United States and Its Territories and Canadian Provinces

United States and Territories					
Alabama	AL	Kentucky	KY	Ohio	OH
Alaska	AK	Louisiana	LA	Oklahoma	OK
American Samoa	AS	Maine	ME	Oregon	OR
Arizona	AZ	Marshall Islands	MH	Palau	PW
Arkansas	AR	Maryland	MD	Pennsylvania	PA
California	CA	Massachusetts	MA	Puerto Rico	PR
Colorado	CO	Michigan	MI	Rhode Island	RI
Connecticut	CT	Minnesota	MN	South Carolina	SC
Delaware	DE	Mississippi	MS	South Dakota	SD
District of Columbia	DC	Missouri	MO	Tennessee	TN
Federated States of Micronesia	FM	Montana	MT	Texas	TX
Florida	FL	Nebraska	NE	Utah	UT
Georgia	GA	Nevada	NV	Vermont	VT
Guam	GU	New Hampshire	NH	Virgin Islands	VI
Hawaii	HI	New Jersey	NJ	Virginia	VA
Idaho	ID	New Mexico	NM	Washington	WA
Illinois	IL	New York	NY	West Virginia	WV
Indiana	IN	North Carolina	NC	Wisconsin	WI
Iowa	IA	North Dakota	ND	Wyoming	WY
Kansas	KS	Northern Mariana Islands	MP		
Canadian Provinces					
Alberta	AB	Northwest Territories	NT	Quebec	QC
British Columbia	BC	Nova Scotia	NS	Saskatchewan	SK
Manitoba	MB	Nunavut	NU	Yukon Territory	YT
New Brunswick	NB	Ontario	ON		
Newfoundland and Labrador	NL	Prince Edward Island	PE		

STOP AND THINK CASE SCENARIO

Practice Mail Security

SCENARIO: You are opening mail for Practon Medical Group, Inc., and come across a piece of mail that looks like it has been opened and resealed with tape.

CRITICAL THINKING: How would you proceed? List several things that you might do to verify the safety of the mail.

1. _____
_____

2. _____
_____

3. _____
_____

STOP AND THINK CASE SCENARIO
Classify Outgoing Mail

SCENARIO: You are preparing outgoing mail and need to classify each piece.

CRITICAL THINKING: Refer to the guidelines for mail classifications in the *Handling Outgoing Mail* section and use critical thinking skills to determine the mail classification for the following items:

1. Medical supply catalogue issued in the spring, summer, fall, and winter

   _____

2. Unsealed letter from Practon Medical Group, Inc., with one-page advertisement for free blood pressure testing

   _____

3. Diagnostic codebook (package, 9 inches long, 6 inches wide, 2¼ inches thick, 3 pounds)

   _____

4. Consultation letter (envelope, 9½ inches long, 4⅛ inches wide, 6 ounces)

   _____

5. Referral letter that must be received the following day (envelope, 9½ inches long, 4⅛ inches wide)

   _____

6. Medical reports in a sealed envelope (9½ inches long, 4⅛ inches wide, 16 ounces)

   _____

7. Postcards (standard size), sent with a "Happy Birthday" wish to patients whose birthdays are this month

   _____

8. Package (18 inches long, 10 inches wide, and 10 inches high; weighs 50 pounds)

   _____

STOP AND THINK CASE SCENARIO
Select the Best Communication Method

SCENARIO: Following are several situations where communication is necessary.

CRITICAL THINKING: Determine what the best form of communication is for the following scenarios and indicate by writing one of the following:

LETTER   MEMO   TELEPHONE   FAX   EMAIL

1. The physician wants to send a note of condolence to a patient.

_____

2. The insurance billing specialist wants to send a copy of a claim form that was already submitted to the insurance company today.

_____

3. The office manager wants to notify all office staff of an emergency meeting that will take place next week.

_____

4. The office manager wants to notify all office staff of a local medical society meeting that will take place next month.

_____

5. Drs. Fran and Gerald Practon want to ask another physician group in the community whether they will be on call while the Practons go on vacation.

_____

FOCUS ON CERTIFICATION*

CMA (AAMA) Content Summary

- Modalities for incoming and outgoing mail
- Prioritizing incoming and outgoing mail
- Keyboard fundamentals and functions (envelopes)
- Equipment operation (computer, fax machine)
- Computer applications (electronic mail)
- Screening and processing mail
- U.S. Postal Service classifications and types of mail services
- Postal machine/meter
- Processing incoming mail
- Preparing outgoing mail (labels, OCR)

RMA (AMT) Content Summary

- Compose correspondence employing acceptable business format
- Employ effective written communication skills adhering to ethics and laws of confidentiality
- Identify and understand application of basic software

CMAS (AMT) Content Summary

- Process incoming and outgoing mail
- Possess fundamental knowledge of word processing
- Employ email applications

*This textbook *and the accompanying* Workbook *meet the entry-level administrative and general competencies for the CMA outlined by the AAMA Examination Content Outline and Occupational Analysis and for the RMA and CMAS outlined by the AMT Competencies, Construction Parameters, and Examination Specifications (see Competency Grid in Appendix B).*

1. In the ZIP + 4 code, the four-digit add-on number is important because it identifies:
   a. a particular city block
   b. the floor of a building
   c. a department within a company
   d. a group of post office boxes
   e. all of the above are correct

2. Metered mail must be deposited:
   a. at the nearest post office to the office address
   b. at any post office
   c. at the post office where the permit was issued
   d. on Mondays only
   e. anywhere regular mail is accepted

3. The *forever stamp:*
   a. has a value that will remain that of a first-class stamp
   b. can be used on a mail piece weighing from 1 to 3 ounces
   c. has a value that lasts until the end of the year in which it was purchased
   d. can only be used on personal mail, not on business mail
   e. has a value that lasts until postage prices increase

4. When the medical assistant reads correspondence and either underlines or highlights important words and phrases or makes explanatory notes in the margin, this is referred to as:
   a. proofreading
   b. editing
   c. annotating
   d. commenting
   e. paraphrasing

5. If mail to the physician marked "Personal and Confidential" is opened by mistake, how should it be handled?
   a. Put it on the physician's desk by itself.
   b. Reseal with transparent tape.
   c. Personally hand it to the office manager.
   d. Reseal with transparent tape and label it "Opened by mistake."
   e. Ignore the error and place it with the other mail.

6. Letters, cards, flats, bills, statements, and small parcels are typically sent by:
   a. first-class mail
   b. second-class mail
   c. third-class mail
   d. priority mail
   e. express mail

7. Priority mail usually reaches its destination in:
   a. 1 day
   b. 2 days
   c. 1 to 3 days
   d. 1 to 5 days
   e. 24 hours

8. Using priority mail flat-rate boxes:
   a. mail items are charged according to their weight
   b. mail items are charged according to their size
   c. you can purchase insurance up to $50
   d. arrival is guaranteed within 1 week
   e. mail items cannot be tracked

9. Domestic registered mail can be insured for a value up to:
   a. $1,000
   b. $10,000
   c. $15,000
   d. $25,000
   e. $35,000

10. When the medical office sends an important letter notifying patients of the pending office relocation and wants to ensure its arrival, which USPS special service would be used?
    a. Certified Mail
    b. Certificate of mailing
    c. Registered Mail
    d. Express mail
    e. Priority mail

11. A *Return Receipt* form:
    a. can be requested for evidence of delivery
    b. can be purchased for a small fee
    c. is free upon request
    d. is available for all classes of mail
    e. both a and b

12. Select the correct statement regarding mail addressed to a post office box *and* to a street address.
    a. Mail is delivered to the address appearing directly below the name.
    b. Mail is delivered to the address that appears directly above the city–state–ZIP code line.
    c. Mail is always delivered to the post office box.
    d. Mail is always delivered to the street address.
    e. Mail cannot be delivered if two addresses appear.

13. In regard to legal issues about ownership of electronic communication systems, court cases have indicated that email is a property of:
    a. the person who sends the email
    b. the person who receives the email
    c. both the sender and receiver
    d. the company, which owns the computer in which the message is sent
    e. all of the above are correct

14. Select the correct statement regarding email and the Health Insurance Portability and Accountability Act.
    a. HIPAA does not directly address email in their standards; therefore, no rules apply.
    b. Only HIPAA security rules apply to email.
    c. Only HIPAA privacy rules apply to email.
    d. If email involves PHI, HIPAA privacy and security rules apply.
    e. None of the above is correct.

15. Select the correct statement regarding the fax machine.
    a. Fax machines are typically used less frequently than email.
    b. Fax machines are typically used more frequently than email.
    c. Fax machines send electronic messages more quickly than email.
    d. Fax machines are no longer needed since the development of email.
    e. Fax machines are useful for sending letters of appreciation, apology, or condolence.

WORKBOOK ASSIGNMENT

To develop competency-based job skills, refer to the *Workbook* and complete the:
- Abbreviation and Spelling Review
- Review Questions
- Critical Thinking Exercises
- Job Skill activities, which are listed at the beginning of the chapter under *Performance Objectives in the Workbook.*

RESOURCES

Internet

To obtain answers to questions and get up-to-date information on mailing and shipping regulations, go to the following Internet websites.

DHL Worldwide Express
    Shipping services
Federal Express
    Shipping services
The United States Postal Service (USPS)
    Top USPS sites:
- Calculate Postage
- Change of Address
- Click-N-Ship
- Online Postal Store
- Track and Confirm
- ZIP Code Lookup

Telephone: (800) ASK-USPS (275-8777)
Website: http://www.usps.com
United Parcel Service (UPS)
    Select location and type of service
Offline Postage and Online Postage Software
- Click-N-Ship®
- Endicia™
- Pitney Bowes
- Stamps.com™

Publications

MailPro
    Free digital online bimonthly publication
    U.S. Postal Service

Unit 5

FINANCIAL ADMINISTRATION

CHAPTER 13

THE REVENUE CYCLE: FEES, CREDIT, AND COLLECTION

LEARNING OBJECTIVES

After reading this chapter and learning step-by-step procedures to gain job skills,* you should be able to:

- Communicate the importance of the revenue cycle.
- Name the types of fee schedules and fee discounts.
- Discuss fees with patients and communicate fee policies.
- Understand billing methods.
- Report how billing services are used in the medical office.
- Interpret an Explanation of Benefits (EOB) form.
- Define credit and collection terminology and use collection abbreviations.
- Describe credit laws.
- List the services of a credit bureau.
- State the importance of aging accounts and dun messages.
- Pursue telephone debt collection tactfully.
- Outline important items in a collection letter.
- Determine when to seek and how to select a collection agency.
- Decide when to use small-claims court.
- Explain federal bankruptcy and garnishment laws.
- Trace a debtor who has moved and left no forwarding address.

PERFORMANCE OBJECTIVES (PROCEDURES) IN THIS TEXTBOOK

- Explain professional fees in an itemized billing statement (Procedure 13-1).
- Separate and prepare monthly itemized billing statements (Procedure 13-2).
- Establish a financial agreement with a patient (Procedure 13-3).
- Perform debt collection using a telephone (Procedure 13-4).
- Select a collection agency (Procedure 13-5).

This textbook and the accompanying Workbook meet the educational components for entry-level administrative and general competencies outlined by CAAHEP and ABHES.

- Take collection action; send an account to a collection agency (Procedure 13-6).
- File an uncollectible account in small-claims court (Procedure 13-7).
- Trace a skip (Procedure 13-8).

PERFORMANCE OBJECTIVES (JOB SKILLS) IN THE WORKBOOK

- Use a physician's fee schedule to determine correct fees (Job Skill 13-1).
- Complete cash receipts (Job Skill 13-2).
- Interpret an explanation of benefits form (Job Skill 13-3).
- Role-play collection scenarios (Job Skill 13-4).
- Compose a collection letter and prepare an envelope (Job Skill 13-5).
- Complete a financial agreement (Job Skill 13-6).

KEY TERMS

accounts receivable (A/R)	dun message	open accounts
aging accounts	explanation of benefits (EOB)	participating fee
assignment	fee schedule	participating physician
bankruptcy	garnishment	physician's fee profile
bill	ledger card	professional courtesy
coinsurance payment	limiting charge	*quantum merit*
collection ratio	Medicare Remittance Advice (RA)	revenue cycle
copayment (copay)	Medicare Summary Notice (MSN)	skip
credit	multipurpose billing form	usual, customary, and reasonable (UCR)
cycle billing	nonparticipating fee	value-based reimbursement (VBR)
debit card	nonparticipating physician (nonpar)	

HEART OF THE HEALTH CARE PROFESSIONAL

Service

Communicating fees tactfully during a first encounter establishes patient responsibility. Answering questions and explaining fees is a courtesy to the patient and offering payment options and arranging monthly payments may be of great assistance to the patient who is having financial difficulties.

INTRODUCTION TO FEES, CREDIT, AND COLLECTION

The physician's primary aim is to provide health care for those who require it; however, it would be unrealistic to ignore another reason for practicing medicine, that is, to provide a livelihood for the physician and the physician's family. This livelihood depends on the good **credit** of those the physician serves. The word *credit* comes from the Latin *credere*, which means "to believe" or "to trust." In today's world, it simply means a trust in a person's integrity and in his or her financial ability to meet all obligations when they come due.

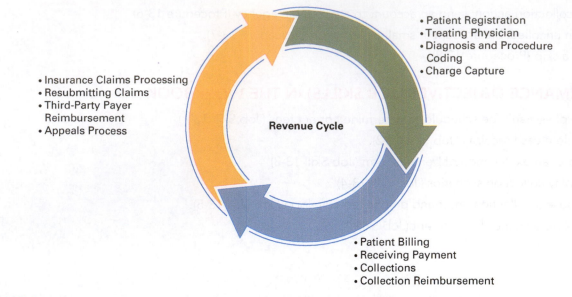

- Insurance Claims Processing
- Resubmitting Claims
- Third-Party Payer Reimbursement
- Appeals Process

- Patient Registration
- Treating Physician
- Diagnosis and Procedure Coding
- Charge Capture

Revenue Cycle

- Patient Billing
- Receiving Payment
- Collections
- Collection Reimbursement

FIGURE 13-1 Revenue cycle showing three phases of the life cycle of patient accounts

THE REVENUE CYCLE

The **revenue cycle** includes the life of patient accounts from creation to payment. The total amount owed to the medical practice appears in the **accounts receivable (A/R)** log. Managing the revenue cycle includes ways in which the health care provider ensures financial viability by capturing charges, improving cash flow, and increasing revenue. All processing points in the revenue cycle need to be executed correctly in order to produce revenue flow.

Processing points in the revenue cycle are shown in Figure 13-1 and presented in various chapters in this *textbook*. This chapter focuses on patient billing, receiving payment, credit, and collections. Following is a brief explanation of each step of the revenue cycle and where additional information may be found.

1. **Patient registration:** Questionnaire designed to provide identifying data to open an account (Chapter 5).
2. **Treating physician:** Provider who renders service to patients (Chapter 9).
3. **Diagnosis and procedure coding:** Diagnosis is the determination of the nature of the disease and substantiates medical necessity for procedures and services; procedures are medical services provided to diagnose or treat a patient (presented in Chapter 9 and discussed in Chapters 16 and 17).
4. **Charge capture:** Recording and posting of all encounters, that is, procedures and services (presented in Chapter 9 and discussed in Chapters 15 and 16).

5. **Patient billing:** Sending itemized statements to patients who have outstanding balances; presented and discussed in this chapter.
6. **Receiving payment:** Incoming monies paid for services and procedures; presented and discussed in this chapter.
7. **Collections:** Taking action on money owed in delinquent accounts in order to receive payment; presented and discussed in this chapter.
8. **Collection reimbursement:** Receiving money from collection action (presenting in this chapter and further described in Chapter 15).
9. **Insurance Claims processing:** Submitting insurance claims to federal and private insurance carriers for reimbursement (Chapter 18).
10. **Resubmitting claims:** Follow up procedures for unpaid insurance claims (Chapter 18).
11. **Third-party payer reimbursement:** Receiving payment from insurance companies; presented and described in this chapter and in Chapter 15.
12. **Appeals process:** Sending unpaid insurance claims to insurance carriers with additional documentation requesting reconsideration for payment (Chapter 18).

Obtaining Billing and Collection Information

The first step to ensure payment is to obtain a complete and accurate registration of the patient at the time of the first visit, securing enough personal and financial history to be able to effectively collect on an account or trace a patient who moves. Verify the patient's identity (see Red Flags Rule in Chapter 5), and review the information on the form before the patient leaves the office to make sure it is legible and complete. Figure 5-5 in Chapter 5 is an example of a patient registration record, which covers in detail the information that should be obtained from a patient. A comprehensive registration form lays the groundwork for a good flow of information that will help in sending statements, billing the insurance company, and collecting. Be sure the registration form includes spaces for a street address in addition to a post office box, an apartment number, a business telephone number with extension, and a statement regarding interest charged on accounts. If a patient invokes the privacy laws and refuses to divulge any information, it should be policy to require payment for services at the time care is rendered.

It is important to update this form regularly, so data is current. This can be done by having the patient review a copy of the original registration form and inserting changes in red ink. This will be vital when follow-up on a delinquent account is necessary.

FEE SCHEDULES

A **fee schedule** is a list of services or procedures and the specific dollar amount that will be charged by the physician or paid by the insurance company for each service. Fee schedules will vary depending on the state where medicine is practiced. A fee schedule is often organized by *CPT®* procedure code numbers (Example 13-1).

As mentioned in Chapter 2, a method of payment called *fee-for-service (FFS)* is one in which the patient pays the physician according to a set schedule of fees. **Quantum merit**, which means "as much as he deserves," is a common-law principle on which fees are based. Literally, this term translates as the promise by the patient to pay the doctor as much as he or she deserves for labor.

The fee schedule must be available to all patients, and under federal regulations, a sign to this effect must be posted in the office. This schedule can be used to quote prices to patients. Practices may have more than one fee schedule except in those states with fair pricing laws that allow only one schedule, which states standard fees. For states that allow multiple fee schedules, there may be separate schedules for workers' compensation, managed care contracts, Medicare, and private pay patients depending on the specialty of the practice and the type and number of signed contractual insurance agreements.

Sometimes a physician charges a fee for a service that is not on the fee schedule, such as an uncanceled "no show" appointment, interest charges for delinquent accounts, or annual summary sheets of the patient's account for income tax purposes. It is wise to tactfully inform a patient before billing for any such services; otherwise, the patient-physician relationship may be adversely affected.

Physician's Fee Profile

As each insurance claim is received by the insurance company, the payment data are entered into permanent computerized records. This is called a **physician's profile** or *fee profile* and becomes a statistical summary of the fee pattern (cost for services) of each physician for a defined population of patients. It is collected over time and compared with other practice patterns. The physician's profile is used to make periodic fee adjustments by insurance carriers.

Usual, Customary, and Reasonable

Reimbursement under the **usual, customary, and reasonable (UCR)** method is based on individual physician charge profiles and customary charge screens for similar groupings of physicians within a geographic area and with similar expertise. UCR definitions include:

- *Usual fee*—The fee normally charged for a given professional service by an individual physician (i.e., the physician's usual fee)

EXAMPLE 13-1

Fee Schedule

Evaluation and Management Services

OFFICE VISIT		New Patient
99201	Level I	$33.25
99202	Level II	$51.91
99203	Level III	$70.92
99204	Level IV	$106.11
99205	Level V	$132.28

- *Customary fee*—The fee that is in the range of usual fees charged by physicians of similar training and experience for the same services within the same specific and limited socioeconomic area
- *Reasonable fee*—The fee that meets the two preceding criteria or is considered justifiable by responsible medical opinion, considering any special circumstances of the particular case in question

Relative Value Studies

Relative value studies, also referred to as a *Relative Value Scale (RVS)*, consist of a list of five-digit *CPT®* procedure codes. Each code is weighted with a number that represents a unit value indicating the relative value for that service.

When using this system, a higher number of units are assigned to services requiring greater resources and, therefore, a higher fee. For example, a 60-minute office visit would carry more value than a 15-minute office visit, or a heart procedure would carry a higher value than an appendectomy. The number representing the weighted value of each service or procedure is multiplied by a *conversion factor (CF)*, which is based on historical cost experience (Example 13-2).

Periodically, the values are updated to reflect increases in actual expenses. Medicare uses its own RVS listings to establish fee schedules and workers' compensation uses either the UCR fees or the RVS fee schedule (Example 13-3).

Capitation

As mentioned in Chapter 2, under managed care plans, the physician is paid by *capitation*, a method of payment for health services by which a health group is prepaid a fixed, per capita amount for each patient enrolled without considering the actual amount of service provided to each patient. This per capita amount is usually paid on a monthly basis.

EXAMPLE 13-2

Relative Value Scale Fee Formula

Procedure Code	Description	Units
10000	Incision and drainage of cyst	0.8

Using a hypothetical figure of $153/unit, this procedure would be valued at $122.40.

Math: $153.00 × 0.8 = $122.4

EXAMPLE 13-3

Workers' Compensation RVS Fee Schedule

Price per Unit	Section of *CPT®*
$7.15/unit	Evaluation and Management section
$6.15/unit	Medicine section
$34.50/unit	Anesthesia section
$153.00/unit	Surgery section
$1.50/unit	Pathology section
$12.50/unit	Radiology section (total unit value column)
$1.95/unit	Radiology section (professional component unit value column)

The unit value is multiplied with the relative value amount for each procedure to determine the actual payment.

Individual Responsibility Program

In some states, a program has been established whereby physicians accept all patients but refuse to accept reimbursement from any third-party, private, or government program. Instead, physicians choose to "opt out" of insurance programs and bill the patient directly; the patient then applies to the carrier or program for reimbursement. This is called an *individual responsibility program (IRP)*.

Concierge Fees

Similar to the individual responsibility program, in concierge medicine, also referred to as *retainer-based medicine*, primary care physicians opt out of insurance programs and decrease their patient load, but instead of billing patients directly they charge a monthly or annual fee for services. Additional fees may be charged for tests and procedures as well as hospital care.

Medicare Fee Schedule

The Centers for Medicare and Medicaid Services (CMS) pays all covered benefits for physicians' services based on the Medicare fee schedule, which is determined by a *Resource-Based Relative Value System (RBRVS)*. Annually, the CMS posts the new local Medicare fee schedule for each area or region on the Medicare website. In a RBRVS

EXAMPLE 13-4

Medicare Formula Calculation for Payment

Code		Work	Overhead	Malpractice
91000	RVUs	1.04	0.70	0.06
	GAF	× 0.975	× 9.26	× 0.378
		1.014 +	0.6482 +	0.02268 = Total adjusted RVUs 1.68488

The 2016 conversion factor for nonsurgical care is $35.8043 × 1.68 = $60.15 allowed amount.

---

system, payment amounts are calculated by taking into account the relative value for:

1. Work done by the physician (work RVU)
2. Practice expense (overhead RVU)
3. Malpractice insurance (malpractice RVU)

The RVU is adjusted by each Medicare local carrier, which determines a *Geographic Adjustment Factor (GAF)* according to the cost of living in its region by using *geographic practice cost indices (GPCIs*—pronounced "gypsies"). To determine a payment amount, a *conversion factor (CF)* is used that is updated each year and published in Medicare newsletters and the *Federal Register* each November. The formula is RVU × GAF × CF = $ amount of Medicare service (Example 13-4).

RVUs are also helpful when negotiating the best contract available with managed care plans, so it is important for office managers or individuals assisting physicians to know and understand RBRVS data.

The Medicare fee schedule lists three columns of figures for each procedure code number: (1) participating physician fees, (2) nonparticipating physician fees, and (3) limiting charge. Following is an explanation of these three fees.

Participating Physician Fees

A **participating fee** is the amount paid to physicians who have contracts with Medicare. When a **participating physician** signs up in the Medicare program, the physician agrees to accept payment from Medicare (*80% of the approved charges/allowed amount*) plus payment from the patient (*20% of the approved charges/allowed amount*) after the deductible has been met. When a physician participates, this is referred to as accepting **assignment** and the Medicare payment is sent directly to the physician. It is permissible but less confusing not to collect the Medicare copayment up front. The deductible should be collected after the claim has been paid.

Nonparticipating Physician Fees

A **nonparticipating fee** is the amount paid to physicians who do not have a Medicare contract. Generally a **nonparticipating physician (nonpar)** does not accept assignment—payment goes directly to the patient, and the patient is responsible for paying the bill in full. A nonparticipating physician has two options, either not accepting assignment for all services or accepting assignment for some services and not accepting assignment for others. An exception to this policy is mandatory assignment for clinical laboratory tests and services.

Limiting Charge

A **limiting charge** is a percentage limit on fees that nonpar physicians may bill Medicare beneficiaries above the fee schedule allowed amount; therefore, no charges are to be submitted to Medicare that are greater than this. Medicare pays 80% of the nonpar allowable fee. The physician can collect 20% of the nonpar allowable fee from the patient and the difference between the allowable fee amount and the limiting charge amount. For assignment claims, nonpar physicians may submit usual and customary fees; thus, two fee schedules are often maintained, one with usual fees and the other with limiting charges. Refer to Example 13-5 for a brief illustration of the three types of Medicare fees and the Mock Fee Schedule shown in Appendix A of the *Workbook* to view a comprehensive listing.

Diagnosis Relate Group (DRG)

Medicare reimbursement to hospitals is based on *Medical Severity Diagnosis-Related Groups (MS-DRGs)*. This system classifies patients who are medically related in regard to diagnosis and treatment and statistically similar in length of hospital stay; in other words, it relates patients treated to the resources they consume. Instead of a fee-for-service system, the hospital receives a lump-sum, fixed-fee payment that is based on the diagnosis rather than on time or services rendered.

Medicare Part B Fee Schedule*

Procedure Code	Participating Fee	Nonparticipating Fee	Limiting Charge
99211	$18.58	$17.65	$20.13
62270	$148.40	$140.98	$162.13

*2016 Fee schedule is for the state of Nebraska for services performed in an outpatient setting

Certain cases or cost outliers (extraordinarily high costs) that cannot be assigned to a DRG because they are considered atypical, such as leaving the hospital against medical advice, rare condition, death, and so forth, are paid the full DRG rate plus an additional amount.

Although DRGs affect Medicare hospital inpatients, the medical assistant plays an important role in DRG assignment when relaying the *admitting diagnosis* to the hospital. All of the diagnoses must be given if there is more than one and the hospital staff can sequence them. If a hospital representative calls with questions about tests, length of hospital stay, or treatment ordered by the attending physician, the medical assistant should be prepared to furnish answers; this information will help determine the amount of the bill presented to Medicare by the hospital. The physician should be asked to review the treatment or procedure if there are questions.

There are various regulations (e.g., 1-Day Rule, 3-Day Rule) that bundle payment for preadmission testing (PAT) with the DRG amount, if they occur in a certain time frame before the hospitalization. At present, seven different DRG systems have been developed in the United States; the Medicare MS-DRG (or CMS-DRG) is just one of them.

Value-Based Reimbursement

Historically, health care providers have been paid on a fee-for-service (FFS) basis regardless of whether treatment improved a patient's condition or not. Essentially, the FFS model rewards volume and intensity of service—the more testing, procedures, treatments, and hospital admissions a provider delivers, the more money earned; this is referred to as *volume-based medicine*. Managed care also thrives on volume-based medicine because the more patients enrolled, the more capitated payment the physician receives. However, managed care programs limit utilization of medical services, especially specialty care. Because of this, the

fee-for-service payment model is expected to decrease over the next 5 years and various models of **value-based reimbursement (VBR)**, also called *value-driven reimbursement*, will emerge. The VBR model is centered around providing the minimum number of services necessary to improve a patient's condition—thus reducing the expense to treat a patient.

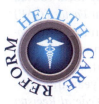

With the onset of the Affordable Care Act, payment reform for both state and government payers has taken place. Through Healthcare Innovation Awards, CMS has provided $1 billion to organizations implementing the most compelling new ideas to (1) deliver better health care, (2) ensure improved outcomes, and (3) lower costs to the public. Pilot programs are being tested around the United States, which are monitored for measurable improvements in quality of care and generated savings (e.g., accountable care organizations, coordinated care organizations, and patient-centered medical homes discussed in Chapter 2).

Regardless of what VBR model is used, documentation must be ensured so that performance measures, quality standards, and indicators of acute and severe illnesses can be tracked. For example, treating a chronically ill patient may generate less revenue and net loss for the practice because those patients require more time and resources than other patients. In a VBR model, the same attention must be given to controlling chronically ill care as to providing care for others.

Discounting Fees

Some doctors give discounts for cash payment. Such discounts must be offered to *all* patients, posted in the office, and outlined in a patient brochure. If fees are raised, a message to patients explaining the increase should accompany the monthly billing, and the assistant should post a notice in the reception room. Following are various types of fee discounts offered.

EXAMPLE 13-6

Sliding Fee Schedule

Family Size	Pay $25 per Visit		Pay 20% of Charges		Pay 40% of Charges		Pay 60% of Charges		Pay 80% of Charges		Pay 100% of Charges
	From:	To:	From:	To:	From:	To:	From:	To:	From:	To:	Income Over
1	0	11,170	11,171	13,365	13,366	16,755	16,756	19,550	19,551	22,340	22,341
2	0	15,130	15,131	18,900	18,901	22,695	22,696	26,478	26,479	30,260	30,261
3	0	19,095	19,096	23,865	23,866	28,635	28,636	33,410	33,411	38,180	38,181
4	0	23,050	23,051	28,815	28,816	34,575	34,576	40,338	40,339	46,100	46,101

Hardship Discounts

Hardship discounts may be granted dependent on the income level. Patients should be asked to verify their level of need by filling out an asset disclosure form or by bringing in their income tax returns. Document the reason for the fee reduction in the patient's financial record.

Hill-Burton Act—Most metropolitan areas have certain hospitals that have received federal construction grants to enlarge their facilities, in exchange for which they must care for indigents needing medical care. This obligation falls under the Hill-Burton Act of 1946. By contacting the local department of health, the assistant can obtain the names of hospitals participating in this service and send patients to these outpatient departments. Generally, the patients must complete financial applications to determine eligibility.

Sliding Fee Schedule

Federally funded programs as well as clinics and physician practices may offer a *sliding fee schedule* to all income-eligible uninsured or under-insured patients. Criteria to be considered for such discounts are household's gross income (e.g., between 101% and 200% of the poverty level), employment status, and special circumstances. Discounts may apply only to specific services, such as office visits, and not to all services provided. A discounted fee schedule must be developed according to local fee standards, appear in writing, and be applied consistently and evenly. Discounted fees apply only to direct patient charges, not to third-party coverage (Example 13-6).

Professional Courtesy

The term **professional courtesy** is a euphemism for a discount or a no-charge exemption extended to certain people by the physician. This policy has a long tradition; however, in today's legal climate, the decision to provide professional courtesy to colleagues and their families is not an easy decision. The physician must use sound judgment in deciding whether to waive or reduce the fees and must document the reason in the medical record. Currently, the trend among physicians is toward billing their colleagues; psychiatrists bill all patients including fellow doctors. The medical assistant must know the physician's policy so as not to bill in error. Computerized systems allow accounts to be coded, so no statements are sent to the patient.

Hospitals and many surgeons have largely given up the practice of free care, especially since most physicians have health insurance coverage for medical expenses. If one physician does not bill another for services

---

COMPLIANCE

Professional Courtesy

The Office of the Inspector General's compliance program guidelines state that professional courtesy arrangements may violate fraud and abuse laws, but this depends on two factors:

1. How the recipients of the professional courtesy are selected
2. How the professional courtesy is extended

If recipients are selected in a manner that directly or indirectly affects referrals, it may implicate the antikickback statute.*

*Section 1320a-7b of the Antikickback Statute prohibits the offer or receipt of certain remuneration in return for referrals for or recommending purchase of supplies and services reimbursable under government health care programs.

rendered, a result is that a third-party payer is relieved of its contractual obligation; this may fall under the False Claims Act (see Chapter 18).

Copayment Waiver

In the past, to reduce the cost of medical care for some patients, a physician who accepted assignment (received payment directly from the insurance company) might waive the copayment amount. However, the physician could be accused of not treating everyone with the same insurance coverage equally.

In most situations, both private insurers and the federal government ban waiving the copayment. It is, therefore, not recommended. There is one exception to this rule: Medicare recognizes a credit adjustment for this purpose on a doctor-to-doctor basis.

Fee Splitting

When one physician offers to pay another physician for the referral of patients, this is referred to as *fee splitting*. It is considered unethical and a felony in several states. Antifraud and abuse provisions in the Medicare and Medicaid programs state that "anyone who receives or pays money directly or indirectly for the referral of a patient for service under Medicare or Medicaid is guilty of a felony punishable by five years' imprisonment or a $25,000 fine, or both."

Discussing Fees

Physicians generally prefer not to discuss financial matters (e.g., insurance deductibles, unpaid bills) with their patients. The job of discussing and collecting fees is the responsibility of the medical assistant.

If the physician is charging fee-for-service, it is important to tell patients when they call for appointments that the office policy is to collect the fee at the time services are given. This type of practice increases collections and decreases the number of billing statements sent. It has been shown that a policy of stating fees up front also improves public relations and reduces patient complaints, business-office turnover, accounts receivable, and write-off amounts. The percentage of patients who pay their bills and return the next time they need health care will increase.

A patient who is a member of a managed care plan should be advised that the copayment will be collected at the time of the visit. In some instances (e.g., elective surgery) and in some types of specialty practices, the policy may be to collect for services as they are rendered

EXAMPLE 13-7

Obstetric Fees

An obstetrician may collect at each prenatal visit a portion of the charge for delivering a baby so that the entire patient responsibility for the obstetric bill is paid before the child is born. This eliminates having to ask the patient to pay a lump sum after delivery or after the insurance company has paid its portion.

while also requiring payment of a small amount toward the performance of future services. Obstetric fees are a case in point (Example 13-7).

There is a right time and a wrong time for everything, including the discussion of medical fees. Most patients who come to the office seeking medical care are more concerned with their health problem than with the expense incurred by their office visit. The assistant begins by listening to the patient's chief complaint but is prepared to discuss the expense. After the patient explains the medical problem, the assistant should tactfully ask about the patient's health insurance coverage. It is wise to ask, "Would you like to know something about the expense?" because occasionally a patient is emotionally unable to handle a discussion of fees. If a patient is elderly and someone in the family is responsible for the bill, the fee discussion should take place with both the *guarantor* (paying party) and the patient.

Never assume anything about a patient's financial status, and do not judge by outward appearance. Even if someone appears poorly dressed, or conveys the impression that they cannot afford to pay, the medical assistant must refrain from asking embarrassing questions. Tact is called for in all inquiries, whether dealing with credit (the ability to pay) or with other decisions. To eliminate psychologically misleading statements about "credit," it is best to use the terminology "patient accounts

COMPLIANCE

Discussion of Patient Fees and Accounts

It is important that any conversation regarding fees be private, so discussion of patients' accounts is not overheard by others and patients feel free to talk about any financial problems. A mature, courteous, tactful, firm, and business-like approach is vital.

department" when referring to the credit department. "Our payment policy" is preferable to "our credit policy." Terms that project a positive tone, such as *fee* instead of *charge*, will be reflected in patients' attitudes.

Guidelines for Communicating Fees

Fees for medical service should be stated clearly and accurately. A misquoted cost may make a patient angry. Every patient coming to the medical office should have heard about the practice's financial policy at least three times: (1) when scheduling an appointment, (2) when confirming the appointment, and (3) when receiving a new patient letter or communication via snail mail, email, patient portals, or the practice website.

The medical assistant should neither hesitate when stating the approximate amount nor apologize for the fee. Practice appropriate phrases and use an approach that makes it easier for the patient to pay than to avoid payment (see Example 13-8). If the patient cannot pay at the time of service, do not reward such behavior by letting him or her leave quickly.

If a patient is having financial difficulties, this may come out during the initial interview. Then the assistant can discuss a payment plan or a discount if it is warranted. Physicians expect patients to make acceptable monthly payments on their accounts regardless of pending payments by insurance companies.

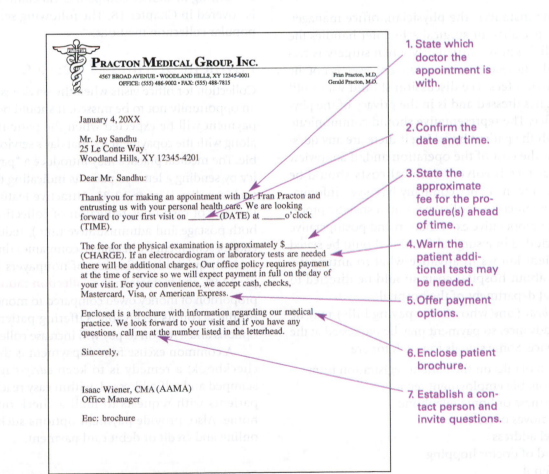

FIGURE 13-2 New patient confirmation letter

EXAMPLE 13-8

Positive Expressions When Asking for Payment

1. When a patient calls for an appointment:

   "Copayment is expected at the time of service."

   "The office visit will be approximately $_____. We accept cash, checks, and credit cards for your convenience."

2. When the patient checks in at the front desk:

   "Your copayment will be $_____ today."

3. When the patient checks out:

   "The office visit is $_____. Would you like to pay by cash, check, or credit card?"

   "I see your deductible has been met and your insurance pays 80%. Your portion of the bill comes to $_____."

In some instances, the physician, office manager, insurance specialist, or surgical scheduler handles the financial discussion, particularly when surgery is recommended. The examination room, however, is not the place to discuss fees. Fee discussion should wait until the patient has dressed and is in the privacy of the physician's office. The representative should communicate directly with the patient by asking if there are any questions about the cost of the operation and, if so, review the surgical fees involved. Surgical costs should be quoted after the insurance company has given information on how much the policy pays on a specific procedure. If the preoperative examination and postoperative care are included in a surgical fee, this should be stated so the patient knows in advance what to anticipate. Questions about hospital costs should be directed to the financial department of the hospital.

A *deadbeat* (one who evades paying bills) may be spotted in advance, so payment may be requested at the time of service. Some signals to watch for are:

1. Unfilled blanks on the patient registration form
2. Questionable employment record
3. No business or home telephone
4. Many moves of residence
5. A motel address
6. A record of doctor hopping
7. No referral
8. No insurance

PATIENT BILLING

Each office has its own policy for fee collection based on whether the patient is (1) insured and a fee-for-service contract is in place, (2) enrolled in a managed care plan with copayment requirements, or (3) not insured.* Collection of fees may also depend on the specialty of the physician, the amount of the average bill, and the patient load. A motivated billing department keeps the following on hand:

- Contracted insurance company's provider-relations contact information
- Copy of the state's prompt-pay law (if applicable)
- List of deadlines that must be met by each payer to submit insurance claims and successfully resubmit denied claims
- Matrix of contracted payers listing what each has agreed to pay for procedure codes the practice submits
- Policy that details when to write off an account or submit it to a collection agency

Billing insurance companies via claim submission is covered in Chapter 18. The following section covers popular collection methods.

Payment at Time of Service

Collection for office visits when the service is rendered is an opportunity not to be missed. It should be stated that payment will be expected when the patient checks in, along with the copayment for that day's service, if applicable. The medical practice may introduce a "pay now" policy by sending a letter to patients indicating the need for such a policy (Figure 13-3). Attractive features include increase of cash flow, reduction of collection costs (in both postage and administrative time), reduced billing chores, settlement by insurance companies directly to the patient, quick identification of nonpayers (see Example 13-9), and increase in the collection ratio, that is, the proportion of money owed compared to money collected on the accounts receivable. Offering patient payment options and a reason to pay will increase collections.

A common excuse for nonpayment is the forgotten checkbook; a remedy is to keep *early-pay envelopes*, stamped and self-addressed, within easy reach to give to patients with requests to mail a check on arrival at home. Also, provide payment options such as paying online and credit or debit card payment.

---

*As of 2014, the Affordable Care Act mandates insurance for all Americans.

PRACTON MEDICAL GROUP, INC.
4567 BROAD AVENUE • WOODLAND HILLS, XY 12345-4700
OFFICE: (555) 486-9002 • FAX: (555) 488-7815

Fran Practon, M.D.
Gerald Practon, M.D.

February 6, 20XX

Mrs. Lupe Centeno
369 Everly Court
Woodland Hills, XY 12345-4201

Dear Mrs. Centeno:

We find that we are confronted with increasing costs for our medical ◄── **1. State the reason why a new policy is required.**
services and supplies used in rendering professional care to our patients.

Rather than raise our fees, we are asking for your help in a new cost
cutting plan. Beginning on (DATE- one to two months in advance),
we will ask you to pay at the time of your office visit. With your ◄── **2. Ask for the patient's cooperation.**
cooperation, we may significantly reduce the costs of billing and
bookkeeping.

Perhaps there may be an occasion when it will be necessary for you
to request a statement rather than pay at the time of service. We will ◄── **3. Give options for other types of situations.**
continue to recognize that need as well as those instances when
payment plans need to be set up for patients who require extensive
treatment.

We hope that this explanation of our new system made well in
advance will lead to your full understanding and willingness to
participate. If you have questions about this or any of our office ◄── **4. Leave the door open for questions the patient may have.**
policies, we will be pleased to discuss them with you. We value you
as our patient and will continue to provide you with our best
professional care.

Sincerely,

Gerald Practon, MD

lf

FIGURE 13-3 Pay now policy letter

EXAMPLE 13-9

Payment Incentives at Time Services Are Rendered

1. Accepting cash, checks, or credit/debit cards offers patients convenience.

2. Paying at the time of service helps the practice avoid further billing costs, which contribute to rising health care costs.

3. Paying insurance deductibles and copayment fees at the time of service allows the insurance company to take care of the entire balance after billing.

4. Paying in monthly installments to a credit card company eases monthly debt.

5. Avoiding collection agencies decreases bad credit reports.

Meeting with the Patient

Meeting face to face with the patient at the time of service regarding outstanding balances is often more successful than telephoning or sending statements. However, an appointment reminder call can be combined with an account call to inform him or her of any balance due.

The day before the visit, the patient appointment schedule can be printed from the computer or copied from the appointment book. Each patient's account balance is reviewed and balances over 60 days are flagged. Upon arrival, the patient is courteously escorted into a private room to discuss the bill. The patient can see how committed the assistant is in regard to solving the collection problem, and the chance of a mutually satisfactory resolution is greatly improved. Although the physician does not perform credit and collection work, he or she can make patients aware of their outstanding debt. The realization that the physician is aware of the delinquency is often effective in encouraging payment.

Multipurpose Billing Form

The **multipurpose billing form** is a combination bill, insurance form, and routing document, which may be given to the patient at the time of the office visit (Figure 13-4). It is also referred to as a *charge slip*, *communicator*, *encounter form*, *fee ticket*, *patient service slip*, *routing form*, *superbill*, and *transaction slip*. The form has been used in a manual (pegboard) bookkeeping system (Chapter 15), but can also be used in an EHR system. It contains the patient's name, date, services rendered, procedure codes, diagnostic codes, the physician's identifying data, and a section to indicate the patient's next appointment. It may also include an assignment of benefits, other insurance requirements, and a section for the patient to complete.

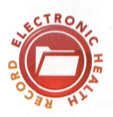

When using an EHR system, a paperless encounter form is available to the physician in the treatment room and when using a paper-based system it is clipped to the front of patients' charts. The form contains all services and procedures typically performed in the physician's office and about 25 to 50 of the practices' most common diagnoses—precoded. Some diagnostic codes may have a short blank line following the code. This is to allow entry of additional characters, so specific diagnostic codes can be reported. The physician indicates procedures that are performed during the office visit, checks off or enters all applicable diagnoses, and at the bottom of the slip indicates if the patient should return for an appointment.

The transaction slip is routed back to the receptionist to make a return appointment and to be totaled for payment. It is designed to facilitate coding for common services and procedures, encourage payment immediately after services have been rendered, provide insurance billing information, and eliminate paperwork.

In some states, private insurance programs still accept a multipurpose billing form from the patient and in some cases the insurance benefits can be assigned to the physician directly; the physician's signature is not

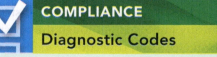

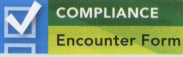

necessarily required. It may be used as a *receipt* if the patient paid for services at the time they were rendered, or a receipt may be printed from the computer.

This form is, in some respects, an attending physician's statement. It is one of the most important tools in the medical practice and should be prenumbered, filed in numerical and chronological order with the most recent first, and used for audit control. A multipurpose form should be annually reviewed and updated to include new or revised procedure and diagnostic codes and any other changes in the practice. All fees and payments should be posted daily by either entering them into the patient's electronic financial account or to a ledger and daysheet.

Computer-Generated Encounter Forms

Some computer software programs offer a "check-in" process, which runs through a series of screens that has practice-specific alerts designed so that the receptionist can view details about the patient's account prior to printing an encounter form—for example, checking the patient's appointment status, demographics (active/inactive), insurance plan, account status (paid in full/bad debt), and producing a balance due summary. By viewing these screens, the receptionist can quickly be brought up to date about each patient at the time of check-in.

Monthly Itemized Statement

Most practices generate an itemized statement or computerized **bill** on a monthly basis, indicating fees owed for services rendered. The same information is found on a ledger card, which is illustrated in Figure 13-5. A **ledger card** is a paper-based financial record showing charges, payments, adjustments, and balance owed and is created for each patient when he or she first receives medical services. Although ledger cards are obsolete in EHR systems, they contain the same information as electronic patient accounts and are presented here to enable a better understanding of the computations that occur on financial accounts. Paper-based medical offices sometimes copy ledgers as monthly itemized statements.

STATE LIC. # C1503X
SOC. SEC. # 000-11-0000
PIN # _____

Practon Medical Group, Inc.
4567 Broad Avenue
Woodland Hills, XY 12345-4700

Phone: 555-486-9002

1. Physician's identifying data

☐ PRIVATE	☐ BLUECROSS	☐ IND.	☐ MEDICARE	☐ MEDI-CAL	☐ HMO	☑ PPO

PATIENT'S LAST NAME	FIRST	ACCOUNT #	BIRTHDATE	SEX ☐ MALE	TODAY'S DATE
Chang	Kim	2936	10 / 05 / 41	☑ FEMALE	03 / 05 / XX

INSURANCE COMPANY	SUBSCRIBER	PLAN #	SUB. #	GROUP
Aetna	self		463-XX-3699	

2. Patient and insurance data

ASSIGNMENT: I hereby assign my insurance benefits to be paid directly to the undersigned physician. I am financially responsible for non-covered services.
SIGNED: (Patient, or Parent, if Minor)   DATE: /   /

RELEASE: I hereby authorize the physician to release to my insurance carriers any information required to process this claim.
SIGNED: (Patient, or Parent, if Minor)   DATE: /   /

3. Assignment of benefits and authorization to release information

✔	DESCRIPTION	CODE		FEE	✔	DESCRIPTION	CODE	FEE	✔	DESCRIPTION	CODE	FEE
	OFFICE VISITS	**NEW**	**EST.**			Venipuncture	36415			**OFFICE PROCEDURES**		
	Blood Pressure Check		99211			TB Skin Test	86580			Anoscopy	46600	
	Level II	99202	99212			Hematocrit	85013			Ear Lavage	69210	
✔	Level III	99203	99213	70.92		Glucose Finger Stick	82948			Spirometry	94010	
	Level IV	99204	99214			**IMMUNIZATIONS**				Nebulizer Rx	94664	
	Level V	99205	99215			Allergy Inj. X1	95115			EKG	93000	
	PREVENTIVE EXAMS	**NEW**	**EST.**			Allergy Inj. X2	95117			**SURGERY**		
	Age 65 & Older	99387	99397			Trigger Pt. Inj.	20552			Mole Removal (1st)	17000	
	Age 40 - 64	99386	99396			Therapeutic Inj.	96372			(2nd to 14th)	17003	
	Age 18 - 39	99385	99395			**VACCINATION PRODUCTS**				Flat Warts (1st - 14th)	17110	
	Age 12 - 17	99384	99394			DT < 7 yrs	90702			15 or More	17111	
	Age 5 - 11	99383	99393			DT 7 yrs & older	90714			Biopsy, 1 Lesion	11100	
	Age 1 - 4	99382	99392			MMR	90707			Addt'l. Lesions	11101	
	Infant	99381	99391			Polio Inj	90713			Endometrial Bx	58100	
	Newborn Ofc		99432			Flu (IIV3)	90654			Skin Tags to 15	11200	
	OB / NEWBORN CARE					Flu (IIV4)	90630			Each Addt'l. 10	11201	
	OB Package		59400			Hib	90647			I & D Abscess	10060	
	Post-Partum Visit N/C					Hepatitis B Vac	90746			**SUPPLIES / MISCELLANEOUS**		
	LAB PROCEDURES					Pneumovax (13)	90670			Surgical Tray	99070	
	Urine Dip		81000			Pneumovax (23)	90732			Handling Charge	99000	
✔	UA Qualitative		81005	15.00		**VACCINE ADMINISTRATION**				Special Report	99080	
	Pregnancy Urine		81025			Age: Through 18 yrs. (1st inj.)	90460			**DOCTOR'S NOTES:**		
	Wet Mount		87210			Age: Through 18 yrs. (ea. addt'l. inj.)	90461					
	KOH Prep		87220			Adult (1st inj.)	90471					
	Occult Blood		82270			Adult (ea. addt'l. inj.)	90472					

4. Codes for professional services

DIAGNOSES	**ICD-10-CM**

___ Abdominal Pain/unspec. .R10.9	___ Colitis/unspec. K51.90	___ FUO R50.9	___ Osteoarthritis (site) . . . .M19._
___ Abscess, Cutaneous . . . .L02._	___ Confusion R41.0	___ Gastritis K29.70	___ Otitis Media H66.9
___ Allergic Reaction . . . . .T78.40_	___ CHF I50.9	___ Gastroenteritis (Colitis) .K52.9	___ Parkinson's Disease . .G20
___ Alzheimer's Disease . . .G30	___ Constipation K59.00	___ G.I. Bleed K92.2	___ Pharyngitis, Acute J02.9
___ Anemia/unspec. D64.9	___ COPD J44.9	___ Gout/unspec. M10.9	___ Pleurisy R09.1
___ Angina/unspec. I20.9	___ Cough R05	___ Headache R51	___ Pneumonia J18.9
___ Anorexia R63.0	___ Crohn's Disease/unspec. K50.90	___ Health Exam . . . . .Z00._	___ Pneumonia, Viral J12.9
___ Anxiety/unspec. F41.9	___ CVA I63.9	___ Hematuria/unspec. . . .R31.9	___ Prostatitis/unspec. N41.9
___ Apnea, Sleep G47.30	___ Decubitus Ulcer . . . . . .L89._	___ Herpes Simplex B00.9	___ PVD I73.9
___ Arrhythmia, Cardiac . . .I49.9	___ Dehydration E86.0	___ Herpes Zoster B02.9	___ Radiculopathy . . . . . . .M54.1_
___ Arthritis, Rheumatoid . .M06.9	___ Dementia/Senility R41.81	___ Hiatal Hernia K44.9	___ Rectal Bleeding K62.5
___ Asthma/unspec. J45.909	___ Depression, Major/unsp. .F32.9	___ HTN (HBP) I10	___ Renal Failure N19
___ Atrial Fibrillation, Parox .I48.0	___ Diab I, no complications .E10.9	___ Hyperlipidemia/unspec. .E78.5	___ Sciatica . . . . .M54.3_
___ B-12 Deficiency E53.8	___ Diab II, no complications E11.9	___ Hypothyroidism/unspec. .E03.9	___ Shortness of Breath . . .R06.02
___ Back Pain, Low M54.5	___ w/Kidney complic. . .E11.2_	___ Impotence . . . . .N52._	___ Sinusitis, Chr./unspec. . .J32.9
___ BPH N40	___ w/Ophthalmic compl. E11.3_	___ Influenza, Respiratory . .J11.1	___ Syncope R55
___ Bradycardia/unspec. . . .R00.1	___ w/Neurolog. compl. .E11.4_	___ Insomnia G47.0	___ Tachycardia/unspec. . . .R00.0
___ Bronchitis, Acute . . . . .J20._	___ w/Circulatory cmpl. .E11.5_	___ IBS, Diarrhea K58.0	___ Tachy., Supraventric. . .I47.1
___ Bronchitis, Chronic . . .J42	___ Insulin Use Z79.4	___ Lupus, Systemic Erythem. M32.9	___ Tendinitis/unspec. M77.9
___ Bursitis/unspec. M71.9	___ Diarrhea/unspec. R19.7	___ MI, Acute . . . . .I21._	___ TIA G45.9
___ CA, Breast . . . . .C50._	___ Diverticulitis K57.92	___ MI, Old I25.2	___ Ulcer, Duodenal/unspec. K26.9
___ CA, Lung . . . . .C34._	___ Diverticulosis K57.90	___ Migraine . . . . .G43.9_	___ Ulcer, Gastric/unspec. . .K25.9
___ CA, Prostate C61	___ Dizziness R42	___ Myalgia M79.1	___ Ulcer, Peptic/unspec. . .K27.9
___ Cellulitis . . . . .L03._	___ Dysuria R30.0	___ Neck Pain M54.2	___ URI/unspec. J06.9
___ Chest Pain/unspec. . . .R07.9	___ Edema/unspec. R60.9	___ Neuropathy G62.9	✔ UTI N39.0
___ Cirrhosis, Liver/unspec. .K74.60	___ Endocarditis I38	___ Nausea R11.0	___ Vertigo R42
___ Cold, Common J00	___ Esophageal Reflux K21.0	___ Nausea/Vomiting R11.2	___ Weight Gain R63.5
	___ Fatigue (Lethargy) R53.83	___ Obesity/unspec. E66.9	___ Weight Loss R63.4

5. Diagnostic codes

6. Additional diagnoses

DIAGNOSIS / ADDITIONAL DESCRIPTION:	DOCTOR'S SIGNATURE / DATE
	Fran Practon, MD

RETURN APPOINTMENT INFORMATION:	-WITH WHOM	SELF/OTHER	REC'D. BY:	
DAYS _____ WKS. 2 MOS. _____			☐ CASH	TOTAL TODAY'S FEE: 85.92
PLEASE REMEMBER THAT PAYMENT IS YOUR OBLIGATION, REGARDLESS OF INSURANCE OR OTHER THIRD PARTY INVOLVEMENT.			☐ CHECK # _____	AMOUNT REC'D. TODAY: 0

7. Appointment information

8. Total charges and payments received

INSUR-A-BILL ® BIBBERO SYSTEMS, INC. • PETALUMA, CA • © 7/90 (BM1092)   (REV. 01/12)

FIGURE 13-4 Multipurpose billing form; procedure codes for professional services are taken from the *Current Procedural Terminology (CPT)** codebook and diagnostic codes are taken from the *International Classification of Diseases, 10th revision, Clinical Modification (ICD-10-CM) codebook*

PRACTON MEDICAL GROUP, INC.

4567 BROAD AVENUE • WOODLAND HILLS, XY 12345-4700
OFFICE: (555) 486-9002 • FAX: (555) 488-7815

Fran Practon, M.D.
Gerald Practon, M.D.

Mr. Marius Popa
1325 Bunsen Street
Woodland Hills, XY 12345-0001

Phone No.(H) 555-320-7145 **(W)** 555-452-8581 **Birthdate** 06-05-1976
Insurance Co. United PPO Insurance **Policy No.** 3467X

DATE	REFERENCE	DESCRIPTION	CHARGES	CREDITS PYMNTS.	ADJ.	BALANCE
		BALANCE FORWARD ➜				
7-4-XX	99202	OV, Level 2	51 91			51 91
7-4-XX	93000	ECG	34 26			86 17
7-14-XX	99212	OV, Level 2	28 55			114 72
7-14-XX	7/4 to 7/14	United insurance billed				114 72
8-30-XX	Voucher #7504	ROA United insurance		91 78		22 94
8-30-XX	7/4 to 7/14	Billed pt 20% copay				22 94
NOTE: YOUR INSURANCE HAS PAID, PLEASE REMIT BALANCE DUE						22 94
9-12-XX	Ck #2087	ROA Pt pmt		22 94		0

RB40BC-2-96   PLEASE PAY LAST AMOUNT IN BALANCE COLUMN ➜

THIS IS A COPY OF YOUR ACCOUNT AS IT APPEARS ON OUR RECORDS

1. Itemized fees for professional services with line-by-line description.

2. Insurance claim submitted showing dates of service billed.

3. Payment received on account from insurance, listing voucher number. Insurance paid 80 percent.

4. Billed patient 20 percent copayment.

5. Patient's payment check received, listing check number.

FIGURE 13-5 Ledger card illustrating posting of professional service descriptions, fees, payments, and balance due

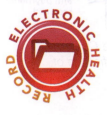

In an EHR system, the computer can be directed to search the database and print financial account records for patients who have outstanding balances. An individual or an entire family can be listed on the account and the insurance claim submission date indicated. The statement usually shows a breakdown of the amounts that are due or delinquent, and how many days they are delinquent. This information is called *aging analysis* and is a feature usually not found in a manual bookkeeping system (see Aging Accounts presented later in this chapter).

In the event an insurance company sends a check and the patient has already paid, a credit balance will appear indicating an overpayment on the account and the patient should be sent a statement showing that there is a credit balance (see Chapter 15). The patient has the right to request a refund for the credit amount. A phrase or message can appear on the statement to

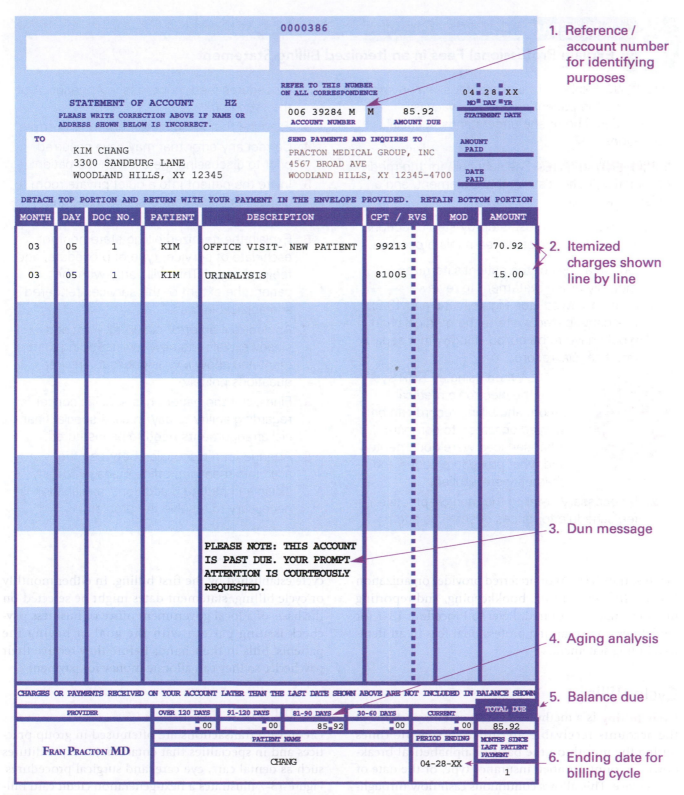

FIGURE 13-6 Computer-generated monthly itemized billing statement showing a dun message

promote payment. This is referred to as a *dun message*, which is described in more detail later in this chapter (Figure 13-6). Statements should be sent to patients on a regular basis about the same time each month. Such

statements are usually not generated for patients on the Medicaid or workers' compensation programs, because there is no patient responsibility. If a patient belongs to a managed care plan, such as a health maintenance

PROCEDURE 13-1

Explain Professional Fees in an Itemized Billing Statement

OBJECTIVE: Explain professional fees in a private setting, so the patient's right of privacy is observed and he or she understands financial obligations.

EQUIPMENT/SUPPLIES: Fee schedule for the medical practice, patient's monthly statement, and a quiet private room.

DIRECTIONS: Follow these step-by-step directions, which include rationales, to learn this procedure.

1. Obtain a copy of the patient's itemized monthly billing statement to review amounts owed (see Figures 13-5 and 13-6). In a paper-based system, the medical chart would have to be pulled along with a separate financial record.

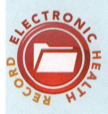

   When using an EHR system, the electronic medical record and billing record can be viewed onscreen to compare what services were documented and what procedure codes and charges were applied.

2. If necessary, refer to the medical practice's fee schedule for prices of services and

procedures (see mock fees in Appendix A of the *Workbook*).

3. Examine the billing statement for any errors.

4. Correct any error that may have occurred prior to discussing the bill with the patient.

5. Invite the patient into a quiet private room to discuss financial matters, observing the patient's right to privacy.

6. Explain the itemized billing statement for each date of service, type of procedure, and fee(s) charged. This will verify with the patient the extent of the services rendered and applicable fees.

7. Apologize if an error occurred. Print and clearly explain the new revised billing statement and show a willingness to answer questions politely.

8. Find out if the patient has specific concerns regarding ability to pay, in case special financial arrangements need to be instituted.

9. Arrange for a discussion between the accounts manager, office manager, or physician and patient if additional explanation is necessary to resolve the problem.

organization (HMO) or preferred provider organization (PPO), different billing, bookkeeping, and reporting methods may be required. Refer to Procedure 13-1 for guidelines on explaining professional fees in an itemized billing statement.

Cycle Billing

Cycle billing is a method in which certain portions of the accounts receivable are billed at specific times during the month on the basis of alphabetical breakdown, account number, insurance type, or the date of first service. This allows continuous cash flow throughout the month, relieves the pressure of having to mail all statements at one time, and distributes patient telephone calls regarding account questions. Cycle billing, based on date of first service, enables the first patient statement to be in the mail within days of the first visit; subsequent billings are then mailed monthly in the

cycle established by the first billing. In either monthly or cycle billing, statement dates might be selected on the basis of a local government office or business paycheck-issuing pattern with the goal of having the patients' bills in their hands before they receive their paychecks, so they can allocate money for payment.

Credit Card Billing

Credit card transactions are often used in group practices and in specialties that entail major expenditures such as dental care, eye care, and surgical procedures. Figure 13-7 illustrates a next-generation credit card billing machine. After swiping a card, the card and amount are verified by the credit card company. The patient makes payment directly to the credit card company, which sends the payment to the physician. Always check with the credit card company for specific procedures and written instructions for completing telephone

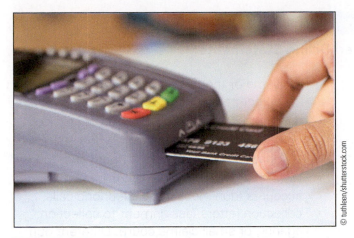

FIGURE 13-7 Next generation chip-enabled credit card machine

transactions. Credit card companies (e.g., Visa, Master-Card, Discover) charge a minimum monthly fee per location as well as a percentage based on the charges submitted. This method reduces office overhead and collection costs. However, under certain circumstances, banks may hold participating merchants or professionals liable for the collection of credit card accounts. For instance, if the bank previously circulated a list of card numbers that should not be honored and if the physician accepted one, the physician could be responsible for the amount charged.

A record of the credit card number should always be kept with the patient's financial records and may be useful if the patient needs to be traced or if collection action is necessary. If the patient is reluctant to charge a large amount to a credit card, a payment plan may be instituted, which allows monthly payments via credit card (Figure 13-8).

Debit Cards

A **debit card**, also known as a *check card*, is used by bank customers to either withdraw cash from any affiliated automated teller machine (ATM) or make electronic transfers of cash from a customer's bank account to a merchant's account. A small fee may be charged to the customer's checking account when the card is used; however, this fee is usually applied once a month regardless of how many times the card is used during the month. Since these cards accompany checking accounts and are easy to use, more patients will have these. Cards are issued either by banks or through credit card companies (e.g., Visa or Master-Card debit card).

PRACTON MEDICAL GROUP, INC.
4567 BROAD AVENUE • WOODLAND HILLS, XY 12345-0001
OFFICE: (555) 486-9002 • FAX: (555) 488-7815
Fran Practon, M.D.
Gerald Practon, M.D.

AUTHORIZATION TO CHARGE CREDIT CARD

Patient Name _Sylvia Kostenbauer_

Cardholder Name _Sylvia Kostenbauer_

Credit Card Company _VISA_

Card Number _7144322152087XX_   Expiration Date _08/XX_

I authorize _Fran Practon MD_ to charge my credit card $ _50.00_ on the _5th_ of each month until my balance of $ _200.00_ is paid in full. I understand that if the charge is not accepted by my credit card company, I will immediately make the monthly payment to the practice.

I understand that I may cancel this authorization at any time, but by doing so I acknowledge that the balance owing will be due and payable in full.

Sylvia Kostenbauer   _2/19/XX_
Signature   Date

FIGURE 13-8 Authorization to charge credit card form

There are two types of debit cards: off-line and on-line. Off-line debit cards do not require a personal identification number (PIN) and generate an electronic check that is debited in about 1 to 3 days against the bank account like a handwritten check. On-line debit cards require a PIN and withdraw money immediately from the holder's account.

If the office processes credit cards electronically, then it can usually use the same electronic credit card machine to swipe the debit card for verification and approval (see Figure 13-7). The bank that issued the debit card is responsible for paying the funds that were approved, so there are no checks returned for nonsufficient funds.

Smart Cards

A *smart card*, like a debit card, is used as an ATM/debit/credit card but is embedded with a programmable microchip that is able to hold much more information. They can be used for banking, electronic cash, government identification, and wireless communication; to purchase goods and services; and to access medical, financial, and other records. They can also store receipts electronically but require special equipment to read the microchip. They improve the convenience and security of any transaction and prevent fraud because data stored on the card is encrypted. They are popular in

PROCEDURE 13-2

Separate and Prepare Monthly Itemized Billing Statements

OBJECTIVE: Separate delinquent accounts and prepare monthly itemized billing statements.

EQUIPMENT/SUPPLIES: Computer, patient accounts, and billing statement forms or ledger cards.

DIRECTIONS: Follow these step-by-step directions, which include rationales, to learn this procedure.

1. Gather all patient accounts or ledger cards with outstanding balances.

2. Separate the accounts/ledgers that have been marked as delinquent. The computer will automatically sort accounts according to the "age" of the account.

3. Prepare the itemized billing statements for the monthly billing, verifying the following information:
   a. Date of the billing statement
   b. Name and address of the person responsible for payment

   c. Name of the patient if different from the person responsible for payment
   d. Itemized dates of procedures or services and charges
   e. Unpaid balance carried forward and due

4. Determine action to take on delinquent accounts (dun messages, telephone calls, collection letters, assignment to collection agency, or small-claims court). Different dun messages can be selected to appear on accounts, according to the "age" of the account.

5. Document on each account the action taken, in case further follow-up is necessary. Most software programs have a comment area attached to the financial account so that notes may be left when action has been taken (e.g., telephone calls).

Europe but have not been used to their potential yet in the United States. American Express offers "blue cards," which are similar.

Online Payment

Medical practices that offer a secure online communication tool to pay for medical services increase collection costs and reduce billing expenses. Patients welcome this option, especially those who already use the Internet to take care of other financial transactions, such as banking, retail shopping, travel expenses, and so forth.

Billing Services

Some medical practices employ billing services to prepare and mail patient bills. These services have a number of advantages over billing done by office personnel, on office time, using office equipment and supplies:

- Patient understanding of statements is improved because all charges and payments are shown.
- Prompt billing is ensured, because sending out statements is the business of the service; the medical practice is free of office disruptions while billing.

- Billing services save the medical office money because expensive billing equipment is not required and valuable space need not be allocated for billing supplies.
- Collection calls to patients do not disrupt the practice, because they are handled by the billing service.
- Patient questions regarding charges are answered by the service.

Most billing services use professional computerized monthly statements generated with dun messages, if required. These billing services either pick up copies of multipurpose forms or receive account information electronically to produce statements and complete insurance claims. Refer to Procedure 13-2 for guidelines on preparing monthly billing statements.

RECEIVING INSURANCE PAYMENT

After a patient has had services rendered, a clean insurance claim is processed (Chapter 18) and payment is received from an insurance plan or program. The assistant then posts the payment to the patient's account in an EHR system, or to a ledger card and daysheet in a paper-based system. Details about posting are discussed in Chapter 15, *Bookkeeping*. In order to understand the amount received by insurance companies, it is necessary to interpret the document that accompanies the insurance check or voucher, referred to as the *explanation of benefit*.

Explanation of Benefits

Accompanying the insurance check, an **explanation of benefits (EOB)** form is generated and transmitted electronically or sent on paper to the physician's practice. If the patient is insured with two companies, assignment should have been obtained for both insurance carriers and the primary carrier billed. When the primary carrier pays, an electronic crossover claim is transmitted to the secondary carrier, or when processing a paper claim, it is submitted to the secondary carrier with an attached photocopy of the primary carrier's EOB. If payment is reduced or the claim is not paid, a code on the EOB will indicate the status of the claim. The following terms are commonly used on the EOB document:

- *Billed amount (charged amount, fee)*—The amount the physician charges the patient and insurance company according to the fee schedule
- *Allowed amount (approved amount, covered amount, covered charges)*—The amount the insurance company will pay under contract with the physician
- *Write off (adjustment, contract adjustment, courtesy adjustment)*—For contracted physicians, the difference between the billed amount and the allowed amount; it is deducted from the books, that is, patient account or ledger
- *Copayment (copay)*—A flat fee that the patient owes (up front) prior to services being rendered
- *Coinsurance payment (coinsurance copay, cost share)*—The amount the patient is responsible for after insurance payment; it may be a percentage of the allowed amount, for example, 20%
- *Payment (insurance payment, contract payment, payment voucher, adjudication)*—Amount of monies received from the insurance carrier, plan, or program
- *Notes (glossary, codes)*—Codes with definitions describing action taken on the claim (e.g., R1TFP—"your other health insurance was considered in the final disposition of this claim").

For an example of an explanation of benefits form, see Figure 13-9.

Medicare Remittance Advice

The **Medicare Remittance Advice (RA)** is a document, similar to the EOB, that accompanies the payment check from the Medicare carrier, showing the breakdown of the amounts charged, allowed, paid, and denied (Figures 13-10A and 13-10B). It may be sent electronically to the provider and the check may be automatically deposited in the medical practice's bank account.

Medicare Summary Notice

Within 30 days of processing a claim, Medicare contractors issue a **Medicare Summary Notice (MSN)** to each beneficiary (Example 13-10). The summary, written in laymen's terms, indicates the disposition of the claim including the status of the deductible, services received, and appeal rights. If a claim was processed but no payment was made, the MSN is issued on a quarterly (90-day) basis.

HISTORY OF CREDIT

Credit for medical services and credit cards grew out of the Depression of the 1930s. Through the Depression years and before, when a patient was unable to pay cash, the doctor was paid in chickens, vegetables, or other material or by an exchange of labor. In societies, such as ancient China, the doctor regularly visited the patient every 3 to 6 months in order to keep the patient healthy and was paid when the patient was well; payment was suspended when the patient became ill, until the patient was cured or much improved.

Times have changed; today in Western society, payment is now expected at the time of service even when an insurance contract is in place. Patients frequently use some type of debit or credit card and in large clinics or a hospital setting, patients may use a *patient record card* that when passed through an electronic terminal will give a printout of their medical history, insurance coverage, and financial information. Patients may authorize via the card the billing of the insurance company or their credit card, so the doctor receives payment quickly.

CREDIT AND COLLECTION LAWS

Credit laws govern the way fees are collected. To keep well informed, the assistant needs to be aware of federal laws that regulate the entire nation and should obtain information about state laws from the state attorney general's office.

EXPLANATION OF BENEFITS

XYZ INSURANCE COMPANY
P.O. BOX 1000
LOS ANGELES, CA
91470-0001

| ISSUE DATE | PAGE E026780 |
| November 16, 20XX | 0001 of 0002 |

PRACTON MEDICAL GROUP, INC.
4569 BROADWAY AVENUE
WOODLAND HILLS, XY 12345-4700

SUBSCRIBER NAME:	Winesberry, Wayne
IDENTIFICATION NUMBER:	1234567
GROUP NUMBER:	G555
GROUP NAME:	Small Group PPO
PRODUCT:	PPO $40 Copay Plan

Patient's Name:	Winesberry Wayne	Sequence Number:	953766324 200400475
Claim Number:	678-000-9439	Provider of Service:	Fran T. Practon, MD
Claim Processed Date:	11/09/XX	Place of Service:	Office
Claim Received Date:	11/08/XX		
Paid Amount:	$14.77	To: Fran T. Practon MD	
It is your responsibility to pay:	$40.00	It is not your responsibility to pay: $40.23	

SERVICE DATE(S)	TYPE OF SERVICE	TOTAL BILLED	AMOUNT NOT ALLOWED	PATIENT SAVINGS	APPLIED TO DEDUCTIBLE	COINSURANCE COPAYMENT AMOUNT	CLAIMS PAYMENT
10/27/XX	Medical Visit	70.00		15.23/01		40.00/02	14.77
10/27/XX	Supplies & Materials	25.00	25.00/03				0.00
TOTAL THIS CLAIM		95.00	25.00	15.23	0.00	40.00	14.77

DETAIL MESSAGE:

01- This is the amount in excess of the allowed expense for a participating provider. The member, therefore, is not responsible for this amount.

02 - This amount is the Home and Office copayment amount specified by the terms of the member's benefit agreement.

03 - CPT Code 99070 is no longer accepted. It is requested that the provider of service please rebill the service(s) for this claim using the appropriate HCPCS code(s). The member is not responsible for this amount.

FOR INFORMATION CALL:	CUSTOMER SERVICE DEPARTMENT AT: (800) 627-0000
MAIL ALL INQUIRIES OR CLAIMS TO:	XYZ INSURANCE COMPANY
	P.O. BOX 1000
	LOS ANGELES, CA
	91470-0001

WE SUGGEST THAT YOU RETAIN THIS COPY FOR INCOME TAX RECORDS.

FIGURE 13-9 Example of Explanation of Benefits form from XYZ Insurance Co. showing claim payment of $14.77 (billed amount [95.00] minus not-allowed amount [25.00] minus amount over allowed amount [15.23] minus patient copayment amount [40.00] equals physician payment [14.77])

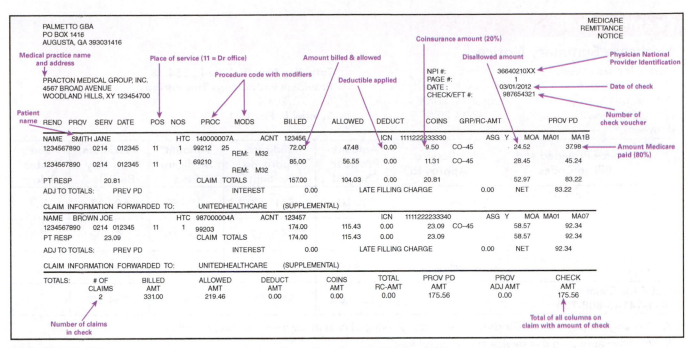

FIGURE 13-10A   Example of an electronic Medicare Remittance Advice (RA)

GLOSSARY	GROUP REASON MOA AND REASON CODES
45	Charges exceed your contracted/legislated fee arrangement. This change to be effective 6/1/07: Charge exceeds fee schedule/maximum allowable or contracted/legislated fee arrangement. (Use Group Codes PR or CO depending upon liability.)
CO	Contractural Obligations
M32	Alert: This is a conditional payment made pending a decision on this service by the patient's primary payer. This payment may be subject to refund upon your receipt of any additional payment for this service from another payer. You must contact this office immediately upon receipt of an additional payment for this service.
MA01	Alert: If you do not agree with what we approved for these services, you may appeal our decision. To make sure that we are fair to you, we require another individual that did not process your initial claim to conduct the appeal. However, in order to be eligible for an appeal, you must write to us within 120 days of the date you received this notice, unless you have a good reason for being late.
MA07	Alert: The claim information has also been forwarded to Medicaid for review.
MA18	Alert: The claim information is also being forwarded to the patient's supplemental insurer. Send any questions regarding supplemental benefits to them.
PR	Patient Responsibility

FIGURE 13-10B   Example of glossary of remarks and reason codes attached to an electronic Medicare Remittance Advice

EXAMPLE 13-10

Medicare Summary Notice

Notice for Troy Wells

Medicare Number	XXX-XX-XXXXA
Date of This Notice	August 14, 20XX
Claims Processed Between	5/20–8/14 20XX

Total You May Be Billed $34.38
Providers with Claims This Period
May 20, 20XX
Samuel R. Fox MD

Service Provided and Billing Codes	Service Approved?	Amount Provider Charged	Medicare-Approved Amount	Amount Medicare Paid	Maximum You May Be Billed	See Notes Below
Established patient office visit (99214)	Yes	$120.00	$115.63	$90.65	**$23.13**	A, B, C
Air and bone conduction assessment of hearing loss (92557)	Yes	$65.00	$40.42	$31.69	**$8.08**	A, B, C
Eardrum testing using ear probe (92567)	Yes	$30.00	$15.84	$12.42	**$3.17**	A, B, C
Total for Claim #11-14148-808-730		$215.00	$171.89	$134.76	**$34.38**	

A A change in payment methods has resulted in a reduced or zero payment for this procedure.

B We have approved this service at a reduced level.

C After your deductible and coinsurance were applied, the amount Medicare paid was reduced due to Federal, State, and local rules.

Fair Debt Collection Practices Act

Although the FDCPA is not designed to govern most medical collection activities, it does affect anyone who collects a debt in the same manner as a collection agency. The following guidelines will help avoid negative patient relations and enhance collections:

1. Debtors may be contacted only once a day.
2. Calls may be placed after 8 a.m. and before 9 p.m.
3. Debtors may not be contacted on a Sunday or a day the debtor recognizes as the Sabbath.
4. Contact the debtor at work only if attempts to contact the debtor elsewhere have failed; if the employer disapproves, no contact should be made.
5. Collectors must identify themselves and the medical practice they represent; they must not mislead the patient.
6. The physician or representative may not contact the debtor except to convey the message that there will be no further contact if the debtor states in writing that the physician is not to contact him or her.
7. An action must be taken, such as turning the patient over to a collection agency, if the physician or representative states that a certain action will be taken.
8. All contact must be made through the attorney if an attorney represents the debtor.
9. The medical assistant may contact other people for tracing purposes only; the nature of the call should not be disclosed to another party.
10. Postcards are not allowed for collection purposes.
11. Collectors should not threaten or use obscene language.
12. Collectors are obligated to send the patient written verification of the name of the creditor and the amount of the debt within 5 days of the initial contact.

Equal Credit Opportunity Act

Under the Federal Equal Credit Opportunity Act, which became law in 1975, if the physician agrees to extend credit to one patient, the same financial arrangement must be extended to all patients who request it. Refusal can be based only on ability or inability to pay, and the physician must either tell the patient the reason for a credit refusal or give the patient notice that no credit will be granted. The patient then has 60 days to request the reason in writing why credit was denied. Once the physician has granted credit, the Equal Credit law coverage applies.

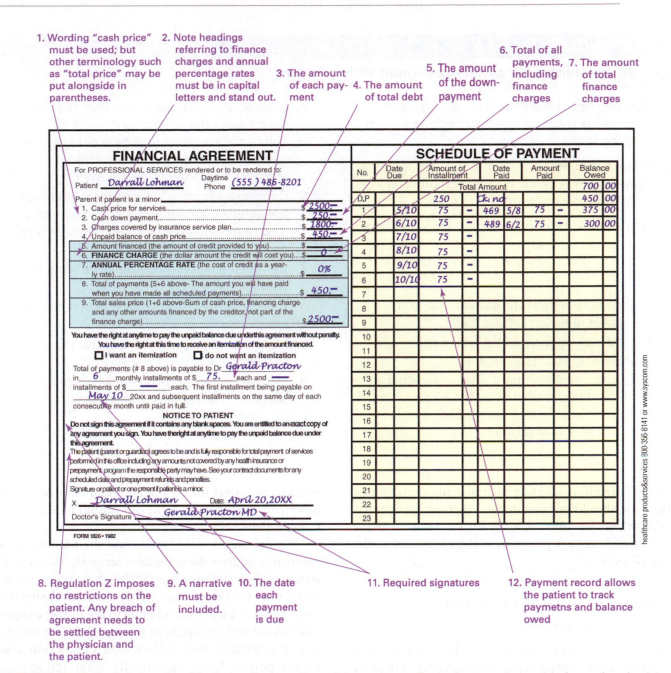

FIGURE 13-11 Truth in Lending Disclosure Form or Financial Agreement Form. By completing this form, the physician provides all information on full disclosure required by the Truth in Lending Act Regulation Z.

Federal Truth in Lending Act

The Federal Truth in Lending Act, which became law on July 1, 1960, governs anyone who charges interest or agrees to more than four payments for a given service. If the physician charges interest rates, the rates may be governed by state laws; therefore, it is important to check with the appropriate agency before beginning such charges.

Regulation Z requires that a disclosure form (Figure 13-11) be completed and signed when a payment plan is instituted; one copy goes to the patient and one to the office files (see Procedure 13-3). According to the Federal Trade Commission (FTC), the Truth in Lending Act does not apply and no disclosures are required if a patient offers to pay in installments or whenever convenient. In discussing an installment plan with a patient, the assistant would cover the amount of the total debt, the down payment, the amount and date of each installment, and the date of final payment. However, if a patient has a delinquent account, the courts have said that continued medical care implies an extension of credit, even if the old account remains

PROCEDURE 13-3

Establish a Financial Agreement with a Patient

OBJECTIVE: Assist the patient in making credit arrangements by completing and signing a Truth in Lending form.

EQUIPMENT/SUPPLIES: Patient's account or ledger, calendar, Truth in Lending form, computer, calculator, and quiet private room.

DIRECTIONS: Follow these step-by-step directions, which include rationales, to learn this procedure. Job Skill 13-6 is presented in the *Workbook* for practice.

1. Discuss the patient's balance due and answer questions about credit.
2. Inform the patient of the office policy about extending credit payments.
3. Discuss an installment plan, including the amount of the total debt, the down payment, amount and date of each installment, and the date of final payment.

4. Subtract the down payment from the total debt. Divide the remaining amount by the number of months the debt is being carried to determine the monthly installment amounts and date of final payment.
5. Complete a Truth in Lending form after mutually agreeing on the terms if the payments require more than four installments. This procedure complies with Regulation Z.
6. Review the completed Truth in Lending form with the patient.
7. Ask the patient to sign the Truth in Lending form.
8. Make a photocopy of the form for the patient to retain.
9. File the original Truth in Lending form in the patient's financial files in the office.

unpaid. Therefore, referring such patients elsewhere for their care should be considered. When the patient has paid the overdue amount, he or she can return with the understanding that payment will be required at the time of service.

Truth in Lending Consumer Credit Cost Disclosure

The Truth in Lending Consumer Credit Cost Disclosure is similar to the Federal Truth in Lending Act. It requires that providers disclose *all* costs including interest, late charges, and so on, *prior* to the time of service. If interest is charged on monthly billing, the amount of each payment, due date, unpaid balance at the beginning of the billing period, finance charge, and date balance due must be included on each statement.

Fair Credit Billing Act

The Fair Credit Billing Act states that patients have 60 days from the date the statement is mailed to complain about an error. The complaint must be acknowledged and documented within 30 days of receiving it. The provider has two billing cycles (maximum of

90 days) to correct the error if an actual error occurred; otherwise, the accuracy of the bill should be explained to the patient.

If a collection call is made and the patient has a complaint, address the complaint seriously. Listen with an open mind, and note specifically what the complaint is and what the person wants to do. Do not sidestep the issue, because it will only add fuel to the fire. Apologize whether the patient is right or wrong. Be sincere and do not try to interject humor. Decide on a resolution, and let the patient know specifically what action will be taken.

Fair Credit Reporting Act

The Fair Credit Reporting Act (FCRA) became law in 1971 and was amended in the Budget Bill of 1996. Consumer reporting agencies (CRAs) gather and assemble information on private individuals to evaluate and determine the credit standing and credit capacity of consumers; they sell consumer reports that detail the information for future creditors, employers, insurers, and other businesses. The FCRA, enforced by the Federal Trade Commission, is designed to promote accuracy and ensure the privacy of the information used in consumer reports. In most cases, a prospective employer is prohibited from using a credit report for hiring purposes.

Credit Bureaus

The most common type of consumer reporting agency is the credit bureau. The industry is divided into two branches. The first branch consists of companies that issue noninvestigative consumer credit reports when someone applies for credit.

The second branch consists of companies that issue consumer investigative reports requested by insurance companies, employers, prospective employers, credit grantors, and others who show a legitimate business need. Some also operate a collection department, receiving delinquent accounts from participating businesses.

As a member of a credit bureau service, a physician may obtain information about a consumer over the telephone. The information may consist of the patient's residence or previous residence (which will show if the patient is transient), the patient's employment verification, approximate salary, number of dependents, how the patient pays on other merchant accounts, and derogatory information, such as bankruptcy, use of an alias, and so forth.

The FCRA permits a person to check the credit report for mistakes, outdated information, disputed information, and negative credit information from earlier years. If there are inaccuracies, the consumer can have them corrected. If a physician joins a credit bureau and uses its services, the medical assistant may be designated to check new patients for information on their credit history.

If a credit refusal is based in whole or in part on a report from a credit bureau or similar agency, then the medical assistant must provide the patient with the name and address of the agency, although the exact nature of the information obtained does not have to be revealed. The procedure is to send a letter courteously informing the patient that the credit has been denied because credit requirements have not been met. The name and address of the bureau that supplies credit information should be given and a copy of the letter should go in the files.

COLLECTIONS

In order to have a successful medical practice, you need to have knowledgeable and dedicated staff that is aware of state laws and insurance contracts. It is often said that, "If the doctor does not get paid, neither does anyone else."

There is a *statute of limitations*, which varies from state to state, establishing the maximum time during which a legal collection suit on a delinquent account may be rendered against a debtor. Table 13-1 lists a summary of the time limits for collections in the various states. The statutes also vary according to oral and written contracts; there are three kinds of accounts:

1. *Open-book account* (also called **open accounts**)— Record of business transactions on the books that represents an unsecured account receivable where credit has been extended without a formal written contract; payment is expected by a specific period. The physician's patient accounts are usually of this type. Open accounts fall under the "oral contract" time limit.
2. *Written-contract account*—Agreement a patient signs to pay the bill in more than four installments under the Truth in Lending provisions.
3. *Single-entry account*—Account with only one charge listed and generally for a small amount.

Aging Accounts

To follow up on accounts in a timely manner, it is important to know when an account begins to become delinquent. A system called **aging accounts** is an analysis of accounts receivable indicating a breakdown of the length of time (30, 60, 90, and 120 days) the account is overdue.

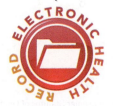

In a practice employing an EHR system, accounts are located using the patient's name or medical record number and charges and payments are entered into the computer; the balance is automatically calculated and aged. Insurance payments are applied to specific charges, and patient payments are applied to the oldest unpaid charge unless specifically directed to a particular date of service. Computerized collection reports are a valuable tool used to monitor patient and insurance payments and to evaluate the staff on their collection efficiency.

In a manual accounting system, some offices use removable, self-adhesive, color-coded labels on ledgers to indicate the age of accounts that are delinquent. They are inexpensive, allow quick identification, and can be used several times.

Regardless of the system used, the key to success is working the accounts receivable regularly, keeping accurate records on aging accounts, and updating notes consistently. See Chapter 15 for further information about financial management using a computer.

TABLE 13-1 Summary of Individual State Time Limits (Statute of Limitations, in Years, on Civil Actions) for Collection of Oral/Written Contracts

State	Contracts: Oral/Written	State	Contracts: Oral/Written
Alabama	6	Montana	3/8
Alaska	6	Nebraska	4/5
Arizona	3/6	Nevada	4/6
Arkansas	5	New Hampshire	3
California	2/4	New Jersey	6
Colorado	6	New Mexico	4/6
Connecticut	3/6	New York	6
Delaware	3	North Carolina	3
D.C.	3	North Dakota	6
Florida	4/5	Ohio	6/15
Georgia	4/6	Oklahoma	3/5
Hawaii	6	Oregon	6
Idaho	4/5	Pennsylvania	4/6
Illinois	5/10	Rhode Island	10
Indiana	6/10	South Carolina	3
Iowa	5/10	South Dakota	6
Kansas	3/5	Tennessee	6/4
Kentucky	5/15	Texas	4
Louisiana	10	Utah	4/6
Maine	6	Vermont	6
Maryland	3	Virginia	3/6
Massachusetts	6	Washington	3/6
Michigan	6	West Virginia	5/15
Minnesota	6	Wisconsin	6
Mississippi	3	Wyoming	8/10
Missouri	5/10		

Note: This information is abstracted from the 2015 Credit Infocenter Statutes of Limitation on Debts and is intended as a brief overview of state statute of limitation laws and requirements; listed in years.

Office Collection Problem Solving

A patient under the physician's care may fall deep into debt and find it impossible to pay bills. In a discussion to find the cause of the problem, the patient may ask the administrative assistant to suggest a solution.

Credit Counseling

Patients with financial problems may be directed to a consumer credit counseling service that can be found in most communities; it is a nonprofit agency that assists people in paying off their debts. Or the debtor may contact his or her own bank or labor union, either of which may provide counseling at no charge. If these suggestions do not help, then a budget consultant might be

the solution. A budget consultant is a financial planner who recommends solutions for a debt by itemizing income and expenses for a projected time period. Commercial debt consolidators charge high fees and should be sought only as a final resort. The assistant must be careful to give only legitimate recommendations and referrals, because if the patient is dissatisfied, the medical assistant or the physician may be blamed.

Verifying Checks

A *check* is a written order to pay a sum of money. When accepting checks, always ask to see two sources of identification. Call to verify checks drawn on out-of-state bank accounts. Examine the check to be sure it is made out to the correct party, it is for the correct amount, and the signature matches other identification. Verify the address and telephone number on the check with the patient's account.

Nonsufficient Funds—When notice is received from a bank indicating a check was not honored because of nonsufficient funds (NSF), call the bank and patient to see if they suggest redepositing it. If it is not worthwhile or if a second NSF notice is received, call the person who wrote the check and tell him or her to bring in payment to the office immediately. Accept only cash, a certified check, a money order, or in certain cases a credit or debit card. Be courteous but straight to the point. If restitution is not received within 3 days, notify the patient in writing to start the legal process. An NSF demand letter (Figure 13-12) should be sent certified mail with return receipt requested and should include the following:

1. Check date
2. Check number
3. Bank the check is drawn on
4. To whom the check was payable
5. Check amount
6. Any allowable service fee
7. Total amount due
8. Number of days the check writer has to take action

In most states, if the debtor has not responded within 30 days, a claim may be filed in small-claims court. It may be possible to collect an additional $100 in damages, and in some states, the person can be sued for three times the amount of the check. Section 1719 of the State Civil Code addresses penal sanctions for individuals who pass checks on nonsufficient funds. The district attorney, district justice, state attorney, or other government official may also help with the collection of a bad check.

The patient must be informed that the medical facility will no longer be able to accept checks as a payment on future services. Future payments need to be in the form of cash, money order, cashier's check, or debit or credit card if office policy permits. Refer to Chapter 15 for step-by-step directions on posting returned checks.

Bad Check Preventive Measures—Larger medical facilities may want to consider a check authorization system. With this type of system, a company supplies a terminal that gives an approval number for each check and guarantees payment on those that are authorized.

To help discourage bad checks, charge a penalty for returned checks. This information should be detailed in the new patient brochures and posted in the office for all patients to see.

PRACTON MEDICAL GROUP, INC.
4567 BROAD AVENUE • WOODLAND HILLS, XY 12345-4700
OFFICE: (555) 486-9002 • FAX: (555) 488-7815

Fran Practon, M.D.
Gerald Practon, M.D.

July 5, 20XX

Miss Leslee Zimmer
9908 Chelan Lane
Woodland Hills, XY 12345-4700

Dear Miss Zimmer:

Your check number 4229 dated June 14, 20XX made payable to Fran Practon, MD in the amount of $41.54 drawn on Woodland City Bank has been dishonored by the bank with a statement marked "Nonsufficient funds."

Payment needs to be received within 15 days from today's date or we will turn this matter over to our attorney for legal action.

Please come to the address listed above to make payment in cash or by money order. We appreciate your immediate attention to this matter.

Sincerely,

Linda Franco

Linda Franco
Accounts Receivable

FIGURE 13-12 Nonsufficient funds (NSF) demand letter

Use of debit cards will also eliminate bad checks. Additional information on payment disputes regarding NSF, misdated checks, incorrect payee's name on check, missing payer's signature, variable amounts, payment-in-full checks, third-party checks, and forged checks appears in Chapter 14, *Banking*.

Dun Messages

If a payment has not been made after rendering professional services, then an itemized billing statement is sent every 30 days. The statement should be simple and to the point. Patients should be able to open a statement, peruse it, and understand the date of service, service rendered, amount owed, and how long past due the account is; see an account that is 81 to 90 days delinquent in Figure 13-6. At the time of the second billing, a reminder in the form of a written note (dun message) on a statement is appropriate.

"Dun" comes from the Old English word *dunnen*, which means "to make a loud noise." A **dun message** is a phrase used to remind a patient with a delinquent account about payment (see Figure 13-5 and Example 13-11). Brightly colored self-adhesive collection labels are also available for this purpose. If a

TABLE 13-2 Collection Abbreviations

Abbreviations	Definitions
B	bankrupt
BLG	belligerent
EOM	end of month
EOW	end of week
FN	final notice
H	he or husband
HHCO	have husband call office
HTO	he telephoned office
L1, L2	letter one, letter two (sent)
LB	line busy
LD	long distance
LMCO	left message, call office
LMVM	left message voice mail
N1, N2	note one, note two (sent)
NA	no answer
NF/A	no forwarding address
NI	not in
NLE	no longer employed
NR	no record
NSF	not sufficient funds (check)
NSN	no such number
OOT	out of town
OOW	out of work
Ph/Dsc	phone disconnected
POW	payment on way
PP	promise to pay
S	she or wife
SEP	separated
SK	skip or skipped
SOS	same old story
STO	she telephoned office
T	telephoned
TB	telephoned business
TR	telephoned residence
U/Emp	unemployed
UTC	unable to contact
Vfd/E	verified employment
Vfd/I	verified insurance

patient's primary language is not English, a dun message should be written in the suitable language.

A notation indicating the type of dun message sent should be inserted in the computer comment area, on the back of the patient's ledger card, or in the accounts receivable log, such as "N1" or "N2" (see Table 13-2), along with the date the notice was mailed. When a payment is received, post it immediately. Patients who send a check and subsequently receive a bill with a stern dun message may decide to look elsewhere for care.

Telephone Collections

Generally if an account remains delinquent for over 60 days, it is important to make personal contact by telephone. First, arrange the accounts according to aging parameters (e.g., 30, 60, 90, 120 days) and select all accounts in the 60-day range. Next prioritize the calls that need to be made according to the amounts owed; take action on accounts that may be difficult to collect first. It is best to prepare thoroughly for the call by outlining what is going to be said. A telephone that allows privacy should be used and the call should be made at a time when there will be no interruptions. According to surveys, the best times to call are between 5:30 and 8:30 p.m., Tuesdays and Thursdays, and between 9:00 a.m. and 1 p.m. on Saturdays. It may be prudent to add one evening per week to the practice schedule for collection purposes or offer the medical assistant a flexible schedule to make collection calls during these hours.

The longer an account remains delinquent, the harder it will be to collect. Although the assistant may hear the same excuses over and over, it is important to convey an understanding of the circumstances. When a patient is talking nonstop, use a "bridge" in the conversation such as *Yes, I understand that, and we do need to talk, but . . . the collection agency picks up our accounts on Friday,* or *Our accountant won't allow a payment plan over 90 days, so you probably need to take out a loan,* or *In order to keep your account current, we need to have your check in the office this week,* and so forth. Refer to Procedure 13-4 for guidelines on telephone debt collection.

Insurance Check Sent to Patient

If the "assignment of benefits" has been signed and the insurance check has gone to the patient, it is the insurance company's responsibility to generate a new check to the physician and collect the amount of the check directly from the patient. Follow up immediately in such situations.

PROCEDURE 13-4

Perform Debt Collection Using a Telephone

OBJECTIVE: Make a telephone call to request payment from a patient who has a delinquent account balance.

EQUIPMENT/SUPPLIES: Telephone, patient's account or ledger, and pen or pencil.

DIRECTIONS: Follow these step-by-step directions, which include rationales, to learn this procedure. Twenty role-playing scenarios are presented in *Workbook* Job Skill 13-4 to practice this skill.

1. From the point that the patient incurs a debt, be clear about how and when payment is expected.

2. Telephone patients who are slow payers shortly before their scheduled appointments. Remind them of the date and time of their appointment, and at the same time ask them to bring in their payment or suggest they use their debit/credit card.

3. Follow the Fair Debt Collection Practices Act when making a telephone call.

4. State the name of the caller and the practice represented, and identify the patient.

5. Verify the patient's address and any telephone numbers listed.

6. Ask for full payment, stating the total amount owed when speaking to a patient about an overdue amount. Ask for payment courteously but firmly, conveying a sense of urgency and requesting that the patient keep payments prompt.

7. Speak slowly in a low voice; staying calm and polite prevents quarreling.

8. Elicit grievances, answer questions, ask why there has not been a payment, give the patient a choice of action, and then set immediate deadlines for payment.

9. Pause for effect and do not assume that if the patient does not respond immediately it is a "no." Some questions to ask include, *How much are you short? When do you get paid?* and *Do you have a checking account?* Asking for a postdated check is another option if allowed per office policy.

10. Make positive instead of negative statements such as *We will NOT send your account to our collection agency as long as we receive payment by (date)* instead of *If we do not receive payment by (date), we WILL send your account to our collection agency.*

11. Treat patients who owe money as you would want to be treated in the same situation. Be assertive and empathetic instead of aggressive.

12. Tune in to the feelings and concerns of patients, showing patience and openness. Respond to patients instead of reacting to them.

13. Ask the patient to write down the payment agreement when an agreement is reached, and read it back to be sure there has been no misunderstanding.

14. Write a short note outlining the conversation and the agreement that was made as a follow-up to the telephone call (Figure 13-13).

15. Make abbreviated notations (see Table 13-2 for abbreviations) in the computer system, on the back of the patient's ledger card, or on the accounts receivable log, and also indicate the date any telephone calls were made. It is vital to be consistent in follow-up procedures and policies.

Solutions for Payment Excuses

The following are some patient tactics used for stalling payment and solutions the medical assistant may use:

1. *Situation:* Saying the check is in the mail.
   Solution/Response: Get a check number, amount, and mail date. Call in 3 days if not received.

2. *Situation:* Broken promise by patient.
   Solution/Response: Follow up within 48 hours. Determine the reason for the broken promise. Get immediate payment.

3. *Situation:* Sending unsigned checks that must be returned.
   Solution/Response: Have the patient come to the office to sign.

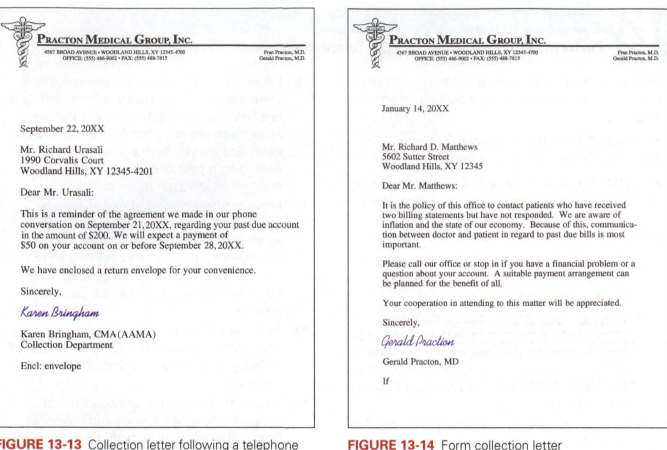

FIGURE 13-13 Collection letter following a telephone agreement

FIGURE 13-14 Form collection letter

4. *Situation:* Paying an incorrect amount.
   Solution/Response: Have the patient come to the office and exchange a new check for the one made out in error.
5. *Situation:* Saying, "I never received your bill."
   Solution/Response: Verify name and address, and resend the bill the same day. Call in 3 days to see if the patient received it.

Collection Letters

If regular statements have been sent, 2 or 3 months have elapsed since the service, and the patient cannot be reached by telephone or a promised payment has not been received, then it is time to send a collection letter. There are a number of letter formats to consider, such as a form letter (Figure 13-14), a letter with a checklist (Figure 13-15), or a personally composed letter. The letter in the chosen format should always be typed and may be sent either in a plain envelope or in a brightly colored one to attract attention. A debtor is more likely to open the envelope and read the contents if it does not look like a bill. If the patient has moved and left a forwarding address, the post office will forward the letter. For a small fee, the post office will also supply a card indicating the new address if "Address Service Requested" or "Forwarding Service Requested" is printed on the envelope as described in Chapter 12 and illustrated in Figure 12-6.

A collection letter should be brief and direct. It should mention how much is owed for a specific service; what the patient should do about the delinquency; when, where, and why the patient should remit; and how the patient can facilitate payment. Enclosing a self-addressed, stamped envelope may help obtain a response. A letter written over the physician's signature rather than the medical assistant's may be more successful in prompting a payment. Collection letters may also

---

COMPLIANCE

Email Collection

Patients may communicate with the medical practice via email and ask questions about their bill. However, email letters CANNOT be used to collect on a debt—this is in violation of HIPAA privacy laws.

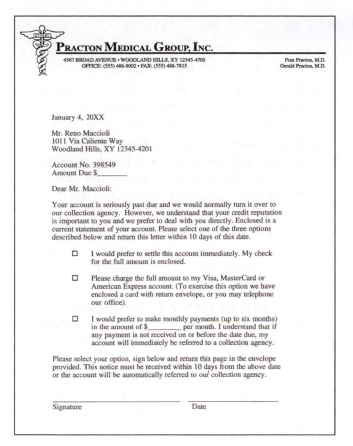

PRACTON MEDICAL GROUP, INC.
4567 BROAD AVENUE • WOODLAND HILLS, XY 12345-4700
OFFICE: (555) 486-9002 • FAX: (555) 488-7815

Fran Practon, M.D.
Gerald Practon, M.D.

January 4, 20XX

Mr. Reno Maccioli
1011 Via Caliente Way
Woodland Hills, XY 12345-4201

Account No. 398549
Amount Due $_____

Dear Mr. Maccioli:

Your account is seriously past due and we would normally turn it over to our collection agency. However, we understand that your credit reputation is important to you and we prefer to deal with you directly. Enclosed is a current statement of your account. Please select one of the three options described below and return this letter within 10 days of this date.

☐ I would prefer to settle this account immediately. My check for the full amount is enclosed.

☐ Please charge the full amount to my Visa, MasterCard or American Express account. (To exercise this option we have enclosed a card with return envelope, or you may telephone our office).

☐ I would prefer to make monthly payments (up to six months) in the amount of $_____ per month. I understand that if any payment is not received on or before the date due, my account will immediately be referred to a collection agency.

Please select your option, sign below and return this page in the envelope provided. This notice must be received within 10 days from the above date or the account will be automatically referred to our collection agency.

_____   _____
Signature   Date

FIGURE 13-15 Multipurpose form collection letter with checklist

be purchased for a small price and the collection follow-up is left in the medical assistant's hands.

When mailing a collection letter toward the end of the year, it might be helpful to remind the patient that medical expenses, if large enough, could qualify as an income tax deduction if the account is settled before the year-end deadline. A message, such as *The medical expense listed on this statement may be used as a deduction on your 20__ income tax, provided it is paid by December 31, 20__*, could be used as an incentive.

Patients can also be encouraged to pay their debts with income tax refunds. Arrangements can be made for patients to make small payments January through March and a large payment when they get their refund in April. Suggest that patients file their income tax returns electronically to expedite the refund. Whenever a letter is sent, it should be noted in the computer comment area, on the back of the ledger card, or on the accounts receivable log as L1, L2, and so on, with the date on which it was mailed.

Depending on the policy of the office, when the account has aged 120 days, a decision needs to be made

whether to (1) send another bill with a dun message, (2) turn the account over to a collection service, or (3) file in small-claims court. After a certain amount of time, some physicians prefer to write off a small debt (e.g., $25) rather than to increase administrative collection costs. From a medicolegal standpoint, a consideration regarding a small-claims suit would be not to file until a counterclaim by the patient alleging negligence is barred by the statute of limitations.

Collection Agencies

Seeking the services of a collection agency should be a last resort; however, do not hold onto an account too long. For best collection results, agencies like to get the delinquent accounts at a maximum of 5 or 6 months after the debt has occurred. When an account has been turned over to a collection agency, the patient's financial record should be removed from the regular file and marked with the date and name of the agency. It is illegal for the physician's office to send a bill to a patient after the account has been turned over to a collection agency. If an agency has an account and payment is directed to the physician's office instead of the agency, the assistant must notify the agency immediately, because a percentage of this payment may be due the agency.

When an account is assigned to an agency, it is suggested that the doctor send the patient a letter of discharge by certified mail for liability protection. Refer to Chapter 3 for sample letters of discharge or withdrawal from a case.

Management consultants recommend that the patient's account balance be written off the accounts receivable (A/R) when an account is turned over to a collection agency. When money is received, the charged amount is reposted (debited/added back) to equal the payment received (refer to Chapter 15 for posting guidelines).

Before seeking the services of a collection agency, the medical assistant needs to determine the type of agency that best meets the office needs. As mentioned, the agency typically takes a percentage of the bill owed, which can be as much as 50%. National agencies that have local and regional branches have advantages when tracking an individual with a debt who moves and leaves no forwarding address. The agency should be licensed and bonded. Procedure 13-5 offers guidelines for the medical assistant seeking to employ a collection agency.

Refer to Procedure 13-6 for step-by-step directions when taking collection action and sending an account to a collection agency.

PROCEDURE 13-5

Select a Collection Agency

OBJECTIVE: Select a reputable collection agency.

EQUIPMENT/SUPPLIES: Telephone and pen or pencil.

DIRECTIONS: Follow these guidelines when seeking to employ a collection agency for the physician's office.

1. Check with physicians who have used the agency for over 2 years to determine the agency's rate of accomplishment. A collection rate of 30% to 60% of the accounts assigned to it is considered successful.

2. Look for an agency that charges on a sliding scale, usually between 33% and 50%, with the higher rate applied to older and smaller accounts.

3. Find out if there is a minimum fee charged if nothing is collected.

4. Make sure the agency does not hold partial payments until the account is collected in full.

5. Ask the agency to provide the form letters sent to patients, so the physician can approve or disapprove of their tone.

6. Keep a record of the money that the agency actually collects. If it is more than 25% to 30% of what is owed, the assistant's own collection procedures need strengthening.

7. Ask whether accounts are forwarded to another collection office if a debtor moves and whether there are penalties for withdrawing an account.

8. Find out if the agency is covered by errors and omissions insurance that would protect both the agency and physician in the event of a lawsuit.

9. Check the agency's policy for a hold harmless clause, which protects the physician from being sued if the agency is accused of harassing a debtor.

PROCEDURE 13-6

Take Collection Action; Send an Account to a Collection Agency

OBJECTIVE: Follow-up on an unpaid account with statements, telephone calls, and collection letters, and then send the account to a collection agency.

EQUIPMENT/SUPPLIES: Patient account or ledger card with applicable data; pen.

DIRECTIONS: Follow these step-by-step directions, which include rationales, to learn this procedure.

1. Send statements for at least three billing cycles (90 days). It is important for the patient to receive consistent statements, with appropriate dun messages, itemizing the amount owed.

2. Contact the patient by telephone. Several attempts should be made by telephone to try to find out why the patient has not paid and/or get a promise to pay.

3. Send a collection letter if unable to reach the patient or if the patient is not interested in paying the debt.

4. Send a collection notice. The notice should state clearly when the account will be turned over to a collection agency if payment is not received (e.g., 10 days).

5. Send the account to the collection agency and post on the account/ledger (see Chapter 15).

6. Flag the patient's electronic account and EMR or chart and financial record (ledger) so that all staff members know that the account has gone to collection. Make a note in computerized accounts in the comment sections of the financial statement, medical record, and appointment schedule. If using a paper-based system, a brightly colored piece of paper with "COLLECTION" written on it, placed in the front of the chart alerts all employees; write "COLLECTION" across the front of the ledger.

7. Post monies received from the collection agency (see Chapter 15).

Small-Claims Court

A physician may decide to file a claim for a delinquent bill in small-claims court rather than turn it over to a collection agency (Figure 13-16). Small-claims court proceedings are an inexpensive collection method; but after the judgment is made, the physician still has to pursue the money. Sometimes that is not easy. To be eligible for small-claims court, the bill must be within the limit the state has set on the amount. This figure varies from $300 to $25,000 state to state and, in some instances, within the state. The majority of states have increased maximum amounts from $2000–$3000 to $5000–$10,000. There may also be limits on the number of claims over specific dollar amounts per year, and other dollar limits regarding claims filed against a guarantor of a debt. In many states, lawyers are not permitted to represent litigants; however, an incorporated physician must usually be represented by an attorney. For large balances when small-claims court is no longer a viable choice, collection attorneys are the second highest choice in alternative enforcement.

If the account has been turned over to a collection agency, the debt cannot be filed in small-claims court. Such agencies have different filing protocols. Refer to Procedure 13-7 when filing an uncollectible account in small-claims court.

Federal Wage Garnishment Law

Title III of the Consumer Credit Protection Act, which became effective on July 1, 1970, set down the legislation affecting garnishment. **Garnishment** means attaching a debtor's property and wage by court order, so monies can be obtained to pay debts. Personal earnings include wages, salary, tips, commissions, bonuses, and income from pensions or retirement programs. Enforcement is carried out by the compliance offices of the Wage and Hour Office, U.S. Department of Labor, which are located across the United States. Two basic provisions of the garnishment law are:

1. It limits the amount of employee earnings withheld for garnishment in a workweek or pay period.
2. It protects the employee from being dismissed if his or her pay is garnished regardless of the number of levies included in the garnishment.

The garnishment law is a continuous garnishment judgment. In other words, if the debt is not paid within 90 days, the garnishment can be continued for another 90 days. The garnishment law does not apply to federal government employees, or court orders in personal bankruptcy cases. The amount of wages subject to garnishment is based on the patient's disposable earnings. This is the amount left after deductions for federal, state, and local taxes and Social Security. Union dues, health and life insurance, assignment of wages, and savings bonds are not considered in disposable earnings. Garnishment is limited to the lesser of 25% of disposable earnings in any workweek or the amount by which disposable earnings for that week exceed 30 times the highest current federal minimum wage.

When state garnishment laws conflict with federal laws, the statute resulting in the smaller garnishment applies. For further information, the assistant can contact the local Wage and Hour Office listed in most telephone directories under U.S. Government, Department of Labor, Employment Standards Administration.

Estate Claims

There are various state time limits and statutes governing the filing of a claim against an estate. First, an itemized billing statement (or in some states, a special form) is completed for the collection of a deceased patient's account. This is mailed in duplicate to the estate administrator by certified mail with return receipt requested. The name of the estate administrator can be obtained by calling the probate department of the superior court or the county recorder's office. The administrator of the estate will either accept or reject the claim. If accepted, an acknowledgment of the debt will be sent to the physician. If rejected, the physician should file a claim against the administrator within a time specified by state law.

Bankruptcy

Bankruptcy laws are federal laws, and a patient who files for **bankruptcy** becomes a ward of the federal court and is thereby protected by the court. If a patient writes or telephones stating bankruptcy has been declared, under the law the medical assistant must not send monthly statements or make an attempt to collect; a creditor can be fined for contempt of court for failing to follow the law. If the account has been turned over to a collection agency and the agency has been notified of the bankruptcy, it is the same as if the physician has been notified.

Bankruptcy laws are organized in sections called *chapters*. The chapters applicable to patients' debts in a medical practice are as follows:

- *Chapter 7, straight petition in bankruptcy*—Allows a person, family, or small business to liquidate

PROCEDURE 13-7

File an Uncollectible Account in Small-Claims Court

OBJECTIVE: File a delinquent or uncollectible account in small-claims court.

EQUIPMENT/SUPPLIES: Small-claims court filing form and instructional booklet, check for filing fee, and photocopies of financial records for cases to be presented.

DIRECTIONS: Follow these step-by-step directions, which include rationales, to learn this procedure skill.

1. Obtain a form from the clerk's office located at the municipal or justice court; there are booklets and material to help guide the claimant through the process.

2. Fill out the forms providing a written signed statement, describing the loss (debt).

3. Pay the filing fee. Filing fees vary by state, by county within some states, and by the amount of the claim.

4. File the initiating papers, either in the county where the defendant lives or the county where the loss occurred.

5. When the clerk accepts the fee and statement of claimed damages, the case will be entered on the small-claim court docket.

6. The clerk will then send a proper notice to the defendant by certified mail, with information about the lawsuit.

7. If the defendant does not receive the notice by certified mail, it may be necessary to make arrangements to have the notice served personally. If the summons is served on the patient by a sheriff or court-appointed office, a fee plus mileage for the officer who serves it is necessary. There must be a street address where the patient can be found. The person serving the defendant completes the proof of service form.

8. After being served, a patient has one of several options:

   a. Contact the physician—try to settle the dispute and reach an out-of-court agreement without going to trial.

   b. Pay the claim—to the court clerk. This will be forwarded to the physician, but the

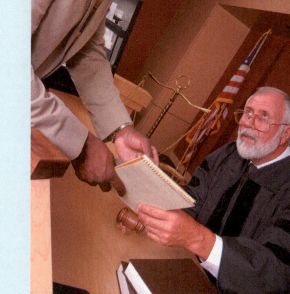

FIGURE 13-16 Medical assistant in a courtroom presenting a small-claims case

filing fee or service charge will not be refunded.

c. Contest the claim—an answer must be filed with the court specifying the basis for the denial.

b. Ignore the claim—the physician will win by default. In some states, a judgment may be requested in writing, but in other states the physician or the medical assistant must appear on a specified date. If the patient does not appear, the judgment is granted in the physician's favor and usually court costs are included in the judgment.

(continues)

   c. Request a small-claims hearing—the court clerk will let both parties know when to appear. The patient may file a counter-claim against the physician at this time.

   d. Demand a jury trial—the case will be taken out of small-claims court. The physician will be notified by the court clerk to file a formal complaint in a higher court, and an attorney must represent the physician.

9. Appear in court (physician or the medical assistant) on the specified date, or the claim will be dismissed and cannot be refilled.

10. Basic information required by the court is:

   a. Physician's name, address, and telephone number

   b. Patient's name and address

   c. Delinquent amount

   d. Summary of the claim including the date the physician's bill was due, date of the last visit, date of the last payment, unpaid amount, and all records of telephone contacts and letters sent

11. Determine what the judge needs to hear to decide a favorable case. Good preparation for the trial can make the difference between success and failure.

12. Organize all the exhibits in a notebook, in chronological order. A timeline showing the sequence of events can be useful.

13. Take a business-like professional approach at the hearing, giving concise and accurate answers to the judge's questions, and speaking slowly and clearly. The physician or assistant must bring any witnesses, statements, receipts, contracts, notes, dishonored checks, or other evidence to court. The judge will question the medical assistant or physician and the patient, review the evidence, and then make a ruling.

14. Put a lien on the debtor's wages, automobile, bank or personal assets, or real property if the judgment, which is usually effective for many years, is in the physician's favor. This is the physician's legal right. The small-claims office will show the medical assistant or physician how to execute a judgment.

15. Pay a small fee if the physician decides to execute against the patient's assets. It is recoverable from the patient.

all debts and to restart with a clean financial slate. First, the patient declares bankruptcy to those to whom money is owed. If the physician is listed, since there is no collateral, he or she will be the last person paid. If the physician is not listed and the patient wishes to make payments, then this is allowed. In this bankruptcy process, a court-appointed trustee takes charge of the patient's assets, subject to certain exemptions, and then sells them and distributes the collected money among the creditors. If the court determines there are assets to be distributed, the physician will be notified to file a creditor's claim.

If a patient files a straight petition in bankruptcy, the physician should file a proof-of-claim form available from an attorney, county clerk's office, or local stationery store. Copies of the patient's outstanding bill are attached to the form and it is mailed to the bankruptcy court. Physician debts are "unsecured" and often go unpaid in bankruptcy cases. However, the physician will never be paid if a claim is not filed. Once a patient has declared bankruptcy, he or she cannot do so again for 6 years. The only exception to this is a Chapter 13, or wage earner's bankruptcy.

- *Chapter 13, wage earner's bankruptcy*—A milder proceeding in which a federal district court acts as a consumer counseling service. The object is to protect wage earners from bill collectors and to make arrangements for the wage earner to pay bills over time. The court fixes a monthly amount that the debtor can pay, collects that sum, and parcels it out among the creditors according to an extended repayment plan that may take as long as 5 years. The plan often includes a reduced repayment of debts. To be paid, the physician must file a claim as directed by the debtor's attorney.

Sometimes patients may file for bankruptcy but do no follow-through to completion. It is wise to verify with the court system to make sure a judgment has been made.

Tracing a Skip

A patient who owes a balance and moves, leaving the physician's office no forwarding address, is called a skip. A skip is discovered when a statement goes out and is returned unopened and marked by the post office "Returned to Sender, Addressee Unknown." This problem can often be avoided by having envelopes printed with "Address Service Requested" or "Forwarding Service Requested" below the physician's return address as discussed in Chapter 12. If the address is a rural delivery box number, go to the post office and fill out a Freedom of Information Act form, pay a nominal search fee, and the United States Postal Service will give the physical location of the person's residence.

It is important to begin tracing a skip as soon as possible. Move quickly in these efforts to locate the patient. If unable to trace and contact the patient, turn the skip over to a collection agency immediately. Time is an important factor. Some agencies offer customized skip tracing. Various levels of tracing are offered for specific dollar amounts. As each level increases, more time is spent trying various tactics to locate the patient. The more time spent, the more money the agency charges. When using such a service, the medical assistant should choose a specific level for each account depending on what dollar amount is owed. Determine how much to spend tracing each debtor. Depending on the amount owed and the time estimated to locate the patient, there may be a decision to write off the balance.

Also, online information services can be used for skip tracing via the Internet. A search is made of the database that contains millions of records. If a match is made with the given data, helpful information may be discovered.

To make locating a skip easier, remember to keep records updated and verify information each time the patient visits the office. Refer to Procedure 13-8 when

tracing a patient who has moved and left no forwarding address (skip).

Search via Computer

When using the Internet for a search, it is important to remember that information is not secure and the patient's right to privacy must never be violated. Some excellent methods of skip tracing using electronic databases or online services to locate a debtor are:

- *Surname scan*—Searches are based on data that have been compiled from public source documents, locally, regionally, or nationally
- *Address search*—Gives property search and any change of address from all suppliers of data to the database, including the U.S. Postal Service; names of other adults in the household, who may have the debtor's telephone number listed under their name, may also be included
- *Electronic directory*—Gives access to the regional telephone operating company's screen of information
- *Credit holder search*—Used to discover occupation
- *Phone number search*—Allows access to the names of other adults in the same household who have a telephone number
- *Neighbor search*—Shows names, addresses, and telephone numbers of the debtor's former neighbors
- *ZIP code search*—Provides names, addresses, and telephone numbers of everyone within that zip code who has the same last name as the debtor
- *City search*—Finds everyone with the same last and first name within a given city
- *State search*—Locates all individuals with the same last and first name within the state, and lists their addresses and telephone numbers
- *National search*—Operates the same way as the state search; use for people with unusual last names
- *Business search*—Lists the names of businesses in the neighborhood of the patient's last known residence; may help find where the patient has relocated or will help verify the patient's place of employment

Refer to the *Resources* section at the end of this chapter for websites used in skip tracing.

PROCEDURE 13-8

Trace a Skip

OBJECTIVE: Use search techniques to trace a debtor who has moved leaving no forwarding address and owes a balance on his or her account.

EQUIPMENT/SUPPLIES: Telephone, patient's electronic account or ledger card, and pen or pencil.

DIRECTIONS: Follow these step-by-step directions, which include rationales, to learn this procedure.

1. Check the address on the returned statement against the patient's registration form, account, or ledger to make sure all match and it was mailed correctly.

2. Check the ZIP code directory to see if the zip code corresponds with the patient's street address or post office box.

3. Telephone the patient's nearest relative, neighbor, or emergency references given on the patient information record, using utmost discretion.

4. File a request with the local post office to try to get a new or corrected address.

5. Look in the local telephone directory or call information, and check for a new or current listing or for the same name. Telephone and ask for the patient by name if the patient has an unusual last name; the person who answers might be a relative. If directory assistance says the number is unpublished, the patient could still be in town.

6. Telephone the primary care physician for updated information when investigating for a physician specialist or any referring practice.

7. Call the patient's employer without disclosing to coworkers the reason for the call. If the patient is no longer employed, ask to speak to the personnel department to inquire if they have a lead.

8. Find out if the Department of Motor Vehicles has been notified of a change of address, if the driver's license number is available.

9. Look in the street directories, city directories, and cross-index directories (available at the public library or via the Internet), and locate a neighbor, relative, or landlord to inquire what happened to the patient.

10. Call the bank and ask if the account was transferred or is still open, if the patient information record contains information about the patient's bank.

11. Call the local hospital's inpatient admission office to see if they have a forwarding address, if the patient was hospitalized.

12. Look in the patient's medical record for referrals or reports from other physicians or laboratory, radiology, or physical therapy reports, and call other facilities.

13. Search other sources of information, such as court records, death and probate records, credit bureau reports, other creditors, marriage licenses, and the police department.

14. Obtain the services of a local credit bureau to check reports and notify you if the patient's Social Security number appears under a different name or the party is listed at a new address.

STOP AND THINK CASE SCENARIO

Tackle Payment Obstacles

SCENARIO: An established patient, Martha Gay, is leaving the office after her appointment and stops by your desk. You state today's fee and she says, "Oh, I forgot my checkbook."

CRITICAL THINKING: Determine what your response should be.

_____

_____

_____

_____

STOP AND THINK CASE SCENARIO

Handle Collection Problems

SCENARIO: Harold Benger's account has become delinquent. You telephone the patient and he says, "I sent in the payment."

CRITICAL THINKING: Formulate questions to ask the patient and state what action you will take.

_____

_____

_____

_____

FOCUS ON CERTIFICATION*

CMA (AAMA) Content Summary

- Charges, payments, and adjustments
- Fee schedules (methods for establishing)
- Contracted fees
- Accounts receivable
- Billing procedures (itemization/billing cycles)
- Aging/collection procedures
- Collection agencies
- Consumer protection acts
- Processing accounts receivable
- Capitation
- Prepaid HMO, PPO, POS
- Applying managed care policies and procedures
- Methods of establishing fees
- Relative Value Studies
- Resource-based Relative Value Scale (RBRVS)
- Diagnosis-Related Groups (DRGs)
- Contracted fees

RMA (AMT) Content Summary

- Process insurance payments and contractual write-off amounts
- Generate aging reports
- Maintain and explain fee schedules
- Collect payments
- Understand and prepare Truth in Lending Statements
- Prepare and mail itemized statements
- Understand and employ available billing methods

- Understand and employ billing cycles
- Collections
- Prepare aging reports and identify delinquent accounts
- Understand and evaluate explanation of benefits
- Perform skip tracing
- Understand application of the Fair Debt Collection Practices Act
- Identify and understand bankruptcy and small-claims procedures
- Understand and perform appropriate collection procedures
- Financial mathematics
- Understand and perform appropriate calculations related to patient and practice accounts

CMAS (AMT) Content Summary

- Perform financial computations
- Manage accounts receivable
- Understand professional fee structures
- Understand physician/practice owner compensation provisions
- Understand credit arrangements
- Understand health care terminology (deductible, copayment, preauthorization, capitation, coinsurance)
- Manage patient accounts/ledgers
- Manage patient billing (methods, cycle billing procedures)
- Manage collections in compliance with state and federal regulations

* _This textbook and the accompanying Workbook meet the entry-level administrative and general competencies for the CMA outlined by the AAMA Examination Content Outline and Occupational Analysis and for the RMA and CMAS outlined by the AMT Competencies, Construction Parameters, and Examination Specifications (see Competency Grid in Appendix B)._

REVIEW EXAM-STYLE QUESTIONS

1. The revenue cycle:
   a. includes the life of the patient account from creation to collection action
   b. includes the life of all patient accounts from creation to payment
   c. is another term for the "money wheel"
   d. starts when a patient is first seen and completes when the patient no longer sees the physician
   e. starts when an insurance company is billed and ends when the insurance company pays

2. The accounts receivable is:
   a. the total amount of money collected
   b. the amount of money received in a day, week, month, and/or year
   c. the total amount of money billed and collected
   d. the total amount of money owed to the medical practice
   e. both a and b

3. Select the correct statement regarding fee schedules.
   a. Some practices may have more than one fee schedule.
   b. The doctor may charge for something that is not on the fee schedule.
   c. Multiple fee schedules are not allowed.
   d. A fee schedule is typically organized alphabetically by type of service.
   e. Both a and b.

4. Select the correct statement regarding physicians giving cash discounts.
   a. The physician has the right to determine who he or she can offer cash discounts to.
   b. Discounts can only be offered to patients with insurance coverage.
   c. If cash discounts are offered, they must be offered to all patients.
   d. Cash discounts can only be offered to patients without insurance coverage.
   e. Cash discounts should never be offered in a medical practice.

5. Certain hospitals have received federal construction grants to enlarge their facilities in exchange for caring for indigent patients; this obligation falls under the:
   a. Medicare program
   b. federal Medicaid program
   c. state Medicaid program
   d. Hill-Burton Act
   e. Indigent-Care Act of 1946

6. The most important collection practice to increase collections, improve public relations, and reduce patient complaints, business-office turnover, accounts receivable, and write-off amounts is:
   a. stating fee-for-service and collecting fees at the time services are given
   b. sending timely billing statements every 30 days
   c. utilizing a collection agency early in the collection process
   d. sending friendly collection letters
   e. telephoning patients who have overdue accounts

7. Cycle billing:
   a. allows billing at certain times of the month based on alphabetical breakdown, account number, insurance type, or date of first service
   b. allows continuous cash flow, relieves mailing statements all at once, and distributes billing telephone calls
   c. distributes statements during the month based on dollar amounts; those with the highest amount due are billed first
   d. is not recommended for the medical office
   e. both a and b

8. What is the name of the credit law that states, "Collectors must identify themselves and the medical practice they represent; they must not mislead the patient?"
   a. Equal Credit Opportunity Act
   b. Fair Debt Collection Practices Act
   c. Federal Truth in Lending Act
   d. Truth in Lending Consumer Credit Cost Disclosure
   e. Fair Credit Billing Act

9. If a physician denies credit to a patient, according to the Equal Credit Opportunity Act, how many days does the patient have to request the reason in writing?
   a. 10 days
   b. 30 days
   c. 60 days
   d. 90 days
   e. 120 days

10. Regulation Z of the Federal Truth in Lending Act applies to:
    a. patients who decide to pay (on their own) their debt in more than four installments
    b. patients who do not pay all of their debt in one payment, but spread it out over time
    c. patients who offer to pay in installments
    d. patients who agree to pay in more than four installments
    e. all of the above are correct

11. Breaking down accounts into lengths of time that money is owed is called:
    a. account divisions
    b. separating accounts
    c. aging accounts
    d. analyzing accounts
    e. maturation of accounts

12. Select the correct statement regarding collections.
    a. Use a public telephone to make collection calls.
    b. Be flexible about interruptions when making collection calls.
    c. The best times to make collection calls are prior to and after regular working hours.

d. Collection letters to obtain payment are better than telephone calls.
e. The longer an account remains delinquent, the harder it will be to collect.

13. When interviewing a collection agency, what collection rate would be considered realistic and good?
    a. 25% to 45%
    b. 30% to 60%
    c. 50% to 75%
    d. 60% to 80%
    e. 75% or above

14. After a judgment is made in favor of the medical practice in small-claims court:
    a. the physician still has to pursue the money
    b. the money is always exchanged in the courtroom and turned over to the physician
    c. the court follows up to make sure payment is made
    d. the court, if necessary, attaches the patient's wages to ensure payment in full
    e. a court representative follows up to make sure payment is made

15. Garnishment is:
    a. limited to 10% of disposable earnings in any workweek
    b. limited to 15% of disposable earnings in any workweek
    c. limited to 25% of disposable earnings in any workweek
    d. limited to 30% of disposable earnings in any workweek
    e. unlimited on the amount that can be garnished

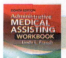

WORKBOOK ASSIGNMENT

To develop competency-based job skills, refer to the *Workbook* and complete the:
- Abbreviation and Spelling Review
- Review Questions
- Critical Thinking Exercises

- Job Skill activities, which are listed at the beginning of the chapter under *Performance Objectives in the Workbook*.

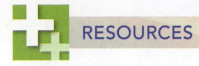

RESOURCES

Collection Resources

American Medical Billing Association (AMBA)
Online billing seminars, billing conferences, and billing resources

Debt Collection
Understanding Your Debt Collection Rights
Frequently asked debt questions

Insurance Companies
Search for an insurance company (e.g., Blue Cross Blue Shield). Click "Ask Blue" for frequently asked health care and billing questions (FAQ).

Credit Bureaus

Equifax
Credit monitoring
Credit report questions

Experian
Credit report and scores

TransUnion
Free credit score

Fee Schedules

Medicare Physician Fee Schedule
Specific downloadable files

Free Medical and Hospital Care

Free Medical Care
Search the Internet: "Free medical care," then the name of your state

Free Hospital Care
Search the Internet: "Free hospital care," then the name of your state

Internet Skip Tracing

Search using the following websites:
- Anywho
- Bigfoot Directions
- InfoSpace
- InfoUSA
- SearchBug
- Yahoo People Search
- 411Locate

Newsletters

The Doctor's Office
HCPro: Newsletter articles

The Health Care Collector
Aspen Publications

CHAPTER 14

BANKING

LEARNING OBJECTIVES

After reading this chapter and learning step-by-step procedures to gain job skills,* you should be able to:

- Define common banking terms.
- List different types of checking accounts.
- Name several types of checks.
- Explain the difference between a blank, a restrictive, and a full endorsement.
- Discuss reasons to make prompt bank deposits.
- State precautions when using an automated teller machine.
- Illustrate how to write a check and perform checkbook management.
- Articulate features of online banking.
- Understand the steps used in reconciling a bank statement.

PERFORMANCE OBJECTIVES (PROCEDURES) IN THIS TEXTBOOK

- Prepare a bank deposit (Procedure 14-1).
- Write a check using proper format and calculate a running balance (Procedure 14-2).
- Reconcile a bank statement (Procedure 14-3).

PERFORMANCE OBJECTIVES (JOB SKILLS) IN THE WORKBOOK

- Prepare a bank deposit (Job Skill 14-1).
- Write checks (Job Skill 14-2).
- Endorse a check (Job Skill 14-3).
- Inspect a check (Job Skill 14-4).
- Reconcile a bank statement (Job Skill 14-5).

---

* This textbook *and the accompanying* Workbook *meet the educational components for entry-level administrative and general competenciesoutlined by CAAHEP and ABHES.*

KEY TERMS

ABA routing number	electronic funds transfer system (EFTS)	postdated check
automated teller machine (ATM)	endorsement	reconciliation
automatic transfer of funds	forgery	service charges
bank statement	money order	signature card
bearer	nonsufficient funds (NSF)	stale check
checking account	overdraft	stop payment orders
currency	payee	voucher
deposits	payer	warrant
direct deposit service		withdrawal

HEART OF THE HEALTH CARE PROFESSIONAL

Service

A medical assistant who is knowledgeable about financial transactions can assist the patient when payments are made for professional medical services.

FINANCIAL INSTITUTIONS

Banks are financial institutions that receive deposits into accounts, lend money, and render other services. It is important to select a financial institution that offers services that can be tailored to the particular needs of a medical practice. Such services as free online banking and a safety deposit box; lines of credit that include a wide variety of loans and equipment financing; and face-to-face interaction with decision makers are all important considerations when choosing a financial institution.

Similar services are offered by credit unions, savings and loan associations, and other financial institutions. By comparing these services and making the most effective use of them for the medical practice, a knowledgeable medical assistant can be a financial asset to an employer.

Every financial transaction between a medical practice and a bank concerns some form of money (e.g., cash, checks, money orders). Therefore, the medical assistant must understand fundamental banking procedures and common banking terms.

ACCOUNTS

Premier accounts, money market accounts, and both personal and business accounts are offered at financial institutions. The most common types of accounts are savings and checking accounts.

Savings Account

A *savings account* is an interest-bearing account into and from which deposits and withdrawals may be made; there is no stated maturity date. Generally, savings accounts have debit restrictions to discourage frequent withdrawals, so they typically do not offer check-writing capabilities; however, some may offer limited check writing (e.g., three checks per month). A physician's office may have a savings account into which regular deposits are made to accrue interest, then money may be transferred into the checking account monthly or as the need arises to pay practice expenses, including payroll.

COMPLIANCE

Identity Theft

Privileged Information

Bank transactions involve privileged information, such as account numbers and signatures. Medical assistants must be aware of the importance of confidentiality in financial matters; for example, they should keep financial documents in locked files and shred documents as their retention period expires.

Checking Account

A **checking account** may or may not be interest bearing; it is subject to withdrawals of funds on deposit by check, debit cards, automatic clearing house (ACH) debits, electronic funds transfers, and online bill paying.

Types of Checking Accounts

The medical assistant may be responsible for making deposits into and withdrawals from a checking account and reconciling the bank statement at the end of each month. There are various types of checking accounts, but the most common are individual or joint checking accounts and business or commercial checking accounts:

- *Individual or joint checking account*—The depositor purchases a supply of checks and places money in the checking account to cover the amount of checks written. A joint checking account is owned by two or more people and requires signatures either singly or jointly for withdrawals or check writing, depending on how the account is set up. The bank keeps a **signature card** on file for each account, showing those authorized to sign or endorse and cash checks. There may be no fee with a specified minimum balance, a flat monthly fee, or a per-check charge.

- *Business or commercial checking account*—A large number of checks are purchased or furnished by the bank to the depositor. Typically, if the account has a minimum balance, there is no charge, but if the balance of the account falls below a set minimum amount (e.g., $10,000), a service charge may be levied.

Electronic Funds Transfer System—A system by which preauthorized transfers are electronically made from one account to another is called an **electronic funds transfer system (EFTS)**. The physician can arrange with the bank to have money automatically transferred on a certain day of the month from an interest-paying savings account into a noninterest-paying checking account. This is called **automatic transfer of funds**. Instead of writing checks, the EFTS may be used for *automatic bill payments* for such things as mortgage payments, utility bills, and insurance premiums. There is often no charge for this service. Payroll can also be handled with an EFTS. Benefits of using an EFTS are security, efficiency, and cost savings because processing electronic payments is less expensive than paper checks.

Pay-by-Phone System—The *pay-by-phone* system is a substitute for check writing whereby the medical assistant telephones the bank or savings and loan association to initiate payments by asking for a transfer of funds. Secure passwords and/or security questions are used to verify the caller and access the account. There may be a nominal fee for the service, which is usually less than the postage to mail a check; some financial institutions provide this as a free service if a minimum balance is maintained.

Point-of-Sale Banking System—A point-of-sale (POS) banking system brings banking to the business location. It allows instant transfer of funds from a patient's bank account at the time services are received. The system uses an electronic terminal and a plastic debit card plus an identification number (PIN), which is known only to the owner.

CHECKS

A large percentage of the money received in a physician's office are payments made by checks. A *check (CK)* is a written order to a bank to pay money on demand. The check illustrated in Figure 14-1A is a business check from Practon Medical Group, Inc. The check register, or stub (Figure 14-1B), is filled out at the time the check is written and the amount of the check is subtracted from the current balance to calculate the checking account's running balance, which is also referred to as the *balance forward*. If a deposit is made, it is added to the balance forward.

Financial software (e.g., Quicken®, QuickBooks™) and medical software programs offer computerized checks with the business name imprinted. They are usually preformatted but unnumbered and sequential check numbers are recorded on each check and the check register at the time of printing, along with the payee's name and amount. If personal information (e.g., gross pay with deductions) or notes (e.g., refund to insurance company) are recorded, that area appears white and the information does not show on the completed check.

Each check is numbered in the top right corner. The check sequence number is also imprinted by the bank as the last number at the bottom, along with a first series of numbers, which identifies the financial institution, and a second series of numbers, which identifies the checking account number. The American Bankers Association code number, called the **ABA routing number**, appears as a fraction and is located on the face of

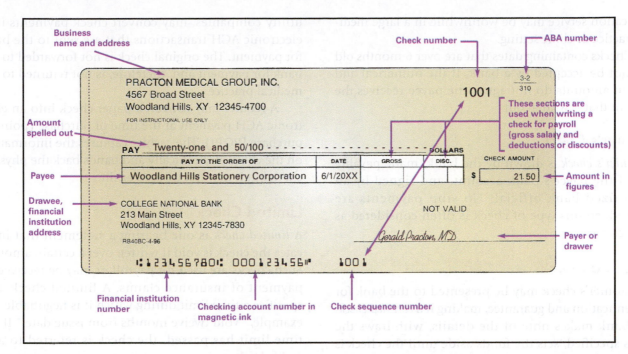

FIGURE 14-1A Completed check with its various parts identified. In an ABA routing number (i.e., 3-2/310), numbers 1 through 49 before the hyphen designate the cities where Federal Reserve banks are located or other key cities, and numbers 50 through 99 designate the states or territories. The number after the hyphen is the bank's assigned number. The denominator (310) is the number of the Federal Reserve district where the bank is located.

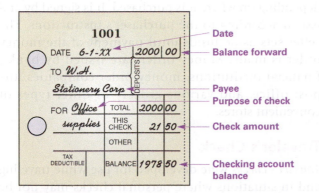
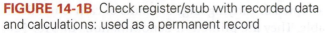

FIGURE 14-1B Check register/stub with recorded data and calculations: used as a permanent record

the check in the top right area. The name and address of the owner of the checking account appears in the top left portion of the check. The blank areas to be completed include the date, name you are writing the check to (payee), amount of the check (written in figures and spelled out), and signature of payer. Three parties are involved when a check is written:

1. The *drawer*/**payer** (or depositor) who orders the bank to pay
2. The *drawee* (or financial institution) where the money is deposited

3. The **payee** (or person) who is directed to receive the money

A check is negotiable, that is, legally transferable, to another person by endorsement when it meets the following requirements. It must be:

1. Written
2. Signed by the drawer, or *maker*
3. An unconditional order to pay a specific amount of money
4. Payable to the order of the bearer
5. Payable on demand or on a definite date
6. Written to the payee

The payee endorses the check, thereby transferring the right to receive the money.

Types of Checks

Various types of checks may be presented in a medical practice. Always inspect a check to be sure it is properly completed. Obtain a state driver's license number and a second form of identification so that they may be compared against existing records before accepting a check for payment. Request additional information for all out-of-state or suspicious checks. Use of a check authorization system or private company that offers a check verification service may be worthwhile in a large medical practice or clinic setting.

Checks containing dates that are over 6 months old will not be accepted by a bank. If the numerical and written amounts do not agree, the payee receives the amount that is written out.

Cashier's Check

A *cashier's check* is drawn by the bank, made payable out of the payee's bank account, and signed by an authorized bank official. No stop payments are allowed, so this type of check is often considered as good as cash.

Certified Check

A customer's check may be presented to the bank for authentication and guarantee, making it a *certified check*. The bank makes note of the details, withdraws the funds specified, sets the funds aside until the check is presented for payment, stamps "certified" on the check face, and has the check signed by an authorized bank official. This check is not used very often.

Counter Check

A *counter check* is one available at the bank for the depositor to draw funds from his or her own account. The wording on the check, "Pay to the Order of Myself Only," makes the counter check nonnegotiable. A counter check can also be a blank check used to transact a payment when a person does not have checks with him or her. The name of the bank must be written in as well as other standard information.

Electronic Check

An *electronic check* is a check created from digital images of the original. The *21st Century Act,* known as "*Check 21,*" is a federal law that went into effect October 28, 2004, and allows the use of electronic checks. Instead of the bank transporting checks physically, they can now transport them electronically to other banks in the check collection process. The reproductions are called *substitute checks.* Both the front and back of the check are copied and a legend that states "This is a legal copy of your check" appears; the substitute check serves all uses of the original check and may or may not be returned with the bank statement.

Some companies will take a paper check that has been sent by the medical office and convert it into an electronic transaction that is processed via the ACH system. Also, regular billers, such as telephone and utility companies, may convert check payments into electronic ACH transactions that are sent to the bank for payment. The original check is not forwarded to the bank for payment and, therefore, is not returned to the medical practice.

A retailer may convert a paper check into an electronic ACH payment at the time of purchase (point of purchase [POP]). The cashier captures the information on the check electronically and hands back the physical check but it may not be used again.

Limited Check

A *limited check* is one bearing a statement that indicates the check is void if written over a certain amount. Such checks are used for payroll or may be received as payment of insurance claims. A limited check also specifies a time limit during which it is negotiable, for example, "Void twelve months from issue date." If the time limit has passed, the check is referred to as a **stale check**.

Money Order

A **money order** is an instrument similar to a check purchased for face value plus a fee, which may vary depending on where it is purchased. It is signed by and issued according to the purchaser's instructions. The seller sets aside funds until payment of the money order is made. Money orders are issued by banks, financial institutions, money order companies, the post office, and various grocery or other types of convenient stores.

Traveler's Check

Traveler's checks were developed for use while traveling and in situations where personal checks may not be accepted or carrying large amounts of cash is not desirable. They are printed in denominations of $10, $20, $50, and $100. The checks, purchased from banks or traveler's clubs, are signed on their face in the presence of a witness at the time of purchase. Then, when cashing a check, the owner fills in the name of the payee and signs his or her name again on the face of the check. The second signature must be done in the presence of the person cashing the check, who can then compare the two signatures for authenticity. Copies of travel check numbers are provided to the purchaser and must be kept separate from the original checks. This provides protection against loss or theft. When a bank deposit slip is completed, traveler's checks are listed as checks, not cash.

Voucher Check

A *voucher check* is a check that is available in a variety of styles. Some medical offices order the style that is bound with three checks to a page. A perforation divides the actual check from that portion that outlines written details of the payment. Another style is unbound checks in assembled packs with a copy that is retained as a record of the transaction. Insurance plans and programs often issue voucher checks as payment for insurance claims.

Warrant

A **warrant** is a check that is not considered negotiable until it is converted into a *negotiable instrument*, that is, a written order promising to pay a specific sum. A warrant shows that a debt is due because services have been rendered, entitling the bearer to payment. Government and civic agencies may issue warrants. An insurance adjuster issues *drafts*, also known as warrants, that order the insurance company to pay a claim. Warrants do not have ABA numbers (see previous section and Figure 14-1A). To receive payment on a warrant, it must be submitted to the bank that has the funds for collection and final payment. A warrant can be subjected to a lengthy delay before funds are available from the source bank.

Check Fraud Prevention

A check written with the knowledge that there is not sufficient money in the account to cover the check is considered an *intent to defraud* and is unlawful. Businesses are more vulnerable during the following times:

- Friday afternoons
- Evenings
- Weekends
- Holidays

Be cautious when receiving checks. Do not give out bank or credit card information over the telephone, and ask the bank about fraud prevention features when checks are ordered.

Check Endorsements

Checks and money orders must be endorsed on the back by the payee (the person or company the check is made out to) exactly as written. If the endorser's name is incorrect on the face of the check, it should be endorsed twice—first as it appears on the face of the check and then as it appears on the account signature card. If a check is made out to "**bearer**" or "cash," it is considered a negotiable instrument and requires no endorsement, although banks may require a signature as evidence of who received the money.

To endorse a check, the payee or the payee's authorized agent writes, types, or stamps his or her name and other pertinent matter on the back of the check within the specified area, 1½ inches from the *trailing edge*. The trailing edge is the left end of the check that has the payee's name and address printed on it. An authorized agent may be the physician, office manager, bookkeeper, or administrative medical assistant in charge of bank deposits. After the check is properly endorsed, it may then be deposited in a bank or cashed.

The most commonly used **endorsements** in a physician's practice are *blank*, *restrictive*, and *full endorsements* (Figure 14-2).

Blank Endorsement

The blank endorsement is the most common way of endorsing a check. The payee simply signs his or her name on the back of the check near the left end. A check so endorsed should be cashed or deposited immediately. The medical assistant is most likely to use a blank endorsement when the physician's office manager or bookkeeper writes a check to "cash" or "petty cash," and the assistant endorses the check, thereby verifying who received payment.

Restrictive Endorsement

In the restrictive endorsement, besides signing the company's name or the endorser's signature, words are added, such as "For deposit only," to indicate that the check cannot be used for any purpose other than that stated. This custom is widely used in medical practices because it protects payment to the payee by preventing a **forgery** (fraudulent endorsement). Use a rubber stamp to stamp the check with a restrictive endorsement immediately on receipt to safeguard it from being negotiable should it be lost or stolen. Sometimes insurance checks require a personal signature endorsement, in which case a stamped endorsement may not be accepted; this is stated on the back of the check. The payee must endorse such checks with his or her signature, and the assistant then stamps the restrictive endorsement immediately below the signature.

Full Endorsement

A full endorsement, sometimes called a *special endorsement*, is used when a check is to be transferred to another person or company. This is referred to as a *third-party check*, mentioned later in this chapter.

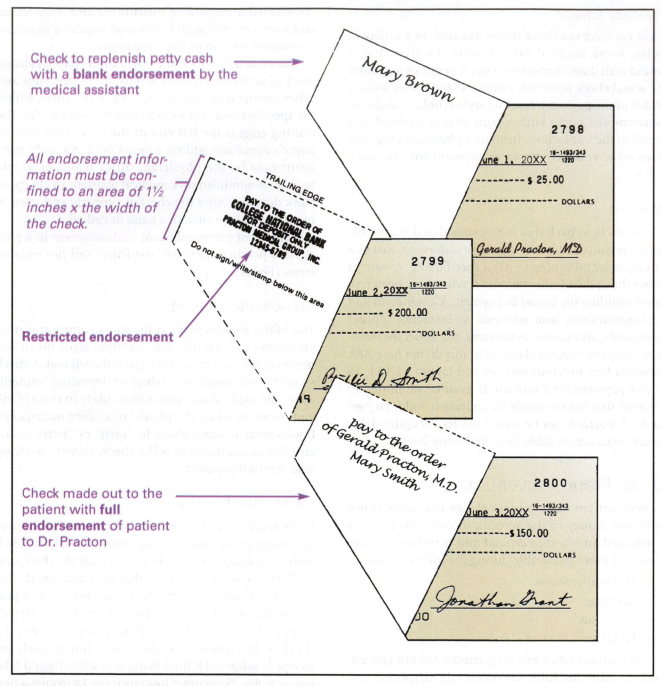

Check to replenish petty cash with a **blank endorsement** by the medical assistant

All endorsement information must be confined to an area of 1½ inches x the width of the check.

Restricted endorsement

Check made out to the patient with **full endorsement** of patient to Dr. Practon

TRAILING EDGE

PAY TO THE ORDER OF
COLLEGE NATIONAL BANK
FOR DEPOSIT ONLY
PRACTON MEDICAL GROUP, INC.
12345-6789

Do not sign/write/stamp below this area

Mary Brown

2798

June 1, 20XX   16-1493/343
1220

$ 25.00

DOLLARS

Gerald Practon, MD

2799

June 2, 20XX   16-1493/343
1220

$ 200.00

DOLLARS

By Mlii D. Smith

pay to the order
of Gerald Practon, M.D.
Mary Smith

2800

June 3, 20XX   16-1493/343
1220

$150.00

DOLLARS

Jonathan Grant

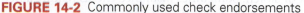

FIGURE 14-2 Commonly used check endorsements

BANK DEPOSITS

Preparing daily bank deposits is one of the routine chores usually handled by the administrative medical assistant. Deposits of checks and currency (paper money) should be made promptly to prevent payments being lost, misplaced, or stolen. Timely deposits reduce the possibility of a check being returned due to insufficient funds.

Some computerized financial software programs create a daily deposit slip when payments are posted to accounts. Manual bookkeeping systems (e.g., pegboard) include a deposit slip that the bank will accept if it is stapled to the physician's *deposit slip*. Such slips have the account number printed in magnetic ink, so they may be "read" by magnetic ink character recognition (MICR) equipment. An itemization lists the types of money included in the deposit (e.g., checks and cash) along with each check's ABA number (Figure 14-3). Since checks are read electronically, banks no longer mandate that the ABA routing number be recorded. Some medical offices prefer to write the patient's last name or check number on the deposit slip instead of the ABA number. Computerized software programs often track the actual check number, which is input when posting payment. Refer to Procedure 14-1 for instructions on preparing a bank deposit.

Banking by Mail

A bank service whereby deposits are mailed by the customer to the bank is known as *bank by mail.* Banks provide special mail deposit slips and envelopes with either preprinted account numbers or with space to record them. This saves the medical assistant considerable time, but cash cannot be deposited by this method unless it is sent by registered mail and all checks should include restrictive endorsements. The bank will send the depositor a receipt along with another envelope and deposit slip, or some banks use a duplicate deposit slip system, whereby the depositor keeps the duplicate as the receipt.

Direct Deposit Program

A **direct deposit service** is the automatic electronic deposit of wages or benefits (e.g., payroll/Social Security check) into a customer's bank account explained earlier as an electronic funds transfer. This expedites the deposit of a check and the availability of funds. It also eliminates mailing expenses or going to the bank to accomplish the transaction.

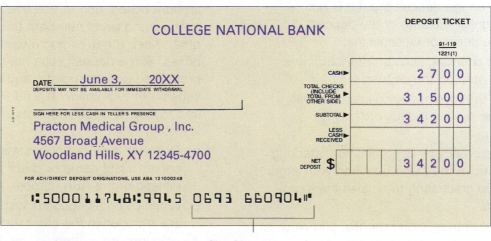

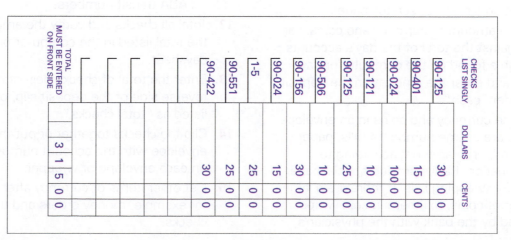

FIGURE 14-3 Both sides of a completed deposit slip showing ABA routing numbers and boxed areas where itemized checks and totals are entered

PROCEDURE 14-1

②③

Prepare a Bank Deposit

OBJECTIVE: Prepare a bank deposit slip for the day's receipts (cash and checks), complete financial records related to the deposit, and deposit the day's receipts into a bank account.

EQUIPMENT/SUPPLIES: Items for deposit (currency, money orders, checks, bank deposit slip), endorsement stamp (optional), computer, envelope, and pen.

DIRECTIONS: Follow these step-by-step directions, which include rationales, to learn this procedure. Job Skill 14-1 is presented in the *Workbook* to practice this skill. Refer to Figure 14-3 for a visual example.

1. Write the name and address of the physician on the deposit slip if it is not preprinted; list the date of the deposit. Never use pencil or erasable ink.

2. Insert the checking account number if it is not preprinted on the deposit slip.

3. Organize the receipts by dividing the bills, coins, checks, and money orders into separate piles.

4. Sort the currency by denomination, stacking bills face up in the same direction with larger bills on top graduating to smaller ones or vice versa.

5. Total the currency (paper money) and write this amount on a piece of scratch paper.

6. Total the amount of coins and write this amount on a piece of scratch paper.

7. Total the amount of currency and coins, verify it against the total of the day's accounts receivable found on the computer or daysheet, and enter the amount on the deposit slip under "cash."

8. Place the currency and coins in an envelope. If there are a large number of bills, paper clip, band, or wrap them according to denomination. Banks provide special paper bands for wrapping bills. If there are a large number of coins, roll them in coin wrappers supplied by the bank with the physician's

name and account number written or stamped on each wrapper.

9. Verify that a restrictive endorsement has been placed on the back of all the checks and money orders.

10. Examine each check to be deposited to ensure it is properly drawn. Watch for **postdated checks** (dated for sometime in the future) and discrepancies between written amounts and figures. If a check is written improperly, the payer must be contacted.

11. List each check separately on the deposit slip, including the top portion of the ABA number (see Figures 14-1A and 14-3) and the amount. Write all numbers inside the amount boxes, do not use fractions or dashes, and avoid numbers touching each other. Keep other writing away from amount boxes. Some deposit slips may not have preprinted decimal points, and others may appear printed. Follow the bank's directions as to whether decimal points should be inserted.

    a. *Optional:* If office policy states, insert the patient's last name or check number instead of the ABA number.

    b. When using a pegboard system, checks are arranged in the order received and amounts are written on the deposit slip listing the names of the patients and the ABA transit numbers.

12. Total all checks and verify the amount with the total listed in the computer or on the daysheet.

13. Enter the total of checks deposited on the reverse side of the deposit slip, or in an area listed as "total checks."

14. Clip the checks together or put them in an envelope with the account number written on each envelope or wrapper.

15. List other items of currency after the checks, for example, money orders and traveler's checks.

(continues)

PROCEDURE 14-1 (continued)

16. Subtotal the amount of cash and currency and verify this amount with the amount listed in the computer or on the daysheet.

17. Recalculate the "net deposit total" for verification (total amount of currency, coins, and checks) and enter this on the deposit slip. Banks accept a date-stamped adding machine tape indicating the amounts of the checks, cash, and change. The tape should be duplicated and the original stapled to the deposit slip; the duplicate should be stapled to the duplicate deposit slip or daysheet.

18. Make a photocopy of the deposit slip, if needed, to retain in the office.

19. Enter the amount of the deposit (preferably with red ink so deposits can be quickly

located) in the checkbook register and add it to the current balance, indicating the new balance.

20. Place coins, currency, checks, and the deposit slip in a large envelope or bank deposit bag to transport it to the bank in person. Or if mailing the deposit, put them in a bank-by-mail envelope and send by registered mail.

21. Obtain a *deposit record* or receipt from the bank at the conclusion of the transaction for deposits made in person. File it for later reference when reconciling the monthly bank statement. *Note:* To guard against embezzlement, have one person collect money and another person prepare the bank deposit.

In a physician's practice, payroll may be deposited directly into an employee's bank account or arrangements can be made for regular insurance payments (e.g., Medicare) to be deposited into the physician's bank account.

After-Hours Deposits

If the physician's office closes after banking hours, a depositor may use the after-hours depository service of a bank. The deposit is placed in an envelope and dropped through a slot located on the outside of the bank. The deposit is processed by the bank the following morning or held unopened until the depositor can get to the bank personally to make the deposit; then during banking hours, it is necessary to obtain a replacement envelope and a deposit receipt. A double-locked security bag is available from banks for a small fee for this purpose. Always double-check that the deposit bag has gone into the evening deposit drawer properly by reopening the drawer.

AUTOMATED TELLER MACHINES

An **automated teller machine (ATM)** is a computerized terminal that enables a customer to make a deposit, withdraw cash, transfer funds, or obtain other bank services (Figure 14-4). Automated teller

machines are accessible 24 hours a day, 7 days a week, and are installed in the outer wall of a bank. Additional terminals can be found in airports, train stations, shopping centers, college campuses, and supermarkets. Depositors are given a debit card and select a personal identification number (PIN) that

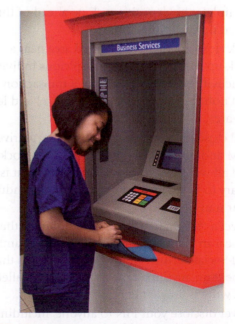

FIGURE 14-4 Medical assistant depositing money in an ATM

gives them access to their own computerized bank accounts. If cash is needed and the bank is not open or located in a convenient area, a debit card allows **withdrawal** (removal of funds) at an ATM. The card may also be used at other locations (e.g., restaurants, stores) to make cashless purchases from funds on deposit. Banks may charge retailers and customers for the use of debit cards. Do not keep a copy of the checking account number and ATM personal identification number in the same place; if found together, these numbers make it easy for a thief to steal from an account even without a check.

Basic Rules of Precaution

ATM "skimming" has led to billions of dollars in yearly losses. Thieves have used portable card reading devices that fit over the card slot to record data on a card's magnetic strip. They have also used tiny cameras that videotape customers entering their PINs into the machine, or a transparent sheet placed over the ATM keyboard that can record PINs. Thieves have even placed a framed laptop computer on top of an ATM screen with a look-alike screen featuring the bank logo and instructions for transactions and used it to duplicate debit cards with PINs written on the back and later sold on the black market.

Because ATMs dispense cash, it is wise to use the machines with caution and awareness. Consider these guidelines:

- Complete the deposit envelope ahead of time to speed up the transaction.
- Park close and in a well-lighted area near a walk-up ATM and look for suspicious individuals or activity nearby. If you begin a transaction and notice something unusual, cancel and leave the area.
- Pull close to the machine when using a drive-up ATM and be sure your vehicle doors are locked and all windows are closed except when it is necessary to lower the driver's window to conduct your transaction.
- Select a PIN that does not have numbers that appear in birthdates, addresses, phone numbers, and Social Security numbers, or numbers that appear on anything that is carried in a wallet. Do not write it down; memorize it.
- Never disclose your PIN to anyone, including merchants, bank employees, government officials, or police officers.

- Use your hand or body as a shield to protect the PIN secret code and prevent others from seeing the PIN code input. Stand directly in front of the panel containing the push buttons. If someone is using the ATM ahead of you, allow that person room for privacy by remaining a few steps back.
- Avoid ATMs with new equipment protruding from or near the card slot or signs noting new equipment.
- Retain the transaction receipt or ATM statement to keep the account information confidential. Do not leave it at the machine or throw it into a nearby trash receptacle. Receipts should be checked against the monthly bank statement.
- For night use, it is preferable to use an ATM that is indoors at a market or shopping mall or to locate a well-lit ATM. If using an enclosed ATM, close the vestibule entry door completely after entering the ATM and do not open the vestibule door to any unknown person(s) at any time.
- Never count or display money at the ATM. Put it away immediately and count it later, in a safe place.
- Put away your cash, card, and receipt and leave immediately upon completion of your transaction. Look around as you prepare to leave the ATM.
- Ask your bank what the ATM withdrawal limit is on your account and lower it if it is too high.
- Keep track of your account balance and report any discrepancies to the bank immediately.
- Never accept offers of help from anyone not associated with the bank.
- Call 911 if emergency assistance due to criminal activity or medical emergency is needed.

Prepaid Cards

Patients who do not have bank accounts may offer to pay the physician using a *prepaid card*. These cards are used to pay bills or buy merchandise in the same places a bank-issued debit card can be used. Cards may be bought at supermarkets, drugstores, and big box retailers (e.g., Walmart) and come with logos (e.g., Visa, MasterCard). Prepaid cards are the fastest growing payment method in the United States because they are now being used instead of checking accounts. Fees are charged to customers to activate, reload, and maintain the cards and merchants also pay a fee every time a card is swiped.

CHECKBOOK MANAGEMENT

At the time a check is written, the assistant should complete the **voucher** or *check stub* attached to the check or designated area in the checkbook, referred to as the *check register* (Figure 14-5). This routine reduces the possibility of forgetting to record information and prevents incorrect calculations. The bank balance should be known at all times, so a check is not written for an amount greater than the balance, causing an **overdraft**. A continuous record of the bank balance is kept on the stub or posted in a check register.

Deposits are added to the balance (preferably in red ink) and checks are subtracted to compute the new balance. Other bank charges, such as service charges for handling checks returned by the bank for insufficient funds, must also be subtracted in the check register to keep the balance accurate. If a check is not written properly, financial responsibility for any loss is borne by the drawer. Refer to Procedure 14-2 for step-by-step directions when writing a check.

Check Writer Machine

Some offices use a check writer machine that imprints the figures on a check so that they cannot be changed. First, the date, the name of the payee, and the amount (in figures) are typed on the check. Then, the check is inserted into the check writer machine. Next, the dollar and cent amounts of the check are set on the machine, and a lever is pressed down. In one operation, the check is imprinted and embossed with the dollar amount. Some machines also imprint over the payee's name, so it cannot be altered. Always double-check the figures before imprinting the check; incorrect checks must be voided. The check should be signed by the physician.

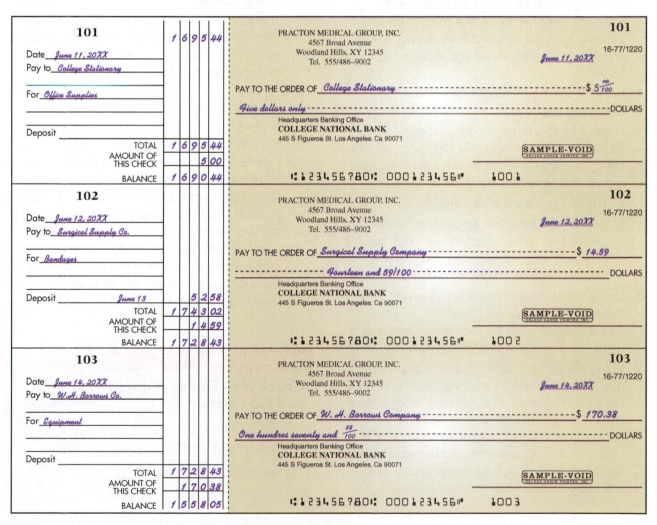

FIGURE 14-5 Handwritten checks with completed check stubs

PROCEDURE 14-2

Write a Check Using Proper Format and Calculate a Running Balance

OBJECTIVE: Write a check, record it in the checkbook, and calculate a new balance.

EQUIPMENT/SUPPLIES: Blank check, checkbook, calculator, and pen.

DIRECTIONS: Follow these step-by-step directions, which include rationales, to learn this procedure. Job Skill 14-2 is presented in the *Workbook* to practice this skill.

1. Balance the checkbook, so it is up to date and be sure there are sufficient funds to cover the check to be written.

2. Complete the check register showing the date the check is being written, the payee's name, the amount of the check, and the purpose for which payment is being made.

3. Subtract the amount of the check from the balance brought forward (running balance) and list the new balance (balance carried forward).

4. Indicate the new balance forward in the check register.

5. Handwrite the information on the check in ink; do not use an erasable ballpoint pen. If a check is made out and an error is made, you can do either one of the following:

   a. Correct the error and initial it.

   b. Draw a diagonal line across the face of the check and write "void." Write "void" on the stub or in the register, and then file the voided check with the canceled checks.

6. Use a check-printing device to prevent tampering. Checks can be "washed" or altered by a skilled crook if ink that is not indelible is used.

7. Enter the current date, including the month, day, and year (checks may be dated on Sundays and holidays). A postdated check can be issued only with permission from the person accepting the check, because this practice may result in an overdraft, embarrassing the physician and reflecting poorly on the financial soundness of the medical practice.

8. Enter the payee's full name without title such as Mr. or Mrs. and begin writing to the extreme left. Draw a line from the name to the dollar sign at the right to protect the check against alteration. Use abbreviations only when instructed to do so or when space is limited. If the payee is an officer of an organization, include this on the check (e.g., "John Doe, Treasurer.")

9. Write the amount of the check in figures, placing them close to the dollar sign and close to each other.

   a. If typing, use the hyphen or asterisk key to fill in all blank spaces.

   b. If handwriting, draw a line in any remaining spaces.

   The amount should agree with the check stub or register. Use commas if the amount of the check is four figures or higher; for example, $4,500.50.

10. Write the amount of the check in words on the line that typically appears below the payee's name; begin at the extreme left of the line so that no additional words can be inserted to increase the amount, and draw a line from the end of the written amount to the printed word *Dollars*. Separate the cents amount from the dollar amount by writing the word *and*, and write the cents as a fraction; for example, 50/100. If there are no cents, write the word *no* as the numerator or the word *only* in place of the fraction (see Example 14-1).

EXAMPLE 14-1

Check with Dollar Amount and No Cents

Ten dollars only

Ten dollars and no/100

Ten dollars and no cents

(continues)

PROCEDURE 14-2 (continued)

11. If there are no dollars, only cents, the figures following the dollar sign should be circled; for example: $.75; the printed word *Dollars* should be crossed out (see Example 14-2).

12. Keep the checkbook in a secure place out of the reach and sight of unauthorized persons.

13. Write the purpose of the check on the face of the check on a memo line, if included.

14. Obtain the physician's or other authorized person's signature on each check.

EXAMPLE 14-2

Written Amounts on Checks

Only seventy-five cents _____ ~~Dollars~~

No and ⟨75/100⟩ _____ ~~Dollars~~

Note: The written words on a check always represent the correct amount no matter what is expressed in figures.

Banking Online

An optional banking method, called online banking or *Internet banking*, that benefits both the financial institution and the client is offered by banks, credit unions, savings and loan associations, and other financial institutions. The physician must have a computer with Internet access. To bank online, you have to have an eligible account (e.g., checking, savings, certificates of deposit, loans), a user identification number, and an online bank password. Usually there is no monthly fee for accessing accounts, but fees may apply to services ordered online. Access is available 24 hours a day, 7 days a week.

Features that are available with this type of communication include viewing account balances; reviewing transaction history; viewing the front and back of a paid item; transferring money between accounts; printing a statement; searching for specific transactions by date, check number, or amount; placing a stop payment on a check; and many other benefits. It is possible to send electronic mail messages to the financial institution and obtain a response.

Payment Disputes and Check-Writing Errors

A normal check endorsement constitutes acceptance. If a patient writes on a statement "paid in full," but the check amount is for less than the balance due, do not return the check to the patient. For legal protection, do not cross out "payment in full," instead write the words *without prejudice, under protest, received as payment on account, endorsement disputes payment in full,* or *endorsed under protest as per UCC 1-207; payment not in full.* Write "balance due" and the amount above your

endorsement and make a copy of this endorsement to be kept in the files for future reference. Send a copy to the patient along with a request for payment in full, or telephone the patient to discuss the unpaid balance before sending a bill. The check may be deposited if bank policy allows acceptance of a conditional endorsement—in this way any disputed balance may be collected. If not resolved, you might consider referring this account to a professional collector.

Correction notices or **stop payment orders** are sent from the bank if a bookkeeping error has been made, if a deposit did not include as much money as shown on the deposit slip, or if a check was uncashable for any of several reasons. The following section lists examples.

Nonsufficient Funds

When the payer did not have sufficient money in the account to cover the check, this is referred to as **nonsufficient funds (NSF)**. First, call the patient and then call the bank to verify the balances, or ask the patient to pay in cash or by money order or credit card. Keep a record of patients who habitually write such checks, and accept only cash, money order, or credit/debit cards from them for future payments.

Misdated Check

If a bank clerk spots a postdated check or an old check dated 3 to 6 months before the day of deposit, it is usually not honored—that is, it is "bounced" by the bank. Look at the date of every check you receive. Federal collection law states that if a check dated more than 5 days in advance is accepted, the patient must be notified no more than 10 days and no less than 3 days before the check is deposited. State laws vary, and some states add regulations in addition to those mandated by federal law. When a check bounces, both the check writer and the person to whom the check is written are usually charged a fee.

Incorrect Payee's Name

If the physician's name or practice's name on a check is incorrect, many banks will refuse to accept the check. For accuracy and to save time, offer the patient a rubber stamp containing the account name. If the name is written incorrectly, correct it and have the patient initial by the correction.

Missing Payer's Signature

Glance over each check to be sure it is signed. If you receive an unsigned check from a patient, first try to obtain a signature by asking the patient to come to the office and sign the check or send a new one. If unable to reach the patient or if there is a transportation or time limitation problem, write "over" on the check where the customer normally signs, then write "lack of signature guaranteed," your physician's name, and your name and title on the back of the check, leaving space above your name. Then sign your name in the space above the written version. When the check is deposited, your bank is assured that if the patient's bank does not honor the check, you will take it back as a charge against your account. This is the normal procedure for a dishonored check. Some banks will process the check if funds are available in the customer's account but other banks will process only if there is a written authorization on file. However, a debtor can protest a check that is deposited without a signature.

Variable Amounts

If the numerical amount and the written-out amount are different, the bank will credit only the written-out amount. Make sure the two amounts agree before accepting the check.

Third-Party Checks

Third-party checks include paychecks, government checks, and insurance checks made out to one party (e.g., the patient) and fully endorsed over to the physician. The bearer to which the check is made out to writes "Pay to the order of," followed by the name of a specified person or company, and signs his or her name, further protecting the check from improper use. Only the new payee can endorse it for further processing. Acceptance of a third-party check made out in an amount over that which is being collected may entail handing out so much cash that the cash drawer is

depleted. Many banks do not process third-party checks, and good office policy is to inform patients that third-party checks are not accepted.

Forged Checks

Accept checks only from patients who are known or, if from an unfamiliar person, obtain two forms of identification such as a driver's license, bank and employee identification cards, or a U.S. passport. Forgers are more likely to have national cards, for example, MasterCard, Visa, and American Express. Identifications that are insufficient are Social Security cards, library cards, voter registration cards, and unfamiliar credit cards.

BANK STATEMENTS

Every month, banks mail each depositor a statement of his or her checking account. Canceled checks or substitute checks that have been debited from the account during the month may or may not be included (Figure 14-6). The **bank statement** lists the date and amount of each deposit and of each withdrawal by date presented for payment, not by the date written. The statement also lists electronic transfers of money to the checking account, payments made via electronic banking (debit cards), and deposits made by mail. **Service charges** for processing transactions and account maintenance, along with interest paid and corrections are also listed, and check numbers are shown. The statement should be compared with the checkbook register immediately to determine the cause of any disparity in figures. The balance on the statement and the balance on the checkbook stub or register may not agree due to outstanding checks, so each month the two balances must be reconciled. It is an act of courtesy to cash checks promptly, so payers' bank statements can be more easily reconciled at the end of the month.

PATIENT EDUCATION
Payment Options

Educate patients about different types of payment accepted by the medical practice. If patients are aware that the office accepts debit and credit cards, the problem of returned checks will be minimized.

College National Bank
700 West Main Street
Woodland Hills, XY 12345

**COLLEGE NATIONAL BANK
ACCOUNT ACTIVITY**

(800) 540-5060

STATEMENT PERIOD: May 17, THROUGH
June 16, 20XX

PRACTON MEDICAL GROUP, INC   140
4567 BROAD AVENUE
WOODLAND HILLS XY   12345

ACCOUNT
12345-6789
ACCESS# 0082

PAGE   1

ITEM COUNT   30

CHECKING   ACCOUNT 12345-6789

SUMMARY			
	BEGINNING STATE BALANCE ON 5-17-20XX	$	633.87
	TOTAL OF 4 DEPOSITS/OTHER CREDITS		1414.75
	TOTAL OF 25 CHECKS PAID		271.53
	5 WITHDRAWALS/OTHER CHARGES		73.00
	ENDING STATEMENT BALANCE ON 6-16-20XX		1704.09

**CHECKS/
WITHDRAWALS/
OTHER CHARGES**

CHECKS:

NUMBER	DATE	AMOUNT	NUMBER	DATE	AMOUNT
0317	06-08	17.40	0328	06-10	29.90
1319	05-25	30.00	0329	05-26	32.05
0320	05-30	7.59	0330	06-02	2.75
0321	05-27	9.00	0331	06-02	30.79
0322	05-24	1.00	0332	06-02	11.47
0323	06-03	6.13			
0324	05-30	1.78			
0325	06-02	67.50			
0326	05-25	21.92			
0327	06-03	2.25			

TOTAL OF 25 CHECKS PAID $271.53–

WITHDRAWALS/OTHER CHARGES:

DATE	TRANSACTION DESCRIPTION	AMOUNT
06-10	SURGICAL SUPPLY PAYMENT AT ELECTRONIC BANKING	34.30
06-07	STAR FREE PRESS PAYMENT AT ELECTRONIC BANKING	2.00
06-07	MARINER'S MAIL PAYMENT AT ELECTRONIC BANKING	1.00
06-07	CELLULAR ONE PAYMENT AT ELECTRONIC BANKING	16.00
06-03	CLINT PHARMACY PAYMENT AT ELECTRONIC BANKING	19.70

**DEPOSITS/
OTHER CREDITS**

DEPOSITS:

DATE	TRANSACTION DESCRIPTION	AMOUNT
06-07	BRANCH DEPOSIT	250.24
06-09	BRANCH DEPOSIT	1000.00
06-15	BRANCH DEPOSIT	156.69
06-16	CHECK DEPOSIT AT BANK BY MAIL	7.82

DAILY BALANCES

DATE	BALANCE	DATE	BALANCE	DATE	BALANCE
05-24	632.87	06-02	418.02	06-09	1605.78
05-25	580.95	06-03	389.94	06-10	1573.88
05-26	548.90	06-07	623.18	06-15	1730.57
05-27	539.90	06-08	605.78	06-16	1704.09
05-30	530.53				

FIGURE 14-6 Bank statement illustrating date and amount of each deposit and withdrawal, service charges, interest, credits, corrections, check numbers, electronic transfers of money, payments made via electronic banking, and deposits made by mail

Bank Statement Reconciliation

As soon as a bank statement is received, the process of **reconciliation** should be performed (see Procedure 14-3 and Example 14-3). A form on the reverse side of the bank statement can be used for this purpose (Figure 14-7).

Balance Differences

If the checkbook balance and bank statement balance do not agree, all details must be rechecked to locate the error, which may result from:

1. Omission of a debit card transaction, a written check, or one or more outstanding checks, which may have been written without recording the information on the register. This could occur if the physician wrote a check without the medical assistant's knowledge.

2. Omission of a deposit in the checkbook register

3. Check drawn for a different sum than that recorded on the register

4. Check that has cleared for a different amount than what is shown in the checkbook

5. Addition or subtraction error(s) in the checkbook register while recording, calculating, or carrying figures forward

6. Transposition of figures on the register (divide the amount by nine to pinpoint a transposition error)

7. Canceled check omitted on the bank statement in error

FOUR EASY STEPS TO HELP YOU BALANCE YOUR CHECKBOOK

1. UPDATE YOUR CHECKBOOK
   - Compare and check-off each transaction recorded in your check register with those listed on this statement. These include checks, direct deposits, direct debits, deposits, ATM transactions, etc.
   - Add interest and subtract service charges.

2. DETERMINE OUTSTANDING ITEMS
   - Use the charts below to list transactions shown in your check register but not included on this statement.
   - Include any from previous months.

OUTSTANDING CHECKS OR OTHER WITHDRAWALS				DEPOSITS NOT CREDITED		
CHECK NO.	AMOUNT	CHECK NO.	AMOUNT	DATE	AMOUNT	
248	$ 2 50		$	6/21/XX	$ 52 58	
318	14 59					
337	5 00					
338	6 15					
339	170 38					
340	5 00					
		TOTAL	$ 203.62	TOTAL	$	

3. BALANCE YOUR ACCOUNT
   - Enter Ending Statement Balance shown on this statement. $ 1704.09
   - Add deposits listed in your register and not shown on this statement.   +   52.58
   - Subtract outstanding checks/withdrawals.   –   203.62
   - **ADJUSTED TOTAL** (should agree with your checkbook balance). $ 1553.05

4. IF THE BALANCE IN YOUR CHECKBOOK DOES NOT AGREE WITH THE ADJUSTED TOTAL, THEN
   - Check all addition and subtraction.
   - Make sure all outstanding checks, withdrawals and deposits have been listed in the appropriate chart above.
   - Compare the amount of each check, withdrawal and deposit in your checkbook with the amounts on this statement.

FIGURE 14-7 Reverse side of a bank statement showing account reconciliation form

If an error is found, mark the register where the error occurred with a reference to the check number or register line where the correction is made. Enter the correction after the last entry, together with a cross-reference to the check number or place in the register where the error occurred.

Refer to Example 14-3 for a simple illustration of the reconciliation formula.

PROCEDURE 14-3

Reconcile a Bank Statement

OBJECTIVE: Verify that all bank deposits and withdrawals agree with the medical practice's financial records of deposits and withdrawals.

EQUIPMENT/SUPPLIES: Ending balance of previous bank statement, current bank statement, reconciliation worksheet, deposit receipts, red pencil, checkbook register, canceled or returned checks, calculator, and pen or pencil.

DIRECTIONS: Follow these step-by-step directions, which include rationales, to learn this procedure. Job Skill 14-7 is presented in the *Workbook* to practice this skill.

1. Compare the opening balance on the current bank statement with the previous month's ending balance. They should agree.

2. Organize the canceled checks (if enclosed) in numerical order or refer to a separate list of canceled checks on the bank statement and compare the entries to the listing of credits on the statement to make sure the numbers and amounts are correct. Make sure that all checks are from the medical office and are for the statement period. Place a red check mark next to the amount of each returned check that has cleared the bank as it is verified.

3. Verify the amount of all electronic checks and place a red check mark next to the amount of each one that has cleared the bank as it is verified.

4. Compare the deposits listed on the bank statement with the amounts of the deposits listed on the check stubs or check register; place a red check mark next to the amount of each deposit as it is verified.

5. List the outstanding checks not returned with the statement on the bank reconciliation form. If a check has been outstanding for an unusual length of time (e.g., for two monthly statements), it may be lost. Call the payee to see if it has been received. Certified checks are not listed as outstanding because the amount has already been deducted from the account.

6. Total all outstanding checks and record the figure in the proper area—it may be titled: "Balance Your Account," "How to Balance Your Checkbook," or "Reconcile Your Checkbook with This Statement."

7. List all deposits in transit, that is, those that were made since the last entry on the bank statement.

8. Total all deposits made and not included on the statement and record this amount in the proper area.

9. Record the ending statement balance and add the total amount of deposits in transit and subtract the total amount of outstanding checks from the ending statement balance. *The result is the adjusted bank statement balance.*

10. Enter on the checkbook register and subtract from the checkbook balance any fees appearing on the bank statement, such as service charges, automatic withdrawals, or payments. *The result is the adjusted checkbook balance.*

11. *The two adjusted balances should agree.* If not in agreement, recheck each step to locate the error. The most common errors are missing an outstanding check and mathematical calculations.

12. When the checkbook is balanced, circle or highlight the balance and insert your initials to indicate who reconciled the statement; include the date it was reconciled.

EXAMPLE 14-3

Reconciliation Formula

Checkbook			Statement
Checkbook ending balance	$ _____	$ _____	Ending balance on bank statement
Subtract service charge and any other charges shown on bank statement; also enter these in your check register	−	+	Add any deposits made after the date of the bank statement
Subtotal	$ _____	$ _____	Subtotal
Add interest earned; also enter in your check register	+	−	Subtract total of outstanding checks and withdrawals listed above
	$ _____	$ _____	
Adjusted checkbook balance	$ _____	$ _____	Adjusted bank account ending balance

These two should agree.

STOP AND THINK CASE SCENARIO

Determine What Type of Checks to Write

SCENARIO A: The physician has asked you to send away to the American Medical Association for a very expensive continuing education video series. The physician left on vacation, and you do not have access to a business credit card. You are completing the order form and note that it states "personal checks" are not accepted. You have check-signing authority on the business account.

SCENARIO B: The physician is purchasing a used automobile from a private party for his eldest son to drive back and forth to college. The seller wishes to meet with the physician and deliver the car to the office tomorrow afternoon at which time payment will be required.

CRITICAL THINKING: Study the differences in cashier's checks, certified checks, counter checks, electronic checks, limited checks, money orders, traveler's checks, voucher checks, and warrants and determine the type of check you should obtain for payment for each scenario; state the reasons for your choice.

A. _____

_____

_____

_____

_____

_____

_____

_____

_____

B. _____

_____

_____

_____

_____

_____

_____

_____

_____

STOP AND THINK CASE SCENARIO
Answer Payment Question

SCENARIO: One of Dr. Practon's patients, Walter Knott, wants to pay an outstanding balance ($100) at the end of an office visit. He hands you a check in the amount of $200 that is made out to him and signed by someone unknown to you.

CRITICAL THINKING: Respond to the situation stating what type of check this is, how you would proceed, and the reason for your answer.

_____

_____

_____

_____

_____

FOCUS ON CERTIFICATION*

CMA (AAMA) Content Summary

- Banking procedures
- Preparing bank deposits

RMA (AMT) Content Summary

- Banking procedures
- Prepare and make bank deposits
- Reconcile bank statements
- Understand check processing procedures and requirements

- Nonsufficient funds (NSF)
- Endorsements

CMAS (AMT) Content Summary

- Understanding banking services and procedures
- Bank accounts
- Lines of credit
- Checking endorsements
- Bank deposits
- Bank reconciliation and statements

REVIEW EXAM-STYLE QUESTIONS

1. A joint checking account requires:
   a. the signature of both parties
   b. the signature of only one party
   c. the signature of a bank employee and the owner of the account
   d. the signature of one or both parties depending on how the account is set up
   e. the signature of a bank employee only

2. A system by which preauthorized transfers can be made from one account to another and automatic bill payments or payroll payments can be made is known by the abbreviation:
   a. EFT
   b. EFTS

   c. AFT
   d. AFTS
   e. PAT

3. The "drawee" is:
   a. the person who orders the bank to pay
   b. the person who is directed to receive the money
   c. the financial institution where the money is deposited
   d. the maker of the check
   e. the bearer to whom the check is written

This textbook and the accompanying Workbook meet the entry-level administrative and general competencies for the CMA outlined by the AAMA Examination Content Outline and Occupational Analysis and for the RMA and CMAS outlined by the AMT Competencies, Construction Parameters, and Examination Specifications (see Competency Grid in Appendix B).

4. If the numerical and written amounts of a check do not agree:
   a. the bank will not accept it
   b. the payee receives the amount that is spelled out
   c. the bank will hold it until the writer of the check verifies the correct amount
   d. the payee receives the numerical amount
   e. the check will be returned unpaid

5. If the endorser's name is written incorrectly on the face of a check:
   a. the incorrect name should be used to endorse the check
   b. the correct name should be used to endorse the check
   c. the incorrect and correct name should both be used to endorse the check
   d. the bank will always refuse the check
   e. the check should be voided

6. All checks received in a medical office should:
   a. be stamped with a restrictive endorsement upon receipt
   b. include a blank endorsement
   c. include a full endorsement
   d. be placed in a safe until they are deposited
   e. be turned over to the physician for safe keeping

7. Select the correct statement about bank deposits.
   a. Bank deposits are routinely prepared by the administrative medical assistant.
   b. Bank deposits should be made promptly to prevent payment from being lost, misplaced, or stolen.
   c. Timely deposits reduce the possibility of a check being returned due to insufficient funds.
   d. Never use pencil or erasable ink to write on a bank deposit slip.
   e. All of the above are correct.

8. ATM PIN numbers:
   a. should include either telephone numbers, address numbers, birthdates, or Social Security numbers so that they can be easily memorized
   b. should be shared confidentially with bank employees in case you forget them
   c. should not be disclosed to anyone except police officers in the case of an investigation
   d. should be written down and kept in a secret place for easy access
   e. should be memorized and shared with no one

9. If an error is made on a check when it is written, you can:
   a. correct the error and initial it
   b. draw a diagonal line across the face of the check and write "void"
   c. erase it, then make the correction
   d. use white out, then make the correction
   e. both a and b

10. Checks made out to one party and fully endorsed over to the physician are called:
    a. fraudulent checks
    b. third-party checks
    c. two-party checks
    d. forged checks
    e. nonsufficient fund checks

11. If a check is not written properly, financial responsibility for any loss is borne by the:
    a. drawee
    b. drawer
    c. payee
    d. depositor
    e. financial institution

12. When reconciling a bank statement:
    a. first start with the beginning balance from the bank statement
    b. subtract all deposits made after the date of the bank statement
    c. add the total of outstanding checks and withdrawals
    d. subtract the total of outstanding checks and withdrawals
    e. add the service charge to the checkbook balance

WORKBOOK ASSIGNMENT

To develop competency-based job skills, refer to the *Workbook* and complete the:
- Abbreviation and Spelling Review
- Review Questions

- Critical Thinking Exercises
- Job Skill activities, which are listed at the beginning of the chapter under *Performance Objectives in the Workbook.*

RESOURCES

Internet

Bank News
Resources, publications, directories, newsletters

How to Balance a Checkbook
Ten-step process to balance your checkbook

National Consumers League Fraud Center
Consumer help desk

Safe Checks
Fraud prevention

CHAPTER 15

BOOKKEEPING

LEARNING OBJECTIVES

After reading this chapter and learning step-by-step procedures to gain job skills,* you should be able to:

- Name four accounting systems and compare their differences and similarities.
- Define bookkeeping terminology and use proper abbreviations.
- Determine components of an account or ledger card.
- State posting procedures on a ledger and on a computerized account.
- Explain posting procedures on a daysheet.
- Describe accounts receivable control procedures.
- Discuss several ways bookkeeping errors can be located.
- Identify two types of cash funds typically used in a medical office.
- Perform bookkeeping procedures.

PERFORMANCE OBJECTIVES (PROCEDURES) IN THIS TEXTBOOK

- Prepare and post to a patient's account (Procedure 15-1).
- Prepare the pegboard; post charges, payments, and adjustments; and balance the daysheet (Procedure 15-2).
- Establish, record, balance, and replenish the petty cash fund (Procedure 15-3).

PERFORMANCE OBJECTIVES (JOB SKILLS) IN THE WORKBOOK

- Post entries to ledger cards and calculate balances (Job Skill 15-1).
- Prepare ledger cards (Job Skill 15-2)
- Bookkeeping Day 1—Post to patient ledger cards and prepare cash receipts (Job Skill 15-3).
- Bookkeeping Day 1—Prepare the daily journal (Job Skill 15-4).
- Bookkeeping Day 1—Post charges, payments, and adjustments using a daily journal (Job Skill 15-5).
- Bookkeeping Day 1—Balance the daysheet (Job Skill 15-6).

This textbook and the accompanying Workbook meet the educational components for entry-level administrative and general competencies outlined by CAAHEP and ABHES.

- Bookkeeping Day 2—Prepare the daily journal (Job Skill 15-7).
- Bookkeeping Day 2—Post charges, payments, and adjustments to patient ledger cards and to the daily journal; prepare cash receipts and the bank deposit (Job Skill 15-8).
- Bookkeeping Day 2—Balance the daysheet (Job Skill 15-9).
- Bookkeeping Day 3—Prepare the daily journal (Job Skill 15-10).
- Bookkeeping Day 3—Post charges, payments, and adjustments to patient ledger cards and to the daily journal; prepare cash receipts and the bank deposit (Job Skill 15-11).
- Bookkeeping Day 3—Balance the daysheet (Job Skill 15-12).
- Bookkeeping Day 4—Set up the daysheet for a new month (Job Skill 15-13).

KEY TERMS

account	bookkeeping	liabilities
accounting	capital	open accounts
accounts payable (A/P) ledger	credits	petty cash fund
accounts receivable control	daysheet	posts
accounts receivable (A/R) ledger	debits	proprietorship
adjustment	double-entry accounting	single-entry accounting
assets	general ledger	
balance	ledger card	

HEART OF THE HEALTH CARE PROFESSIONAL

Service

Confidence is communicated and mistakes are minimized when the medical assistant is knowledgeable about financial matters. All charges, payments, and adjustments should be posted precisely and figures computed accurately. It is the medical assistant's responsibility and an important part of customer service to display a concerned attitude when handling financial accounts, performing bookkeeping skills, answering account questions, and trying to locate and correct an error.

ACCOUNTING

Accounting is defined as the system of recording and summarizing business and financial transactions and analyzing, verifying, and reporting the results. A *bookkeeper* is the one who does the recording.

The combination of private and managed care patients who are insured under a variety of contracts makes accounting in a physician's office a complex and challenging task. Because managed care plans vary in their financial reimbursement structure, a variety of accounting procedures are required. Such plans can range from fee-for-service, using a variety of fee schedules to capitation, where fixed amounts are paid for each enrollee in the plan; usually monthly. Many contracts require either a fixed-dollar copayment amount or a percentage to be paid by the patient for each office visit. Some contracts have a *stop loss* section, which means that if the patient's services go over a certain amount, the physician can begin asking the patient to pay. In such cases, the patient's accounts would need monitoring. Managed care contracts may also retain a portion of the monthly capitation payment called a *withhold* until the end of the year. This serves as an incentive to reduce overutilization.

Bookkeeping Process

Most medical practices rely on the medical assistant to have competent **bookkeeping** skills and to record and manage the financial affairs of the medical practice.

TABLE 15-1 Explanation of Debits and Credits

Debit Is Anything That:	Examples	Credit Is Anything That:	Examples
Increases assets	Items of value owned by the practice: Cash, money owed by patients (receivables), real estate (building, land), equipment, supplies, office furniture	Decreases assets	Sale of equipment, building, furniture
Decreases liabilities	Bills owed by the medical practice	Increases liabilities	Monies owed for business expenditures, mortgage, supplies, equipment, furniture
Decreases earnings	Money that is outstanding, because it is owed by patients	Increases earnings	Payments made by patients for medical services rendered

This enables the physician to have a clear daily picture of the income derived from patient accounts, detailed information on office expenditures, and the necessary figures for income tax purposes.

This chapter begins by defining various accounting systems and then explains basic bookkeeping guidelines and terminology, posting procedures, and the use of cash funds. Chapter 20 gives additional information about financial responsibilities for office managers such as accounts payable and payroll procedures.

Although computerized bookkeeping is commonly used in an electronic health record (EHR) system, manual bookkeeping skills are explained and taught in this chapter to help increase understanding of the basic computations a computerized system automatically performs, as well as the various steps needed to balance books.

Accounting Systems

In a medical practice, one of four accounting systems is usually chosen based on the complexity of the physician's practice, whether it is a group or single physician office, and on elements of the physician's other personal income. Whichever system is chosen—single-entry, double-entry, pegboard, or computerized—it will include a record of daily income (receipts) and payments (disbursements), showing amounts owed to the physician by patients and amounts paid for expenses.

When these transactions are recorded completely, the books will reflect where all money comes from and where it goes.

The terms *debit* and *credit* are basic bookkeeping terms used in all accounting systems (see Table 15-1). Increases in assets are termed **debits**. Decreases in assets are called **credits**.

Single-Entry Accounting

Single-entry accounting is relatively easy to learn and use and is acceptable to both federal and state authorities as a basis for filing tax returns. In this system, records include:

1. The **general ledger**, called a *daysheet, daily log,* or *charge journal,* in which all fees for services rendered and payments are recorded every day
2. An **accounts receivable (A/R) ledger**, which consists of all of the patients' accounts showing the amounts owed for services rendered, should be insured against fire or flood damage
3. An **accounts payable (A/P) ledger** (check register or checkbook), which shows amounts paid out for the expenses of the business practice
4. The **petty cash fund**, which contains records showing monies that are available for minor office expenses and monies that have been disbursed
5. The payroll records, which indicate salaries and wages paid and deductions made

Single-entry accounting is neither self-balancing nor well formulated. It does not rely on equal debits or credits; therefore, errors are not obvious in this system.

Mistakes can be easily made because entries must be registered on one sheet and then transferred onto other journals and ledgers. The medical assistant handles these books of original entry. Many physicians hire accountants, who keep the general ledgers (books of final entry). The assistant gives the accountant the information from the books of original entry, which the accountant then turns into a double-entry system.

Double-Entry Accounting

Double-entry accounting is an exact science because the books must **balance**. Advanced accounting skills are necessary, so most medical offices do not require the administrative assistant to record entries using double-entry bookkeeping. However, it is advisable for the assistant to understand the basics of this system, including related terminology such as *assets, capital, liabilities,* and *proprietorship.*

Assets are anything owned by the business, such as equipment, furniture, bank accounts, buildings, accounts receivable, and so on. The physician may own some of the assets outright and may have some that are not completely paid for. **Capital** is original investment money and other property of a corporation that is owned. **Liabilities** are monies that are owed for business expenditures (debts). **Proprietorship**, also called *owner's equity,* is the owner's net worth, which consists of the amount by which the fair market value of all assets exceeds liabilities (see Example 15-1).

For recording the transactions, a general ledger sheet is divided in half, with the assets on the left side and the liabilities and capital on the right side. These two sides should balance; that is, the totals of all columns would be the same if no errors occur. The bookkeeper **posts** (records) each transaction to the daily ledger, a book of original entry, and then records totals into this general ledger.

Places of business that offer merchandise for sale keep accounts on an *accrual basis;* that is, income is considered earned when the merchandise is sold. Physicians' accounts are kept on what is called a *cash basis,* indicating only what happens to the money taken in. Earned money is not considered income until the patient pays, and purchases are not recorded as expenses until the physician actually pays the bills. Therefore, only two journals are required, one for cash receipts and one for cash disbursements.

Accounts payable, the cash receipt journal, and check writing are discussed in Chapter 20.

Pegboard Accounting

Pegboard accounting has been a popular bookkeeping method used in physicians' offices for decades. Although computerized accounting is used in the majority of medical practices, many educators feel that learning the manual pegboard system provides students an excellent foundation in bookkeeping and helps them understand the underlying concepts of a computerized system. The principles of the pegboard system can be transferred easily when adapting to an electronic computerized accounting program. If the computer system crashes, or if you have an electronic system that is accessed via the Internet and you cannot gain online access, you will need to know the mechanisms of basic bookkeeping to track all transactions while the electronic system is down.

The pegboard system is accurate, easy to learn, and uses a "write-it-once" process for recording daily office transactions. It minimizes errors and saves clerical writing time. The system uses a lightweight board with pegs on the left side and often on the top and right side too. Various forms (e.g., transaction slips, cash receipts, ledgers, deposit slips) have holes to affix over the pegs, thus aligning them to post a transaction. Using this method, several forms may be layered, one on top of the other, and held in place on the board (Figures 15-1A and 15-1B). Usually the layered forms are printed on no-carbon-required (NCR) paper or card stock.

To begin the day's transactions, a new daysheet **(A)** is placed on the pegboard. Then a series of prenumbered, shingled perforated transaction slips, known by many names **(B)**, are aligned so that the posting line is directly over the first available line on the daysheet near the top. Use of these slips increases cash flow because they are presented to the patient at the time the service is rendered. Each slip acts as a receipt if payment is made, indicates the balance owed, and can be used as an insurance billing statement or to input information into a computerized system; a portion of the slip can be removed and given to the patient to show the next appointment date. If an error is made on the slip, it is

---

EXAMPLE 15-1

Formula Explaining Assets and Proprietorship

The following equation can help you remember:

Assets − Liabilities = Proprietorship
(Owner's Equity)

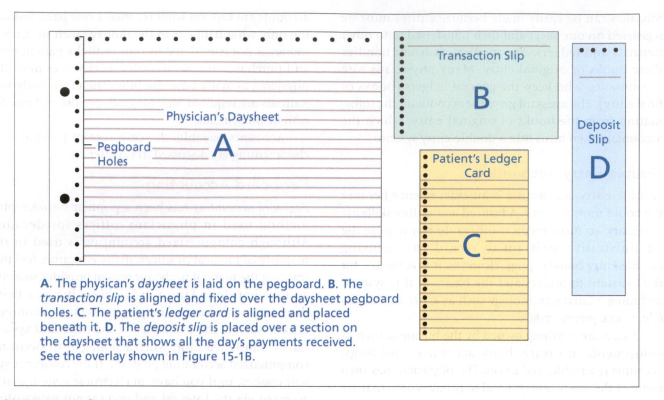

A. The physican's *daysheet* is laid on the pegboard. B. The *transaction slip* is aligned and fixed over the daysheet pegboard holes. C. The patient's *ledger card* is aligned and placed beneath it. D. The *deposit slip* is placed over a section on the daysheet that shows all the day's payments received. See the overlay shown in Figure 15-1B.

FIGURE 15-1A Component parts of a pegboard bookkeeping system

voided and retained. Embezzlement is prevented because the slips are prenumbered and must be accounted for at the end of each day. This is called an *audit control*.

As each patient arrives, his or her ledger card, also referred to as an **account** (C), is slipped between the daysheet and the transaction slip. When an entry is written, it registers simultaneously on all three items—the daysheet, the patient's ledger card, and the transaction slip, thus decreasing posting errors. After each patient has left the office, the ledger card is removed and the next patient's card is inserted.

All monies (cash and checks) are totaled and recorded on a *bank deposit slip* (D) at the same time that they are recorded on the daysheet, using overlapping forms in the same manner. A *cash control log* is usually included, which tracks beginning cash on hand, total daily receipts, cash paid out, the bank deposit, and closing cash on hand.

At the end of the day, the daysheet is balanced using a proof of posting area, so if an error has been made it can be corrected the same day; this reduces the chance of an error being discovered at the end of the month. Daily totals are then added to the previous day's totals, providing month-to-date figures. An accounts receivable control and proof of accounts receivable are performed to ensure that the books are balanced.

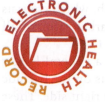

Computerized Accounting

Computerized accounting is a method adopted by medical practices to expedite posting, reduce paper, increase accurate accounting, and incorporate electronic billing capabilities. The computer automatically adds all debits, subtracts all credits, and computes a running balance. It also generates data that calculate overhead costs and compare monthly billings, payments from insurance carriers, percentage of adjustments (amount written off), and percentage of accounts receivable assigned to each insurance carrier. The computer replaces all manual systems, such as pegboard bookkeeping, and has the capability of generating hard copies (paper printouts) of financial data. Basic computerized accounting elements are further discussed in Chapter 20.

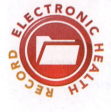

From Manual Bookkeeping to Electronic Bookkeeping—It is easy to understand how the components of a manual bookkeeping system compare to an electronic system. Instead of having to post on a separate account (ledger), daysheet

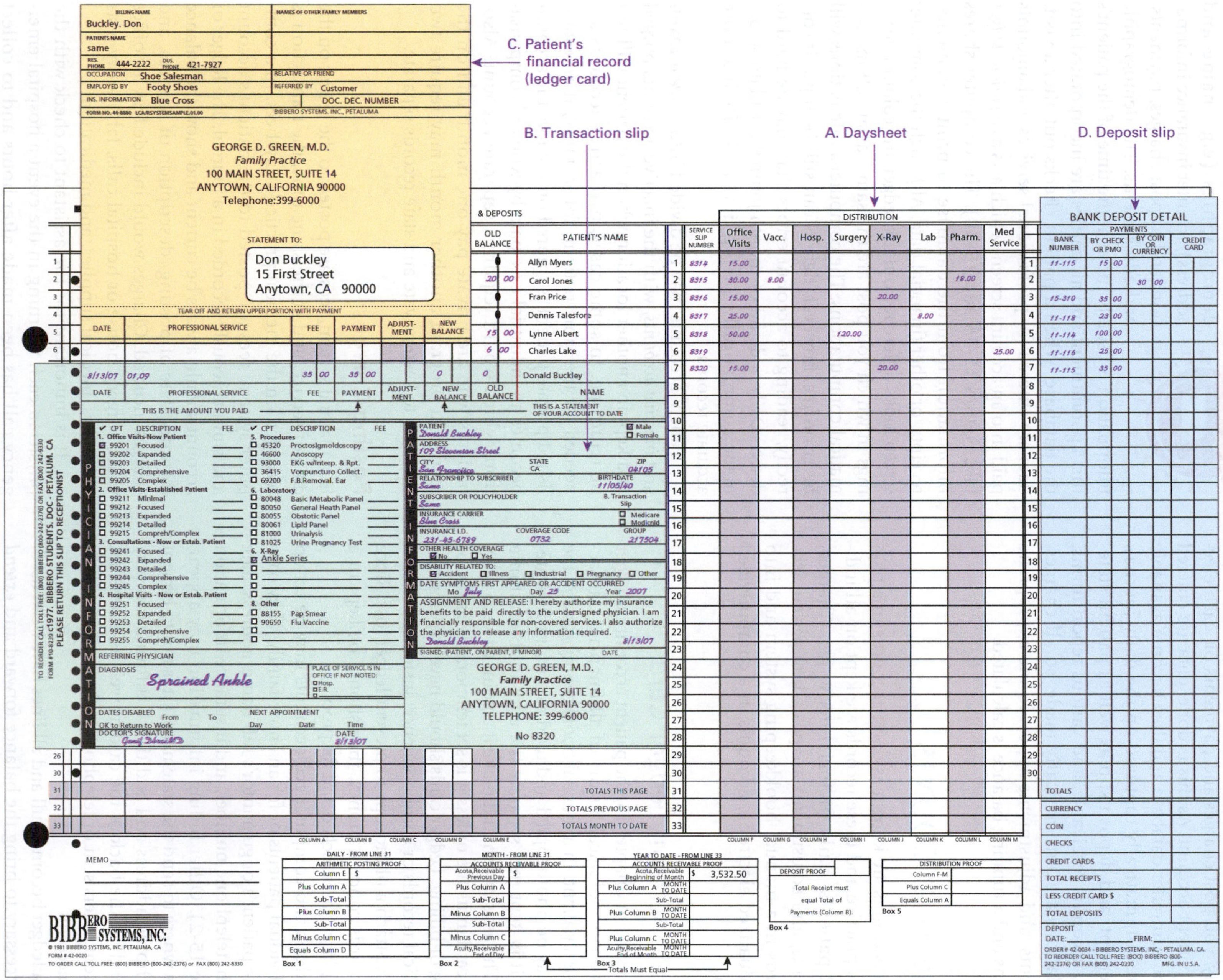

Reprinted with permission of Bibbero Systems, Inc., Petaluma, CA, Telephone: (800) 242-2376; Fax: (800) 242-9330; Website: http://www.bibbero.com.

FIGURE 15-1B Pegboard bookkeeping system complete with overlays. In some pegboard systems, an overlay for the deposit slip is not used

(daily journal), cash receipt, and deposit slip, or having to layer each on a pegboard so they are posted simultaneously, you post charges and payments on each electronic patient account. As this is done, data are entered into the computer database and they become available and are automatically captured on the daily journal, cash receipt, and deposit slip as well as patient statements, accounts receivable, and various report forms. Calculations are automatically made, so all charges, payments, and adjustments appear in the appropriate columns and a running balance is calculated.

PATIENT ACCOUNTS

Patient accounts are known as **open accounts** in a physician's practice and these records are kept on all individual patients' daily financial activities. Charges, payments, and adjustments are posted on patient ledger cards in a manual bookkeeping system and into individualized electronic accounts in a computerized system.

Patient Account/Ledger Card

As presented in Chapter 13, the patient account or **ledger card** is a chronological history of all financial transactions for a patient. In a manual bookkeeping system, the card may be photocopied and used as a monthly statement. It is kept in a separate file and not bound in a book. The assistant should make it a point to keep every ledger card in its file unless it is set temporarily aside for posting or billing. Ledger cards should never be attached to medical records or correspondence; instead, the assistant can attach a photocopy to prevent ledger loss. Since ledger cards concern money, they should be kept in a secure place that is locked and fireproof.

Ledgers and computerized accounts may be set up for individual patients or for an entire family. They contain the patient's or guarantor's full name, address, date of birth, telephone number, and insurance information (Figure 15-2). Other billing information may appear, such as where to send the statement if it is not to be sent to the home address and additional information may be found on the back of the card as well as dates that document letters sent or telephone calls made to collect on an account.

If a ledger becomes full and all lines have been used, it is necessary to bring the balance forward and *extend* the account. To do this, the first entry on the reverse side or on a new card is called the *balance forward* amount. See the first posted entry of $20 on the ledger shown in Figure 15-2.

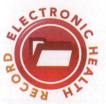

In an EHR system, separate screens are used to input patient demographics (e.g., name and address); to enter insurance information; and to post charges, payments, and adjustments. The demographic information is usually input at the time of the patient's first appointment and all entries are incorporated into the database. When a patient checks out after a visit, data are entered for professional services and amounts paid into an account screen, which acts as a *patient ledger* (see Figures 15-3A and 15-3B). The computer shares information from the database to print statements, receipts, or other financial data. Although the computer screen looks different from the ledger, the column headings in which you post are the same, as are all mathematical computations. The computer's calculations will be error-free; however, figures can still be input incorrectly, leading to account errors that may be hard to detect. Daily and end-of-month journal calculations are made automatically, saving time and offering more accurate records.

Patient accounts may be divided into *active accounts* and *inactive accounts*, with the inactive accounts purged and kept in another location when the patient will not be returning. In some cases, two active accounts are needed for the same patient, for instance, if an established private patient is injured on the job, the account becomes an industrial case paid by workers' compensation, which would require a separate account. Also, patients who are private pay one month and on the Medicaid program another month may require two accounts to keep private and state records separate.

Posting Charges

In a manual system, fees are posted to the ledger on the date of service, and at the same time, the transaction is recorded on the medical practice's daysheet. In a computer system, fees are posted to the patient's account and simultaneously recorded in a journal. The ledger or account should always be current and show the balance forward, date of posting, description of services, and charges incurred. Charges would include fees for office visits, surgery, house or hospital calls, laboratory tests and x-rays, medical supplies, and medication.

It is important for the assistant to check with the physician each morning in the event a hospital emergency call has been made after hours and to collect information on other services provided. The services are often abbreviated (e.g., office visit = OV, hospital visit = HV) to fit into the description area. The level of office visit recorded corresponds with the last digit of the

PRACTON MEDICAL GROUP, INC.

4567 BROAD AVENUE • WOODLAND HILLS, XY 12345-4700
OFFICE: (555) 486-9002 • FAX: (555) 488-7815

Fran Practon, M.D.
Gerald Practon, M.D.

Mr. Jeffrey Brown
230 Main Street
Woodland Hills, XY 12345-0001

Phone No.(H) __555-201-3762__ (W) __555-611-2001__ Birthdate __10-02-1936__
Insurance Co. __Medicare__ Policy No. __XXX-XX-9766A__

DATE	REFERENCE	DESCRIPTION	CHARGES	CREDITS PYMNTS.	ADJ.	BALANCE
		BALANCE FORWARD ⟶				20 00
1-13-XX	ck #398	ROA Pt pmt		20 00		0 00
2-1-XX	99202	NP OV, Level 2	51 91			51 91
2-14-XX	99222	Adm. hosp	120 80			172 71
2-15-XX	99231	HV	37 74			210 45
2-16-XX	99231	HV	37 74			248 19
2-17-XX	99238	Discharge	65 26			313 45
2-17-XX	2/1/to 2/17	Medicare billed				313 45
4-15-XX	voucher #766504	ROA Medicare pmt		250 76		62 69
NOTE: YOUR INSURANCE HAS PAID, PLEASE REMIT BALANCE OF $62.69						
5-1-XX	ck #540	ROA Pt pmt		62 69		0

RB40BC-2-96

PLEASE PAY LAST AMOUNT IN BALANCE COLUMN ⟶

THIS IS A COPY OF YOUR ACCOUNT AS IT APPEARS ON OUR RECORDS

FIGURE 15-2 Ledger card illustrating how charges and payments are posted

procedure code. For example, a new patient office visit coded 99202 would be recorded as NP OV, level 2.

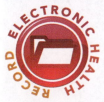

In a computerized system, when the procedure code is input it links to the correct description and the charge for that procedure is automatically posted. The diagnostic code may also be input at this time and later used on the computerized claim form. The account may be called up on the screen at any time if a patient makes an inquiry, or it can be printed as hard copy and sent as a statement (Figure 15-4).

Posting Multiple Procedures—When posting several procedures on the same day, these are input as separate transactions in a computerized system (Figure 15-5); however, when using a manual system, the same line is often used on the ledger to record all charges (see Example 15-2).

Posting Payments

Payments at the time of service or payments received by mail must be recorded daily. Payments are posted on the date received to the patient's account using the

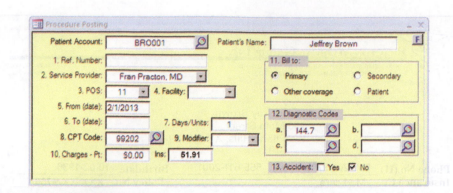

FIGURE 15-3A The top portion of procedure posting screen where charges are input in an EHR practice management system

FIGURE 15-3B The first charge posted to Jeffrey Brown's computerized account (as seen on the ledger in Figure 15-2), is shown in the Posting Detail on the bottom portion of the procedure posting screen after posting is completed in an EHR practice management system

EXAMPLE 15-2

Posting Multiple Procedures

DATE	REFERENCE	DESCRIPTION	CHARGES	CREDITS		BALANCE
				Pymts	Adj	
7-10-XX	99202, 36415,	NP-OV, Venipuncture,	66 91			66 91
	99000	Handling fee				

Note: (99202) $51.91 + (36415) $10.00 + (99000) $5.00 = total charge $66.91

GREGORY REINHARDT
16952 BLANCHE PL
WOODLAND HILLS XY 12345-0000

ACCOUNT NUMBER	356-001127
PHONE NUMBER	363-0677
PERIOD ENDING	12/31/XX
ACCOUNT TYPE	1

LEDGER

DATE	CODE	DESCRIPTION	FAMILY MEMBER	DR NO	AMOUNT
01-01		BALANCE AS OF 12 31 XX			26.00
01-23	00030	CHECK	GREG		15.00–
02-06	00030	CHECK	GREG		11.00–
04-14	99214	OFFICE VISIT	KAREN	02	35.00
04-14	71020	CHEST TWO VIEWS	KAREN	02	35.00
04-14	80112	PROFILE PANEL	KAREN	02	30.00
04-14	99000	VENIPUNCTURE, TRANSFER	KAREN	02	9.00
04-28	99213	OFFICE VISIT	KAREN	02	28.00
05-29	00020	INS PAYMENT AETNA	GREG		87.20–
06-09	99213	OFFICE VISIT	KAREN	02	28.00
06-12	00020	INS PAYMENT AETNA	GREG		22.40–
06-16	00030	CHECK	GREG		60.00–
07-08	00260	REFUND	GREG	02	4.60
09-10	99282	E.R. VISIST	GREG	02	65.00
09-11	99215	OFFICE VISIT	GREG	02	45.00
09-11	93000	ECG W/REPORT	GREG	02	35.00
09-11	93225	HOLTER 24 HR	GREG	02	250.00
09-16	99213	OFFICE VISIT	GREG	02	28.00
09-16	80061	LIPID PANEL	GREG	02	30.00
09-16	99000	VENIPUNCTURE, TRANSFER	GREG	02	9.00
09-23	99213	OFFICE VISIT	GREG	02	28.00
10-10	99212	OFFICE VISIT	KAREN	02	18.00
10-20	99212	OFFICE VISIT	GREG	02	18.00
10-28	00020	INS PAYMENT AETNA	GREG		42.10–
11-06	00020	INS PAYMENT AETNA	GREG		181.75–

OVER 120 DAYS	90.120 DAYS	60–90 DAYS	30–60 DAYS	CURRENT	MONTHS SINCE LAST PAYMENT ---------	TOTAL DUE
.00	266.15	36.00	.00	.00		302.15

FIGURE 15-4 Computer printout of a patient account

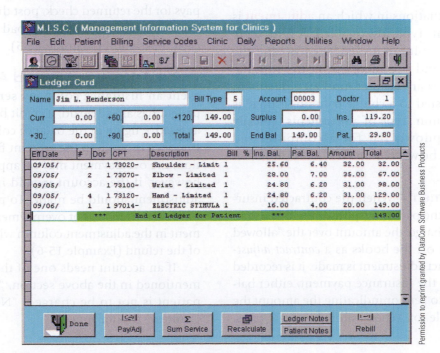

FIGURE 15-5 Sample patient account record illustrating the posting of multiple procedures on same day; generated from an EHR practice management system

abbreviation "ROA," received on account. If the payment is received by the patient, the abbreviation "pt" is used, and if received by an insurance company the name of the company must be recorded. The method of payment is also listed as cash, check (ck), voucher, money order, and so forth along with the check number—these choices may appear in a dropdown menu in a computerized program. All payments are credited (subtracted) from the account balance.

Posting Adjustments

There are several situations in which an **adjustment** is made on an account. Typically, on a ledger card, there is an "Adjustment" column under "Credits" and the amount is posted and subtracted from the running balance. Parentheses are used around an adjustment entry when it is posted to a charge column, if there is no adjustment column. Type of adjustments typically appears in a dropdown list for a computerized account and would be written under "Description" on a ledger card.

Contract Adjustment—When the contracted insurance payment plus the patient responsibility is *less* than the amount of the charge, the amount over the "allowed amount" is written off the books as a *contract adjustment*. When a contract adjustment is made, it is recorded at the same time as the insurance payment, either balancing the account to zero or indicating the amount the patient is responsible for. When billing Medicare cases,

a "courtesy adjustment" is made after receiving the Medicare payment if the charged amount is over the allowed amount. The word *courtesy* implies that Medicare patients are treated well and is preferred to phrases like *not allowed* or *write off* (see Example 15-3).

Uncollectible Debt Adjustment—It may also be necessary to record the adjustment of a small amount on an uncollectible debt (e.g., amounts under $25). Any adjustment to an account other than the known contractual write-off amounts should be authorized by the office manager before being posted (e.g., bad debt write-off, adjustment for an unhappy patient). Document the individual who authorizes the adjustment on the patient's account.

Account Sent to Collection Agency—When an account is sent to a collection agency, write off the entire balance of the account in the adjustment column and indicate a zero balance. When the collection agency collects and sends a check to the physician's office, post the monies back onto the account as a payment and reverse the adjustment (e.g., 50.00 in the payment column, and <50.00> in the adjustment column); the balance remains zero (Example 15-4).

Returned Check for Nonsufficient Funds—When a check is returned for nonsufficient funds (NSF), post the NSF's bank charge in the charge column, which will be added to the balance. Reverse the amount of payment in the payment column (e.g., <45.00>), which will also be added to the balance. When the patient pays for the returned check, post the amount in the payment column, including the bad check charge with a clear description (Example 15-5).

Credit Balance and Refund Adjustment—In the event an insurance company sends a check and the patient has already paid, a credit balance will appear as a negative figure in the balance column (e.g., <41.53>). If money is owed on the account from another transaction, the overpayment may be applied to that amount; however, if the account is paid in full then a refund adjustment should be made. To post this transaction, indicate the amount of overpayment as a reverse adjustment in the adjustment column with a clear description of the refund (Example 15-6).

If an account needs one of the adjustment entries mentioned in the above section, "adj" is noted; or if a patient is not to be charged, "NC" or "Professional Courtesy" should appear.

EXAMPLE 15-3

A. Private Insurance Contract Adjustment

Date	Reference	Description	Charges		Credits				Balance	
					Pymts		Adj			
3/12/XX	99205	NP OV level 5	132	28					132	28
3/30/XX	Voucher No. 63905	ROA ABC Ins			101	20			31	08
3/30/XX	ABC Ins	Contract adj					5	78	25	30

ABC insurance allowed amount is 126.50. MATH: Charged amount minus allowed amount equals contract adjustment (132.28 – 126.50 = 5.78). Insurance paid 80% of allowed amount (.80 × 126.50 = 101.20). Patient is responsible for 20% of allowed amount (.20 × 126.50 = 25.30).

B. Medicare Courtesy Adjustment

Date	Reference	Description	Charges		Credits				Balance	
					Pymts		Adj			
3/12/XX	99205	NP OV level 5	132	28					132	28
3/30/XX	Voucher 100051	ROA Medicare			96	86			35	42
3/30/XX	Medicare	Courtesy adj					11	20	24	22

Medicare participating fee (allowed amount) is 121.08. MATH: Charged amount minus allowed amount equals Medicare courtesy adjustment (132.28 – 121.08 = 11.20). Medicare paid 80% of allowed amount (.80 × 121.08 = 96.86]. Patient is responsible for 20% of allowed amount (.20 × 121.08 = 24.22).

EXAMPLE 15-4

Write Off an Uncollectible Account; Post Monies from a Collection Agency

Date	Reference	Description	Charges		Credits				Balance	
					Pymts		Adj			
6/13/XX	30520	Septoplasty	660	88					660	88
7/15/XX	6/13/XX	Billed pt							660	88
8/15/XX	6/13/XX	Billed pt							660	88
9/15/XX	6/13/XX	Billed pt							660	88
10/1/XX 10/2/XX 10/5/XX	6/13/XX	Telephoned pt re: collections— UTC X 3							660	88
10/15/XX	6/13/XX	Sent collection notice							660	88
11/1/XX	6/13/XX	Sent acct to XYZ Collection Agency					660	88	0	00
12/15/XX	Ck # 8970	XYZ Collection Agency pd			250	00	<250	00>	0	00

EXAMPLE 15-5

Returned Check

| Date | Reference | Description | Charges | | Credits | | Balance | |
					Pymts	Adj		
5/23/XX	99383	NP Preventive OV	45	00			45	00
5/23/XX	Ck #101	ROA Pt mother			45	00	0	00
6/3/XX	Rtn Ck #101	NSF + bank charge	10	00	<45	00>	55	00
6/5/XX	ROA Cash	NSF + bank charge, pt mother			55	00	0	00

Posting an Explanation of Benefits

When an insurance company sends payment and an explanation of benefits (EOB) form is received, pull the insurance claim or view the computerized account to verify that the payment is correct. Payment figures will occur for each line of service; some services on the claim may or may not be paid. If the claim is paid, post the amount of money received, referencing it and applying it to each line of service. If there is a question about the amount of payment, or if a line of service is not paid for, refer to the reference code on the EOB (see Figure 13-10B in Chapter 13). If questions still occur, call the insurance company for further clarification.

After posting payments and the applicable contract or courtesy adjustments, file each EOB in a file folder with a reference to the date that payments were posted.

Some offices staple paper claims to an EOB for a single payment, or for multiple claims, copy the EOB, highlight the lines of service that apply to that claim, and staple them accordingly. EOBs are typically filed by date of posting, month received, or payer—depending on office policy.

When an electronic EOB is received, it is easier to print it so that you can track and record payments and adjustments. Automatic, electronic posting of a EOB that synchronizes with electronic claims is possible in some practice management systems. Refer to Chapter 13 for information on reading an EOB and Figures 13-9, 13-10A, and 13-10B for illustrations of an EOB and Medicare Remittance Advice (RA).

All financial transactions should be recorded in bookkeeping codes as shown in Table 15-2. Refer to Procedure 15-1 to setup and post to a patient's account.

EXAMPLE 15-6

Credit Balance/Refund Adjustment

| Date | Reference | Description | Charges | | Credits | | Balance | |
					Pymts	Adj		
3/12/XX	99202	OV level 2	51	91			51	91
3/12/XX	Ck #189	ROA pt			51	91	0	00
3/13/XX	3/12/XX	ABC Insurance billed (51.91)					0	00
4/15/XX	Check #8954	ABC Insurance payment 80%			41	53	<41	53>
5/1/XX	Check #2389	Refund pt credit balance				<41	53>	0	00

TABLE 15-2 Bookkeeping Abbreviations and Definitions

Abbreviation	Definition	Abbreviation	Definition
AC or acct	account	J/A	joint account
A/C	account current	LTTR	letter
adj	adjustment	MO	money order
A/P	accounts payable	mo	month
A/R	accounts receivable	msg	message
B/B	bank balance	NC, N/C	no charge
Bal fwd, B/F	balance forward	NF	no funds
BD	bad debt	NSF	nonsufficient funds
BSY	busy	PD, pd	paid
c/a, CS	cash on account	pmt	payment
cc	credit card	pt	patient
ck	check	PVT CK	private check
COINS	coinsurance	recd, recv'd	received
Cr	credit	ref	refund
CXL	cancel	Req	request
DB	debit	ROA	received on account
DED	deductible	Snt	sent
def	charge deferred	T	telephoned
disc, discnt	discount	TB	trial balance
EC, ER	error corrected	UCR	usual, customary, and reasonable
Ex MO	express money order	w/o	write off
FLW/UP	follow-up	$	money/cash
fwd	forward	0	no balance due (zero balance)
IB	itemized bill	○	posted
I/F	in full	<$56.78>	credit symbols
ins, INS	insurance		
inv	invoice		

DAYSHEET

In single-entry or pegboard bookkeeping, the **daysheet** is known by various names, such as a *daily log*, *charge journal*, or *daily record* but all have the same basic components (Figure 15-6). The daysheet is a cumulative listing of each patient seen in the office, services rendered, fees charged, payments made, and adjustments calculated on one day, with each patient's current daily balance indicated. As patients receive services, the assistant posts the fee to each patient's ledger and to the current daysheet, totaling the charges for each patient's account. All payments and adjustments recorded to a patient's ledger are also simultaneously recorded to the daysheet.

At the end of the day, all charges, payments, and adjustments are totaled along with the total of all previous and current balances. These final figures are recorded on a monthly summary of charges and receipts appearing at the bottom of the daysheet in the proof of posting area. Previous day totals are added to these figures to give month-to-date totals for each item. It is important for the assistant to check that the total of each day's cash and check receipts equals the day's total bank deposit. To assure that there is no misappropriation of funds (fraud), it is wise to have one person receive checks and money and another verify the money collected and the bank deposit. Refer to Procedure 15-2 when preparing the daysheet in a pegboard system and when posting charges, payments, and adjustments; recording deposits; and balancing the daysheet.

PROCEDURE 15-1

Prepare and Post to a Patient's Account

OBJECTIVES: Prepare, insert descriptions; post charges, payments, and adjustments; and calculate a running balance to a patient's account.

EQUIPMENT/SUPPLIES: Computer or pencil, patient accounts or ledger cards, and calculator.

DIRECTIONS: Follow these step-by-step directions, which include rationales, to learn this procedure. Job Skills 15-1, 15-2, 15-3, 15-5, 15-8, and 15-11 are presented in the *Workbook* for practice.

PERSONAL DATA:

1. Insert the patient's name, address, and pertinent information on the ledger card. On a computerized account, this information is stored in the data bank and automatically populates patient accounts and statements.

DATE:

2. In the first column on the first available line, post the current date (date service, procedure, or transaction took place); this date is usually the same as the date of service (DOS). If the DOS differs from the posting date, list the DOS in the reference column. This date column should never be left blank.

REFERENCE:

3. Write a reference to the transaction being posted.
   a. *Charges:* List the *CPT®* procedure code.
   b. *Payments:* List the type of payment (cash, check, debit/credit card, or money order) and check or voucher number (e.g., voucher no. 543).
   c. *Adjustments:* List the DOS the adjustment is being made on.
   d. *Billing Comments:* List the dates of service(s) billed. Note: The balance at the end of the line depicts a running balance and may not coincide with the amount being billed to the insurance company.

DESCRIPTION:

4. Write a brief description of the transaction that is being posted.

a. *Charges:* Use a key at the bottom of the ledger or standard abbreviations to indicate charges posted (e.g., OV [office visit], HV [hospital visit]). Indicate the Evaluation and Management service levels (1 through 5) using the last digit of the E/M code (e.g., 99205 5 level 5). Abbreviate the name of other services or surgical procedures (e.g., ECG, vaccine, T & A).

b. *Payments:* Indicate ROA (received on account), and who made the payment (e.g., pt [patient] or name of insurance company).

c. *Adjustments:* Indicate the type of adjustment (e.g., insurance plan adj., contract adj., courtesy adj.).

d. *Billing Comments:* Indicate the name of the insurance company billed or that a patient statement was sent and amount due if different from the current balance (e.g., patient billed $50.00 balance after insurance payment).

e. *Other Comments:* Indicate other comments that pertain directly to the account (e.g., account sent to XYZ Collection Agency, account scheduled for small-claims court).

CHARGES:

5. Refer to the mock fee schedule in Appendix A of the *Workbook* and post each fee on a separate line in the "charge" column. Charges *increase* the account balance, so they are debited (added) to the balance.

PAYMENTS:

6. Enter the amount paid in the "payment" column. Payments *decrease* the account balance, so they are credited (subtracted) from the balance.

ADJUSTMENTS:

7. Enter the amount adjusted off the account in the "adjustment" column. Adjustments *decrease* the account balance, so they are credited (subtracted) from the balance. (See previous Example 15-3.)

(continues)

PROCEDURE 15-1 *(continued)*

CURRENT BALANCE:

8. Line by line, add (increase or debit) and subtract (decrease or credit) each posting to the running balance to determine the amount for the "current balance" column. If a line is used to indicate a date an action was taken (e.g., insurance company or patient billed, account sent to collection), bring down the running balance from the previous line. This column must always contain an amount and should never be left blank. On a computerized account, totals are automatically calculated.

ACCOUNT SENT TO COLLECTION:

9. When an account is sent to a collection agency:
   a. *Date:* Post the date stated in the collection notice.
   b. *Reference:* Indicate date(s) of service for amounts owed.
   c. *Description:* Record "Sent account to collection agency," naming the agency.
   d. *Adjustments:* Post the total amount owed in the adjustment column.
   e. *Balance:* Subtract the adjustment amount from the balance; the entire amount should have been written off leaving a zero balance (Example 15-4).

POST MONIES RECEIVED FROM COLLECTION AGENCY:

10. When the collection agency pays the physician's office:
    a. *Date:* Post the date payment is received.
    b. *Reference:* Indicate the check or voucher number.

    c. *Description:* Record the name of the collection agency.
    d. *Payment:* Post the amount of the check.
    e. *Adjustment:* Post the amount of payment as a reverse adjustment <20.00>; thereby adding it back onto the account— the balance remains zero (Example 15-4).

RETURNED CHECKS:

11. When a check is returned:
    a. *Date:* Enter the date of the nonsufficient fund (NSF) notice.
    b. *Reference:* Indicate "Rtn" for returned check and the check or voucher number.
    c. *Description:* List "NSF and "bank charge."
    d. *Charge:* Post the NSF fee in the charge column, which will be added to the balance.
    e. *Payment:* Reverse the amount of payment in the payment column (e.g., <37.00>), which will also be added to the balance. When the patient pays for the returned check, post the amount including the check charge in the payment column (Example 15-5).

12. *Credit Balances:* If an overpayment or double payment is received:
    a. Enclose the credit balance with a symbol (e.g., <20.00>); some offices post these in red ink.
    b. List the refund amount in either the "Payment" or "Adjustment" column as a negative < > number; the amount is added back into the balance (Example 15-6).

ACCOUNTS RECEIVABLE CONTROL

The **accounts receivable control** is a daily summary of dollar amounts that remains unpaid on all accounts. Statements are sent every month to patients who have outstanding balances and to ensure the balance of all outstanding accounts equals the total monies owed, it is important to have an accounts receivable control for verification of the records. To accomplish this, at the end of each month the medical assistant would:

1. Total the balances of all patient account records (ledgers) that indicate a balance due.
2. Compare that total with the month-end total A/R figure on the daysheet (general ledger). If these

two figures do not agree, there is an error in calculation or a ledger may be missing. The error must be found and corrected.

In a computerized system, a trial balance can be obtained by generating a *monthly summary report*.

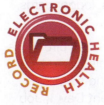

Computerized Reports

A variety of reports that provide a summary of the information stored in the database can be produced by an EHR system. The same information that appears on a daysheet can be printed to view the day's activities and to balance the bank deposit. Patient accounts, containing the same information as a

DAY SHEET (RECORD OF CHARGES AND RECEIPTS)   PAGE NO 1 OF 1   DATE 3/1/XX   RECORD OF DEPOSITS

DATE	REFERENCE	DESCRIPTION	CHARGES	CREDITS PYMNTS	CREDITS ADJ.	BALANCE	PREVIOUS BALANCE	NAME		RECEIPT NUMBER	DATE: 3/1/XX ABA	CASH	CHECKS
3/1/XX	142	992.03	70 92			70 92	0	Black, Harriet	1				
3/1/XX	143	992.12	28 55			38 55	10 00	Emery, John	2				
3/1/XX	144	90702 & 992.11	50 07			75 07	25 00	Farrel, William	3				
3/1/XX	145	992.05	132 28			132 28	0	Antrum, Jerry	4				
3/1/XX	146	99396 & 93000	69 26			109 26	40 00	Potter, Sylvia	5				
3/1/XX	147	992.14	61 51			86 51	25 00	Kaufman, Roger	6				
3/1/XX	148	992.13	40 20			140 20	100 00	Ryan, Wilbur	7				
3/1/XX	149	99213 & 96372	44 97	44 97		35 00	35 00	Meadows, Terri	8	142			44 97
3/1/XX	150	992.03	70 92			70 92	0	Smith, Harold	9				
3/1/XX	151	992.11	14 70			76 21	61 51	Morris, Don	10				
3/1/XX	152	99385	50 00			78 55	28 55	Blake, Leona	11				
3/1/XX	153	992.13	40 20			73 45	33 25	Ohta, Pat	12				
3/1/XX	154	992.21	73 00			113 20	40 20	Goodman, Anne	13				
3/1/XX	155	992.21	66 82			103 62	36 80	Lopez, George	14				
3/1/XX	156	992.17	61 22			117 53	56 31	Nason, Sarah	15				
3/1/XX	157	992.32	55 56			75 56	20 00	Davis, Baby Katy	16				
3/1/XX	1/20/XX	Blue Cross/Blue Shield		49 21		12 30	61 51	Barnes, Helen	17	91-119			49 21
3/1/XX	2/3/XX	Industrial Indemnity		50 00		1150 00	1200 00	LaMacchia, Maria	18	90-270			50 00
3/1/XX	1/7/XX	Medicare voucher #2.7611		51 94	6 00	12 98	70 92	Kh	19				51 94

CASH CONTROL

Beginning Cash On Hand	$	100.00
Receipts Today (Col. B-1)	$	44.97
Total	$	144.97
Less Paid Outs	$	
Less Bank Deposit	$	44.97
Closing Cash On Hand	$	100.00

	Col. A	Col. B-1	Col. B-2	Col. C	Col. D			
TOTALS THIS PAGE	930 18	196 12	6 00	2572 11	1844 05	BY	TOTAL CASH	44 97
PREVIOUS PAGE	968 00	1020 00	145 00	3259 03	3456 03	m+f	TOTAL CHECKS	151 15
MONTH-TO-DATE	1898 18	1216 12	151 00	5831 14	5300 08		TOTAL DEPOSIT	196 12

PROOF OF POSTING		ACCOUNTS RECEIVABLE CONTROL		ACCOUNTS RECEIVABLE PROOF	
COL. D TOTAL	$ 1844.05	PREVIOUS DAY'S TOTAL	$ 3259.03	ACCTS. REC. 1ST OF MONTH	$ 3456.03
PLUS COL. A TOTAL	$ 930.18	PLUS COL. A	$ 930.18	PLUS COL. A - MONTH TO DATE	$ 1898.18
SUB TOTAL	$ 2774.23	SUB TOTAL	$ 4189.21	SUB TOTAL	$ 5354.21
LESS COLS. B-1 & B-2	$ 202.12	LESS COLS. B-1 & B-2	$ 202.12	LESS B-1 & B-2 MO. TO DATE	$ 1367.12
MUST EQUAL COL. C	$ 2572.11	TOTAL ACCTS. REC.	$ 3987.09	TOTAL ACCTS. REC.	$ 3987.09

FIGURE 15-6 Completed daysheet, a record of charges, adjustments, and receipts

PROCEDURE 15-2

Prepare the Pegboard; Post Charges, Payments, and Adjustments; and Balance the Daysheet

OBJECTIVE: Set up a daysheet; post charges, payments, and adjustments; verify that entries are correct and totals balance.

EQUIPMENT/SUPPLIES: Pegboard, calculator, pencil, transaction slips, daysheet, receipts, ledger cards, and balances from the previous day.

DIRECTIONS: Follow these step-by-step directions, which include rationales, to learn this procedure. Job Skill 15-1 has a variety of posting scenarios. Job Skill 15-2 through 15-6 represent Day 1; Job

Skills 15-7, 15-8, and 15-9 represent Day 2; and Job Skills 15-10, 15-11, and 15-12 represent Day 3 in the *Workbook* so that you can practice bookkeeping procedures.

PREPARE THE PEGBOARD:

1. Prepare the pegboard by placing a daysheet on the pegs located on the left side of the board.

2. Fill in the information at the top of the day-sheet (current date and page number) and

(continues)

PROCEDURE 15-2 (*continued*)

insert your name at the bottom (Prepared by). When posting in a computerized system, the program will automatically track the user so if mistakes are made they can be linked to a specific computer at a specific time.

3. Enter the previous page totals and cumulative balance in the correct "Previous Page" columns (A–D).

4. Refer to the bottom section of the daysheet and list the "Previous Day's Total" in the "Accounts Receivable Control." This figure is picked up from the entry in "Previous Page" Column D.

5. List "Accounts Receivable 1st of Month" in the "Accounts Receivable Proof" section. This amount does not change during the calendar month because it always shows the A/R balance from the first day of the month.

6. Pull ledger cards for patients scheduled to be seen in the office, placing them in the order that each patient will arrive.

7. Place transaction slips over the pegs. Be careful to align the posting line on the top slip with the first writing line on the daysheet.

POST CHARGES AND PAYMENTS TO THE DAYSHEET:

8. Place the first patient's ledger card under the first transaction slip; align it to the first writing line so that the correct posting entry occurs on the transaction slip and transfers to the ledger and daysheet.

9. Enter the date, transaction slip number, and patient's name—last name first.

10. Remove the transaction slip from the pegboard and clip it to the front of the patient's medical record to be seen that day. The physician will check off the services and procedures, indicate the diagnostic codes, and list any future appointments.

11. Before the transaction slip is replaced on the pegboard, enter the appropriate fee from the fee schedule next to each procedure if it is not already indicated; calculate and write the total for today's services on the front of the transaction slip.

12. Replace and carefully realign the transaction slip on the pegboard, matching the transaction slip number, and insert the patient's ledger card under the last page of the transaction slip.

13. Post fees in the charge column and add to any previous balance indicated on the ledger and record the current balance.

14. Post payments and adjustments in the credit column subtracting from any previous balance indicated on the ledger and record the current balance.

15. Record all payments on the "Record of Deposits" slip in the correct column (cash or check). List the receipt number for cash payments and the ABA number for all checks.

16. Remove the completed transaction slip and give to the patient as a receipt.

17. Refile the patient's ledger card.

18. Repeat Steps 8 through 17 for each patient seen that day.

BALANCE THE DAYSHEET:

19. Total Columns A, B-1, B-2, C, and D of the daysheet at the end of the day in pencil. Use a calculator with paper strip and keep the printout.

20. Complete "Proof of Posting" by entering all figure totals from the "Totals This Page" column boxes to that section of the worksheet. Follow the directions of addition and subtraction to obtain subtotals and totals.

EXAMPLE 15-7

Proof of Posting

Proof of Posting	
COL B TOTAL	$ 1,844.05
PLUS COL A TOTAL	$ 930.18
SUBTOTAL	$ 2,774.23
LESS COLS B-1 & B-2	$ 202.12
MUST EQUAL COL C	$ 2,572.11

(*continues*)

BALANCE THE MONTH-TO-DATE SECTIONS OF THE DAYSHEET:

21. Note the "Previous Day's Total" on the "Accounts Receivable Control." This amount is brought forward from the previous day.

EXAMPLE 15-8

Accounts Receivable Control

Accounts Receivable Control	
PREVIOUS DAY'S TOTAL	$ 3,259.03
PLUS COL A	$ 930.18
SUBTOTAL	$ 4,189.21
LESS COLS B-1 & B-2	$ 202.12
TOTAL ACCTS REC	$ 3,987.09

22. In the "Accounts Receivable Proof," enter figures from the "Month-to-Date" column boxes. Then, add, subtract, subtotal, and total as directed. If posted amounts, additions, and subtractions are correct, the "Total Accounts Receivable" figure in the "A/R Control" and "A/R Proof" boxes will match, indicating the daysheet is balanced.

EXAMPLE 15-9

Accounts Receivable Proof

Accounts Receivable Proof	
ACCTS REC 1ST OF MONTH	$ 3,456.03
PLUS COL A MONTH TO DATE	$ 1,898.18
SUBTOTAL	$ 5,354.21
LESS B-1 & B-2 MONTH TO DATE	$ 1,367.12
TOTAL ACCTS REC	$ 3,987.09

23. Verify the deposit section of the daysheet by totaling the cash column and the checks column. Enter the sum of both columns in the space marked "Total Deposit."

24. Verify that the "Total Deposit" amount and the total payments received in Column B-1 match.

CASH CONTROL:

25. Count and enter the amount of beginning cash on hand in the "Cash Control" section. List and add *cash payments* from Column B-1 and enter the subtotal. Subtract any amounts paid out and the amount of cash that will be deposited in the bank.

26. Total the "Closing Cash on Hand"; the closing cash on hand should match the amount of beginning cash on hand.

EXAMPLE 15-10

Cash Control

Cash Control	
Beginning Cash on Hand	$ 100.00
Receipts Today (Col B-1)	$ 44.97
Total	$ 144.97
Less Paid Outs	$
Less Bank Deposit	$ 44.97
Closing Cash on Hand	$ 100.00

AFTER THE DAYSHEET IS BALANCED:

27. Obtain a new daysheet, transfer balances to the new sheet, and begin with Step 1 to set up the sheet for the following day.

ledger, can be printed to verify activity on individual accounts. And, a variety of other reports can be produced to track the money flow in and out of the office. At the end of the day, print the daily journal and crosscheck the day's transaction forms against the charges, payments, and adjustments on the journal to verify that all entries have been made correctly. Refer to Chapter 20 for closer look at a variety of computerized financial status reports.

Locating Errors

To search for an error in posting, the assistant would look for a figure that was missed, a miskeyed number,

or a transposition in figures; for example, a check for $830 may have been posted as $803. An amount divisible by nine may indicate a transposed number. Errors also occur when amounts are placed in wrong columns—for example, a credit in the debit column or vice versa. An amount divisible by two may indicate posting in the wrong column. Another type of error occurs from sliding a number; that is, writing 500 for 50 or writing 80 for 800. To minimize this possibility when posting, the assistant can eliminate writing zeros if there are no cents; for example, write $15 rather than $15.00.

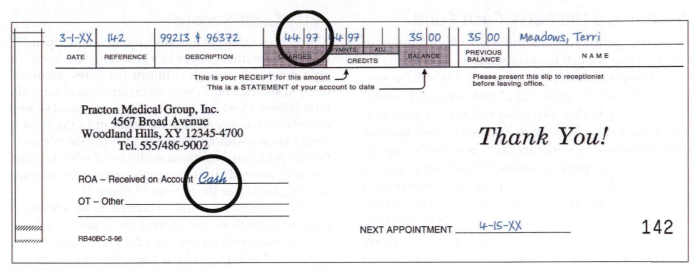

FIGURE 15-7 Completed receipt for a patient who paid cash on account

CASH FUNDS

A medical practice has various needs for dispensing *cash* (currency, coins) on a daily basis. It is important to have two sources for access to cash and to keep them separate—a change drawer and a petty cash fund.

Change Drawer

Medical practices collecting copayments from patients may need to make change when patients pay by cash. This type of transaction should involve a *change drawer*, and a receipt should be issued (Figure 15-7).

At the beginning of each day, the change drawer typically contains from $50 to $200 in small bills, depending on the size of the practice. At the conclusion of each day after cash payments are received and change is made, the cash received should equal the cash amount on the deposit slip; the remaining amount in the change drawer should be the same as the beginning amount (see Example 15-10 and 15-11).

When payment is made by the patient, write the word *check* or *cash* next to ROA on the receipt. If a payment is received by mail from the patient's insurer, list the name of the insurance carrier by OT (other).

For good bookkeeping practice, cash is usually handled by one individual. However, if the responsibility for the change drawer is shared by several individuals—more than one receptionist or bookkeeper—each person should reconcile the drawer and the monies received from patients during his or her shift.

Petty Cash

The term *petty* means small or little; hence, the purpose of a *petty cash fund* is to provide cash to make small, unanticipated purchases, such as coffee, small quantities of office

supplies, postage-due fees, CODs, office refreshments, or an employee's parking expense while on an errand for the physician. Use a petty cash fund only for minor expenses. Major expenses would always be paid by check.

The medical assistant may be responsible for the office petty cash and must account for each disbursement from the fund. Maintaining good cash procedures with firm control of funds is important to prevent cash being used in an unauthorized manner. Balancing, maintaining, and replenishing the cash drawer as well as the petty cash fund is accomplished by keeping proper records for all transactions. Employees handling cash receipts should be bonded (see Chapter 3).

EXAMPLE 15-11

Cash/Change Drawer

Drawer contents: $100: five $10 bills, six $5 bills, and twenty $1 bills.

Patient's copayment: $15. The patient gives the receptionist a $20 bill, and the cashier places the $20 in the change drawer and gives the patient $5 in change.

End-of-day change drawer: If no other cash transactions take place, at the end of the day, the change drawer would add up to $115 ($15 goes to the bank deposit and $100 remains in the drawer).

Cash proof: The day's cash received must match the cash control on the daysheet.

Bank deposit: The individual who does the banking should replenish the small bills from the larger ones in the drawer. It is best to separate the payments into an envelope and keep them apart from the money in the cash drawer. In this scenario, the receptionist would place $15 in an envelope.

Setting Up the Petty Cash Fund

Set up the petty cash fund initially with an amount of money large enough to cover small cash payments for 2 to 4 weeks—perhaps $100. A check is written payable to "Cash" or "Petty Cash," endorsed, and cashed. The currency is then placed in a drawer or cash box. When the fund is depleted to a predetermined amount, perhaps $25 or $50, another check is written to replenish it to the original amount of $100. Sometimes a fund is replenished weekly, if there is continuous demand for the funds, or monthly regardless of the amount of expenditures. Judgment must be used not to allow the fund to become so low that it is entirely depleted before new funds can be obtained. A good rule is to replenish the fund when it goes below 25% of its full value. The medical assistant would reconcile the petty cash account and arrange for the fund to be replenished.

Petty Cash Record

A petty cash record of amounts received and expended may be permanently kept in a standard cash book, or on a memo sheet with columns for dates, amounts received and expended, with an explanation of expenditures (Figure 15-8). An additional column could show a cumulative balance so that the amount in the fund is always known without having to total the list of expenditures. Additional columns would be of value for categorizing expenditures for each petty cash account showing totals (see the bottom of Figure 15-8).

The memo sheet could be printed on or attached to a manila envelope containing the cash, vouchers, receipts, and receipted bills for a defined period of time. This should be kept in a locked box, desk, or file, preferably fireproof. Borrowing from the petty cash fund should *not* be permitted. If the physician requests cash from the fund, a personal check or petty cash voucher should be written in exchange for the cash. Refer to Procedure 15-3 when dealing with a petty cash fund.

PROCEDURE 15-3

②③

Establish, Record, Balance, and Replenish the Petty Cash Fund

OBJECTIVE: Establish, maintain a record of expenditures for, balance, and replenish a petty cash fund.

EQUIPMENT/SUPPLIES: Calculator, petty cash record form, receipts (vouchers) for expenditures, check record (disbursement journal), checks, list of expenditures, and petty cash box.

DIRECTIONS: Follow these step-by-step directions, which include rationales, to learn this procedure.

1. Determine the amount needed in the petty cash fund.
2. Write a check to "Petty Cash" in the amount determined to establish the fund.
3. Cash the check and put the money in the petty cash box.
4. Enter the beginning and ending dates on the petty cash record form.
5. Post the beginning balance (office fund amount) on the petty cash record to indicate the original amount in the fund.
6. Post the amount of each petty cash receipt on the petty cash record, listing the date, receipt number, to whom paid, item purchased, name of account, and amount.

7. Label the headings at the bottom of the petty cash record and post the expenditure under the appropriate heading.
8. Add the "Amount" column and enter the total for "Receipts Paid."
9. Total all columns listed under the "Distribution of Petty Cash" on the petty cash record.
10. Count the cash available and enter the amount in "Cash on Hand."
11. Add the "Receipts Paid" plus the "Cash on Hand" and list the "Total." This total should equal the amount established for the fund.
12. Enter the "Total of Receipts and Cash" (on hand) and subtract it from the original "Office Fund Amount" to determine if there is an overage or shortage.
13. Prepare a check made out to "Cash," "Petty Cash," or the name of the bank cashing the check for the shortage amount. Write a check only for the amount that was used to bring the fund back to the original petty cash amount. Insert the check number on the petty cash record form.
14. Cash the check and add the money to the petty cash box.

PETTY CASH RECEIPT ENVELOPE

From ___Sept 1___ **20XX** To ___Sept 30___ **20XX** Paid by Check No. ___100___

Entered	Audited	Approved	Paid

Date	No.	Paid to:	Item	Account	Amount	
9/1	45	ABC Drug Store	1 box rubber bands	ofc. supp	1	56
9/4	46	US Postal Service	stamps	postage	3	32
9/16	47	Bank Parking Downtown	parking 1 hour	misc	1	50
9/20	48	ABC Drug Store	3 boxes tissue	med supp	2	51
9/29	49	US Postal Service	50 stamps	postage	24	50
					33	39

Office Fund Amount	$ 100.00	Receipts Paid	$ 33.39
Total Receipts and Cash	$ 100.00	Cash on Hand	$ 66.61
(Over or Short)	$ 0	TOTAL	$ 100.00

DISTRIBUTION OF PETTY CASH

Ofc. Supp	Postage	Med. Supp	Misc.								Totals
1 56	3 32	2 51	1 50								
	24 50										
1 56	27 82	2 51	1 50								33.39

FIGURE 15-8 Completed monthly petty cash record printed on, or attached to a small manila envelope

STOP AND THINK CASE SCENARIO

Determine an Accounting System

SCENARIO: The physician is establishing a new medical practice and consults you regarding what type of accounting system to use.

CRITICAL THINKING: State what questions you would ask to obtain necessary information to make this decision. Name the advantages and disadvantages of each.

Questions to ask:

_____

_____

_____

_____

1. Single-Entry System:

_____

_____

_____

_____

2. Double-Entry System:

_____

_____

_____

_____

3. Pegboard System:

_____

_____

_____

4. Computerized System:

_____

_____

_____

_____

STOP AND THINK CASE SCENARIO

Obtain Change for a Patient

SCENARIO: You are the receptionist working at the front desk and have had to make change several times today. Your change drawer is depleted to one $10 bill and some coins. The deposit envelope has $200 cash. The petty cash drawer has been replenished and has three $20 bills, three $10 bills, and two $5 bills. A patient comes to the front desk to pay for the services he has received. The charge is $75 and he hands you a $100 bill; you cannot make change from the change drawer.

CRITICAL THINKING: What would you do? Consider the suggestions listed and comment on each choice, stating which action you would take and why.

1. Make change from the deposit if possible.

_____

_____

_____

_____

_____

2. Make change from the petty cash drawer and write an invoice indicating what you have done.

_____

_____

_____

_____

_____

_____

3. Ask coworkers in the office if anyone has $25 or change for $100.

_____

_____

_____

_____

_____

4. Ask the patient to make a quick trip to the bank or go next door to the pharmacy to obtain change and then return.

_____

_____

_____

_____

_____

FOCUS ON CERTIFICATION*

CMA (AAMA) Content Summary

- Bookkeeping principles
- Daily reports, charge slips, receipts, ledgers
- Charges, payments, and adjustments
- Identifying and correcting errors
- Petty cash
- Reconciling third-party payments

RMA (AMT) Content Summary

- Process insurance payments and contractual write-off amounts
- Understand terminology associated with medical financial bookkeeping
- Collect and post payments
- Manage patient ledgers and accounts
- Employ appropriate accounting procedures (pegboard/double entry, computerized)

- Perform daily balancing procedures
- Prepare monthly trial balance
- Apply accounts receivable principles
- Understand and manage petty cash account
- Understand and maintain disbursement accounts
- Financial mathematics

CMAS (AMT) Content Summary

- Perform bookkeeping procedures including balancing accounts
- Perform financial computations
- Manage accounts receivable
- Manage patient accounts/ledgers
- Manage petty cash
- Use computer for billing and financial transactions

REVIEW EXAM-STYLE QUESTIONS

1. In a medical office, day-to-day bookkeeping tasks are usually performed by:
   a. the medical assistant
   b. the office manager
   c. an outside accountant
   d. a CPA
   e. the physician

2. Manual bookkeeping skills are:
   a. not needed since all physician's offices are computerized
   b. outdated and no longer apply
   c. helpful because they increase understanding of the basic computations a computerized system automatically does
   d. not related in any way to how debits and credits are recorded in a computerized system
   e. never used in the new millennium

3. Physician accounts are kept on a/an:
   a. accrual basis
   b. cash basis
   c. income basis
   d. credit basis
   e. appreciation schedule

4. Which accounting system requires the transfer of information onto journals and ledgers?
   a. single-entry accounting
   b. double-entry accounting
   c. triple-entry accounting
   d. pegboard accounting
   e. computerized accounting

5. The accounts receivable is a/an:
   a. asset
   b. capital
   c. liability
   d. proprietorship
   e. equity

---

* This textbook *and the accompanying* Workbook *meet the entry-level administrative and general competencies for the CMA outlined by the AAMA Examination Content Outline and Occupational Analysis and for the RMA and CMAS outlined by the AMT Competencies, Construction Parameters, and Examination Specifications (see Competency Grids in Appendix B).*

6. In a physician's practice, patient accounts are known as:
   a. restricted accounts
   b. open accounts
   c. closed accounts
   d. inactive accounts
   e. public accounts

7. A record that contains a cumulative listing of each patient seen in the office, services rendered, fees charged, payments made, and adjustments calculated on one day is called a/an:
   a. ledger or account
   b. accounts payable log
   c. accounts receivable log
   d. daysheet or daily journal
   e. check register

8. Select the correct statement regarding debits, credits, posting, and calculations on a ledger card.
   a. Credits are added and debits are subtracted from the account balance.
   b. Fees are posted in the credit column; payments and adjustments are posted in the charge column.
   c. Fees are posted in the charge column; payments and adjustments are posted in the credit column.
   d. Credits are fees charged by the physician.
   e. Debits are payments made by patients for services rendered.

9. To locate a transposition error, you would:
   a. divide the amount by 2
   b. divide the amount by 3
   c. divide the amount by 9
   d. look for an extra or missing zero
   e. round all numbers to the highest dollar amount

10. Totaling the balances of all patient accounts that indicate a balance due and comparing that total with the ending total A/R figure on the daysheet is referred to as:
    a. double-entry bookkeeping
    b. aging accounts
    c. ledger card balancing
    d. accounts receivable control
    e. end-of-month carryover procedures

11. Money kept in a physician's office for the purpose of making small cash purchases is called:
    a. a petty cash fund
    b. a change drawer
    c. a bank deposit
    d. patient payments
    e. payables

12. A change drawer would typically have:
    a. $50
    b. $75
    c. $100 to $200
    d. $50 to $200
    e. $500

WORKBOOK ASSIGNMENT

To develop competency-based job skills, refer to the *Workbook* and complete the:
- Abbreviation and Spelling Review
- Review Questions

- Critical Thinking Exercises
- Job Skill activities, which are listed at the beginning of the chapter under *Performance Objectives in the Workbook.*

RESOURCES

Books

Medical Office Procedures with Medical Pegboard, 5th edition
Flores, Eleanor
Cengage Learning, 2013
Website: http://www.cengagebrain.com

Organizations

The American Institute of Professional Bookkeepers (AIPB)
Bookkeeping tips
Certification information

CHAPTER 16

PROCEDURE CODING

LEARNING OBJECTIVES

After reading this chapter and learning step-by-step procedures to gain job skills,* you should be able to:

- Outline items to address in a coding compliance program.
- Explain the standard code set and its components and purpose.
- Name codebooks used to code professional services.
- List advantages and disadvantages of encoders and computer-assisted coding.
- Discuss codebook terms and identify symbols in the *Current Procedural Terminology (CPT)* codebook.
- Determine code edits and define reimbursement terminology.
- Describe sections and subsections of *CPT* and recount unique coding practices within each section.
- Summarize the concept of surgical package rules, follow-up days, and Medicare's global surgery policy.
- State reasons procedure modifiers are used and explain how to apply add-on codes.
- Review items found in *CPT* codebook appendices.
- Code professional services and procedures using *CPT* and *HCPCS II.*

PERFORMANCE OBJECTIVES (PROCEDURES) IN THIS TEXTBOOK

- Select correct procedure codes (Procedure 16-1).
- Determine code selections from an operative report (Procedure 16-2).

PERFORMANCE OBJECTIVES (JOB SKILLS) IN THE WORKBOOK

- Review *Current Procedural Terminology* codebook sections (Job Skill 16-1).
- Code evaluation and management services (Job Skill 16-2).
- Code surgical services and procedures (Job Skill 16-3).
- Code radiology and laboratory services and procedures (Job Skill 16-4).
- Code procedures and services in the Medicine section (Job Skill 16-5).
- Code clinical examples (Job Skill 16-6).

* This textbook and the accompanying Workbook meet the educational components for entry-level administrative and general competenciesoutlined by CAAHEP and ABHES.

KEYTERMS

add-on codes

bundled code

closed fracture

coding compliance program

complementary and alternative
   medicine (CAM)

computer-assisted coding (CAC)

concurrent care

consultation

counseling

critical care

downcoding

emergency care

encoder

HCPCS Level II codes

manipulate

National Correct Coding Initiative
   (NCCI)

natural language processing (NLP)

open fracture

patient status (new/est)

place of service (POS)

qualitative analysis

quantitative analysis

separate procedure

surgical approach

type of service (TOS)

unbundling

upcoding

HEART OF THE HEALTH CARE PROFESSIONAL

Service

When you accurately code procedures and process insurance claims in a timely manner, you help gain maximum reimbursement for the physician and patient.

COMPLIANCE

Coding Regulations

The Health Insurance Portability and Accountability Act (HIPAA), Occupational Safety and Health Administration (OSHA), Stark Regulations, and Anti-Kickback Act of 1986 all address coding regulations. Although a compliance program is not mandated, it is recommended, and a practice's focus on patient care can be enhanced by the adoption of a voluntary compliance program.

INTRODUCTION TO PROCEDURE CODING

Procedure coding involves looking up and selecting correct codes for all services, procedures, tests, and surgeries performed by the physician. Procedure codes are then entered on the CMS-1500 health insurance claim, which is sent to third-party payers to bill for services. To meet coding and billing standards, coding guidelines should be adhered to and a **coding compliance program** implemented. Items to address would include:

- Coding and documentation review sessions for physicians and staff
- Current coding manuals and updated encounter forms
- Documentation Guidelines for Evaluation and Management Services (1995 and 1997)
- Education in coding and compliance—ongoing for physicians and staff
- Employee confidentiality statements—reviewed and re-signed yearly
- Internal audit plan for medical records to substantiate correct code usage

- Current payer policy and procedure manuals, outlining coding requirements
- Practice policy manual that includes incorrect billing practices and fraud prevention
- Reference coding documents (e.g., advisory resources, bulletins, newsletters, samples)
- Staff meetings scheduled regularly with physicians to discuss practice management issues

CODING FOR PROFESSIONAL SERVICES

The codes listed on insurance claims are tied to the physician's reimbursement. The diagnosis code will determine whether the physician gets paid (Chapter 17), and the procedure code will determine how much the practice receives. Codes from a standard code set should be used, which has been developed by the Centers for Medicare and Medicaid Services (CMS) and mandated by HIPAA (Figure 16-1).

Standard Code Set

The American National Standards Institute (ANSI) sponsors the Health Information Technology Standards Panel (HITSP) that works between public and private sectors to establish standards to support local, regional, and national health information networks. The standardization of coded information allows sharing all health care information in an electronic format resulting in less paperwork, an increase in efficiency, and more accurate information. In Chapter 18, you will be learning more about HIPAA X12 Version 5010 of the transaction code set that must be used by all covered entities (i.e., health care providers, health plans, and clearinghouses) that conduct electronic transactions named under HIPAA regulations.

Codes within this standard that apply to billing outpatient medical claims include:

- *Current Procedural Terminology (CPT)* (also referred to as *HCPCS Level I* codes for procedures and services)
- *Healthcare Common Procedure Coding System (HCPCS) Level II* codes for services, procedures, drugs, products, and supplies not listed in *CPT*
- *International Classification of Diseases, 10th Revision, Clinical Modification (ICD-10-CM)* (diagnostic codes)—see Chapter 17

CPT Codebook

The most common reference used to code procedures is the annual publication entitled *Current Procedural Terminology (CPT)** published by the American Medical Association (Figure 16-1). This code system uses five-digit code numbers with two-digit modifiers. New codes are added, codes are deleted, and descriptions are revised each October, so it is important to obtain the current edition to code accurately. Mini *CPT* codebooks

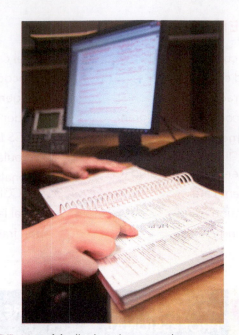

FIGURE 16-1 Medical assistant at the computer completing and coding an insurance claim

are available for specialty practices, and coding software may be purchased to assist in the assignment of codes.

Encoders

An **encoder** is a computerized or Web-based software program that is used instead of coding books to search for, locate, and verify code selections (e.g., Optum EncoderPro, TruCode, EpiCoder, Flash Code). The program presents code choices and additional questions to help assist the coder match the service or procedure with the correct code. Encoder edits can be performed to ensure inconsistencies do not take place. For example, if a code for a tubal ligation is entered for a male patient, an error message would appear. Prompts may also appear to help check for documentation requirements prior to code assignment.

Computer-Assisted Coding (CAC)

Computer-assisted coding (CAC) is a software program that goes a step further than encoder programs and automatically assigns codes to clinical procedures and services. CAC can integrate with other systems like document imaging and transcription, making remote coding a possibility; however, as this has become

---

COMPLIANCE

Transaction Code Sets

As part of HIPAA, the transaction code sets are just the start of standardization of coded information within the health care industry. Watch and be prepared for the changes this standardization effort produces.

integrated in medical offices, the coder's responsibilities have changed to include such things as editing and analyzing data, outcomes, and coding trends. There are two models used by CAC to produce codes: (1) structured software and (2) natural language processing software.

Using CAC-structured software, the data entry screen features point-and-click fields, pull-down menus, and structured templates, which are presented to the physician who is prompted for more information as necessary. Words and phrases selected are linked to codes that are automatically generated after the physician fills out the required fields. All codes must be validated by a coder prior to integrating the codes into a medical claim.

When using unstructured, or **natural language processing (NLP)**, software, the physician dictates as usual. Artificial intelligence technology, which is built into the software, scans the document and singles out important terms, converting them into codes. Accurate documentation in a free-text format is vital to have this type of system produce the right codes. As with the structured software, a coder must validate that all codes are correct prior to transmission to the billing department.

CAC programs may include special features, such as Correct Coding Initiative (CCI) edits, the Medicare Physician Fee Schedule (MPFS), Medicare coding rules and policies, anatomical illustrations, and links to other coding resources. Advantages of using CAC include increased productivity, consistent and comprehensive code assignment, and an audit trail that tracks steps taken to obtain final code choices. Even though electronic coding programs are considered a vital tool to assist in today's coding world, it is prudent to remember that errors may occur and electronic medical record coding engines can degrade the accuracy of the coding process.

Electronic hand-held mobile devices are also being used in the coding and billing process. They can easily capture, store, and manipulate a variety of information, helping to secure charges and track, record, and access patient data while reducing paperwork. Use of the *CPT* codebook will be emphasized in this chapter.

HCPCS Level II Codebook

HCPCS Level II codes are used to code those services, products, supplies, drugs, and procedures generally not fully listed in the *CPT* codebook. There are both temporary and permanent codes. This second-level coding system is composed of alphanumeric codes from A through V (e.g., A0225 = ambulance; neonatal

transport) and is used by all regional Medicare fiscal agents or carriers along with many other insurance programs. Special alpha modifiers (e.g., AA = anesthesia services performed personally by anesthesiologist) and alphanumeric modifiers (e.g., A1 = dressing for one wound) have been developed by the CMS to clarify unusual services or procedures not fully described by *HCPCS* codes. A list of *HCPCS* code examples with alpha modifiers may be found at the end of the Mock Fee Schedule shown in Appendix A of the *Workbook*.

Code Edits

Part of learning to code procedures, services, and diagnoses is to understand how codes interact with other components in the billing process. The CMS developed the **National Correct Coding Initiative (NCCI)** edits that relate to *CPT* and *HCPCS* codes for outpatient and physician services—another set is utilized for hospital reporting. These edits, found on the Medicare website, list procedure codes in tables that may be referred to in order to verify a particular code's usage with other codes and with modifiers. They are used by Medicare carriers to process professional claims and curtail improper coding practices, detect incorrect reporting of codes, eliminate unbundling of services, and prevent payments from being made due to inappropriate code assignments. *Code edits* are performed by computer software programs and along with Medicare, other federal programs, state Medicaid programs, and private payers use code editing software.

RVS Codebook

Another code system commonly used in workers' compensation billing is the relative value studies (scale/schedule), or RVS. This code system falls outside the standard code set mandated via HIPAA. Five-digit codes and two-digit modifiers are also used with this coding system, but it includes unit values for each service and procedure. As described in Chapter 13, the unit value indicates the relative value for each service performed, taking into account the time, skill, and overhead cost required (see Example 16-1). The units in this scale are based on median charges of all physicians during the period in which the *RVS* was published. Conversion factors are used to translate the abstract units in the scale to dollar fees for each service. A commonly used annual publication is entitled *Relative Values for Physicians* by Optum.

EXAMPLE 16-1

Relative Value Scale Fee Formula

Procedure Code	Description	Units
10060	Incision and drainage of cyst	0.8

Using a hypothetical figure of $153/unit, this procedure would be valued at $122.40.

Math: $153.00 × 0.8 = $122.40

ABC Codebook

Complementary and alternative medicine (CAM) is offered by a group of diverse medical practitioners whose practices and products are not presently considered to be part of conventional medicine in the United States. Complementary medicine is used in conjunction with conventional medical treatments, while alternative medicine is used in place of existing therapies or products. CAM includes five major categories:

- Alternative medical systems (e.g., homeopathic/naturopathic)
- Biologically based therapies (e.g., dietary supplements)
- Energy therapies (e.g., biofield therapies/bioelectromagnetic-based therapies)
- Manipulative and body-based methods (e.g., chiropractic manipulation/massage)
- Mind-body interventions (e.g., meditation/mental healing)

The *Alternative Billing Coding (ABC) Manual for Integrative Healthcare* was developed to help assign appropriate codes, establish billing systems, justify claims, and provide a common language for insurance carriers and health care researchers. CAM codes consist of five alpha characters that describe services, remedies, or supplies (e.g., NAAGN: pain management or control; initial 60 minutes). These basic codes are followed by two-character alphanumeric code modifiers that describe the various types of licensed health care practitioners (e.g., 1A Doctor of Chiropractic; 1B Licensed Massage Therapist; 1C Doctor of Oriental Medicine). Although *ABC* codes are not recognized in HIPAA's standard code set, they can be used to bill insurance carriers who have approved CAM services and supplies on their benefit list. For information on where to obtain all codebooks mentioned, refer to the *Resources* section at the end of this chapter.

CODING TERMINOLOGY

The medical assistant needs to be familiar with terminology used in codebooks as well as medical and reimbursement terminology used to process and follow up on insurance claims. Acronyms, symbols, and abbreviations must be interpreted for efficient coding—coding is an art, not an exact science.

CPT Codebook Terms

The *Current Procedural Terminology* codebook uses medical and surgical terminology to accurately describe professional services, so correct codes can be assigned and maximum payment from insurance carriers can be obtained.

Codebook terms also relate to the type of care the patient receives and it is important to differentiate between a new and established patient when selecting Evaluation and Management codes. As mentioned in Chapter 7, a *new patient* is one who has not received any professional services from the physician, or another physician of the same specialty who belongs to the same group practice, within the past 3 years. An *established patient* is one who has received professional services from the physician, or another physician of the same specialty who belongs to the same group practice, within the past 3 years. If a patient has registered at a hospital as an outpatient or inpatient within the past 3 years prior to seeing a physician in an outpatient setting, the patient would be considered established for that visit according to the CMS definition.

Concurrent care is the provision of similar services (e.g., hospital visits) to the same patient by more than one physician on the same day. The physicians are typically from different specialties, taking care of different medical problems. When concurrent care is provided, each physician is cross-referenced on the insurance claim.

Critical care is the care of an unstable, acutely ill, or injured patient requiring constant bedside attention by a physician (e.g., cardiac arrest, shock, bleeding, respiratory failure, postoperative complications, a seriously ill neonate, and so forth). Critical care may sometimes but not always be rendered in a critical care area, such as the coronary care unit, intensive care unit, respiratory care unit, or emergency care facility. Critical care requires high-complexity decision making by the physician and careful documentation of work performed and time spent, both with the patient and the family (if a family member is operating as a surrogate decision maker). Neonatal and pediatric critical care codes are age-specific and provided for initial and subsequent encounters.

Emergency care differs from critical care in that it is provided to prevent serious impairment of bodily functions or a serious dysfunction to a body part or organ (see Chapter 6). It is typically provided in an emergency department and codes 99281—99285 are used. Code 99288 is used when advanced life support is required during emergency care. If office services are provided on an emergency basis, some insurance carriers accept code 99058 from the medicine section in addition to a code from the evaluation and management section.

Counseling is a discussion with a patient and family concerning one or more of the following:

1. Diagnostic results, impressions, and recommended studies
2. Prognosis
3. Risks and benefits of treatment options
4. Instructions for treatment and/or follow-up
5. Compliance with treatment options
6. Risk factor reduction
7. Patient and family education

It may be billed separately if time is documented and a complete history and physical examination does not take place.

Consultations can occur in a home, office, hospital, extended care facility, and so forth. A physician consultant gives a second opinion regarding a condition or need for surgery and may initiate diagnostic or therapeutic services. Remember the three Rs when coding consultations: Services must be *requested* by another physician, findings and recommendations must be *recorded*, and a *report* must be sent to the referring physician. Codes for consultations are as follows:

- Office or other outpatient consultations (new or established patient) 99241—99245
- Initial inpatient consultations (new or established patient) 99251—99255

If an insurance company states that a second opinion is necessary prior to approval for a surgery, modifier -32 (mandated services) should be applied to the consultation code. If a physician performs a follow-up consultation in a hospital setting, the appropriate subsequent hospital care code should be selected. For each admission, only one initial consultation should be reported. If a physician performs a follow-up consultation in an office setting, the office consultation codes may be used again. If follow-up visits in the consultant's office take

place, the appropriate new patient or established patient evaluation and management code should be used.

Medicare has eliminated the use of consultation codes for inpatient and outpatient services. For medical claims, inpatient hospital codes (99221–99223), previously used only by admitting physicians, will also be used to bill inpatient consultation services. Outpatient consultations will be billed using new and established office/clinic codes (99201–99205 and 99211–99215), according to new and established patient rules. If consultative services are provided in the emergency room, emergency department codes 99281–99285 are used as long as the patient is not admitted.

A *referral* is the transfer of the total or specific care of a patient from one physician to another (see Chapters 2 and 7). It is not a consultation. However, a patient may be referred from one physician to another for a consultation.

Codebook Symbols

With each annual edition of *CPT*, there are new codes and description changes indicated by the use of symbols, as seen in Figure 16-2. Other symbols are used to alert the coder when codes can or cannot be used in certain situations. It is important to be mindful of these symbols and become familiar with the new codes and any description changes. Appendix B in the *CPT* codebook gives a summary of the additions, deletions, and revisions.

Reimbursement Terminology

When processing insurance claims and when code edits are made, certain terms are used to communicate situations when services and procedures may be suspended, paid less than charged, or denied because of the codes selected or missing medically necessary criteria. Following are common situations and terminology used when they occur.

Downcoding

When **downcoding** occurs, the computer system changes the submitted code to a lower level code. This can occur in the following instances:

- When the coding system used on the insurance claim does not match the coding system used by the insurance carrier. The computer converts the code submitted to the closest code in use. Payment generated is typically less.

Current Procedural Terminology Codebook Symbols

New code (Appendix B)

● 43327   Esophagogastric fundoplasty partial or complete; laparotomy

Revised code (Appendix B)

▲ 43605   <u>Biopsy of stomach</u>, by laparotomy

New or revised text (other than the procedure descriptors)

▶◀ 88334   Pathology consultation during surgery; cytologic examination
              ▶(Use 88334 in conjunction with 88331, 88333)◀

Reinstated/Recycled code (Appendix B)

○ 0058T   Cryopreservation; reproductive tissue, ovarian

Add–on code (Appendix D)

+11732   Avulsion of nail plate; each additional nail plate (list separately in addition
              to code for primary procedure)

Modifier -51 exempt (Appendix E)

⊘ 17004   Destruction (e.g., laser surgery), 15 or more lesions

Moderate (Conscious) Sedation (Appendix G)

⊙ 33222   Relocation of skin pocket for pacemaker

Product Pending FDA Approval (Appendix K)

⚡ 90664   Influenza virus vaccine, pandamic formulation, live, for intranasal use

Code listed out of numerical sequence (Appendix N)

87623   Human Papillomavirus, low risk types

Reference to *CPT Assistant, CPT Changes: an Insider's View,* and *Clinical Examples in Radiology*

47000   Biopsy of liver, needle; percutaneous
     ● *CPT Assistant* Fall 93:12

2017 *Current Procedural Terminology* © 2016 *American Medical Association. All rights reserved.*

FIGURE 16-2 *Current Procedural Terminology** codebook symbols

- When the claims examiner in a workers' compensation case must convert the submitted *CPT* code to an RVS code. The claims examiner will select the lowest-paying code. Before billing, find which RVS system is used by the carrier and find the best match for the *CPT* code.

- When a claims examiner reviews an attached document and compares the code used with the written description of the procedure. If the two do not match, the insurance carrier will reimburse according to the lowest-paying code that fits the stated description.

To detect downcoding and prevent further occurrences, always monitor reimbursement and become knowledgeable about which codes are affected. Call the insurance carrier and verify that the standard code set is being used.

Upcoding

The term **upcoding** is the practice of coding and billing a health plan for a procedure that reimburses the physician at a higher rate than the procedure actually done; this is also known as *code creep, overcoding,* or *overbilling*. Because computer software has built-in edits referred to as *post-payment screens* in the Medicare program, this may be easily spotted and can lead to an audit and penalties.

Bundled Codes

A **bundled code** contains a grouping of one or more services that are related to a procedure, so coding and billing for these individual services should not be done. Sometimes a payment notice will state, "Benefits have been combined." The Medicare program has many procedures considered bundled. For example, a sterile tray (99070) is typically bundled with surgical procedures unless a second tray is needed due to complications, so it is not billed separately. Services such as telephone calls, surgical dressings, and reading of test results are typically bundled into evaluation and management codes. Major surgical procedures often bundle other procedures even when not mentioned in the code description. For example, a total abdominal hysterectomy (corpus and cervix), with or without removal of tube(s), with or without removal of ovary(s) (58150), includes a dilation and curettage (57800 D & C canal, instrumental [separate procedure]). The term **separate procedure** means that the procedure, if not performed alone, is an integral part of another procedure and is bundled into other procedures; it should not be billed and will not be paid for.

Unbundling

Unbundling is breaking down a procedure into separate billable codes with charges to increase reimbursement; this is also known as *fragmentation, exploding,* or *à la carte medicine*. To code a bilateral procedure using two codes when one code includes it in the description is a good example of unbundling (see *CPT* code 77056, bilateral mammogram). There are unbundling reference books (see the *Resources* section at the end of this chapter), and insurers use special software to detect unbundling. This practice is considered fraud and can lead to an audit and costly penalties. The use of out-of-date codes often results in unbundling, so it is important to use current codebooks.

CODEBOOK SECTIONS

There are six main sections in *CPT*. Within each section, there may be subsections, categories, and subcategories divided according to anatomic body system, procedure, condition, description, and specialty.

At the beginning of each section are guidelines relating to that portion of the codebook. Read these thoroughly prior to coding as they contain helpful definitions and directions. *CPT* codes are considered Category I codes. At the end of all Category I codes are Category II and III codes, which have been developed to improve the coding system. Category II codes are supplemental tracking codes that can be used for performance measurements. They are optional and are used to help decrease the need for record abstraction and chart review. Category III codes are temporary codes used for emerging technologies and new services or procedures.

Table 16-1 lists the main sections for the 2017 edition of *CPT*.

Evaluation and Management Section

The Evaluation and Management (E/M) section has subsections, categories, and subcategories that have codes with three to five levels for reporting purposes. These levels are represented by the last digit (e.g., 99201 = level I) and are based on key components and contributory factors. To code, first determine the following:

- **Place of service (POS)**—Where is the service taking place?

☑️ **COMPLIANCE**

Overutilized Codes

A list of overutilized codes was published by the Centers for Medicare and Medicaid Services (CMS) that included the following codes, listed in order of upcoding frequency: 99310, 99205, 99204, 99255, 99245, and 99211. Each code was insufficiently documented.

TABLE 16-1 Sections of the *Current Procedural Terminology* Codebook with Code Ranges

Section	Code Range
Evaluation and Management (E/M)	99201 to 99499
Anesthesia	00100 to 01999
	99100 to 99140
Surgery	10021 to 69990
Radiology	70010 to 79999
Pathology and Laboratory	80047 to 89398
Medicine	90281 to 99607

- **Type of service (TOS)**—What type of service was provided?
- **Patient status (new/est)**—Is the patient new or established?

Then familiarize yourself with the section divisions by looking at the Table of Contents at the beginning of the E/M section. Once you have located the right POS, TOS, and patient status, read the description thoroughly to match the *key components:*

- History
- Physical examination
- Medical decision making

Note the *contributory factors,* counseling, coordination of care, nature of presenting problem, and face-to-face time for the service. For detailed information about the key components and contributory factors, refer to the following sections in Chapter 9: "Patient Medical History," "Physical Examination," and "Complexity of Medical Decision Making."

For a new patient, all three of the key components must be met or exceeded to assign a code; otherwise, code to the lowest key component documented by the physician. For an established patient, two out of three key component levels must be met to assign a code.

An additional subsection on preventive medicine is categorized according to new or established patients and patient ages to be used for such services as routine physical examinations and well-baby checkups.

In the majority of E/M services where counseling or coordination of care dominates (more than 50%) the face-to-face physician-patient encounter, *time* is considered the key component to qualify for a particular level of service (see Example 16-2).

EXAMPLE 16-2

When Time Is the Determining Factor

Scenario: Dr. Practon sees a patient for an initial outpatient consultation. After the evaluation, he decides that the patient requires a surgical procedure and spends a considerable amount of time discussing the risks, possible complications, alternative treatments, and possible lifestyle accommodations that may be necessary as a result of the surgery.

Description	Time
Total face-to-face time spent	35 minutes
Total counseling time spent	25 minutes
Level of care code selected	99243* (40 minutes)

*The counseling time amounted to more than 50% of the total time (1/2 of 35 = 17.5 min.); therefore, it can be used as the key component in determining the level of service.

As learned in Chapter 9, documentation is required in the patient's record to substantiate the chosen level.

A longtime adage within the coding community states, "If it is not documented, it did not happen. If it is not legible, it is not valid. And, if it is not signed, it does not exist." Tables 16-2, 16-3, and 16-4 give a concise view of the components for the most common E/M code numbers. The American Medical Association (AMA) publishes a concise *CPT Express Reference Tables* pamphlet that can be used as a quick guide when deciding levels of E/M services. A similar guide may be found in the front of the professional edition of the *CPT* codebook.

Hospital Admits and Observation Status

When the physician admits a patient to the hospital for either a planned surgery or via the emergency room, you will be coding the hospital admit, subsequent visits, and hospital discharge. If your physician sees the patient in the emergency room, you will also code for those services.

In 2014, as part of the *Inpatient Prospective Payment System (IPPS)*, the CMS initiated a "Two-Midnight Rule" which states that if a patient stays fewer than two midnights, the hospital will be paid on observation (outpatient) status, rather than inpatient status; this applies to the majority of cases. Formal admittance as an inpatient is presumed to be "reasonable and necessary" for inpatient status if a patient's stay spans two or more midnights. Table 16-2 outlines various coding scenarios when a patient is on observation status.

TABLE 16-2 Observation Status and Code Selections

Observation Status	Code Selections
Observation lasting fewer than 8 hours	99218-99220
Observation lasting more than 8 hours	99234-99236
Observation status; admission and discharge on same day	99234-99236
Observation status with discharge on next day	99218-99220
Observation status, when admitted on same day	99221-99223
Observation status, when admitted on next day	99218-99220 and 99221-99223
Observation status for 3 or more days: Initial date of service	99218-99220
Subsequent observation care (days in between, e.g., day 2, day 3)	99224-99226
Final date of service	99217

TABLE 16-3 Selection of E/M Codes for Office/Other Outpatient and Inpatient Services

E/M Code	History	Exam	Medical Decision Making	Problem Severity	Coordination of Care; Counseling	Time Spent (avg.)
Office or Other Outpatient Services						
New Patient*						
99201	Problem-focused	Problem-focused	Straightforward	Minor or self-limited	Consistent with problem(s) and patient's needs	10 min. face to face
99202	Expanded problem-focused	Expanded problem-focused	Straightforward	Low to moderate	Consistent with problem(s) and patient's needs	20 min. face to face
99203	Detailed	Detailed	Low complexity	Moderate	Consistent with problem(s) and patient's needs	30 min. face to face
99204	Comprehensive	Comprehensive	Moderate complexity	Moderate to high	Consistent with problem(s) and patient's needs	45 min. face to face
99205	Comprehensive	Comprehensive	High complexity	Moderate to high	Consistent with problem(s) and patient's needs	60 min. face to face

(*continues*)

TABLE 16-3 **Selection of E/M Codes for Office/Other Outpatient and Inpatient Services** *(continued)*

E/M Code	History	Exam	Medical Decision Making	Problem Severity	Coordination of Care; Counseling	Time Spent (avg.)
Office or Other Outpatient Services						
Established Patient*						
99211	—	—	Physician supervision but presence not required	Minimal	Consistent with problem(s) and patient's needs	5 min. face to face
99212	Problem-focused	Problem-focused	Straightforward	Minor or self-limited	Consistent with problem(s) and patient's needs	10 min. face to face
99213	Expanded problem-focused	Expanded problem-focused	Low complexity	Low to moderate	Consistent with problem(s) and patient's needs	15 min. face to face
99214	Detailed	Detailed	Moderate complexity	Moderate to high	Consistent with problem(s) and patient's needs	25 min. face to face
99215	Comprehensive	Comprehensive	High complexity	Moderate to high	Consistent with problem(s) and patient's needs	40 min. face to face
Hospital Inpatient Services: Initial Care*						
99221	Detailed or comprehensive	Detailed or comprehensive	Straightforward or low complexity	Low	Consistent with problem(s) and patient's needs	30 min. unit/ floor
99222	Comprehensive	Comprehensive	Moderate complexity	Moderate	Consistent with problem(s) and patient's needs	50 min. unit/ floor
92223	Comprehensive	Comprehensive	High complexity	High	Consistent with problem(s) and patient's needs	70 min. unit/ floor
99231	Problem-focused interval	Problem-focused	Straightforward or low complexity	Stable, recovering, or improving	Consistent with problem(s) and patient's needs	15 min. unit/ floor
99232	Expanded problem-focused interval	Expanded problem-focused complication	Moderate complexity	Inadequate response to treatment; minor complication	Consistent with problem(s) and patient's needs	25 min. unit/ floor
99233	Detailed interval	Detailed	High complexity	Unstable; significant new problem or complication	Consistent with problem(s) and patient's needs	35 min. unit/ floor
99238	Hospital discharge day management	—	—	—	—	30 min. or less
99239	Hospital discharge day management	—	—	—	—	More than 30 min.

*Key component: For new patients with initial office and other outpatient services, all three component levels (history, exam, and medical decision making) are essential in selecting the correct code. For established patients, at least two of these three component levels are required.

TABLE 16-4 Code Selection Criteria for Consultations

E/M Code	History	Medical Decision Exam	Problem Making	Severity	Coordination of Care; Counseling	Time Spent (avg.)
			Consultations			
Office and Other Outpatient						
99241	Problem-focused	Problem-focused	Straightforward	Minor or self-limited	Consistent with problem(s) and patient's needs	15 min. face to face
99242	Expanded problem-focused	Expanded problem-focused	Straightforward	Low	Consistent with problem(s) and patient's needs	30 min. face to face
99243	Detailed	Detailed	Low complexity	Moderate	Consistent with problem(s) and patient's needs	40 min. face to face
99244	Comprehensive	Comprehensive	Moderate complexity	Moderate to high	Consistent with problem(s) and patient's needs	60 min. face to face
99245	Comprehensive	Comprehensive	High complexity	Moderate to high	Consistent with problem(s) and patient's needs	80 min. face to face
Initial Inpatient*						
99251	Problem-focused	Problem-focused	Straightforward	Minor or self-limited	Consistent with problem(s) and patient's needs	20 min. face to face
99252	Expanded problem-focused	Expanded problem-focused	Straightforward	Low	Consistent with problem(s) and patient's needs	40 min. face to face
99253	Detailed	Detailed	Low complexity	Moderate	Consistent with problem(s) and patient's needs	55 min. face to face
99254	Comprehensive	Comprehensive	Moderate complexity	Moderate to high	Consistent with problem(s) and patient's needs	80 min. face to face
99255	Comprehensive	Comprehensive	High complexity	Moderate to high	Consistent with problem(s) and patient's needs	110 min. face to face

*Key component: For initial care, all three component levels (history, exam, and medical decision making) are essential in selecting the correct code. For subsequent care, at least two of these three component levels are required.

Anesthesia Section

The anesthesia section is divided into subsections according to the anatomic site where the surgery is performed. After locating the correct site, you must determine what type of anesthetic was administered and by whom (e.g., anesthesiologist, nurse anesthetist).

After the code selection is made, anesthesia modifiers are assigned to indicate patient status (e.g., P3 = patient with severe systemic disease). Special add-on codes are used in addition for qualifying circumstances if they exist, such as + 99100, "Anesthesia for patient of extreme age, under 1 year and older than 70." These modifiers and add-on codes are found at the beginning of the Anesthesia section.

Surgery Section

The Surgery section is the largest section in *CPT.* It is divided into many subsections according to body systems (e.g., integumentary, musculoskeletal). When coding from the Surgery section, always go to the index first. Following are rules that apply to the Surgery section and instructions on how to code.

Surgical Supplies

Typically, the surgical tray is included in the procedure code for the surgery being performed. However, if a sterile surgical tray is used for office surgery and the materials are over and above those usually included for such a surgery, *CPT* code 99070 from the medicine section may be used and supplies may be itemized on an attachment and given a separate fee.

Surgical Code Language

Surgical coding language appears in the *CPT* codebook, in various insurance carrier billing guidelines, and in other resource material used to code. Surgical code descriptions may define a correct coding relationship when one code is part of another (see Example 16-3). Following are several rules that apply when coding surgery.

EXAMPLE 16-3

Descriptive Surgical Code Language

- *Partial or complete,* which means the partial procedure is included in the complete procedure.

    56620   Vulvectomy simple; *partial*

    56625   *complete*

- *Partial or total,* which means the partial procedure is included in the total procedure.
- *Unilateral and bilateral,* which means the unilateral procedure is included in the bilateral procedure.

    58940   Oophorectomy, *partial* or *total,* *unilateral or bilateral*

- *Single and multiple,* which means the single procedure is included in the multiple procedure.

    49321   Laparoscopy, surgical; with biopsy (*single or multiple*)

Surgical Package Rules—Surgical package rules apply to major and minor surgical procedures and include bundled services with the surgery code. A full description of *CPT* surgical package rules may be found in "Surgery Guidelines" at the beginning of the Surgery section of the codebook. This concept means the surgical code includes the operation, local infiltration, digital block or topical anesthesia, and normal, uncomplicated postoperative care, such as follow-up hospital visits, hospital discharge, and follow-up office visits, for a number of designated follow-up days. This is referred to as a "package" for surgical procedures, and one fee covers the entire package. Preoperative services, such as consultations, office visits, and initial hospital care, are usually billed and paid for separately if they occur more than 24 hours prior to surgery; otherwise, they are included. The CMS and the AMA provide different definitions of what is included in the package fee, so it is wise to determine whether the carrier is following CMS or AMA guidelines.

Follow-up Days—A variable number (10, 30, or 90) of follow-up days after surgery is included in the surgical code depending on whether it is minor or major surgery. Postoperative services pertaining to the surgery may not be billed separately during this period. Since the codebook does not specify how many follow-up days should be given to a specific surgery, a separate reference is needed. A source that lists the follow-up days, also referred to as the *global fee period,* for each surgical procedure is the Medicare fee schedule published annually in the *Federal Register* (see the *Resources* section at the end of this chapter). Refer to surgical codes listed in the fee schedule in Appendix A of the *Workbook* (right column) for an example of follow-up days.

Medicare Global Package Rules*—The surgical package concept is used by Medicare (CMS) with varying rules. It applies in all settings and is referred to as the "Medicare Global Surgical Package"; it includes the following:

1. *Preoperative*—E/M office visit or hospital visit 1 day (24 hours) prior to hospital admit for major surgery and preoperative visits on day of surgery for minor procedures
2. *Intraoperative*—Services that are a usual and necessary part of a surgical procedure, such as local infiltration, digital block, or topical anesthesia

---

*Beginning in 2017, Medicare plans to eliminate global follow-up days (10, 90) so that all surgical procedures will have zero (0) days. They will, no doubt, adjust all surgical fees and establish new rules for coding and billing pre- and postsurgical care.

3. *Postoperative*—Routine postoperative care and any complications not requiring return to the operating room 10 or 90 days after surgery
4. *Supplies*—All supplies needed for surgery, except those identified as exclusions
5. *Miscellaneous Services*—Services such as dressing changes; local incision care; removal of sutures, staples, wires, tube, drains, casts, and splints; and so forth

Services provided for a Medicare patient NOT included in the global surgery package are:

1. Initial consultation or evaluation that prompted the decision for major surgery regardless of when it occurs (apply modifier -57 if within 24 hours prior to surgery)
2. Services of other physicians related to the surgery, except if there is an agreement on the transfer of care
3. Postoperative visits unrelated to the diagnosis for which the surgical procedure was performed (modifier -24 would apply)
4. Treatment required to stabilize a seriously ill patient before surgery
5. Diagnostic tests and procedures performed more than 20 hours prior to surgery
6. Clearly distinct surgical procedure occurring during the postoperative period; not reoperations or treatment for complications
7. Related procedure for postoperative complications that requires a return trip to the operating room (modifier -78 would apply)
8. Immunosuppressive therapy following transplant surgery
9. Critical care services for reasons unrelated to the surgery

Global surgery has the following three classifications:

1. Zero-Day Postoperative Period
   - No preoperative period
   - No postoperative days
   - Visit on day of procedure generally not payable
2. 10-Day Postoperative Period
   - No preoperative period
   - Visit on day of procedure generally not payable
   - Total global period of 11 days (day of surgery plus 10 days following)
3. 90-Day Postoperative Period
   - 1 day preoperative included
   - Day of procedure generally not payable
   - Total global period of 92 days (1 day prior to surgery, day of surgery, plus 90 days following)

When keying in services and procedures, some computer programs will automatically send an alert if the service/procedure being entered is within the global period of a previous procedure. The warning states, "this may be bundled" and prompts the medical assistant to check prior codes and the time frame for any follow-up days.

How to Code Using the *Current Procedural Terminology Codebook*

The *CPT* codebook has a wealth of information that can be used to help locate correct codes for procedures and services. Refer to Procedure 16-1 to select correct procedure codes using the *Current Procedural Terminology* codebook.

How to Code from an Operative Report

To code surgical procedures from an operative report, obtain a copy of the report; read and review it carefully. Do not code only the "operation performed" listed at the beginning of the report. Look for key terms within the body of the report to ensure that the codes selected reflect what was actually performed. The report may be a single page or several pages long and contains specific information in the physician's documentation about the surgery and how it was performed.

Look for and highlight key words that may change the code or determine the need for the assignment of a modifier, such as "very difficult," "extensive," "complicated," "hemorrhage," "blood loss of over 600 mL," "unusual findings or circumstances," "multiple," "ordinary," "simple," "uncomplicated," "unilateral," or "bilateral." If the physician verbally says "extensive complications," make sure these are described in the report to validate the codes chosen.

If unsure about the terminology or a code assignment, ask the physician to clarify the case. Medical terminology is very technical and can puzzle even the most knowledgeable medical assistant. A good medical dictionary can help. If the case is complex, send copies of the operative report, discharge summary, or any test results to the insurance carrier. Refer to Procedure 16-2 for step-by-step directions when coding from an operative report.

Integumentary Subsection (Surgery Section)

The Integumentary System subsection lists a variety of procedures performed on the skin. Local treatment of burns is listed according to the percentage of total body

PROCEDURE 16-1

Select Correct Procedure Codes

OBJECTIVE: Accurately locate and select codes for procedures and services.

EQUIPMENT/SUPPLIES: *Current Procedural Terminology* codebook, medical dictionary, and pen or pencil.

DIRECTIONS: Follow these step-by-step directions to learn this procedure. Job Skills 16-2 through 16-6 are presented in the *Workbook* for practice.

1. Read the introduction section at the beginning of the codebook. This information may change with each annual edition.

2. Select the term to look up and use the index at the back of the codebook. First look under the *procedure* or *service* performed. If it is not listed, check for the *organ* or *anatomical site* involved. If the procedure or organ is difficult to find, look up the *condition*. Keywords, such as synonyms or eponyms, and abbreviations may also help you find the appropriate code.

3. Next look up the subterms until you identify the procedure or service. You will find a single code, several codes listed, or a code range (see Example 16-4).

4. Mark down and look up all codes listed. Page numbers are not listed.

5. Turn to the beginning of the section for the code(s) given in the index and read the guidelines. They give general information and instructions on coding certain procedures within each section.

6. Look at the size of the title to find out the area you are in. Some codebooks have color-coded titles, making this determination easier. In the surgery section, each subsection is further divided into categories based on anatomic site. Within each category are subcategories listed by type of procedure (e.g., excision, repair, destruction, graft) or condition (burn, fracture).

EXAMPLE 16-4

Procedure Codes Listed in the Index

Bone Marrow (anatomic site)

Aspiration (procedure)	38220	→ Single code
Biopsy (procedure)	38221, 88305	→ Multiple codes
Transplant Preparation (procedure)	38207–38215	→ Code range

7. Turn to the correct section, subsection, category, or subcategory, and thoroughly read through all notes pertaining to that area.

8. Read all code descriptions carefully.

9. Notice punctuation and indentations. Descriptions for parent codes begin at the left margin and have a full description (see Example 16-5, code 11055). Read the description of an indented code (e.g., 11056) by reading the portion of the description of the parent code that appears above it and comes before the semicolon (;)—then continue reading the description after the semicolon. No matter how many indented codes are listed, always go back to the parent code to begin reading the description.

10. Select and write down the code. Remember, the service or procedure description should match the code's narrative description before an assignment is made.

11. Determine if one or more modifiers are needed to give a more accurate description of the services rendered or the circumstances in which they were performed.

12. Enter a five-digit code(s) and modifier (if applicable) in the proper field(s) on the insurance claim for each procedure or service rendered (24D for paper claims). Take care not to transpose numbers.

EXAMPLE 16-5

Reading *CPT* Code Descriptions

11055	**Paring or cutting of benign hyperkeratotic lesion;** single lesion	→	parent code
11056	two to four lesions	→	indented code
11057	more than four lesions	→	indented code

PROCEDURE 16-2

Determine Code Selections from an Operative Report

OBJECTIVE: Review an operative report and accurately locate and select codes for a surgical procedure.

EQUIPMENT/SUPPLIES: Operative report, *Current Procedural Terminology* codebook, medical dictionary, highlighter, and pen or pencil.

DIRECTIONS: Follow these step-by-step directions to learn this procedure.

1. Identify the type of surgery.

EXAMPLE 16-6

Type of Surgery

Code Range	49491–49659
Surgery Types	Hernias: Inguinal, lumbar, femoral, incisional, ventral, epigastric, umbilical, spigelian, and omphalocele

2. Identify the surgical approach:

EXAMPLE 16-7

Surgical Approach

Code Range	Approach
49491–49611	Open incision
49650–49659	Laparoscopic

3. Define the episode of care.

EXAMPLE 16-8

Episode of Care

Initial	One that has not been previously repaired
Recurrent	One that appears at the site of a previous hernia

4. Verify the clinical presentation.

EXAMPLE 16-9

Presentation

Reducible	Hernia sac contents return to normal location spontaneously or by gentle manipulation
Incarcerated or Strangulated	Herniated tissue is trapped and cannot be pushed back to normal position (reduced)

5. Determine patient's age at time of surgery or postconception.
6. Apply the steps to an operative note.

EXAMPLE 16-10

Operative Note

A *7-year-old male* was prepped and draped in sterile fashion. An infraumbilical *incision* was formed and taken down to the fascia. The *umbilical hernia* carefully *reduced* back into the cavity. The fascia was closed with interrupted vertical mattress sutures to approximate the fascia. The wounds were infiltrated with 0.25% Marcaine. The skin was reattached to the fascia with 2-0 Vicryl. The skin was approximated with 2-0 Vicryl subcutaneous, and then 4-0 Monocryl subcuticular stitches. The wound was dressed with Steri-Strips and 4 × 4s. Patient was extubated and taken to the recovery area in stable condition.

Code Assignment:	49586
Code Description	*Repair umbilical hernia, age 5 years or older; reducible*

surface area—see Chapter 17 for measurement determinations. Breast procedures are also listed in this subsection (e.g., breast biopsy, mastectomy).

Included are several types of lesion removals. The official guidelines for coding and reporting neoplasm states, "To properly code a neoplasm it is necessary to determine from the record if the neoplasm is benign, in-situ, malignant, or of uncertain histologic behavior." Following are brief definitions for these terms found in a pathology report and in the *CPT* codebook:

- Benign—not containing cancer cells
- In-situ—early-stage tumor that has not metastasized
- Malignant—cancerous tumor (either primary or secondary)
- Uncertain behavior—atypia or dysplasia

When selecting the code, be sure to distinguish the type of removal:

- Paring or cutting
- Biopsy
- Ligature strangulation, electrosurgical or chemical destruction, electrocauterization
- Shaving
- Excision

There are three types of closures of lacerations or wounds:

- Simple repair—used to close superficial tissue
- Intermediate repair—involves subcutaneous tissue and requires layered closure
- Complex repair—requires more than one layered closure (e.g., debridement, scar revision, reconstructive surgery)

Repairs are coded according to the type of repair, site-specific location, and size—length in centimeters (cm) rather than inches measured by the greatest diameter plus the margin required for excision. When multiple wounds of the same type (e.g., simple) occur in the same area listed in the codebook (e.g., scalp, neck, axillae), add together the lengths of all lacerations and report them with a single code (Example 16-11).

If the wound repairs are not of the same type, or are not in the same anatomic grouping, list the most complex first or that with the highest dollar value. The first code will be given the highest payment, and the payments for the subsequent codes will be substantially decreased. An easy way to remember this is, "the harder the procedure, the higher the code" (Example 16-12).

EXAMPLE 16-11

Coding Multiple Lacerations of Same Type in Same Anatomic Regions

Scenario: The physician repaired three simple lacerations. The first was located on the patient's scalp and measured 2.8 cm. The second was located on the patient's neck and measured 7.7 cm. The third was located on the patient's right hand and measured 3.9 cm.

Location	Measurement	
Scalp	2.8 cm	All wounds are the same type (simple) and
Neck	7.7 cm	occur in the same area, as defined in the
Hand	3.9 cm	codebook.
Total	14.4 cm	**Code 12005**

Description: Simple repair of superficial wounds of scalp, neck . . . extremities (12.6 to 20.0 cm)

Musculoskeletal Subsection (Surgery Section)

The Musculoskeletal System subsection is arranged by anatomic site—starting at the head and moving downward toward the feet. Under the anatomic categories are subcategories that include:

- Incision
- Excision
- Introduction/Removal
- Repair/Revision/Reconstruction
- Fracture/Dislocation
- Arthrodesis
- Amputation
- Unlisted Procedures

Treatment for sprains, strains, fractures, and spinal problems are just a few of the listings that orthopedic surgeons frequently use from this subsection of the codebook. When coding a fracture, be sure to note whether it is a **closed fracture** (with unbroken skin), or an **open fracture** in which the bone has broken the skin (also referred to as a *compound fracture*). Also note whether the fracture has been **manipulated** (i.e., stretched or realigned with manual pressure, traction, or angulation); this is also referred to as a *reduction*. These key terms will help determine the correct code.

EXAMPLE 16-12

Coding Multiple Lacerations of Different Types in Different Anatomic Regions

Scenario: The physician repaired three lacerations. The first was a simple repair located on the patient's face and measured 2.7 cm. The second was an intermediate repair located on the patient's scalp and measured 4.5 cm. The third was an intermediate repair located on the patient's left foot and measured 5.1 cm.

Location	Measurement	Type of Repair	Code	Description
Face	2.7 cm	Simple	12001	Simple repair of superficial wounds of *face*, ears, eyelids, nose, lips, and/or mucous membranes; 2.6 cm to 5.0 cm
Scalp	4.5 cm	Intermediate	12032	Repair, intermediate, wounds of *scalp*, axillae, trunk, and/or extremities; 2.6 cm to 7.5 cm
Foot	5.1 cm	Intermediate	12042	Repair, intermediate, wounds of neck, hands, *feet*, and/or external genitalia; 2.6 cm to 7.5 cm

Sequencing of codes: 12042, 12032–59, 12001–59

Note: The most difficult intermediate repair is listed first. Although the scalp repair is also intermediate, it is smaller and appears in a different anatomic grouping so it needs to be listed separate. The second and third codes are appended with modifier -59, which indicates that each is a distinct surgical procedure.

Respiratory Subsection (Surgery Section)

The Respiratory System subsection is arranged by anatomic site, then procedure. It includes procedures of the nose, sinuses, larynx (voice box), trachea (windpipe), and various parts of the lung. Endoscopic procedures are commonly performed to view the interior tube that passes from the nose to the lung. If the endoscope is passed into the bronchi, it is referred to as a bronchoscopy (31622), which may involve an injection, biopsy, scraping, and so forth. A surgical endoscopy may also include an incision, repair, or excision. The farther the scope is passed into the body, the more complex the procedure—the code selected should reflect the farthest area of visualization. A diagnostic endoscopy is bundled into a surgical endoscopy and may not be billed separately.

Cardiovascular Subsection (Surgery Section)

The Cardiovascular System subsection is arranged by anatomic site. Procedures are listed after each site, starting with pericardiocentesis (33010). Pacemaker implantation is included with a table that lists the procedure (e.g., insert transvenous single lead only without pulse generator), the pacemaker code (33216), and the implantable defibrillator code (33216).

Other procedures include valvular procedures and *coronary artery bypass graft (CABG)*. The vascular system is included here with codes for arteries and veins including a Central Venous Access Procedures Table. However, all cardiovascular procedures are not located in this subsection. The Medicine section contains noninvasive studies of the heart, such as electrocardiogram, angiography, and cardiac catheterization. Coding of the cardiovascular system is thought to be one of the more challenging areas, even for an experienced coder.

The *Hemic and Lymphatic Systems* as well as the *Mediastinum and Diaphragm* are small subsections that follow this subsection.

Digestive Subsection (Surgery Section)

Codes are arranged in the Digestive System subsection by anatomic site, starting with the lips and mouth and continuing through the digestive tract according to the route food travels. Organs include the stomach, small intestines (duodenum, jejunum, ileum), large intestine (colon), and accessory organs (liver, pancreas, gallbladder). Endoscopic procedures are listed throughout this subsection and are coded according to the anatomic site examined. It is important to note the **surgical approach** used when the physician performs an abdominal procedure. The less invasive procedure, a *laparoscopy*, is performed by making a small incision in the abdominal wall. The laparoscope penetrates several layers of tissue and then enters the abdominal cavity. When a large incision is made, it is referred to as a *laparotomy*.

Urinary Subsection (Surgery Section)

Codes are arranged in the Urinary System subsection according to anatomic site—starting with the kidney and progressing to the ureter (the tube leading from the kidney to the bladder), then to the bladder (the sac that holds the urine), and ending at the urethra (the tube leading from the bladder to the outside). Major procedures include excision of these organs and renal (kidney) transplant. There are many endoscopic procedures listed which include:

- *Cystoscopy*—Visualization of the bladder
- *Cystourethroscopy*—Visualization of the urethra and bladder
- *Renal endoscopy*—Visualization of the kidney through a small incision
- *Ureteral endoscopy*—Visualization of the ureters through a small incision
- *Urethroscopy*—Visualization of the urethra

Urodynamic procedures (e.g., cystometrogram, voiding pressure studies, uroflowmetry) are used to measure how well the bladder holds urine and the rate at which urine moves out of the bladder. These are often performed in the physician's office and include all necessary supplies.

Male Genital Subsection (Surgery Section)

The Male Genital System subsection lists anatomic sites such as the penis, testis, scrotum, and prostate. Codes for lesion removal, such as condyloma and herpetic vesicle, are found in this subsection and should be used instead of codes located in the Integumentary System subsection. Methods of removal should be noted to find the correct code assignment (Example 16-13). *Reproductive System Procedures* and *Intersex Surgery* are separate subcategories following the Male Genital System subsection that have one and two codes, respectively.

EXAMPLE 16-13

Male Genital System: Destruction of Lesions

Diagnosis:	Penis, Lesions
54050	Destruction of lesion(s), penis, simple; chemical
54050	Electrodesiccation
54050	Cryosurgery
54050	Laser surgery
54050	Surgical excision

Female Genital Subsection (Surgery Section)

Many codes in the Female Genital System subsection are used in physicians' offices by family practitioners, general practitioners, and obstetric-gynecology (OB-GYN) specialists. Codes are arranged according to anatomic sites starting at the vulva (perineum/introitus) and continuing upward to the vagina, uterus (corpus uteri), oviduct (fallopian tubes), and ovary. The last category is In Vitro Fertilization. Some incision and drainage codes are included in this subsection (56405–56442), while notes refer you to the Integumentary System subsection for other specific types. As with the Male Genital System subsection, there are a few codes for destruction of lesions (57061, 57065) and there are also some endoscopic/laparoscopic procedures. Many procedures are bundled together and performed at the same operative session (Example 16-14), so it is important to read code descriptions carefully.

Another example of bundling is the code for vaginal delivery (59400). It includes routine obstetric care (i.e., antepartum care), vaginal delivery (with or without episiotomy, and/or forceps), and postpartum care.

The *Endocrine System* is a short subsection that follows and includes procedures on the thyroid, parathyroid, and thymus glands.

EXAMPLE 16-14

Bundled Hysterectomy Code

Code	Description
58150	Total abdominal hysterectomy (corpus and cervix), with or without removal of tube(s), with or without removal of ovary(s)

Included in code 58150 is any one of the following:

- Removal only of the uterus
- Removal of uterus and one or both tubes
- Removal of uterus and one or both ovaries
- Removal of uterus and one tube and one ovary
- Removal of uterus and both tubes and both ovaries

Note: A hysterectomy can also be performed vaginally (e.g., 58260) and laparoscopically (e.g., 58541) with many variances on what other organs are removed at the same time or procedures performed.

Nervous Subsection (Surgery Section)

Codes representing procedures on the brain and nerves (both autonomic and peripheral) are found in this subsection arranged according to the anatomic site. There are various methods used to open the skull (twist drill, burr hole, trephine, craniotomy) and there are codes to inject, drain, biopsy, or excise brain lesions as well as surgeries of the skull base. Injection procedures of the spine and spinal cord, as well as drainage, aspirations, and catheter implants (e.g., 62350), are listed with detailed descriptions.

Eye and Ocular Adnexa Subsection (Surgery Section)

Surgical codes of the eye and related visual structures are categorized in the Eye and Ocular Adnexa subsection. The eye is divided into anterior and posterior segments/chambers with all anatomic parts (e.g., cornea, iris, lens) subcategorized separately. Codes pertaining to various procedures (e.g., insertion, destruction, repair, removal) are found within these subcategories.

The *Auditory System* is a short subsection that follows the eye. It is divided into the External Ear, Middle Ear, Inner Ear, and Temporal Bone, Middle Fossa Approach. *Operating Microscope* is the last subsection of the surgery section with one add-on code (69990). It can be used with codes from any subsection in the surgery section. Be sure to read the coding notes because they list procedure codes where the operating microscope is an inclusive component of the procedure and is not to be coded separately.

Radiology Section

Diagnostic radiology, ultrasound, radiation oncology, and nuclear medicine are listed in the Radiology section but are coded separately. When coding x-rays, take into consideration the part of the body viewed, number of views, and type of view, such as AP (anteroposterior), Lat (lateral), Obl (oblique), and so on. Also note whether procedures are done with contrast, or without contrast (e.g., MRI, CT), and which side x-rays are taken so that an HCPCS II modifier can be added (i.e., right = RT and left = LT).

Pathology and Laboratory Section

A pathologist working in a hospital or freestanding laboratory will use codes from this section which are arranged according to tests performed. When the physician performs laboratory work in a *physician office laboratory* (POL), it is coded separately from office visits. Locate codes in subsections that describe the type of test (e.g., urinalysis, chemistry, hematology).

At the beginning of this section, you will find *test panels*. Various tests (e.g., calcium, chloride, glucose) are grouped together under a single code (e.g., basic metabolic panel). These are the most common tests done to investigate a specific disease or organ. If any single test named as part of the panel is not performed, report the codes to describe the individual tests performed, rather than the panel code. You cannot report two or more panel codes that include any of the same component tests. If other tests are performed that are not listed in the panel, they must be coded separately.

Read notes carefully because tests in this section may be performed on blood or urine (e.g., pregnancy test), and are either automated or performed manually (e.g., urine tests). A qualitative analysis, which determines the presence of an agent within the body, is much less time consuming and expensive to run than a quantitative analysis, which measures how much of the agent is within the body (e.g., drug tests). If the physician collects a specimen, such as a pap smear, biopsy, or throat culture, and sends it to an outside laboratory, assign code 99000 from the medicine section for collection and handling of a specimen. If the medical assistant performs a phlebotomy and obtains a blood sample, assign code 36415 (venipuncture) from the surgery section.

Medicine Section

The Medicine section includes a wide range of codes representing diagnostic and therapeutic services that are generally not surgically invasive. These codes may be used in conjunction with codes from all different sections of *CPT*. The *CPT* table of contents may be reviewed to determine various subsections (e.g., vaccines, toxoids, psychiatry, ophthalmology, and so forth). Examples of other codes found in this section have to do with cardiology testing, allergy testing, physical therapy modalities, chiropractic manipulative treatment, and sleep studies.

Injections are found in the Medicine section. The type of injection (therapeutic, prophylactic, diagnostic), as well as the route—IA (intra-arterial), IM (intramuscular), IV (intravenous), SC or SQ (subcutaneous), ID (intradermal), or parent (parenteral)—needs to be determined prior to code assignment. When documenting injections, record the name of the medication, the amount of substance to be injected in cubic centimeters or grams, the lot number from the bottle, and the route of administration. Each medically necessary injection can be billed separately, except when a single preparation exceeds the volume safely injected at a single site.

When coding injections, use one code for the *product* and one for the *administration*. These two types of codes are not always found in the same location. For instance, there are separate subsections for the vaccine codes (90476–90749) and the immunization administration for vaccines/toxoids (90460–90474). Refer to the *Resources* section at the end of this chapter for information on "Commonly Administered Pediatric Vaccines" with procedure and diagnostic codes found on the Internet.

The therapeutic, prophylactic, and diagnostic injection and infusion products are in another area and listed separately from the administration codes (e.g., 96372), which need to be billed with them. Note that injection codes may list more than one substance and some list patient age ranges (Example 16-15).

EXAMPLE 16-15

Coding Vaccine Injections

Code	Description
90707	Measles, mumps, and rubella virus vaccine, live, for subcutaneous use **(product code)**
90471	Immunization administration (includes percutaneous, intradermal, subcutaneous, or intramuscular injections); 1 vaccine (single or combination vaccine/toxoid) **(administration code)**

Near the end of this section is the *Special Services, Procedures and Reports* subsection. Under this category, miscellaneous services are listed; some have been mentioned earlier:

- *99000*—Handling and/or conveyance of specimen for transfer from office to a laboratory
- *99070*—Supplies and materials, provided by the physician or other qualified health care professional over and above those usually included with the office visit or other services rendered
- *99080*—Special reports such as insurance forms, more than the information conveyed in the usual medical communications or standard reporting form
- *99090*—Analysis of clinical data stored in computers

Code Modifiers

A modifier is used in addition to the procedure code to indicate circumstances in which a procedure as performed differs in some way from that described by the *CPT* five-digit code. In some billing scenarios, it is necessary to use two-digit modifiers to give a more accurate description of the services rendered. Use of modifiers prevents a physician's fee profile from being affected. Refer to Table 16-5 at the end of this section for a complete list of *CPT* modifiers, descriptions of when to use them, and examples. Modifiers may also be found in Appendix A of the *Current Procedural Terminology* codebook.

Add-On Codes

Certain five-digit *CPT* codes have been designed to be used with primary procedure codes, also referred to as *parent codes*. These **add-on codes** are indicated by a plus symbol (+) and cannot stand alone as separately reportable services. A complete list can be found in *CPT* Appendix D. Add-on code descriptions usually start with, "each additional," "list separately," or "second lesion" and may sometimes be used more than once. Before applying an add-on code, read the *CPT* notes following the parent code you wish to apply it to. There you will find the codes listed that are applicable. Refer to Example 16-16 for an illustration of add-on codes found in various sections in the *CPT* codebook.

EXAMPLE 16-16

Add-On Codes

Code	Description
11730	Avulsion of nail plate, partial or complete, simple; single (parent code)
+11732	each additional nail plate (add-on code)
15786	Abrasion; single lesion (parent code)
+15787	each additional 4 lesions or less (list separately in addition to code for primary procedure) (add-on code)
33533	Coronary artery bypass, using arterial graft(s); single arterial graft (parent code)
+33518	2 venous grafts (add-on code)
59510	Routine obstetric care including antepartum care, cesarean delivery, and postpartum care (parent code)
+59525	Subtotal or total hysterectomy after cesarean delivery (add-on code)

Codebook Appendices

The *CPT* codebook has appendices located after Category III codes and before the index. Following is a brief list of each appendix and what it includes for the 2017 edition of *CPT*:

- *Appendix A*—Complete list of modifiers with descriptions
- *Appendix B*—Summary of additions, deletions, and revisions
- *Appendix C*—Clinical examples for evaluation and management codes
- *Appendix D*—Summary of add-on codes
- *Appendix E*—Summary of codes exempt from modifier -51
- *Appendix F*—Summary of codes exempt from modifier -63
- *Appendix G*—Codes that include moderate (conscious) sedation
- *Appendix H*—Alphabetical clinical topics listing
- *Appendix I*—Genetic testing code modifiers
- *Appendix J*—Electrodiagnostic medicine listing of sensory, motor, and mixed nerves (with coding chart)
- *Appendix K*—Codes for products pending FDA approval
- *Appendix L*—Vascular family branches
- *Appendix M*—Crosswalk to deleted codes
- *Appendix N*—Summary of resequenced *CPT* codes
- *Appendix O*—Multianalyte assays with algorithmic analyses (with coding chart)
- *Appendix P*—Codes that may be used for synchronous telemedicine services

Unlisted Procedures

When a service is rendered and a code number cannot be found for the procedure, check Category III codes found after the medicine section. These are temporary codes and may be assigned, if available. If no Category III code is found, proceed to the end of the appropriate category, subsection, or section and locate a five-digit code for "unlisted procedures." Use this code with the description stating "unlisted" (see Example 16-17). Send in a report that details the nature and extent of the procedure and the supporting diagnosis.

EXAMPLE 16-17

Unlisted Services and Procedures

99499	Unlisted preventive medicine service (E/M section)
19499	Unlisted procedure, breast (integumentary subsection)

TABLE 16-5 **Current Procedural Terminology Modifier Codes**

Modifier Code	Brief Description, Explanation, and Example
-22	*Increased procedural services*
	Explanation: Use when work required to provide a service is substantially greater than typically required; attach documentation. Use cautiously; it increases payment.
	Example: Removal of foreign body from stomach, which was expected to take about 45 minutes, took 2 hours due to an internal genetic malformation. Append modifier -22 to surgical code.
-23	*Unusual anesthesia*
	Explanation: Occasionally, because of an unusual situation, a procedure that does not require anesthesia will require general anesthesia.
	Example: A proctoscopy usually requires no anesthesia; however, the patient recently experienced a violent rape attack and the physician decided to use general anesthesia for the examination **(46614–23)**.
-24	*Unrelated evaluation and management service by the same physician or other qualified health care professional during a postoperative period*
	Explanation: Use when the patient requires the service of the physician for the treatment of an unrelated condition during the postoperative period.
	Example: A patient seen for a postoperative visit after an appendectomy complains of a lump on her leg. The physician takes a history and examines the site, and a biopsy is scheduled. The appropriate E/M code is used for the unrelated postsurgery examination and the modifier is added for unrelated service rendered during a postoperative period **(99213–24)**.

(continues)

TABLE 16-5 **Current Procedural Terminology Modifier Codes** *(continued)*

Modifier Code	Brief Description, Explanation, and Example
-25	*Significant, separately identifiable evaluation and management service by the same physician or other qualified health professional on the day of a procedure or other service*
	Explanation: Use when a patient is in the office for a minor procedure and requires an E/M service above and beyond that normally provided.
	Example A: Patient is seen for a diabetic follow-up and the physician discovers a suspicious mole on the patient's neck (0.4 cm), which is removed. The physician makes an adjustment of the oral diabetes medication and goes over the patient's diet and exercise program.
	99213–25 Significant E/M service
	11420 Removal of the benign lesion
	Example B: Patient is seen for a PT/INR lab test and complains of increased appetite, change in diet, and weight gain. The patient takes 4 mg Coumadin 7 days a week and has not changed any medication. The medical assistant takes the patient's vital signs and performs a finger stick for prothrombin time; the results are documented. The MA discusses an exercise program and encourages the patient to eat more fruits and vegetables. The patient is aware to continue the same dosage of Coumadin and repeat the PT in 4 weeks.
	85610 **PT/INR**
	36416 **Finger stick**
	99211-25 **E/M service for separately identifiable/significant nurse visit**
	Note: This modifier is not used to report an E/M service that resulted in a decision to perform major surgery. See modifier -57.
-26	*Professional component*
	Explanation: The professional component comprises only the professional services performed by the physician during radiologic, laboratory, and other diagnostic procedures. These services include a portion of a test or procedure that the physician does, such as interpretation of the results. The technical component includes personnel, materials, and equipment (excludes the cost of radioisotopes). When billing for the technical component, check with the insurance carrier to see if modifier -TC is required.
	Example:
	70450-26 Computerized axial tomography, head or brain; without contrast material (physician interpreted this test only)
	70450-TC Computerized axial tomography, head or brain; without contrast material (facility is billing only for the use of the equipment, and technician)
-32	*Mandated services*
	Explanation: Service, such as a consult, required by insurance carrier, government, or regulatory agency.
	Example: A patient is referred to the physician by an insurance company for an unbiased opinion regarding permanent disability after a year of treatment following an accident. Clearly document who requested the service and why, then add modifier -32 to the E/M code **(99244-32)**.
-33	*Preventive services*
	Explanation: This modifier allows the provider to report a service as preventive that is not already listed as "preventive" in *CPT* to indicate that no cost-sharing has been collected (e.g., deductible, copay); a mandate of the Patient Protection and Affordable Care Act.
	Example: Screening colonoscopy that leads to a polypectomy.
	45378 Screening colonoscopy
	45383-33 Polypectomy (no cost-share required)

(continues)

TABLE 16-5 Current Procedural Terminology Modifier Codes *(continued)*

Modifier Code	Brief Description, Explanation, and Example
-47	*Anesthesia by surgeon* **Explanation:** Surgeon provides and administers anesthesia other than local; do not use for anesthesia procedures 00100 through 01999. **Example:** A gastroenterologist performs an endoscopy for removal of esophageal polyps using the snare technique. The physician needs to use general anesthesia because the patient does not tolerate moderate sedation; append to surgical code **(43217-47)**.
-50	*Bilateral procedure* **Explanation:** Used if procedure is not defined as bilateral. It is important to read each surgical description carefully to look for the words "one, both, or bilateral." **Example A:** **73080-50** Radiologic examination, elbow, complete, minimum of three views (x-ray was performed on both elbows) **Example B:** **19305-50** Mastectomy, radical (bilateral procedure)
-51	*Multiple procedures* **Explanation:** This modifier indicates the same physician performed multiple procedures and is exempt from certain procedures (see *CPT* Appendix E) and should not be appended to designated "add-on" codes (see *CPT* Appendix D). Always list the procedure of highest dollar value first. **Example A:** Patient had a herniated disk in the lower back with stabilization of the area where the disk was removed. **63030** Laminectomy with disk removal; 1 interspace, lumbar **22612-51** Arthrodesis; lumbar (modifier used after the lesser of the two procedures) **Example B:** Patient had removal of a malignant skin lesion on the trunk (0.5 cm). A layered closure of the wound is performed at the same time. **12031** Repair, intermediate, wounds of . . . trunk; 2.5 cm or less **11600-51** Excision, malignant lesion . . . excised diameter 0.5 cm or less
-52	*Reduced services* **Explanation:** Medicare requires an operative report and a statement as to how the reduced service is different from the standard procedure. **Example:** The provider orders an x-ray of the right wrist, but only requests one view. **73100-52** Radiologic examination, wrist; two views (reduced service)
-53	*Discontinued procedure* **Explanation:** This modifier is not used to report the elective cancellation of a procedure before the patient's anesthesia induction and/or surgical preparation in the operating suite; send an operative report and statement as to how much of the original procedure was accomplished. **Example:** At 5:30 a.m., a patient arrives at the hospital for a laparoscopic cholecystectomy, which is scheduled for 8:00 a.m. He registers and is escorted to a pre-op room where he undresses and the nurse takes his vital signs. The anesthesiologist visits him and fills out a questionnaire. Around 7:30 a.m., he is being transferred to the operative suite where he will receive anesthesia prior to the surgery, when an earthquake of great magnitude occurs and the electricity is shut off. The backup generator comes on and electricity is restored; however, because of the disarray in the operative suite, the physician decides to discontinue the surgery **(47562-53)**.

(continues)

TABLE 16-5 **Current Procedural Terminology Modifier Codes** (continued)

Modifier Code	Brief Description, Explanation, and Example
-54	*Surgical care only* **Explanation:** Physician provides surgical care only; other physicians provide pre- and postoperative care. Use of modifiers -54 and -55 apply when physicians agree on the transfer of care during a global period. **Example:** A patient presents in the emergency department with severe abdominal pain. Dr. A, the on-call surgeon, examines the patient and performs an emergency appendectomy. Dr. A is leaving on vacation the next morning, so he calls his friend and colleague, Dr. B. He asks him to visit the patient in the hospital the following day and take over the postoperative care. Dr. A bills using the appendectomy procedure code modifier **(44950-54)**.
-55	*Postoperative management only* **Explanation:** Physician provides postoperative care only. The fee would be approximately 30% of the surgeon's fee. **Example:** The Dunmires are relocating to Memphis, Tennessee, when she discovers a lump on her arm. She visits her family physician, Dr. A, who tells her it needs to be excised. She wants her physician (Dr. A) to do the surgery and he agrees if she promises to arrange for a physician in Memphis to follow her postoperatively. She makes arrangements with Dr. B in Memphis. Dr. B bills using the excision code that he obtained from Dr. A and modifies it with -55.
-56	*Preoperative management only* **Explanation:** Physician provides preoperative care only. **Example:** Dr. A performs a detailed history and physical examination on Mrs. Jones and determines she needs to have a lung biopsy. He admits her to the hospital and becomes ill. Dr. B is called in and performs the surgery. Dr. A bills for the preoperative care using the surgical code he obtained from Dr. B and modifies it with -56.
-57	*Decision for surgery* **Explanation:** Use this modifier only if the E/M service occurs within 24 hours of major surgery. **Example:** A patient is referred to a surgeon for a consultation to determine whether surgery is necessary. The patient consents to surgery for the following day. The surgeon bills the E/M consultation code and adds modifier -57. By adding this modifier, the third-party payer is informed that the consultation is not part of the global surgical procedure **(99245-57)**.
-58	*Staged or related procedure or service by the same physician or other qualified health care professional during the postoperative period* **Explanation:** Use when another service/procedure is: • planned or anticipated • more extensive than the original procedure • therapy following a surgical procedure **Example:** The physician removed a breast tumor and billed for the excision. It was determined that a mastectomy was necessary so the following week the entire breast was removed. Note: Another postoperative period began when the second procedure took place. **19120** Excision of cyst, fibroadenoma, or other benign or malignant tumor . . . **19307-58** Mastectomy, modified radical. . .
-59	*Distinct procedural service* **Explanation:** Used to indicate a: • Different session or encounter • Different procedure or surgery • Different site or organ • Separate incision, excision, lesion, injury, or body part

(continues)

TABLE 16-5 Current Procedural Terminology Modifier Codes *(continued)*

Modifier Code	Brief Description, Explanation, and Example
	Note: Several HCPCS Level II codes are used by Medicare to define subsets of Modifier -59 (see -XE, -XP, -XS, and -XU) **Example:** The patient is scheduled for a hysterectomy. She asks the physician if he will remove a lipoma (2.2 cm) from the right upper thigh area while she is under anesthesia. The surgeon bills for the hysterectomy and for the lipoma with a modifier. **58150** Total abdominal hysterectomy **11403-59** Excision benign lesion . . . legs; excised diameter 0.5 or less
-62	*Two surgeons* **Explanation:** Used when two surgeons work together as primary surgeons performing distinct parts of a procedure. If the co-surgeon acts as an assistant in the performance of additional procedure(s) during the same surgical session, those services may be reported using separate procedure code(s) with modifier -80 or -81. **Example:** An 8-hour procedure for scoliosis is performed by a thoracic surgeon who does the anterior approach and monitors the patient's heart and lungs. An orthopedic surgeon does the posterior approach and repair. Each surgeon bills his or her portion of the surgery with modifier -62.
-63	*Procedure performed on infants less than 4 kg* **Explanation:** Unless otherwise designated, this modifier may only be appended to procedures/services listed in the 20005–69990 code series. Modifier -63 should not be appended to any *CPT* codes listed in the Evaluation and Management, Anesthesia, Radiology, Pathology and Laboratory, or Medicine sections. **Example:** A premature neonate has heart surgery for tetralogy of Fallot **(33692-66)**.
-66	*Surgical team* **Explanation:** Use when a team of surgeons is required for complicated surgery. **Example:** A kidney transplant requires a vascular surgeon, urologist, and nephrologist. Each surgeon bills using the modifier -66.
-76	*Repeat procedure by same physician or other qualified health care professional* **Explanation:** Used to indicate a service or procedure was repeated. Do not use modifier -76 with an E/M service. **Example:** A femoral-popliteal bypass graft is performed, the graft clots later that day, and the entire procedure is repeated. The original procedure is reported, and the repeat procedure is reported using the same code with modifier -76. A report should be attached to the insurance claim when using this modifier. 35556 Initial procedure for bypass graft reported 35556-76 Repeat procedure reported with modifier
-77	*Repeat procedure by another physician or other qualified health care professional* **Explanation:** Similar to modifier -76, a second procedure is required, but done by a different physician. Do not use modifier -77 with an E/M service. **Example:** A femoral-popliteal graft is performed in the morning by Surgeon A and in the afternoon it becomes clotted. The original surgeon is not available and Surgeon B performs the repeat operation later in the day. **35556** Bypass graft, with vein; femoral-popliteal (performed by original Surgeon A) **35556-77** Bypass graft, with vein; femoral-popliteal (performed by second Surgeon B with modifier)

(continues)

TABLE 16-5 Current Procedural Terminology Modifier Codes *(continued)*

Modifier Code	Brief Description, Explanation, and Example
-78	*Unplanned return to the operating/procedure room by the same physician or other qualified health care professional following initial procedure for a related procedure during the postoperative period* **Explanation:** Return trip to the operating room for same or related procedure, usually due to complications. **Example:** A patient has an open reduction with fixation of a fractured elbow. It appears that the pin has caused an allergic reaction because while still hospitalized the patient develops an infection. The patient is returned to surgery for removal of the pin. **24635** Open treatment of Monteggia type of fracture dislocation at elbow, includes internal fixation **20680-78** Removal of implant; deep (e.g., pin) (procedure performed during the postoperative period)
-79	*Unrelated procedure or service by the same physician or other qualified health care provider during the postoperative period* **Explanation:** Typically, the patient undergoes a primary procedure, then during the postoperative period has an unrelated procedure performed. **Example:** A patient in the hospital has colon resection surgery and is discharged home. After 7 days, the patient develops acute renal failure, is hospitalized, and does not recover renal function. Hemodialysis is ordered. A nephrologist inserts a cannula for the dialysis. When billing for the nephrologist, the code for hemodialysis is shown with a -79 modifier indicating that this is unrelated to the initial surgery.
-80	*Assistant surgeon* **Explanation:** Complex operative procedures require an assistant surgeon who is a medical doctor to help the primary surgeon. Some insurance policies do not include payment for assistant surgeons, such as for 1-day surgery, but do pay for major or complex surgical assistance. Medicare will not pay assistant surgeons for operations that are not "life threatening." Therefore, Medigap would also consider this service nonallowable. Assisting surgeons usually charge 16% to 30% of the primary surgeon's fee. **Example:** The primary surgeon performs a right ureterectomy with the help of an assistant surgeon. **50650-RT** Ureterectomy, with bladder cuff—right side (primary surgeon) **50650-RT-80** Ureterectomy, with bladder cuff—right side (assistant surgeon)
-81	*Minimum assistant surgeon* **Explanation:** Payment for this modifier is made to physicians but not registered nurses or technicians who assist during surgery. **Example:** A primary surgeon plans to perform a surgical procedure, but during the operation circumstances arise that require the services of an assistant surgeon for a relatively short period of time. In this scenario, the second surgeon provides minimal assistance and may report using the procedure code with -81 modifier appended.
-82	*Assistant surgeon (when qualified resident surgeon is not available.)* **Explanation:** This modifier is used for procedures rendered at a teaching hospital. **Example:** A resident surgeon is scheduled to assist with an anorectal myomectomy. Surgery is delayed due to the previous surgery, the shift rotation changes, and the resident (nor any other resident) is not available. A nonresident assists with the surgery and reports the surgeon's procedure code appending it with modifier -82. **45108-82** Anorectal myomectomy (nonresident assistant surgeon)
-90	*Reference (outside) laboratory* **Explanation:** Use this modifier when the physician bills the patient for the outside laboratory work and the laboratory is not doing its own billing. **Example:** Dr. Input examines the patient, performs venipuncture, and sends the specimen to an outside laboratory for a lipid panel. The physician has an arrangement with the laboratory to bill for the test, and, in turn, he bills the patient for all three services. **99203** E/M services **36415** Venipuncture **80061-90** Lipid panel

(continues)

TABLE 16-5 **Current Procedural Terminology Modifier Codes** *(continued)*

Modifier Code	Brief Description, Explanation, and Example
-91	*Repeat clinical diagnostic laboratory test* **Explanation:** This modifier may not be used when tests are rerun to confirm initial results; due to testing problems with specimens or equipment; or for any other reason when a normal, one-time, reportable result is all that is required. This modifier may not be used when other code(s) describe a series of test results (e.g., glucose tolerance tests, evocative/suppression testing). This modifier may only be used for laboratory test(s) performed more than once on the same day on the same patient. **Example:** A patient is scheduled for a nonobstetrical dilation and curettage for dysfunctional uterine bleeding. When the patient arrives at the office, a routine hematocrit is obtained. During the procedure, the patient bleeds excessively. After the procedure, the physician orders a second hematocrit to check the patient for anemia due to blood loss. **85014** Hematocrit (initial) **85041-91** Hematocrit (second, follow-up test)
-92	*Alternative laboratory platform testing* **Explanation:** Used for tests performed using a kit or transportable instrument. **Example:** HIV testing for antibodies **(codes 86701–86703).**
-95	*Synchronous telemedicine service rendered via real-time interactive audio and video telecommunications system* **Explanation:** Used when a real-time interaction takes place between a physician or other qualified health care provider and a patient who is located at a distant site, which meets the same key components of the same service when rendered face-to-face (see Appendix P for codes used for telemedicine services). **Example:** A patient located on St. Lawrence Island has a deep untreated wound on his lower right leg which appears to be infected and needs debridement. A nurse contacts the physician in Anchorage Alaska and uses both audio and video to access the situation.
-99	*Multiple ,odifiers* **Explanation:** Two or more modifiers may be necessary to delineate a service completely. **Example:** See Example 16-18.

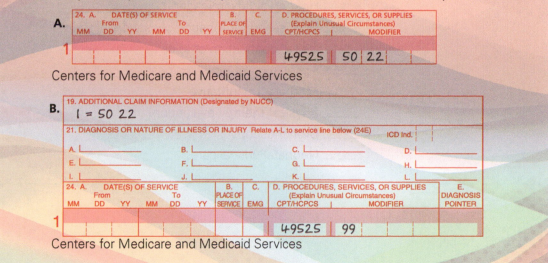

EXAMPLE 16-18

Multiple Modifiers

The patient is grossly obese, and the operative report states that a bilateral sliding-type inguinal herniorrhaphy was performed. The procedure took 3 hours, 15 minutes to perform.

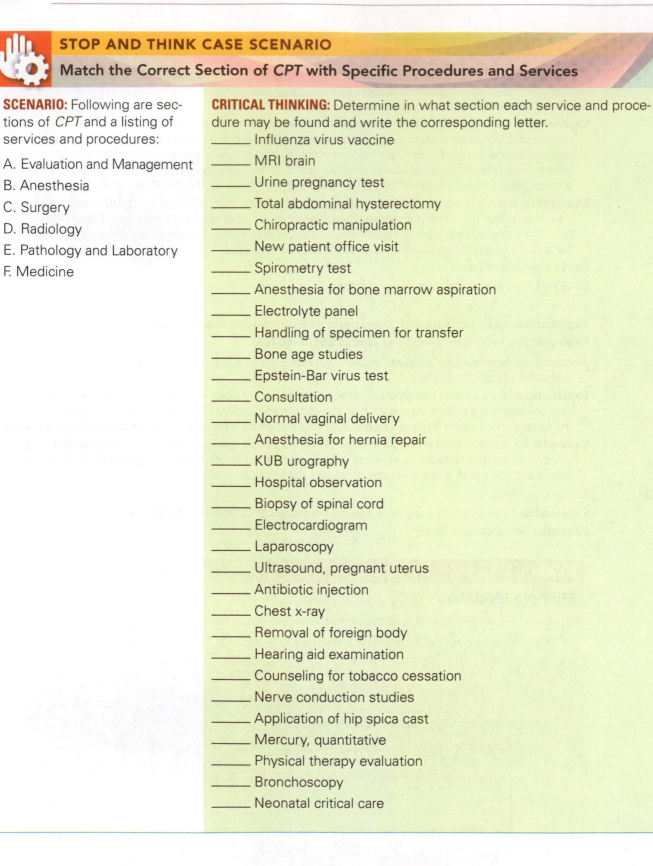

STOP AND THINK CASE SCENARIO

Match the Correct Section of *CPT* with Specific Procedures and Services

SCENARIO: Following are sections of *CPT* and a listing of services and procedures:

A. Evaluation and Management
B. Anesthesia
C. Surgery
D. Radiology
E. Pathology and Laboratory
F. Medicine

CRITICAL THINKING: Determine in what section each service and procedure may be found and write the corresponding letter.

_____ Influenza virus vaccine

_____ MRI brain

_____ Urine pregnancy test

_____ Total abdominal hysterectomy

_____ Chiropractic manipulation

_____ New patient office visit

_____ Spirometry test

_____ Anesthesia for bone marrow aspiration

_____ Electrolyte panel

_____ Handling of specimen for transfer

_____ Bone age studies

_____ Epstein-Bar virus test

_____ Consultation

_____ Normal vaginal delivery

_____ Anesthesia for hernia repair

_____ KUB urography

_____ Hospital observation

_____ Biopsy of spinal cord

_____ Electrocardiogram

_____ Laparoscopy

_____ Ultrasound, pregnant uterus

_____ Antibiotic injection

_____ Chest x-ray

_____ Removal of foreign body

_____ Hearing aid examination

_____ Counseling for tobacco cessation

_____ Nerve conduction studies

_____ Application of hip spica cast

_____ Mercury, quantitative

_____ Physical therapy evaluation

_____ Bronchoscopy

_____ Neonatal critical care

STOP AND THINK CASE SCENARIO
Determine Where to Look for Codes

SCENARIO: A 28-year-old male sustained an acute injury to his right knee while playing tennis. The physician examined his leg and took right knee x-rays, which were negative for a fracture or bone disease. He has no history of knee problems. His knee is extremely painful and swollen, so the doctor applied a long-leg immobilizer and asked him to return in 1 week.

CRITICAL THINKING: What codebooks would you use to code for the services the doctor performed?

a. _____

b. _____

To code for the professional services, where in the codebook(s) would you look? List each procedure or service and approximate section of the codebook(s).

a. _____

b. _____

c. _____

FOCUS ON CERTIFICATION*

CMA (AAMA) Content Summary

- *Current Procedural Terminology (CPT)* coding system
- Modifiers
- Upcoding
- Bundling charges
- *Healthcare Financing Common Procedural Coding System (HCPCS Level II)*
- Diagnostic and surgical procedures

RMA (AMT) Content Summary

- Laws, regulations, and acts pertaining to the practice of medicine

- Identify HIPAA-mandated coding systems and references
- *ICD-10-CM*
- *CPT*
- *HCPCS*

CMAS (AMT) Content Summary

- Understand procedure codes
- Employ *Current Procedural Terminology (CPT)* and Evaluation and Management codes appropriately
- Employ *Healthcare Financing Administration Common Procedure Coding System (HCPCS)* codes appropriately

REVIEW EXAM-STYLE QUESTIONS

1. A coding compliance program is:
   a. mandated by HIPAA
   b. mandated by OSHA
   c. mandated by both HIPAA and OSHA
   d. part of Health Care Reform
   e. voluntary

2. The standard code set:
   a. is mandated by HIPAA
   b. includes codes found in *CPT*
   c. includes codes found in *HCPCS Level II*
   d. includes codes found in *ICD-10-CM*
   e. all of the above are correct

---

* *This* textbook *and the accompanying* Workbook *meet the entry-level administrative and general competencies for the CMA outlined by the AAMA Examination Content Outline and Occupational Analysis and for the RMA and CMAS outlined by the AMT Competencies, Construction Parameters, and Examination Specifications (see Competency Grids in Appendix B).*

3. *CPT* codes are revised each:
   a   January
   b.   March
   c.   July
   d.   October
   e.   December

4. CAC natural language processing software uses:
   a.   point-and-click fields
   b.   pull-down menus
   c.   structured templates
   d.   artificial intelligence technology
   e.   all of the above are correct

5. Care of an unstable, acutely ill, or injured patient requiring constant bedside attention by a physician is referred to as:
   a.   emergency care
   b.   critical care
   c   concurrent care
   d.   advanced life support
   e   mental health care

6. The "three Rs" to remember when coding consultation services are:
   a.   request, review, and respond
   b.   review, recite, and recommend
   c.   request, record, and report
   d.   review, revise, and report
   e.   request, record, and recommend

7. Consultation codes are no longer used by:
   a.   private insurance carriers
   b.   Medicare
   c.   Medicaid
   d.   workers' compensation
   e.   Blue Cross/Blue Shield

8. How many sections are there in *Current Procedural Terminology*?
   a.   3
   b.   5
   c.   6
   d.   8
   e.   10

9. When coding Evaluation and Management services, first determine:
   a.   past history, family history, social history
   b.   place of service, type of service, patient status
   c.   history, physical examination, medical decision making

d.   counseling, coordination of care, nature of presenting problem
   e.   time, counseling, diagnosis

10. Three key components needed to code evaluation and management services are:
    a.   past history, family history, social history
    b.   place of service, type of service, patient status
    c.   history, physical examination, medical decision making
    d.   counseling, coordination of care, nature of presenting problem
    e.   time, counseling, diagnosis

11. When coding from the surgery section of *CPT*, the first thing you should do is:
    a.   start at the beginning
    b.   go to the index
    c.   go to the table of contents
    d.   go to the appendices
    e.   determine the section the procedure or service is in

12. According to *CPT*, a surgical package:
    a.   applies only to major procedures with a 90-day follow-up
    b.   applies only to minor procedures with a 30-day follow-up
    c.   applies to hospital surgeries only
    d.   includes the operation, certain types of anesthesia, and normal uncomplicated postoperative care within designated follow-up days
    e.   includes all pre- and postoperative visits, surgery, and follow-up days

13. The sums of multiple laceration repairs can be added together if:
    a.   they are in the same body area, as defined in *CPT*
    b.   they are the same "type" of wound
    c.   they are under 1 cm
    d.   they can never be added; each repair has to be reported separately
    e.   both a and b

14. In *CPT*, descriptions for "indented codes" always relate back to the:
    a.   master code
    b.   primary code
    c.   parent code
    d.   main code
    e.   principal code

15. Starting at the beginning of the following subsections in the Surgery section (Musculoskeletal, Respiratory, Cardiovascular, Digestive, and Urinary), codes are arranged by:
    a. type of procedure
    b. anatomic site
    c. complexity
    d. surgical approach
    e. alphabetical listing

WORKBOOK ASSIGNMENT

To develop competency-based job skills, refer to the *Workbook* and complete the:
- Abbreviation and Spelling Review
- Review Questions

- Critical Thinking Exercises
- Job Skill activities, which are listed at the beginning of the chapter under *Performance Objectives in the Workbook.*

RESOURCES

Codebooks and Resources

American Academy of Professional Coders
    Search: *Current Procedural Terminology* Resources
3-2-1 Code It, 4th edition
    Green, Michelle
    Cengage Learning, 2014
    Website: http://www.cengagebrain.com
2015 Coding Workbook for the Physician's Office
    Covell, Alice
    Cengage Learning, 2016
    Website: http://www.cengagebrain.com
Coding Surgical Procedures: Beyond the Basics
    Smith, Gail
    Cengage Learning, 2011
    Website: http://www.cengagebrain.com
Current Procedural Coding Expert, 1st edition
    Optum, 2015
    Website: http://www.cengagebrain.com
Current Procedural Terminology (CPT)
    American Medical Association (published annually)
Health Care Financing Administration Common Procedure Coding System (HCPCS) National Level II Codes
- American Medical Association
- Optum
- Practice Management Information Corporation (PMIC)
- Wasserman Medical Publishers, Limited

Optum Learning: Understanding E/M Coding, 1st edition
    Optum, 2015
    Website: http://www.cengagebrain.com
Procedure Coding and Reimbursement for the Physician Services: Applying CPT and HCPCS
    Kuehn, Lynn
    American Health Information Management, 2014
Understanding Health Insurance: A Guide to Billing and Reimbursement, 12th edition
    Green/Rowell
    Cengage Learning, 2015
    Website: http://www.cengagebrain.com
Understanding Medical Coding: A Comprehensive Guide, 3rd edition
    Johnson, Sandra
    Cengage Learning, 2013
    Website: http://www.cengagebrain.com
Understanding Procedural Coding: A Worktext, 2nd edition
    Bowie, Mary Jo
    Cengage Learning, 2015
    Website: http://www.cengagebrain.com

Coding and Billing Questions

Part B News
    Subscribe to listserv, ask questions, and communicate with insurance billers via email

Coding Guidelines

National Correct Coding Initiative (NCCI) Edits

Centers for Medicare and Medicaid Services (CMS)

Search: NCCI Edits

Internet

Commonly Administered Pediatric Vaccines/Toxoids

American Academy of Pediatrics

Vaccine *CPT* code, name, manufacturer, brand name, diagnostic code

Search: Commonly administered pediatric vaccines

Medical Dictionaries

- *Fordney's Medical Insurance Dictionary for Billers and Coders*

Fordney, Marilyn

Saunders/Elsevier

- *Merriam-Webster*

Medical Encyclopedia

Atlas of the Human Body

American Medical Association

Transaction and Code Set Standards

Rules and information for electronic claim submission

Search: CMS—Electronic billing

Surgical/Global Package Books

- *Correct Coder for Unbundling Book*

Wasserman Medical Publishers, LTD, 2015

- *Global Surgery Fact Sheet*

Medicare Learning Network

Media

Critical Thinking for Medical Assistants, 1st edition

Online Video Series—Program 5

Insurance and Coding: Individual access

Delmar Learning, 2005

ISBN13: 978-1-4354-0182-2

DIAGNOSTIC CODING

LEARNING OBJECTIVES

After reading this chapter and learning step-by-step procedures to gain job skills,* you should be able to:

- Name the codebook used to code diagnostic services.
- Discuss the history and development of diagnostic coding.
- Compare *ICD-9-CM* to *ICD-10-CM* and state changes and advantages of the new system.
- Describe the format and organization of the *ICD-10-CM* codebook.
- Explain principal and primary diagnoses.
- Define a qualified diagnosis.
- Understand codebook terms, abbreviations, and punctuation used in *ICD-10-CM*.
- List coding steps used to locate codes in the Alphabetic Index (Volume II) of *ICD-10-CM*.
- List coding steps used to verify codes in the Tabular List (Volume I) of *ICD-10-CM*.
- Follow coding guidelines and apply general and chapter-specific rules to code diagnoses using *ICD-10-CM*.

PERFORMANCE OBJECTIVES (PROCEDURES) IN THIS TEXTBOOK

- Select correct diagnostic codes using *ICD-10-CM* (Procedure 17-1).
- Select burn and corrosion codes (Procedure 17-2).
- Select diagnostic codes from the Table of Drugs and Chemicals (Procedure 17-3)

PERFORMANCE OBJECTIVES (JOB SKILLS) IN THE WORKBOOK

- Code diagnoses from Chapters 1, 2, 3, 4, and 5 in *ICD-10-CM* (Job Skill 17-1).
- Code diagnoses from Chapters 6, 7, 8, 9, and 10 in *ICD-10-CM* (Job Skill 17-2).
- Code diagnoses from Chapters 11, 12, 13, 14, and 15 in *ICD-10-CM* (Job Skill 17-3).
- Code diagnoses from Chapters 16, 17, 18, 19, and 20 in *ICD-10-CM* (Job Skill 17-4).
- Code diagnoses from Chapter 21 and the Table of Drugs and Chemicals in *ICD-10-CM* (Job Skill 17-5).
- Code diagnoses from chart notes using *ICD-10-CM* (Job Skill 17-6).

---

* *This* textbook *and the accompanying* Workbook *meet the educational components for entry-level administrative and general competencies outlined by CAAHEP and ABHES.*

KEY TERMS

benign	malignant	principal diagnosis
code linkage	morbidity	qualified diagnoses
combination code	mortality	remote coder
comorbidity	neoplasm	scribe
etiology/manifestation	placeholder	
first-listed condition	primary diagnosis	

HEART OF THE HEALTH CARE PROFESSIONAL

Service

Diagnostic codes are input into a nationwide central computer database, which is accessed by all insurance companies and used to make policy decisions. Codes are also used for international statistical reporting. Precise coding ensures that each patient's condition is reported correctly; therefore, insurance records and statistics are accurate. The average person may not know that by reporting diagnoses correctly you are serving them and an important worldwide need.

DIAGNOSTIC CODING USING *ICD-10-CM*

After the medical assistant has learned procedure coding rules and experienced how to code basic procedures, the next step is to learn how to code diagnoses.

Diagnostic Coding History

In 1893, the French physician Jacques Bertillon introduced a Classification of Causes of Death at the International Statistical Institute in Chicago. It was recommended for adoption by the United States and other countries, with revisions every 10 years. The following revisions contained minor changes until the 6th revision, published in 1949, which was followed by the 7th revision in 1958, the 8th revision in 1968, and the 9th revision in 1979. The book was originally adopted to classify diseases and health conditions using numerical codes, and to report morbidity and mortality rates—it was never designed as part of a reimbursement system; gradually, it began to be used for such purposes.

Although the *World Health Organization (WHO)* began work on *ICD-10* in 1983, it was not completed until 1992. *ICD-10* was implemented outside of the United States long before the *clinical modification (ICD-10-CM)* prerelease version became available, around the year 2000. It is easy to understand how a system that has been around so long had become obsolete; it could not keep up with the clinical or technical changes, nor offer accurate reporting to other nations. In 2003, the prerelease draft was posted on the Internet, and pilot tests were conducted to move toward implementation in the United States.

COMPLIANCE

ICD-10-CM Implementation Date

October 1, 2015 was the implementation compliance date of *ICD-10-CM* code set to report diagnoses for all HIPAA-covered entities, including large and small health care providers. The Department of Health and Human Services concluded that, "It would be in the health care industry's best interest if all entities were to comply with the *ICD-10-CM/PCS* code set standards at the same time to ensure the accuracy and timeliness of claims and transaction processing."

Entities that are not covered under HIPAA, such as auto insurance companies and workers' compensation carriers, do not have to adopt the new coding system—they can continue using *ICD-9-CM*. However, coding updates for the *ICD-9-CM* coding system have been discontinued as of October 1, 2014 and that system is longer maintained. Since it is in the best interest of all carriers to implement *ICD-10-CM*, both property and casualty carriers and workers' compensation insurance carriers plan to utilize *ICD-10-CM* regardless of state mandates. Regular updates to *ICD-10-CM* will be made annually.

ICD-9-CM versus ICD-10-CM: Comparisons and Advantages

The number of codes represented in *ICD-9-CM* is approximately 13,600 compared to 69,000 in *ICD-10-CM*.* This comparison makes it easy to see the benefits of the new system—over 55,000 additional codes represent many more diseases and conditions physicians need to report. The new coding system also has room for expansion, and codes are better grouped with more complete descriptions (e.g., laterality; left, right, bilateral), updated terminology, and additional notes to guide the coder. There is a reduced need for attachments to explain the patient's condition because the coder will be able to substantiate the medical necessity of diagnostic and therapeutic services using the physician's documentation. Also, research studies, and clinical trials, as well as financial and administrative performance, will be improved. View Example 17-1 for a brief look at the differences between *ICD-9-CM* and *ICD-10-CM*.

A variety of *crosswalks* that guide the coder from *ICD-9-CM* codes to *ICD-10-CM* codes were developed during the transition period. A *General Equivalence Mapping (GEM)* system, designed by the National Center for Health Statistics and further developed by the Centers for Medicare and Medicaid Services

COMPLIANCE
Codified Diagnostic Data

Codified diagnostic data will impact clinical outcome measurements; consistent health care delivery; and the tracking of medical errors, *morbidity* (diseased conditions), *comorbidity* (coexisting medical conditions), and *mortality* (deaths in a population).

(CMS), is available on the CMS website (see the *Resources* section at the end of this chapter). Caution must be used when relying on mapping systems because they do not consider medical record information and some do not include code descriptions; there may be more than one code in *ICD-10-CM* that maps to *ICD-9-CM*.

THE *ICD-10-CM* CODEBOOK

The *International Classification of Diseases, 10th Revision, Clinical Modification (ICD-10-CM)*, Volumes 1 and 2 are used to code diagnoses in outpatient settings. See the *Resources* section at the end of this chapter for information on where to obtain this codebook. The diagnosis is determined by the health care professional providing medical care. It can be found in a variety of sources in the medical record, such as the clinical progress notes, laboratory tests, radiologic results, and so forth.

Volume 3, the *Procedure Coding System (PCS)*, is used to code procedures in the hospital setting. Psychiatric disorders are coded using the *Diagnostic and Statistical Manual of Mental Disorders*, Fourth Edition (DSM IV),** which is not discussed in this text.

The Encounter Form

In a paper-based system, most diagnoses are written or checked-off on an encounter form, then coded if necessary and entered into a computer system (see Figure 13-4 in Chapter 13). The average superbill is 8 ½" × 11" (front and back). This translates into 20 pages using *ICD-10-CM* codes, so space becomes an issue.

EXAMPLE 17-1

ICD-9-CM versus ICD-10-CM

ITEMS	ICD-9-CM	ICD-10-CM
No. of codes	13,600	69,000
Format	3–5 digits	3–7 alphanumeric
Level of detail	Minimal	Extensive
Specificity	Limited	Extensive
Laterality	Lacking	Present
Placeholders	None	Uses x when necessary as 4th, 5th, or 6th digit
New code additions	Limited	Extensive
Interoperability	U.S. only	United States & most countries internationally

---

*American Academy of Professional Coders. Other sources have estimated that there are up to 80,000 codes in *ICD-10-CM*, Volumes 1 and 2; 155,000 total including Volume 3.

**American Psychiatric Press, Inc., Washington, D.C.

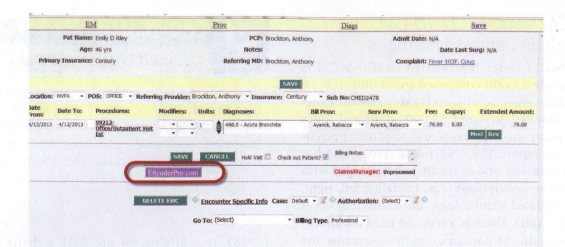

FIGURE 17-1 Electronic Medical Record (EMR) software showing EncoderPro Button used to select diagnostic codes

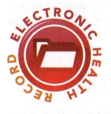

When using an electronic medical record (EHR) system, a paperless encounter form can be customized to save time and space. Start with a list of the most frequently used diagnostic codes based on the specialty of the medical practice. Typically, the most frequently used codes make up 80% of diagnoses coded. When listing codes, insert a dash (-) if more digits are needed for specificity; documentation may need to be referred to, to determine the correct 4th-, 5th-, 6th-, and 7th-digit extensions where applicable. Determine what additional information is needed to arrive at the correct code (e.g., L/R, acute/chronic, trimester) and list these, so they can be easily circled. Always leave space to write the diagnoses that are not listed. To complete an insurance claim, abstract the correct diagnosis from the patient's transaction slip or medical record, code it, and insert the code in the computer system (use Field 21 on a paper claim).

Encoders and Computer-Assisted Coding

As with procedure coding, a computer or Web-based *encoder* can be used instead of the codebook to search for, locate, and verify diagnostic code selections (Figure 17-1).

Computer-assisted coding (CAC) software uses "natural language intelligence" and "clinical language understanding" to read and analyze the medical record, then interpret it and calculate which codes should be assigned. The record is first scanned and applicable phrases are highlighted. This allows the coder to view where the supporting documentation exists in the medical record. CAC can also be used to increase diagnostic coding productivity. When using computer-generated codes, all codes need to be verified prior to applying them to an insurance claim. CAC cannot assign a code to a greater level of specificity than it finds, so documentation remains the key to coding accurately.

Codebook Official Guidelines

ICD-10-CM Official Guidelines for Coding and Reporting have been developed by two agencies within the U.S. federal government's Department of Health and Human Services (DHHS).[1] These guidelines have been approved by four organizations[2] to correspond with the official conventions and instructions provided within the *ICD-10-CM* codebook. The medical assistant needs to become familiar with these guidelines and work with the physician to achieve accurate documentation so that correct reporting and code assignment can be achieved. A comprehensive list of the guidelines can be found on the Internet (see *Resources* section at the end of this chapter) and are included in the *ICD-10-CM* codebook.

Coding Terminology

It is imperative to have a working knowledge of medical terminology to become an efficient diagnostic coder.

---

[1] The Centers for Medicare and Medicaid Services (CMS) and the National Center for Health Statistics (NCHS).
[2] The American Hospital Association (AHA), the American Health Information Management Association (AHIMA), the CMS, and the NCHS.

Principal versus Primary Diagnosis

In an inpatient setting, the condition established after study that prompts the hospitalization is the **principal diagnosis**; this is documented in the medical record and coded.

In an outpatient setting, the condition, problem, or other reason for the health encounter that is chiefly responsible for the services provided is recorded and coded. This is called the **first-listed condition** or **primary diagnosis** and is usually related to the *chief complaint*. A *secondary diagnosis*, which may contribute to the condition or define the need for a higher level of service may be listed subsequently. It is important to note that the secondary diagnosis is not the underlying cause of the condition; this will be discussed later. In the medical record, the physician may list "IMP" (impression) or "DX" (diagnosis) when recording the diagnosis.

Linking Codes for Medical Necessity

All diagnoses that affect the current status of the patient must be assigned a code and the diagnoses must agree with the treatment rendered. Therefore, each procedure or service that is performed needs to be linked to the reason it was done, which means that each procedure code needs to be connected to a diagnostic code. The insurance carrier's computer software cross-checks claims to match procedure codes with diagnostic codes; this is referred to as **code linkage**. If there are discrepancies, the insurance claim is held up and payment becomes questionable. The new CMS-1500 claim form (02/12) and the 5010 electronic format will allow 12 diagnostic codes, four of which may be linked to each *CPT* code listed. Refer to Example 17-2 for an illustration of code linkage.

Code Edits and Audits—As mentioned in Chapter 16, the *National Correct Coding Initiative (NCCI)* was implemented by CMS to promote correct coding and control the improper assignment of codes that result in inappropriate reimbursement. Computerized edits are automatically performed to catch diagnostic codes that do not substantiate medical necessity for the services or procedures they are linked to. The NCCI Coding Policy Manual for Medicare Services is a general reference tool that explains the rationale for NCCI edits. It is updated yearly and should be utilized by physician practices.

Frequent internal audits can help catch coding problems early and avoid the denial of claims. Following are some common coding errors:

- Assigning too few or too many codes
- Assuming a diagnosis without definitive documentation of a condition
- Carelessness brought on by worrying about productivity instead of accuracy

---

EXAMPLE 17-2

Code Linkage

The patient comes into the physician's office for a diabetic check. The doctor performs a blood test to check his blood sugar level and adjusts his oral diabetic medication. The patient mentions a lump on his cheek. The physician inspects and palpates the lump and diagnoses it as a sebaceous cyst. The doctor recommends monitoring it and rechecking it on the next office visit.

Procedure/Service Description	Procedure Code (CPT)	Diagnosis Description	Diagnostic Code (ICD-10-CM)
Return office visit, level III	99213	Diabetes mellitus, type II (primary diagnosis)	E11.9
		Sebaceous cyst (secondary diagnosis)	L72.3
Venipuncture	36415	Diabetes mellitus, type II	E11.9
Blood sugar test	82947	Diabetes mellitus, type II	E11.9

- Coding two conditions when a combination code should have been used
- Coding a symptom or sign when there is a definitive diagnosis
- Coding a qualified diagnosis (e.g., rule-out)
- Depending on the Alphabetic Index to code—not going to the Tabular List to verify code selections
- Encoder errors that occur because the pathway used to determine the code was not substantiated
- Forgetting to code conditions that coexist
- Incomplete/inadequate documentation resulting in selection of unspecified codes
- Incorrect primary diagnosis coded
- Missing secondary diagnosis code
- Misunderstanding, misinterpreting, ignoring, or incorrectly applying coding guidelines
- Not coding to the highest level of specificity—using too few digits
- Sequencing codes improperly
- Using old editions of the codebook

Combination Codes

Sometimes two or more codes are necessary to completely describe a given diagnosis unless a combination code exists. A combination code is a single code used to classify (1) two diagnoses, (2) a diagnosis with a secondary process, or (3) a diagnosis with an association complication. Combination codes may be found in any chapter of *ICD-10-CM*; however, there are many combination codes in Chapter 19, *Injury, Poisoning, and Certain Other Consequences of External Causes*. Assign a combination code when it is available and the code description identifies the diagnostic conditions involved (Example 17-3).

EXAMPLE 17-4

Qualified Diagnosis

Scenario: Breast lump, right upper, outer quadrant; rule out malignant tumor

Code	Description
N63	Unspecified lump in breast (includes nodules)

Note: Look up "mass," "breast" in the Alphabetic Index to code this sign; do not code malignant tumor.

Qualified Diagnoses

If the final diagnosis is qualified by any of the terms *suspected, suspicion of, questionable, likely, probably,* or *possible,* do not code these conditions as if they existed or were established; these are called qualified diagnoses. Instead, code signs, symptoms, abnormal test results, or other reasons for the encounter. Signs or symptoms that are routinely associated with a disease process should not be coded. If the statement "rule out" is used, DO NOT CODE. This refers to a condition that is suspected and is being ruled out after tests are performed (see Example 17-4).

Abbreviations

The *ICD-10-CM* codebook frequently uses the following abbreviations. These may be found in the code description area.

NEC   Not Elsewhere Classifiable (in the codebook): The category number for a diagnosis that includes NEC is used only when the coder cannot find the description necessary to code the

---

EXAMPLE 17-3

Combination Codes

Examples	Conditions	Combination Code	Code Description
1. Two diagnoses	Atherosclerotic heart disease Unstable angina pectoris	I25.110	Atherosclerotic heart disease of native coronary artery with unstable angina pectoris
2. Diagnosis with secondary process	Type 1 diabetes Diabetic nephropathy	E10.40	Type 1 diabetes mellitus with diabetic nephropathy, unspecified
3. Diagnosis with associated complications	Toxic liver disease Chronic active hepatitis Ascites	K71.51	Toxic liver disease with chronic active hepatitis with ascites

diagnosis in a more specific category. An NEC entry in the Index directs the coder to an *other specified code* in the Tabular List.

NOS Not Otherwise Specified: This term means "unspecified" by the physician. The coder may need to ask the physician for more specific information; if it is available, details needs to be added as an addendum to the documentation. When additional clinical evidence is not available to assign a specific code, an unspecified code may be assigned.

Punctuation

Study the following types of punctuation that are used in the Tabular List or Alphabetic Index:

[ ] Brackets are used in the Tabular List to enclose synonyms, alternative wording, or explanatory phrases. Brackets are used in the Alphabetic Index to identify *manifestation codes* (explanation to follow).

( ) Parentheses are used in both the Tabular List and Index to enclose supplementary words that may be present in the statement of a disease or condition without affecting the code number to which it is assigned; also called *non-essential modifiers*.

: Colons are used in the Tabular List after an incomplete term that needs one or more of the modifiers that follow to make it assignable to a given category.

- Dash appearing after a code in the Alphabetic Index indicates that an additional character(s) is required; the Index does not always provide the full code (see "Dislocation, hip" in the Index for code S73.00-). Never code only from the Index, always use both Volumes 1 and 2 when assigning a code.

.- Point dash (e.g., F17.-), is used in the Tabular List to indicate a code that needs one or more digits to be considered a complete code; refer to the three-digit category or subcategory to view options for the additional digit(s).

Codebook Terms

Following are terms used in the codebook that will help you understand code descriptions and guidelines:

Acute, sub-acute, chronic	Look for these terms, which describe if the disease/injury has a sudden onset or is ongoing. If two terms appear in the same record (e.g., the patient has chronic tonsillitis and an acute phase occurred last night), code both terms; list acute first, then chronic.
and	When you read the term "and" in a narrative statement it represents "and/or."
code also	When you see "code also," it means that two codes may be required to fully describe a condition.
default code	A "default code" is an unspecified code that represents the condition most commonly associated with a main term. It appears next to the main term.
degree	Mild, moderate, or severe.
etiology/ manifestation	Some conditions have an underlying cause (etiology) with manifestations (disease) that occur due to the underlying condition (Example 17-5). In these situations, code the underlying condition first; code the manifestation second. Next to the etiology code you will see the instructional note "use additional code," and by the manifestation code you will see the note "code first" to help in sequencing codes. The manifestation code title will also have the note "in diseases classified elsewhere" because these codes can never be used in the first position; they must be used in conjunction with an underlying condition code. In the Index, both codes are listed with the etiology code first followed by the manifestation code in brackets.
dominant/ nondominant	Refers to side of the body affected for all paralytic syndrome codes, such as hemiplegia, monoplegia, and hemiparesis.

EXAMPLE 17-5

Etiology/Manifestation

Scenario: While the chief complaint is being taken, the patient's husband states that his wife, who has multiple sclerosis, is developing dementia and her behavior is changing rapidly; that is why they are at the doctor's office today.

Alphabetic Index
Dementia, multiple sclerosis, with behavioral disorders G35 [F02.81]

Tabular List
G35 multiple sclerosis
F02.81 dementia in other diseases classified elsewhere, with behavior disturbances

Note: When coding dementia, the codebook directs the coder to the underlying cause, multiple sclerosis, which is coded first

episode of care	This is a reference to when the disease or injury happened, was treated, or what state it is in (e.g., today, yesterday, last week, initial, subsequent, acute, chronic, healed).
excludes 1	An "excludes 1" note means *not coded here*; it should never be used at the same time as the code that it refers to because the two conditions cannot occur together.
excludes 2	An "excludes 2" note means *not included here*. In other words, the condition is not a part of the condition represented by the code that is referred to.
includes note	Appearing under a three-digit code title, this term further defines or gives an example of the category content.
includes term	Terms, listed under some codes that represent conditions for which the code is to be used.
initial encounter	Regarding an injury: Any encounter while the patient is receiving active treatment.
intermittent/ persistent	Reference to infrequent/mild symptoms versus ongoing/regular symptoms (e.g., intermittent asthma).
laterality	Included in some code descriptions, refers to left and right sides of the body in which a neoplasm or injury has occurred (e.g., joint pain, fracture, sprains, arthritis).
main term	Terms found in the diagnostic statement that typically includes a/an: (1) admission, (2) condition, (3) defect, (4) disease, (5) disorder, (6) disturbance, (7) history of, (8) syndrome, (9) test, or (10) eponym; name of a disease or syndrome derived from the individual's name who discovered it (e.g., Lou Gehrig's disease).
other	When the medical record provides detail for a specific disease, but a specified code does not exist, the term *other* or *other specified* appears.
see/see also	You will find the terms *see* and *see also* in the Alphabetic Index when other codes are referenced. Go to the main term referenced to locate the correct code.
sequela	Used for complications or conditions that arise as a direct result of an injury (e.g., scar formation).
stage	Period or phase in the course of a disease; degree or involvement in the development of a disease (e.g., Stage III cancer, Stage IV decubitus ulcer).
stage of care	Seventh digit assignment appearing in the Numeric Index used to identify the stage of care the patient is receiving (e.g., A = initial encounter for closed fracture, B = initial encounter for open fracture).
subsequent encounter	Regarding an injury: Encounter after the patient has received active treatment of an injury and is receiving routine care during the healing or recovery phase.
syndrome	When coding syndromes, follow directions found in the Alphabetic Index. If no guidance is given, code the documented manifestations of the syndrome.

unspecified When information in the medical record is insufficient to assign a specific code, an "unspecified" code may be selected.

with In the Alphabetic Index, the term *with* follows the main term. After it is a listing of conditions that may accompany the disease or condition.

Codebook Organization

To become familiar with the format and organization of the coding manual, it is important to review some basic information and then have a "hands-on" session where you can actually follow coding steps to locate diagnostic codes. Although the format may vary slightly among publishers, all use common terms and have the same basic organization. Volume I of *ICD-10-CM* is divided into chapters according to specific diseases. Volume II contains an Alphabetic Index, which is referred to first when looking up codes. Refer to Table 17-1 for an outline of the chapters in Volume I and divisions in Volume II.

The Alphabetic Index (Volume II)

To code using *ICD-10-CM*, always start in Volume II, the Alphabetic Index. In some codebooks, the Alphabetic Index may be labeled with the number "2" and located in the front; others have it in the back. You will find "guide words," in boldface at the top right and left of each page, similar to those found when locating words in a dictionary. Look through the alphabetical listing until you locate the *main term* of the disease or condition. You will then look for sub-terms and sub-subterms that further identify the disease or condition (e.g., type [congenital/acquired], specific body part).

The Tabular List (Volume I)

After locating the code(s) in Volume 2, turn to Volume I, the Tabular List, also called the *Alphanumeric Index* (which may be labeled "1"). As mentioned, this section is divided into chapters based on body system or condition and codes are listed in alphanumeric order—for example, Chapter 1: A00–B99, Chapter 2: C00–D49.9, Chapter 3: D50—D89.9, and so forth.

The Tabular List contains categories, subcategories, and codes comprising three to seven digits. You should code each health care encounter to the level of certainty that is known and documented. All code categories use three alphanumeric digits (e.g., **M65**). If there are no further subdivisions you may use this code. Subcategories are either four or five digits (M65.**22**), and sub-subcategories may have six or seven alphanumeric characters (M65.**221**)—so, you can code using three, four, five, six, or seven digits as long as you *use all applicable characters*. A code is invalid if it has not been coded to the full number of characters required for that code, including the 7th character.

A **placeholder** character (x*) is used as a 4th, 5th, or 6th digit placeholder with certain seven-character codes to allow for future expansion. Where a placeholder exists, it must be used in order for the code to be considered valid (Example 17-6).

EXAMPLE 17-6

Understanding Code Digits and Placeholders

Code	Hierarchy	Description
T36	Category	Poisoning by, adverse effect of and underdosing of systemic antibiotics
T36.0	Subcategory	Poisoning by, adverse effect of and underdosing of penicillins
T36.0x	Subcategory (note Placeholder in 5th digit)	Poisoning by, adverse effect of and underdosing of penicillins
T36.0x1	Sub-subcategory (Note: Maximum digits listed in this category is 6)	Poisoning by penicillins, accidental (unintentional)
T36.0x1A	Add 7th digit (Note: Category T36 requires a 7th digit—see note after 3rd-digit category T36)	Poisoning by penicillins, accidental, unintentional, initial encounter

*In various codebooks, the placeholder may be seen as a capital (X) or lower case (x) letter; either may be used.

TABLE 17-1 Chapter Outline of Volume 1 and Divisions in Volume 2 of the *International Classification of Diseases, 10th Revision, Clinical Modification (ICD-10-CM)*, 2017)

Front Matter

- How to Use *the ICD-10-CM* for Physicians
- *ICD-10-CM* Official Conventions
- Summary of Code Changes
- *ICD-10-CM* Official Guidelines and Reporting

Volume 1 Tabular List of Diseases and Injuries (Numeric Index)

Chapter Titles	Code Ranges
1. Certain Infectious and Parasitic Diseases	A00–B99
2. Neoplasms	C00–D49
3. Diseases of the Blood and Blood-Forming Organs	D50–D89
4. Endocrine, Nutritional and Metabolic Diseases	E00–E89
5. Mental, Behavioral, and Neurodevelopmental Disorders	F01–F99
6. Diseases of the Nervous System	G00–G99
7. Diseases of the Eye and Adnexa	H00–H59
8. Diseases of the Ear and Mastoid Process	H60–H95
9. Diseases of the Circulatory System	I00–I99
10. Diseases of the Respiratory System	J00–J99
11. Diseases of the Digestive System	K00–K95
12. Diseases of the Skin and Subcutaneous Tissue	L00–L99
13. Diseases of the Musculoskeletal System and Connective Tissue	M00–M99
14. Diseases of the Genitourinary System	N00–N99
15. Pregnancy, Childbirth, and the Puerperium	O00–O9A
16. Certain Conditions Originating in the Perinatal Period	P00–P96
17. Congenital Malformations, Deformations and Chromosomal Abnormalities	Q00–Q99
18. Symptoms, Signs and Abnormal Clinical and Laboratory Findings, Not Elsewhere Classified	R00–R99
19. Injury, Poisoning and Certain Other Consequences of External Causes	S00–T88
20. External Causes of Morbidity	V00–Y99
21. Factors Influencing Health Status and Contact with Health Services	Z00–Z99

Appendices

The Appendix varies according to publisher. Some examples include:

- Coding Exercises/Scenarios
- Illustrations

Volume 2 Alphabetic Index to Diseases and Injuries

- Index to Diseases and Injury
- Neoplasm Table
- Table of Drugs and Chemicals
- Index to External Causes

EXAMPLE 17-7

7th Character Extensions

Scenario: Mrs. Black, 86 years old, returns to the office to have her back reexamined; it is healing well.

Dx: (1) Pathologic fracture; vertebra (2) Osteoporosis

Code	Description
M84	Disorder of continuity of bone
M84.4	Pathological fracture, not elsewhere classified
M84.48	Pathological fracture, other site

The appropriate 7th character (extension) needs to be added to each code from category M84.4:

A   initial encounter for fracture

D   subsequent encounter for fracture with routine healing

G   subsequent encounter for fracture with delayed healing

K   subsequent encounter for fracture with nonunion

P   subsequent encounter for fracture with malunion

S   sequela (used for complications or conditions that arise as a direct result of an injury, e.g., scar formation)

Code assignment: M84.48xD (note placeholder digit [x] in the 6th position)

Some code subcategories have mandatory 7th digits (called *extensions*) that may not be located by the applicable code. Extensions have different meanings depending on the section where they are located (e.g., accidents, injuries, babies). Always apply the 7th digit if it is available within a category. If a code requiring a 7th digit is not six characters, a placeholder (x) must be used to fill the empty character space(s) (Example 17-7). Refer to Procedure 17-1 for step-by-step instructions to select correct diagnostic codes.

CHAPTER-SPECIFIC CODING GUIDELINES

Following are specific coding guidelines pertaining to certain chapters in *ICD-10-CM*. These represent some of the more common coding situations encountered in a physician's office.

Human Immunodeficiency Virus (HIV)

In the evolution of the disease process for HIV, you will be using codes for HIV, ARC *(AIDS- related conditions)*, and AIDS. A patient may test positive for HIV but be *asymptomatic*, that is, not have any symptoms. When symptoms occur, it is a signal that the disease is in a state of transition, referred to as ARC. Patients with symptoms that occur due to a comprised immune system or opportunistic infections are considered to have AIDS.

Code only confirmed cases of HIV according to the physician's statement using code B20 from Chapter 1. Also use this code when the patient has an encounter for a *related condition* (including hospital admission), followed by the disease or condition that prompted the visit/admission. If the patient is seen for an *unrelated condition*, code the condition first followed by the HIV code B20 and any other HIV-related conditions. The following codes are used in other HIV coding scenarios:

- *Z21*—Use this code if the patient does not have HIV symptoms, as long as the patient is known to have HIV.
- *Z20-6*—Use this code when the patient has had contact with and (suspected) exposure to HIV.
- *Z11.4*—Use this screening code when a patient is seen to determine his or her HIV status; use additional codes for associated high-risk behavior. If the patient presents for testing with signs or symptoms, code the signs or symptoms first; the additional counseling code (Z71.7) is used in the second position.
- *Z71.7*—Use this counseling code when the patient returns to find out his or her HIV status when negative.

PROCEDURE 17-1

Select Correct Diagnostic Codes Using *ICD-10-CM*

OBJECTIVE: Accurately select diagnostic codes for insurance claims.

EQUIPMENT/SUPPLIES: *ICD-10-CM* diagnostic codebook (Volumes 1 and 2), medical dictionary, and pen or pencil.

DIRECTIONS: Follow these step-by-step directions to learn this procedure. Job Skills 17-1 through 17-5 are presented in the *Workbook* for practice.

1. Locate the *main term* or condition (not anatomic site) in the diagnostic statement that relates to the patient's condition, that is, What is wrong with the patient?

2. Next, locate the *main term* in the Alphabetic Index (Volume 2). See Example 17-8.

3. Look for subterms and sub-subterms indented under the main term (see Example 17-9).

4. If the condition or disease is not listed, rearrange the root portions of the medical terms (see Example 17-10).

5. Refer to any notes or instructions under the main term closed in parentheses and read them.

6. Follow any cross-reference instructions.

7. Write the code number(s).

8. Verify the code selection in Volume I (Tabular List).

9. Read any instructional terms in the Tabular List.

10. Determine if additional digits/characters need to be added to the code.

11. Check to see if *laterality* is applicable; if so, assign an extension.

12. Do not arbitrarily use a zero as a filler character when listing a diagnostic code number. This may nullify the code or indicate a different disease. The codebook includes decimal points after the 3rd digit, but these are not required on insurance claims.

13. Code to the highest level of specificity; that is, code to the highest digit available in the classification.

14. Always use both Volume 2 (Alphabetic Index) and Volume 1 (Tabular/Numeric List) of *ICD-10-CM* before assigning a code.

15. Assign the code.

EXAMPLE 17-8

Main Terms

Diagnostic Statement	Main Term	Additional Terms	Code Selection
Muscle atrophy	Atrophy	Where?—muscle	M62.50
Chronic bronchitis	Bronchitis	Time frame?—chronic	J42
Allergic conjunctivitis (chronic)	Conjunctivitis	Type?—allergic	H10.45
Nasal (bone) fracture	Fracture	Where?—nose	S02.2

EXAMPLE 17-9

Identifying Terms

Scenario: Newly diagnosed pathologic fracture of the right humerus

Main Term	Subterm	Sub-Subterm	Code Assignment
↓	↓	↓	↓
fracture,	pathologic	humerus (right)	M84.421A

EXAMPLE 17-10

Medical Terminology Components

Scenario: Newly diagnosed pathologic fracture of the right humerus

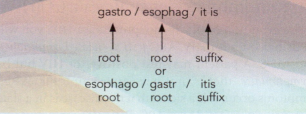

gastro / esophag / it is
↑ ↑ ↑
root root suffix
or
esophago / gastr / itis
root root suffix

- *R75*—Use this code if the patient has had an inconclusive HIV laboratory serology test.
- *098.7*—Use this code for a pregnant patient with HIV, which will complicate the pregnancy, childbirth, and the puerperium.

Neoplasms

A **neoplasm** is a spontaneous new growth of tissue, often referred to as a tumor. **Benign** neoplasms are noninvasive and do not *metastasize* (spread to other tissue). **Malignant** neoplasms spread and invade other tissue if not treated and are often called *cancerous tumors*. Neoplasms are found in Chapter 2, and the Table on Neoplasms may be found following the Alphabetic Index to Diseases. When coding, first examine documentation to determine if the neoplasm is benign or malignant. If malignant, determine if it is a/an:

- *Primary malignancy*—Original site of a tumor
- *Secondary malignancy*—Additional tumor that appears at the site of metastasis
- *Carcinoma in situ*—Localized or confined to the site of origin
- *Neoplasm of uncertain behavior*—Properties of the tumor are not recognizable as benign or malignant
- *Unspecified neoplasm*—Status of tumor not documented by physician or pathologist

In the Alphabetic Index, neoplasms are classified according to the type, then the anatomic site. In the Neoplasm Table, they are listed according to the site affected in the left column; the other columns represent the way they behave (Example 17-11). You can use the Neoplasm Table to quickly locate a tumor; however, it is important to then turn to the Tabular List, confirm the code, and view instructional notes. Report only those codes that represent the current status of the neoplasm. Sequencing the codes depends on which site is being treated. Following are some coding tips with examples:

- If the patient comes in for treatment that is directed at the malignancy, code first the malignancy.
- If the patient has metastasis to a secondary site and comes in for treatment of that site, code the secondary neoplasm first, even if the primary tumor is still present.
- If the tumor has been excised and the patient is still undergoing treatment (chemotherapy or radiation), code the neoplasm.
- If the patient presents for an encounter for administration of chemotherapy or radiation treatment, assign a "Z" code from Chapter 21 (Factors Influencing Health Status and Contact with Health Services). The primary diagnosis would be Z51.-- and the secondary diagnosis would be the reason for which the service is being performed.
- If the patient comes in for follow-up care but the tumor is no longer present or the patient is not receiving treatment, assign a "Z" code from Chapter 21.
- If the patient has multiple neoplasms of the same site that are not contiguous, code each neoplasm (e.g., tumors in different quadrants of the same breast).
- If the patient has a neoplasm of *ectopic tissue*, that is, tissue that has relocated to another part of the body, code to the site of origin.

EXAMPLE 17-11

Neoplasm Table

Anatomic Site	Malignant Primary	Malignant Secondary	Carcinoma In Situ	Benign	Uncertain	Unspecified Behavior
Neoplasm bone (periosteum)*	C41.9	C79.51	-	D16.9	D48.0	D49.2
limb NEC	C40.9-	C79.51	-	D16.9-	-	-
lower (long bones)	C40.2-	C79.51	-	D16.2	-	-
short bones	C40.3-	C79.51 -	-	D16.3-	-	-

*Note: Carcinomas and adenocarcinomas of any type other than intraosseous or odontogenic of the site listed under "neoplasm, bone" should be considered as constituting metastatic spread from an unspecified primary site and coded to C79.51 for morbidity coding and to C80.1 for underlying cause of death coding.

There are additional guidelines for other circumstances where a neoplasm is present.

Diabetes Mellitus (DM)

Diabetes mellitus (DM) codes are *combination* codes that include the type of diabetes, the body system affected, and the complications affecting that body system. They are found in Chapter 4 and include the following:

- *Type I diabetes mellitus* (E10)
- *Type II diabetes mellitus* (E11)
- *Type II diabetes mellitus with complications* (e.g., kidney complications, neuropathy E11.21)
- *Type II diabetes mellitus with complications affecting a body system* (e.g., chronic kidney disease E11.22)
- *Diabetes mellitus due to drugs or chemicals* (E09)
- *Diabetes mellitus due to underlying condition* (E08)
- *Other specified diabetes mellitus* (E13)
- *Unspecified diabetes mellitus* (E15)

If the type of diabetes is not documented, assign a default code for type 2 diabetes (E11.-). If it is documented that the patient regularly uses insulin, also assign code Z79.4 (long-term/current use of insulin). The reason for the encounter will determine the primary code. Use as many codes as necessary to identify all associated conditions.

Secondary diabetes is always caused by another condition (e.g., due to pancreatitis, cystic fibrosis, adverse effect of drug). Be aware of "code first" and "use additional code" instructions in the Tabular List when assigning these codes.

Pain

If acute or chronic pain is documented in the medical record, codes from category G89 (pain not elsewhere classified) may be used. Do not use these codes if an underlying definitive diagnosis is known unless the code description provides further information. Codes from category G89 may be the first-listed code when pain management is the reason for the encounter. Site-specific pain codes may be found in other chapters and may be sequenced with pain codes as seen in Example 17-12.

Routine postoperative pain should not be coded. However, postoperative pain associated with a complication should be assigned a code from Chapter 19 (Injury, Poisoning, and Certain Other Consequences of External Causes)—additional codes from category G89 may also be used. If the postoperative pain is not associated with a specific complication but is more than routine pain expected from the procedure, assign a pain code from category G89.

EXAMPLE 17-12

Site-Specific Pain Codes

Scenario: Patient sees a physiologist for pain management. She fell down a flight of stairs and is experiencing acute back pain, which radiates down her right leg.

Code	Description
G89.11	Acute pain due to trauma (identifies intensity of pain)
M54.41	Lumbago with sciatica, right side (identifies site of pain)

Hypertension

There are several kinds of hypertension and codes that apply to this disease. *Essential primary hypertension* (I10) includes high blood pressure and many basic types: arterial, benign, essential, malignant, and systemic hypertension, regardless of whether the patient's hypertension is controlled or uncontrolled. Following are some of the more common forms:

- *Transient hypertension*—Unless the patient has the diagnosis of "hypertension" assign code R03.0 (elevated blood pressure reading without the diagnosis of hypertension).
- *Secondary hypertension*—Use the primary code to identify the cause of, or underlying condition and a second code from category I15 to identify the hypertension.
- *Gestational hypertension*—For transient hypertension in pregnancy, code 013.- is used if the patient does not have proteinuria.
- *Hypertension with heart disease*—Code the heart condition from category I50 (heart failure) and I51 (complications and ill-defined descriptions of heart disease) and include a code from I11 (hypertensive heart disease) when the chart note implies or states, "due to hypertension."

Myocardial Infarction

Acute myocardial infarction (AMI) codes identify the site that is affected (e.g., anterolateral wall). Subcategories identify two types of AMIs:

- ST elevation myocardial infarction (STEMI)
- Non-ST elevation myocardial infarction (NSTEMI)

Code descriptions further differentiate the time of the MI as follows:

- Encounters occurring while the MI is equal to, or less than, 4 weeks old (I21)
- Encounters occurring after the 4-week time frame while the patient is still receiving related care; do not use codes from category I21
- Older, healed MIs not requiring further care (I25.2)

Respiratory failure may be coded in the second position if it occurs after admission, or if it occurs at admission and does not meet the criteria for the principal diagnosis.

Influenza

When a patient presents with influenza, the medical record will indicate if the physician states a specific kind of influenza, for example, influenza due to avian virus J09.0-, or swine flu J09.1-. Documentation of different types of flu does not have to be verified by positive laboratory serology. Influenzas are also coded according to various manifestations (e.g., sinusitis J01.0, myocarditis J10.82). When patients come in for a flu shot, use code Z23 (encounter for immunization).

Pregnancy and Childbirth

Chapter 15, Pregnancy, Childbirth, and the Puerperium, provides obstetric codes that have sequencing priority over codes from other chapters. Additional chapter codes may be used to further specify conditions. With many of the codes, the final character indicates the trimester of pregnancy for the current encounter (e.g., O26.91—pregnancy related condition, unspecified, first trimester). Look at the beginning of the codebook chapter for trimester indications (see Example 17-13).

When working in an OB-GYN office, the most common code assigned will be O80 (encounter for full-term uncomplicated delivery). If the patient was admitted for a cesarean procedure, code the condition that prompted the C-section. When complications arise, a seventh character may be assigned for certain categories: (1) To identify the fetus affected (e.g., 7th character "0" for single gestation), (2) when documentation is insufficient to make a determination regarding the affected fetus, or (3) when it is not clinically possible to determine the affected fetus.

For routine prenatal outpatient visits, select a code from category Z34; these should not be used in conjunction with codes from Chapter 15. For routine prenatal outpatient visits for patients with high-risk pregnancies, select a code from category O09; secondary codes from

---

EXAMPLE 17-13

Pregnancy Terms

Trimesters are counted from the first day of the last menstrual period:

1st Trimester: Less than 14 weeks, 0 days

2nd Trimester: 14 weeks (0 days) to less than 28 weeks (0 days)

3rd Trimester: 28 weeks (0 days) until delivery

Normal delivery gestation: 40 weeks

Postpartum period: Immediately after to 6 weeks following delivery

Peripartum period: Last month of pregnancy to 5 months postpartum

---

Chapter 15 may be used with these codes. If the patient is seen for a reason other than pregnancy, assign code Z33.1 (pregnant state, incidental).

Use a code from Chapter 20 to indicate the outcome of delivery on the mother's record (e.g., Z37.0—single live birth). If working for a pediatrician, do not use this code on the newborn record, instead use a code from the Z38 category (e.g., Z38.0—single liveborn infant, born in hospital).

Sprains, Strains, and Fractures

In Chapter 19 you will find "S" codes for a multitude of sprains, strains, and fractures (see Example 17-14).

Fractures are listed in the Alphabetic Index under "fracture, traumatic." As with procedure codes, if documentation does not state "open fracture" or "closed fracture," code it as closed. The same is true with displaced

---

EXAMPLE 17-14

Sprains, Strains, Fractures

Diagnosis	Code	Description
Lower back strain	S39.012A	Strain of muscle, fascia, and tendon of lower back; initial encounter
Left sprained ankle	S93.402D	Sprain of unspecified ligament of left ankle; subsequent encounter
Colles' fracture, right wrist	S52.351A	Colles' fracture right radius; initial encounter, closed fracture

and not displaced fractures; if not indicated, code as not displaced. When coding fractures, look for the following:

- Site
- Laterality
- Type
- Location

Current, acute injuries should be coded from Chapter 19 (Injury, Poisoning, and Certain Other Consequences of External Causes). Use a separate code for each injury unless there is a combination code (e.g., multiple site codes). Sequence the most serious injury first, as described by the provider. Most categories in this chapter have the following 7th character extensions that are required for each applicable code:

- *A—Initial Encounter for Fracture*: Use as long as the patient is receiving *active* treatment.

    EXAMPLE: ER encounter, evaluation and continuing ongoing treatment by same or different physician

- *D—Subsequent Encounter for Fracture*: Use for routine healing—after the patient has completed *active* treatment.

    EXAMPLE: X-ray to check healing status, cast change or removal, removal of internal/external fixation device, medication adjustment, follow-up visits

- *S—Sequela*: Use when complications or conditions arise as a direct result of an injury or condition. Sequence the sequela first, followed by the injury code with an "S" extension in the 7th position.

    EXAMPLE: Scar formation

    Refer to Example 17-15 for a fracture scenario.

If there are other conditions associated with the healing process, other 7th digits can be applied (e.g., "P" subsequent encounter for fracture with malunion). If the patient experiences superficial injuries at the same site as a more severe injury (abrasions/contusions), they should NOT be coded.

Chapter 13, Diseases of the Musculoskeletal System and Connective Tissue, contains codes pertaining to bone, joints, and muscles with conditions that are the result of *healed injuries* in those areas. When coding pathologic fractures (M80), you will find a listing in the Alphabetic Index under "fractures, pathologic." Do not code these as traumatic fractures, even if the patient falls, if the fall would not usually break a normal, healthy bone.

Burns and Corrosions

There is a distinction in *ICD-10-CM* between thermal burns that come from a heat source (e.g., fire or hot appliance), or those that result from electricity or radiation, and "corrosions" that are chemical burns;

EXAMPLE 17-15

Fracture Scenario

Scenario: A 12-year-old boy was *playing football*. As he *caught the ball*, he *jammed his left middle finger*. He is experiencing pain with movement and the finger is red and swollen. An x-ray is taken and the physician diagnosed a *nondisplaced traumatic fracture of the left middle phalanx, not involving the growth plate*. He is fitted with an aluminum splint to stabilize the finger and instructed to ice it 20 to 30 minutes three times a day. He is to avoid activities that would cause further injury and return in 1 week for a recheck.

Questions to Ask	Documentation	*ICD*-10-CM Alpha Index	Code with Description
What is the injury and what body part is affected? (specific site, laterality, depth/degree/severity)	Jammed—left, middle finger	Fracture, finger, middle, proximal, phalanx, nondisplaced	S62.643A Nondisplaced fracture of proximal phalanx of left middle finger
How did it occur?	Struck by football	Striking against, object, sports equipment	W21.01XA Struck by football; initial encounter
What activity was he doing at the time the injury occurred?	Playing football	Football (American) NOS	Y93.61 American tackle football

however, coding rules are the same. Code category T20–T32 in Chapter 19 describes burns and corrosions. Sunburn (L55.-) is excluded from this section.

Burns of the eye and internal organs are classified by site but not by degree (e.g., T26.11, burn of cornea and conjunctival sac, right eye). All other burns are classified by:

- *Depth*—First degree (erythema), second degree (blistering), third degree (full-thickness involvement)
- *Extent*—Amount of body surface involved*
- *Agent*—Caused from exposure to smoke, fire, and flames (see Chapter 20, code category X00)

Follow the directions in Procedure 17-2 when selecting burn and corrosion codes.

Poisoning and Adverse Effects

Although there is a Table of Drugs and Chemicals located following the Alphabetic Index, all codes should be verified in the Tabular List. Codes in categories T36–T65 are combination codes that include the substance taken and the intent. No additional *external cause code* is required when coding poisonings, toxic effects, adverse effects, and underdosing.

Code all drugs, medicinal or biological substances that relate to the patient's condition, and if there are two or more, code each individually unless there is a combination code. Following are definitions for terms in Chapter 19 that will help you understand coding language used in this section:

- *Adverse effect*—When a drug is applied or properly administered but the patient has an adverse effect, apply an "adverse effect" code. Use additional codes for manifestations (e.g., respiratory failure, tachycardia, vomiting).
- *Poisoning*—When an overdose occurs, a wrong substance is given or taken in error, or the wrong route of administration is used, determine the intent (accidental, intentional self-harm, assault,

---

PROCEDURE 17-2

Select Burn and Corrosion Codes

OBJECTIVES: Accurately select burn and corrosion codes from *ICD-10-CM*.

EQUIPMENT/SUPPLIES: *ICD-10-CM* diagnostic codebook (Volumes 1 and 2), medical dictionary, and pen or pencil.

DIRECTIONS: Follow these step-by-step directions to learn this procedure.

1. Turn to Volume 2, the Alphabetic Index, and look under the *main term* "burn."
2. Identify the *subterm*, which will be the *site* of the burn. You may be directed to a more specific site (e.g., arm, see upper limb; upper limb, above elbow; right or left). Follow the instructions until you come to the exact burn site.
3. Locate the degree of the burn (first, second, or third).
4. Write down the code.
5. Turn to Volume 1, the Tabular List, locate the code, and read the complete description.

6. Look at the code category to see if a 7th character extension needs to be applied. If so, apply the 7th digit using a placeholder (x) as necessary.
7. In certain circumstances, an external cause code from Chapter 20 ("X") can be used to explain how the burn happened (e.g., X00.1xxD "exposure to uncontrolled fire in building or structure; subsequent encounter").
8. Read these guidelines to learn how to code the following situations:

MULTIPLE BURNS ON BODY
Always assign separate codes for each burn; unspecific codes in category T30 should be rarely used. When more than one burn is present, sequence the burn with the highest degree first.

MULTIPLE BURNS AT SAME SITE
When there is more than one burn at the same site, code the burn with the highest degree.

(continues)

---

*For diagnostic coding, the "Rule of Nines" is used to estimate body surface area (head/neck 9%, each arm 9%, each leg 18%, anterior trunk 18%, posterior trunk 18%, genitalia 1%).

PROCEDURE 17-2 *(continued)*

NONHEALING BURNS

Code nonhealing burns as acute burns (e.g., necrosis of burned skin).

INFECTED BURNS

Use an additional code for infected burns.

EXTERNAL AND INTERNAL BURNS

The first-listed diagnosis, determined by the circumstance, will govern the sequencing of codes.

THIRD-DEGREE BURNS

Use codes from category T31 when there is a third-degree burn involving 20% or more of the body surface.

MORTALITY CODES

Apply codes from category T31 (Burns Classified According to Body Extent Involved) when working in a burn unit to provide data and evaluate mortality.

LATE EFFECTS OF BURNS

Apply the 7th character "S" to indicate late effects when the patient encounter is for treating a sequela (e.g., scarring).

ADMIT/ENCOUNTER FOR BURNS AND OTHER RELATED CONDITIONS

The circumstances of the admit or encounter govern the first-listed diagnosis (e.g., burns with smoke inhalation and/or respiratory failure).

---

or undetermined) and assign a code from category T36–T50. If abuse or dependence is also documented, assign an additional code.

- *Intoxication*—When an accumulation of a substance (e.g., alcohol) or medication (e.g., Coumadin intoxication) collects in the patient's bloodstream, it is considered a *poisoning*.

- *Toxic effect*—When a harmful substance comes in contact with a person or is ingested, select a code from category T51–T65. These codes have an associated intent (accidental, intentional, self-harm, assault, undetermined).

- *Underdosing*—When the patient takes less medication than prescribed by the physician and has a relapse of the medical condition for which the drug was prescribed, code first the condition the patient is experiencing and code second the underdosing (T36–T50). Noncompliance codes (Z91.12-, Z91.13-) or complication of care codes (Y63.6–Y63.9) may be used with an underdosing code to indicate intent, if known.

Refer to Procedure 17-3 for step-by-step directions when using the Table of Drugs and Chemicals.

External Causes

External causes of *morbidity codes* are used after the primary diagnosis to explain the mechanism for an injury; never use these codes in the first position. They also provide data for injury research and evaluation of injury prevention strategies (formerly called "E" codes

in *ICD-9-CM*). They help tell a story about (1) how the injury or health condition happened; (2) whether the event was intentional (e.g., assault, suicide), unintentional, or accidental; (3) the place where the event occurred; (4) the activity of the patient at the time of the event; and (5) the person's status (e.g., civilian, military).

These secondary "V, W, X, Y" codes are combination codes that can be used with codes from any chapter in *ICD-10-CM* that describe an accident, disease, or condition that is due to an external cause; however, they are most frequently used with injury codes. These codes identify sequential events that result in an injury, but unlike other *ICD-10-CM* codes they do not produce revenue. First, turn to the separate Index to External Causes found after the Alphabetical Index to Diseases and determine the main external cause code, then sequence the place of occurrence, activity, and external cause status codes. Assign as many codes as necessary to describe the circumstances as long as the claim format allows.

☑ COMPLIANCE

External Cause Codes

There is no national requirement for mandatory use of *ICD-10-CM*'s external cause codes for outpatient services. However, there are some states and insurance payers who may require their use.

PROCEDURE 17-3

Select Diagnostic Codes from the Table of Drugs and Chemicals

OBJECTIVE: Select diagnostic codes from the Table of Drugs and Chemicals and confirm in the Tabular List.

EQUIPMENT/SUPPLIES: *ICD-10-CM* diagnostic codebook (Volumes 1 and 2), medical dictionary, and pen or pencil.

DIRECTIONS: Follow these step-by-step directions to learn this procedure.

1. Go to the Table of Drugs and Chemicals, located after the Tabular List, and follow the steps below that relate to various scenarios.

POISONING OR TOXIC EFFECTS

2. Find the medicinal, chemical, or biological substance (e.g., drug, alcohol, or harmful agent) in the first column; each will be listed in alphabetical order.

3. Next, determine the cause for the poisoning or toxic effect: accidental (unintentional), intentional self-harm, assault, or undetermined. Select a code from that column.

4. Code each substance documented in the medical record as a cause for the medical condition.

5. Next, code the result (manifestation) of the poisoning or toxic effect. Note: Codes in this category are combination codes that include

the substance related to the poisoning as well as the external cause; no additional external cause code is needed.

ACCUMULATIVE AFFECT OF A MEDICATION

6. Assign the manifestation code first (e.g., dizziness, nausea, vomiting).

7. Assign a code from the adverse effect column second.

ADVERSE EFFECTS

8. When a drug has been correctly prescribed and properly administered and an adverse effect occurs, *code the nature of the adverse effect first* (e.g., delirium, hepatitis, renal failure).

9. Next, code the chemical substance causing the adverse effect, found in the Adverse Effect column.

10. Assign codes for all adverse effects documented as a cause and all substances listed that contribute to the condition.

UNDERDOSING

11. Code first the medical condition for which the drug was prescribed.

12. Code second the chemical substance found in the Underdosing Column (T36 through T50).

13. Verify ALL codes in the Tabular List.

Factors Influencing Health Status and Contact with Health Services

Factors Influencing Health Status and Contact with Health Services codes are found in Chapter 21. These "Z" codes can be used in any health care setting (formerly called "V" codes in *ICD-9-CM*). They can be sequenced in the first or second position depending on the circumstance. Following are some of the more common uses for Z codes with examples:

- *Contact/Exposure*—When an asymptomatic patient is suspected to have been exposed to a communicable disease or is in an area where a disease is epidemic, use Z codes in the second position to indicate the suspected exposure and

potential risk. These codes may be used in the first position to explain an encounter for testing. Such codes are referred to as *status codes* because they are informative but do not describe an active diagnosis. There are many uses for status codes; some examples are: Z22 Carrier of infectious disease, Z67 Blood type, Z89 Acquired absence of limb, and Presence of prosthetic or mechanical devices.

- *Counseling*—When a patient or family receives counseling in the aftermath of an illness or injury, or when counseling is needed to direct and support during a social crisis, use Z codes to describe the reason for the service (e.g., Z32.3—encounter for childcare instruction).

- *Diagnostic services*—When patients receive diagnostic services only, code the condition, problem, or reason for the encounter first. Codes for secondary diagnoses may be applied.

- *History of*—When a patient has a condition that no longer exists and is not receiving treatment but a potential for reoccurrence exists, personal history codes (Z85–Z91.5) and family history codes (Z80–Z84) are used to describe risk factors, which may alter the treatment plan for the existing condition. Regardless of the reason for the visit, they can be used on any medical record.

- *Inoculations and vaccinations*—Use code Z23 in the first position if the vaccine is the reason for the visit, and in the second position if the patient has an inoculation as a routine part of preventive health care (e.g., annual physical examination, well-baby visit).

- *Observation*—When a patient is being observed for a suspected condition, use code Z03. When a patient is examined and observed for other reasons, use code Z04. These codes are used as a first-listed diagnosis; additional codes may be used but only if they are unrelated to the suspected condition being observed. Do not use these codes if a condition is confirmed.

- *Prenatal visits*—Report a code from *ICD-10-CM* category Z34 as the first diagnosis for routine outpatient prenatal visits. Do not report this code in combination with Chapter 15 codes. If the pregnancy is high-risk, report a code from category O09 as the first diagnosis; a code from Chapter 15 may also be reported as a secondary diagnosis.

- *Preoperative evaluations*—When patients come in for their pre-op visit, use a code from subcategory Z01.81 to describe the consultation. The patient's condition or reason for the surgery should be coded in the second position as well as any findings that relate to the preoperative evaluation. If any findings are discovered during the preoperative evaluation, they may also be coded.

- *Screening*—Early detection of disease is offered via screening tests so that early treatment may take place. When a patient has a screening examination, a code from categories Z11–Z36 may be billed in the first position (e.g., Z12.31 Encounter for screening mammogram for malignant neoplasm of breast). If the patient is being seen for other health problems and a screening takes place, apply the code in the second position. If screening is part of a routine examination (e.g., pap smear during a routine pelvic exam), the screening code should not be used. Testing to rule out or confirm a qualified diagnosis is not screening; instead use codes that reflect the patient's signs and symptoms.

- *Therapeutic services*—When patients receive therapeutic services only, code the diagnosis, condition, problem, or other reason for the visit that is documented in the medical record. Also assign codes to other conditions that are being treated or medically managed or that would affect the patient's receipt of the therapeutic services. *Exception:* When a patient is receiving chemotherapy or radiation treatment, assign the appropriate Z code in the first position and the problem or diagnosis in the second position.

SUMMARY

As you may have discovered, procedure and diagnostic coding is a specialty all of its own. Both training and experience will help the coder to find and abstract all the elements needed to code correctly. Becoming a certified coder will increase professional status and help with employment opportunities. Refer to Table 1-2 in Chapter 1 for a listing of various coding certifications.

A new position has surfaced in medical offices, that of a **scribe**. As previously mentioned in Chapter 9, a medical scribe follows (shadows) the physician into treatment rooms and records, according to the direction of the physician, all the elements of the history, physical examination, and medical decision-making process that are needed for evaluation and management services, as well as details about tests, surgical procedures, and diagnoses. There is a close relationship between a scribe and a coder—they both need to glean key terms that are required to substantiate medical necessity and code services, procedures, and diagnoses. There are scribe companies that recruit, train, and employ workers interested in the medical field.

There are also **remote coders**, that is, coders who work at locations other than in the physician's office (e.g., home or billing service). Companies outside of the United States may provide coding and billing services. When a medical practice, clinic, or hospital sends its records to such a company, this is called *outsourcing*. Offshore coding is taking place in several countries, India being the most prevalent.

STOP AND THINK CASE SCENARIO
Practice Code Linkage

SCENARIO: You have received a patient's encounter form with multiple procedures checked off, tests to be scheduled, and diagnoses.

CRITICAL THINKING: Determine which diagnosis should be linked to which procedure for the services billed and for the requisition slip that you are filling out for tests. Write the letter for the service or procedure by the diagnosis; there may be more than one that applies.

SERVICES/PROCEDURES

A. Evaluation and Management services
B. Electrocardiogram
C. CT brain
D. X-ray knee
E. Fasting blood sugar
F. Urinalysis

DIAGNOSES

Painful right knee: _____
Numbness and tingling in feet: _____
Heart arrhythmia: _____
Burning with urination: _____
Diabetes: _____
Lump on neck: _____
Chronic headaches: _____

STOP AND THINK CASE SCENARIO
Verify Service and Diagnosis

SCENARIO: You are responsible for coding professional services, procedures, and diagnoses in the physician's office. You receive a fee ticket that has the highest level evaluation and management code (Level V) checked off with the diagnosis "sunburn." You know that the diagnosis would not substantiate this level of service.

CRITICAL THINKING: What would you do to verify that the procedure code for the encounter and diagnosis are correct?

_____
_____
_____
_____
_____
_____
_____

FOCUS ON CERTIFICATION*

CMA (AAMA) Content Summary

- *International Classification of Diseases, 10th Revision, Clinical Modifications (ICD-10-CM)* coding system
- Relationship between procedure and diagnostic codes

RMA (AMT) Content Summary

- Identify HIPAA-mandated coding systems and references
- ICD-10-CM

CMAS (AMT) Content Summary

- Understand diagnoses codes
- Employ *International Classification of Diseases (ICD-10-CM)* codes appropriately

*This textbook and the accompanying Workbook meet the entry-level administrative and general competencies for the CMA outlined by the AAMA Examination Content Outline and Occupational Analysis and for the RMA and CMAS outlined by the AMT Competencies, Construction Parameters, and Examination Specifications (see Competency Grids in Appendix B).

REVIEW EXAM-STYLE QUESTIONS

1. *ICD-10-CM* has replaced *ICD-9-CM* on:
   a. January 1, 2014
   b. October 1, 2014
   c. January 1, 2015
   d. October 1, 2015
   e. January 1, 2016

2. Coexisting medical conditions are referred to as:
   a. morbidity
   b. comorbidity
   c. dual-morbidity
   d. mortality
   e. comortality

3. When coding diagnoses, start by looking:
   a. in Volume I
   b. in the Tabular List
   c. up the anatomic body part
   d. in Volume II
   e. in the Table of Contents

4. In an inpatient setting, the condition established after study that prompted the hospitalization is called the:
   a. primary diagnosis
   b. first-listed diagnosis
   c. principal diagnosis
   d. chief complaint
   e. both a and b

5. Checking a diagnostic code against a procedure code to ensure medical necessity is referred to as:
   a. cross-checking
   b. proofreading
   c. code linkage
   d. code correlation
   e. spot-checking

6. When a single code exists that can classify two diagnoses, a diagnosis with a secondary process, or a diagnosis with an associated complication, it is referred to as a:
   a. dual code
   b. double code
   c. binary code
   d. combination code
   e. complex code

7. A "qualified diagnosis" is a:
   a. diagnosis that is waiting for a second opinion to substantiate it
   b. diagnosis that is not found in the codebook
   c. sign or symptom
   d. condition coded as if it existed but has not been proven
   e. confirmed diagnosis

8. The coding rule for etiology and manifestations is to:
   a. only code the etiology of a disease
   b. only code the manifestation of a disease
   c. code the etiology in the first position and the manifestation in the second position
   d. code the manifestation in the first position and the etiology in the second position
   e. code only the condition the patient is being seen for

9. All categories in *ICD-10-CM*:
   a. have 3 alphanumeric digits
   b. have 3 alpha digits
   c. have 3 numeric digits
   d. have 5 digits
   e. have 7 digits

10. In diagnostic coding, the following symbol is used as a "placeholder" when a subcategory does not have a fourth, fifth, or sixth digit and a seventh digit needs to be applied.
    a. 0 (zero)
    b. 1 (one)
    c. x (ex)
    d. – (dash)
    e. 1 (plus)

11. Tables listed in *ICD-10-CM* are:
    a. Hypertension Table and Neoplasm Table
    b. Hypertension Table and Table of Drugs and Chemicals
    c. Neoplasm Table and Table of Drugs and Chemicals
    d. Neoplasm Table and Pain Table
    e. Table of Drugs and Chemicals and Diabetes Table

12. A *carcinoma in situ* is a tumor:
    a. appearing at its original site
    b. that has spread to a second site
    c. that has metastasized
    d. in which the properties are not recognizable
    e. localized or confined to the site of origin

13. When a patient presents with influenza, the type of flu documented in the medical record:
    a. does not have to be verified by positive laboratory serology
    b. needs to be verified by positive laboratory serology
    c. needs to be verified by a laboratory serology of >125
    d. needs to be verified by a laboratory serology of >275
    e. is not coded

14. If documentation in a patient's medical record does not state "open fracture," code it as:
    a. open, if you think it is open
    b. closed
    c. unspecified
    d. undermined fracture type
    e. NOS

15. Burns are classified by:
    a. depth, extent, agent
    b. size, extent, agent
    c. degree, extent, agent
    d. depth, size, agent
    e. depth, extent, type

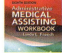

WORKBOOK ASSIGNMENT

To develop competency-based job skills, refer to the *Workbook* and complete the:
- Abbreviation and Spelling Review
- Review Questions
- Critical Thinking Exercises

- Job Skill activities, which are listed at the beginning of the chapter under *Performance Objectives in the Workbook*.

RESOURCES

Codebooks and Resources

American Academy of Professional Coders
    Search: *ICD-10-CM* resources
2015 Coding Workbook for the Physician's Office
    Covell, Alice
    Cengage Learning, 2016
    Website: http://www.cengagebrain.com
3-2-1 Code It, 4th edition
    Green, Michelle
    Cengage Learning, 2014
    Website: http://www.cengagebrain.com
Coding from the Operative Report for ICD-10-CM and PCS, 1st edition
    Optum, 2015
    Website: http://www.cengagebrain.com
Detailed Instructions for Appropriate ICD-10-CM Coding
    Optum, 2015
    Website: http://www.cengagebrain.com

Diagnostic and Statistical Manual of Mental Disorders, 4th edition
    American Psychiatric Press, Inc.
International Classification of Diseases, Tenth Revision, Clinical Modification (ICD-10-CM)
- American Medical Association
- Channel Publishing, Ltd.
- Optum
- Practice Management Information Corporation (PMIC)
Understanding Health Insurance: A Guide to Billing and Reimbursement, 12th edition
    Green/Rowell
    Cengage Learning, 2015
    Website: http://www.cengagebrain.com
Understanding ICD-10-CM and ICD-10-PCS: A Worktext
    Bowie/Schaffer
    Cengage Learning, 2015
    Website: http://www.cengagebrain.com

Understanding Medical Coding: A Comprehensive Guide,
3rd edition
> Johnson, Sandra
> Cengage Learning, 2013
> Website: http://www.cengagebrain.com

Coding and Billing Questions

Part B News
> Subscribe to listserv, ask questions and communicate
> with insurance billers via email

National Correct Coding Initiative (NCCI) Edits
> Centers for Medicare and Medicaid Services (CMS)
> Search: NCCI Edits

Internet

Commonly Administered Pediatric Vaccines/Toxoids
> American Academy of Pediatrics
> Vaccine *CPT* code, name, manufacturer, brand name,
> *diagnostic code*
> Search: Commonly administered pediatric vaccines

General Equivalence Mapping (GEM)
> Search: CMS.gov website

Human Diseases, **4th Edition**
> Neighbors/Tannehill-Jones
> Cengage Learning, 2015
> Website: http://www.cengagebrain.com

ICD-10-CM Official Guidelines for Coding and Reporting
- American Academy of Professional Coders (AAPC)
  > Search: ICD-10 Documentation Training for
  > Physicians
- American Health Information Management Association (AHIMA)
  > Search: Clinical Documentation for ICD-10 Training
- American Hospital Association (AHA)
  > Search: ICD-10 Central Office (reference material)
- Centers for Disease Control and Prevention (CDC)
  > Search: New ICD-10 Draft Guidelines

- Centers for Medicare and Medicaid Services
  > Search: *ICD-10-CM* Documentation Guidelines
  > Road to 10: The Small Physician's Practice route to
  > ICD-10
  > The Provider Perspective (Focus on cost and quality)
- Physicians Practice
  > Search: ICD-10 Resources (multiple articles)
- World Health Organization (WHO)
  > Search: ICD-10 Interactive Self Learning Tools

ICD-10-CM **Implementation Date**
> Federal Register
> Search: Final rule

Medical Dictionaries

- *Fordney's Medical Insurance Dictionary for Billers and Coders*
  > Fordney, Marilyn
  > Saunders/Elsevier
- **Merriam-Webster**
  > English Dictionary, Thesaurus, Medical, Spanish

Medical Encyclopedia

Atlas of the Human Body
> American Medical Association

Standard Code Set

Rules and information for electronic claim submission
> Search: Electronic billing

Media

Critical Thinking for Medical Assistants, **1st Edition**
> Online Video Series—Program 5
> Insurance and Coding: Individual access
> Delmar Learning, 2005
> ISBN13: 978-1-4354-0182-2

HEALTH INSURANCE SYSTEMS AND CLAIM SUBMISSION

LEARNING OBJECTIVES

After reading this chapter and learning step-by-step procedures to gain job skills,* you should be able to:

- Define frequently used insurance terms and abbreviations.
- Identify third-party payers and types of insurance.
- Understand insurance policies, plans, and basic benefits.
- Describe Medicaid and Medicare Parts A, B, C, and D.
- Indicate the three main types of TRICARE coverage.
- Discuss different types of workers' compensation disability coverage.
- Become familiar with data fields on the health insurance claim form.
- State claim submission guidelines and time limits for various insurance programs.
- Name the differences between electronic and paper claim submissions.
- Complete health insurance claims.**
- Determine claim status and follow-up procedures.
- Trace unprocessed insurance claims and describe the appeals process.

PERFORMANCE OBJECTIVES (PROCEDURES) IN THIS TEXTBOOK

- Verify Insurance Coverage (Procedures 18-1).
- Complete the CMS-1500 Health Insurance Claim Form using OCR guidelines (Procedure 18-2).
- Complete an Advance Beneficiary Notice (ABN) Form (Procedure 18-3).

PERFORMANCE OBJECTIVES (JOB SKILLS) IN THE WORKBOOK

- Complete a managed care authorization form (Job Skill 18-1).
- Complete a health insurance claim form for a commercial case (Job Skill 18-2).
- Complete a health insurance claim form for a Medicare case (Job Skill 18-3).
- Complete a health insurance claim form for a TRICARE case (Job Skill 18-4).

---

*This textbook *and the accompanying* Workbook *meet the educational components for entry-level administrative and general competencies outlined by CAAHEP and ABHES.*

**International Classification of Diseases, 10th Revision, Clinical Modification *codes in this chapter are from the 2017* ICD-10-CM.*

KEY TERMS

adjudicate	exclusions	permanent disability (PD)
adjuster	fiscal intermediary	preexisting condition
Advance Beneficiary Notice (ABN)	grace period	premium
beneficiary	insurance agent	provider
benefit list	insurance application	temporary disability (TD)
birthday rule	insured	third-party payer
claim	limitations	time limit
clearinghouse	major medical	total disability
conversion privilege	Medicare Administrative	veteran
coordination of benefits (COB)	Contractor (MAC)	waiting period (w/p)
deductible (deduc)	National Provider Identifier (NPI)	waiver
dependents	partial disability	

HEART OF THE HEALTH CARE PROFESSIONAL

Service

By processing claims accurately, taking care of insurance requests promptly, and solving insurance problems in an efficient and expedient manner, you will serve both the physician and the patient.

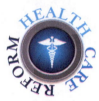

INTRODUCTION TO INSURANCE

In March 2010, the Patient Protection and Affordable Care Act (ACA) was signed. It was designed to insure millions of poor and middle-income Americans in public and private programs. In 2014, Americans started signing up and the number of uninsured dropped by 16.5 million and reached the lowest number in four decades. This was due to the health care law's provision of new affordable state insurance exchanges, the expansion of Medicaid across America, and the requirement for business with 100 or more employees to provide health insurance to 70% of their workers.*

---

*In 2016, companies with 50 or more employees are required to provide health insurance to 95% of their workers; however, some employers are dropping their coverage and instead offering "raises" to help employees buy coverage from state insurance exchanges.

Table 18-1 shows a brief overview of the types of health insurance held among 18- to 64-year-olds in the United States. Reports for the year 2015 indicate the number of uninsured dropped to 12.9%.

With the majority of reimbursement coming into physicians' offices through insurance contracts, the importance of understanding various types of health insurance cannot be overemphasized. The insurance **claim** is the tool used to request insurance payment under an insurance contract. Since the claims process has developed into one of the most sophisticated and complex tasks an administrative medical assistant performs, it is more important than ever for the health care professional to understand how to process claims accurately. A thorough knowledge of all types of insurance and the ability to handle patients' insurance claims competently will not only increase the income and cash flow for the physician's practice but will also enhance the medical assistant's position in a medical office.

Some medical assistants specialize and become insurance claims and coding specialists. Detailed information about procedure coding was discussed in Chapter 16 and diagnostic coding in Chapter 17. For information about the organizations that have certification programs for this fast growing field, refer to Table 1-2 in Chapter 1.

In general, private health insurance and managed care claims follow similar patterns, with variations; therefore, this chapter will cover what the assistant needs to know about (1) insurance terminology; (2) types of insurance and common plans and programs; (3) eligibility and *deductible (deduc)*, coinsurance, or

TABLE 18-1 Types of Health Insurance Coverage in the United States

Types of Health Insurance	2013 3rd Quarter	2013 4th Quarter	2014 1st Quarter	2014 2nd Quarter	2014 3rd Quarter	2014 4th Quarter
Employer	44.4%	44.2%	42.5%	43.5%	43.3%	43.4%
Self-paid	16.7%	17.6%	19.3%	20.7%	20.7%	20.6%
Medicaid	6.8%	6.9%	7.9%	8.4%	8.7%	8.6%
Medicare	6.4%	6.1%	6.3%	6.9%	7.1%	7.5%
Military/veterans	4.3%	4.6%	4.8%	4.7%	4.9%	4.7%
Unions	2.89%	2.5%	2.6%	2.5%	2.4%	2.6%
Other insurance	3.8%	3.5%	3.7%	3.8%	3.6%	4.1%
No insurance	21.2%	20.8%	19.0%	16.2%	16.2%	15.5%

Age 18 to 64 years old (Gallup-Healthways Well-Being Index).

copayment (copay) requirements for each program; (4) basic format and input requirements for claims processed electronically and manually; and (5) claim submission time limits and follow-up procedures.

The medical assistant is not usually expected to interpret fine points in health insurance policies and managed care plans. If questions arise, patients may be instructed to contact their insurance representative.

Insurance Terminology

As with all chapters, you will find key terms that pertain to the chapter subject listed at the beginning of this chapter. They are also boldfaced with definitions within the chapter and listed in the glossary at the end of the textbook. To keep the list of key terms to a reasonable length, you will find numerous italicized terms within this chapter. These terms are also commonly used within the insurance industry, and it is important to take note of their definitions and usage.

THIRD-PARTY PAYERS

The phrase third-party payers comes from the fact that three entities are involved in health care reimbursement:

1. *Patient*—One who receives medical care
2. *Provider*—Physician or supplier who provides medical care and supplies

3. *Public or private payer*—Entity that bears the costs of medical services, such as the insurance company, government program, self-insured employer, or managed care plan

In other words, third-party payers are private insurance companies and insurance programs that pay personal liability claims, workers' compensation claims, and claims for patients seen under the government programs known as Medicaid, Medicare, TRICARE, and CHAMPVA.

America's Health Insurance Plans (AHIP) is a national association that represents health insurers on federal and state regulatory issues. They are a political advocacy group and trade organization with about 1300 member companies that sell insurance to millions of Americans. AHIP publishes research and provides statistical information and data to inform the public and policy makers about health care financing and delivery.

Types of Insurance

A person may purchase health insurance through a private commercial or indemnity contract and pay premiums on an individual basis, or insurance may be purchased where many individuals are covered in one master policy, called a *group contract*. A person can be included in a prepaid managed care health plan, such as a health maintenance organization (HMO), or may be a beneficiary under state or federal government programs such as Medicare, Medicaid, TRICARE, or workers' compensation.

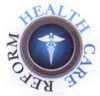

The Affordable Care Act is not just one program, instead it is a series of mandates, regulations, subsidies, and programs that fill areas not previously addressed in the health insurance system. The United States spends trillions of dollars each year on health care and has the highest per capita health care expenditure rate in the world. An estimate for the year 2019 predicts that 19 cents of every dollar will be spent on health care. The cost of health insurance premiums has also doubled over the last decade and has become unaffordable to many Americans. The ACA addressed these problems by shifting the focus to value-based medicine and by devising a new system for Americans to purchase affordable health insurance.

Effective 2015, physician payments will be tied to the quality of care they provide. The insurance-for-all mandate says that most individuals must have minimum essential health insurance coverage or pay a tax penalty. Some individuals will be exempt from the penalty while others may receive financial assistance to help pay for the cost of health insurance coverage. Since the inception of this mandate in 2014, affordable health insurance may be purchased through "marketplaces," called state insurance exchanges. Each type of insurance contract will be discussed in this chapter along with the process of filing a health insurance claim, both manually and electronically.

Commercial Insurance

Commercial insurance plans are owned and run by private companies. Private plans consist of traditional indemnity benefit plans, self-insured plans, and managed care plans, which have been discussed in Chapter 2. Some examples of commercial plans are Aetna Casualty, Allstate, BlueCross/BlueShield, Farmers Insurance, and United American.

Indemnity Insurance—Traditional *indemnity insurance*, also called "fee-for-service plans," offers protection against injury or loss of health and covers a preset number of services. It may only cover hospital costs or pay when an individual is ill or injured. These plans offer flexibility of choice for health care providers or facilities and usually include a **deductible** and copayment amount. The deductible is the amount the insured must pay in a calendar or fiscal year before policy benefits begin.

Self-Insurance—*Self-insurance* is an arrangement in which an employer or other group, such as a labor union, assumes risk and pays for health care expenses usually covered by insurance. This is also known as *self-funding*. Some examples are the Procter & Gamble Company and the Teamsters Union. Self-insured employer groups are regulated by the federal government under the *Employee Retirement Income Security Act of 1974 (ERISA)*. This act protects the interests of workers and their beneficiaries who participate in private pension and welfare plans and also allows an employee not covered by a pension plan other than Social Security to put money aside on a tax-deferred basis to be used for health care expenses. Self-insured employers usually contract with an administrator who processes the claims.

High-Deductible Health Plans—As the name indicates, a *high-deductible health plan (HDHP)* has a higher deductible than traditional plans, for example, an annual deductible of $1100 for an individual or $2200 for self and family coverage. Typically, there are annual out-of-pocket limits (e.g., $5000 for self and $10,000 for self and family), and often those who select this plan will have one of the following:

- *Health Savings Account (HSA)*—Tax-sheltered trust account to which individuals make tax-deferred contributions and tax-free withdrawals for medical expenses (e.g., deductibles and out-of-pocket expenses). Unused funds and interest, without limit, are carried over from year to year.
- *Health Care Flexible Spending Account (HFSA)*—An employer-sponsored benefit where fixed amounts of pretax wages are set aside for qualified expenses (e.g., child care or uncovered medical expenses). The money cannot be rolled over from year to year.

All of the aforementioned plans would be considered *consumer-driven health care (CDHC),** that is, a range of products from which employees can choose that help motivate patients to take charge of their health care budget as well as their health (see Chapter 2).

Group Insurance

Most group insurance is obtained through an employer. However, a patient may be eligible to obtain group insurance through an association or club to which he or she belongs (e.g., American Association for Retired Persons—AARP). If an individual with group coverage

---

*Also referred to as consumer-directed health care.

leaves the employer or organization or the group contract is terminated, the insured may continue with the same or lesser coverage under an individual policy if the group contract has a **conversion privilege**.

The Consolidated Omnibus Budget Reconciliation Act

The *Consolidated Omnibus Budget Reconciliation Act of 1985 (COBRA)* applies to employees who have left their place of employment and requires that an extension of group health insurance be offered to the employee and his or her dependents at group rates for limited periods of time. This federal law applies to employees working for a company with 20 or more workers in certain circumstances, such as a reduction of work hours, transition between jobs, voluntary or involuntary job loss, death, divorce, and other life events. The COBRA premium rates are higher than rates previously paid by the employee for the same insurance, so often this option becomes unaffordable. Those seeking COBRA insurance may find better rates through their state insurance exchanges.

State Insurance Exchanges

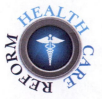

Starting in 2014, new entities called "State Insurance Exchanges," approved by the United States Department of Health and Human Services (HHS), started offering a variety of certified health insurance plans to the general public. These plans will offer four levels of coverage—bronze, silver, gold, and platinum. All plans will include basic benefits such as office visits, maternal and newborn care, pediatric care, laboratory tests, preventive care, prescription drugs, emergency services, hospitalization, rehabilitation care, as well as mental health and substance abuse treatment.

The vast majority of those who already have health insurance can keep their plans; however, insurance carriers are increasing premiums, starting to cap the amount they pay for procedures, and refusing to cover dependents. Those without insurance can use these exchanges as a *marketplace* to compare health care overage and benefits. Health insurance premiums will no longer be based on gender but will vary based on age as well as local and state regulations. To make coverage more affordable, the federal government subsidizes premium costs for certain individuals through a type of federal tax credit called "premium credits." The exchanges also provide information and education services to help consumers understand their options. Not all states have developed their own exchanges. Following are options that were available for states to satisfy this new law:

- Establish one or more exchanges
- Partner with the federal government to run an exchange
- Merge with other state exchanges
- Opt out and have a federal government-run exchange

See *Resources* section at the end of this chapter to determine which option your state selected.

Under the ACA, noncitizens who are "lawfully present" in the United States qualify to participate in, and are subject to, the health insurance mandate. In order to qualify, they must be lawfully present in the United States for the entire term of the insurance policy, that is, 12 months.

In order for this mandate to be effective, every person needs to purchase health insurance so that the overall insurance risk will decrease; however, many of the uninsured are opting to go without health insurance and paying the penalty instead. Penalties for the year 2014 were $95 or 1% of income. This increased to $325 or 2% of income for 2015 and $695 or 2.5% of income for 2016—with additional increased penalties scheduled each year.

Low-cost laboratory services for uninsured patients is another option that is now available (see Any Lab Test Now® in the *Resources* section at the end of this chapter).

Health Insurance Identification Card

The patient's health insurance identification card provides much of the needed data to complete an insurance claim. It is important to verify that the patient presenting at the front desk is the same one named on the card. Refer to Chapter 5 for details on the Red Flags Rule, which can be followed to prevent identity theft.

Ask the patient to show his or her insurance card, and note the effective date and pertinent information. Scan or photocopy both sides of the card and write the current date on the copy for future reference. Figure 18-1 illustrates a health insurance identification card for a private carrier. Cards for other carrier types may be found later in this chapter.

Insurance Benefits

Medical health insurance was originally designed to assist the patient with expenses incurred for medical treatment, not to cover all costs associated with health care. Although basic health insurance coverage provides protection for illness, injury, and disease and includes benefits for hospital and surgical care, it now may also help pay the cost of staying well, which is referred to as *preventive medicine*.

Major medical or *extended benefits* policies are created to help with compensation when an individual encounters large medical expenses caused by long illness or serious injury. Each plan will have a **benefit list** from which coverage determinations are made. Calling the insurance carrier to "precertify" and find out if a service or procedure is covered, or verifying high-dollar procedures with the "predetermination" process, will help inform patients about covered expenses and assist the physician when collecting reimbursement.

Genetic Information Nondiscrimination Act

The *Genetic Information Nondiscrimination Act* of 2008 (GINA) prohibits discrimination in health coverage based on genetic information. GINA defines genetic information as: (1) individual genetic testing, (2) family member genetic testing—up to and including fourth-degree relatives, (3) fetus genetic testing, (4) manifestation of a disease in an individual or family member, and (5) any request for, or receipt of, genetic services or participation in clinical research that includes genetic services by an individual or family member.

The Insurance Policy

The **insured** is the individual who contracts for a policy of insurance coverage; the insured is also known as a *member, policyholder, subscriber,* or *recipient* and may or may not be the patient seen for medical services. For example, if a child is covered by a parent's insurance plan the parent is the insured.

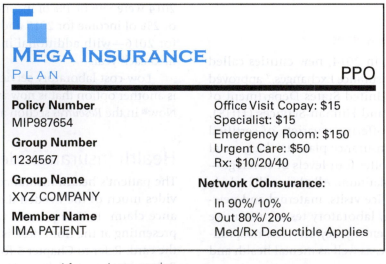

FIGURE 18-1 Health insurance card for a private carrier

To obtain an insurance policy, the individual contacts an **insurance agent** who represents the insurance company and helps the candidate complete an **insurance application**. The *insurance carrier* is an organization that offers a *contract* to protect against losses in exchange for a dollar amount. The application is a signed statement of facts used to determine whether to insure the individual. It becomes part of the health insurance contract if a policy is issued. Before a policy is written, the insurance company may ask the applicant to undergo a physical examination. Information is obtained about the applicant, so the company can decide whether to accept the risk.

An *insurance policy* is a legally enforceable agreement, or contract. If a policy is issued, the applicant becomes part of the insurance contract or plan. Some policies may have a **waiting period (w/p)** (*excepted period* or *elimination period*), which is a time frame after the beginning date of a policy before benefits for illness or injury become payable. A policy might include **dependents** of the insured, which typically are children, spouses, and domestic partners. The policy becomes effective after the company offers it and the person accepts it and then pays the initial **premium**, which is the payment made periodically to keep the policy in force. When a policy includes more coverage, the premiums are higher, but out-of-pocket expenses are reduced. When a policy has less coverage, premiums are lower, but out-of-pocket expenses are increased.

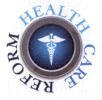

Prior to health care reform, some policies had **exclusions** or **limitations**, which prohibited benefits for certain conditions such as pregnancy and self-inflicted injury, and other policies had **waivers**, which excluded certain illnesses or disabilities that would otherwise be covered. Health care reform ensures that (1) health insurance can no longer be canceled if you get sick, (2) limitations on coverage cannot be imposed when treatment costs go up due to sickness, (3) the lifetime maximum benefit will be eliminated, (4) adult children will be able to stay on their parents health plan until the age of 26, and (5) patients with **preexisting conditions**, that is, conditions that existed and were treated before the policy was issued, cannot be denied insurance.

Since 2010, when you join a new plan, or when your current plan's next coverage year begins, health plans must provide certain preventive services, screenings, and vaccinations free of charge. New health insurance contracts are now written so that no one is denied insurance based on a history of illness, an accident, or disease. At the time these changes were made, approximately 5 million people were considered "uninsurable" due to preexisting conditions.

Verification of Insurance Coverage

Information on the insurance card will be the source document used to verify insurance coverage. This can be done in one of the following ways, by using a/an:

- Online tool, such as the insurance program's website
- Dedicated telephone line
- Point-of-service device, similar to a credit card machine

Refer to Procedure 18-1 for step-by-step instructions when verifying insurance coverage.

Coordination of Benefits

A **coordination of benefits (COB)** statement is included in most policies. If a patient has more than one insurance policy, this prevents duplication of benefits for the same medical expense and is called *nonduplication of benefits*.

Birthday Rule—When a child is covered by both parents, most states honor the **birthday rule**, which helps determine the primary insurance plan. The health plan of the person whose birthday (month and day, *not year*) falls earlier in the calendar year will pay first, and the plan of the other person covering the dependent will be the secondary payer. If both parents have the same birthday, the plan of the person who has had coverage longer is the primary payer. Most states have adopted this law; however, if one of the two plans has not, the plan not abiding by the birthday law determines which plan is primary and which is secondary.

In situations of divorce, the plan of the parent with custody of the child is the primary payer unless the court determines differently and it is so stated in the divorce settlement.

Companies that self-insure their employees and unions do not fall under this law. The states that do not have birthday laws are Georgia, Hawaii, Idaho, Massachusetts, Mississippi, Vermont, and Virginia; also Washington, D.C.

Information about primary versus secondary coverage for specific types of insurance will be discussed under each type of insurance plan.

PROCEDURE 18-1

Verify Insurance Coverage

OBJECTIVE: Verify if the patient has insurance coverage.

EQUIPMENT/SUPPLIES: Insurance card, patient record or other source document, insurance eligibility and benefit form, and computer with Internet connection, point-of-service device, or telephone, and pen.

DIRECTIONS: Follow these step-by-step directions, which include rationales, to learn this procedure.

1. Obtain the insurance card from the patient and scan or copy both sides.
2. Identify the patient's insurance plan or managed care program and verify that the physician's practice participates in the plan.
3. Fill in the demographic and insurance information on the insurance eligibility and benefit form, noting the:
   a. patient's full name and date of birth
   b. subscriber's name
   c. insurance identification number
   d. group's name or number
   e. effective date
   f. insurance company's provider telephone number

4. Contact the insurance carrier and verify the:
   a. patient's name and date of birth
   b. effective date of insurance coverage
   c. basic benefits, exclusions, and noncovered items
   d. specific procedures or surgeries in the patient's treatment plan
   e. patient's financial responsibility for the deductible, copayment, and out-of-pocket expenses
   f. requirements for preauthorization
   g. coordination of benefit rules, if more than one policy is held by the patient
   h. address for sending the insurance claim or payer identification number for electronic claims
5. Document the name, title, and phone extension number of the person giving the information.
6. Document all information received on the insurance eligibility and benefit form, including the date that the insurance eligibility was verified.
7. Notify the patient of eligible and noneligible insurance benefits and any restrictions that apply.

Provider Contracts

Physicians contract with a multitude of insurance plans and programs. Developing a list of payers the medical practice accepts will be invaluable when scheduling new patients, verifying benefits, and answering insurance questions.

The National Alliance of Medical Accreditation Services offers a Certified Professional Managed Care Negotiator (CPMCN) program to learn the most effective strategies to negotiate profitable managed care contracts. The entire contract should be read before agreeing to it. Make sure the contract discloses their full fee schedule and includes a covered services list. Look for vague language and withhold provisions and understand time limitations on filing claims and appeals. Make sure unilateral changes or unlimited

overpayment recovery is not included, and avoid provisions that give the payer the right to arbitrarily adjust and pay claims at a lower level than submitted.

INSURANCE PLANS AND PROGRAMS

To answer patient questions and process insurance claims, a thorough understanding of the various types of insurance plans and programs is necessary. Following is an overview of managed care plans previously presented in Chapter 2, and a discussion of government programs such as Medicaid, Medicare, TRICARE, and CHAMPVA as well as state disability and workers' compensation plans.

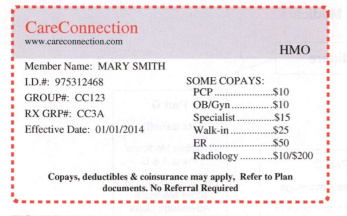

FIGURE 18-2 Managed care (HMO) insurance card showing copayment amounts for various services

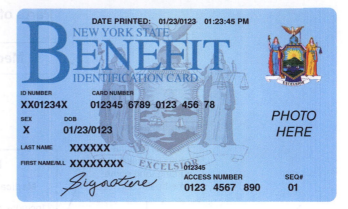

FIGURE 18-3 Medicaid insurance identification card for the state of New York

Managed Care Plans

As discussed in Chapter 2, numerous managed care plans operate under many different contracts with physicians and health facilities. These plans are called *prepaid health plans*. Collecting copayments up front (Figure 18-2) and using network facilities are two important aspects to remember when treating patients using manage care insurance. Although reimbursement is made via monthly capitation checks sent to the medical practice for all participants registered with the physician and the plan, insurance claims (CMS-1500 or electronic version) may be required by the organization for tracking and auditing purposes.

Medicaid

Medicaid is a plan sponsored by federal, state, and local governments. It is an *assistance program* rather than an insurance program. Each state operates its own Medicaid program; however, coverage and benefits vary widely among states. In California, this program is known as Medi-Cal.

In 1967, some states began bringing managed care to their Medicaid programs. Many states have adopted managed care systems as an effort to control escalating health care costs. When the last state, Arizona, joined Medicaid, it started with prepaid care rather than following the way most states had structured their programs.

Individuals with Medicaid have fewer doctors to choose from and may end up in the ER because they do not know where else to go. Because of this, some states have increased the share-of-cost a Medicaid patient pays for office visits (from $1 to $5), emergency room visits,

and hospitalizations as well as limited the number of office visits per year. Check your state's guidelines to verify details about the Medicaid program in your state.

Medicaid Eligibility and Enrollment

Eligibility requirements vary from state to state, but historically the Medicaid program was designed for certain needy and low-income people including people who are blind or disabled, the elderly, pregnant women, and members of families receiving aid to dependent children.

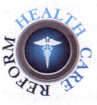

Effective January 2014, the Patient Protection and Affordable Care Act expanded the Medicaid program for millions of nonelderly low-income adults to include 133% of the federal poverty level and made numerous improvements to both Medicaid and the Children's Health Insurance Program (CHIP). States that have implemented Medicaid expansion have seen increased enrollment through the modernized, simpler enrollment process that offers multiple options such an enrollment by phone, mail, or online. Patients may enroll directly to Medicaid or through an insurance exchange marketplace. In many cases, immediate determination of eligibility is possible via an electronic telecommunication system or special computer software program.

A plastic or paper Medicaid identification card (Figure 18-3)—or in some states, coupons is issued either monthly or at other intervals depending on state laws. Scan or photocopy the front and backsides of the card, and carefully check the expiration date and eligibility for the month of service *each time the patient visits*.

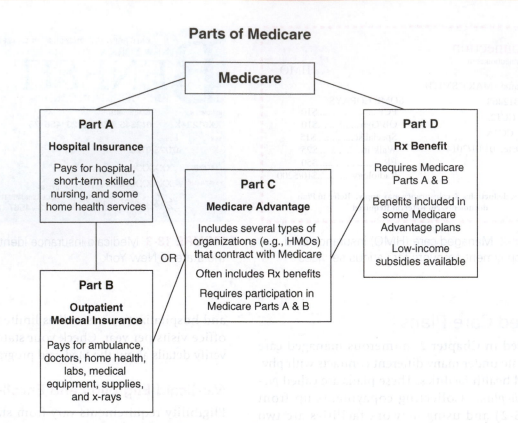

FIGURE 18-4 Brief overview of Medicare Parts A, B, C, and D benefits

The provider's name may also appear on the card, and if so, it would need to be verified monthly. Look to see if the patient has other insurance, copayment requirements, or restrictions (eligible for only certain types of service). Obtain any copayment when the patient comes in for the appointment.

In some instances, prior authorization is required before the service is rendered, unless it is a bona fide emergency. This may be done either via telephone, if urgent, or by completing a special request form (e.g., treatment authorization form [TAR]) and transmitting it electronically or sending it by mail.

Medicare

Medicare is funded by the federal government and administered by the *Centers for Medicare and Medicaid Services (CMS)*. There are several parts of Medicare and Figure 18-4 provides a quick overview of Medicare Parts A, B, C, and D coverage.

Medicare Eligibility and Enrollment

Depending on eligibility, a person may qualify for only Part A, only Part B, or both. At the time of enrollment, a choice is made about how the health care coverage is delivered. The original Medicare plan is a fee-for-service plan, or coverage can be obtained by signing up for Part C, a Senior Advantage plan. Part D offers prescription drug coverage.

A person is eligible for Medicare health insurance coverage at age 65 and when enrolled receives a Medicare health insurance card; application is made through local Social Security Administration (SSA) offices. Medicare is also available to dependent widowers between ages 50 and 65; people who are blind; workers with disabilities of any age including widows, children, and adults who have amyotrophic lateral sclerosis (ALS, Lou Gehrig's disease), chronic kidney disease requiring dialysis, or end-stage renal disease (ESRD) requiring transplant; and kidney donors. Computerized offices can check eligibility online or by calling an interactive voice recognition (IVR) system.

Part A—Medicare Part A covers hospital costs, short-term skilled nursing facility and home care, hospice care, and blood for transfusions. The funds to furnish these health services come from the special contributions of employees and the self-employed and from employers

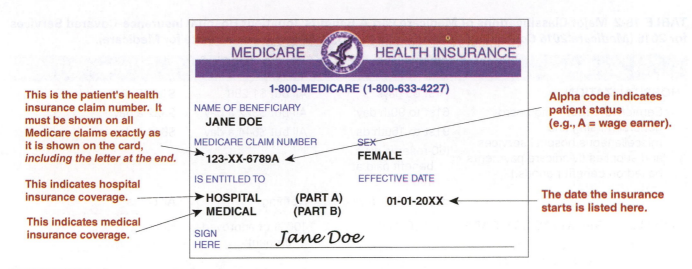

This is the patient's health insurance claim number. It must be shown on all Medicare claims exactly as it is shown on the card, *including the letter at the end.*

This indicates hospital insurance coverage.

This indicates medical insurance coverage.

Alpha code indicates patient status (e.g., A = wage earner).

The date the insurance starts is listed here.

FIGURE 18-5 Medicare health insurance claim card

who pay an amount equal to employees. The contributions are collected as Federal Insurance Contributions Act (FICA) contributions from wages and self-employed income earned during a person's working years.

A hospital *benefit period* begins the day a patient enters a facility and ends when the patient has not been a bed patient in any facility for 60 consecutive days. Each time a patient begins a new benefit period, hospital insurance protection is renewed. Refer to Table 18-2 for information on inpatient Medicare Part A benefits, including benefit periods, what Medicare pays, and what patients' cost-sharing responsibility is.

Part B—Medicare Part B covers outpatient medical services and is referred to as supplementary medical insurance because it supplements Part A, hospital coverage. The funds for this program come from premiums paid by those who sign up for it and from the federal government. The insurance premiums are deducted monthly from Social Security checks, from railroad retirement benefits, and from payments made to those receiving civil service annuities. Others not receiving Social Security benefits pay premiums directly to the Social Security Administration. When working in a physician's office, you will be billing Part B.

Refer to Table 18-3 for information on outpatient Medicare Part B benefits, including benefit periods, what Medicare pays, and what patients' cost-sharing responsibility is.

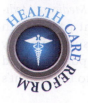

For 2016, the minimum Medicare Part B premium is $104.90 per month. Higher Medicare premiums based on income earnings (starting at $121.80) will be paid by eligible beneficiaries

earning above $85,000 for a single person and $170,000 for married couples filing joint returns; all income levels will be frozen until 2020.

Medicare National and Local Coverage Determinations—Coverage for Medicare services is determined by law, regulation, or *national coverage determinations (NCDs)*. In some situations, local Medicare contractors are authorized to develop *local coverage determinations (LCDs)*, which specify under what conditions a service or item is considered to be "reasonable and necessary." All physician offices billing Medicare patients should be familiar with NCDs and LCDs, which can be found on the CMS website (see *Resources* section at the end of this chapter).

Medicare Opt-Out Providers—According to Section 4507 of the Balanced Budget Act of 1997, "Certain Medicare physicians and practitioners are permitted to 'opt out' of Medicare for two years for all covered items and services that he or she furnishes to Medicare beneficiaries." At the beginning of each calendar quarter, the participating physician may terminate his contract with Medicare Part B. In order for patients to continue seeing the same physician, they have to agree to pay the physician's charges, without regard to any Medicare limits that would otherwise apply (see Chapter 2 under Concierge Medical Care).

Part C—The Balanced Budget Act of 1997 created *Medicare + Choice*, which offers more health care options by allowing Medicare beneficiaries to join managed care plans. These plans provide Parts A and B overage as well as Part D (prescription drug coverage) and are

TABLE 18-2 Major Classifications of Medicare Part A Benefits: Inpatient Hospital Insurance-Covered Services for 2016 (*Medicare 2016 Costs at a Glance.* The Official U. S. Government Website for Medicare).

Services	Benefit	Medicare Pays	Patient Pays
HOSPITALIZATION Semiprivate room and board, general nursing and miscellaneous hospital services and supplies (Medicare payments based on benefit periods.)	First 60 days 61st to 90th day 91st to 150th day (60-reserve-days benefit paid at 100%)[1] Beyond 150 days	All but $1,288 All but $322 a day All but $644 a day Nothing	$1,288 deductible $322 a day $644 a day All costs
SKILLED NURSING FACILITY CARE Patient must have been in a hospital for at least 3 days and enter a Medicare-approved facility generally within 30 days after hospital discharge.[2] (Medicare payments based on benefit periods.)	First 20 days 21st to 100th day Beyond 100 days	100% of approved amount All but $161 a day Nothing	Nothing Up to $161 a day All costs
HOME HEALTH CARE Part-time or intermittent skilled care, home health aide services, durable medical equipment and supplies, and other services	Unlimited as long as Medicare conditions are met and services are declared "medically necessary"	100% of approved amount; 80% of approved amount for durable medical equipment	Nothing for services; 20% of approved amount for durable medical equipment
HOSPICE CARE Pain relief, symptom management, and support services for people who are terminally ill	If patient elects the hospice option and as long as doctor certifies need	All but copay for outpatient drugs and 95% of approved amount for inpatient respite care	Up to $5 copay for outpatient drugs and 5% of approved amount for inpatient respite care
BLOOD	Unlimited if medically necessary	All but first 3 pints per calendar year	For first 3 pints[3]

[1]This 60-reserve-days benefit may be used only once in a lifetime.
[2]Neither Medicare nor private Medigap insurance will pay for most nursing home care.
[3]To the extent the blood deductible is met under Part B of Medicare during the calendar year, it does not have to be met under Part A.

referred to as *Senior Advantage Plans.* Out-of-pocket costs vary as well as rules pertaining to network physicians and referrals.

Prior to health care reform, Medicare paid a larger amount for enrollees in Medicare Advantage plans. Starting in 2014, plans must spend at least 85% of the money they take in from premiums on medical care; copayment amounts are now regulated. People enrolled in Medicare Advantage plans that earn higher incomes will pay higher premiums. Medicare Advantage plan benefits may change each year as well as the size of provider and pharmacy networks. Patients can change

plans during the Annual Election Period each year, so it proves best to compare plans.

If a Medicare patient elects to join a Medicare + Choice managed care plan, there is no need for secondary coverage (e.g., Medigap). The patient agrees to go to doctors, hospitals, and other facilities on the plan's approved list.

Another Medicare + Choice plan is a *Medicare Medical Savings Account (MSA).* The patient pays a high annual deductible for a catastrophic insurance policy approved by Medicare. Premiums for the policy are paid by the patient and deposits are made into the patient's

TABLE 18-3 Major Classifications of Medicare Part B Outpatient Benefits: Medical Insurance-Covered Services for 2016 (*Medicare 2016 Costs at a Glance*. The Official U. S. Government Website for Medicare).

Services	Benefit	Medicare Pays	Patient Pays
MEDICAL EXPENSES Doctor's services, outpatient medical and surgical services and supplies, diagnostic tests, ambulatory surgery center facility fees for approved procedures, and durable medical equipment (such as wheelchairs, hospital beds, oxygen, and walkers). Also covers second surgical opinions, outpatient mental health care, and outpatient physical and occupational therapy, including speech-language therapy.	Unlimited if medically necessary	80% of approved amount (after $166 deductible); reduced to 50% for most outpatient mental health services	$166 deductible, plus 20% of approved amount or limited charges
PREVENTIVE MEDICINE SERICES Selected Preventive Medicine Services	See benefit list for (1) all adults, (2) women, (3) pregnant women, and (4) children (frequency parameters apply)	100% of approved amount	Nothing for services
Physical Examinations	One-time "Welcome to Medicare" physical exam within 12 months of joining Part B. Yearly "Wellness" exams every 12 months	100% of approved amount	Nothing for services
CLINICAL LABORATORY SERVICES Blood tests, urinalyses, and more	Unlimited if medically necessary	100% of approved amount	Nothing for services
HOME HEALTH CARE Part-time skilled nursing care, physical therapy, speech language therapy, home health aide services, medical social services, durable medical equipment (such as wheelchairs, hospital beds, oxygen, and walkers), medical supplies, and other services	Unlimited as long as patient meets conditions and benefits are considered medically necessary	100% of approved amount; 80% of approved amount for durable medical equipment	Nothing for services; 20% of amount for durable medical equipment
OUTPATIENT HOSPITAL TREATMENT Services for the diagnosis or treatment of illness or injury	Unlimited if medically necessary	Medicare payment to hospital based on hospital cost	$166 deductible, plus 20% of the hospital charges
BLOOD	Unlimited if medically necessary	80% of approved amount (after deductible and starting with 4th pint)	First 3 pints plus 20% of approved amounts for additional pints (after deductible)[2]
AMBULATORY SURGICAL SERVICES	Unlimited if medically necessary	80% of predetermined amount (after $166 deductible)	$166 deductible, plus 20% of predetermined amount

[1]Once the patient has had $166 of expenses for covered services in the year, the Part B deductible does not apply to any further covered services received for the rest of the year.
[2]To the extent the blood deductible is met under Part A of Medicare during the calendar year, it does not have to be met under Part B.

MSA equaling the dollar amount difference between what is paid for the average beneficiary in the patient's area and the cost of the premium. The patient uses the money from the MSA to pay medical expenses until the high deductible is reached. Out-of-pocket payments may be necessary if the MSA money runs out before the deductible is met. Unused funds roll over to the next calendar year.

Part D—Medicare Part D is voluntary prescription drug coverage that became effective January 1, 2006. Private insurance companies offer a variety of plans; however, basic standardized benefits are set by the federal government and must be adhered to. Companies can offer benefits that exceed the basic standard, so premiums depend on the particular plan selected and income level of the patient.

The patient may pay an annual deductible, and will pay part of the cost of his or her prescriptions. Each plan has a drug formulary that lists covered generic and brand-name drugs categorized in four "tiers" according to the drug cost and copayment amount (e.g., Tier 1—generic drugs, Tier 2—preferred brand-name drugs). A certain drug may be listed in Tier 1 in one plan and in Tier 2 in another plan, so comparing plans is important. Using preferred network pharmacies provides the lowest prices. Drugs are paid for by Medicare as follows:

- *Part A*—Pays for medications related to hospital stays, skilled nursing facility stays (unless place of residence), and hospice care
- *Part B*—Covers medications that are administered by (or under the supervision of) the physician in the physician's office that cannot be self-administered; oral anti-cancer drugs, hemophilia clotting factors, drugs furnished by dialysis facilities, medication given as part of an outpatient procedure, intravenous immune globulin provided in the home; flu, pneumonia, and hepatitis B vaccines
- *Part D*—Is designed to cover drugs available only by prescription (exceptions apply)

An individual is eligible for Part D prescription drug coverage provided that he or she is entitled to Part A and/or enrolled in Part B and lives in an area where the Part D plan is offered. Enrollment is not automatic unless the patient is dual eligible, that is, enrolled in both Medicare and Medicaid. If the patient is eligible and does not enroll, a late enrollment penalty will be applied that equals 1% per month added to the premium. Those in original fee-for-service Medicare plans can enroll in a Part D Prescription Drug Plan (PDP) that contracts with Medicare. This is considered a stand-alone drug plan. Those who are in Medicare Advantage managed care plans can enroll in that plan's Part D *Medicare Advantage Prescription Drug (MAPD)* plan for combined medical and drug coverage. An annual election period is set aside for patients to change plans if desired.

Part D plans are designed in three levels (see Example 18-1). The first level lists what the patient pays per prescription (copayment amount) up to a dollar

---

EXAMPLE 18–1

Part D Coverage Example

Plan XYZ Premium: $27/Month Deductible: $320/Annually	Tier 1 Generic Drugs	Tier 2 Preferred Brand Drugs	Tier 3 Nonpreferred Brand Drugs	Tier 4 Specialty Brand Drugs
LEVEL I Payment per prescription. *Total yearly drug cost up to $2960	$5 copay	$25 copay	$45 copay	25% coinsurance
LEVEL II Payment per prescription after reaching $2960 total yearly drug costs until annual out-of-pocket expenses reach $4550	100% out of pocket	50% out of pocket	100% out of pocket	100% out of pocket
LEVEL III	The Greater of . . .			
Payment per prescription after yearly out-of-pocket drug costs reach $4550	$2 or 5%	$5 or 5%	$5 or 5%	$5 or 5%

*This amount is when all drug costs reach $2960; not the total of all copayments.

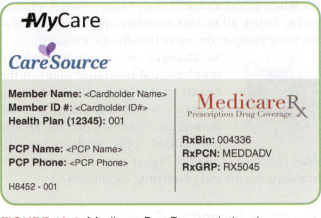

FIGURE 18-6 Medicare Part D prescription drug insurance card

amount (e.g., $2960) for total drug costs. The second level is a coverage gap called the "donut hole" because the patient pays 100% of the cost of all prescriptions until the established yearly out-of-pocket drug cost is met (e.g., $4700*). The third level is a reduced amount that the patient pays per prescription (copay or percentage) *after* the yearly out-of-pocket drug costs have been met, until the year's end. Refer to Figure 18-6 for an illustration of a Medicare Part D prescription drug insurance card.

Medicare Cost Containment

The need to hold down rising health care costs was recognized by the government in the late 1970s, so a number of laws were passed to address cost containment and are discussed here. Provisions in the ACA also address various cost-savings measures and are discussed throughout this chapter.

Tax Equity and Fiscal Responsibility Act—In 1982, the Tax Equity and Fiscal Responsibility Act (TEFRA) was passed. It implemented a *prospective payment system (PPS)* for all hospitalization under the Medicare program (see Chapter 13, Diagnosis-Related Groups).

In 1997, the Balanced Budget Act granted authority to CMS to establish a hospital *Outpatient Prospective Payment System (OPPS)*, which uses ambulatory payment

classifications (APCs) to assign codes for reimbursement of hospital outpatient health care services according to the resources required. This system was modified and refined in 1999 and is used today for hospital outpatient reimbursement.

Peer Review Organization—Under the *Prospective Payment System*, responsibility for maintaining quality of care is given to *Peer Review Organizations (PROs)*. PROs are composed of licensed doctors of medicine or osteopathy actively engaged in the practice of medicine or surgery. PROs review cases and focus on patient admission, readmission, transfer review, and review of procedures. They also study clinical data in cases for additional Medicare reimbursement, day outlier assignments (short and long lengths of hospital stay), the medical necessity of all services rendered, and cost outlier assignments for extraordinarily high costs.

Civil Monetary Penalties Law—To further contain costs, the government passed the *Civil Monetary Penalties Law (CMPL)* in 1983 to prosecute cases of Medicare and Medicaid fraud. A physician may be penalized for every requested payment that violates a Medicare participating or nonparticipating physician agreement. If an assistant submits false billings that the physician knows nothing about, the physician may be held liable. Incorrectly coded procedures can cause penalties to be imposed on a physician. It is the medical assistant's responsibility to keep up to date on all Medicare policies and perform related responsibilities capably and honestly.

Stark I, II, and III Regulations*—In 1992, Stark I was enacted, prohibiting a physician or any member of a physician's family who has a financial relationship with a laboratory from referring patients to that facility. Then in 1995, an amendment, Stark II, was put into effect to expand prohibiting payments for other services where ownership interest is established, such as physical or occupational therapy, durable medical equipment, radiation therapy, and many other ancillary facilities and health-related services.

Stark III became effective in 2007 to reduce the regulatory burden on the health care industry. It addresses both Stark I and II regulations and focuses on physician group practices, modifying previous regulations and

---

*Prescription drug health care reform mandates started in 2011. If the coverage gap is reached, a 50% discount applies to covered brand-name prescription drugs. There will be additional savings in the coverage gap each year through 2020, at which time the gap will disappear and the patient will pay no more than 20% for all prescriptions.

*There are numerous exceptions in the Stark statute and regulations. To read the final rule, search "Stark III final rules, information and regulations."

listing a number of exceptions that apply. Sanctions for violations of the law include denial of payment, required refunds to patients, civil monetary penalties, and exclusion from participation in the Medicare and Medicaid programs.

Physician Quality Reporting System—The Center for Medicare and Medicaid Services (CMS) has requested the reporting of "quality measures" to improve the value received for health care expenditures (see "Meaningful Use," Chapter 9). The Physician Quality Reporting System (PQRS) was developed to serve this purpose and relies on "measures" reported over the course of a patient's treatment. For the development of these measures, clinical input and evidence-based medicine was used, whenever possible.

Medicare/Medicaid

In certain instances, some people qualify for both Medicare and Medicaid, simultaneously. In some states, this coverage is referred to as *Medi-Medi.* Usually these people are disabled, blind, or over age 65 and are entitled to Medicaid benefits, such as *Old Age Security (OAS)* assistance benefits. When patients are covered by both programs, Medicare is considered primary and Medicaid covers the residual not paid by Medicare. On such claims, the physician *must always accept assignment* or the payment goes directly to the patient and the Medicaid program does not pick up the residual.

Senior-Assisted Programs—Pilot and regional Medicaid Senior-Assisted Programs, such as *Doctors Assisting Seniors at Home (DASH)* may be available in your local. DASH is funded by a Health Care Innovation Award from CMS. It is fully covered by Medicare for seniors 60 years and over who live in low-income housing or receive Medicaid benefits. DASH provides rapid response medical treatment to seniors in their own homes—it is a supplement to, not a replacement for, their own doctors. Other program may exist in your area under different names that provide various functions.

Medicare/Medigap

Many Medicare beneficiaries purchase insurance policies regulated by the federal government to assist in paying their portion of medical costs, such as deductibles and copayment amounts. Such policies are referred to as Medigap coverage; they are offered by private insurance companies and controlled by the federal government. Many plans are available and are named using

the letters of the alphabet (e.g., Plan A, Plan B, Plan G, and so forth). All include Medicare-approved benefits—the more you pay, the more benefits are included.

No changes were made to Medigap supplemental insurance plans in the health care reform bill. If Medigap insurance is purchased outside of the limited time frames when full federal protections apply, insurers can still deny coverage or require higher premiums because of health problems and preexisting conditions.

Medicare Secondary Payer

Individuals age 65 years or over who are still employed may have insurance through an employer's health plan, which may be a private or managed care plan. If the employer has 20 or more employees, the employer's sponsored plan is considered primary (first) and Medicare is considered second. These situations are referred to as a *Medicare Secondary Payer (MSP).* Payments for these types of policies may not necessarily go to the physician but may go to the insured. When an employee retires, Medicare becomes the primary coverage and the company's group health plan coordinates benefits with Medicare. These are conversion policies and are not considered "Medigap" as defined by federal law.

Another instance of an MSP claim is when liability insurance is primary to Medicare because the contractual agreement exists between the injured party and the liability insurance company, not Medicare. There are other situations that apply.

TRICARE

TRICARE is a comprehensive health benefits program offering three (TRI) main types of plans for dependents of men and women in the uniformed services (military). To control escalating medical costs and to standardize benefits for regions across the United States and Hawaii, TRICARE has also phased in managed care programs for eligible persons. The three basic plans are:

- *TRICARE Standard*—Fee-for-service cost-sharing plan
- *TRICARE Extra*—Preferred provider organization plan
- *TRICARE Prime*—Health maintenance organization plan with a point-of-service (POS) option

In addition to the three main plans, other plans are offered; the following additional plans are covered in this section:

- *TRICARE Young Adult*—Premium-based plan for qualified dependents who have aged out of TRICARE and are under age 26
- *TRICARE for Life*—Supplemental Medicare plan
- *TRICARE Plus*—Primary care program available at selected military treatment facilities

TRICARE Eligibility

One who qualifies for TRICARE is known as a **beneficiary**. The active duty service member is referred to as the *sponsor*. Beneficiaries entitled to medical benefits under this government program are:

- Spouse and unmarried children up to age 21* (or 23 if full-time student) of uniformed service members who are in (1) active duty,**(2) the United States Coast Guard, (3) Commissioned Corps of the U.S. Public Health Service, or (4) the National Oceanic and Atmospheric Administration
- Eligible children over age 21 with disabilities
- Uniformed service retirees and their eligible family members
- Unremarried spouses and unmarried children of deceased, active, or retired service members
- Former spouses of uniformed service personnel who meet certain length-of-marriage criteria and other requirements
- Physically or emotionally abused spouses, former spouses, or dependent children of uniformed service personnel who were found guilty and discharged for the offense
- Spouses and children of North Atlantic Treaty Organization (NATO) nation representatives (outpatient services only)
- Disabled beneficiaries younger than 65 years of age who have Medicare Parts A and B

Those *not* eligible for TRICARE are:

- Medicare-eligible beneficiaries age 65 and over not enrolled in Medicare Part B
- Veterans eligible for CHAMPVA

---

*See "TRICARE Young Adult" for eligibility beyond age 21 (or 23 if full-time student).
**Active duty service members are entitled to medical benefits in a program called TRICARE Prime Remote.

- Uniformed service member parents or parents-in-law (unless eligible under Supplemental Health Care Program)
- Secretarial designees who are entitled to care at a military treatment facility (MTF) or from a civilian provider

Defense Enrollment Eligibility Reporting System—The sponsor's responsibility is to make sure all TRICARE-eligible persons in his or her family are enrolled in the *Defense Enrollment Eligibility Reporting System (DEERS)* computerized database. The sponsor's Social Security number (SSN) or Department of Defense (DOD) number is used to access DEERS and file claims. Before processing claims, TRICARE claims processors check DEERS to verify beneficiary eligibility.

Providers do not access DEERS; instead, they verify a TRICARE beneficiary's eligibility by reporting the sponsor's SSN or DOD number when logging onto the TRICARE administrator's website, or by using the *Voice Response Unit (VRU)* system, which is manned 24 hours a day. To use this system, call the toll-free number and follow the commands, which will connect to DEERS and provide eligibility information.

Identification Cards—The medical assistant should scan or copy both sides of the beneficiary's identification card and check the expiration date. Although the TRICARE card does not prove eligibility, it has important information (Figure 18-7). The following program cards are not required to obtain medical care: TRICARE Prime, TRICARE Prime Remote, TRICARE Reserve Select, and TRICARE Retired Reserve.

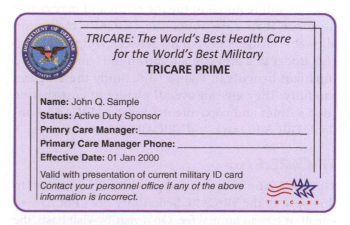

FIGURE 18-7 TRICARE Prime health insurance identification card

TRICARE Standard

The TRICARE program is designed to provide families of uniformed services personnel and service retirees with comprehensive health care coverage in military and civilian health care facilities. All those who qualify are automatically enrolled in the TRICARE Standard program with no enrollment fee.

TRICARE Benefits—Those on the TRICARE Standard program may receive a wide range of civilian health care services with a portion of the cost paid by the federal government. Patients usually seek care from a military hospital near their home. In certain areas or in certain situations, they can seek care through a private physician's office. The patient pays a deductible for outpatient care and cost-sharing percentages. If the provider signs a contract, accepts assignment, and files a claim, he or she accepts the TRICARE allowable fee as the full amount for the services rendered.

If the provider does not accept assignment, the physician is still required to file the claim and may charge no more than 15% above the TRICARE maximum allowable charge for his or her services. Outpatient benefits under this program are shown in Figure 18-8 and inpatient benefits in Figure 18-9. Study these figures carefully. They give an overall picture of cost-sharing (deductibles and copayments) for the TRICARE Standard, TRICARE Extra, and TRICARE Prime programs.

TRICARE Extra

TRICARE Extra is a preferred provider organization. In this option, the TRICARE beneficiary does not have to enroll or pay an annual fee. On a visit-by-visit basis, the individual may seek care from a provider who is part of the TRICARE Extra network and receive a discount on services and reduced cost-shares. Therefore, a beneficiary may bounce back and forth between network and nonnetwork providers on a visit-by-visit basis and receive benefits from both TRICARE Standard and TRICARE Extra options. No identification card is issued, because the individual presents a military identification card when receiving care. Eligibility still needs to be verified online or by using the VRU system.

TRICARE Prime

TRICARE Prime coverage options include TRICARE Prime, TRICARE Prime Remote, and TRICARE Prime Remote for Active Duty Family Members. These are all managed care (HMO-type) options offering the most affordable and comprehensive coverage. Retirees, family members, and survivors pay an annual fee per person or per family but active duty service members and their families do not. As shown in Figures 18-8 and 18-9, benefits and covered services include preventive and primary care. Medical care is rendered from within a Prime network of civilian and military providers. The beneficiary has the option of choosing or being assigned a *primary care manager (PCM)* for each family member. This provider furnishes and manages all aspects of the patient's health care, including referrals to specialists. For *active duty service members (ADSMs)* and their families who work and live more than a 60-minute drive from an MTF, the TRICARE Prime Remote program is available, which enables these individuals to receive care from any TRICARE-certified civilian provider.

Active duty service members are enrolled automatically in TRICARE Prime and use local military providers and, when directed, the civilian portion of the TRICARE network. There are no annual deductibles, and copayments vary (see Figure 18-8). A dental plan is available for an additional monthly premium. Outpatient or ambulatory surgery must be verified against the approved procedure list in the TRICARE Policy Manual before it is performed.

Enrollees are issued a TRICARE Prime identification card (Figure 18-7), but this does not guarantee eligibility. Providers must call the automated Voice Response Unit system to verify eligibility. Photocopy both sides of the military identification card and the TRICARE Prime card, and retain them in the patient's file. Check both cards at every visit. Beneficiaries who are not enrolled as members in TRICARE Prime may continue to receive services through TRICARE Extra from network providers or through TRICARE Standard using nonnetwork providers.

ADFM = active duty and family members RFMS = retires (under 65), family members and survivors	**Benefit and Coverage Chart**					
OUTPATIENT SERVICES	**Programs and Beneficiary Costs**					
Program and Classification	**TRICARE Prime**		**TRICARE Extra**		**TRICARE Standard**	
	ADFM	**RFMS**	**ADFM**	**RFMS**	**ADFM**	**RFMS**
Annual Enrollment Fee* (per fiscal year)	None	$282.60/person $565.20/family	None ———————→		None ———————→	
Annual Deductible (per fiscal year 10/1 to 9/30) (applied to outpatient services before cost-share is determined)	None (except when using point-of-service option)		E-4 and below $50/person $100/family E-5 and above $150/person $300/family	$150/person $300/family	E-4 and below $50/person $100/family E-5 and above $150/person $300/family	$150/person $300/family
Physician Services	None	$12	15% of contracted fee	20% of contracted fee	20% of maximum allowable charge	25% of maximum allowable charge
Ambulance Services	None	$20				
Durable Medical Equipment (greater than $100)	None	20% cost-share				
Emergency Services (network and non-network)	None	$30 copayment				
Outpatient Behavioral Health (limitations apply)	None	$25 copayment $17 group visits				
Ambulatory Surgery (same day)	None	$25 copayment (applied to facility charges only)	$25 copayment for hospital charges	20% of contracted fee	$25 copayment for hospital charges	*Professional:* 25% of maximum allowable charge *Facility:* 25% of maximum allowable charge OR billed charges, whichever is less

*No enrollment fee for those who are eligible for Medicare (enrolled in Part B) on the basis of disability or end–stage renal disease

NOTE:TRICARE Prime Remote–benefits are similar to TRICARE Prime program; however, ADSMs have no copayment, costshare, or deductible

Program for Persons with Disabilities–no deductible; monthly cost-share varies from $25 to $250, depending on sponsor's rank

FIGURE 18-8 TRICARE Prime, Extra, and Standard Outpatient Service Benefits and Coverage Chart

Nonavailability Statement—A Nonavailability Statement (NAS) is a certification by a *Uniformed Services Medical Treatment Facility (USMTF)*, usually a hospital, when a specific type of nonemergency care is not available at that facility, at a specific time, to a patient who needs care and who lives within the hospital's ZIP code service area. For all *outpatient* services from civilian sources, patients do not need *Nonavailability Statements*.

NASs are required for nonemergency *inpatient* care from civilian sources for those people who live within the service areas of one or more uniformed services hospitals and who get their civilian care under TRICARE Standard or TRICARE Extra. An inpatient NAS is not required for persons enrolled in TRICARE Prime or who use the POS option and live within the service area of a uniformed services hospital.

The only exception is that in areas where TRICARE contracts are in operation, providers who see TRICARE-eligible persons must obtain preauthorization for

ADFM = active duty and family members RFMS = retires (under 65) family members and survivors	**Benefit and Coverage Chart**					
INPATIENT SERVICES	**Programs and Beneficiary Costs**					
Program and Classification	**TRICARE Prime**		**TRICARE Extra**		**TRICARE Standard**	
	ADFM	**RFMS**	**ADFM**	**RFMS**	**ADFM**	**RFMS**
Hospitalization*	No copayment	$11/day or $25 min charge per/admission, whichever is greater	$18.00/day or $25 min charge per/admission, whichever is greater	$250/day or 25% cost-share whichever is less, plus 20% for separately billed professional charges	$18.00/day or $25 min charge per/admission, whichever is greater	$810/day or 25% cost-share whichever is less, plus 25% cost-share for separately billed professional charges
Skilled Nursing Care			$25/admission, or $18.00/day whichever is greater	$250/day or 20% cost-share + 20% cost-share for separately billed charges	$25/admission, or $18.00/day whichever is greater	25% cost-share (billed charges), plus 25% cost-share for separately billed professional charges
*Preauthorization required						

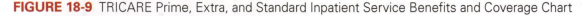

FIGURE 18-9 TRICARE Prime, Extra, and Standard Inpatient Service Benefits and Coverage Chart

certain procedures, or the amount of payment may be reduced by 10% or more.

Call the *health benefits advisor (HBA)* at the nearest military medical facility to verify the procedures, the approved facility, and the need for an NAS before scheduling surgery. If no preauthorization is obtained, a POS option is available featuring an annual outpatient deductible and 50% cost-share. Patients may need prior authorization for nonemergency care received while away from the area in which they are enrolled.

TRICARE Young Adult

TRICARE Young Adult (TYA) is a premium-based plan available for purchase by qualified dependents who are no longer eligible for TRICARE.

TYA Eligibility—Eligibility for TYA is established by the uniformed service sponsor. Young adult dependents must prove their eligibility by being enrolled in the Defense Enrollment and Eligibility Reporting System (DEERS). They may purchase TYA coverage if they:

- Are a dependent of an eligible uniformed service sponsor
- Are under age 26

- Have "aged out" of TRICARE at age 21 or 23 and are a full-time college student
- Are not married
- Are not a member of the uniformed services
- Do not qualify for an employer-sponsored health plan
- Are not eligible for other TRICARE coverage

TRICARE for Life

TRICARE for Life (TFL) is a health care program funded by the Department of Defense (DOD) offering additional TRICARE benefits as a supplementary payer to Medicare.

TFL Eligibility—Those eligible are uniformed service retirees, their spouses, and survivors age 65 and over. Most beneficiaries must be eligible for Medicare Part A and enrolled in Medicare Part B to qualify for TFL. An exception is Uniformed Services Family Health Plan (USFHP) members. TFL beneficiaries do not have to enroll, but they do need to be enrolled in DEERS. Beneficiaries who qualify for TFL do not need a TRICARE enrollment card. There are no preauthorization requirements for the TFL program. For coverage, all services and supplies must be a benefit of the Medicare program, TRICARE program, or both.

TRICARE Payment Guidelines—Payment guidelines for primary versus secondary coverage are as follows:

1. *Services covered under Medicare and TRICARE*— Medicare pays the Medicare rate and TRICARE covers the beneficiary's deductible and cost-share. No copayment, cost-share, or deductible is paid by the TFL beneficiary.
2. *Services covered under Medicare, but not TRICARE*— Medicare pays the Medicare rate and the beneficiary pays the Medicare cost-share and deductible amounts.
3. *Services covered under TRICARE, but not Medicare*— TRICARE pays the TRICARE-allowed amount and Medicare pays nothing. The beneficiary is responsible for the TRICARE cost-share and the deductible amounts.

TRICARE Plus

TRICARE Plus is a military treatment facility (MTF) primary care program available at selected MTFs. Persons who normally get care at an MTF and are not enrolled in TRICARE Prime or a commercial HMO are eligible. There is no enrollment fee.

Enrollees of TRICARE Plus receive an identification card and are identified in the DEERS.

CHAMPVA

The *Civilian Health and Medical Program of the Veterans Administration (CHAMPVA)*, now known as the Department of Veterans Affairs, is a service benefit program; therefore no premiums are paid. A **veteran** is anyone who has served in the United States Armed Forces and has received an honorable discharge.

CHAMPVA Eligibility

The Veterans Health Care Expansion Act of 1973 (PL93082) authorized a TRICARE-like program for the spouses and children of veterans with total, permanent, service-connected disabilities, and for the surviving spouses and children of veterans who die as a result of service-connected disabilities.

CHAMPVA Benefits

CHAMPVA covers most medically necessary health care services. A comprehensive list of preventive services and noncovered services is provided in the CHAMPVA handbook, which can be found online. Typically, prior authorization is not needed, except for select services

U.S. Department of Veterans Affairs Veterans Health Administration Chief Business Office Purchased Care **VA** CHAMPVA	**Open Access No Referral Required**

Beneficiary Name

Include this <u>Member Number</u> on all claims and letters
"Patient SSN"
This is your Identification Card

Effective Date	Expiration Date	**CHAMPVA** 1- 800 -733 - 8387 www.va.gov/hac

CHAMPVA pays after most other health plans. Include an explanation of benefits from other insurers. CHAMPVA is primary to Medicaid.

Once you become eligible for Medicare part A, you must obtain and maintain Medicare part B to remain eligible for CHAMPVA.

For Electronic Claims Filing please follow the instructions at: **www.va.gov/hac/forproviders** under "How to File a Claim."

For Mental Health/Substance Abuse Authorization Call 1-800-424-4018—Authorization is required: • After 23 outpatient mental health visits in a calendar year • For all other mental health/substance abuse services **For Durable Medical Equipment (DME) Authorization** Call 1-800-733-8387—Authorization is required: • For DME purchase or rental over $2,000

FIGURE 18-10 Front and back sides of a CHAMPVA insurance identification card

(e.g., durable medical equipment [DME], hospice care, mental health).

When a CHAMPVA beneficiary presents in the office, scan or copy both sides of the patient's CHAMPVA identification card (Figure 18-10). There is a $50 annual deductible ($100 per family) for outpatient services and if the provider agrees to accept assignment, 75% of the allowable fee is paid by CHAMPVA and 25% is collected from the patient. Ninety days prior to a beneficiary turning 65 years old, CHAMPVA automatically enrolls the patient in Medicare Parts A and B. To continue CHAMPVA eligibility, the patient must enroll in, and remain enrolled in, Medicare Part B.

State Disability Insurance

State Disability Insurance (SDI) is insurance that gives coverage for off-the-job injury or sickness and is paid for by deductions from a working individual's paycheck. This program is administered by a state agency and is sometimes known as *Unemployment Compensation Disability (UCD)*. SDI programs are available in five states (California, Hawaii, New Jersey, New York, and Rhode Island) and Puerto Rico. SDI deductions are discussed briefly in the payroll section of Chapter 19.

Benefits begin after the seventh consecutive day of disability. An employee is also entitled to disability benefits from a previous disability or illness if he or she has returned to work for 15 days and then becomes ill with the same ailment. Most states mentioned have maternity benefits that may be applied for when maternity leave is taken. There are some limitations, so it is important for the medical assistant to contact the state agency regarding current regulations. With the exception of Hawaii and Puerto Rico, most states' programs do not allow hospital benefits. If you do not live in one of the above-mentioned states, short- or long-term disability benefits may be purchased privately or from an employer prior to getting pregnant, injured, or sick.

The definition of total disability varies in each of the five states, but a general definition might be that the insured must be unable to perform the major duties of his or her specific occupation. This may be temporary or permanent. The term partial disability may be defined as when an illness or injury prevents an insured person from performing one or more of the functions of his or her regular job either temporarily or permanently.

Workers' Compensation

An industrial accident or disease is an unforeseen, unintended event arising out of one's employment. Workers' compensation is a form of insurance paid by the employer and provides cash benefits to a worker injured or disabled in the course of his or her employment. The worker is also entitled to benefits for some or all of the medical services necessary for treatment and restoration to resume a useful life, and in some instances, the worker is rehabilitated and trained for a new job.

Workers' Compensation Laws

Workers' compensation (WC) programs are mandatory under state laws in all states. Some of their goals are to provide the best medical care to achieve maximum recovery, to get the ill or injured individual back to work, and to provide income to prevent the injured from having to go on welfare. The following are a number of federal workers' compensation laws that have been enacted:

1. *Workmen's Compensation Law of the District of Columbia* provides benefits for workers in Washington, D.C.

2. *Federal Coal Mine Health and Safety Act* provides benefits to coal miners
3. *United States Longshoremen's and Harbor Workers' Compensation Act* provides benefits for private or public employees engaged in maritime work
4. *Federal Employees' Compensation Act (FECA)* provides benefits for on-the-job injuries to all federal workers

In industrial injury (WC) cases, the contract exists between the physician and the insurance carrier. The insurance company adjuster is an employee of the WC carrier who handles the case, gives verbal authorization for testing, procedures, surgeries, and referrals, and follows the case until it is "adjusted" or settled. When an adjuster telephones for information on a case, the medical assistant should verify who the adjuster is before providing medical information. Such cases do not require a signed consent from the patient to release information.

If the patient is a private patient of the physician, a separate medical record and financial account should be maintained for the industrial accident or illness. If the injured or ill person has several different industrial accidents on different dates, separate financial accounts and medical records are required for each situation.

Types of Disability

There are three types of workers' compensation claims: nondisability, temporary disability, and permanent disability. A *nondisability* claim is one in which the patient is seen by the physician but may continue to work. Temporary disability (TD) claims are those in which the injured cannot perform all the functions of his or her job for a limited period of time. Weekly TD benefits are based on the employee's earnings at the time of the injury. Permanent disability (PD) claims are those in which the injured worker is left with residual disability. Sometimes, such a person can be rehabilitated in another occupation; however, recent reforms in workers' compensation in some states replaced vocational rehabilitation with a voucher system that is not issued until after the case is settled. When the employee's condition becomes *permanent and stationary (P & S)* and no further improvement is expected, the industrial case is rated as to the percentage of permanent residual disability and adjudicated so that a monetary settlement (payment) can be made, called a *compromise and release (C & R)*. This settlement can be awarded as a lump sum or in the form of monthly payments.

Notification of an Injury and Sending the Doctor's Report

The employee must inform the employer promptly should a work-related injury occur, preferably within 48 hours; however, some state laws require notification within 21 to 45 days. In some states, an oral notification is accepted but in other states the notification must be in writing. The notice should include the date, time, location, and circumstances surrounding the accident. It is the employer's responsibility to pay for all first aid and emergency services, two treating physicians, surgeons or hospitals of the employee's choice, and any additional medical providers to whom the employee is referred by the two physicians, surgeons, or hospitals. When seeing a patient in the office for an industrial injury, services provided may be for an initial visit, consultation, or second opinion.

In most states, an initial report is submitted by both the employer and the physician; it is a requirement of the law. The form and time limit to submit the report vary with each state. Copies of the first report (Figure 18-11) go to the insurance carrier, the state, and the employer, and one copy is retained by the physician. The initial report contains the history of the accident, present complaints (subjective information), past history, findings on physical examination (objective observations), laboratory and x-ray results, diagnosis, recommended treatment, disability (type and length), and prognosis.

Subsequent reports informing the carrier of the progress of the injured or ill worker are submitted each time the patient is seen or every 30 to 45 days. If the patient is seen more than once in a 30-day period, there needs to be a significant change in his or her condition in order for the provider to get paid. These reports entail either completing forms, writing a letter, or copying the patient's chart. Refer to the *Resources* section at the end of this chapter for information about the employer or physician reporting schedule for various states, and for information on where to find the Doctors' First Report of Injury or Illness for your state.

GENERAL GUIDELINES FOR HANDLING INSURANCE CLAIMS

To process insurance claims, it is important to understand the path that must be traveled to obtain information that ultimately will be incorporated in the claim. Refer to Figure 18-12 to review important points along the information-gathering pathway.

Patient Registration Process

The complete, accurate, and up-to-date information obtained on the patient registration form discussed in Chapter 5 and illustrated in Figure 5-5 is the same data abstracted and included on an insurance claim form. The importance of obtaining complete and accurate source information cannot be overstressed. This information needs to be reverified frequently for claims to be processed efficiently.

Assignment and Consent

The CMS-1500 claim form includes an assignment of benefits (Field 12 for government programs and Field 13 for private insurance). If the physician has a contract with the insurance company or wishes to have the insurance check sent to the office, the patient is asked to sign the assignment of benefits statement either on the form or on a separate form kept in his or her file.

Scan or photocopy the assignment of benefits and attach it to every insurance claim when (1) submitting a workers' compensation claim, (2) submitting a personal injury insurance claim, or (3) if you know a payer tends to send the insurance check to the patient.

A consent to release medical information statement also appears in Field 12 of the CMS-1500 claim form. As mentioned in Chapter 3, patients may sign an informed consent to release medical information for treatment, payment, and operations but this is no longer mandated by HIPAA. Although this statement appears on the claim form, if a consent is obtained it is best to use a separate *consent form* that is kept in the patient's file.

Medicare Lifetime Beneficiary Claim Authorization and Information Release

Medicare states that "To insure informed consent of Medicare beneficiaries to release information and Medicare payment information to third-party carriers, physicians and suppliers must have their patients and customers sign and date an authorization statement." A lifetime authorization form containing a *signature on file* may be used—it must contain the specific language found in Figure 18-13.

THE HEALTH INSURANCE CLAIM

When all of the source data has been collected, the life cycle of the insurance claim goes through four major stages: (1) claim submission, (2) claim processing, (3) claim adjudication, and (4) payment (Figure 18-14).

STATE COMPENSATION INSURANCE FUND

DOCTOR'S FIRST REPORT OF OCCUPATIONAL INJURY OR ILLNESS STATE OF CALIFORNIA

Within 5 days of your initial examination, for every occupational injury or illness, send original and one copy of this report to the employer's workers' compensation insurance carrier or the self-insured employer. Failure to file a timely doctor's report may result in assessment of a civil penalty. In the case of diagnosed or suspected pesticide poisoning, send a copy of this report to Division of Labor Statistics and Research, P.O. Box 420603, San Francisco, CA 94142-0603, and notify your local health officer by telephone within 24 hours.

	PLEASE DO NOT USE THIS COLUMN
1. INSURER NAME AND ADDRESS STATE COMPENSATION INSURANCE FUND P.O. BOX 9045, OXNARD, CA 93031-9045	Case No.
2. EMPLOYER NAME Tri Color Paint Company Policy # 189-2467-344	
3. Address: No. and Street 4200 Main Street, City Woodland Hills, XY Zip 12345-0000	Industry
4. Nature of business (e.g., food manufacturing, building construction, retailer of women's clothes) commercial painting company	County
5. PATIENT NAME (First name, middle initial, last name) Jack P. Hiner 6. Sex ☒ Male ☐ Female 7. Date of Birth Mo. Day Yr. 11 - 02 - 55	Age
8. Address: No. and Street City Zip 789 Stanton Avenue, Woodland Hills, XY 12345-0000 9. Telephone number (555) 509-8760	Hazard
10. Occupation (Specific job title) house painter 11. Social Security Number XXX- XX - 1298	Disease
12. Injured at: No. and Street 5409 West First Street City Woodland Hills, County Los Angeles	Hospitalization
13. Date and hour of injury or onset of illness Mo. Day Yr. 10 - 20 - 20XX a.m. 4:00 p.m. Hour 14. Date last worked Mo. Day Yr. 10 - 20 - 20XX	Occupation
15. Date and hour of first examination or treatment Mo. Day Yr. 10 - 20 - 20XX a.m. 5:30 p.m. Hour 16. Have you (or your office) previously treated patient? ☐ Yes ☒ No	Return Date/Code

Patient please complete this portion, if able to do so. Otherwise, doctor please complete immediately. Inability or failure of a patient to complete this portion shall not affect his/her rights to workers' compensation under the California Labor Code.

17. DESCRIBE HOW THE ACCIDENT OR EXPOSURE HAPPENED (Give specific object, machinery or chemical. Use reverse side if more space is required.)

While painting a room ceiling, I slipped and fell from a ladder and hit the left side of my body and my head.

18. SUBJECTIVE COMPLAINTS (Describe fully. Use reverse side if more space is required.)

Left shoulder pain, head pain, dizziness, blurred vision

19. OBJECTIVE FINDINGS (Use reverse side if more space is required.)

A. Physical Examination

Abrasions, multiple contusions and sprain of the left shoulder, 2.5 cm head laceration; 2 views each AP & lat of lt hip, lt femur, and cervical spine, all negative.

B. X-ray and laboratory results (State if none or pending.)

20. DIAGNOSIS (If occupational illness, specify etiologic agent and duration of exposure.) Chemical or toxic compounds involved? ☐ Yes ☒ No

Abrasions, multiple contusions, and sprain of the left shoulder. Head laceration.   ICD-10 Code M 2 5 5 1 2*

21. Are your findings and diagnosis consistent with patient's account of injury or onset of illness? ☒ Yes ☐ No   If "no", please explain.

21A. Based on your evaluation, is the injury/illness work related? ☒ Yes ☐ No ☐ Further investigation needed

22. Is there any other current condition that will impede or delay patient's recovery? ☐ Yes ☒ No   If "yes", please explain.

23. TREATMENT RENDERED (Use reverse side if more space is required.) Examination, x-rays, treated for abrasions and contusions, 2.5 cm head laceration sutured, to be kept under observation in hospital to rule out head trauma.

24. If further treatment required, specify treatment plan/estimated duration. Hospital observation

25. If hospitalized as inpatient, give hospital name and location. College Hospital, 4500 Broad Ave., Woodland Hills   Date admitted Mo. Day Yr. 10-20-20XX   Estimated stay 1 day

26. WORK STATUS – Is patient able to perform usual work? ☐ Yes ☒ No If "no", date when patient can return to: Regular work 11 / 1 / 20XX Modified work 10 / 29 / 20XX   Specify restrictions No lifting

Doctor's Signature *Gerald Practon, MD* Date 10-22-20XX   CA License Number C 4821X
Doctor Name and Degree (please type) Gerald Practon, MD   IRS Number 95-366402XX
Address 4567 Broad Avenue, Woodland Hills, XY 12345-0000   Telephone Number (555) 486 9002

wtf
SCIF 3110 (REV. 2-93)   FORM 5021 (Rev. 4) 1992

FIGURE 18-11 Example of a completed Doctor's First Report of Occupational Injury or Illness form from the state of California for a workers' compensation case

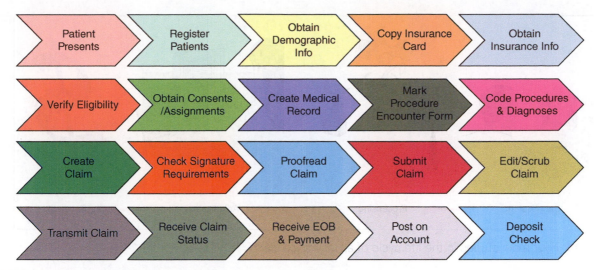

FIGURE 18-12 Path of information collected and traveled during the claims process

---

PRACTON MEDICAL GROUP, INC.

4567 BROAD AVENUE • WOODLAND HILLS, XY 12345-4700
OFFICE: (555) 486-9002 • FAX: (555) 488-7815

Fran Practon, M.D.
Gerald Practon, M.D.

LIFETIME BENEFICIARY CLAIM AUTHORIZATION AND INFORMATION RELEASE

Patient's
Name __Busaba McDermott__ Medicare I.D. Number __329-XX-6745__

I request that payment of authorized Medicare benefits be made either to me or on my behalf to (name of physician/supplier) for any services furnished me by that physician/supplier. I authorize any holder of medical information about me to release to the Health Care Financing Administration and its agents any information needed to determine these benefits or the benefits payable to related services.

I understand my signature requests that payment be made and authorizes release of medical information necessary to pay the claim. If other health insurance is indicated in Item 9 of the CMS-1500 claim form or elsewhere on other approved claim forms or electronically submitted claims, my signature authorizes releasing of the information to the insurer or agency shown. In Medicare assigned cases, the physician or supplier agrees to accept Medicare's allowed amount. The carrier pays 80% of the allowed amount and the patient is responsible for the deductible, 2090 coinsurance, and noncovered services. Coinsurance is based upon the allowed amount of the Medicare carrier.

__Busaba McDermott__   __May 15, 20XX__
Patient's Signature   Date

FIGURE 18-13 Medicare Lifetime Beneficiary Claim Authorization and Information Release form. The patient's signature field on the CMS-1500 claim form should be submitted with this notation: "Signature on File" (SOF)

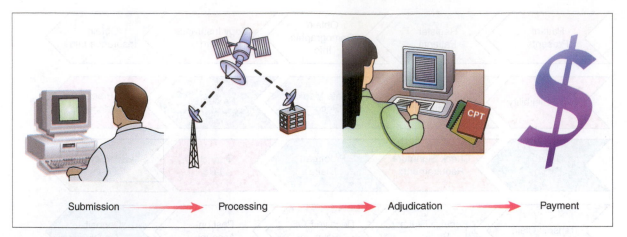

FIGURE 18-14 Four main stages in the life cycle of an insurance claim

Two methods are used to complete health insurance claims for submission to insurance carriers. The electronic claim is the recommended method and has many advantages that will be discussed later in this chapter. The longstanding method, the paper claim, referred to as the CMS-1500 claim form is submitted manually and although this method is being phased out, it is still in use. Learning the field requirements of paper claims will help you understand various data elements that need to be completed, proofread, and edited in an electronic format.

The CMS-1500 Claim Form

The CMS-1500 Health Insurance Claim Form (02/12) is accepted by most health insurers for outpatient services. It is the basic form prescribed by the Centers for Medicare and Medicaid Services (CMS), and it has received the approval of the American Medical Association (AMA) Council on Medical Services. The Health Insurance Association of America (HIAA) endorses the CMS-1500 and recommends that their members (private insurance companies) accept the form. TRICARE also approves the form and in some states, the CMS-1500 claim form can be used for industrial claims. Ambulatory Surgery Centers (ASCs) use a combination of physician and hospital billing for outpatient surgical services. Some third-party carriers will accept the CMS-1500 form and others request the hospital billing form, UB04.

The red printed version of the CMS-1500 form was developed, so insurance carriers could process claims by optical character recognition (OCR) for speed and efficiency. The scanner transfers the data on the insurance claim directly to a computer's memory, thus eliminating the need to key it separately. Quantities of the CMS-1500 can be purchased from the United States Government Printing Office, the AMA, or large medical office supply companies (see the *Resources* section at the end of this chapter). The forms may be personalized to the medical practice. All insurance claims should be submitted as soon as possible after the service is performed.

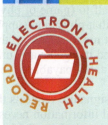

COMPLIANCE
Transaction Code Set

The Health Insurance Portability and Accountability Act (HIPAA) developed standards for the electronic transmission of protected patient information; this is known as the Transaction Code Set. The code set specifies the format to be used by insurance carriers when submitting electronic claims, referred to as the HIPAA X12 Version 5010 Health Care Claim: Professional. All entities (i.e., providers, clearinghouses, vendors, and health insurance carriers) that transmit protected health information are required to comply with HIPAA law and use this standard. The various fields on a CMS-1500 paper claim closely parallel electronic transmission standards and each data element field has a number and a name that correspond to a field on the CMS-1500 claim form (see Example 18-2).

EXAMPLE 18-2

CMS-1500 and Version 5010 Data Field Comparison

Field No. for CMS-1500	Field Name for CMS-1500	Data Element No. for Version 5010	Data Element Name for Version 5010
2	Patient name	2010BA, NN1/IL, 03 2010BA, NN1/IL, 04	Patient last name
3	DOB Sex	2010BA, DMG, 02 2010BA, DMG, 03	Patient date of birth Patient gender code
12	Patient or authorized person's signature	2300, CLM, 10	Patient's signature
25	Provider SSN# or EIN#	2010AA, REF, 02 R	Rendering provider identification

*For a complete crosswalk of all fields on the CMS-1500 Claim Form, Google: CMS-1500 Claim Form Crosswalk to ANSI 837 v5010

Completing the Claim

If it is office policy to complete and submit the insurance claim for the patient, the assistant should do so even in situations when coverage of specific services is in question. An official rejection from the carrier may be the best explanation to present to the patient. Electronic submission is preferred; however, if paper claims are being processed, the assistant should use the CMS-1500 Health Insurance Claim Form.

Instructions for individual fields on the CMS-1500 claim form for the major programs are included in Appendix A of this *textbook*: (1) commercial carriers, (2) Medicare, (3) Medicare/Medicaid, (4) Medicare/Medigap, (5) Medicare Secondary Payer, and (6) TRICARE.

Information is color-coded, so you can quickly locate data related to a specific program or plan. Only general guidelines are stated since claim requirements may differ between private carriers and from state to state. Templates are provided in this chapter to illustrate data that have been entered properly in each field (see Figures 18-15, 18-17, and 18-18 later in this chapter). A template makes it easier to learn which fields to complete and which to ignore (screened fields). By learning field requirements on paper claims, these learned components can be used while inputting information into a computerized system for electronic submission. Following are instructions relating to specific fields on the claim form followed by Procedure 18-2, which presents guidelines to follow when completing the CMS-1500 form for OCR processing.

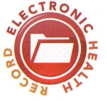

Signatures for Electronic Claims

Each medical practice must have a signed agreement with individual carriers so that claims can be submitted electronically. The physician's signature on the agreement is a substitute for his or her signature on the electronic claim.

Each patient must have a signature on file (SOF) in his or her medical record if the patient's claims are to be processed by electronic claims transmission (ECT). This consent authorizes information to be sent electronically to the insurance carrier and is indicated by a code in the electronic format.

Signatures on Paper Claims

A signature on the insurance claim form indicates that the signee agrees and approves all content entered on

✓ COMPLIANCE
Requesting Signatures

Inform the patient of his or her right to know how health information is used when asking for a signature on a consent/authorization form. Never ask a patient to sign a form without explaining what the form is for. Refer to Chapter 3 for a complete discussion on this HIPAA requirement.

PROCEDURE 18-2

Complete the CMS-1500 Health Insurance Claim Form Using OCR Guidelines

OBJECTIVE: Manually complete the CMS-1500 claim form.

EQUIPMENT/SUPPLIES: CMS-1500 claim form (02/12), computer and printer, procedural and diagnostic codebooks, medical dictionary, and pen or pencil.

DIRECTIONS: Follow these step-by-step directions, which include rationales, to learn this procedure. Job Skills 18-2, 18-3, and 18-4 are presented in the *Workbook* to practice this skill.

1. Use original claim forms printed in red ink; photocopies cannot be scanned.

2. Enter data in uppercase (CAPITAL) letters using a computer; this is the preferred method, although the scanner can now read lowercase letters and punctuation.

3. Use alpha or numeric symbols. Do not use symbols such as $, #, -, /, periods, commas, ditto marks, or parentheses. Do not use decimals in the money columns.

4. Select number 10 font, which is preferred for OCR claims. Do not handwrite information on the document.

5. Leave the field blank when information is not applicable. Do not use N/A or DNA and do not insert data in the shaded areas, as shown in claim templates.

6. DO NOT strike over any errors or use correction tape or correction fluid, highlighter pens, colored ink, or rubber stamps; OCR equipment will not pick these up.

7. DO NOT use stickers or rubber stamps such as those that indicate "tracer," "resubmitted," or "corrected billing."

8. *Optional*: Have patients sign a consent form or Field 12, the consent to release information, so data may be given to a third party.

9. Obtain patient's signature when assigning benefits to the physician, either on a separate form or in Field 13.

10. Indicate in Field 19 "See attachment" and name the type of attachment when documents are included. Accompanying documents must include the patient's name, claim number, and insurance identification number keyed near the top. Do not use paper clips, cellophane tape, or staples to affix attachments to the left upper corner of the form.

11. List diagnostic codes in Field 21 and include reference pointer(s) in Field 24E.

12. Enter date using 8-digit format in Field 24A (050120XX) and procedure codes in Field 24D (lines 1 through 6). Do not use narrative descriptions of diagnoses, procedures, or modifiers.

13. Have the physician sign the claim (first and last name with credential) and keep the signature within Field 31. Rubber stamps may be used if they are accepted by the insurance company and produce complete, clean images without smudges or missing letters.

14. Use laser or ink jet printer; clean line printers frequently.

15. Align the printer correctly, so characters appear in the proper fields. Run a test sample first in order to keep the characters within the borders of each field; do not touch the box lines.

16. If using continuous forms, use care when separating them. Do not overtrim or undertrim forms when bursting them apart.

17. Mail forms in large manila envelopes. Do not fold forms because they will not properly feed into OCR equipment if creased.

the claim. The provider should sign the form in Field 31 using his or her first and last name and credential; in some instances a stamped signature is allowed. Some insurance carriers accept the signature of the physician's representative; however, if the medical practice is audited and fraud or embezzlement is discovered, then the individual who had signature authorization can be held liable as well as the physician.

The assistant keys the physician's name above or below the signature if the name is not preprinted on the form. A removable adhesive indicator tab may be placed where the physician should sign the claim. The medical assistant inserts his or her initials in the bottom lower left corner of the claim to eliminate confusion as to who completed the form in case a claim is returned because of errors.

Insurance-Related Identification Numbers

Several types of identification numbers are used to identify providers and health plans when processing insurance claims.

Employer Identification Number—The physician's or medical group's Internal Revenue Service *employer identification number (EIN)* or Social Security number (SSN) must be listed on the insurance contract for electronic billing or appear on the insurance claim (Field 25) for tax purposes.

National Provider Identifier—A standard unique health identifier for health care providers is called the National Provider Identifier (NPI). The NPI requirement applies by law to covered entities such as health care providers, clearinghouses, and health plans in the United States when exchanging electronic transactions for which a national standard has been adopted under HIPAA.

The NPI is an all-numeric intelligence-free identifier consisting of 10 digits (9 plus a check digit in the last position). The NPI is a lifetime number that will not change if the provider changes location or specialty. Use of this number allows transmission to any health plan in the United States; however, some Medicare specialties do not require this number for such things as mass immunization roster billing. Transactions such as the remittance advice and referral authorizations also reference this number with transmissions.

Taxonomy Codes—In order for a physician to obtain a National Provider Identifier (NPI), a 10-digit specialty designation *taxonomy code* must be submitted with the application. This code set represents medical specialties (e.g., family practice [207Q00000X], oncology [207Rx0202X]) that may impact payments to the performing physician according to the health program payer's contract. Taxonomy codes are published twice a year—in July with an implementation date of October 1, and in January with an implementation date of April 1.

Health Plan Identification Number—A 10-digit standard unique *health plan identification (HPID)* number is being assigned to each health plan that processes

COMPLIANCE
NPI

All HIPAA-covered health care providers, whether individuals (e.g., physicians, nurse practitioners, chiropractors) or organizations (e.g., hospitals, home health agencies, clinics, group practices), must obtain an NPI for use to identify themselves in HIPAA standard transactions.

electronic claims. Use of this number will increase automation for offices that bill and perform insurance-related tasks electronically. Covered entities will be required to us HPIDs on or after Number 7, 2016.

Proofreading Claims

Proofread every claim on screen or in paper form, especially longer and more complex claims, as they involve larger sums of money and are more difficult to input or complete. Try to be as accurate as possible when inputting data. Review the data, and check for transposition of numbers (group, policy, claim, physician's identification, diagnostic and procedural codes), misspelled name(s), incorrect gender, missing date of birth, and blanks appearing in mandatory fields.

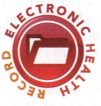

Posting to the Account

When using an EHR system, charges are posted automatically when each procedure code is input that identifies the service performed.

For paper claims, charges are posted individually on the patient's account or ledger with the date and a brief description of the service. An entry is made with the current date indicating when the insurance company was billed and stating the name of the carrier (see Chapter 15, Figure 15-2). Inclusive dates of service should also be cross-referenced, so money received can be applied accurately.

CLAIMS SUBMISSION AND TIME LIMITS

Insurance claims can be sent on paper using the revised CMS-1500 claim form (02/12) or electronically using a modem.

Paper Submission

The paper claim form (CMS-1500) is only accepted from physicians and suppliers who are excluded from mandatory electronic claim submission as required by law.

There are a number of methods for submitting paper insurance claims after they have been either manually completed (typed) or printed (generated) via computer. The medical practice may send them by mail, transmit them via fax machine, or employ a billing service for submitting insurance claims.

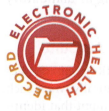

Electronic Submission

To submit claims using *electronic claims transmission (ECT)*, a computer needs to communicate directly with the insurance carrier's computer via the Internet using a cable or telephone modem. The electronic claim, also called an *electronic media claim*, is constructed from digital files, that is, files that were created from data that were input into the system during the information-gathering pathway. Electronic claims are not printed on paper but are transmitted using *encryption*, so they cannot be opened and read if intercepted.

Electronic transactions must be formatted and sent in a particular way using compatible software to facilitate automated processing by the payer. The American National Standards Institute (ANSI) developed the electronic format used to transmit insurance information. Each type of transaction is identified and referred to by a three-digit number preceded by "ASC X 12," which stands for the "American Standards Committee." For example, ASC X 12 **837** refers to the electronic claim transaction and **837P** refers to the CMS-1500 paper claim. These national standards apply to all government and private payers. Besides electronic transactions for claim submission and reimbursement, following are some other uses for electronic transactions in the health care industry:

- Additional information inquiry and response for claim completion
- Authorization for referral
- Claim attachments
- Claim remittance advice and payment
- Claim status inquiry and response
- Coordination of benefits information
- Eligibility status for health care insurance plans
- Enrollment and disenrollment in health care plans
- Premium payment for health care plans
- Workers' compensation first report of injury

The following data populate the claim form automatically in the software program:

- Patient demographic information is abstracted from the initial data file that was set up when the patient's information was entered into the system.
- Physician information, including EIN and NPI numbers, is abstracted from the physician profile that was initially set up in the practice management software system.
- Payer information is abstracted from the insurance plan's file that was set up when the contract was signed with the carrier.
- A financial account is set up in the practice management system for each patient. Then, procedure codes for professional services are picked up, as marked on the encounter form or coded by an administrative medical assistant, and selected from a list in the procedure code data file. Corresponding charges, which are automatically abstracted from the fee schedule and linked to a procedure code are then assigned and populate the electronic claim as appropriate to the individual insurance carrier.
- Diagnostic codes are selected from the encounter form, or written on the encounter form by the physician and coded by the administrative medical assistant and then selected from the diagnostic code database, or if not found entered into the system.
- Other data populate the claim form, for example, place of service codes are found in a separate data file and abstracted according to where the procedure is done.

Claims are located according to dates of service, and batches (or data packets) of claims are then selected by an insurance biller and electronically transmitted to insurance carriers. An electronic digital file is automatically formed by the system of all batches sent. An *Attachment Control Form* (*ACF*) is available on government websites to assist with the process of linking paper attachments to electronic claims.

Electronic transmission can occur in several ways. An insurance biller on site can transmit; the physician can employ a billing service to input information, transmit, and follow up; or the practice can employ a **clearinghouse**. A clearinghouse is a service that receives electronic claims in a central location and sorts them, processes them through a computer claims error check, and electronically transmits claims to the appropriate insurance carriers. Charges for this service may be calculated per claim, by month, or by amount billed. This service may also be used by offices that are not computerized or do not have a modem for electronic billing.

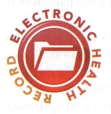

Advantages and Disadvantages of Electronic Transmission

This paperless method decreases administrative costs because fewer hours are needed to prepare forms and mail envelopes, pay for and apply postage, gather signatures, and store claim forms. It also allows for fewer errors and omissions when compared with manual processing and provides a quicker turnaround time from submission to payment; this increases cash flow. When submitting electronically, software code edit checks (in the physician's, clearinghouse, or insurance company's computer) can identify invalid codes, age conflicts, gender conflicts, procedure and diagnostic code linkage conflicts, and other problematic data before claims are processed or paid. These can be corrected quickly and a clean claim resubmitted electronically. The physician receives automatic tracking reports, noting the claim's arrival or problems and the insurance carrier automatically issues a check (i.e., *adjudicates* the claim) unless an error or omission occurs causing the claim to be set aside for manual review.

Some disadvantages would be the setup cost for the hardware, software, and Internet service; the time it takes to train office staff to use the computerized system; and dealing with technical problems that occur with power failures and all computerized equipment.

Regardless of the system used, all claims must comply with national electronic standards. Sometimes claims are outsourced to different states or countries. Refer to the transcription section in Chapter 11 and the "Summary" in Chapter 17 for more information on *outsourcing* claims and coding.

Claim Scrubbers

Most electronic billing systems have built-in edits, called *claim scrubbers*, that review the claim information and search for inconsistencies and missing data. They then prompt the biller to change or enter information on claims. Each payer has its own internal processing editors, so these systems cannot accomplish complete edits for all payers—they do not take the place of strong billing skills. The medical insurance biller needs to be knowledgeable about multiple payer requirements.

Medicaid Claim Completion and Submission

January 2012 was the compliance date for Medicaid programs to transmit electronic claims using the Standard Code Set Version 5010. If using paper claims, the CMS-1500 claim form must be adopted in all states that optically scan their claims for payment. Always refer to the local Medicaid intermediary for guidelines on how the form should be completed. Claims must be signed by the physician and then be submitted either to a **fiscal intermediary**, an insurance carrier who contracts to pay claims, or to the local department of social services, depending on the rules of the state.

Medicaid Time Limit

Every state has a time limit for the submission of Medicaid claims; it can vary from 2 months from the date of service to 1 year. If submitted after the time limit, payment can be reduced by percentages according to how late it is, or the claim can be rejected unless there is valid justification recognized by state laws. Drugs and dental services may be billed to a different intermediary than services performed by a physician. The medical assistant can contact the local state department of public health or department of social services for further information.

Medicare Claim Completion and Submission

Medicare claims for a physician's office are submitted to a **Medicare Administrative Contractor (MAC)** for Part B services. MACs (formerly called fiscal agents) are insurance carriers who contract to pay claims. The United States is divided into approximately 20 MAC jurisdictions, each covering several states. Patients are not allowed to send in claims for reimbursement.

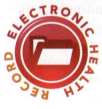

As stated earlier, the Standard Code Set Version 5010 is used when submitting electronic claims. If the provider is exempt from this mandate and submits paper claims, physician offices complete the CMS-1500 claim form. Charging for completing and submitting the claim form on an assigned basis violates the terms of the assignment. A template (Figure 18-15) may be used for reference when completing claims for patients on Medicare. Proper signatures need to be obtained prior to submitting the form (see earlier *Assignment and Consent* section). If the physician accepts assignment, an authorized person may sign the form or use a rubber stamp with the physician's signature.

Advance Beneficiary Notice

When Medicare is not likely to pay for a service or supply because medical necessity parameters have not been met, the patient's signature on an **Advance Beneficiary Notice (ABN) form** of noncoverage needs to be obtained by the provider (Form CMS-R-131). This form is provided by the physician's office and should be signed by the patient *prior* to the service being rendered,

so the beneficiary can make an informed decision regarding services Medicare may not pay for, but for which he or she may be financially responsible (see Figure 18-16).

A list of diagnoses that support medical necessity may be found on the Medicare website; refer to NCDs and LCDs in the following section. Ask the physician what diagnosis will be used prior to performing a procedure or service, and if it is not listed get an ABN. There are also frequency parameters, which are time frames stating how often a patient may have a procedure. Become familiar with these parameters that apply to procedures performed in your medical office prior to scheduling patients, so the claim will not be rejected. If the provider delivers a noncovered service without obtaining an ABN, the physician cannot bill the patient and must write off the charge.

When sending in an insurance claim for services listed on an ABN, HCPCS level II modifier–GA (waiver of liability on file) needs to be appended to the *CPT* procedure code. Medicare then informs the patient that he or she is responsible for the bill.

Do not confuse noncovered services with services that are excluded from the Medicare program. Physicians may bill Medicare patients for benefits that are not listed as covered; it is best to determine this and ask for payment in advance. For such services, the provider does not have to obtain an ABN but may voluntarily have the patient sign a "Notice of Exclusions from Medicare Benefits" (NEMB) form.

An ABN is in effect for 1 year from the date of signature, providing there are no changes to the information recorded on the form. Copies must be retained for 5 years from the date of service; electronic retention via a scanned form is acceptable. Refer to Procedure 18-3 for step-by-step directions when filling out an ABN form.

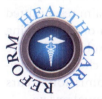

Medicare Time Limit—Basic standards for timely filing of Medicare claims were part of the Patient Protection and Affordable Care Act of 2010. Timely filing rules state that claims must be submitted within 1 year from the date of service. For example, claims having a date of service of February 29 must be filed by February 28 of the following year—if received on or after March 1, the claim would be denied.

Late filing of Medicare claims may be subject to a 10% reduction in payment.

HEALTH INSURANCE CLAIM FORM

MEDICARE Claim

APPROVED BY NATIONAL UNIFORM CLAIM COMMITTEE (NUCC) 02/12

CARRIER

| PICA | | | | | | | PICA | |

1. MEDICARE [X] (Medicare#)   MEDICAID ☐ (Medicaid#)   TRICARE ☐ (ID#/DoD#)   CHAMPVA ☐ (Member ID#)   GROUP HEALTH PLAN ☐ (ID#)   FECA BLK LUNG ☐ (ID#)   OTHER ☐ (ID#)

1a. INSURED'S I.D. NUMBER (For Program in Item 1)
524XX1981A

2. PATIENT'S NAME (Last Name, First Name, Middle Initial)
Munoz, Pedro, B

3. PATIENT'S BIRTH DATE   MM 03 DD 15 YY 1946   **SEX** M [X] F ☐

4. INSURED'S NAME (Last Name, First Name, Middle Initial)

5. PATIENT'S ADDRESS (No., Street)
4302 Century Street

6. PATIENT RELATIONSHIP TO INSURED
Self [X] Spouse ☐ Child ☐ Other ☐

7. INSURED'S ADDRESS (No., Street)

CITY Woodland Hills   **STATE** XY

8. RESERVED FOR NUCC USE

CITY   **STATE**

ZIP CODE 12345-4700   **TELEPHONE** (Include Area Code) (555) 4780299

ZIP CODE   **TELEPHONE** (Include Area Code) ( )

PATIENT AND INSURED INFORMATION

9. OTHER INSURED'S NAME (Last Name, First Name, Middle Initial)

10. IS PATIENT'S CONDITION RELATED TO:

11. INSURED'S POLICY GROUP OR FECA NUMBER
NONE

a. OTHER INSURED'S POLICY OR GROUP NUMBER

a. EMPLOYMENT? (Current or Previous) ☐ YES [X] NO

a. INSURED'S DATE OF BIRTH MM DD YY   **SEX** M ☐ F ☐

b. RESERVED FOR NUCC USE

b. AUTO ACCIDENT? ☐ YES [X] NO   PLACE (State)

b. OTHER CLAIM ID (Designated by NUCC)

c. RESERVED FOR NUCC USE

c. OTHER ACCIDENT? ☐ YES [X] NO

c. INSURANCE PLAN NAME OR PROGRAM NAME

d. INSURANCE PLAN NAME OR PROGRAM NAME

10d. CLAIM CODES (Designated by NUCC)

d. IS THERE ANOTHER HEALTH BENEFIT PLAN? ☐ YES ☐ NO   If yes, complete items 9, 9a, and 9d.

READ BACK OF FORM BEFORE COMPLETING & SIGNING THIS FORM.

12. PATIENT'S OR AUTHORIZED PERSON'S SIGNATURE I authorize the release of any medical or other information necessary to process this claim. I also request payment of government benefits either to myself or to the party who accepts assignment below.

SIGNED _Signature on ÿle_   DATE _____

13. INSURED'S OR AUTHORIZED PERSON'S SIGNATURE I authorize payment of medical benefits to the undersigned physician or supplier for services described below.

SIGNED _____

14. DATE OF CURRENT ILLNESS, INJURY, or PREGNANCY (LMP) MM DD YY   QUAL.

15. OTHER DATE QUAL.   MM DD YY

16. DATES PATIENT UNABLE TO WORK IN CURRENT OCCUPATION FROM MM DD YY   TO MM DD YY

17. NAME OF REFERRING PROVIDER OR OTHER SOURCE DN Thomas Stanton MD
17a.
17b. NPI 40315107XX

18. HOSPITALIZATION DATES RELATED TO CURRENT SERVICES FROM MM 11 DD 08 YY 20XX   TO MM 11 DD 12 YY 20XX

19. ADDITIONAL CLAIM INFORMATION (Designated by NUCC)

20. OUTSIDE LAB? ☐ YES [X] NO $ CHARGES

21. DIAGNOSIS OR NATURE OF ILLNESS OR INJURY Relate A-L to service line below (24E)   ICD Ind. 0
A. K4040   B.   C.   D.
E.   F.   G.   H.
I.   J.   K.   L.

22. RESUBMISSION CODE   ORIGINAL REF. NO.

23. PRIOR AUTHORIZATION NUMBER

24. A. DATE(S) OF SERVICE						B. PLACE OF SERVICE	C. EMG	D. PROCEDURES, SERVICES, OR SUPPLIES (Explain Unusual Circumstances) CPT/HCPCS MODIFIER	E. DIAGNOSIS POINTER	F. $ CHARGES		G. DAYS OR UNITS	H. EPSDT Family Plan	I. ID. QUAL.	J. RENDERING PROVIDER ID. #
From MM 11	DD 08	YY 20XX	To MM	DD	YY	21		49520	A	615	00	1		NPI	46278897XX
1														NPI	
2														NPI	
3														NPI	
4														NPI	
5														NPI	
6														NPI	

25. FEDERAL TAX I.D. NUMBER SSN ☐ EIN [X]
208765432

26. PATIENT'S ACCOUNT NO.

27. ACCEPT ASSIGNMENT? (For govt. claims, see back) [X] YES ☐ NO

28. TOTAL CHARGE $ 615 00

29. AMOUNT PAID $

30. Rsvd for NUCC Use

31. SIGNATURE OF PHYSICIAN OR SUPPLIER INCLUDING DEGREES OR CREDENTIALS (I certify that the statements on the reverse apply to this bill and are made a part thereof.)
Gerald Practon MD
Gerald Practon MD
SIGNED   112220XX   DATE

32. SERVICE FACILITY LOCATION INFORMATION
College Hospital
4500 Broad Avenue
Woodland Hills XY 12345-4700
a. 54378601XX   b.

33. BILLING PROVIDER INFO & PH # (555) 4869002
Practon Medical Group Inc
4567 Broad Avenue
Woodland Hills XY 12345-4700
a. 36640210XX   b.

NUCC Instruction Manual available at: www.nucc.org   **PLEASE PRINT OR TYPE**   APPROVED OMB-0938-1197 FORM 1500 (02-12)

PHYSICIAN OR SUPPLIER INFORMATION

Courtesy of the Centers for Medicare and Medicaid Services

FIGURE 18-15 Example of a completed CMS-1500 Health Insurance Claim Form for a basic Medicare case with no other insurance coverage. Screened blocks do not need to be completed. The physician has accepted assignment. See Appendix A for step-by-step instructions on how to complete this form

A. Notifier: *Gerald Practon, MD*

B. Patient Name: *Frances Campbell*

C. Identification Number: *DOB 04/04/1944*

Advance Beneficiary Notice of Noncoverage (ABN)

<u>NOTE:</u> If Medicare doesn't pay for **D.** *hemoglobin A1c* below, you may have to pay.

Medicare does not pay for everything, even some care that you or your health care provider have good reason to think you need. We expect Medicare may not pay for the **D.** *hemoglobin A1c* below.

D.	E. Reason Medicare May Not Pay:	F. Estimated Cost
Hemoglobin A1c	*Medicare does not pay for this test as often as this.*	*$66.00*

WHAT YOU NEED TO DO NOW:
- Read this notice, so you can make an informed decision about your care.
- Ask us any questions that you may have after you finish reading.
- Choose an option below about whether to receive the **D.** *hemoglobin A1c* listed above
  Note: If you choose Option 1 or 2, we may help you to use any other insurance that you might have, but Medicare cannot require us to do this.

G. OPTIONS: Check only one box. We cannot choose a box for you.

☑ **OPTION 1.** I want the **D.** *hemoglobin A1c* listed above. You may ask to be paid now, but I also want Medicare billed for an official decision on payment, which is sent to me on a Medicare Summary Notice (MSN). I understand that if Medicare doesn't pay, I am responsible for payment, but **I can appeal to Medicare** by following the directions on the MSN. If Medicare does pay, you will refund any payments I made to you, less co-pays or deductibles.

☐ **OPTION 2.** I want the **D.** *hemoglobin A1c* listed above, but do not bill Medicare. You may ask to be paid now as I am responsible for payment. **I cannot appeal if Medicare is not billed**.

☐ **OPTION 3.** I don't want the **D.** *hemoglobin A1c* listed above. I understand with this choice I am **not** responsible for payment, and **I cannot appeal to see if Medicare would pay.**

H. Additional Information:

This notice gives our opinion, not an official Medicare decision. If you have other questions on this notice or Medicare billing, call **1-800-MEDICARE** (1-800-633-4227/**TTY:** 1-877-486-2048). Signing below means that you have received and understand this notice. You also receive a copy.

I. Signature: *Frances Campbell*	**J. Date:** *3/16/20XX*

According to the Paperwork Reduction Act of 1995, no persons are required to respond to a collection of information unless it displays a valid OMB control number. The valid OMB control number for this information collection is 0938-0566. The time required to complete this information collection is estimated to average 7 minutes per response, including the time to review instructions, search existing data resources, gather the data needed, and complete and review the information collection. If you have comments concerning the accuracy of the time estimate or suggestions for improving this form, please write to: CMS, 7500 Security Boulevard, Attn: PRA Reports Clearance Ofÿcer, Baltimore, Maryland 21244-1850.

Form CMS-R-131 (03/11)   Form Approved OMB No. 0938-0566

FIGURE 18-16 Example of a completed Advance Beneficiary Notice of Noncoverage (ABN) for the Medicare program

PROCEDURE 18-3

Complete an Advance Beneficiary Notice (ABN) Form

OBJECTIVE: Complete an Advance Beneficiary Notice (ABN) form.

EQUIPMENT/SUPPLIES: Patient's upcoming service or procedure that is in question of payment, Advance Beneficiary Notice of Noncompliance form, and pen.

DIRECTIONS: Follow these step-by-step directions, which include rationales, to learn this procedure.

1. Complete the following sections:
   A. Physician's name, credentials, address, and telephone number.
   B. Patient's full name as it appears on his or her Medicare card.
   C. *Optional:* Date of birth or medical record number.
   D. General description of service or procedure you believe will not be covered. Note: The letter "D" occurs and needs to be filled in, in several places on the form.
   E. Explanation of why Medicare will not pay for the service or procedure, such as:
      • Medicare will not pay for this condition.
      • Medicare will not pay for this test or service this often.
   F. Estimate of the cost of the service or procedure. A dollar range (e.g., between $150 and $200) may be given if the actual cost is not known.
   G. Have the beneficiary select one of the following options:
      (1) Go ahead and have the service and ask the provider to bill Medicare for an official decision (collect or bill the patient for the cost of the service).
      (2) Have the service without billing Medicare (collect or bill the patient for the cost of the service).
      (3) Decide not to have the service; the patient will have no payment responsibility.
   H. Insert any comments, clarification, or information that may be beneficial to the beneficiary.
   I. Instruct the patient to sign the form to indicate that he or she understands its contents.
   J. Have the patient or beneficiary's representative date the form.

Medicare and Medigap/Medicaid Claim Completion and Submission

Completing a claim for a patient who has Medicare and another insurance plan can be confusing. First, find out whether Medicare is the primary or secondary payer, and then follow the directions on what information to enter in each field of the software program or form according to the primary payer. Refer to Figure 18-17 for a Medicare/Medigap CMS-1500 claim form template.

Medicare/Medigap Time Limit—Medicare claims that have Medigap as a secondary payer should be submitted according to Medicare rules.

Medicare/Medicaid Time Limit—Medicare/Medicaid claims should be submitted according to the time limit designated by the state Medicaid program. These claims are referred to as *crossover claims* because if they are sent electronically they automatically cross over from the Medicare system to the state Medicaid system. In some states, the Medicare Administrative Contractor (MAC) for a Medi/Medi claim may have a different address from that used for the processing of a Medicare-only claim. The assistant can contact the nearest MAC for guidelines pertinent to the state or region.

TRICARE Claim Completion and Submission

The TRICARE program is administered by the Department of Defense's TRICARE Management Activity (TMA) in Aurora, Colorado; however, all TRICARE network providers must submit electronic claims to their regional administrator; nonnetwork providers still have the option to submit paper claims. For TRICARE

HEALTH INSURANCE CLAIM FORM

APPROVED BY NATIONAL UNIFORM CLAIM COMMITTEE (NUCC) 02/12

MEDICARE/MEDIGAP Claim

PICA | | | | | | | PICA

1. MEDICARE	MEDICAID	TRICARE	CHAMPVA	GROUP HEALTH PLAN	FECA BLK LUNG	OTHER	1a. INSURED'S I.D. NUMBER (For Program in Item 1)
X (Medicare#)	(Medicaid#)	(ID#/DoD#)	(Member ID#)	X (ID#)	(ID#)	(ID#)	419XX7272A

2. PATIENT'S NAME (Last Name, First Name, Middle Initial)	3. PATIENT'S BIRTH DATE / SEX	4. INSURED'S NAME (Last Name, First Name, Middle Initial)
Barnes, Agusta, E	MM 08 DD 29 YY 1927 M X F	

5. PATIENT'S ADDRESS (No., Street)	6. PATIENT RELATIONSHIP TO INSURED	7. INSURED'S ADDRESS (No., Street)
356 Encina Avenue	Self X Spouse Child Other	

CITY		STATE	8. RESERVED FOR NUCC USE	CITY		STATE
Woodland Hills		XY				

ZIP CODE	TELEPHONE (Include Area Code)		ZIP CODE	TELEPHONE (Include Area Code)
12345-4700	(555) 4672646			( )

9. OTHER INSURED'S NAME (Last Name, First Name, Middle Initial)	10. IS PATIENT'S CONDITION RELATED TO:	11. INSURED'S POLICY GROUP OR FECA NUMBER
SAME		NONE

a. OTHER INSURED'S POLICY OR GROUP NUMBER	a. EMPLOYMENT? (Current or Previous)	a. INSURED'S DATE OF BIRTH SEX
MEDIGAP 419XX7272	YES X NO	MM DD YY M F

b. RESERVED FOR NUCC USE	b. AUTO ACCIDENT? PLACE (State)	b. OTHER CLAIM ID (Designated by NUCC)
	YES X NO	

c. RESERVED FOR NUCC USE	c. OTHER ACCIDENT?	c. INSURANCE PLAN NAME OR PROGRAM NAME
	YES X NO	

d. INSURANCE PLAN NAME OR PROGRAM NAME	10d. CLAIM CODES (Designated by NUCC)	d. IS THERE ANOTHER HEALTH BENEFIT PLAN?
CALFCA002		YES NO If yes, complete items 9, 9a, and 9d.

READ BACK OF FORM BEFORE COMPLETING & SIGNING THIS FORM.

12. PATIENT'S OR AUTHORIZED PERSON'S SIGNATURE I authorize the release of any medical or other information necessary to process this claim. I also request payment of government benefits either to myself or to the party who accepts assignment below.

SIGNED *Agusta E. Barnes*   DATE 11/21/20XX

13. INSURED'S OR AUTHORIZED PERSON'S SIGNATURE I authorize payment of medical benefits to the undersigned physician or supplier for services described below.

SIGNED *Agusta E. Barnes*

14. DATE OF CURRENT ILLNESS, INJURY, or PREGNANCY (LMP) MM DD YY QUAL.	15. OTHER DATE QUAL. MM DD YY	16. DATES PATIENT UNABLE TO WORK IN CURRENT OCCUPATION FROM MM DD YY TO MM DD YY

17. NAME OF REFERRING PROVIDER OR OTHER SOURCE	17a.	18. HOSPITALIZATION DATES RELATED TO CURRENT SERVICES
DN Gaston Input MD	17b. NPI 32783127XX	FROM MM DD YY TO MM DD YY

19. ADDITIONAL CLAIM INFORMATION (Designated by NUCC)	20. OUTSIDE LAB? $ CHARGES
	YES X NO

21. DIAGNOSIS OR NATURE OF ILLNESS OR INJURY Relate A-L to service line below (24E) ICD Ind. 0	22. RESUBMISSION CODE ORIGINAL REF. NO.
A. R0789 B. C. D.	
E. F. G. H.	23. PRIOR AUTHORIZATION NUMBER
I. J. K. L.	

24. A. DATE(S) OF SERVICE From MM DD YY	To MM DD YY	B. PLACE OF SERVICE	C. EMG	D. PROCEDURES, SERVICES, OR SUPPLIES (Explain Unusual Circumstances) CPT/HCPCS MODIFIER	E. DIAGNOSIS POINTER	F. $ CHARGES	G. DAYS OR UNITS	H. EPSDT Family Plan	I. ID. QUAL.	J. RENDERING PROVIDER ID. #
1 11 21 20XX		11		93350	A	146 83	1		NPI	65499947XX
2									NPI	
3									NPI	
4									NPI	
5									NPI	
6									NPI	

25. FEDERAL TAX I.D. NUMBER SSN EIN	26. PATIENT'S ACCOUNT NO.	27. ACCEPT ASSIGNMENT? (For govt. claims, see back)	28. TOTAL CHARGE	29. AMOUNT PAID	30. Rsvd for NUCC Use
208765432 X	060	X YES NO	$ 146 83	$	

31. SIGNATURE OF PHYSICIAN OR SUPPLIER INCLUDING DEGREES OR CREDENTIALS (I certify that the statements on the reverse apply to this bill and are made a part thereof.)	32. SERVICE FACILITY LOCATION INFORMATION	33. BILLING PROVIDER INFO & PH # (555) 4869002
Fran Practon MD 112220XX		Practon Medical Group Inc 4567 Broad Avenue Woodland Hills XY 12345-4700
Fran Practon MD SIGNED DATE	a. NPI b.	a. 36640210XX b.

NUCC Instruction Manual available at: www.nucc.org   **PLEASE PRINT OR TYPE**   APPROVED OMB-0938-1197 FORM 1500 (02-12)

Sidebar labels: CARRIER — PATIENT AND INSURED INFORMATION — PHYSICIAN OR SUPPLIER INFORMATION

Courtesy of the Centers for Medicare and Medicaid Services

FIGURE 18-17 Template of a CMS-1500 Health Insurance Claim Form (02/12) indicating Medicare as primary payer and Medigap as the supplemental insurance policy. Shaded fields do not need to be completed.

providers who submit less than 150 TRICARE claims per month, an online electronic claims system called *Xpress-Claim* is offered via the Internet. Figure 18-18 illustrates a completed TRICARE claim, so you may view various fields that correspond to an electronic claim.

The TRICARE fiscal year is from October 1 to September 30, so medical assistants collecting deductibles and copayments need to post reminder notices to TRICARE patients in the waiting room prior to October 1.

The beneficiary does not file claims under TRICARE Standard, TRICARE Extra, or TRICARE Prime, so the physician must agree to accept assignment, thereby consenting to accept what TRICARE states are "reasonable charges," plus the 20% or 25% portion from the patient after the deductible has been met—the payment goes to the physician. If the physician does not participate on a claim (accept assignment), the payment goes directly to the patient and the patient pays the total bill.

TRICARE and Other Insurance Claim Completion and Submission

When patients have other insurance in addition to TRICARE, by law TRICARE is last to pay except when the other insurance is:

1. A plan administered under Title XIX of the Social Security Act (Medicaid)
2. Coverage specifically designed to supplement TRICARE benefits

If the patient has TRICARE and Medicare and you are submitting a TRICARE for Life claim, submit the claim to Wisconsin Physicians Service who has signed an agreement with Medicare carriers allowing direct, electronic transfer of claim information.

If the patient is in an automobile accident or receives an injury that may have third-party involvement, TRICARE Form 691 (Statement of Personal Injury—Possible Third-Party Liability) must be sent with the regular claim for cost sharing of the civilian medical care.

TRICARE Time Limit—TRICARE claims must be filed on time—within 1 year from the date of service or, for inpatient care, within 1 year from the patient's date of discharge from the inpatient facility.

CHAMPVA Claims Submission and Time Limit

For CHAMPVA claims, the CMS-1500 claim form is completed and submitted to the VA Health Administration Center in Denver, Colorado. For clean claims, the time limit is 1 year from the date of the service or discharge from a hospital. The provider cannot seek payment from the beneficiary when the provider fails to meet timely filing requirements and a waiver for late filing is not granted.

CHAMPVA is always the secondary payer when other health insurance is involved *except* when the beneficiary is also insured through one of the following programs:

- Medicaid
- State Victims of Crime Compensation Programs
- Indian Health Services
- CHAMPVA supplemental insurance

State Disability Claim Completion and Submission

State disability claim forms are supplied by each state and may appear in two or three parts to be completed by the claimant, employer, and physician. The claim must be documented with the signatures of both the patient and the physician before the claimant can begin receiving benefits. It is important for the Social Security number of the patient to be accurate because without it the claim cannot be properly researched to establish wages earned in the last quarter. Claims are submitted to:

California	Branch Office of Employment Development Department
Hawaii	Department of Labor and Industrial Relations Disability Compensation Division
New Jersey	Department of Labor and Industry Division of Unemployment and Disability Insurance
New York	Workers' Compensation Board Disability Benefits Bureau
Puerto Rico	Department of Labor and Human Resources Bureau of Employment Security Disability Insurance Division
Rhode Island	Department of Labor and Training Temporary Disability Insurance Division

Addresses of these offices can be found online or in the telephone directory. Those working in states that do not have disability programs may contact a local private insurance carrier about disability coverage. Some state laws provide that a voluntary plan may be adopted instead of the state plan if a majority of company employees consent to private coverage.

HEALTH INSURANCE CLAIM FORM

APPROVED BY NATIONAL UNIFORM CLAIM COMMITTEE (NUCC) 02/12

TRICARE Claim

PICA			PICA

1. MEDICARE ☐ (Medicare#) | MEDICAID ☐ (Medicaid#) | TRICARE ☒ (ID#/DoD#) | CHAMPVA ☐ (Member ID#) | GROUP HEALTH PLAN ☐ (ID#) | FECA BLK LUNG ☐ (ID#) | OTHER ☐ (ID#)

1a. INSURED'S I.D. NUMBER (For Program in Item 1)
1234567890

2. PATIENT'S NAME (Last Name, First Name, Middle Initial)
Forbes, Susan, M

3. PATIENT'S BIRTH DATE MM 03 DD 16 YY 1997 SEX M ☐ F ☒

4. INSURED'S NAME (Last Name, First Name, Middle Initial)
Forbes, William, O

5. PATIENT'S ADDRESS (No., Street)
882 Sharp Street

6. PATIENT RELATIONSHIP TO INSURED
Self ☐ Spouse ☒ Child ☐ Other ☐

7. INSURED'S ADDRESS (No., Street)
SAME

CITY
Woodland Hills
STATE
XY

8. RESERVED FOR NUCC USE

CITY
STATE

ZIP CODE
12345-4700
TELEPHONE (Include Area Code)
(555) 7899698

ZIP CODE
TELEPHONE (Include Area Code)
( )

9. OTHER INSURED'S NAME (Last Name, First Name, Middle Initial)

10. IS PATIENT'S CONDITION RELATED TO:

11. INSURED'S POLICY GROUP OR FECA NUMBER

a. OTHER INSURED'S POLICY OR GROUP NUMBER

a. EMPLOYMENT? (Current or Previous)
YES ☐ NO ☒

a. INSURED'S DATE OF BIRTH MM 06 DD 12 YY 1994 SEX M ☒ F ☐

b. RESERVED FOR NUCC USE

b. AUTO ACCIDENT?
YES ☐ NO ☒
PLACE (State)

b. OTHER CLAIM ID (Designated by NUCC)
USN

c. RESERVED FOR NUCC USE

c. OTHER ACCIDENT?
YES ☐ NO ☒

c. INSURANCE PLAN NAME OR PROGRAM NAME
TRICARE

d. INSURANCE PLAN NAME OR PROGRAM NAME

10d. CLAIM CODES (Designated by NUCC)

d. IS THERE ANOTHER HEALTH BENEFIT PLAN?
YES ☐ NO ☒ If yes, complete items 9, 9a, and 9d.

READ BACK OF FORM BEFORE COMPLETING & SIGNING THIS FORM.

12. PATIENT'S OR AUTHORIZED PERSON'S SIGNATURE I authorize the release of any medical or other information necessary to process this claim. I also request payment of government benefits either to myself or to the party who accepts assignment below.

SIGNED SOF   DATE

13. INSURED'S OR AUTHORIZED PERSON'S SIGNATURE I authorize payment of medical benefits to the undersigned physician or supplier for services described below.

SIGNED

14. DATE OF CURRENT ILLNESS, INJURY, or PREGNANCY (LMP) MM 09 DD 19 YY 20XX QUAL. 484

15. OTHER DATE QUAL. MM DD YY

16. DATES PATIENT UNABLE TO WORK IN CURRENT OCCUPATION FROM MM 06 DD 28 YY 20XX TO MM 08 DD 09 YY 20XX

17. NAME OF REFERRING PROVIDER OR OTHER SOURCE
DN Port Hueneme Naval Base MTF

17a.
17b. NPI 6657832XX

18. HOSPITALIZATION DATES RELATED TO CURRENT SERVICES FROM MM 06 DD 28 YY 20XX TO MM 07 DD 01 YY 20XX

19. ADDITIONAL CLAIM INFORMATION (Designated by NUCC)

20. OUTSIDE LAB? YES ☐ NO ☒ $ CHARGES

21. DIAGNOSIS OR NATURE OF ILLNESS OR INJURY Relate A-L to service line below (24E) ICD Ind. 0

A. O80 | B. | C. | D.
E. | F. | G. | H.
I. | J. | K. | L.

22. RESUBMISSION CODE | ORIGINAL REF. NO.

23. PRIOR AUTHORIZATION NUMBER

24. A. DATE(S) OF SERVICE From MM DD YY	To MM DD YY	B. PLACE OF SERVICE	C. EMG	D. PROCEDURES, SERVICES, OR SUPPLIES (Explain Unusual Circumstances) CPT/HCPCS / MODIFIER	E. DIAGNOSIS POINTER	F. $ CHARGES	G. DAYS OR UNITS	H. EPSDT Family Plan	I. ID. QUAL.	J. RENDERING PROVIDER ID. #
1	06 28 20XX		21		59400	A	1864 30	1		NPI	C1503X
2										NPI	
3										NPI	
4										NPI	
5										NPI	
6										NPI	

25. FEDERAL TAX I.D. NUMBER 208765432 SSN ☐ EIN ☒

26. PATIENT'S ACCOUNT NO. 080

27. ACCEPT ASSIGNMENT? (For govt. claims, see back) YES ☒ NO ☐

28. TOTAL CHARGE $ 1864 30

29. AMOUNT PAID $ 1864 30

30. Rsvd for NUCC Use

31. SIGNATURE OF PHYSICIAN OR SUPPLIER INCLUDING DEGREES OR CREDENTIALS (I certify that the statements on the reverse apply to this bill and are made a part thereof.)
Fran Practon MD
Fran practon MD
SIGNED   062920XX DATE

32. SERVICE FACILITY LOCATION INFORMATION
College Hospital
4500 Broadway Avenue
Woodland Hills XY 12345-4700
a. 54378601XX b.

33. BILLING PROVIDER INFO & PH # (555) 4869002
Practon Medical Group Inc
4567 Broadway Avenue
Woodland Hills XY 12345-4700
a. 208765432 b.

NUCC Instruction Manual available at: www.nucc.org   **PLEASE PRINT OR TYPE**   APPROVED OMB-0938-1197 FORM 1500 (02-12)

Courtesy of the Centers for Medicare and Medicaid Services

FIGURE 18-18 Template of a CMS-1500 Health Insurance Claim Form for a TRICARE Standard case when billing for professional services

TABLE 18-4 State Disability Information Summary for Five States and Puerto Rico

State	Name of State Law	Maximum Weekly Payments in Benefit Year	Time Limit for Filing Claims	Benefits
California	California Unemployment Insurance Code	52	9–49 days from disability	Based on 55% earnings in the highest quarter of base period
Hawaii	Temporary Disability Insurance Law	26	No specific timeframe listed; however, must be filed in "timely" manner within a week or so	Based on 58% of average weekly wage
New Jersey	Temporary Disability Benefits Law	26	30 days from disability	Based on 66 2/3 of average weekly wage for base period
New York	Disability Benefits Law	26	30 days from disability	Based on 50% of average weekly wage
Puerto Rico	Disability Benefits Act	26	30 days from disability	Based on 65% of weekly earnings
Rhode Island	Temporary Disability Insurance Act	30	30 days from disability	Based on 4.62% of highest base period quarter wages

State Disability Time Limit

A claim for disability insurance should be filed within the time limit for your state—there is a grace period of 7 to 8 days after the deadline. Maximum payments in a benefit year, time limits for filing claims, deductions from salaries, and a listing of what the benefits are based on appear in Table 18-4.

Workers' Compensation Claim Completion and Submission

An itemized billing statement is usually submitted at the time the first or supplemental report is sent to the workers' compensation insurance company (see Figure 18-11). The physician must sign all forms and letters in ink—a stamped signature is not acceptable. If payment is not received, the assistant should contact the insurance carrier to find out if the claim has been assigned to an adjustor. Each state has a waiting period before income and medical benefits are paid. Refer to the *Resources* section at the end of this chapter for state

workers' compensation reporting schedules and waiting periods.

Physicians accept payment from workers' compensation insurance carriers as payment in full. The physician does not bill the patient directly unless the insurance carrier will not accept the claim as an industrial case. If the status of the claim is questionable, there is a 90-day period in which a determination can be made. If the case does not turn out to be a workers' compensation claim, the insurance carrier is still obligated to pay a stated amount (e.g., the first $10,000).

Workers' Compensation Time Limit

Each state has a different time limit and forms for reporting an accident or illness. Timely filing of claims will keep the carrier informed about the ongoing cost of medical care. Contact the Workers' Compensation Board to inquire about your state's time limit for sending supplemental reports and filing claims.

CLAIM STATUS

Each claim can be designated according to the claim status, which is indicated by a code on the explanation of benefits (EOB) as described:

- *Clean Claim*—Completed insurance claim submitted within the program time limit containing all necessary data to process and pay promptly
- *Denied Claim*—Claim received and payment rejected because of a technical error or payment policy issue (e.g., noncovered benefit)
- *Dirty Claim*—Claim submitted with errors or one that requires manual processing
- *Incomplete Claim*—Medicare claim missing required information; may be resubmitted
- *Invalid Claim*—Medicare claim that contains complete, valid information but is illogical or incorrect; may be resubmitted
- *Pending Claim*—Claim held in suspense owing to review or other reason; may be cleared for payment or denied
- *Rejected Claim*—Claim submitted but discarded by the system because of technical errors; may be returned to the provider for investigation, correction, and reprocessing
- *Suspended Claim*—Claim held by insurance company as pending because of error or additional information needed

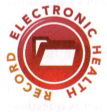

Claim Adjudication and Payment

When an electronic claim is received by the insurance carrier, it is downloaded into a special administrative software program to verify the subscriber and determine benefits.

When a paper claim is received, it is scanned and information keyed into the payer system. The *adjudication* process, which involves decision making, begins when the patient's demographic data are cross-checked against the subscriber file and benefits are confirmed. Procedure codes are electronically matched with the policy's master benefit list and diagnostic codes are compared to medical necessity parameters. After determination is made for the charges submitted, the deductible amount is automatically subtracted first, and then copayment or coinsurance requirements are determined. If the claim meets all the parameters, an explanation of benefits and insurance payment is generated and sent to the physician, as described in Chapter 13. The following section will cover various aspects of claim follow-up for insurance claims that were not paid.

Claim Follow-Up

Each office needs to institute a claim follow-up process. For electronic claims, the medical practice software billing program creates a log of transmitted claims according to the date of submission. A report can be printed for nontransmitted or unpaid claims by dates of service, dates of submission, or insurance carrier name. All outstanding claims can then be followed up in batches according to each carrier's filing time limit. An aging accounts receivable report can also be used to obtain the total amounts outstanding.

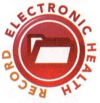

For most electronic claims, their status can be viewed online. Use payer websites to verify patient eligibility, check claim status, confirm the insurer's billing address, examine coverage criteria, look at payment policies, and submit claim corrections and appeals as necessary.

For paper claims, when an insurance form is completed and sent to the carrier, it can be chronologically filed according to dates of service in an accordion file. Each major carrier (e.g., Medicare, Medicaid, Blue Plans) would have its own file and some private carriers may be combined. As claims are paid, they are pulled from these pending files and stapled to the explanation of benefits then placed in a "Paid Claim" file according to dates of service. Every week, or once a month for smaller offices, the outstanding claims can be pulled according to the dates of service and follow-up procedures performed. An insurance log is another way of tracking unpaid claims. This can be kept manually or by using a computerized spreadsheet. When using this system, information would have to be input and dates noted when claim follow-up is made or when payment is received. When using the United States Post Office to resubmit "lost" paper claims to the same address, use certified mail to prove timely filing deadlines.

Billing Errors

The Office of Inspector General has targeted several areas where frequent billing errors take place:

- *Duplicate billing*—Filing claims more than once for the same service

- *Medical necessity*—Level of service provided not supported with documentation
- *NPI placement*—Incorrect placement of the NPI (see claim field instructions)
- *Place of service*—Service provided in outpatient facility but billed indicating that it was performed in the physician's office
- *Stark violations*—Patients being referred to services in which the physician or a family member has a financial interest

Comprehensive Error Rate Testing Program—

The Medicare Comprehensive Error Rate Testing (CERT) program was established in 2003 as part of the Improper Payments Information Act. In an attempt to reduce improper and overpayments, Medicare randomly selects claims to determine if each claim submission and payment is correct under Medicare's coverage, coding, and billing rules. Documentation must verify all coverage criteria and be submitted according to Medicare's plan limits (i.e., 75 days). CERT focuses on the following primary error types:

- No or insufficient documentation
  - Missing or illegible physician signature
  - Missing or incomplete orders
- Medical necessity
  - Not enough documentation
  - Physician intent to order tests missing
- Incorrect coding
  - See Chapters 16 and 17
- "Other" errors

Recovery Audit Contractor Review—Medicare's

Recovery Audit Contractors (RAC) review claims on a postpayment basis. Auditor's may go back 3 years from the date of initial determination made on a claim and focus on finding improper payments by detecting and recovering overpayments, identifying underpayments, and developing methods to prevent future improper payments. If a RAC auditor comes to your office, respond quickly to his or her request and appeal his or her determination, if necessary, within 120 days of the audit. Regional RACs publish a list of improper coding and billing issues approved by CMS on the Medicare website.

Tracing Insurance Claims

Many states require insurers to respond to clean claims and either pay or deny within 45 days. Become familiar with your state's *prompt payment laws* to verify response

time limits (see *Resources* section at the end of this chapter). When sufficient time has passed and no payment has been received, according to the patterns of payment from various insurance plans, look at, print, or pull all outstanding claims for one carrier and send an electronic inquiry, place a telephone call, or write a letter addressing the multiple claims. A form letter can be used for this purpose and one letter to an insurance carrier each month rather than placing multiple calls or submitting many letters covering individual claims is a time-efficient way of following up.

Unprocessed Claims

Medicare defines an "unprocessable claim" as a claim that contains incomplete or invalid information. For private payers, this may also include a lost claim or a claim that has been suspended because of an error, or which needs additional information.

Missing or Incorrect Information—Claims received by insurance carriers may have simple errors or lack the information required to properly adjudicate the claim. This may result in claim rejection or denial. In such situations, you will be notified either electronically or receive a form letter indicating what information is needed. If Medicare sends an *Additional Documentation Request (ADR)*, you have 45 days in which to respond; otherwise, the claim will be denied. Substantiate the information in question on the claim, and then send the correction in a timely manner.

On a Medicare claim, if a simple question needs to be answered or if information is incorrect (e.g., mathematical error, transposed diagnostic code), the carrier may ask for a "telephone reopening." Call the dedicated "Medicare Reopening line" and state the reason for the correction and provide the information needed to correct the claim. You may call for a maximum of three claims. If Medicare requests information using the *Automated Development System (ADS)*, answer the request as soon as possible (within 45 days maximum) and return the original development letter as the first page of your response. This could be for such things as a missing provider's signature, incorrect dates of service, or no patient name recorded on each page of the medical record.

When you do not know why the claim has not been processed, follow these recommendations:

- Telephone the insurance carrier to inquire about the claim.
- Send an inquiry letter; a form letter or template can be used.

- Fax or send an electronic claim noting "second submission."
- Respond immediately to additional document requests (ADRs) made by the insurance carrier.

Unpaid or Denied Claims

For unpaid or denied claims, it is important to study the exact reason the payer has not paid the claim. It may be due to a lapse in or cancellation of medical coverage, noncovered benefits, services performed that needed prior authorization or were not medically necessary, or another carrier's involvement (e.g., coordination of benefits issue, personal injury claim, or workers' compensation case). Following are recommendations for a denied claim:

- Resubmit only rejected lines of service.
- Gather documentation, which might include history of similar claims that have been paid.
- Present logic for time spent and skill of the physician.
- Obtain "position papers" from a specialty society (e.g., OB-GYN) or FDA regarding procedure or service.
- Send letter from physician giving summary of circumstances that relate directly to the patient.

It is important to keep detailed records of all follow-up efforts, including dates of contact and names of people you have dealt with. It may be necessary to get the patient involved. Let them know the status of the delayed payment and ask for additional information; a form letter or template can be used for this purpose.

False Claim Act

The False Claim Act (FCA) is a federal statute that covers fraud involving any federally funded contract or program (e.g., Medicare, Medicaid). Liability is established for any worker who knowingly presents a false or fraudulent claim to the government for payment. "Knowingly" is defined to mean that a person, with respect to information, (1) has actual knowledge of falsity of information in the claim, (2) acts in deliberate ignorance of the truth or falsity of the information in a claim, or (3) acts in reckless disregard of the truth or falsity of the information in a claim.

The act does not require proof of a specific intent to defraud the government. A health care practice or physician may be held liable for the conduct of its individual employees, or even the conduct of associates or other entities with which it contracts (e.g., billing

service), even when the health care facility or group practice has no knowledge that its employee or contracted entity is engaged in the preparation or submission of false claims. If found guilty, the offending party can be held liable*.

Liability under the False Claims Act can lead to civil monetary penalties ranging from $5500 to $11,000 for every fraudulent claim filed, as well as three times the amount of actual damages to the federal government. Current proposals would increase this amount up to $100,000 in certain circumstances. Categories of fraud and abuse include:

- Billing for service not rendered
- Billing for services not medically necessary
- Billing separately for services that should be bundled (see coding, Chapter 16)
- Duplicate billing
- Failure to report overpayments (credit balances)
- Falsifying certificates of medical necessity
- Falsifying diagnoses or treatment plans to gain payment
- Offering health care providers inducements in exchange for referral for services

The Office of Inspector General (OIG) oversees the integrity of federal health care programs and works with providers to resolve program abuses and correct problems leading to program abuse. Adopting proactive practices can minimize the risk of fraudulent activity.

Appeals

If payment is not received after inquires have been made, or if you disagree with a coverage or payment decision, an appeal may need to be filed. Learn all you can about why the claim was not paid and do not be afraid to ask questions. If the insurer states that the services were not medically necessary, request an explanation that includes the insurer's policy language and any information used in making the decision.

Appeals must be written and should be sent by certified mail with a copy of the original claim, the explanation of benefits, and any documentation that would justify the appeal. Submit new and relevant information not previously considered. Write concisely and list details that support the level of service. It may be beneficial to cite the carrier's guidelines as it relates to the claim. Include the physician, if necessary, as he or

---

*There is a 10 year staute of limitation for fraudulant claims.

she may be able to detail how all treatment alternatives were exhausted before starting the care in question, or be able to provide medical journal articles that detail the effectiveness of the treatment.

Refer to guidelines for each carrier's appeal process; some require special forms and each has time limits in which the appeal must be made. For example, a request for reconsideration of a TRICARE claim must be made within 90 days from the issue date on the explanation of benefits, or an appeal must be filed within 90 days from the date of denial. For a CHAMPVA claim, you must submit a request in writing within 1 year of the date on the EOB. Continue to track the status of the claim until it is paid or the appeal process has been exhausted.

A *peer review*, which is an evaluation done by a group of unbiased physicians, may be considered as the next step if the appeal does not bring forth payment. Although individual states offer an external appeals process for health plan decisions, state laws vary.

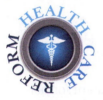

The Affordable Care Act has instituted new federal appeal standards that allow consumers to challenge initial claim denials. This regulations serves to standardize the internal and external appeals process throughout the United States. Experts who help with this type of appeals process say that patients have a 50% chance of having the denial overturned.

Medicare Appeals

All Medicare appeal requests must have the following information:

- Beneficiary name
- Health Insurance Claim (HIC) number
- Exact dates of service

- Specific services requesting reconsideration or review
- Supporting documents and rationale for appealing the denied claim
- Name and signature of party submitting the appeal

There are five levels of Medicare appeals:

1. Redetermination—Use the National Government Services Medicare Determination Request form and transmit electronically or send in writing within 120 days of receiving the remittance advice; no minimum dollar amount is required. Use the same form to request redetermination for all denied services on the claim. Include a full signature on the request form.
2. Reconsideration—If dissatisfied with the redetermination decision, request a reconsideration within 180 days of the notification. Include the name of the contractor that made the determination.
3. Administrative Law Judge (ALF)—File the request within 60 days of the reconsideration decision; minimum dollar amount, $150. A determination will be made within 90 days of receipt of review request.
4. Department Appeals Board Review—File the request within 60 days of receipt of the ALJ's decision; no minimum dollar amount required. The appeals council will issue a decision within 90 days.
5. Federal Court Review—Request this review within 60 days of the Appeals Board decision; minimum dollar amount, $1,500.

Medicare states that appeals are overturned at the rate of 50%. Refer to the *Resources* section at the end of this chapter for the Medicare website where you can find extensive information.

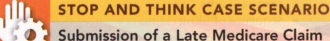

STOP AND THINK CASE SCENARIO
Submission of a Late Medicare Claim

SCENARIO: You have recently begun to work for Dr. Practon's office and discover an old claim that has not been submitted. The date of service on this Medicare claim is May 16, 2014.

CRITICAL THINKING: Using the date November 22, 2016, is it too late to submit this claim?

_____

What is the billing limitation of this claim; in other words, what is the deadline date by which the claim should have been submitted?

_____

STOP AND THINK CASE SCENARIO
Determine TRICARE Coverage and Benefits

SCENARIO: A patient calls the doctor's office and states that she is covered under the TRICARE program; her husband is serving in the United States Air Force, his rank is E4. Doctors Fran and Gerald Practon are contracted physicians with the TRICARE Extra network but do not participate in the TRICARE managed care plan.

CRITICAL THINKING: The patient asks the following questions about how the claim will be processed for outpatient services and what her payment responsibilities will be.

1. Will the physician's office be submitting the claims?
_____

2. What is my responsibility for the deductible?
_____

3. How will my eligibility be checked?
_____

STOP AND THINK CASE SCENARIO
Determine the Responsible Party in an Injury Case

SCENARIO: An established patient has arrived at Dr. Practon's office with an injury to his head.

CRITICAL THINKING: What questions should you ask the patient (or person accompanying the patient) to determine who will be paying the medical bill?
_____
_____
_____

FOCUS ON CERTIFICATION*

CMA (AAMA) Content Summary

- Third-party billing
- Commercial carriers
- Government plans (Medicare, Medicaid, TRI-CARE, CHAMPVA)
- Workers' compensation
- Processing manual claims
- Processing electronic claims
- Tracing claims
- Sequence of filing claims
- Reconciling payments, rejections
- Inquiry and appeal process
- Referrals
- Precertification

---

*This textbook and the accompanying Workbook meet the entry-level administrative and general competencies for the CMA outlined by the AAMA Examination Content Outline and Occupational Analysis and for the RMA and CMAS outlined by the AMT Competencies, Construction Parameters, and Examination Specifications (see Competency Grid in Appendix B).

RMA (AMT) Content Summary

- Insurance terminology
- Insurance plans
- Identify and understand short-term and long-term disability
- Identify and understand workers' compensation (first and follow-up reports)
- Identify and understand Medicare (Advance Beneficiary Notice [ABN])
- Identify and understand Medicaid
- Identify and understand TRICARE and CHAMPVA
- Complete and file insurance claims
- File claims for paper and Electronic Data Interchange
- Understand and adhere to HIPAA Security and Uniformity Regulations
- Evaluate claims rejection and utilize proper follow-up procedures
- Identify and comply with contractual requirements of insurance plans
- Track unpaid claims

CMAS (AMT) Content Summary

- Understand private/commercial health care insurance plans
- Understand government health care insurance plans
- Process patient claims using appropriate forms and time frames
- Process workers' compensation/disability reports and forms
- Submit claims to third-party reimbursements including the use of electronic transmission methods
- Understand health care insurance terminology
- Understand requirements for health care insurance plans
- Process insurance payments
- Track unpaid claims, and file and track appeals
- Understand fraud and abuse regulations

REVIEW EXAM-STYLE QUESTIONS

1. The term *third-party payers* indicates that the following entities are involved in health care reimbursement:
   a. provider and insurance company
   b. provider and patient
   c. patient, provider, and payer
   d. provider and government program
   e. provider and private payer

2. State insurance exchanges:
   a. are also called "marketplaces"
   b. offer insurance based on gender, age, and location
   c. are offered in every state
   d. may be used by all "noncitizens" residing in the United States
   e. all of the above are correct

3. The insured is also known as a:
   a. member
   b. policyholder
   c. subscriber
   d. recipient
   e. all of the above

4. In an insurance contract, the waiting period is:
   a. also called the elimination period
   b. a time frame after the beginning date of a policy before benefits for illness or injury become payable
   c. the time frame during which the applicant is waiting to be approved
   d. in force only if there are preexisting conditions
   e. both a and b

5. The birthday rule states that when a child is covered by both parents, the health plan of the parent:
   a. who is the oldest, according to the calendar year will pay first
   b. whose birthday falls earliest according to the month of the calendar year will pay first
   c. whose birthday, by month and day falls earlier in the calendar year will pay first
   d. who has had the insurance for the shortest time will pay first
   e. who has had the insurance for the longest will pay first

6. Medicaid is sponsored by:
   a. the federal government
   b. the state government
   c. local governments
   d. federal and local governments
   e. federal, state, and local governments

7. When working in a physician's office, you will be billing:
   a. Medicare Part A
   b. Medicare Part B
   c. Medicare Part C
   d. Medicare Part D
   e. all of the above

8. In the TRICARE program, an enrollment fee is sometimes charged for:
   a. TRICARE Standard
   b. TRICARE Extra
   c. TRICARE Prime
   d. all TRICARE programs
   e. none of the TRICARE programs

9. State disability is available in Puerto Rico and in the states of:
   a. California, Hawaii, New Jersey, New York, and Rhode Island
   b. California, Hawaii, Nevada, New Jersey, and New York
   c. Arizona, Florida, New Hampshire, New York, and Texas
   d. Alaska, California, Florida, New York, and Texas
   e. Hawaii, Nebraska, Oregon, New York, and Washington

10. In a workers' compensation case, who does the medical assistant communicate with?
    a. Claims representative
    b. Insurance representative
    c. Adjuster
    d. Authorization desk
    e. Social worker

11. The CMS-1500 claim form has an assignment of benefits for government programs in:
    a. Field 12
    b. Field 13
    c. Field 14
    d. Field 31
    e. Field 33

12. The four main stages in the life cycle of an insurance claim are:
    a. patient registration form, insurance card, code books, explanation of benefits
    b. gathering source information, applying source information, claim submission, payment
    c. claim submission, claim processing, adjudication, payment
    d. verifying insurance eligibility, coding procedures and diagnoses, transmitting the insurance claim, receiving the explanation of benefit and payment
    e. registering the patient, filling out the insurance claim form, sending the claim, depositing the check

13. A standard unique health identifier for health care providers is called a/an:
    a. PIN
    b. UPIN
    c. state license number
    d. ECT
    e. NPI

14. The reason that the CMS-1500 claim form is printed in red ink is:
    a. to make the inserted information stand out
    b. to make it easier to read
    c. to comply with OCR machines
    d. to comply with copyright laws
    e. to make sure no one copies the form

15. When filling out the CMS-1500 claim form and information is not applicable:
    a. insert "not applicable"
    b. insert "does not apply"
    c. insert "N/A"
    d. leave it blank
    e. a, b, and c are all correct

16. When comparing electronic versus paper claim submission, the average processing time is:
    a. 10 to 15 days for paper and 1 to 2 days for electronic claims
    b. 15 to 20 days for paper and 5 to 6 days for electronic claims
    c. 28 to 30 days for paper and 7 to 10 days for electronic claims
    d. 30 to 45 days for paper and 10 to 12 days for electronic claims
    e. 45 to 60 days for paper and 12 to 15 days for electronic claims

17. Some advantages of electronic transmission of insurance claims are:
    a. fewer errors and omissions
    b. quicker turnaround time
    c. increased cash flow
    d. built-in code edit checks
    e. all of the above are correct

18. A claim scrubber is:
    a. someone who manually looks at claims for missing information
    b. someone who manually looks at claims for errors
    c. an electronic eye that is built into computerized billing software to flag all possible problems on an electronic claim
    d. built-in edits in electronic software that prompt the biller to change or enter information on claims
    e. all of the above are correct

19. An Advance Beneficiary Notice:
    a. must be completed when it is suspected that Medicare may not deem a service or supply medically necessary
    b. must be completed when a service or supply is not included on Medicare's benefit list
    c. must only be completed for services and supplies above $500
    d. must be completed for all insurance carriers prior to receiving services
    e. must be completed for all Medicare patients for outpatient services

20. Liability under the False Claims Act can lead to civil monetary penalties for every fraudulent claim filed, ranging from:
    a. $1500 to $5500
    b. $2500 to $7500
    c. $3500 to $8500
    d. $5500 to $11,000
    e. $10,000 to $20,000

WORKBOOK ASSIGNMENT

To develop competency-based job skills, refer to the Workbook and complete the:
- Abbreviation and Spelling Review
- Review Questions

- Critical Thinking Exercises
- Job Skill activities, which are listed at the beginning of the chapter under Performance Objectives in the Workbook.

RESOURCES

Books

A Guide to Health Insurance Billing, 4th edition
    Moisio, Marie
    Cengage Learning, 2014
    Website: http://www.cengagebrain.com
Insurance Directory, 1st edition
    Optum, 2015
Understanding Health Insurance: A Guide to Billing and Reimbursement, 12th edition
    Green, Michelle
    Cengage Learning, 2015
    Website: http://www.cengagebrain.com

Claim Forms

American Medical Association
    Search: CMS-1500
Bibbero Systems, Inc.
    Select: Ordering information
    Website: http://www.bibbero.com
CMS-1500 Claim Form
    Search: Fillable CMS-1500 Form—download and fill out
Medical Arts Press
    Select: Office supplies
Veterans Affairs (VA)
    Search: U.S. Department of Veteran Affairs—government forms

Internet

Advance Beneficiary Notice

U.S. Department of Human Services

Centers for Medicare and Medicaid Services

Search: ABN

Affordable Care Act

Medicaid State Participants

Search: How is the ACA Impacting Medicaid Enrollment?

America's Health Insurance Plans (AHIP)

Represents nearly 1300 members providing health benefits to more than 200 million Americans

Any Lab Test Now®

Lab services for uninsured patients—store locater

Appeal Letter (sample)

Search: Prompt Payment Laws by State

CHAMPVA

Select: Health A–Z topic finder

Department of Insurance

State Insurance Commissioner

Consumer services division

Fraud and Abuse

Search: How to protect your practice

Health Insurance Portability and Accountability Act

Search: Public law

HIPAA Health Savings Account

Search: HSA

Medicaid

Select: Home page

Medi-Cal

Select: Topic of choice

Medicare

Select topic of choice:

- Appeals
- CMS Forms
- HIPAA
- LCDs
- Manuals
- Medicaid
- Medicare Learning Network (MLN)
- Medicare Local Coverage Determinations (LCDs)
- Medicare Secondary Payer Fact Sheet (Search MLN)
- National Coverage Determinations (NCD Manual)
- National Provider Identifier Standard (NPI)
- NCDs
- Physician Fee Schedule

Website: http://www.medicare.gov

Medicare Education and Training

Medicare Learning Network

Medicare Prescription Drug Plans

Search: Part D coverage

Medicare Preventive Services

Department of Health and Human Services: Preventive Services Chart

Guide to Medicare's Preventive Medicine Services

Medicare University

Course List Includes:

- ABN
- Billing Guidance for Items Requiring Span Dates
- Claim Status Inquiry
- Introduction to Medicare Billing Process
- Medicare Secondary Payer

Stark Law

Stark III Final Rules

Information and regulations

State Disability Insurance Programs

Overview

State Prompt Payment Laws

Search: Prompt Payment Laws by State (pdf download)

View your state's regulations

Payment timeframes, penalties, contact information

State-Run Insurance Exchanges

Select: Your state

Website: http://www.ncsl.org

TRICARE

Information or providers

Workers' Compensation

- Comparison of State Workers' Compensation Systems

U.S. Department of Labor

- Workers' Compensation Forms

Select: Workers' compensation home page, workers' compensation forms, select state of your choice

Video

Critical Thinking for Medical Assistants: Online Video Series, Program 5: Insurance and Coding, **1st edition**

Delmar Learning, 2005

Website: http://www.cengagebrain.com

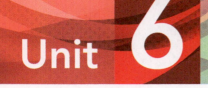
MANAGING
THE OFFICE

CHAPTER 19

OFFICE MANAGERIAL RESPONSIBILITIES

LEARNING OBJECTIVES

After reading this chapter and learning step-by-step procedures to gain job skills,* you should be able to:

- Summarize the rules and responsibilities of an office manager.
- Discuss ways to promote patient satisfaction and communication.
- Describe ways of increasing office productivity.
- List reasons for office staff meetings.
- State components of an employee handbook.
- Understand and apply federal and state employment laws.
- Assemble items for an office policies and procedures manual.
- Identify techniques used for recruitment, screening, interviewing, hiring, and training new employees.
- Write a plan for building and equipment maintenance.
- Select a system for ordering and controlling inventory.
- Design a basic travel itinerary and locate travel help sites on the Internet.

PERFORMANCE OBJECTIVES (PROCEDURES) IN THIS TEXTBOOK

- Develop a complaint protocol (Procedure 19-1).
- Set up a staff meeting (Procedure 19-2).
- Prepare a staff meeting agenda (Procedure 19-3).
- Develop and maintain an employee handbook (Procedure 19-4).
- Prepare an incident report (Procedure 19-5).
- Compile and maintain an office policies and procedures manual (Procedure 19-6).
- Recruit an employee (Procedure 19-7).
- Orient a new employee (Procedure 19-8).
- Manage equipment maintenance (Procedure 19-9).
- Prepare an order form (Procedure 19-10).

---

* This textbook and the accompanying Workbook meet the educational components for entry-level administrative and general competencies outlined by CAAHEP and ABHES.

- Pay an invoice (Procedure 19-11).
- Establish and maintain inventory (Procedure 19-12).
- Prepare a travel expense report (Procedure 19-13).

PERFORMANCE OBJECTIVES (JOB SKILLS) IN THE WORKBOOK

- Document patient complaints and determine actions to resolve problems (Job Skill 19-1).
- Write an agenda for an office meeting (Job Skill 19-2).
- Prepare material for an office procedures manual (Job Skill 19-3).
- Perform inventory control and keep an equipment maintenance log (Job Skill 19-4).
- Abstract data from a catalog and key an order form (Job Skill 19-5).
- Complete an order form for office supplies (Job Skill 19-6).
- Perform mathematic calculations of an office manager (Job Skill 19-7).
- Prepare two order forms (Job Skill 19-8).
- Prepare a travel expense report (Job Skill 19-9).

KEY TERMS

agenda

back ordered (B/O)

employee handbook

human resource
   management

inventory cards

invoice

itinerary

job descriptions

office manager (OM)

office policies and
   procedures manual

packing slip

practice information
   brochure

purchase order (PO)

staff meetings

HEART OF THE HEALTH CARE PROFESSIONAL

Service

The office manager (OM) can set the scene of service within the medical office by exemplifying a responsible and caring attitude. Opportunities to model a professional image and positive work ethic characteristics are numerous and should be observed and adopted by employees.

OFFICE MANAGER

One of the most prestigious yet demanding positions associated with the medical office is that of an **office manager (OM)**. When the medical practice grows to a point where there are several employees or more than one physician sharing a facility, it may be prudent to assign one person to oversee employees and all activities, both administrative and clinical. A variety of skill sets, experience, and proven competence in the role of administrative medical assistant can be rewarded with promotion to OM. If you are ambitious and enjoy a fast-paced atmosphere, ongoing challenges, and unpredictable shifting responsibilities, you may want to consider pursuing management. Managing people and projects takes a creative approach as well as leadership, organizational abilities, and interpersonal skills. A good manager needs to create clear boundaries, establish lines of communication and authority, learn to delegate and motivate employees, manage time wisely, plan for periods of uninterrupted concentration, prioritize responsibilities, and be able to accept that a task may not be completed at the close of the day.

The line of authority is, first, the physician; next, the OM; and finally, the staff members. The OM acts as a *liaison* between employees and physician(s). This is graphically shown in Chapter 2, Figure 2-6. The administrative assistant who has been promoted to this responsible position needs to prepare and implement an effective management plan that will foster a team spirit of cooperation among all employees with an equitable division of the workload. He or she must be able to take the initiative and exercise independent judgment, which reflects accurately the attitude of the physician.

Once the chain of command has been established, the OM should be firm, yet flexible and fair, in his or her decisions to ensure respect, promote teamwork, and avoid friction and tension within the office. Responsibilities may include hiring and training, performance and salary review, supervision, and disciplining or dismissal of employees when necessary.

The OM usually delegates the maintenance of equipment and ordering of supplies to promote the efficient running of the office. Another responsibility might include making travel arrangements for the physician to attend medical conventions. Tracking continuing education units for the physician, sending in documentation to ensure that the physician's state license is current, and maintaining liability coverage for malpractice insurance are also responsibilities of the OM. Other tasks may include generating and analyzing financial reports and preparing payroll; these topics are discussed in the next chapter.

The duties of managing the office are numerous and challenging, but there are rewards and immense personal satisfaction knowing that the office operates efficiently for the physician and serves patient needs. Updating skills, attending seminars, and reading medical periodicals will enable the manager to keep current, excel in his or her position, and possibly attain a higher career goal as an administrator of an outpatient facility or multiphysician clinic.

The Work Environment

It is important for the OM to set the tone for the entire office and create a work atmosphere that is free of barriers and bias. A multicultural staff can help strengthen an office, attract new patients, and connect with a rapidly growing immigrant population that may be wary of seeking medical care.

The OM should be a model to all employees, lead by example, and hold staff members to a high standard. The OM should also set performance goals, seek input from employees, utilize individual talents,

and allow employees to grow and feel an important part of the team. Align desired behaviors with the goals of the practice and maintain an upbeat spirit, always thanking employees for the work they have done while displaying a cooperative attitude.

Be a mentor and coach to those who are learning how to be good employees. Plan strategies together, foster problem-solving skills, delegate responsibility, and ask employees how things are going. Be authentically committed to each person's achievement and support staff members, so they know that help is available if and when they need it.

Promoting Patient Satisfaction and Communication

Promote patient satisfaction by being professional and polite, respecting the opinion of others, maintaining composure in all situations, and providing help and information. Utilize good communication skills and become the communication hub for the entire office, so everyone feels free to contribute ideas to improve patient care. Be observant, listen carefully, and develop a complaint protocol that includes procedures to document the complaint and a mechanism to resolve it (see Procedure 19-1). Think of a complaint as an opportunity for improvement and use a patient complaint form to prompt staff to pay close attention to patient relations and to learn where policies and procedures need to be changed (Figure 19-1). A patient survey form may be another tool used to gain insight regarding problematic areas.

When there is a problem, staff members should feel free to openly discuss their concerns, thus avoiding unexpected confrontations. This is often referred to as having an open-door policy. Problematic situations can be discussed at the staff meeting or privately.

Practice Information Brochure

Management consultants have determined that the easiest way to close the communication gap and reduce the number of patient questions is to present each new patient with a printed **practice information brochure** describing the basic office policies and procedures of the physician's practice (Figure 19-2). It is best designed by the physician's OM and office staff. The brochure should be personalized and avoid technical language as if it were addressed to a friend. Patients could be referred to as "you" and the staff as "we." The brochure is intended to act as an effective instrument for communication and to provide the answers to

PROCEDURE 19-1

Develop a Complaint Protocol

OBJECTIVE: Develop policies and procedures to document a complaint and solve problems.

EQUIPMENT/SUPPLIES: Patient complaint (can use scenario), complaint form (Figure 19-1), and pen or pencil.

DIRECTIONS: Follow these step-by-step directions, which include rationales, to learn this procedure. Job Skill 19-1 is presented in the *Workbook* to practice this skill.

1. Read the complaint document and identify the reason for the complaint. Clarify if there is an underlying issue involved.

2. Practice empathy. Put yourself in the other person's position to better understand his or her viewpoint. Remember, perceptions differ among people and the best solutions satisfy everyone's needs.

3. Brainstorm options and list all possible solutions, evaluating each independently.

4. Determine the best option. This may be done by offering several options to the patient and letting him or her decide.

5. Use active listening skills and offer feedback when necessary.

6. Document the interaction and write down the option that was determined to be the best; this helps clarify the scenario.

7. Determine if a similar complaint is likely to reoccur in the future, and if so, write a protocol (policy and procedure), and then have a staff training session to communicate how to handle the situation to employees.

PRACTON MEDICAL GROUP, INC.

4567 BROAD AVENUE • WOODLAND HILLS, XY 12345-4700
OFFICE: (555) 486-9002 • FAX: (555) 488-7815

Fran Practon, M.D.
Gerald Practon, M.D.

PATIENT COMPLAINT DOCUMENT

Date of complaint ___5/13/XX___   Account number ___006935___

Patient name ___Kevin Skuza___   Account balance ___$750.00___

Complaint ___Pt states authorization was obtained for in network services, but insurance pd as if he went "out of plan" and applied $500 to the deductible. Pt called ofc and "someone" told him to work it out c̄ his insurance.___

Action taken to resolve complaint ___Track autho and rebill insurance c̄ hard copy and explanation.___

___Norma Vasquez___   ___5/13/XX___
Employee signature   Date

FIGURE 19-1 Patient complaint document

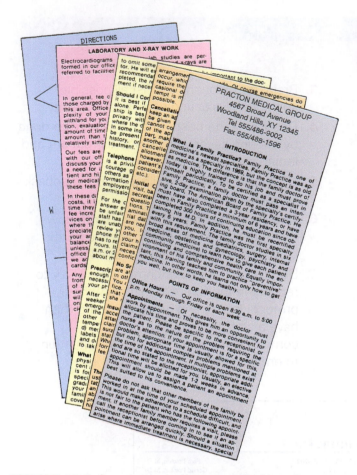

FIGURE 19-2 Sample pages from a medical practice information brochure

"This booklet prepared especially for the ___ family." If booklets are printed, it is advisable to order a 6-month supply at a time, allowing sufficient time for both printing and delivery.

Much of the information detailed in the brochure for new patients is related to that in the office procedures manual. Therefore, any change in the manual will probably necessitate an updating of the patient information brochure. This information helps inform patients of their responsibilities and helps train them to work with the office staff and physician to provide the best medical care possible.

Brochure Headings—Paragraph headings in the patient brochure may include some or all of the following:

- Appointments
  - Cancellations
  - Holiday Schedules
  - House Calls
- Billing and Collection Procedures
  - Past-Due Accounts
  - Payments
- Emergencies
- Managed Care and Insurance Participation
- Maps
  - Transportation
- Medical Records
  - Authorization for Release of Records
  - Consent for Medical Treatment
- Office Hours
- Physician and Staff Information
- Prescriptions

patients' most commonly asked questions. It reduces questions by introducing the physician and the specialty as well as office's policies and procedures—presenting an image of a practice that is professional in every aspect. Physicians who have used information brochures report marked improvement in rapport and have found that the brochure serves as an effective marketing tool because patients often share them with friends and relatives.

Brochure Format—Paragraphs can be typed on 8½-inch by 11-inch letterhead stationery or can be printed in a multipage pamphlet or brochure to fit into a standard office size envelope. If the office has a logo, it can appear on the cover. General information can include office hours, appointment scheduling, telephone procedures, and so forth. In a multiphysician office, a short biography of each doctor might be included. In a family practice, a line on the front of the brochure with a space for the patient's name might read,

- Privacy Policy
- Services and Procedures
- Smoking Policy
- Specialty Information
- Telephone Calls
- Miscellaneous

Distribution of the Brochure—The brochure can be mailed with the patient registration and history forms before the first appointment. Or, the medical assistant may personally hand the brochure to the patient after completing forms in the office, taking that opportunity to review pertinent items. An adequate supply of information brochures should also be available in all examination rooms, in the physician's office, and at the front desk.

Medical Practice Website

A website for the medical practice can be a marketing and communication tool. It should be simply designed so that navigation is easy. It should attract new patients, educate existing patients, answer general questions, and include items mentioned in the medical practice brochure such as office hours, location, and driving directions. Following is a list of basic headings that may be included:

- *About Us*—State who you are. For example: Practon Medical Group is a family practice established in 1987 (list physician biographies and a brief statement about each staff member)
- *Our Mission*—The medical practice's vision and philosophy
- *Our Services*—Primary care, hospital care, surgery, nursing home visits, home visits
- *FAQ*—Frequently asked questions may be included with straightforward answers
- *Our Locations*—Include all office locations and directions from north, south, east, or west and a map
- *Contact Us*—Address, telephone and fax numbers, and email address

A website can streamline or expedite tasks if registration, privacy notices, and history forms can be filled out and printed or emailed to the office.

Designing a Website—After the decision is made to launch a website, a domain name must be selected, registered, and paid for with a nominal fee. This process involves logging onto a domain name registration service and entering the name to be sure it is not already in use. Next, all Web pages must be created and the

information written. Special software programs are designed to help with this task. Services such as Webmonkey, which provide step-by-step authoring procedures and developing tips, can also be used.

If the OM does not have the time or technical skill to design the website, a professional designer may be contacted who has experience creating a clean, attractive-looking site, linking other sites, and offering technical enhancements. Whether a medical office designs a website in-house or outsources the job, all staff members should be asked to contribute some time and effort to the cause.

After the website is created, it needs to be published. Some *hosting services* are free, but it is best to avoid such sites and to instead purchase the service. Finally, maintenance of the site must be considered. Maintenance is an ongoing process in which someone browses the site frequently to make sure all links are working and updates content as needed. See the *Resources* section at the end of this chapter for specific website information.

Increasing Office Productivity

The office manager should strive to boost office productivity so as to improve efficiency and increase income for the physician. To accomplish this goal, suggestions to the physician might include:

1. Promote specialization; for example, assign one person to handle all insurance claims, who, as a result, will acquire expertise, become known personally to claims processors, file claims more efficiently, follow up on unpaid claims, and thus increase reimbursement.

PATIENT EDUCATION

Medical Practice Website

Information sites, pertaining to the medical practice's specialty, can be linked on the website (e.g., American Heart Association, American Diabetes Association, American Cancer Association), and patient education articles may be included and changed periodically. Subjects such as "Healthy Living," "Diabetes," "Obesity," "Women's Health Concerns," "Men's Health Concerns," "Parents and Kids," and "Seniors" could be included.

2. Employ part-time personnel to help during peak hours, file documents, transcribe reports, or assist the insurance biller when there is not enough work to warrant hiring a full-time person.

3. Hire two part-time employees to job *share* (i.e., share one job) to decrease overhead.

4. Initiate *flextime*. Adopt flexible work hours by having some personnel arrive before normal office hours to prepare for the day's patients, while others start later and stay after office hours to handle additional tasks or prepare for the next day. Offer the option of 1-hour lunch breaks to be reduced to 1/2 hour, thus allowing employees to arrive late or leave early. Flextime reduces tardiness and sick time substantially and is an effective recruiting tool and morale booster.

5. Encourage continuing education for the staff by paying fees for attendance at workshops and seminars, and tuition wholly or in part.

6. Ensure employees have the most current knowledge by subscribing to the latest reference material and covering dues for membership in medical societies.

7. Cross-train all staff to allow substitution for each other to reduce boredom, increase efficiency, encourage professional growth, and make the staff more versatile when personnel are absent.

8. Promote in-house expertise in financial matters; for example, develop a follow-up collection routine to handle difficult collection cases or find ways to earn top interest on cash reserves.

9. Suggest that each employee keep a notebook of hints on how to perform office tasks more efficiently and effectively. Items could be shared at a staff meeting.

10. Make clear to all employees that attendance is extremely important and is one of the criteria used in evaluating performance; also reduce absenteeism by paying back unused sick time or giving bonuses to those who have the best attendance records.

11. Minimize distractions in open-space offices by facing desks away from high-traffic areas.

12. Measure the physician's productivity level by determining the patient-per-hour rate. Select 8 to 10 recent half-day office sessions, total the number of patients seen during those sessions, and divide by the total number of office hours in all sessions. This will help determine patient scheduling, staffing needs, and space design.

Staff Meetings

The importance of establishing a pattern of good communication among all members of the staff cannot be overstated. Regularly scheduled **staff meetings** with organized topics for discussion are a necessity; usually a 15- to 30-minute session once a week will provide a pattern of positive staff interaction (Figure 19-3). Start and stop all meetings on time; this is a courtesy to those who are punctual. Proceed at a fast pace so that inattention will not be a problem and discourage repetitious dialogue by using phrases such as "I am sure everyone agrees that . . ." or "We have concluded that. . . ." Involve employees in solving staff problems and generating outcomes or assignments from decisions that have been made. Once a decision is final, it is important for those who may disagree to refrain from carrying their dissatisfaction out of the meeting room. Allow dissatisfied employees to vent their frustration and then move on to other business. Remind everyone that all decisions are made for the good of the whole and they are sometimes restricted by financial limitations or other barriers.

Small or established offices may schedule meetings less often than large or new offices that have multiple staff members or start-up concerns. Monthly meetings around the noon hour, either in a private meeting room of a restaurant or in the office with catered food—with the physician occasionally paying for lunch—can create an atmosphere of informality and camaraderie. Emphasize a team attitude by using the word *we* instead of *you*, offer praise for jobs well done, and say thank you to boost performance.

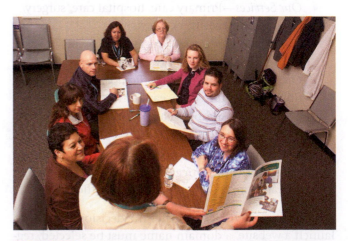

FIGURE 19-3 Routine staff meetings between the office manager and coworkers help improve patient care and maintain good rapport

PROCEDURE 19-2

Set Up a Staff Meeting

OBJECTIVE: Arrange a staff meeting for the physician's employees.

EQUIPMENT/SUPPLIES: Physician, employees, meeting place, purpose, agenda, and computer.

DIRECTIONS: Follow these step-by-step directions, which include rationales, to learn this procedure.

1. Verify the proposed date and time for the meeting to ensure the room will be available.
2. Arrange for the meeting room.
3. Gather details for the meeting, such as:
   a. Purpose (goals) of the meeting
   b. Attendees
   c. Program agenda
   d. Expected duration of the meeting
4. Prepare the agenda (see Procedure 19-3).
5. Obtain necessary equipment; for example, microphone, computer/projector, screen, and handouts.
6. Compose a memo to the employees and physician to notify them of the following:
   a. Date
   b. Time
   c. Place of the meeting
   d. Program agenda

Meetings can also be used to educate or to share information acquired at workshops and seminars with a free interchange of ideas as they relate to office matters. Effective training can take place with a captive audience, and outside experts can be invited to speak or demonstrate use of new equipment or software. Refer to Procedure 19-2 when arranging a staff meeting for physician employees.

Agenda

Even though staff meetings are usually informal, a solid agenda will speed discussion and diffuse office conflicts. When a time has been set for a staff meeting, the OM is usually assigned to compose an agenda with input from the staff and physician. The agenda outlines topics to be reviewed at the meeting to create a plan of action. The agenda should focus on specific points but be open-ended to allow for changes. After it has been written, copies are distributed to everyone in the office for review 2 or 3 days before the meeting. A well-organized agenda will improve the quality of a staff meeting because it will provide sufficient time for a new proposal to be studied, keep topics well focused, enable participants to prepare for discussion of office concerns, and provide time to research various aspects of office functions. Figure 19-4 shows a sample agenda.

Refer to Procedure 19-3 to prepare a staff meeting agenda.

Brainstorming Session

In a *brainstorming session*, all attendees express ideas, no matter how far-out or wild they may be. This technique may be utilized when solving problems or when starting a new venture (e.g., redecorating the office). After everyone has been heard, start the process of elimination by listing the pros and cons of each idea. Top suggestions should be summarized and a plan on how to carry out the recommendations documented. Brainstorming or informal sessions should have agendas to provide direction and to make sure time is used wisely in accomplishing goals.

Minutes

Often the administrative assistant will be asked to take minutes at staff or professional meetings. Notes have to be taken even if everyone at the meeting is in agreement that the discussion can be taped. Generally, the minutes will follow the outline of the agenda with the assistant noting decisions made, actions to be taken, and the most important information. As soon as possible after the meeting, the minutes should be typed concisely and accurately while fresh in mind to avoid any omissions.

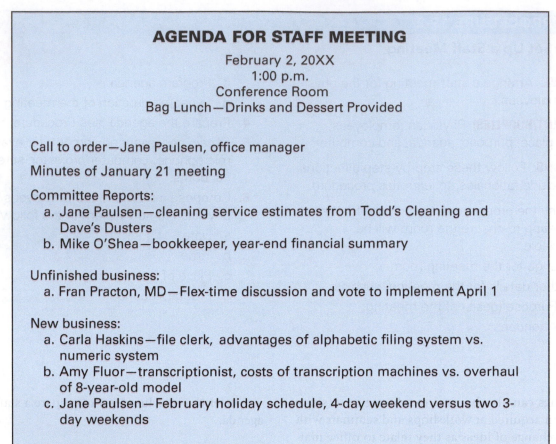

AGENDA FOR STAFF MEETING

February 2, 20XX
1:00 p.m.
Conference Room
Bag Lunch—Drinks and Dessert Provided

Call to order—Jane Paulsen, office manager

Minutes of January 21 meeting

Committee Reports:
    a. Jane Paulsen—cleaning service estimates from Todd's Cleaning and
       Dave's Dusters
    b. Mike O'Shea—bookkeeper, year-end financial summary

Unfinished business:
    a. Fran Practon, MD—Flex-time discussion and vote to implement April 1

New business:
    a. Carla Haskins—file clerk, advantages of alphabetic filing system vs.
       numeric system
    b. Amy Fluor—transcriptionist, costs of transcription machines vs. overhaul
       of 8-year-old model
    c. Jane Paulsen—February holiday schedule, 4-day weekend versus two 3-
       day weekends

Adjournment until February 25 meeting

FIGURE 19-4 Example of a computer-generated agenda for a staff meeting

---

PROCEDURE 19-3

Prepare a Staff Meeting Agenda

OBJECTIVE: Prepare a staff meeting agenda to be discussed and acted on for the smooth and efficient operation of the medical practice.

EQUIPMENT/SUPPLIES: Minutes from previous meeting, order of business, names of individuals giving reports, notes for rough draft of agenda, new business items, and computer.

DIRECTIONS Follow these step-by-step procedures, which include rationales, to learn this procedure. Job Skill 19-2 is presented in the *Workbook* to practice this skill.

1. Review the previous meeting's minutes to determine which old business topics need to be included.

2. Check with employees for reports on various job duties.

3. Identify new business subjects.

4. Compose a rough draft of the agenda with the gathered information.

5. Ask the physician to view the agenda for content and to make sure the agenda is correct and complete.

6. Key the final draft of the agenda.

7. Email or print copies of the final agenda to be distributed to the staff meeting participants so that each one can prepare for the meeting by completing any required tasks and preparing necessary documentation for reports.

Appropriate terminology, content, and format for taking minutes can be found in *Robert's Rules of Order Newly Revised*. If no action was taken on an item discussed, reference to the discussion should be omitted. Copies of the minutes should be distributed to those who attended the meeting and kept with the agenda and any handouts in a file. They serve to remind attendees of events and actions. Acceptable content and sequence of topics for writing minutes would be:

- Name of parties holding meeting
- Type of meeting (staff) and interval (weekly, monthly) with time, date, and place indicated
- Name of chairperson
- Names of people present and absent (sign-in sheet can be used)
- Reading of minutes of previous meetings
- Reports of committees, departments, or individuals
- Old, unfinished business
- New business
- Adjournment, with date and place of next meeting indicated
- Signature of chairperson or person recording minutes

If the office staff has part-time employees who seldom come together at one time, keep everyone informed on office matters by distributing minutes from the meeting, outlining decisions or action taken. A "communications book" with "need-to-know" information can be set up where each entry would be dated and addressed to specific staff members, who initial it after it has been read.

OFFICE GUIDEBOOKS

Office guidebooks are used in a medical practice as reference books for employer policies and procedures and to outline job descriptions, describe office routines, and detail job tasks. Everything an employee needs to know about the place of employment should be included in an employee handbook.

Employee Handbook

An **employee handbook**, also known as a *personnel manual*, is a compilation of data that provides standards and guidelines for work conditions such as attendance, compensation, and payroll files; work schedules and break policies; holiday, vacation, and sick leave policies;

as well as personnel records and training files. Each policy (rule or regulation) should be clearly stated and needs to have a procedure that describes how to implement the policy. Persons affected by the policy should be listed according to job title. The manual should also include a glossary of definitions (e.g., abbreviations, acronyms) in the back to clarify unfamiliar terms.

In a separate section, **job descriptions** are listed with the responsibilities of each position and the qualifications needed to fulfill them. This can be used as a guide for each staff member's work assignments and is an excellent hiring and evaluation tool for practice management. Figure 19-5 shows the importance of a job description in various areas of office management. It assists in training, enhances morale, and fosters a cooperative spirit by making clear to employees exactly what their jobs entail. A generic job description for an entry-level administrative medical assistant may be found in Chapter 1, Figure 1-3. A job description can also be useful when candidates are interviewed for a position because it effectively ensures that the applicant will understand the individual tasks and responsibilities of the position.

All employees should sign a statement indicating the handbook has been read. See Table 19-1 for suggested contents of an employee handbook. Refer to Procedure 19-4 to develop and maintain an employee handbook.

Office Policies and Procedures Manual

An **office policies and procedures manual** is a written guide describing office routines and practices. It is maintained separate from the employee handbook and may contain a compilation of sample forms to be used for reference when executing office tasks. It can be used

---

PATIENT EDUCATION

Promote Public Relations

Promote the medical practice through positive public relations by offering quality medical care and an efficient business environment with staff members that express the four Cs (care, concern, compassion, and competence). This will have a domino effect and patients will tell others.

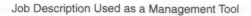

Job Description Used as a Management Tool

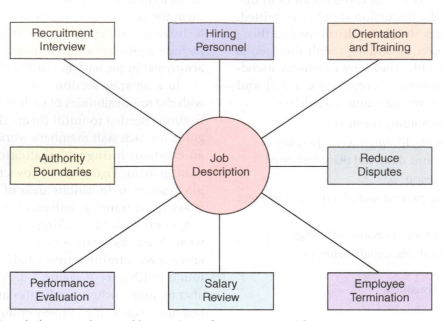

FIGURE 19-5 Job descriptions can be used in a variety of ways as a tool for good practice management

TABLE 19-1 Recommended Contents of an Employee Handbook (Not All-Inclusive)

Introduction: Welcome to Practon Medical Group, Inc.	Email, Internet (Facebook, Tweeting), and Intranet Policies	Performance Reviews
Absenteeism and Tardiness	Employment Application	Personal Telephone Calls
Americans with Disabilities Act	Equal Opportunity Employment	Personnel Records
Benefit Plans	Equipment and Facility Use Policy	Privacy Policy
Bereavement	Family and Medical Leave Act Policy	Probationary Period
Cash Shortage	Forms	Promotions
Code of Ethics	Full-Time/Part-Time Schedule	Resignations, Terminations, Grounds for Dismissal
Confidentiality Rules and Privacy Laws	Grievance Procedure and Discipline	Retirement Plan
Conflict Resolution Plan	Health Insurance (COBRA rights)	Safety Policy
Continuing Education and Tuition Reimbursement	Holidays	Salary/Wage Increases
Disability: Short-Term, Long-Term, and Disability Insurance Benefits	Hours of Work, Lunch, Rest Breaks	Security Guidelines
	Job Descriptions	Sexual Harassment Policy
Disciplinary Policies	Jury Duty	Smoking Policy
Discrimination Issues	Leaves of Absence: Condolence, Sick Leave, Emergency, Maternity, Family	State Disability Insurance
Dress Code and Regulations		Time Cards and Time Clocks
Drug Abuse, Alcoholism, and Smoking Policies	Orientation Period and Training	Vacations: Eligibility, Accrual, Capping
	OSHA Compliance	Work-Related Injury (Workers' Compensation) (procedures and forms)
	Overtime Policy	
	Paychecks and Paydays	*Right to Revise Policy*
	Payroll Deductions	

PROCEDURE 19-4

Develop and Maintain an Employee Handbook

OBJECTIVE Develop and maintain a comprehensive, up-to-date employee handbook to establish employment guidelines to be followed.

EQUIPMENT/SUPPLIES: Computer, three-ring binder, paper, job descriptions, and employee handbook.

DIRECTIONS: Follow these step-by-step directions, which include rationales, to learn this procedure.

1. Compile information and compose detailed step-by-step guidelines with rationales for each employment policy. These policies help staff understand the office rules and procedures pertaining to employees.

2. Write detailed and comprehensive job descriptions for each position in the medical practice.

3. Distribute appropriate job descriptions to employees within the office.

4. Title each item and key the data into a computer file, which can be easily modified when updates are needed.

5. Print the file, then alphabetize, collate, and place the pages into a three-ring reference binder. The binder format lends itself to periodic updates as changes are made.

6. Identify sections by placing colored indexing tabs, and use transparent sheet covers to protect all pages.

7. Add examples where appropriate to facilitate understanding and act as a reference guide.

8. Put the employee handbook in an easily accessible location to all employees; it is only relevant if it is used as a reference.

9. Review the employee handbook annually. Keep it current by adding any new policies and deleting or modifying as necessary.

10. Indicate a revision date at the top or bottom of each new policy when added; for example, "Rev. 11/14/16." This shows that the handbook is being maintained and is up to date.

---

for orientation of new employees and as a handbook for people substituting for absent personnel. Figure 19-6 shows a sample page from an office policies and procedures manual.

For some offices, a more limited manual may be desirable—one that contains task lists only, covering the work assignments of each assistant, and arranged in the sequence in which the duties are performed during a typical office day. These can be easily updated and modified in a computerized file and can also be printed in hardcopy. Refer to Procedure 19-5 for step-by-step instructions on how to compile and maintain an office policies and procedures manual.

Employment Laws and Management Plans

Employers must adhere to many statutes and regulations that are administered by the Department of Labor (DOL) and other federal agencies*. The

Employer Law Guide published by the DOL is a resource that can be used to determine which statutes apply to a particular business. Some content areas of an employee's handbook are described next in more detail, including the laws that relate to them. An attorney should review the handbook for wording and content to avoid future legal problems. See the *Resources* section at the end of this chapter for website information on agencies mentioned. Office safety and emergency preparedness are found in Chapter 5. Laws pertaining to wages, hours worked, and payroll are covered in Chapter 20.

---

*Also check with your state's employment laws; some have enacted new state laws that cover such things as credit checks, dress codes, social media, classification of workers, and discussion of workplace hours, wages, and conditions.

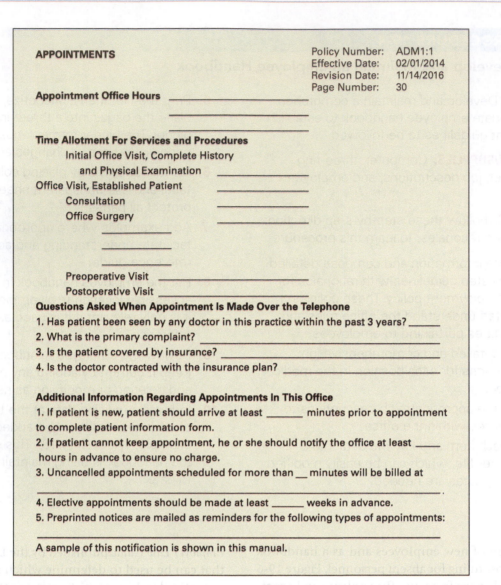

APPOINTMENTS

Policy Number: ADM1:1
Effective Date: 02/01/2014
Revision Date: 11/14/2016
Page Number: 30

Appointment Office Hours _____

_____

_____

Time Allotment For Services and Procedures

Initial Office Visit, Complete History
and Physical Examination _____
Office Visit, Established Patient _____
Consultation _____
Office Surgery _____

_____

_____

_____

Preoperative Visit _____
Postoperative Visit _____

Questions Asked When Appointment Is Made Over the Telephone

1. Has patient been seen by any doctor in this practice within the past 3 years? _____
2. What is the primary complaint? _____
3. Is the patient covered by insurance? _____
4. Is the doctor contracted with the insurance plan? _____

Additional Information Regarding Appointments In This Office

1. If patient is new, patient should arrive at least _____ minutes prior to appointment to complete patient information form.
2. If patient cannot keep appointment, he or she should notify the office at least ____ hours in advance to ensure no charge.
3. Uncancelled appointments scheduled for more than __ minutes will be billed at
_____.
4. Elective appointments should be made at least _____ weeks in advance.
5. Preprinted notices are mailed as reminders for the following types of appointments:
_____

A sample of this notification is shown in this manual.

FIGURE 19-6 Appointment page for an office procedure manual

American with Disabilities Act

The Americans with Disabilities Act of 1990 (ADA) is legislation that provides open access to facilities and nondiscriminatory care for all patients as it addresses the needs of employees or patients with physical or mental problems. A disabled person is a person who has a physical or mental condition that limits at least one major life activity such as walking, seeing, learning, and breathing, or a person who has a history of disability resulting from such things as a stroke or severe burns.

This law affects medical offices, hospitals, and nursing homes that employ 15 or more persons. To accommodate disabled employees, for example, job descriptions and work schedules might need to be modified to fit the person's limitations. Structural changes might include making drinking fountains and bathrooms easily accessible, widening aisles, raising the desk height to accommodate a wheelchair, and equipping telephones for use by the deaf. Steps taken to comply with the act would include training staff members with a fundamental knowledge on how to accommodate and communicate with patients from all walks of life so that full access for health care services may be provided. Document actions taken to erase employee biases, revise job applications, and create detailed job descriptions.

PROCEDURE 19-5

Compile and Maintain an Office Policies and Procedures Manual

OBJECTIVE: Develop and maintain a comprehensive, up-to-date policies and procedures manual for each administrative procedure performed in the medical office, with step-by-step instructions and rationales for performing each task to establish consistent guidelines to be followed.

EQUIPMENT/SUPPLIES: Computer, three-ring binder, paper, and procedure manual.

DIRECTIONS: Follow these step-by-step directions, which include rationales, to learn this procedure. Job Skill 19-3 is presented in the *Workbook* to practice this skill.

1. Ask each staff member to outline detailed instructions for work assignments. The job instructions can be reviewed by the OM and all office personnel for modification before being written as office policy. Clinical assistants' tasks can provide guidelines on patient care, contents of an emergency or crash cart, sterilizing procedures, laboratory and x-ray techniques, ECG procedures, and so forth. See Table 19-2 for contents of a front-office policies and procedures manual.

2. Compose and compile complete, detailed step-by-step instructions with rationales for each administrative function. These policies help maintain organized, efficient, and effective operation of the office, and employees understand why a task is performed in a specific manner.

3. Title each job assignment.

4. Key data into a computer file and print on loose-leaf sheets.

5. Alphabetize each task under assignment headings.

6. Collate and place into a reference three-ring binder. This lends itself to periodic updating as changes are made.

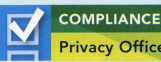

COMPLIANCE

Privacy Officer

To adhere to the Health Insurance Portability and Accountability Act of 1996 (HIPAA), a medical practice must have an appointed privacy official who drafts privacy policies and procedures and implements a program to educate and train physicians and all employees to the mandates of HIPAA—this person could be the OM. These policies and procedures become part of the office procedure manual, which may be used as a resource to train employees and physicians. Revisions need to be made as necessary and documentation retained for a minimum of 6 years.

7. Identify sections by placing colored indexing tabs.

8. Use transparent sheet covers to protect all pages.

9. Add samples or examples where appropriate to facilitate learning and act as a reference guide.

10. Put one office policies and procedures manual in an easily accessible location to all employees because it is only relevant if it is used.

11. Distribute appropriate sections to various departments within the office.

12. Review the office policies and procedures manual annually. Keep it current by adding any new procedures and deleting or modifying as necessary. This should be the task of one person.

13. Indicate a revision date at the top or bottom of each new assignment when added, for example, "Rev. 11/14/2016," because this shows that the manual is being maintained and is up to date.

TABLE 19-2 Front-Office Procedures Manual Assignment Headings

Areas That Might Be Discussed in a Front-Office Procedures Manual Are:			
Accounts payable	Dismissal of patient letter	Laboratory procedures	Professional courtesy
Agenda samples	Emergency and referral telephone list	Letter samples	Recycling
Appointment scheduling, cancellations, and recalls	Equipment and maintenance	Mail incoming/outgoing	Security measures
Authorization forms	Fee schedule and financial policy	Medicolegal forms	Staff meetings
Banking	Filing guidelines	Memo samples	Statements
Billing	Financial accounts	Narcotic records	Supply order book
Bonding	Hospital admission sheet	Patient information form	Telephone protocol
Bookkeeping instructions	Housekeeping duties	Petty cash	Travel information
Cash and check policy	Insurance claim forms	Photocopy policy	Waste management
Collection follow-up	Inventory	Physician's bibliography	
		Prescriptions	

Benefit Plans

Title I of the *Employee Retirement Income Security Act (ERISA)* covers most employee benefit plans in the private sector. Such plans are voluntary and ERISA sets uniform minimum standards to ensure the plans are maintained in a fair and financially sound manner. Benefits are ensured via the statutes and authority of the *Employee Benefits Security Administration (EBSA)* and the Internal Revenue Service (IRS).

Equal Employment Opportunity

The federal *Equal Employment Opportunity Act (EEOA)* prohibits job discrimination based on race, color, religion, sex*, or national origin. The *Equal Pay Act of 1973* protects men and women who perform the same type of work in the same establishment from sex-based wage discrimination. Protection for age discrimination for individuals 40 years or older is provided by the Age Discrimination in *Employment Act of 1967*.

Family and Medical Leave Act

The Family and Medical Leave Act was adopted in 1993 and applies when there are more than 50 employees on staff. A few policies that would affect hospital or medical facilities are:

- Employers must offer as much as 12 weeks of unpaid leave after childbirth, adoption, or serious illness or when it is necessary to care for a seriously ill child, spouse, or parent.
- A doctor must verify a serious illness and indicate the planned duration of medical treatment.
- Health care insurance covering the employee at the time of an illness must be continued during the leave, including employee contributions.
- Employees will be able to return to the same or a comparable position.
- Employees may be exempt from leave if they have not worked at least a year or 1250 hours or 25 hours a week in the previous 12 months.
- Employees are required to give 30 days' notice for a future planned leave.

Genetic Information Nondiscrimination Act

The Genetic Information Nondiscrimination Act (GINA) of 2008 is a federal law that prohibits discrimination in employment based on genetic information. GINA defines genetic information as: (1) individual genetic testing, (2) family member genetic testing—up to and including fourth-degree relatives, (3) fetus genetic testing, (4) manifestation of a disease

*Some states have passed laws that address "gender identity" and "gender expression." Check with your state to learn if any new discrimination laws are in place.

in an individual or family member, and (5) any request for, or receipt of, genetic services or participation in clinical research that includes genetic services by an individual or family member.

Code of Conduct

In creating a healthy workplace, a code of conduct may be established to eliminate unfavorable behavior against patients or between coworkers, managers, or physicians. Following is a brief list of some unfavorable behaviors, which are not accepted in a medical office setting:

- Bullying
- Coercion
- Discourteous or rude behavior
- Disrespectful words or actions
- Intimidation
- Threats

The legal term for "bullying" is *lateral violence*, which means belittling, harassment, or shaming. If bullying is allowed to exist in the workplace, it decreases productivity, increases stress, undermines relationships, and weakens the work team. Examples are constant criticism, intimidation, verbal abuse, as well as subtle actions such as ignoring a coworker, intruding on a person's privacy, removing areas of responsibility without cause, and assigning an unreasonable workload. An employee's actions should not be tolerated who fails to cooperate with a coworker in the normal course of business or interferes with office procedures.

Code of conduct policies should be clearly stated and all employees made aware of conduct expectations. Employee observation allows the office manager to catch undesired behavior and deal with employees who breach the code of conduct. It is important to make workers feel comfortable reporting violations, so an open door policy and reporting protocol should be in place.

Sexual Harassment

Any conduct in the workplace that occurs because of a person's gender is sex discrimination, and is prohibited by Title VII of the Civil Rights Act of 1964. If an employee regards the conduct as undesirable or offensive and does not solicit or initiate the conduct, then it is considered unwelcome. If employment conditions are altered so an abusive work environment is created by sexual harassment, then the work environment is considered hostile. The legal definition of sexual harassment includes several types of sexual conduct in the workplace:

EXAMPLE 19-1

Sexual Harassment

Sexual Advances by a Manager
The physician said repeatedly, "You look good in those tight white pants" to Jeanne each time she walked passed him in the office. Jeanne ignored the statement, hoping he would stop.

Sex as a Condition for Promotion
An administrator of a large group medical practice called female subordinates while they were at work and bragged about sexual encounters he supposedly had with several other female workers. One time he stated, "Maggie will get the promotion because she really knows how to make me feel good."

- *Quid pro quo harassment* (something for something)—Someone in authority offers a benefit in return for something else (e.g., a boss says, "Come to dinner with me if you want to get that raise"—see Example 19-1).
- *Hostile environment*—Continual, relentless, and unwelcome sexual conduct in the workplace that interferes with an employee's work performance or creates an abusive, intimidating, and hostile work environment (e.g., sexual flirtation, vulgar language).
- *Sexual favoritism*—Sexual favors are granted by an employee to a boss in exchange for a promotion. A second employee can claim harassment because of the favoritism.
- *Harassment by nonemployees*—Customers, suppliers, or other third parties perform some form of sexual harassment and the employer has some degree of control to stop the improper behavior but does not.

The OM should take every complaint seriously. All complaints should be documented in an *incident report* and investigated. Never assume or make judgments based on reputation or looks. Everyone is at risk for sexual harassment, not just women. If a case should go to court, the following questions may be asked:

- Did the practice know or should it have known that harassment was taking place?
- Did the practice take any action to stop the harassment?

To reduce liability, the medical practice should establish a written policy prohibiting harassment. The language of the policy should:

- State that sexual harassment will not be tolerated.
- Define various types of harassment.
- Outline complaint procedures and list the person of authority with whom to file the complaint.
- Guarantee that all complaints will be treated confidentially.
- Guarantee that employees who file a complaint will not suffer adverse job consequences.
- State that any employee who engages in sexual harassment is subject to discipline and possible discharge.

Plan a staff meeting to present and explain the policy and have employees sign a form indicating they have read and understand it. The OM should seek training on how to enforce the policy and establish an effective complaint procedure. In some states, sexual harassment training for management is mandatory. Refer to Example 19-2 for key features to include in an incident report and Procedure 19-6 for step-by-step directions when preparing such a report.

EXAMPLE 19-2

Key Features of an Incident Report

An incident is an unusual experience, occurrence, happening, or accident that takes place in the medical office. An incident report should include the following:

- Date of report
- Date, time, and location of incident
- Name, address, and telephone number of injured party
- Brief description of incident
- Action (e.g., first aid, telephone call) at time of incident
- Name of witnesses present at time of incident
- Signature of reporting party

EMPLOYER RESPONSIBILITIES

This section of **human resource management** includes recruiting and hiring new employees, conducting personal interviews, maintaining employee

---

PROCEDURE 19-6

Prepare an Injury and Illness Incident Report

OBJECTIVE: Report details of an office incident using an incident report form.

EQUIPMENT/SUPPLIES: Incident report form, or OSHA Form 301 for work-related injury or illness, patient medical record (when applicable), employee file (when applicable), and pen.

DIRECTIONS: Follow these step-by-step directions, which include rationales, to learn this procedure.

1. Obtain an incident report form and fill in the date, time, and place of the incident and the injured party's name, address, and telephone number. Complete the report in a timely manner to comply with office policy and state regulations.

2. Use OSHA Form 301 (Injury and Illness Incident Report) for a work-related injury or illness.

3. Interview the injured party and document a brief summary of the stated facts; do not include opinions or judgments. It is important to be objective and not become emotionally involved in the incident.

4. Interview witnesses and document their statements; be brief and to the point.

5. Document the action taken at the time of the incident, if any. For example, "walked away from an angry patient," "left the room when the off-color remarks were made," "called 911," or "administered first aid."

6. Proofread the completed report and review the document with the injured party.

7. Sign and date the report.

8. Make sure that the physician is aware of the report and file it.

records, orientation, training, and staff development. Strategies for working with various personality types are discussed as well as disciplining employees, handling employee evaluations, and terminating employees.

Recruitment and Hiring

A key responsibility of the OM is locating a qualified individual to fill a job that has become vacant or finding the right person for a new position. When résumés are received and application forms are completed, then the job of screening the applicants is performed. This is followed by doing initial interviews of the individuals chosen. Refer to Procedure 19-7 when recruiting an employee.

Applicant Screening

Applicants may send in a résumé or complete an application form. Review résumés and applications carefully by looking at handwriting, spelling, and sentence structure in addition to education, work experience, and skills. Read through those received to see if they are correctly typed, include essential information, and contain the qualifications needed to fill the open position. Can you read the handwriting on the application? Is the form thoroughly or partially completed? Did the applicant follow the form's instructions?

Screen all the applicants according to those most suited to the open position and then arrange personal interviews. If you telephone the applicant to schedule an appointment, you will have the opportunity to critique his or her telephone voice, which may be helpful if the position requires that skill. If a prospective candidate stops by the office to personally hand in an application or résumé, take the opportunity to see how the person is dressed and determine whether he or she projects a professional image.

Personal Interview

Prepare for interviewing an applicant by composing a standard list of questions you wish to ask—every person interviewed should be asked the same questions. Be careful not to make inquiries that would be prohibited by the Equal Employment Opportunity Act of 1972, such as an applicant's race, color, country of origin, sex, religion, medical history, debts, arrest records, former drug use, sexual preference, whether married, or has children. Example 19-3 illustrates legal questions to ask and obtain needed information.

PROCEDURE 19-7

Recruit an Employee

OBJECTIVE: Fill a new position or replace a vacant position.

EQUIPMENT/SUPPLIES: Job description, computer, telephone, paper, and pen.

DIRECTIONS: Follow these step-by-step directions, which include rationales, to learn this procedure.

1. Discuss with the physician and staff members the required skills of the new position, or, if filling a vacancy, review the existing job description to make sure it meets the needs and is current.

2. Discuss the hourly rate for the open position with the physician even though it may be listed in the job description.

3. Compose an advertisement describing the job and submit it online or to the classified section of the local newspaper; indicate what response is to be made (e.g., mail résumé, fill out application).

4. Telephone the local college or technical school and inquire from the career placement service or instructor of the medical assisting courses if he or she has any suitable candidates.

5. Attend local job fairs to let attendees know about the available position.

6. Call a local employment agency to obtain help in getting applicants interested in the open position.

7. Network with colleagues to inquire if they know of someone who might be qualified for the open position.

EXAMPLE 19-3

Illegal versus Legal Interview Questions

Illegal Question (Do Not Ask . . .)	Legal Question (Instead Ask . . .)
Where did you grow up?	Are you legally eligible for employment in the United States?
When did you graduate from college?	Do you have a college degree?
How many children do you have?	Do you have any commitments that could prevent you from meeting the work schedule that was discussed?
Do you have a car?	Is there anything that could interfere with your ability to get to our office every morning?
Have you ever been arrested?	Have you ever been convicted of a crime?

Use open-ended questions that cannot be answered with a simple "yes" or "no" answer, such as:

- What were the duties at your last job?
- What challenges have you encountered when trying to get to work on time, and how have you dealt with the situation?
- What kind of experience have you had handling multiple tasks at once without getting frustrated or losing your temper with patients and coworkers?
- How are you qualified to perform this job?
- What are two of your strengths and two weaknesses?

Refer to online Chapter 21* for a list of interview questions for the job seeker, which could be used as a reference aid in developing the office manager's interview dialogue.

Another list to be developed would pertain to the observation of the applicant's grooming, eye contact, interest in and motivation for the position, mannerisms, and so on. Explain the office policies regarding working hours, pay scale, future raises, and mention sick leave, time off, vacations, fringe benefits, and dress code; detail expected duties.

---

*Chapter 21, Seeking a Position as an Administrative Medical Assistant, *may be found online at www.cengagebrain .com with student and instructor resources.*

Ask the applicants for the names and telephone numbers of references you may have permission to call. Research at least two references and compose a list of questions prior to telephoning. You may also obtain a signed release form for a complete background check, including criminal and DMV record, and details from past employment. Background checks may not be used to discriminate against potential employees and must adhere to the Fair Credit Reporting Act. Check state laws to obtain information on which background checks are legal.

Let the applicants ask you questions also. This may give you some idea of their communication style. Conclude the interview on a positive note if you are seriously considering an applicant for the position.

Testing

After selecting several prospective employees, test their knowledge and skills to determine whether they are capable. For grammar, spelling, composition, and tact, have them compose a letter discharging a patient from the practice. For 10-key and computer skills, give a timed test. For telephone etiquette, prepare several brief role-playing situations; you can be the patient and the applicant the receptionist. For an insurance and coding position, devise a quiz asking specific questions about insurance carrier billing policies and create a coding test that has scenarios requiring both procedural *(CPT)* and diagnostic *(ICD-10-CM)* coding.

Employment Verification

When hiring an employee, ask for picture identification and a Social Security card. A newly revised *Employment Verification Form I-9* is now required within 3 days of hiring to ensure both citizens and noncitizens are eligible to legally work in the United States. A completed I-9 form must be kept for 3 years or for 1 year after the person leaves employment. Fines for "simple" or "technical" violations can range from $110 to $1100 per violation and go much higher for substantive violations.

A list of acceptable documents that establish both identity and employment authorization can be found on the last page of the I-9 document, or you can use an Internet E-Verify tool that compares information from an employee's I-9 form to data from the U.S. Department of Homeland Security and Social Security Administration records to confirm employment eligibility.

PROCEDURE 19-8

2 **Orient a New Employee**

OBJECTIVE: Direct a new employee through job orientation and initial training of procedures required in a medical office.

EQUIPMENT/SUPPLIES: Office policies and procedure manual, timesheet, paper, and pen.

DIRECTIONS: Follow these step-by-step directions, which include rationales, to learn this procedure.

1. Meet with the new employee; be friendly and courteous, and introduce him or her to all employees.
2. Familiarize the new employee with the entire facility, showing location of coat closets, supply cabinets, staff meeting room, laboratory, physician offices, restrooms, lunchroom, and so on.
3. Inform the new employee of the duties he or she is expected to perform.
4. Give the new employee a copy of the office policies and procedures manual and advise him or her to read it. Ask the employee to

note any questions down on paper for discussion at a later time.
5. Conduct training sessions appropriate to the job. This may involve having the new hire shadow a person working in a similar position.
6. Periodically check with the new employee during the first 2 weeks to find out if the work is going smoothly or if there are additional questions.
7. Meet weekly during the probationary period (typically the first 3 months) to address any problems or concerns and to give positive feedback on duties performed.
8. Check with the physician and other staff members to find out how the new employee is doing with the required job duties and working as a team member.
9. Note items discussed at any meetings with the new employee and comments from other staff members. This may be of some help when the employee comes up for job performance evaluation.

Employee File

File the original application, I-9 form, and résumé, noting the hire date. Hand out all job descriptions that pertain to the position and obtain a signed policies and procedures agreement form. Make copies of all certificates of training, document dates of tuberculosis and hepatitis tests, and note any exposure to bloodborne pathogens. Obtain the employee's emergency contact information and give the insurance enrollment form to the new employee for completion. Obtain signatures on other forms such as sign-off sheets for office keys and the confidentiality agreement. Financial forms related to payroll are discussed in Chapter 20.

Orientation and Training

The new employee should be introduced to everyone in the office and given a tour of the facility. An explanation of the types of patients seen gives the employee some

insight into who to expect to interact with as well as how to handle some of the problems that might occur. The employee's immediate supervisor usually walks the employee through the daily routine to make the employee feel more comfortable.

Specific training in use of the office's medical software program should be conducted by the OM or a knowledgeable and patient coworker. The employee should be allowed to take on responsibilities one at a time and not be expected to perform all tasks immediately. Refer to Procedure 19-8 for instructions on how to orient a new employee to the workplace.

Staff Development

Offer staff development opportunities to employees and encourage staff members to attend workshops, seminars, and medical conventions. Provide reading material from newsletters, bulletins, government carriers, and professional publications. Encourage employees to attend continuing education classes at local community colleges and to join professional organizations. The more knowledgeable your staff is, the more pride they will take in their work and the better job they will do.

Working with Various Personality Types

The OM has the opportunity to work with a number of different types of people. Similar communication methods can be used when dealing with patients, coworkers, vendors, and others as long as expectations are made known. Always project a positive attitude and learn to work with different personalities, not against them. Empower employees by giving them encouragement, compliments, recognition, and respect. Although work styles may vary, remember they were hired because they were qualified and have the right attitude to fit into the work team. Allow their differences to become assets.

One way to build morale is to learn what inspires positive action and recognize milestones (e.g., birthdays, anniversaries) and accomplishments (e.g., completion of school courses). Another way is to have a social event outside the office where employees can get to know staff members in a more relaxed atmosphere (e.g., Christmas party, company picnic).

Employee Disagreements and Discipline Approaches

Office morale, staff productivity, and even patient care can be affected when coworkers have slight disagreements. When conflicts do not resolve on their own and are not addressed, these can escalate into major controversies. A mature OM with sensitive leadership skills can intervene in a positive way to help determine a solution. A conflict resolution plan should be incorporated into the employee handbook and open discussions held to hear suggestions on how to handle such issues. Your response to employees who come to you with a disagreement will be directed by the circumstances at hand. By listening and allowing an employee to vent, often the right action will become apparent. If necessary, outline expectations and enforce them with a verbal warning; note in the employee's file of more extreme action is needed. Take the time to learn wise responses. Although there is no guarantee for success, a positive change in employee's attitudes might result. Following

are various examples with approaches that can be used:

- *Advisory Approach*—When an employee complains about a coworker's problematic behavior, try to help the employee solve the problem without intervening. Recall times when the employee acted appropriately and discuss how to reinforce this behavior.
- *Direct Approach*—When an employee leaves the reception desk unattended and another employee has to cover, speak directly to the employee stating, "Please let your coworker know at least 5 minutes in advance if you have to leave your job post so that coverage can be arranged."
- *Dismissive Approach*—When an employee complains about all the foot traffic passing by the door, you may want to let him or her vent and not take any action. A response could be "It sounds like this is disturbing you; however, I see you are trying to work through it and doing a good job of it."
- *Investigative Approach*—If an employee comes to you stating he or she overheard the receptionist talking back to a patient, this may involve improper behavior. Your response may be to formally investigate the situation by asking, "Can you describe how the conversation started and recite what each party said?"
- *Mediation Approach*—When two employees do not see "eye to eye" on how their shared job duties are being carried out, it may be the result of an interpersonal conflict, poor communication, or a lack of clear responsibilities. Your response may be to bring in an objective third person (another experienced employee) to help successfully resolve the disagreement.
- *Performance Approach*—When an employee does not like a coworker's personality and is disgruntled with the way he or she performs the job, try to provide work habit coaching with a performance objective: "Let's discuss three things that can be done to build a more effective working relationship. Then, we will assess your performance in carrying out these actions during your upcoming evaluation."
- *Planning Approach*—When one employee blames another for contributing to a problem at hand, it may be an interpersonal problem, a problem processing the information, or just sloppy work. Try outlining a work plan that requires both

employees to work together to accomplish the task. Let each know that they are responsible for making the plan work and getting the task done.

- *Team Approach*—When two employees disagree on how a new task is to be done, your response might be to put together a team made up of the two employees and two others who will discuss all the possible ramifications of doing the task in several different ways. The team then decides which way will be best.

Evaluation of Performance and Salary Review

Most employers use a 60- to 90-day probationary period to determine whether a new employee is able to work well with patients and as a team member performing all job duties in a satisfactory manner. A date and time should be set at the end of the probationary period to review positive observations as well as areas of deficiency (Figure 19-7). A negative review should not come as a surprise to the employee—any problems should have been addressed as they occurred. The employee may ask questions and be given the opportunity to respond to a negative performance evaluation by giving his or her version of the facts.

The development of employees is an ongoing process and should be continually addressed throughout the year, not just at evaluation time. The evaluation should be candid but constructive. A job description can become a checklist to review attitudes, skills, quality and quantity of work, personal grooming, team spirit, dependability, self-discipline, motivation, and attendance. It is at this time that any problems should be mentioned and a discussion on how to resolve them conducted using problem-solving techniques and helpful criticism. Specific goals should be developed to improve any deficient areas (see Example 19-4).

EXAMPLE 19-4

SMART Goal Assessment Process

Use the acronym **SMART** to set goals:

Specific:	Detail goals for success
Measureable:	Make goals quantifiable
Attainable:	Set realistic goals
Relevant:	Develop objectives for each goal
Timeline:	Set dates for reporting and goal completion

Use formal performance reviews wisely—they protect the employer. Such evaluations should be continued at regular intervals (quarterly or semiannually) because this is helpful for determining increased responsibilities, future promotions, and for reviewing salaries. The evaluation should be signed by one or two appraisers and the employee, so there is proof that the employee received the evaluation. The written evaluation should be kept confidential with one copy given to the employee and the original locked in the personnel file. Online Chapter 21 gives additional information on performance evaluation from an employee's perspective, and Figure 21-11 shows an example of a performance evaluation form. Refer to Table 19-3 for various types of performance appraisals with definitions and examples.

Termination of Employees

An employee who does poorly during the probationary period should be terminated using tact and giving him or her a complete explanation of the reasons for the dismissal during an exit interview.

An employee who has worked in the medical office for some time but is not performing satisfactorily should be fairly evaluated and counseled regarding the problem. A long-term attempt to cure the problem should be well documented—this will reduce the likelihood of retaliatory actions and future legal claims. If

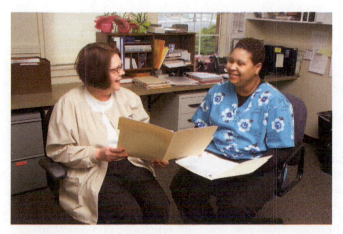

FIGURE 19-7 The office manager and medical assistant have established a good rapport by maintaining open communication during the performance evaluation

TABLE 19-3 Types of Performance Evaluations with Definitions and Examples

Type of Evaluation	Definition	Example
Behavioral Evaluation	Assess specific actions and conduct (on-the-job behavior) to weigh job success	The supervisor sits at the side of the employee while doing computer functions and accesses his or her attitude toward technology
Critical Incident Evaluation	Specific events and actions are used to assess employees' performance	The employee calmed down a patient at the front desk who was out of control. The appraisal focuses on the elements used in the successful encounter.
Duties Evaluation	The job description is used as a basis for assessment	Each duty of the job description is rated, either numerically (1 to 10) or in narrative form
Forced Choice Evaluation	Both employee and OM rate skills and performance	Assessment of the employee's ability to solve problems: Are solutions individually analyzed or are others involved in discussion of the problem?
Management-by-Objective Evaluation (MBO)	Compares actual performance and results against predetermined benchmarks	A certain number of insurance claims should be processed daily; daily results are assessed
Metric Evaluation	Various areas of performance are reduced to quantitative scales or standards and assessed by coworkers	Assessing how well an employee can multitask: Coworkers are asked to rate the employee on a numerical scale (1 to 10)
Performance Review Form	Various statements are included on a form with an area to check off "Excellent," "Satisfactory," "Needs Improvement," or "Unacceptable"	List might include: (1) Conducts self in professional manner with patients, (2) performs well under pressure, and (3) work is neat and legible
Periodic Evaluation	Supervisor appraises the employee's work at regular intervals throughout the year (weekly, monthly) in conference style	Annually, the evaluation is a compilation and summary of previous appraisals
Process Evaluation	Attempts to assess how well the employee follows procedures	Uses standards for such duties as accuracy of computer input or timeliness of submitting authorization requests
Rating Evaluation	Classifies performance on a number of job attributes using a numerical scale with room for comments	(1) Continuing education, (2) efficient use of time, (3) motivation, (4) neatness, (5) punctuality
Self-Appraisal	Employee initially evaluates his or her work by preparing a narrative summary of accomplishments; used as a basis for discussion	Accounts receivable was decreased by 3% during the last quarter
360-Degree Evaluation	Attempts to obtain feedback from everyone who works with the employee	How well does the employee communicate with patients? . . . Handle stress? . . . Interact with coworkers?

he or she does not improve, then dismissal would follow. Causes for dismissal include:

- Willful disobedience
- Violation of company policies
- Business downturn

The office policies and procedures manual should have a section listing the ground rules for terminating an employee. However, the final decision is left to the physician-employer based on recommendations by the OM. The OM is the one who should do the firing if he or she did the hiring. It is recommended by practice consultants that a discussion about termination with the employee be scheduled at the end of the day after all employees have left. When asked by a prospective employer for details about the employee who was terminated, the OM or physician can simply state, "The employee is not eligible for rehire."

According to the Fair Labor Standards Act, severance pay is a matter of agreement between an employer and an employee. It is usually based on how long an employee has been employed when he or she is terminated.

FACILITY OVERSIGHT

The OM is in charge of all aspects of the facility and the medical practice, including building maintenance, service contracts, utilities, insurance, equipment, and supplies. Keeping the office in good running order involves overseeing housekeeping duties and making purchasing decisions, although some tasks can be delegated to staff members.

Going Green

To conserve medical practice resources, which will also save money, "go green" and select products and practices that will help instead of injure the environment. Adopting green strategies involves a new perspective and changed behavior by all employees. Two environmental building rating systems have been developed by *Green Globes* and *Leadership in Energy and Environmental Design (LEED)* that offer "green" certification in several categories for achieving green practices for maximum environmental performance. Hospitals and health care facilities across the United States are now committing to "going green" and are reaping financial benefits and seeing reduced health risks. Assess the medical office and follow these tips to "go green:"

- Avoid incineration of waste products.
- Do not purchase furniture or textiles with "bromated flame retardants."

- Eliminate the use of mercury (e.g., thermometers).
- Increase recycling of all office products.
- Install systems to control lights, so they are turned down or off when not in use.
- Keep blinds open during warm days and let the sun heat the office.
- Landscape with drought-resistant plants where possible and do not use pesticides.
- Purchase PVD-free products (e.g., urinary catheter tubes).
- Recycle electronic equipment.
- Reduce the amount of medical waste generated.
- Select products with less and/or recyclable packaging.
- Set up energy-saving features, which will place computers and monitors in a low-power "sleep mode" after a period of inactivity.
- Use energy-efficient electronic equipment, lighting, doors, and heating/cooling systems that are Energy Star rated (e.g., light bulbs).
- View records and faxes onscreen instead of printing.

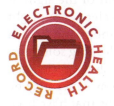

Moving to electronic medical records and e-prescribing has reduced paper and helped the "green movement."

Building Maintenance

Whether the building is owned by the medical practice or rented, it should be well maintained. If owned, the OM will deal directly with outside contractors and should arrange for periodic inspections to check the condition of the water heater, roof, carpet, parking lot, and so forth. Termite and fire inspections will need to be arranged. If the office space is rented, the OM will contact the landlord when problems occur.

Housekeeping

The OM will determine which housekeeping duties will be performed by the staff and which ones will be done by a professional cleaning service. The staff may be asked to pick up loose objects and make sure everything is in its place, dust furniture, wipe glass tables, clean mirrors, spot-clean furniture and carpets, and disinfect portions of the reception area (see Chapter 5).

Before selecting a service, minimum cleaning requirements must be established and standards set. Janitorial duties usually include vacuuming rugs, mopping floors, washing woodwork, scrubbing sinks and toilets, and emptying wastepaper baskets. Cleaning services are often reluctant to wipe treatment room counters and perform cleaning near unfamiliar equipment; these tasks are best left to staff members. The clinical medical assistant is usually assigned to disinfect treatment rooms and the office laboratory. This person should pay particular attention to countertops and doorknobs. Leave a note for the cleaning staff when special tasks need to be done.

Arrange a schedule for additional services such as window washing, laundering drapes, cleaning carpet, and other types of deep cleaning. Before a contract can be negotiated, several price bids should be solicited for comparison. If during the contract period, the service proves to be inadequate and discussion fails to solve the problem, seek new bids and hire a new cleaning service.

Cleaning Equipment and Supplies—Ongoing cleaning of equipment and supplies is performed by staff members so that they can keep the facility clean throughout the day. Protective gloves should be worn as necessary; try to perform tasks out of the sight of patients when possible. A vacuum cleaner (upright with handheld attachments), dust mop, and broom are essential equipment along with cleaning solutions, window cleaner, furniture polish, trash bags, cleaning washcloths, and a bucket. A carpet sweeper may be kept on hand to quickly pick up items that have been dropped or dirt that has been tracked into the office.

Equipment

Office and medical equipment must be serviced and maintained and may periodically need to be replaced. The OM can order new instruments, furniture, or expensive pieces of equipment only with the physician's express approval. Communication equipment, such as a computer, the telephone system, fax machine, and handheld devices, is offered by many vendors, so it is wise to do comparison shopping. Solicit staff input when purchasing such items as dictating/transcribing equipment and calculators. The performance of staff members often depends on the type of equipment used, so it is good to involve them in purchasing decisions.

Photocopy machines receive a lot of use in a medical office, and their selection should be based on the size of the machine needed, as well as function, volume, speed, ease of use, and cost. A postage meter machine/scale proves to be a good investment, saving both time and money. A paper shredder should be available; however, all final decisions to shred documents should be directed by the OM or physician. Computer hardware is considered a major expense and a thorough investigation should take place prior to deciding to purchase this type of equipment. Medical software can be expensive, and it is wise to investigate it thoroughly and spend a day at another facility where the software under consideration is being used. This will allow you to see it in action and ask questions prior to making the decision to buy.

Purchasing

When evaluating a piece of equipment, examine all of its special features and consider the benefits they will provide. Determine which ones are necessary and how easy the equipment is to use. Note the size, weight, appearance, warranty, and price. When replacing equipment, evaluate how the old piece of equipment served the office needs. If the equipment performed well and lasted a long time, consider replacing it with a newer model of the same name brand.

When large pieces of equipment are needed, decide first whether to purchase it outright or lease it. Look in the Yellow Pages, visit local retail stores, and search online for the best prices and sales information. Have sales representatives demonstrate the product and operate it yourself prior to the final purchase. Take time to analyze the product and compare it to others before selecting what you think best meets the needs of the office. You may want to get a recommendation from the physician and or discuss the purchase with him or her.

Each piece of large equipment comes with a limited warranty, usually for 1 year. Find out what is included and what is not, along with the length of time covered. Consider an extended warranty to increase the length of coverage if the item demands frequent service (e.g., copy machine). Consult an accountant about depreciation and tax consequences of all major purchases.

Leasing

Consider leasing equipment if keeping costs low is a priority or if the physician replaces equipment frequently. Before leasing, examine the terms of the lease agreement, find out the initial cost, and determine what the monthly payment will be. Consider how much you will pay over the time frame listed in the agreement and compare it with the outright purchase price. Find out if the lease includes service and if the lease payments are deductible on the physician's income tax return. Weigh the advantages and disadvantages of leasing and buying prior to making a decision.

Equipment Maintenance

Keep office equipment in working order so that it will provide high-quality service. Vacuum dust particles from computer components and the copy machine, change ink cartridges and toner when needed, and treat all equipment as if you owned it personally. Become familiar with each piece of equipment, so simple problems can be resolved without service calls. Solicit the help of a staff member who enjoys technology and put him or her in charge of equipment maintenance.

Repairs may be facilitated by keeping a service file containing maintenance records and operation instructions on all office and medical equipment. Major equipment repairs should be handled by qualified repair professionals. Guarantees, instruction manuals, information pamphlets, and service contracts are placed in the service file folder; and guarantee cards should be mailed as soon as the equipment has been delivered. If the medical assistant performs a well-organized approach to equipment repairs, delays due to downtime will be minimized, and many of the problems that can destroy operating efficiency will be avoided. To manage equipment maintenance, refer to Procedure 19-9.

OFFICE SUPPLIES

Ordering supplies and maintaining an adequate inventory is usually the responsibility of the OM, but the task may be delegated to those who use the supplies daily. The clinical assistant is primarily concerned with keeping on hand medical supplies and equipment related to patient care, whereas the administrative assistant orders clerical supplies, forms, and items used in running the business side of the practice. An inventory control system will help the buyer track actual usage and will discourage waste and theft.

Reducing Supply Expenses

Some suggestions for maintaining inventory and reducing expenses are:

- Establish a baseline amount spent previously on a specific item and then track price trends.
- Set a budget for supplies based on the average amounts spent during the past year or two.
- Comparison shop about twice a year, researching prices on major items.

PROCEDURE 19-9

Manage Equipment Maintenance

OBJECTIVE: Perform routine maintenance of office and medical equipment.

EQUIPMENT/SUPPLIES: Office or medical equipment, service agreement, warranty, service repair file, telephone, and pen or pencil.

DIRECTIONS: Follow these step-by-step directions, which include rationales, to learn this procedure. Job Skill 19-4 is presented in the *Workbook* to practice recording information on an inventory control sheet and equipment maintenance log.

1. Assign one person to request repairs on all equipment, thus eliminating the possibility of everyone, or no one, calling for service.

2. Arrange for equipment to be serviced immediately when failures occur.

3. Deal only with respected service companies that respond quickly to requests for service.

4. Keep an inventory control and maintenance log listing all equipment and repair costs; this information will help determine when the cost of maintaining a piece of equipment might justify its replacement. These figures will be necessary and readily available for making up the operating budget.

5. Understand the warranty and service agreement before the equipment is purchased. A service agreement is a form of insurance against future repair costs and as such contains certain specifications that should be thoroughly understood by the staff person in charge of managing the maintenance of the equipment.

6. Stockpile frequently replaced parts for future use.

- Buy selected items in bulk if storage is available, and consider pooling purchases if there are other physicians in the building.
- Take advantage of special discounts and free shipping incentives.
- Maintain a friendly attitude with the local stationer who can get items immediately even if most items are ordered from catalogs or the Internet.
- Track inventory in the storage room at regular intervals.

Ordering Supplies

The frequency of ordering supplies will depend on storage space and cash flow—availability of products and approximate delivery time also need to be considered. Supplies should be ordered to last for several months, and the ordering should be done on a preset schedule.

Important points to consider when selecting a supplier are quality, price, and service; that is, how the sales representative will work with you to get the item when needed. When the stationery or business supply houses to patronize have been chosen, the assistant should establish and maintain good credit and business relations with the designated firms. If a problem develops, work with the merchant to solve it. There is generally no reason to change to another supplier unless the service has deteriorated, items are inferior in quality, or a better price can be consistently obtained by another retailer. Most firms try to please their established customers by expediting orders and by allowing a new product to be sampled before purchase.

Orders for supplies may be placed directly with a sales representative; by email, fax, or telephone; or by completing and mailing a purchase order form. If necessary, delivery in 1 or 2 days can be arranged with United Parcel Service (UPS) or other delivery services. Typical office supplies ordered are paper goods (e.g., Kleenex, paper towels); copy machine and printer cartridges; paper for printers, fax machines, and copy machines; appointment sheets, daysheets, ledger cards, file folders, and labels if using a paper-based system; and letterhead stationery, envelopes, pens, pencils, rubber stamps, paper clips, and so forth.

Consider ordering online if you are in a remote area or if your storage space is small. Supplies ordered over the Internet can be shipped within 24 hours, less

cash is tied up in inventory, and less space is devoted to storing supplies.

Consider a group purchase organization (GPO) if you manage a small office and are paying high prices for goods. A GPO is an organization joined by a group of businesses to increase negotiating and purchasing power. Experts provide information to its members and handle the purchasing. The limitations of using a GPO might include limited choices of products (usually only one line of each product type is carried) and decreased information on new products.

Purchase Orders

A **purchase order (PO)** is a written authorization to a merchant to deliver merchandise, materials, or services at an agreed-on price. Once accepted by the supplier, the purchase order becomes a legally binding purchase contract. Purchase orders are used by large businesses, such as hospitals and clinics. When supplies are delivered, the purchase order number is included on the invoice as verification of the order.

Smaller offices use an order form (Figure 19-8), which may or may not include a PO number. Refer to Procedure 19-10 for step-by-step instructions when filling out an order form.

Payment of Invoices

Business-like purchasing habits are fundamental to the efficient management of the medical office. Purchasing supplies in bulk and paying invoices within the 10- to 30-day discount period will save the physician money. However, overstocking of items to obtain a discount can mean extra costs if the items become obsolete, deteriorate with age, get dirty on the shelf, or monopolize shelf space; for example, rubber bands stiffen if kept too long, and some liquids evaporate.

If an item is temporarily out of stock, the supplier indicates on the invoice "**back ordered (B/O)**" and returns a copy to the office; then, when shipment is received from the manufacturer, the supplier sends it on to the office. A date may be included to indicate when the back-ordered item will be available. When an order needs a follow-up, an item is defective, or a mistake has been made, notify the supplier and indicate the invoice number, the date of the order or shipment, and the complaint. When an order is received, each item should be checked off on the packing slip, which is a statement of the contents of a container. Then the **packing slip** is

map medical arts press®   **ORDER FORM**   67000_B

| 1-A | BILL TO: | Party responsible for payment. If name and address are not correct, please make changes below. We cannot ship to a P.O. Box. If P.O. Box is shown, please fill in street address in "Ship To" area at right. |

SOURCE CODE	CUSTOMER NUMBER
B2PX	6796030

PRACTON MEDICAL GROUP, INC
4567 BROAD AVENUE
WOODLAND HILLS, XY 12345-4700

Office Phone (555) 486-9002   FAX Phone (555) 488-7815
E-Mail Address: PMGI@AOL.COM

For questions...
Call _____ BECKY _____
Phone (555) 486-9002

To serve you better
Practice Specialty Family/General practice
No. of Doctors 2

1-B SHIP TO: (Fill in only if different from "BILL TO".) For delivery, we must have a street address. We cannot ship to a P.O. Box.

Name(s) _____
Address _____
_____
_____
City _____
State/Zip _____

| **3** | **PLEASE SEND ME:** | Fill in only those areas that apply to your order. | | | | | | | | _Please Fill In As Applicable_ | | | |

QUANTITY	CATALOG NUMBER	DESCRIPTION	MESSAGE	INK COLOR(S)	TYPE STYLE	LAYOUT NO.	LOGO NO.	PRODUCT COLOR	SIZE	YEAR	START NO.	TOTAL AMOUNT
3 ea	36 B	Correction pens										9.75
4 boxes	98IT	Plastic clip ball point pens										15.92
1 pk	337P	Post-it pop-up dispenser pack										12.73
5 reams	811P	16 # White bond paper						white				51.25
3 reams	989J	Yellow second sheet paper						yellow				6.75

COUPON CODE(S)	If you have any coupon or discount codes, please enter them here:			MERCHANDISE TOTAL	96.40

*For Rush Delivery specify: ☐ UPS Next Day   ☐ UPS 2nd Day
Check the box at left if desired. You will be billed for rush shipping and handling charges.

	Handling Fee	FREE
Sales Tax: Medical Arts Press collects tax in all states that have a sales/use tax. Please add tax at applicable rate.		4.82

☐ RX BLANKS (Complete the following information as it pertains to your state requirements.)
DEA No. _____
License No. _____

☐ MEDICAL INSURANCE CLAIM FORMS (Only complete the following if you want it printed on your forms.)
Box 25:
SSN No. _____
or
Group No. _____
Box 33:
PIN No. _____
or
EIN No. _____

*Rush Delivery	
TOTAL	101.22

FIGURE 19-8 Order form for office supplies

filed, awaiting arrival of the **invoice**, a statement of amounts owed that is prepared by the seller of the supplies or services listing quantity, item, shipping date, and price. Refer to Procedure 19-11 for instructions on paying an invoice.

Types of Systems for Controlling Inventory

A continuing ample stock of supplies depends on an effective inventory control system. A good system should include current office supply catalogs, an up-to-date list of all supplies, the number of items on the shelf, the reorder point, and time required to fill an order.

Many supply companies include a reorder form with shipments, so it is important to check the amount of remaining stock each time items are removed from the shelf or storage area in case an order needs to be placed.

Manual System

One method for maintaining adequate office supplies is to apply a label to the shelf of each inventory item on which is written the name of the item and the minimum number of units constituting a safe reserve. Each time stock is withdrawn, the units remaining are checked against the reorder point; when the reserve supply matches the number on the label, an order is placed.

PROCEDURE 19-10

Prepare an Order Form

OBJECTIVE: Prepare an order form for ordering office or medical supplies.

EQUIPMENT/SUPPLIES: Order form, inventory reorder notice, catalog, and computer.

DIRECTIONS: Follow these step-by-step directions, which include rationales, to learn this procedure. Job Skills 19-5, 19-6, and 19-8 are presented in the *Workbook* for practice.

1. Obtain all inventory reorder notices and make a list of all supplies and items low in inventory.

2. Use an order form and insert the "ship to" address where the items ordered should be sent by the supplier.

3. Insert the address where the supplier needs to send the billing statement (invoice) for payment, if the "bill to" address is different from the office location.

4. Note the customer (order) number, which may be preprinted on the order form. This number may be used for tracking a lost order and appear on the invoice when billing.

5. Include, as necessary, the physician's signature, a copy of his or her medical license, or a copy of the doctor's DEA certificate (required for some supplies).

6. Insert the vendor or supplier name and the address (if not provided) where the order needs to be faxed or sent.

7. Insert the date on the order, which is the date on which the order is placed.

8. Insert the method of payment (cash, check, credit card) agreed on under "terms."

9. Enter the agreed-on method of shipping (United Parcel Service, Federal Express, Airborne Express, U.S. Postal Service) and indicate whether express delivery is required.

10. List the quantity of each item ordered and type of unit (e.g., box, ream, package).

11. List the stock, catalog, or item number.

12. Give a brief description of the ordered item to ensure accuracy; the supplier may need to refer to the description if an item number is obsolete or entered incorrectly.

13. Insert special order information (e.g., color, style, size) if applicable, and the unit price in the designated areas on the form, stating whether it is sold individually (each), box, case, dozen, or gross.

14. Calculate and enter the total cost of all units for each item (multiply the number of units ordered by the unit price).

15. Insert a subtotal of all of the items ordered.

16. Calculate and list the sales tax required by the state.

EXAMPLE 19-5

Calculate Sales Tax

Using a sales tax percentage, multiply the total cost by the sales tax rate:

5%	7.25%
$ 125	$ 125
× .05	× .0725
$ 6.25	$ 9.06

17. Enter the shipping and handling fee.

18. Enter the "total amount due" for all items, including tax, shipping, and handling.

19. Either insert the name of the person requesting the item or sign the order.

20. Double-check figures and proofread the order before submitting it to the supplier.

21. Submit the order by fax, telephone, mail, or transmit electronically over the Internet. If ordering by fax, telephone to verify that the order was received and understood, and confirm the delivery date and payment requirements. If ordering by telephone, obtain the order or confirmation number.

22. Indicate on the inventory cards the date the order was placed so as not to duplicate the order.

23. File a copy of the order in the appropriate file for easy access when the merchandise is received.

PROCEDURE 19-11

Pay an Invoice

OBJECTIVE: To verify receipt of an order and pay the invoice using appropriate accounting procedures.

EQUIPMENT/SUPPLIES: Invoice, packing slip, check, envelope, and pen.

DIRECTIONS: Follow these step-by-step directions, which include rationales, to learn this procedure.

EXAMPLE 19-6

Invoice Terms

Term	Meaning
• Terms	Refers to timing of payment
• Net 30 B	Buyer has 30 days in which to pay the total amount
• 1 Percent 10 Days Net 30	A savings of 1% of the total sales amount by paying the balance within 10 days (or 2 to 5 Percent 30 Days Net)
• F.O.B.	"Free on Board" relates to responsibility for paying the carrier
• F.O.B. Point	Customer will have Point responsibility for the charge and claim if the material is lost in transit
• F.O.B. Destination	Vendor will bear the responsibility

1. Acknowledge receipt of merchandise ordered by signing the shipping receipt and listing the date received.

2. Check the original order against the packing slip to determine that all items ordered have been received in good condition.

3. Verify that dated drugs or supplies are current.

4. Compare the invoice with the packing slip and confirm that quantity discounts and discount dates have been observed.

5. Authenticate that invoice calculations and figures are correct; confirm the price.

6. Verify that the invoice has not already been paid.

7. Write a check for the balance due amount of the invoice. "For Deposit Only" may be written on the back of any check to be mailed. Then if the check is stolen, the thief cannot cash it.

8. Write the invoice number in the memo section on the front of the check to provide identification on the canceled check should any question arise at a later date.

9. Present the check to the physician for his or her signature.

10. Post an entry in the check register.

11. Rubber-stamp or write a notation on the invoice that indicates the invoice has been paid ("Pd" or "PIF" for "paid in full") and include the date, amount of payment, check number, and the assistant's or physician's initials.

12. Staple the packing slip to the invoice and file with other accounts payable receipts (in an accordion A-to-Z file folder) to be kept a minimum of 3 years.

A similar system is to put colored reorder reminder cards on shelves between boxes or supplies at the reorder point. A red marker or card might signal that an item needs to be reordered; a yellow marker is substituted to indicate the order has been placed. When staff members remove the item just in front of the marker, they notify the OM so the supplier can be contacted or the card placed in a "to be ordered" envelope. When the order arrives, the yellow marker is removed and a red marker is reinserted at the point where reordering is necessary.

With either manual system you can list each inventory item on **inventory cards** arranged in alphabetic order. Entries should be written in pencil because some data will change (see Example 19-7).

The amount of an item to purchase can be determined by evaluating and comparing information dealing with the consumption rate, cost, and amount of storage space available. If an item proves unsatisfactory, it can be identified by a notation on the card. Orders can be made by placing a call to the supplier's toll-free

INVOICE

No. 1972

Sold to:	Ship to:
Practon Medical Group, Inc. **4567 Broad Avenue** **Woodland Hills, XY 12345-4700**	**Practon Medical Group, Inc.** **4567 Broad Avenue** **Woodland Hills, XY 12345-4700**

Date	Order No.	Terms	Weight	Store No.	Dept No.	Shipped Via
05/01/20XX	97231	C.O.D.		15	23	United Parcel Service

BEST-BUY MEDICAL SUPPLY COMPANY

Quantity	Unit	Size/Color	Description	Unit Price	Amount	Total
12	boxes	medium	Non-latex exam gloves	9.49	113.88	113.88
2	cartons	white	Table paper	34.99	69.98	183.86
					Sales tax	9.19
					TOTAL DUE	**$193.05**

DATE PD   6/2/20XX
CK.#   4289
AMT.   193.05
APPROVED BY: MS

CUSTOMER COPY

FIGURE 19-9 Completed invoice with a paid notation

800 number, by fax or email, or via their website. Preplanning will avoid costly rush orders.

A running-inventory card provides preprinted columnar headings for listing quantity, reorder point, and the location of supplies (Figure 19-10). Each time items are removed from the shelf or storage area, the amount taken is crossed off leaving the correct amount remaining; this provides sufficient warning to reorder. Running-inventory cards should be kept near the supply cabinets.

Computerized Systems

Computer software is available for creating a database of inventory for equipment as well as clinical and office supplies. When an item is purchased, sold, traded, or replaced, the information is keyed into the inventory database. It is easy to add or delete items as necessary. A current inventory list can be printed at any time (Figure 19-11). The computer can be programmed to automatically alert when to order supplies and the order can be placed directly with the supply house via the Internet, which speeds delivery and reduces mistakes.

In a multiphysician practice, supplies are usually checked and stocked in a major supply room once a week, with the OM maintaining control and another staff member assigned as backup. Replenishing items on a regular basis prevents unanticipated shortages.

EXAMPLE 19-7

Inventory Card

Item Name	Manufacturer	Catalog Number	Supplier's Name	Quantity Ordered	Reorder Point	Unit Price	Total Price	Date Ordered	Date Received
Reminder Notice		401-123	ABC Medical Supply	3 rolls (#300/roll)	1 roll	$14.95/ea	$44.85	6/12/XX	
Past Due Notice		401-456		3 rolls (#300/roll)	1 roll	$14.95/ea	$44.85	6/12/XX	
Final Notice		401-789		3 rolls (#300/roll)	1 roll	$14.95/ea	$44.85	6/12/XX	
Dunn Message Labels	Stat Medical Company						Total Order: $134.55 plus tax & shipping		

Comments: Good quality

ITEM	QUANTITY	REORDER POINT	LOCATION
Black felt-tip pens	6 bx. 5 4 3 2 1	2	Drawer #2
9 x 12 manila file folders (center cut)	6 bx. 5 4 3 2 1	2	Cupboard #4
Blue adhesive file folder labels	8 bx. 7 6 5 4 3 2 1	5	Cupboard #4
3" center metal fasteners	6 bx. 5 4 3 2 1	3	Drawer #3

FIGURE 19-10 Running-inventory card for office supplies

Regardless of the inventory system used, all supplies must be counted regularly and labeled with expiration dates when applicable. The scheduling of inventory will be governed by the rate at which items are used.

Storing Office Supplies

When shelves are being restocked, older supplies go in front and newer items at the rear. If a central supply area is not provided, similar items of inventory can be grouped and placed at various locations in the office (Figure 19-12).

The following are tips for storing office supplies:

- Leave all bond paper sealed in original boxes; use older paper first and open new packages only as needed.
- Avoid storing paper products in cold, damp rooms; do not expose to direct sunlight.
- Stack boxes horizontally because standing paper packages on end will cause paper to curl.
- Install wooden dividers to separate items stored on one shelf.
- Store information pamphlets and maintenance brochures vertically to save space.

```
DATE: 09/30/XX    STOCK LIST    PAGE:1
TIME:  01:13 PM


STOCK
NUMBER    DESCRIPTION         AMOUNT
DEPT
....................................................................

3         ACE 1" WRAP              10
2         ACE 3" WRAP              10
1         BANDAGE                  10
5         SHEETS                    3
4         TONGUE DEPRESSORS         2


          5 ITEMS ON FILE
```

FIGURE 19-11 Computer printout of an inventory sheet for office supplies

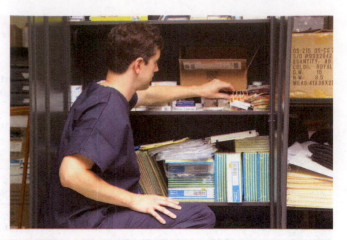

FIGURE 19-12 Medical assistant organizing supplies on a shelf in the medical office

- Position small items at eye level.
- Place large, bulky supplies on lower rear shelves.
- Never keep on hand more than a year's supply of inventory unless space is of no concern and the discount was terrific.
- Check all incoming orders to make certain that items ordered have been received, and then place them beneath or behind other similar items.

Disposable drapes and gowns have virtually eliminated the need for an inventory of linen supplies. If, however, the physician owns linens or contracts to have them cleaned, each item should be labeled with permanent ink. When linen supplies are delivered to the office, the medical assistant is responsible for checking the invoice to be sure that everything sent out has been returned. Refer to Procedure 19-12 for step-by-step instructions when establishing and maintaining inventory.

BUSINESS TRAVEL

The OM may be asked by the physician to formulate and expedite arrangements for business trips or travel to medical conventions held in this country or abroad. A worry-free trip depends on systematic and prudent planning to eliminate the frustrating problems that haphazard arrangements can bring. Regardless of the distance or duration of the trip, the manager should be able to make arrangements when the physician announces his or her plans.

Travel Arrangements

As soon as a convention site is announced and a decision is made to attend, the OM must see that applications for attendance are returned, and if requested make travel and hotel arrangements. Any delay or procrastination in initiating reservations may mean the physician will be unable to stay at the hotel where the convention is being held, and it might affect the chance of securing the most direct transportation at an affordable cost.

Use an atlas or perform an Internet map search if you are unfamiliar with geography and need to familiarize yourself with the location. Accumulate the physician's preferences in a travel file folder noting favorite airlines, hotel/motel accommodations, and car rental agencies. Also included might be discount and credit card identification numbers, passport and visa numbers, frequent flyer numbers, class of travel preferred, airline aisle or window seating choice, and other preferences. The OM can discuss with the physician the purpose of the trip, the dates of departure and arrival, as well as a daily business schedule and the preferred accommodations. When the basic details are obtained, the OM can proceed to make the arrangements via the Internet or telephone, or by contacting a travel agent who will handle all the details for a small fee.

PROCEDURE 19-12
Establish and Maintain Inventory

OBJECTIVE: Establish and maintain an inventory of all expendable supplies and follow an efficient well-organized plan of order control using a card system.

EQUIPMENT/SUPPLIES: File box, inventory control cards, list of supplies on hand, metal tags, reorder tags, and pen or pencil.

DIRECTIONS: Follow these step-by-step directions, which include rationales, to learn this procedure. Job Skill 19-4 is presented in the *Workbook* to practice recording an inventory of office equipment.

1. Compose a list of administrative and clinical supplies and insert a copy in the office policies and procedures manual.

2. Make a file for completed order forms and attach packing slips and supply invoices. These documents must be retained for a minimum of 3 years.

3. Create an inventory system of 3-inch × 5-inch file cards and list the following data on each card.
   a. Name of the item and quantity on hand.
   b. Identification or catalog number.
   c. Name, address, and telephone number for the supplier or sales representative.
   d. Reorder point: Place a reorder tag at the location where the supply should be replenished and place the movable tag over the order section of the file card to act as a reminder when placing the next order.
   e. Quantity ordered: Place the order and note the date and amount ordered in the appropriate location on the file card. Move the metal tag to the "on order" section of the card.
   f. List the price of each item.

4. When the shipment is received, insert the date received and unit cost or price per piece in the appropriate location on the file card, remove the tag, and refile the card. For orders only partially filled, let the tag remain until the order is complete.

5. Take inventory every 1 to 2 weeks to check stock and reorder. Mark the date on your calendar or make a tickler file in the computer each time inventory is checked.

Travel Agent

If the physician plans to be out of town on numerous occasions during the year or is planning a convention trip with multiple stopovers, the OM should select a reputable local travel agent to make the plans. A travel agent has the expertise to assist in all areas of travel (airline, hotel, car rental) and can handle changes or problems if they occur.

To work productively with a travel agent, the assistant should gather all information and determine a basic itinerary, that is a detailed outline of the trip. In addition to making reliable arrangements for transportation and accommodations, a travel agent will arrange for shuttles to and from the airport, procure visa application forms, obtain insurance information, make sight-seeing reservations, and handle any other special arrangements. The final itinerary is supplied by the travel agent, which can be distributed to other physicians and medical personnel who might need to contact the physician in an emergency (Figure 19-13).

Airline Travel Reservations

When making airline reservations via the Internet or by telephone, note the name of the reservation clerk and the confirmation number, which will be used to retrieve the reservation. Connecting flight reservations can be made with the airline through which the trip is initiated. Plane arrival and departure times are stated as local times. Multilegged trips usually require confirmation at every point of departure. A nonstop flight means the airplane makes *no* stops, while a direct flight means a stop or plane change will occur.

Typically, better rates and convenience are offered when booking online. E-tickets are then sent via email and when received, verify arrival and departure dates and times against the information on the itinerary worksheet. It is extremely important to clarify baggage fees and the charge for a cancellation or change when making the reservations. Airline tickets are nontransferable, may not be totally refundable, and have penalties to reuse.

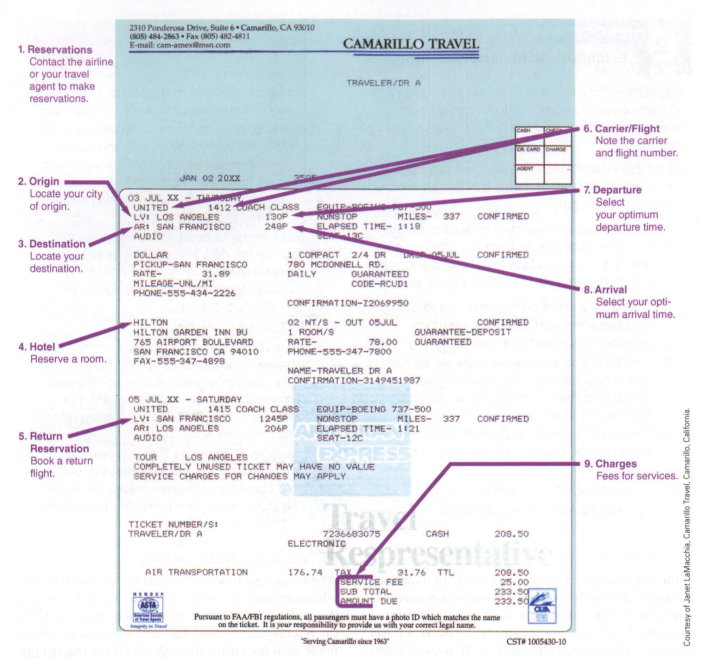

1. Reservations
Contact the airline or your travel agent to make reservations.

2. Origin
Locate your city of origin.

3. Destination
Locate your destination.

4. Hotel
Reserve a room.

5. Return Reservation
Book a return flight.

6. Carrier/Flight
Note the carrier and flight number.

7. Departure
Select your optimum departure time.

8. Arrival
Select your optimum arrival time.

9. Charges
Fees for services.

CAMARILLO TRAVEL
2310 Ponderosa Drive, Suite 6 • Camarillo, CA 93010
(805) 484-2863 • Fax (805) 482-4811
E-mail: cam-amex@msn.com

TRAVELER/DR A

JAN 02 20XX

03 JUL XX - THURSDAY
UNITED   1412 COACH CLASS   EQUIP-BOEING 737-500
LV: LOS ANGELES   130P   NONSTOP   MILES- 337   CONFIRMED
AR: SAN FRANCISCO   248P   ELAPSED TIME- 1:18
AUDIO   SEAT-13C

DOLLAR   1 COMPACT 2/4 DR   DROP 05JUL   CONFIRMED
PICKUP-SAN FRANCISCO 780 MCDONNELL RD.
RATE-   31.89   DAILY   GUARANTEED
MILEAGE-UNL/MI   CODE-RCUD1
PHONE-555-434-2226

                      CONFIRMATION-Z2069950

HILTON   02 NT/S - OUT 05JUL   CONFIRMED
HILTON GARDEN INN BU 1 ROOM/S   GUARANTEE-DEPOSIT
765 AIRPORT BOULEVARD RATE-   78.00   GUARANTEED
SAN FRANCISCO CA 94010 PHONE-555-347-7800
FAX-555-347-4898
                      NAME-TRAVELER DR A
                      CONFIRMATION-3149451987

05 JUL XX - SATURDAY
UNITED   1415 COACH CLASS   EQUIP-BOEING 737-500
LV: SAN FRANCISCO   1245P   NONSTOP   MILES- 337   CONFIRMED
AR: LOS ANGELES   206P   ELAPSED TIME- 1:21
AUDIO   SEAT-12C

TOUR   LOS ANGELES
COMPLETELY UNUSED TICKET MAY HAVE NO VALUE
SERVICE CHARGES FOR CHANGES MAY APPLY

TICKET NUMBER/S:
TRAVELER/DR A   7236683075   CASH   208.50
                      ELECTRONIC

AIR TRANSPORTATION   176.74 TAX   31.76 TTL   208.50
                      SERVICE FEE   25.00
                      SUB TOTAL   233.50
                      AMOUNT DUE   233.50

Pursuant to FAA/FBI regulations, all passengers must have a photo ID which matches the name on the ticket. It is *your* responsibility to provide us with your correct legal name.

"Serving Camarillo since 1963"   CST# 1005430-10

FIGURE 19-13 A travel itinerary and invoice

Most airlines offer 24-hour check-in via the Internet and serve-yourself kiosks at the airport to pay for baggage and/or obtain baggage tags.

Hotel and Motel Accommodations

Most hotel and motel chains have online websites and toll-free 800 numbers that can be used to make and verify reservations. A hotel room is typically "reserved" until 6 p.m. If arrival time is to be after 6 p.m., it is necessary to notify the reservation clerk ahead of time. If the physician is attending a convention, the assistant should convey this to the clerk to obtain special group rates. Before making the room reservation, the OM should be prepared to ask the hotel clerk the following questions:

- Do all rooms have Internet access?
- Is there a "business-center," "media room," or club floor that can be used with Internet access and computer/printer stations?
- Are there express check-in and checkout procedures?

- What is the deadline for cancellation? (Note it in writing.)
- What is the checkout time and is there a charge or penalty for early or late checkout?

When making a room reservation, the assistant should be ready with the following information:

- Type of room desired (single, double, queen, king, suite)
- Specific features desired (kitchenette, tub, shower, safe, refrigerator)
- Special requests such as nonsmoking, away from an elevator, lower floor room
- Number of people in room
- Approximate arrival and departure times based on transportation schedules
- Dates of occupancy
- Price rate desired

Car Arrangements

The physician may request a reservation be made with a local door-to-door shuttle service to eliminate driving and parking a car at the airport. This is listed in the telephone directory under "Airport Transportation Services." When booking, hotel personnel may be able to give you information regarding destination airport shuttle service.

If the physician plans to rent a car in the destination city, car rental discounts are usually given if an American Medical Association (AMA) or other association card is presented at the time the reservation is made. Advance car reservations may be made via the Internet when making the airline or hotel reservation. Reserve the car based on arrival and departure times.

Travel Help on the Internet

You can use the Internet to find the lowest fares. Internet navigational services such as Infoseek, Lycos, or Yahoo (see the *Resources* section at the end of the chapter) can help you locate travel sites. Enter a word or words describing a topic (e.g., air travel, cheap flights); a list of related websites will appear. Click on the address or the underlined or highlighted words to get to a site. Check out sites like the Internet Travel Network, which covers major and some smaller airlines and employs the same booking software that travel agents use. To be safe, use a separate credit card for Internet use only.

Use of a hotel broker (e.g., Hot Rooms, Hotel Reservations Network, Hotwire, Kayak) to compare prices and cut a lodging bill substantially. Hotels use brokers to fill empty rooms. Some brokers make the reservation and the client pays the hotel on checkout. Others require a prepayment fee. The broker may mail a voucher to the client or have one waiting at the hotel on check-in. If the reservation is canceled, a penalty may be issued by the prepaid broker to the client.

Medical Meeting Expenses

Expenses related to the attendance of the physician or medical assistant at medical conferences are considered tax deductible if courses are classified as professional and if credits are granted for attendance. Medical meetings are divided into two categories, those held in the United States and those held in foreign countries. Tax rules covering expenses for meetings held in this country are more lenient than for those held abroad.

The Tax Reform Act of 1986 requires that detailed written records support all deductions and that receipts for expenditures be retained. Basic information to support deductions includes date and time of departure and return, place of the event, the purpose of the event, and the benefit expected from attendance at the event. Travel expenses include lodging and meals subject to the 50% rule, which limits deductions to 50% of the cost. A photocopy of the signed registration sheet and a record of the place, dates, and time spent at each meeting will verify attendance.

The best way to document expenses is to use major credit cards and to complete the reverse side of the voucher each time an expense is incurred, listing the date, name, and location of the establishment, and the reason for the expense.

The rules and requirements for deducting expenses connected with seminars and conventions are complex, and the recordkeeping requirements are demanding. Some type of daily record detailing the expenses of an entire trip should be maintained (Figure 19-14). The tax implications can be attended to by the OM and the accountant. Refer to Procedure 19-13 to learn how to prepare a travel expense report.

TRAVEL EXPENSE REPORT

for _Gerald Practon, MD_

TRIP BEGINNING _June 10, 20XX_   **TRIP ENDING** _June 17, 20XX_

NAME OF EVENT _American Medical Assn. national convention_

DATE	SAT 6/10	SUN 6/11	MON 6/12	TUES 6/13	WED 6/14	THURS 6/15	FRI 6/16	SAT 6/17	TYPE OF EXPENSE TOTALS
LODGING	175.00	175.00	175.00	175.00	175.00	175.00	200.00		$1,250.00
BREAKFAST		15.00	10.00	15.00	9.00	15.00	10.00		74.00
LUNCH		15.00	16.00	15.00	13.00	12.00	15.00		86.00
DINNER		38.00	35.00	39.00	41.00	36.00	35.00		224.00
AUTO FUEL		25.00					25.00		50.00
PARKING FEE		40.00	40.00	40.00	40.00	40.00	40.00		240.00
PHONE/FAX		10.00	10.00	15.00	15.00	10.00	10.00		70.00
ENTERTAINMENT									
TIPS		5.00			5.00		6.00		16.00
MISCELLANEOUS									
AIR TRANSPORTATION								500.00	500.00
DOOR TO DOOR SHUTTLE								200.00	200.00
DAILY SUBTOTAL	175.00	323.00	286.00	299.00	298.00	288.00	341.00	700.00	

GRAND TOTAL $ _2710.00_

Description of business purpose/locations

Attend annual AMA convention (lectured on June 12, 20XX) in Chicago, Illinois. Theme: How Health Care Reform

Affects Physicians

FIGURE 19-14 A completed travel expense report form

PROCEDURE 19-13

Prepare a Travel Expense Report

OBJECTIVE: Complete a travel expense report by listing dates, details of the purpose of the trip, and related business trip expenditures.

EQUIPMENT/SUPPLIES: Travel expense report form (see Figure 19-14) calculator, and pen or pencil.

DIRECTIONS: Follow these step-by-step directions, which include rationales, to learn this procedure. Job Skill 18-9 is presented in the *Workbook* to practice this skill.

1. Insert the name of the individual taking the business trip.

2. Insert the dates of departure and return of the business trip.

3. List the name of the event.

4. State the purpose of the business trip.

5. Describe the benefit expected from attendance at the event to justify the business trip.

6. Insert all of the dates showing itemization of costs for transportation, lodging, meals, parking fees, telephone and fax fees, business entertainment, tips, tolls, and other miscellaneous business expenses.

7. Total each column showing the type of expense as subtotals.

8. Add all expenditures to get a grand total of business expenditures.

STOP AND THINK CASE SCENARIO
Determine the Agenda for a Staff Meeting

SCENARIO: You are preparing for an end-of-year staff meeting and need to establish an agenda.

CRITICAL THINKING: What items might you select to place on the agenda for discussion? List at least three items to talk about.

1. _____

_____

2. _____

_____

3. _____

_____

STOP AND THINK CASE SCENARIO
Calculate Prices for an Order Form

SCENARIO: You are preparing to order the following items from a supply company.

CRITICAL THINKING: (1-10) Calculate the price of each item ordered, (11) add them all together to determine a total price, (12) subtract the discount of 2% if paid in 10 days, (13) calculate sales tax at 5.25%, (14) add the shipping charge of 0.25% of total sale, and (15) calculate a total.

1. Ten cases of paper @ $23.92/case _____

2. Three 6-inch desk rulers @ $0.69/each _____

3. Five packages of transparent tape @ $5.85/package _____

4. Ten glue sticks @ $1.89/each _____

5. Twenty highlight pens @ $1.94/each _____

6. Twenty-five red roller pens, five to a box, @ $6.98/each _____

7. Twelve packages of adhesive flags @ $4.69/each _____

8. Two print cartridges for the laser jet copy machine @ $99.49/each _____

9. Eighteen single ink cartridges for the color copy machine @ $12.99 each _____

10. Fifteen reams of colored paper @ $6.64/ream _____

11. Total of all items ordered: _____

12. Discount: _____

13. Sales tax: _____

14. Shipping charge: _____

15. Total of all items ordered including sales tax and shipping _____

FOCUS ON CERTIFICATION*

CMA (AAMA) Content Summary

- Americans with Disabilities Act
- Employment laws
- Personnel records
- Performance evaluation
- Maintenance and repairs
- Inventory control
- Purchasing
- Personnel manual
- Policy and procedures manual
- Job readiness and seeking employment

RMA (AMT) Content Summary

- Maintain inventory of medical/office supplies and equipment
- Coordinate maintenance and repair of office equipment
- Maintain office sanitation and comfort
- Employ appropriate interpersonal skills with employer, coworkers, vendors, and business associates
- Understand and utilize proper documentation of instruction

CMAS (AMT) Content Summary

- Know basic laws pertaining to the medical practice
- Observe and maintain confidentiality of records
- Facilitate staff meetings and in-service, and ensure communication of essential information to staff
- Manage medical office business functions
- Manage outside vendors and supplies
- Comply with licensure and accreditation requirements
- Manage/supervise medical office staff
- Conduct performance reviews and disciplinary action
- Maintain office policy manual
- Manage staff recruiting in compliance with state and federal laws
- Orient and train new staff
- Manage medical and office supply inventories and order supplies
- Maintain office equipment and arrange for equipment maintenance and repair
- Maintain office facilities environment

REVIEW EXAM-STYLE QUESTIONS

1. Medical assistants:
   a. rarely get promoted to office manager
   b. move into management positions with a variety of skill sets and experience
   c. are not qualified to be office managers
   d. can attain higher career goals only with additional education
   e. make poor office managers

2. A patient complaint:
   a. is always hard to deal with
   b. should always be handled by the OM
   c. should be viewed as an opportunity for improvement
   d. should be taken directly to the physician
   e. both a and b

3. One easy and practical way of closing the communication gap and reducing patient questions is to:
   a. place practice information on Facebook
   b. present each new patient with a practice information brochure
   c. schedule and conduct new patient interviews
   d. maintain a separate telephone line for frequently asked questions (FAQs)
   e. encourage patients to talk to others within the practice

4. Adoption of flextime is one way to:
   a. keep the physician happy
   b. ensure employees come to work on time
   c. increase office productivity
   d. discourage overtime
   e. cross-train staff

---

* *This* textbook *and the accompanying* Workbook *meet the entry-level administrative and general competencies for the CMA outlined by the AAMA Examination Content Outline and Occupational Analysis and for the RMA and CMAS outlined by the AMT Competencies, Construction Parameters, and Examination Specifications (see Competency Grids in Appendix B).*

5. An employee handbook is also knows as a/an:
   a. office policy manual
   b. office procedure manual
   c. office routine's manual
   d. personnel manual
   e. work assignment manual

6. A written guide describing office routines may be found in a/an:
   a. office productivity file
   b. employee handbook
   c. office policy and procedures manual
   d. personnel file
   e. employee guidebook

7. Employment applications should be:
   a. disregarded if a résumé is provided
   b. reviewed by the receptionist when the applicant brings it to the office prior to an interview
   c. reviewed with résumés for handwriting, spelling, and sentence structure
   d. typed
   e. required only if all information is not included on the resume

8. A contract with a cleaning service would fall under:
   a. ordering office supplies and other miscellaneous expenditures
   b. facility oversight performed by the office manager
   c. the office manager's inventory responsibilities
   d. the administrative medical assistant's housekeeping duties
   e. purchasing and leasing

9. The OM should consider leasing equipment if:
   a. the medical practice cannot afford the equipment
   b. the physician has bad credit
   c. the office manager has bad credit
   d. the physician does not agree that a piece of equipment is needed
   e. keeping costs low is a priority or the physician likes to replace equipment frequently

10. A purchase order is:
    a. used by all medical practices
    b. only used by small medical practices
    c. a way to reduce supply expenses
    d. a written authorization that ensures an agreed-on price
    e. used instead of an invoice

11. "Net 30" means:
    a. the vendor is offering a percentage reduction on the purchased goods
    b. the buyer has 30 days in which to pay the total amount of an order
    c. the physician has a 30-month price contract
    d. the vendor will be responsible for delivering the order within 30 days
    e. the price of an item is good for 30 days

12. Business travel is:
    a. often arranged via the Internet
    b. arranged only after seeking the physician's preferences
    c. never handled by the administrative medical assistant
    d. only handled by the physician
    e. both a and b

WORKBOOK ASSIGNMENT

To develop competency-based job skills, refer to the *Workbook* and complete the:
- Abbreviation and Spelling Review
- Review Questions

- Critical Thinking Exercises
- Job Skill activities, which are listed at the beginning of the chapter under *Performance Objectives in the Workbook*.

RESOURCES

Books

Introduction to Medical Practice Management, 1st edition
Montone/Lenzi
Cengage Learning, 2013
Website: http://www.cengagebrain.com

Internet

AllBusiness
Resources for businesses
Management articles
Website: http://www.allbusiness.com

Business Manuals
Search: Medical Office Procedure Manual

Conflict Resolution Information
Browse: Virtual bookshelf

Employment Law Guide
U.S. Department of Labor
Conflict resolution resource

HCPro Healthcare Marketplace
Health management resources

Medical Economics Practice Management
Topics: Career/legal, personal development, malpractice

Medical Group Management Association (MGMA)
Practice Resources

National Labor Relations Board
Employee/Employer rights

Online Library Services
- Digital Library
- Internet Public Library
- Library World
Search: Topics (e.g., Sexual Harassment Manual)

Proofreaders' Marks
Symbols and abbreviations

U.S. Department of Labor
Search: Topics and agencies

U.S. Equal Employment Opportunity Commission (EEOC)
Employer/Employee topics

Medical Supplies—Online Vendors

Esurg
Group purchasing

Green Products
- Energy Star
- Green Electronics
- Healthcare Without Harm
- U.S. Environmental Protection Agency

Medical Buyer.Com
Medical equipment and devices

Organizations

Professional Association of Health Care Office Managers (PAHCOM)
Journal articles

Travel

Airline Travel
Tom Parsons' Best Fares

Complete Trip Information
- American Automobile Association
- American Express
- Expedia
- Priceline.com
- Travelocity

Currency
XE Universal Classic Currency Converter

Food
Zagat-rated restaurants

Inoculations/Traveler's Health
Centers for Disease Control and Prevention

Passport and Visa Information
U.S. Department of State Bureau of Consular Affairs

Transportation Security Administration
Luggage regulations

Travel Accommodations
- Kayak
- Orbitz
- Trivago
- TravelNow

Weather
National and local weather forecasts

Web Design

JKC Publishing
Web design services

Web Development
Search: Top 10 best website builders
- GoDaddy
- Intuit Web builder
- Webmonkey

Website Design
Search: Internet safety

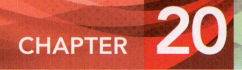

CHAPTER 20

FINANCIAL MANAGEMENT OF THE MEDICAL PRACTICE

LEARNING OBJECTIVES

After reading this chapter and learning step-by-step procedures to gain job skills,* you should be able to:

- Understand the value of a medical office budget.
- Distinguish between types of financial reports.
- Determine various ways to analyze practice productivity.
- List accounts payable categories.
- Explain gross and net income.
- Define payroll terminology.
- Name deductions withheld and state how they are determined when preparing payroll.
- Identify tax reports and forms used in payroll.
- State when quarterly and annual reports are due.
- Discuss components of an employee's earnings record and payroll register.

PERFORMANCE OBJECTIVES (PROCEDURES) IN THIS TEXTBOOK

- Create headings and post entries in an accounts payable system; write checks (Procedure 20-1).
- Create category headings, determine deductions, calculate payroll, and make entries to a payroll register (Procedure 20-2).

PERFORMANCE OBJECTIVES (JOB SKILLS) IN THE WORKBOOK

- Perform accounts payable functions: write checks and record disbursements (Job Skill 20-1).
- Pay bills and record expenditures (Job Skill 20-2).
- Replenish and balance the petty cash fund (Job Skill 20-3).
- Balance a check register (Job Skill 20-4).
- Reconcile a bank statement (Job Skill 20-5).
- Prepare payroll (Job Skill 20-6).
- Complete a payroll register (Job Skill 20-7).

---

* *This* textbook *and the accompanying* Workbook *meet the educational components for entry-level administrative and general competencies outlined by CAAHEP and ABHES.*

- Complete an employee earning record (Job Skill 20-8).
- Complete an employee's withholding allowance certificate (Job Skill 20-9).
- Complete an employee benefit form (Job Skill 20-10).

KEY TERMS

accounts payable

balance sheet

deductions

disbursement record

employee's earning record

Employee's Withholding Allowance Certificate (Form W-4)

employer identification number (EIN)

Employer's Quarterly Federal Tax Return

exemptions

Federal Insurance Contributions Act (FICA)

Federal Unemployment Tax Act (FUTA)

federal withholding tax (FWT)

gross income

net income

payroll

payroll tax

Social Security (FICA) taxes

State Disability Insurance (SDI)

state withholding tax

time card

Unemployment Compensation Disability (UCD)

Wage and Tax Statement (Form W-2)

wage base

HEART OF THE HEALTH CARE PROFESSIONAL

Service

Analyzing practice productivity involves scrutinizing financial reports, assessing medical care, and evaluating patient satisfaction. It takes a well-rounded medical practice to be successful, one that patients will talk about with high regard.

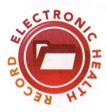

COMPUTERIZED FINANCIAL MANAGEMENT

In previous chapters, you learned about the financial administration of a medical practice, including fee schedules, credit and collection of accounts receivable, banking procedures, posting and balancing patient accounts, petty cash procedures, and processing insurance claims. In this chapter, you will learn how to interpret financial management reports, analyze practice productivity, generate disbursements for invoices and record them in an accounts payable system, calculate payroll, post entries to a payroll register, and understand which tax reports are needed for the employer.

In a medical practice, financial management is the most widely used of all computer applications. It provides an accurate business analysis of a medical practice and improves cash flow by accelerating the collection process. This system can retrieve and organize statistical data into a myriad of reports, which relieves time-consuming activities such as tracking office expenditures, counting the dollar amounts in outstanding accounts, and preparing numerous monthly reports, as well as accelerating the process of preparing billing statements and completing insurance claims. Following is an explanation of accounting systems used to capture data in a medical office.

Accounting Systems

Accounting is the systematic recording, summarizing, analyzing, and reporting of financial transactions of a business. Through the process of accounting, a medical practice can determine if it is making a profit or experiencing a loss for a given period. The following two basic accounting methods are used by medical practices:

- Accrual Method—Revenue is recorded as it is earned, that is, when services are rendered and billed to patients or insurance carriers. The exact payment that will be received from third-party payers is hard to predict; therefore, this method does not show an accurate accounting of cash on hand. Expenses are recorded as they are incurred, whether paid for or not.

- Cash Method—Revenues are recorded when payment is actually received and expenses are recognized when they are paid. Most medical practices use this method because it more accurately reflects the current financial status.

Medical Office Budget

In a medical practice, financial problems may develop and not be realized until it is too late. The office manager (OM) needs to keep an eye on the checkbook balance and have a good idea of how much *cash on hand* is needed for the operations of the practice each month (e.g., rent, utilities, payroll, insurance). Actual cash available is different from monies posted when services are rendered and shown as income on the daily journal. To project the actual cash that will be needed, a written budget is essential. The budget is derived from analyzing the previous year's income and expenses and then projecting the needs of the practice for the upcoming year.

Financial Status Reports

Financial status reports help managers and physicians plan and make corrections to avoid expensive problems. Each medical practice financial management software system generates a variety of reports, but the names of these reports vary depending on the software used. Some vendors provide inferior accounts receivable packages; therefore, the system selected should include the following basic reports.

Periodic Transaction Summary

A periodic transaction summary report presents the financial position of the medical practice at a particular point in time, usually the last day of the accounting period. It may be compiled into an annual report, such as a profit and loss statement, to discover the financial condition of the practice, for the completion of tax forms, for analysis of insurance needs, for loan applications, and for management planning. This report is referred to by other names depending on the medical software program used, such as *practice management report, annual summary sheet,* or **balance sheet**. Although this report may be prepared by the medical practice's accountant, it is important that the OM understand the reason why summaries are kept and why figures must be accurate.

To utilize a computerized periodic transaction summary, the physician circles procedures and diagnoses on each patient's encounter form. At the end of each day, the OM then compares the total charges and payments from the manual forms with those from the computer-generated management report. If they do not agree, the OM should locate and correct any errors and then post the reconciled total to a control log. At the end of the month, charges are added from the control log and compared with the computer's monthly total. This is not to check arithmetic but to reveal other problems. Sometimes after the date a transaction was keyed into the computer, it may have been adjusted incorrectly or the computer itself may be mishandling something.

Profit and Loss Statement

A *profit and loss statement* is a financial report for a specific period of time summarizing income received and expenses paid with an indication of the resulting profit or loss (Figure 20-1). It may also be called an *income and expense statement* or *operating statement*. Generally, this report is required at the end of an accounting period (i.e., fiscal or calendar year) to determine if the business has made a profit or loss, to determine a yearly budget, or to find out the net worth of the business when selling a practice.

Daily Transaction Register

A computer-generated daily transaction register (Figure 20-2) shows all the services posted for one day, including (1) the name of each patient seen, (2) the medical record number, (3) type of insurance, (4) date of service, (5) procedure code number, (6) type of service, (7) fee charged, (8) whether the claim has been paid, and (9) whether assignment has been accepted (AA). This information is critical when analyzing the day-to-day activity in a medial office and when comparing activity for days of the week or specific days in a month.

Accounts Receivable Aging Summary Analysis

A computerized accounts receivable (A/R) management system creates and maintains database files containing demographic and billing information used in the preparation of patient statements, insurance forms, and management reports including a breakdown of the A/R. It is a vital report used in the collection process.

An insurance *aging summary analysis* shows the age of the accounts divided by account type, so the physician can analyze how private pay patients and various insurance carriers are paying and take appropriate action on unpaid accounts (Figure 20-3).

PRACTON MEDICAL GROUP, INC.
4567 BROAD AVENUE • WOODLAND HILLS, XY 12345-4700
OFFICE: (555) 486-9002 • FAX: (555) 488-7815

Fran Practon, M.D.
Gerald Practon, M.D.

PROFIT AND LOSS STATEMENT
(monthly, quarterly, semi-annually)

For the Month of August, 20XX

Year to Date: December 31, 20XX

	2015	2016	Budget	%Last Year	% Budget
Total Income	$890,000	$991,000	$950,000	+8.81%	104.316%
Total Expense	$340,000	$365,000	$375,000	13.6%	99.635%
Net Income/Loss	$550,000	$626,000		+7.2%	

Math: 991,000 − 890,000 = 101,000 difference
890,000 ÷ 101,000 = 8.81% increase in income
991,000 ÷ 950,000 = 104.316% of budget expended

Previous year

Current year

Projected amount of monies for calendar year

Comparison increase or decrease between last year's expenditures and this year's expenditures

Indicates the percentage of the budget that was expended for current year

FIGURE 20-1 Example of a profit and loss statement with budget projection

Insurance Aging Report

Another way a computer software program can separate the accounts receivable is with a breakdown of the length of time (or age) the account is overdue (0–30 days, 31–60 days, 61–90 days, 91–120 days, and 120 days or more) as shown in Figure 20-4. It is also possible for the report to show the percentage of accounts in each category, only the accounts that are delinquent over 90 days, or accounts that are delinquent by a certain dollar amount.

Financial Summary

A *financial summary* is a monthly report that shows in detail the diagnoses and the frequency of cases treated by the physician, the amount of income generated each month, and the percentage of income generated. The cost of treating each diagnosis is listed to help with office management, inventory of supplies, and fee profile studies (Figure 20-5).

ANALYZING PRACTICE PRODUCTIVITY

There are many areas in a medical practice that can be analyzed and various ways to evaluate them. Following are several formulas to obtain information that will help determine whether the medical practice is profitable.

Overhead Expenses

Office expenses can be divided into several categories. Overhead expenses, more commonly referred to as "fixed overhead," include such things as the cost of the building (mortgage or rent), utilities, long-term equipment purchases, leased equipment, janitorial services, and permanent staff payroll. Items such as supplies and staff overtime vary according to the number of patients seen. Physician expenses such as malpractice insurance, automobile costs, and salary all figure into determining how much it costs to run a medical practice.

Cost of Procedures and Services

To find out the cost of performing a specific procedure or service in the office, divide the total expenses for the procedure for 1 month by the number of procedures performed that month (see Example 20-1).

EXAMPLE 20-1

Cost per Procedure Formula

$$\frac{\text{Total expenses for procedure}}{\text{Total number of procedures}} = \text{Cost per procedure}$$

DAILY TRANSACTION REGISTER

Run Date: 01/13/20XX

New patients are marked with *

PRACTION MEDICAL GROUP INC

① Patient Name	② Rec No	③ Ins-Type	④ Date/Ser	⑤ Code	⑥ Tx/Proc	⑦ Chg	⑧ Pd	⑨ AA
BOND MARK	430	Medicaid	12/16/XX	99233	HV L-3	130.00		Y
			12/17/XX	99232	HV L-2	100.00		Y
			12/18/XX	99231	HV-L1	75.00		Y
CHAN ERIC*	431	Medicare	12/16/XX	99204	OV-L4	106.11		Y
ESTRADA JOSE*	146	Medi-Medi	12/16/XX	99202	OV-L2	51.91		Y
NGUYEN KIN*	435	Medi-Medi	12/16/XX	99204	OV-L4	106.11		Y
SCHMIDT CARL	311	PPO	12/16/XX	99233	HV-L-3	130.00		Y
SOUZA JOE	13	Medicare	12/16/XX	99231	HV-L1	75.00		Y
SMITH FRED*	43	HMO	12/16/XX	99203	OV-L3	70.92		Y
TALMAN AL	432	Medicaid	12/16/XX	99291	CC 1st HR	250.00		Y
URICH BUD	509	BC	12/16/XX	99215	OV-L5	96.97		Y
WEST ALAN	213	BS	12/16/XX	99213	OV-L3	40.20		Y
WONG CHI	234	Medicare	12/16/XX	99212	OV-L2	28.55		Y
WYNN KEN	450	PPO	12/16/XX	99211	OV-L1	16.07		Y

Totals	Transaction Type	Patients	Number	Debit Amt	Credit Amt
	Production	12	14	1276.83	
	Collections	0	0		0.00
	Debit Adjustments	0	0	0.00	
	Credit Adjustments	0	0		0.00
	Grand Totals	12	14	1276.83	0.00
	New Change to A/R			1276.83	
	Total New Patients	4			

FIGURE 20-2 Computer printout of a daily transaction register for December 16, 20XX

Managed Care Analysis

While under contract to managed care plans, it is important to track capitated monthly payments with systematic audits. This is done by comparing the actual amount per patient contracted for against the incoming capitation eligibility list of current members. As mentioned previously, monthly *capitation* revenue means what the medical practice receives as a dollar amount per patient whether the patient is seen or not. The contracted rates by benefit plan are matched against the monthly capitated payment received. There may be errors discovered because of retroactivity of membership and inaccurate payments.

It is also important to have certain data available when a medical practice is making a decision to sign a contract to participate in a managed care plan because contracts may operate in a variety of ways, for example,

Run Date: 12/31/20XX

AGING SUMMARY ONLY
FOR PATIENTS INCLUDED IN THIS REPORT (ONLY)

TOTALS FOR FRAN PRACTON MD

INSURANCE TYPE	PATIENTS	DEBITS	CREDITS	BALANCE DUE	CURRENT	AS OF 11/01/20XX	AS OF 10/02/20XX	AS OF 9/02/20XX
NO INS	7	23,850.00	0.00	23,850.00	23,850.00	0.00	0.00	0.00
MEDICARE	43	72,650.00	3,811.97	68,838.03	65,632.86	3,015.17	190.00	0.00
MEDICAID	22	35,880.00	1,000.00	34,880.00	33,140.00	1,740.00	0.00	0
MEDI-MEDI	45	86,785.00	3,567.13	83,217.87	80,080.00	2,715.02	260.00	162.85
PRIVATE	16	20,985.00	5,643.18	15,341.82	11,749.13	3,592.50	0.00	0.00
WORK COMP	1	5,950.00	4,810.00	1,140.00	1,140.00	0.00	0.00	0.00
PPO/HMO	34	45,140.00	17,102.45	28,037.55	25,803.86	2,233.69	0.00	0.00
TOTALS	**168**	**291,240.00**	**35,934.73**	**255,305.27**	**241,396.04**	**13,296.38**	**450.00**	**162.85**

TOTALS FOR GERALD PRACTON, MD

INSURANCE TYPE	PATIENTS	DEBITS	CREDITS	BALANCE DUE	CURRENT	AS OF 11/01/20XX	AS OF 10/02/20XX	AS OF 9/02/20XX
NO INS	2	4,750.00	0.00	4,750.00	4,750.00	0.00	0.00	0.00
MEDICARE	83	100,698.69	82,295.74	18,402.95	6,029.14	66.54	0.00	12,307.27
MEDICAID	34	79,555.00	63,755.00	15,800.00	4,880.00	3,750.00	0.00	7,170.00
MEDI-MEDI	72	131,520.01	108,973.55	22,546.46	2,453.34	0.00	0.00	20,093.12
PRIVATE	40	65,843.75	24,111.87	41,731.88	5,843.86	27,310.00	0.00	8,578.02
WORK COMP	3	5,240.00	3,640.00	1,780.00	790.00	0.00	0.00	950.00
PPO/HMO	30	40,505.07	31,227.59	9,277.48	1,880.00	702.13	0.00	6,695.35
TOTALS	**264**	**428,292.52**	**314,003.75**	**114,288.77**	**26,626.34**	**31,828.67**	**0.00**	**55,833.76**

Includes transactions with posting dates through 12/31/20XX.
Report compiled using all of the patients.
Includes patients with all insurance types.
There were no condition codes selected or de-selected for this report.
Includes the patients of both treating physicians.
Includes patients with all balances.
Aged by date of first billing with an aging date of 12/31/20XX.

FIGURE 20-3 Computer printout of an aging summary report divided by physician and insurance type

Insurance Aging Report

Friday, January 02, 20XX

MEDICAID

Clyde E. Williams (WILLIA0010)   Date of Birth: 03/17/1933   Insured: Self
Insurance: Secondary   Policy: 5133031815   ID: 5133031815

Billing	Date	Code/CPT	Billed	Amount	Current	31 - 60	61 - 90	91 - 120	> 120	Total
Patient Total				95.00	95.00	0.00	0.00	0.00	0.00	95.00

Insurance Total				111.40	111.40	0.00	0.00	0.00	0.00	111.40

MUTUAL—Mutual of Omaha

James K. Froist (FROIST0000)   Date of Birth: 07/11/1972   Insured: Self
Insurance: Primary   ID:CMZX1C-193591-97

Billing	Date	Code/CPT	Billed	Amount	Current	31 - 60	61 - 90	91 - 120	> 120	Total
5170233	12/05/20XX	99204/99204	01/03/20XX	175.00	175.00					175.00
5170233	12/05/20XX	87070/87070	01/03/20XX	35.00	35.00					35.00
5170233	12/05/20XX	36415/36415	01/03/20XX	20.00	20.00					20.00
5170233	12/05/20XX	81002/81002	01/03/20XX	21.00	21.00					21.00
517305	12/11/20XX	99213/99213	01/03/20XX	95.00	95.00					95.00
Patient Total				346.00	346.00	0.00	0.00	0.00	0.00	346.00

Insurance Total				346.00	346.00	0.00	0.00	0.00	0.00	346.00

PAC POS—Pacificare

Dorothy J. Blan (BLAN0000)   Date of Birth: 02/23/1950   Insured: Self
Insurance: Primary   Policy: 90158778   ID: 463808651 01

Billing	Date	Code/CPT	Billed	Amount	Current	31 - 60	61 - 90	91 - 120	> 120	Total
5170434	12/20/20XX	99214/99214	01/03/20XX	150.00	150.00					150.00
5170434	12/20/20XX	93000/93000	01/03/20XX	85.00	85.00					85.00
5170434	12/20/20XX	36415/36415	01/03/20XX	20.00	20.00					20.00
5170434	12/20/20XX	81002/81002	01/03/20XX	21.00	21.00					21.00
5170434	12/20/20XX	Patient co-pay	01/03/20XX	-10.00	-10.00					-10.00
Patient Total				266.00	266.00	0.00	0.00	0.00	0.00	266.00

Alice Oganesyan (OGANES0000)   Date of Birth: 06/17/1960   Insured: Self
Insurance: Primary   Policy: 00010085   ID: 564972684

Billing	Date	Code/CPT	Billed	Amount	Current	31 - 60	61 - 90	91 - 120	> 120	Total
5166555	06/04/20XX	99213/99213	06/13/20XX 08/29/20XX	95.00					95.00	95.00
5166555	06/04/20XX	Patient co-pay		-10.00					-10.00	-10.00
5170283	12/09/20XX	99213/99213		95.00	95.00					95.00
5170283	12/09/20XX	Patient co-pay		-10.00	-10.00					-10.00
Patient Total				170.00	85.00	0.00	0.00	0.00	85.00	170.00

Mona Vargas (VARGAS0001)   Date of Birth: 07/23/1973   Insured: Self
Insurance: Primary   Policy: 00010659   ID: 584-69-5112 01

Billing	Date	Code/CPT	Billed	Amount	Current	31 - 60	61 - 90	91 - 120	> 120	Total
5167164	05/16/20XX	99213/99213	07/12/20XX	95.00					95.00	95.00
5167164	08/07/20XX	IA		-25.69					-25.69	-25.69
5167164	05/16/20XX	Patient co-pay		-15.00					-15.00	-15.00
Patient Total				54.31	0.00	0.00	0.00	0.00	54.31	54.31

Insurance Total				490.31	351.00	0.00	0.00	0.00	139.31	490.31

PRU - Prudential HMO

Patty J. Smith (SMITH0002)   Date of Birth: 09/12/1946   Insured: Robert Smith, Sr. (SMITH0000)
Insurance: Primary   Policy: 23236   ID: 54650875702

Billing	Date	Code/CPT	Billed	Amount	Current	31 - 60	61 - 90	91 - 120	> 120	Total
5166497	04/30/20XX	99213/99213	06/13/20XX	95.00					95.00	95.00
5166497	04/30/20XX	Patient co-pay		-10.00					-10.00	-10.00
5167710	07/09/20XX	99214/99214	07/12/20XX	150.00					150.00	150.00
5167710	07/09/20XX	Patient co-pay		-10.00					-10.00	-10.00
Patient Total				225.00	0.00	0.00	0.00	0.00	225.00	225.00

Insurance Total				225.00	0.00	0.00	0.00	0.00	225.00	225.00

Provider Totals										
Fran Practon, M.D.				45979.01	29743.84	2851.42	1114.13	600.94	11668.68	45979.01
Gerald Practon, M.D.				17885.34	7476.27	1413.79	414.85	805.00	7776.43	17855.34

Report Totals				63864.35	37219.11	4265.21	1528.98	1405.94	19445.11	63864.35

Percent of Total					58.28%	6.68%	2.39%	2.20%	30.45%	100.00%

FIGURE 20-4 Computer printout of an insurance aging analysis report

RUN DATE: 12/31/20XX		FINANCIAL SUMMARY						
ALL DOCTORS	PROC	12/01/20XX TO 12/31/20XX			PROC	YEAR-TO-DATE		
DESCRIPTION	FREQ	% PRACTICE	DOLLARS	% PRACTICE	FREQ	% PRACTICE	DOLLARS	% PRACTICE
OPEN WOUND ABDOMINAL WALL	3	0.2	345.00	0.1	31	0.8	5,005.00	0.7
CANDIDIASIS OF MOUTH	14	1.0	1,940.00	0.8	27	0.7	3,795.00	0.5
ENDOCARDITIS VALVE UNSPFD	10	0.7	2,050.00	0.8	15	0.4	2,700.00	0.4
MYCOBACTERIA DISEASE UNSP	0	0	.00	0	1	0.0	100.00	0.0
EMBOLISM/THROMBOSIS OTHER	2	0.1	260.00	0.1	2	0.0	260.00	0.0
TOXIC EFFECT OF VENOM	1	0.1	130.00	0.1	1	0.0	130.00	0.0
ACUTE FACILITIES								
COLLEGE HOSPITAL	380	25.9	60,795.00	25.0	1,046	25.5	172,615.00	24.0
GRANADA HILLS COMMUNITY HOSP	566	38.6	91,750.00	37.8	1,433	34.9	245,865.00	34.2
CONVALESCENT FACILITIES								
VISTA GRANADA SKILLED NRSG	57	3.9	11,150.00	4.6	79	1.9	16,185.00	2.2
HOLY CROSS HOSPITAL SNF	22	1.5	5,550.00	2.3	23	0.6	5,750.00	0.8
PLACE OF SERVICE CATEGORIES								
INPATIENT HOSPITAL	1,382	94.3	225,520.00	92.8	3,907	95.1	679,030.00	94.4
OUTPATIENT HOSPITAL	0	0	.0	0	2	0.0	380.00	0.1
DOCTOR'S OFFICE	5	0.3	810.00	0.3	55	1.3	7,155.00	1.0
SKILLED NURSING FACILITY	79	5.4	16,650.00	6.9	102	2.5	21,935.00	3.0
INSURANCE TYPES								
NO INSURANCE	43	2.9	9,040.00	3.7	221	5.4	49,900.00	6.9
MEDICARE	439	29.9	69,195.00	28.5	1,135	27.6	176,679.46	24.6
MEDICAID	115	7.8	25,400.00	10.0	458	11.2	106,885.00	14.9
MEDI-MEDI	725	49.5	112,540.00	46.3	1,356	33.0	209,594.18	29.1
PRIVATE INSURANCE	40	2.7	7,775.00	3.2	327	8.0	63,562.99	8.8
WORKMAN'S COMP	6	0.4	1,020.00	0.4	85	2.1	11,500.00	1.6
PPO/HMO	98	6.7	19,010.00	7.8	525	12.8	101,410.07	14.1
REFERRING PHYSICIANS								
NO REFERRING SOURCE	96	6.5	17,490.00	7.2	394	9.6	67,755.44	9.4
66 SINGH DENT MD	84	5.7	14,580.00	6.0	174	4.2	31,825.00	4.4
82 NAHED BALBIR MD	82	5.6	13,715.00	5.6	207	5.5	41,465.00	5.8

FIGURE 20-5 Computer printout of a monthly and year-to-date financial summary of a medical practice. The first part of the summary connects outpatient services to diagnoses indicating the number of cases treated by the physician, amount of income generated, and the percent of each type of case relative to all diagnostic cases. Other parts of the summary show number of patients treated, income generated, and percentage for various places of services, insurance type, and patients referred by other physicians.

monthly capitation amounts, copayments, discounted fees, withholds, and so on. Example 20-2 illustrates helpful ratios for tracking managed care information.

Capitation Stop Loss—*Stop loss* limits are set in the physician contract and limit the dollar amount of pre-paid services that can be incurred by any one patient during the plan year. For example, the plan may have a stop loss limit of $7000 per patient. In addition to the capitated amount paid for this patient, charges beyond this stop loss limit would be paid on a reduced fee-for-service basis. The physician must therefore keep track of all charges incurred for each patient. By maintaining good tracking, the physician knows when to bill on a fee-for-service basis for each patient.

Withhold—When physicians participate in a capitated plan, a percentage of the monthly payment from the

managed care plan is withheld until the end of the year or contract period (see Example 20-3). This is done to create additional incentives to provide efficient care and lower utilization. Physicians who exceed utilization norms will not receive the full amount. Withholds are also used to pay for administrative costs for the plan. To determine the percentage withheld, take the total amount of withhold and divide by the amount paid by the managed care plan that is withholding a part of the payment.

Risk Pools—In addition to withholds, some health plans have created risk pools. These risk pools are used to pay for nonprimary care services and are a further incentive to control utilization. If utilization is controlled, part of the risk pool will be distributed among the referring physicians.

EXAMPLE 20-2

Managed Care Formulas

- *Encounters per Member per Year*—Divide annual total visits of capitated managed care members by the average number of members seen per month:

$$\frac{\text{Annual number of visits by members}}{\text{Average number of members per month}} = \begin{array}{l}\text{Average number} \\ \text{of encounters per} \\ \text{member per year}\end{array}$$

- *Revenues per Member per Month*—Divide total capitation revenues by total number of members seen each month:

$$\frac{\text{Total capitation revenue}}{\text{Total members seen per month}} = \begin{array}{l}\text{Revenues per} \\ \text{member per month}\end{array}$$

- *Revenues per Visit*—Divide total capitation revenues by total capitation visits:

$$\frac{\text{Total revenues}}{\text{Total visits}} = \begin{array}{l}\text{Revenue amount} \\ \text{per visit}\end{array}$$

- *Total Managed Care Revenue*—Add total capitation payments received, total copayment receipts, and any fee-for-service revenues received from capitation members:

$$\begin{array}{l}\text{Total} \\ \text{capitation} \\ \text{payments}\end{array} + \begin{array}{l}\text{Total} \\ \text{copays}\end{array} + \begin{array}{l}\text{Fee-for-} \\ \text{service} \\ \text{receipts}\end{array} = \begin{array}{l}\text{Total} \\ \text{managed} \\ \text{care revenue}\end{array}$$

EXAMPLE 20-3

Withhold

Charges	$100.00
Patient's copayment	$10.00
Payment from plan	$55.00
Withhold	**$5.00**
Physician's adjustment (write-off)	$30.00

Note: The withhold of $5.00 must be tracked until the end of the year or contract period.

EXAMPLE 20-4

Capitation versus Fee-for-Service Plan

Capitation Plan

A specialist physician group may have 90,000 patients in a capitated plan and the group receives $0.81 per patient. The group receives payment of $72,900 each month for all 90,000 patients whether the patients are seen or not.

versus

Fee-for-Service Plan

A patient is seen and the physician is paid for each service delivered. Under the fee-for-service system, expenditures increase only if the fees increase and also if more units of service are charged for or more expensive services are substituted for less expensive ones. A physician group may charge for services worth $90,000 for the month and receive $48,000 (80% of allowed amount or 80% of $60,000) from the insurance company. This requires an adjustment of $30,000 (difference between the charged amount and allowed amount) and patients pay a portion totaling $12,000 (20% of allowed amount or 20% of $60,000).

Capitation to Fee-for-Service Ratio

Divide total capitation revenues by total fee-for-service (noncapitation) revenues:

$$\frac{\text{Total capitation receipts}}{\begin{array}{l}\text{Total fee-for-service} \\ \text{(noncapitation)} \\ \text{revenues}\end{array}} = \begin{array}{l}\text{Capitation to fee-for-} \\ \text{service ratio}\end{array}$$

Capitation versus Fee-for-Service Plan— Example 20-4 illustrates the difference in payment between capitation and fee-for-service and the ratio between the two.

ACCOUNTS PAYABLE

Verifying invoices and writing checks is another major part of running a business. You must learn to perform **accounts payable** procedures by paying bills and recording medical practice expenditures in a **disbursement record**, a separate journal that has many columns used to categorize expenditures (Figures 20-6A to 20-6C).

RECORD OF CHECKS DRAWN ON *College National Bank*

MONTH OF *June* *20XX* PAGE NO. *1*

CHECK REGISTER

	MEMO	PAID TO	DATE	GROSS AMOUNT	DIS-COUNT		AMOUNT OF CHECK	CHECK NO.
							BALANCE FORWARD →	
1		South Coast Medical	6/2/XX	75 00	7 50		67 50	1423
2		Sargeants	6/2/XX				37 90	1424
3		First Church	6/2/XX				100 00	1425
4		Faulkners	6/2/XX				58 87	1426
5		Mary Wells	6/6/XX				349 50	1427
6		Auto Club	6/6/XX				45 00	1428
7		White Motors	6/6/XX				97 85	1429
8		Professional Building Corp	6/6/XX				2200 00	1430
9		Model Laundry	6/6/XX				74 70	1431
10		Cash-Personal	6/6/XX				1000 00	1432
11	Reception chair	Fairfax Store	6/6/XX				206 85	1433
12		Union Oil	6/8/XX				32 90	1434
13		Love to Travel	6/8/XX				245 75	1435
14	Decorator	H. Cain	6/8/XX				305 00	1436
15	Direct Payment	Woodland Hill Light Co.	6/8/XX				138 90	
16		Petty Cash	6/8/XX				63 50	1437
17		Mary Wells	6/13/XX				349 50	1438
18		Woodland Hills County Collector (o/c)	6/13/XX				218 75	1439
19		American Medical Assn.	6/13/XX				549 20	1440
20		Dinner Dr. & Mrs. Ross	6/13/XX				151 50	1441
21		County Line Florist	6/13/XX				52 75	1442
22		Mary Wells	6/20/XX				349 50	1443
23		General Life Ins. Co.	6/20/XX				415 54	1444
24		Community Fund	6/20/XX				200 00	1445
25		First National Bank	6/20/XX				750 00	1446
26		Comp USA	6/20/XX				1175 00	1447
27		Mary Wells	6/27/XX				349 50	1448
28		Home Federal Bank	6/27/XX					
29	Deposit	Security National Bank	6/30/XX				140 00	1449
30		Bell Telephone	6/30/XX				330 00	1450
TOTAL							10,055 46	
					(A)	(B)	(C)	

PROOF FORMULAS: *7.50* *67.50* *75.00*
DISBURSEMENTS – COL'S. (B) + (C) = (A)

COL. (C) TOTAL = TOTAL OF COLUMNS USED FOR EXPENSE DISTRIBUTION.

195.77+
511.85+
1,398+
2,200+
468.90+
32+
218.75+
175.75+
74.70+
204.25+
245.75+
140+
1,175+
549.20+
300+
2,165.54
10,055.46*

FIGURE 20-6A Completed accounts payable disbursement record (part 1)

MONTH OF _June_ _20XX_

(MEMO) BANK BALANCE	LINE NO.	Deposit DATE	Deposit AMOUNT	1 Medical Supplies	2 Office Maint.	3 Salaries	4 Rent Upkeep	5 Utilities	6 Office Supplies	7 Taxes and Licenses	8 Books & Journals	9 Auto Maint.	10 Laundry & Cleaning	11 Promotion & Entertain.
15728 00														
15660 50	1			67 50										
15622 60	2			37 90										
15522 60	3													
15463 73	4			58 87										
15114 23	5					349 50								
15069 23	6											45 00		
14971 38	7											97 85		
12771 38	8						2200 00							
12696 68	9												74 70	
11696 68	10													
11489 83	11				206 85									
11456 93	12											32 90		
11211 18	13													
10906 18	14				305 00									
10767 28	15							138 90						
10703 78	16			31 50					32 00					
10354 28	17					349 50								
10135 53	18									218 75				
9586 33	19													
9434 83	20													151 50
9382 08	21													52 75
9032 58	22					349 50								
8617 04	23													
8417 04	24													
7667 04	25													
6492 04	26													
6142 54	27					349 50								
6365 74	28	6/27/XX	223 20											
6225 74	29													
5895 74	30							330 00						
TOTAL			223 20	195 77	511 85	1398 00	2200 00	468 90	32 00	218 75		175 75	74 70	204 25

PREPARED BY _Marilyn Fordney_

FIGURE 20-6B Completed accounts payable disbursement record (part 2)

Check Controls

The following guidelines will help maintain safe controls over the office checking account:

- Request that the physician maintain a separate checking account; for income tax purposes, this type of recordkeeping clearly separates business expenses from personal expenditures.
- Do not provide blank checks to anyone; maintain control over the stock of blank checks by keeping them under lock and key.
- Use sequentially numbered checks to be sure that none are missing.
- Determine a time each month to write checks. A weekly, biweekly, or monthly schedule will depend on the size of the practice, timing of incoming bills, and cash flow.
- Check purchase orders against packing slips, invoices, and supplies to verify the price, quantity, condition, and promised discount prior to making payment.
- Prepare checks from invoices or other legitimate documents; review statements from suppliers.
- Monitor and compare monthly utility bills.
- Do not abbreviate names or amounts when writing checks; spell everything out.

MONTH OF _June_ _____ _20XX_

	EXPENSE DISTRIBUTION												MISCELLANEOUS	
LINE NO.	12 Business Travel	13 Collections	14 NSF Checks	15 Equip. & Maintenance	16 Prof. Meetings	17 Bus. Insurance	18 Contributions	19	20	21	22		DESCRIPTION	AMOUNT
1														
2														
3							100 00							
4														
5														
6														
7														
8														
9														
10													Personal Cash	1000 00
11														
12														
13	245 75													
14														
15														
16														
17														
18														
19					549 20									
20														
21														
22														
23													Life Ins	415 54
24						200 00								
25													Treasury Notes	750 00
26			1175 00											
27														
28														
29		140 00												
30														
TOTAL	245 75	140 00		1175 00	549 20		300 00							2165 54

FIGURE 20-6C Completed accounts payable disbursement record (part 3)

- Use roller-ball or felt-tip pens to write checks; ballpoint or permanent ink can be washed out by counterfeiters.
- Make notations in the memo area indicating what the check is for.
- Sign all checks yourself; do not use the physician's signature stamps.
- Write or stamp "paid" with the current date, check number, and amount on each invoice or bill that is paid.

- Have someone other than the check writer reconcile the bank accounts.
- Refer to Procedure 20-1 to write checks, create headings, and post entries in an accounts payable system.

Overpayments and Refunds

As of March 2010, if an overpayment—money paid that the provider is not entitled to—is received from

PROCEDURE 20-1

Create Headings and Post Entries in an Accounts Payable System; Write Checks

OBJECTIVE: Create headings and post entries to an accounts payable disbursement journal and write checks.

EQUIPMENT/SUPPLIES: Disbursement journal sheets, invoices, bills, checks, and pen.

DIRECTIONS: Follow these step-by-step directions, which include rationales, to learn this procedure. Job Skills 20-1 and 20-2 are presented for practice in the *Workbook*.

1. Fill in the top of the check register and each page with the name of the bank, date, and page number.

2. Create and write in the names of the column headings under which you will record basic check information, such as name of payee, date, gross amount, discount, amount of check, and check number (see Figure 20-6A).

3. Write in the column headings for the bank balance and bank deposit (see Figure 20-6B).

4. Write in the column headings for each type of business expense. Refer to Figures 20-6B and 20-6C for common category headings.

5. Write the check (see Figure 20-7) for the expenditure indicating:

   a. written paid amount

   b. name and address of who the check is paid to the order of

   c. current date

   d. gross amount (prior to discount or for payroll)

   e. discount amount (or total of deductions for payroll)

   f. check amount (net amount after discount or deductions)

   g. signature (as it appears on the bank signature card)

6. Complete check stub (or register) information and bring balance forward (Figure 20-7).

7. Write "paid," the date paid, the check number, and the amount of the check in the appropriate columns. Review the columns for categorizing each expense and list the amount under the appropriate heading. If, for example, in Figure 20-7 the check was written to pay an electricity bill (Woodland Hills Light Company), it should appear in the "Utilities" column. Follow this procedure for each check written during the month. In some instances, a check may be written that must be divided among two or three categories; for example, a check for $63.50 written to "Petty Cash" and used for medical supplies and office supplies would be entered as $63.50 for the amount of the check, then as $31.50 under "Medical Supplies" and $32 under "Office Supplies."

8. Total each disbursement column at the end of the month.

9. Total the column for the amount of checks written. The total of the check column and the sum of all the disbursement columns should agree (balance).

10. Enter all totals on an annual summary sheet that is maintained monthly to be available for comparison and when tax returns are prepared. This sheet also contains monthly income information, payroll deductions and taxes, and accounts receivable monthly totals.

a government agency (i.e., Medicare, Medicaid), the provider must report the reason for the overpayment and return the money to the Secretary of State, an intermediary, a carrier, or a contractor within 60 days after the overpayment was identified. According to the False Claims Act, the provider is obligated to report and return all overpayments, regardless of the amount.

On the other hand, monies paid by patients in excess of the amount owed may be kept on the books as

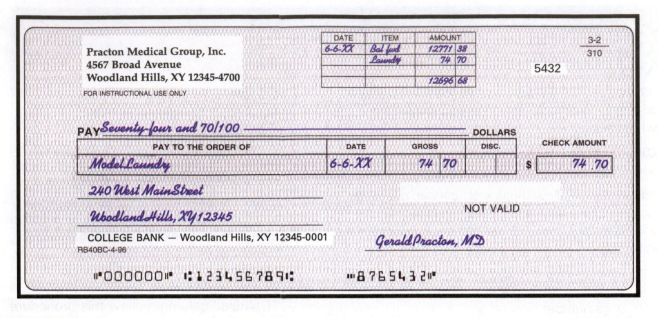

FIGURE 20-7 Completed check for a medical practice expenditure. Check stub superimposed on face of check for reference.

a credit (if the patient is active); however, it is best to inform the patient and offer a refund.

PAYROLL

The office manager or bookkeeper has varying responsibilities for processing **payroll** records and reports. Payroll refers to all wages and salaries paid to employees, including deductions. Since wages, salaries, and benefits constitute a major portion of a practice's expenses, great care should be taken to be sure these functions are done properly. The OM must be familiar with federal and state requirements for wages and hours of work in order to oversee employees and issue payroll.

Wages and Hours of Work

Minimum wage and overtime standards are covered by the *Fair Labor Standards Act (FLSA)*. Rules apply to *nonexempt employees*. An *exempt employee* is one who is released from requirements of federal and state wage and hour laws*. Administrative medical assistants would be nonexempt; however, office managers may fall into the exempt category since their work is "primarily intellectual, managerial, or creative, and which requires exercise of discretion and independent judgment."

A federal minimum wage amount is set for all employees 20 years of age or older. Youth minimum wage applies to workers under 20 years of age during their first 90 consecutive calendar days of employment, after which the youth worker must be paid the full minimum wage. Individual states may have their own minimum wage laws that would supersede federal law and require payment of a higher wage. Special rules cover home workers, child labor, foreign workers, and nonimmigrant workers. Although state laws vary, typically a 30-minute mealtime is required (without pay)

---

*Fines may be imposed in some states for the willful misclassification of workers.

when an employee works greater than 5 hours as well as 10-minute break times for every 4 hours worked.

Some states have legislation in place that require employers to provide a written notice to each new hire that specifies rate of pay, method of payment, classification of employee (salary versus hourly), and any overtime rates.

Overtime

FLSA does not place a limit on the total hours worked; however, it does require that for all covered employees 16 years of age or older, the rate of pay in excess of 40 hours in a workweek be paid at a rate of one and one-half times their hourly wage. Individual states may have laws for employees working in excess of 8 hours a day and rules that apply to double time.

Office Posting Requirements

Employers must clearly post specific Federal Labor Law information. Posting of local laws will vary from state to state. Following are key items included in posting requirements:

- Civil Rights Act of 1964; equal opportunity
- Disability Insurance
- Discrimination Acts: Age, Americans with Disabilities, Title VII
- Employee Polygraph Protection Act of 1988
- Family and Medical Leave Act of 1993 (50 or more employees)
- Federal Minimum Wage (Fair Labor Standards Act)
- Medical Emergency Contact
- No Smoking Policy
- Notification of Employee Rights Under Federal Labor Laws
- Occupational Safety and Health Act of 1970
- Payday Schedule
- Rehabilitation Act of 1973
- Vietnam Era Veterans Readjustment Assistance Act of 1974
- Workers' Compensation Coverage
- Unemployment Benefits
- Uniformed Services Employment and Reemployment Rights Act

Payroll Procedures

Employers must keep records on hours worked, wages, and other information as set forth in the Department of Labor's regulations. Usually a **time card** is kept for each pay period indicating the days and hours worked for each employee. At the end of the pay period, it is signed by the employee and turned in to the person responsible for payroll. Payroll information must be posted on a separate earnings record and employees given an itemized statement with each paycheck. Regular paydays must be set by employers and pay distributed within 10 days of the end of each pay period. If an employee resigns, wages must be paid within 72 hours; if fired or laid off, wages are to be paid immediately.

Practices may hire a bookkeeper or an accountant or utilize payroll software. If the payroll is done by a computer system (e.g., EasyPay Payroll Services), it should have the capabilities to calculate deductions and taxes, print forms and year-end reports, and write checks.

A payroll company may supply the computerized software for a reasonable price and trains employees. Services include calculating the payroll and deductions; printing payroll checks; transmitting federal and state remittances at the required intervals; producing semimonthly, quarterly, and yearly reports; and notifying the employer of tax regulations and changes. Small offices may prefer to use a write-it-once payroll journal, which resembles the pegboard bookkeeping system and combines check writing with an itemized account of all deductions written simultaneously and recorded on the payroll journal.

When the office manager is in complete charge of the payroll, responsibilities might include explaining payroll procedures and policies to new employees, obtaining payroll information, processing payroll checks, and understanding the regulations and forms legislated by the **Federal Insurance Contributions Act (FICA)** (called **Social Security taxes**), the Fair Labor Standards Act, the federal and state unemployment compensation acts, Internal Revenue Service (IRS) income tax laws, and **state withholding tax** laws. Quarterly and annual reports must be filed with the IRS, and in some states reports are also filed with a state agency.

Employer Identification Number

As mentioned in Chapter 18, every physician-employer must have a tax identification number for federal tax accounting purposes. The **employer identification number (EIN)** is a nine-digit number (see Example 20-5).

EXAMPLE 20-5

Employer Identification Number

12-3456789

The physician applies for a number from the Internal Revenue Service, using Form SS-4. The practice may already have a *tax identification number (TIN)* by virtue of being an entity other than a sole proprietorship. In that event, the same TIN is used for payroll purposes. In states that require employers' payroll reports, the state will issue a separate identification number.

Social Security Number

Each person born in the United States is required to obtain a Social Security number by age 2. The card contains a nine-digit tax identification number used by employees and retained for life. The first three digits indicate where the cardholder lived when the card was requested. The middle two numbers follow a pattern known only to government officials and can be used to spot phony cards. The last four numbers are randomly assigned with no two individuals having the same number.

Application may be made at the nearest Social Security office using Form SS-5. Those who are not born in the United States may obtain a Social Security card by proving age, identity, and status. An original birth certificate, other forms of identification, and documents from the Immigration and Naturalization Service (INS) are needed. When in the process of being hired, each person is required to provide his or her Social Security number and the employer then lists the number on all payroll transactions.

Employment Eligibility Verification

The Immigration and Nationality Act requires employers to verify that all employees hired, citizens and noncitizens, are authorized to work. As mentioned in Chapter 19, the Employment Eligibility Verification Form I-9 is completed for this purpose. Any documents presented proving the employee's identity and work eligibility need to be examined by the employer for genuineness prior to being recorded. Some states also require employers to file a "New Employee Registry" (e.g., CA form DE-34). This form is used to quickly identify employees responsible for child support and other state liabilities.

Employers in all states are able to verify Social Security numbers and work eligibility in the United States electronically through the Social Security Number Verification Service (SSNVS). Verification must be made within 3 days of hire.

Employee Withholding Allowance Certificate

Because income taxes are deducted on a pay-as-you-go plan, each new employee must complete an **Employee's Withholding Allowance Certificate (Form W-4)**, stating the number of claimed **exemptions** (Figure 20-8). Each employee is entitled to one exemption for himself or herself and one for each person claimed as a dependent if not claimed by someone else. The employee who takes no exemptions, thereby increasing the amount of withheld tax, may qualify for an income tax refund at the end of the year. An employee who paid no tax last year or expects to pay no tax this year can be exempt from any withholding tax.

Generally, by December 1 of each year, the person doing payroll should ask each employee to file a new W-4 form, requesting any changes such as name, address, marital status, and number of exemptions. Make sure employees also report any name changes to the Social Security Administration and *do not* change payroll records until the employee has obtained a new Social Security card. This can ensure more accurate wage reporting and eliminate earnings being held in a suspense file rather than credited to an employee's earning record.

Payroll Deductions

Payroll deductions are categorized as before-tax and after-tax deductions. Before-tax deductions include all monies that are exempt from income taxes such as flexible spending accounts, medical insurance, and voluntary tax-deferred retirement contributions (e.g., 401K). After-tax deductions are not exempt from taxes. These include long-term disability, union dues, and charitable contributions (e.g., United Way).

Cut here and give Form W-4 to your employer. Keep the top part for your records.

Form **W-4** — **Employee's Withholding Allowance Certificate** — OMB No. 1545-0074 — **2016**

Department of the Treasury Internal Revenue Service

▶ **Whether you are entitled to claim a certain number of allowances or exemption from withholding is subject to review by the IRS. Your employer may be required to send a copy of this form to the IRS.**

1 Your first name and middle initial: Kevin | Last name: O'Brien | 2 Your social security number: XXX: XX: 1963

Home address (number and street or rural route): 2521 Olive Avenue

3 ☒ Single ☐ Married ☐ Married, but withhold at higher Single rate.
Note. If married, but legally separated, or spouse is a nonresident alien, check the "Single" box.

City or town, state, and ZIP code: Woodland Hills, XY 12345-0001

4 **If your last name differs from that shown on your social security card, check here. You must call 1-800-772-1213 for a new card.** ▶ ☐

5 Total number of allowances you are claiming (from line **H** above **or** from the applicable worksheet on page 2) — 5: 1

6 Additional amount, if any, you want withheld from each paycheck — 6: $

7 I claim exemption from withholding for 2006, and I certify that I meet **both** of the following conditions for exemption.
- Last year I had a right to a refund of **all** federal income tax withheld because I had **no** tax liability **and**
- This year I expect a refund of **all** federal income tax withheld because I expect to have **no** tax liability.

If you meet both conditions, write "Exempt" here ▶ 7

Under penalties of perjury, I declare that I have examined this certificate and to the best of my knowledge and belief, it is true, correct, and complete.

Employee's signature (Form is not valid unless you sign it.) ▶ Kevin O'Brien — **Date** ▶ January 2, 20XX

8 Employer's name and address (Employer: Complete lines 8 and 10 only if sending to the IRS.): Practon Medical Group, Inc. 4567 Broad Avenue, Woodland Hills, XY 12345-4700 | 9 Office code (optional) | 10 Employer identification number (EIN): 95 : 36640XX

For Privacy Act and Paperwork Reduction Act Notice, see page 2. Cat. No. 10220Q Form **W-4** (2012)

Internal Revenue Service, www.irs.gov

FIGURE 20-8 Employee's Withholding Allowance Certificate, Form W-4

Federal Insurance Contributions Act Taxes

Under Social Security, the Federal Insurance Contributions Act (FICA) has three separate programs financed from one payroll tax to which employers and employees contribute at a rate specified by law.

1. *Old Age Survivors and Disabilities Insurance (OASDI) (retirement program)*—provides older adults with retirement benefits and their surviving dependents with survivors' benefits.
2. *Medicare Hospital Insurance (HI) program*—provides hospitalization insurance for older adults.
3. *Disability Insurance (DI) program*—provides workers with insurance if they become disabled during their working years.

Tax rates for 2016 are listed in Table 20-1. For example, in 2016, the Social Security tax was 7.65% on each worker's wage. This amount is divided into two rates: a 6.2% **payroll tax** that pays for Social Security benefits and a 1.45% payroll tax that helps finance Medicare's hospital insurance program. Typically, employers pay another 7.65% on each worker's wages. The maximum **wage base**, which is the amount that is subject to tax in 2016, is $118,500.

The employee's percent is withheld from the salary; the employer's contribution and the employee withheld amount are paid by the employer in a monthly federal tax deposit or with a quarterly report on March 31, June 30, September 30, and December 31.

Income Tax Deductions

All physician-employers are required by the federal government to withhold income taxes on employees' earnings. A penalty is imposed if the tax is under withheld.

TABLE 20-1 Federal Insurance Contribution Act (FICA), 2016 Dollar Figures and Percentage Tax Rates Withheld from Salaries

	Employer/Employee Tax Rates*	Maximum Wage Base
FICA**	6.2%	$118,500
Medicare	1.45%	None
Totals	7.65%	$118,500

*These dollar figures and percentage rates are subject to change in subsequent years.
**Typically, both the employee and employer pay the same rates.

Wage Bracket Method Tables for Income Tax Withholding
SINGLE Persons—WEEKLY Payroll Period
(For Wages Paid through December 31, 2015)

And the wages are—		And the number of withholding allowances claimed is—										
At least	But less than	0	1	2	3	4	5	6	7	8	9	10
		The amount of income tax to be withheld is—										
$600	$610	$75	$64	$52	$41	$29	$18	$10	$2	$0	$0	$0
610	620	77	65	54	42	31	19	11	3	0	0	0
620	630	78	67	55	44	32	21	12	4	0	0	0
630	640	80	68	57	45	34	22	13	5	0	0	0
640	650	81	70	58	47	35	24	14	6	0	0	0
650	660	83	71	60	48	37	25	15	7	0	0	0
660	670	84	73	61	50	38	27	16	8	1	0	0
670	680	86	74	63	51	40	28	17	9	2	0	0
680	690	87	76	64	53	41	30	18	10	3	0	0
690	700	89	77	66	54	43	31	20	11	4	0	0
700	710	90	79	67	56	44	33	21	12	5	0	0
710	720	92	80	69	57	46	34	23	13	6	0	0

FIGURE 20-9 Illustration of a federal tax table for a single person, paid weekly, earning $619 in a payroll period, claiming two deductions

The **federal withholding tax (FWT)**, more commonly known as the *federal income tax deduction*, is filed quarterly using Form 941 but the remittance is paid electronically through the *electronic funds transfer system (EFT)* monthly. After an employee files Form W-4 (Figure 20-8) stating the number of exemptions claimed, this information plus the employee's **gross income** (amount earned before deductions) for the payroll period determine the amount to be withheld. Income tax **deductions** (withholding) can be found in standard tax tables. These tables are referred to for weekly, biweekly, semimonthly, monthly, daily, or miscellaneous payroll periods, which appear in *Circular E, Employer's Tax Guide*, available free of charge from the IRS center where the returns are filed (Figure 20-9). The biweekly table is referred to for employees paid every 2 weeks. The semimonthly tables are used for employees paid twice a month, usually on the 15th and 30th. Divorced people are considered single people on federal tax tables and heads of households on state tax tables. If an employee is single but qualifies as head of a household, the single table for federal deductions and head of household table for state deductions are used.

Disability Insurance Deductions

As mentioned in Chapter 18, **Unemployment Compensation Disability (UCD)** deductions, also known as *Temporary Disability Insurance (TDI)* or **State Disability Insurance (SDI)**, are mandatory in five states—California, Hawaii, New Jersey, New York, and Rhode Island—and in Puerto Rico. It is a form of insurance that is part of an employment security program providing temporary cash benefits for employees suffering a wage loss due to nonindustrial illness or injury. A small percentage, about 1%, of the gross pay is deducted from the employee's paycheck each month, although physicians may choose to pay all or part of the cost as a fringe benefit for employees. The money is sent quarterly to the state and put into a special fund. Each state sets a maximum annual amount to be contributed; after the employee has had the maximum amount deducted for the year, no more is deducted.

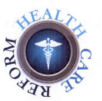

Health Insurance Deductions

Effective 2014, employers with 50 or more employees must provide a comprehensive affordable health plan that costs below 9.5% of an employees' income and pays no less than 60% of health care costs. Depending on the plan, premiums may be made via payroll deductions with pretax or after-tax dollars.

Employers with less than 50 employees may offer health insurance through the Small Business Health Options Program (SHOP) marketplace. Employers with less than 25 employees may quality for a Small Business Tax Credit worth up to 50% of premium costs.

Optional Payroll Deductions or Benefits

Some physicians provide fringe benefits for their employees consisting of partial or full payment of health

EMPLOYEE BENEFITS

Benefit	Employer Pays	Employee Pays
Medical insurance	$ 8,190.00	$ 420.00
Life insurance	$ 210.00	$
Accident insurance	$ 81.00	$
Disability insurance	$	$
Workers' compensation	$	$
Holiday # 7	$ 728.00	$
Vacation # 10	$ 1040.00	$
Sick leave # 6	$ 624.00	$
Personal leave	$	$
Education	$ 100.00	$
Incentive bonus	$	$
Retirement	$	$
Uniforms	$ 420.00	$
Other	$	$
TOTAL BENEFITS	$ 11,393.00	$ 420.00

Hourly wage or salary of employee $ 13/hr

Gross wage for 20X___ $ 24,648.00

Total employment package $ 36,041.00

Employee name: Garth Cartwright   Date: 11/7/XX

FIGURE 20-10 Example of a summary of an employee's benefit package

insurance, life insurance, pension plans, profit-sharing plans, and stock or savings bonds. When the employee is paying for part or all of such benefits, deductions can be made if agreed to by the employee. These deductions may be canceled by the employee during specified times of the calendar year. Other typical optional deductions are credit union deposits and loan payments.

The dollar amount from a benefit package should be considered along with the wages earned by the employee. The federal and Social Security tax on the dollar value of some benefits may be required by law to be reported as wages (see the federal publication *Taxable and Nontaxable Income*); examples might be bonuses, sick or vacation pay, and so on. Other items can be considered *practice expenses* instead of taxable wages, such as uniform allowances, automobile expenses, professional dues, and job-related education. Good benefit packages will attract new employees and add incentives to present staff if the employee realizes the dollar value (Figure 20-10).

Unemployment Taxes

The **Federal Unemployment Tax Act (FUTA)** imposes a federal employer tax used to pay the administrative costs of state workforce agencies and helps fund an extended unemployment benefit program. Along with state employment taxes it provides unemployment compensation to workers who have lost their jobs. In some cases, the employer is required to make payments during the tax year in installments. FUTA applies to employers that pay at least $1500 in wages in any calendar quarter or who have at least one employee on any given day in each of 20 different calendar weeks.

State unemployment taxes vary—some states are governed by the *State Unemployment Tax Act (SUTA)*, some states do not require employers with fewer than four employees to pay unemployment tax, and some states tax both the employer and the employee. Filing dates for state unemployment taxes also vary with penalties imposed on employers who submit late payment.

A form is sent to the employer from the unemployment compensation fund stating the rate the employer is required to pay. State laws frequently change in regard to coverage, rate of contributions required, eligibility to receive benefits, and amounts of benefits payable. The employer's individual claim history is a determinative factor in influencing the rate charged.

Annual Tax Return

Employers must report payments of federal unemployment taxes under FUTA by filing an annual report on Form 940. This should be filed by January 31 of the new year following the taxable year, and any tax still due is paid with the return. If all deposits were paid in full, the return is due on February 10.

Tax Reports

All medical practices are required to prepare and file various payroll records for each employee. The physician is not considered an employee unless the practice is incorporated. If the physician is considered

self-employed, neither income taxes nor FICA taxes are withheld from the amounts withdrawn as earnings. However, as a self-employed person, a tax is paid to provide benefits similar to those that employees receive from FICA deductions.

The office manager should carefully read the information that is included on commonly used forms and consult the medical practice's accountant prior to completing forms. Refer to Circular E, *Employer's Tax Guide,* which is published by the Department of the Treasury, Internal Revenue Service, for current guidelines and requirements in submitting quarterly reports and for making federal tax deposits and unemployment tax payments. The time of year for submitting each form or providing the information to an accountant should be entered on a tickler file, allowing time for completion before each deadline.

Federal Tax Deposits and Receipts

Social Security legislation and the Internal Revenue Code require employers to act as collection agents by obtaining from their employees both the FICA tax and income tax. Each pay period the office manager doing payroll must handle employer and employee taxes that are being withheld for that time frame. The frequency of payments or deposits depends on the amount of taxes involved. The current regulations appear on the reverse side of the **Employer's Quarterly Federal Tax Return**.

Employer's Quarterly Federal Tax Return—

Form 941 must be filed by the physician-employer on or before April 30, July 31, October 31, and January 31, each covering the preceding 3 months' activity. The total of the income tax and the FICA tax withheld are stated on the front of the form. Commercial tax preparation software allows the taxpayer to electronically file (e-file) Form 941 using a personal computer and modem. Attach Voucher 941V with the payment and submit deposits on Form 8109-B (Figure 20-11). The FTD coupons are sent to a Federal Reserve Bank and tax deposits are made via an *electronic funds transfer system (EFTS)*.

Wage and Tax Statement

On or before January 31 of each year, or within 30 days after an employee terminates service, the employer is required to give each employee a **Wage and Tax Statement (Form W-2)** (Figure 20-12). This form is completed,

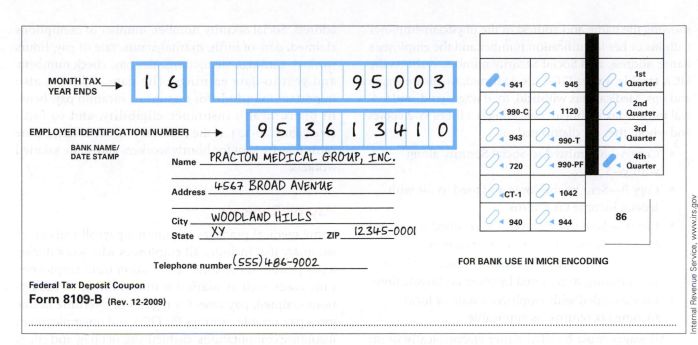

FIGURE 20-11 Federal Tax Deposit (FTD) Coupon, Form 8109-B

22222	Void ☐	**a** Employee's social security number		**For Official Use Only ▶** OMB No. 1545-0008

b Employer identification number (EIN)	**1** Wages, tips, other compensation	**2** Federal income tax withheld
c Employer's name, address, and ZIP code	**3** Social security wages	**4** Social security tax withheld
	5 Medicare wages and tips	**6** Medicare tax withheld
	7 Social security tips	**8** Allocated tips
d Control number	**9**	**10** Dependent care benefits
e Employee's first name and initial Last name Suff.	**11** Nonqualified plans	**12a** See instructions for box 12
	13 Statutory employee ☐ Retirement plan ☐ Third-party sick pay ☐	**12b**
	14 Other	**12c**
		12d
f Employee's address and ZIP code		

15 State Employer's state ID number	**16** State wages, tips, etc.	**17** State income tax	**18** Local wages, tips, etc.	**19** Local income tax	**20** Locality name

Form W-2 **Wage and Tax Statement**   **2015**   Department of the Treasury—Internal Revenue Service

Copy A For Social Security Administration — Send this entire page with Form W-3 to the Social Security Administration; photocopies are **not** acceptable.

For Privacy Act and Paperwork Reduction Act Notice, see back of Copy D.

Cat. No. 10134D

Do Not Cut, Fold, or Staple Forms on This Page — Do Not Cut, Fold, or Staple Forms on This Page

FIGURE 20-12 Wage and Tax Statement, Form W-2

showing the name and address of the physician-employer with his or her identification number and the employee's name, address, and Social Security number. It shows the FICA taxable wages, FICA tax deducted, Medicare wages and tips, Medicare tax withheld, total wages paid, and federal income tax withheld. Following is a list of W-2 copies and whom they are distributed to:

- *Copy A*—Submitted to Social Security along with W-3
- *Copy B*—Sent to employee and used to file with federal income tax returns
- *Copy C*—Sent to employee and retained as a record
- *Copy D*—Retained as a record by employer
- *Copy 1*—Submitted by employer to state or local tax authority, as required by some tax jurisdictions
- *Copy 2*—Filed with employee's state or local income tax returns, as applicable

All wages must be filed either electronically or on paper. Filing on paper requires prior approval and Social Security accepts laser-printed W-2 forms and standard red-ink forms, which can be obtained from the local IRS office. Form W-3 must also be submitted, which is a summary of all W-2 forms completed. Filing electronically is free, fast, and secure. A later filing deadline (last day of March) is used and an immediate receipt for proof of filing is provided. There are three ways to file electronically:

- Create a Wage Report using special software and follow the "Social Security's Specification for Filing Forms W-2 Electronically (EFW2/EFW2C)."
- File W-2 forms online (up to 20), electronically submit them to Social Security, and print copies for distribution to employees.
- Complete W-2c forms (up to 5) on the computer, electronically submit them to Social Security, and print copies for distribution to employees.

A summary and schedule for the payroll, tax forms, and tax withholding responsibilities of the office manager appear in Table 20-2.

Employee's Earning Record

Separate financial records are kept for each employee. An **employee's earning record** shows the total earnings (gross income), the amounts deducted or withheld from gross income, and the **net income**, amount after deductions, also referred to as take-home pay. The information sheet should contain the employee's name, address, Social Security number, number of exemptions claimed, date of birth, marital status, rate of pay, hours worked, earnings, deductions, net pay, check numbers, and year-to-date earnings. The date of hire is also important to include for reasons of vacation pay, benefit plans, health insurance eligibility, and so forth (see Figure 20-13). If the medical practice is large, time cards may be kept for hourly workers and some salaried workers.

Payroll Register

Some medical practices maintain a payroll register, or summary that includes all employees who work during a pay period. It contains information from employees' time cards such as marital status, number of exemptions claimed, pay rates for regular or overtime hours, gross pay, taxable earnings for FICA and unemployment insurance computations, deductions, net pay, and check numbers (Figure 20-14). Refer to Procedure 20-2 for guidelines when creating category headings, determining deductions, calculating payroll, and making entries to a payroll register.

Payroll via Electronic Banking and Paycard

As mentioned previously, besides being able to make federal tax deposits via EFTS, if employees wish to have their paycheck deposited automatically to their bank account, they must give their bank account number and the bank routing number to the employer. Advantages when using this system are that money is available on the day of deposit, the employee cannot lose a paycheck, and he or she does not have to get to the bank before it closes. Employees receive a record with a notification of the deposit, so earnings and deductions can be easily tracked.

Another alternative to the standard paycheck is a payroll debit card called a *paycard*. The plastic cards are loaded electronically with the workers' pay and the employee can use it like a bank debit card to make purchases at retail stores, buy gas, pay bills online, or get money at most bank ATMs. Employees who do not select direct deposit because they do not have a checking account may choose the paycard to avoid fees charged by check-cashing companies; however, there may be monthly fees and other charges attached to using a paycard.

TABLE 20-2 Schedule and Summary of the Medical Assistant's Payroll, Tax Forms, and Tax Withholding Responsibilities*

Qualifying Criteria and Target Dates	Action Taken
If the physician does not have an employer identification number . . .	*Physician-employer identification number*—Fill out a duplicate Form SS-4 and send it to the district director of the IRS.
When new employees are hired . . .	*Income tax withholding*—Ask each new employee to fill out a withholding exemption certification Form W-4. Although the federal government no longer requires the filing of Form W-4, some states require it to be filed. *Social Security* (FICA)—Obtain and record the employees' account numbers as shown on the Social Security card. If an employee has no card, file an application using Form SS-5 with any field office of the Social Security administration. *Immigration and Naturalization Service* (INS)—Complete the Employment Eligibility Verification Form I-9.
On payment of wages to employees . . .	*Income tax withholding*—Withhold tax from each wage payment according to the exemption certificate and the withholding rate given in Circular E, Employer's Tax Guide. *Federal Insurance Contributions Act* (FICA)—Withhold the appropriate percentage from each wage payment; the amount is to be matched by the physician.
By the 15th day of each month or semiweekly . . .	*Payroll tax deposit*—Determine if a deposit needs to be made. The employer's deposit is based on the total tax liability reported on Form 941. There are two deposit schedules. If $50,000 or less was reported in taxes for the lookback period, that is, beginning July 1 and ending June 30 of the two previous years, a deposit would be made monthly. If more than $50,000 was reported for the lookback period, make the deposit semiweekly. When paying on the monthly schedule, deposit Social Security, Medicare, and income taxes paid during the month by the 15th of the following month using Form 941.
On or before April 30, July 31, October 31, and January 31 . . .	*Quarterly tax return*—File Form 941 with the district director of the IRS and pay the full amount of taxes due for the previous quarter on both the income tax withheld from wages and from the physician-employer Social Security taxes.
Before December 1 of each year at the end of employment . . .	*Form W-4*—Request a new form W-4, if employees have any changes in name, address, marital status, or number of exemptions from those recorded the previous year.
On or before January 31 of each year . . .	*W-2 Statements*—Distribute W-2 statements to all employees. Federal *Unemployment Tax Act* (FUTA)—File the annual return on Form 940 and remit the tax to the district director of the IRS.
On or before February 28 of each year . . .	*Income tax withholding*—File Form W-3, Reconciliation of Income Tax Withheld from Wages, together with all district director's copies of withholding statements provided employees on Form W-2 for the preceding year.

*The employer's income tax return reports are not shown in this table.

EMPLOYEE EARNINGS RECORD

Name   Mary Jo Davis   Date of Hire   August 1, 20XX

Address 2200 Sunset Lane   Date of Birth   11-28-70

Woodland Hills, XY   12345   Position Administrative Medical Assistant   PT/FT

Telephone   (555) 438-0900   No. of Exemptions   (1) Single   S/M

Social Security Number XXX-XX-5678   Rate of Pay $13/hour   hr/wk/mo

| Period Ended | Total Hours Worked | EARNINGS | | | DEDUCTIONS | | | | | | Check No. | NET PAY | Year to Date |
		Reg. Pay	Over-time Pay	Gross Pay	FICA	Fed. Inc. Tax	State Inc. Tax	SDI	Medicare	TOTAL DEDUC.			
								--					
								--					

FIGURE 20-13 Example of a completed employee earning record

MONTHLY PAYROLL REGISTER FOR PERIOD ENDING: August 31, 20XX

| EMPLOYEE NAME | No. of Exempts | Hours Worked | Hourly Rate | EARNINGS | | | DEDUCTIONS | | | | | | | |
				Reg. Pay	Over-time	Gross Pay	FICA	Fed. Inc. Tax	State Inc. Tax	SDI	Medicare	TOTAL DEDUC.	Check No.	NET PAY
Mary Jo Davis	1-S	168	13.00	2184.00	78.00	2262.00	140.24	243.00	49.06	–	32.80	465.10	554	1796.90
Beverly Woo	0-S	168	Salary	2500.00	–	2500.00	155.00	317.00	73.72	–	36.25	581.97	555	1918.03
Harold Bohrn	2-M	88	12.00	1056.00	–	1056.00	65.47	1.00	0	–	15.31	81.78	556	974.22
Joan Gonzalez	1-M	168	Salary	2300.00	–	2300.00	142.60	176.00	24.41	–	33.35	376.36	557	1923.64

FIGURE 20-14 Example of a monthly payroll register

PROCEDURE 20-2

Create Category Headings, Determine Deductions, Calculate Payroll, and Make Entries to a Payroll Register

OBJECTIVE: Create category headings, calculate payroll, and post entries to a payroll register (employees' earnings record).

EQUIPMENT/SUPPLIES: Monthly payroll register sheets (see Figure 20-14), employees' time cards, W-4 forms, rate of pay, IRS tax tables, checks, check register, and pen.

DIRECTIONS: Follow these step-by-step directions to learn this procedure. Job Skills 20-6 and 20-7 are presented in the *Workbook* for practice.

SET UP A MONTHLY PAYROLL REGISTER:

1. Insert the names of the three major column headings for the basic payroll check information, such as employee name, earnings, and deductions.

2. Insert the column headings for number of exemptions, hours worked, and hourly rate of pay.

3. Insert the column headings for earnings, such as regular pay, overtime pay, and gross pay.

4. Insert the column headings for the payroll deductions, such as Federal Insurance Contributions Act (FICA) tax, federal income tax, state income tax, state disability insurance (SDI), and Medicare.

5. Insert the column headings for the total deductions, check number, and net pay.

ENTER DATA ON A PAYROLL REGISTER AND CALCULATE PAY:

6. Record employee names, number of exemptions, and hours worked from all employees' time cards under the appropriate columns. Enter rate of pay from confidential records.

7. Calculate the total regular pay by multiplying hourly rate by the regular hours worked—for example, 40 hours per week (including any paid vacation or paid holidays) times $14 per hour, equals $560. Enter the totals under the appropriate headings on the payroll register. If an employee is on salary, list the salary in "Regular Pay."

8. Compute the total overtime pay by calculating the pay rate for overtime pay (e.g., time and a half or double time) and multiplying the number of overtime hours worked by the overtime rate. Enter the totals under the appropriate headings on the payroll register.

9. Add the regular pay and the overtime pay and record the total salary under "Gross Pay" on the payroll register.

10. Determine federal and state tax deductions using IRS and state tax tables and data on the employee earnings record based on the employee's marital status, number of exemptions, and frequency of payroll. Look under the proper heading (single, married, and paid weekly, biweekly, semimonthly, monthly, etc.). Record the amount of tax under the proper heading.

11. Compute the amount of FICA tax to withhold for Social Security and Medicare. Enter the total amount withheld from all employees for FICA under the headings for Social Security and Medicare. The employer must match these amounts.

12. Follow state procedures to determine the amount of state income taxes (if any) to withhold based on the employee's marital status, number of exemptions, and frequency of payroll.

13. Calculate the employer's contributions to FUTA and to the state unemployment fund. Post these amounts to the employer's account.

14. Enter any other deductions, such as health insurance or contributions, to a 401(k) fund.

15. Total the deductions and list the total amount under "Total Deductions."

16. Subtract the total deductions from the gross pay amount and record the total under "Net Pay."

17. Record the deductions on the check stub, if indicated, including the employee's name, date, pay period, gross earnings, deductions, and net pay.

18. Write the payroll check for the "Net Pay" amount and deposit each deduction in a tax liability account.

19. Distribute payroll checks in envelopes to protect privacy.

STOP AND THINK CASE SCENARIO

Prepare an Analysis to Determine the Effectiveness of Capitated Plans

SCENARIO: Your physician asks you to do an analysis of capitated plans in your office and compare their reimbursement totals with the same population of patients as if they had fee-for-service plans.

CRITICAL THINKING:

1. What information do you need to gather before you can start the analysis?

_____

_____

_____

2. What type of formula will you use to make this determination?

_____

_____

_____

3. What additional information, perhaps covered in previous chapters, can you think of that would have an impact on this analysis?

_____

_____

_____

STOP AND THINK CASE SCENARIO

Determine Payroll Category and Frequency for Deductions

SCENARIO: You are a married female administrative medical assistant, and the physician asks you to take over some bookkeeping duties including the preparation of the office payroll. The office manager is a single woman who gets paid by salary at the beginning of the month. A part-time high school boy does the filing and gets paid an hourly rate each week on Friday. Occasionally, the physician's teenage daughter comes in and helps where needed; she gets paid at the conclusion of her workday. The remaining staff gets paid an hourly rate every other week on Fridays; this includes a married woman who does the insurance billing, a single woman who is the receptionist, a divorced woman who is the clinical medical assistant, and a married man who is the x-ray and laboratory technician.

CRITICAL THINKING: Determine the dates you will be making out payroll for each type of employee for next month and circle them on a calendar. Select where you will look to find the deductions from the following choices that appear on the withholding tables. Write your answers by each staff member:

single person—weekly   married person—weekly

single person—biweekly   married person—biweekly

single person—semimonthly   married person—semimonthly

single person—monthly   married person—monthly

single person—daily or   married person—daily or
miscellaneous   miscellaneous

1. Office manager: _____

2. Part-time employee: _____

3. Physician's teenage daughter: _____

4. Insurance biller: _____

5. Receptionist: _____

6. Clinical medical assistant: _____

7. X-ray and lab tech: _____

FOCUS ON CERTIFICATION*

CMA (AAMA) Content Summary

- Document reporting to the Internal Revenue Service (IRS)
- Accounts payable
- Employee payroll
- Calculating payroll and payroll forms
- Practice management software
- Report generation
- Applying managed care policies and procedures

RMA (AMT) Content Summary

- Generate aging reports
- Employ appropriate accounting procedures
- Maintain checking accounts
- Process payables and practice obligations
- Understand and maintain disbursement accounts
- Prepare employee payroll
- Understand hourly and salary payroll procedures
- Understand and maintain payroll records
- Prepare and maintain payroll tax deduction/withholding records
- Prepare employee tax forms
- Prepare quarterly tax forms
- Understand terminology pertaining to payroll and payroll tax
- Understand and perform appropriate calculations related to patient and practice accounts

CMAS (AMT) Content Summary

- Understand basic principles of accounting
- Perform bookkeeping procedures including balancing accounts
- Perform financial computations
- Manage accounts payable
- Prepare monthly trial balance reports
- Understand basic audit controls
- Manage other financial aspects of office management
- Prepare employee payroll and reports
- Maintain payroll tax deduction procedures and records
- Possess fundamental knowledge of computing in the medical office
- Manage staff payroll and scheduling
- Manage employee benefits

REVIEW EXAM-STYLE QUESTIONS

1. The most widely used of all computer applications in a medical practice is:
   a. insurance billing
   b. patient statements
   c. financial management
   d. appointment scheduling
   e. word processing

2. In the "accrual method" of accounting:
   a. revenue is recorded as it is earned
   b. expenses are recorded as they are incurred
   c. revenue is recorded when payment is received
   d. expenses are recognized when they are paid
   e. both a and b

3. When selling a medical practice, what report is used to determine the net worth of the business?
   a. Profit and loss statement
   b. Budget
   c. Periodic transaction summary
   d. Accounts receivable report
   e. Insurance aging report

---

* *This* textbook *and the accompanying* Workbook *meet the entry-level administrative and general competencies for the CMA outlined by the AAMA Examination Content Outline and Occupational Analysis and for the RMA and CMAS outlined by the AMT Competencies, Construction Parameters, and Examination Specifications (see Competency Grid in Appendix B).*

4. In a managed care contract, a "stop loss" is:
   a. a dollar amount of revenues collected per member per month
   b. a limit on how many managed care patients one physician or group can see
   c. monies used to pay for nonprimary care services, used as an incentive to control utilization
   d. a percentage of the monthly payment set aside from the managed care plan until the end of the year or contract period
   e. a dollar limit of prepaid services incurred by any one patient during the plan year

5. When paying bills, the office manager would record expenditures in a/an:
   a. disbursement record
   b. accounts receivable ledger
   c. payroll register
   d. bank register
   e. notebook

6. If an overpayment is received from a government agency, for example, Medicare, the provider must report the reason for the overpayment and return the money within:
   a. 10 days
   b. 30 days
   c. 60 days
   d. 90 days
   e. 120 days

7. An administrative medical assistant is considered a/an:
   a. exempt employee
   b. nonexempt employee
   c. salaried employee
   d. contract employee
   e. pay-for-hire employee

8. If an employee resigns, wages must be paid within:
   a. 24 hours
   b. 36 hours
   c. 72 hours
   d. 1 week
   e. 2 weeks

9. Typically, both the employee and the employer pay the same tax rate for:
   a. FICA
   b. Medicare tax
   c. federal income tax
   d. state tax
   e. both a and b

10. An Employer's Quarterly Federal Tax Return, Form 941, must be filed by the physician-employer on or before:
    a. January 1, April 1, July 1, October 1
    b. January 30, April 30, July 30, October 30
    c. April 30, July 31, October 31, January 31
    d. February 28, May 31, August 31, November 30
    e. March 30, June 30, September 30, December 31

11. When following the medical assistant's payroll and tax schedule, payroll tax deposits in an amount exceeding $50,000 need to be made:
    a. monthly
    b. by the 1st of every month
    c. by the 15th of every month
    d. semimonthly
    e. weekly

12. Information used to calculate pay and record on each employee's payroll register comes from:
    a. the employee's time card
    b. the office checkbook
    c. the employee handbook
    d. the office policy and procedures manual
    e. the employee's resumé

WORKBOOK ASSIGNMENT

To develop competency-based job skills, refer to the *Workbook* and complete the:
- Abbreviation and Spelling Review
- Review Questions

- Critical Thinking Exercises
- Job Skill activities, which are listed at the beginning of the chapter under *Performance Objectives in the Workbook.*

RESOURCES

Booklets

Federal Tax Information

Obtain booklets and forms online or from your local Internal Revenue Service
- IRS Publication 15, Circular E: *Employer's Tax Guide*
- IRS Publication 15A, *Employer's Supplemental Tax Guide*
- State Information: Obtain a booklet from your state tax information office.

U.S. Government

Employment Standards Administration (ESA) Wage and Hour Division

U.S. Department of Labor

Equal Employment Opportunity Commission (U.S.)

Workplace discrimination and harassment

Internal Revenue Service

Forms and publications

Tax and payroll information

Social Security Administration

Frequently asked questions (FAQ)

U.S. Department of Labor

Find it—by topic

CHAPTER 21

SEEKING A POSITION AS AN ADMINISTRATIVE MEDICAL ASSISTANT

ACCESS THIS CHAPTER EXCLUSIVELY ON THE FREE STUDENT COMPANION WEBSITE AT WWW.CENGAGEBRAIN.COM.

Follow instructions to login or create an account. Add *Administrative Medical Assisting* 8th edition ISBN 978-1-305-85917-3 to your bookshelf. You can then access all the free online student resources including the full text for Chapter 21: *Seeking a Position as an Administrative Medical Assistant.*

LEARNING OBJECTIVES

After reading this chapter and learning step-by-step procedures to gain job skills,* you should be able to:

- List employment opportunities.
- Conduct a job search for a position as an administrative medical assistant.
- State advantages of seeking a temporary job.
- Contact an electronic job search database.
- Explain the purpose of an application for employment and a letter of introduction.
- Analyze your educational and vocational background, work experience, and skills.
- Name various types of résumés.
- Prepare appropriate responses to interview questions.
- Assemble items for a portfolio.
- Identify interview questions that are legal and illegal.
- Take follow-up steps after an interview.
- Determine areas considered when an employee's performance is evaluated.

PERFORMANCE OBJECTIVES (PROCEDURES) IN THIS TEXTBOOK

- Answer a classified advertisement (Procedure 21-1).
- Complete a job application form (Procedure 21-2).
- Prepare a résumé (Procedure 21-3).
- Prepare an electronic résumé in ASCII text (Procedure 21-4).
- Prepare and format a scannable résumé (Procedure 21-5).
- Compose and send a thank-you letter (Procedure 21-6).

*This textbook *and the accompanying* Workbook *meet the educational components for entry-level administrative and general competencies outlined by CAAHEP and ABHES.*

PERFORMANCE OBJECTIVES (JOB SKILLS) IN THE WORKBOOK

- Complete a job application form (Job Skill 21-1).
- Compose a letter of introduction (Job Skill 21-2).
- Key a résumé (Job Skill 21-3).
- Prepare a follow-up thank-you letter (Job Skill 21-4).

KEY TERMS

blind letter	electronic job search	network
chronological résumé	employment agencies	performance evaluation
combination résumé	format	portfolio
cover letter	functional résumé	results-oriented résumé
diplomate	human resource department	résumé

APPENDIX A

CMS-1500 CLAIM FORM FIELD-BY-FIELD INSTRUCTIONS AND A COMMERCIAL INSURANCE TEMPLATE

NATIONAL UNIFORM CLAIM COMMITTEE

The American Medical Association (AMA) publishes instructions for the CMS-1500 claim form with cooperation of the National Uniform Claim Committee (NUCC). The NUCC, which took over the responsibility for the development and maintenance of CMS-1500 in 1995, publishes periodic revisions to the form and the standardized national instructions approved by the Centers for Medicare and Medicaid Services (CMS). The NUCC's comprehensive instructions can be found on its website (www.nucc.org) under the "1500 Claim Form" tab.

CMS-1500 CLAIM FORM INSTRUCTIONS

The following instructions contain information needed to complete the CMS-1500 claim form (02/12) using optical character recognition (OCR) guidelines for commercial payers, Medicare (Medicare/Medicaid, Medicare/Medigap, and Medicare Secondary Payer), and TRICARE programs. These instructions follow NUCC, Medicare, and TRICARE guidelines but have been simplified and abbreviated for this *textbook*. Information on specific coverage guidelines, program policies, and practice specialties is not included. Consult your local intermediary or commercial insurance carrier for detailed instructions.

To use these instructions, follow these steps:

1. Locate the field number you need an instruction for. Field numbers match those on the CMS-1500 claim form and include titles that give a brief description of what information is required within the field.

2. Identify the type of insurance program you are completing the claim for; titles appear in bold-face, color-coded capital letters.

3. Read the instructions for specific field requirements. Guidelines for completing *Workbook* exercises are indented and appear in color when there are optional ways of completing a field.

4. Refer to the section of the CMS-1500 claim form shown following each field for a visual example. The field being referred to is highlighted in yellow.

5. Screened areas on insurance templates do not apply to the program examples illustrated and should be left blank. See the templates in Figures A-1, 18-15, 18-17, and 18-18 in Chapter 18.

Program icons and descriptions are as follows:

THIRD-PARTY PAYERS: Guidelines cover all private insurance companies and all federal and state programs, unless another Payer ICON appears indicating separate instructions.

COMMERCIAL PAYERS: Guidelines cover all private insurance companies.

MEDICARE: Guidelines cover federal Medicare programs as well as Medicare/Medicaid, Medicare/Medigap, and Medicare Secondary Payer (MSP).

TRICARE: Guidelines cover TRICARE Standard, TRICARE Prime, and TRICARE Extra programs.

KEY: **Ⓡ** = Required fields that must always be completed

Ⓒ = Conditional fields that may need to be completed depending on the circumstances of the insured

HEALTH INSURANCE CLAIM FORM

APPROVED BY NATIONAL UNIFORM CLAIM COMMITTEE (NUCC) 02/12

Midwest Insurance Company
2515 South O Street
Suite 160
Lincoln NE 68000

CARRIER

| | PICA | | | | | | | | PICA | |

1. MEDICARE (Medicare#)	MEDICAID (Medicaid#)	TRICARE (ID#/DoD#)	CHAMPVA (Member ID#)	GROUP HEALTH PLAN (ID#) [X]	FECA BLK LUNG (ID#)	OTHER (ID#)	1a. INSURED'S I.D. NUMBER (For Program in Item 1) 2984567

2. PATIENT'S NAME (Last Name, First Name, Middle Initial)
Mitchell, Caleb, S

3. PATIENT'S BIRTH DATE MM 04 | DD 18 | YY 1973   **SEX** M [X] F [ ]

4. INSURED'S NAME (Last Name, First Name, Middle Initial)
Mitchell, Caleb, S

5. PATIENT'S ADDRESS (No., Street)
444 Sheridan Way

6. PATIENT RELATIONSHIP TO INSURED
Self [X] Spouse [ ] Child [ ] Other [ ]

7. INSURED'S ADDRESS (No., Street)
444 Sheridan Way

CITY Woodland Hills **STATE** XY

8. RESERVED FOR NUCC USE

CITY Woodland Hills **STATE** XY

ZIP CODE 12345 **TELEPHONE (Include Area Code)** (555) 4862233

ZIP CODE 12345 **TELEPHONE (Include Area Code)** (555) 4862233

9. OTHER INSURED'S NAME (Last Name, First Name, Middle Initial)

10. IS PATIENT'S CONDITION RELATED TO:

11. INSURED'S POLICY GROUP OR FECA NUMBER
F23

a. OTHER INSURED'S POLICY OR GROUP NUMBER

a. EMPLOYMENT? (Current or Previous) YES [ ] NO [X]

a. INSURED'S DATE OF BIRTH MM | DD | YY **SEX** M [ ] F [ ]

b. RESERVED FOR NUCC USE

b. AUTO ACCIDENT? YES [ ] NO [X] PLACE (State)

b. OTHER CLAIM ID (Designated by NUCC)

c. RESERVED FOR NUCC USE

c. OTHER ACCIDENT? YES [ ] NO [X]

c. INSURANCE PLAN NAME OR PROGRAM NAME
Midwest Insurance Company

d. INSURANCE PLAN NAME OR PROGRAM NAME

10d. CLAIM CODES (Designated by NUCC)

d. IS THERE ANOTHER HEALTH BENEFIT PLAN? YES [ ] NO [X] *If yes,* complete items 9, 9a, and 9d.

READ BACK OF FORM BEFORE COMPLETING & SIGNING THIS FORM.
12. PATIENT'S OR AUTHORIZED PERSON'S SIGNATURE I authorize the release of any medical or other information necessary to process this claim. I also request payment of government benefits either to myself or to the party who accepts assignment below.

SIGNED *Caleb S. Mitchell*   DATE 03/20/20XX

13. INSURED'S OR AUTHORIZED PERSON'S SIGNATURE I authorize payment of medical benefits to the undersigned physician or supplier for services described below.

SIGNED *Caleb S. Mitchell*

PATIENT AND INSURED INFORMATION

14. DATE OF CURRENT ILLNESS, INJURY, or PREGNANCY (LMP) MM 02 | DD 16 | YY 20XX QUAL. 431

15. OTHER DATE QUAL. 444 MM 03 | DD 24 | YY 20XX

16. DATES PATIENT UNABLE TO WORK IN CURRENT OCCUPATION FROM MM 03 | DD 24 | YY 20XX TO MM 04 | DD 07 | YY 20XX

17. NAME OF REFERRING PROVIDER OR OTHER SOURCE
DN Thomas Rothschild MD

17a.
17b. NPI 23345678XX

18. HOSPITALIZATION DATES RELATED TO CURRENT SERVICES FROM MM 03 | DD 24 | YY 20XX TO MM 03 | DD 30 | YY 20XX

19. ADDITIONAL CLAIM INFORMATION (Designated by NUCC)

20. OUTSIDE LAB? YES [ ] NO [X] $ CHARGES

21. DIAGNOSIS OR NATURE OF ILLNESS OR INJURY Relate A-L to service line below (24E) ICD Ind. 0

A. A020 B. C. D.
E. F. G. H.
I. J. K. L.

22. RESUBMISSION CODE ORIGINAL REF. NO.

23. PRIOR AUTHORIZATION NUMBER

24. A. DATE(S) OF SERVICE From MM DD YY	To MM DD YY	B. PLACE OF SERVICE	C. EMG	D. PROCEDURES, SERVICES, OR SUPPLIES (Explain Unusual Circumstances) CPT/HCPCS MODIFIER	E. DIAGNOSIS POINTER	F. $ CHARGES	G. DAYS OR UNITS	H. EPSDT Family Plan	I. ID. QUAL.	J. RENDERING PROVIDER ID. #
1	03 24 20XX		21		99223	A	152 98	1		NPI	46278897XX
2	03 25 20XX		21		99233	A	76 97	1		NPI	46278897XX
3	03 26 20XX	03 28 20XX	21		99232	A	166 68	3		NPI	46278897XX
4	03 29 20XX		21		99231	A	37 74	1		NPI	46278897XX
5	03 30 20XX		21		99238	A	65 26	1		NPI	46278897XX
6										NPI	

25. FEDERAL TAX I.D. NUMBER 208765432 SSN [ ] EIN [X]

26. PATIENT'S ACCOUNT NO. MIT123

27. ACCEPT ASSIGNMENT? (For govt. claims, see back) YES [X] NO [ ]

28. TOTAL CHARGE $ 499 63

29. AMOUNT PAID $ 10 00

30. Rsvd for NUCC Use

31. SIGNATURE OF PHYSICIAN OR SUPPLIER INCLUDING DEGREES OR CREDENTIALS (I certify that the statements on the reverse apply to this bill and are made a part thereof.)
Gerald Practon MD
Gerald Practon MD 033020XX
SIGNED DATE

32. SERVICE FACILITY LOCATION INFORMATION
College Hospital
4500 Broadway Avenue
Woodland Hills XY 12345-4700
a. 54378601XX b.

33. BILLING PROVIDER INFO & PH # (555) 4869002
Practon Medical Group Inc
4567 Broad Avenue
Woodland Hills XY 12345-4700
a. 36640210XX b.

PHYSICIAN OR SUPPLIER INFORMATION

NUCC Instruction Manual available at: www.nucc.org   *PLEASE PRINT OR TYPE*   APPROVED OMB-0938-1197 FORM 1500 (02-12)

FIGURE A-1 Commercial payer with no secondary coverage*

COMPLIANCE

Paper Claim Submission

The Administrative Simplification Compliance Act (ASCA) prohibits payment of initial health care claims not sent electronically, except in the following limited situations:

- Small providers required to bill Medicare that have fewer than 25 full-time equivalent employees
- Physicians and suppliers required to bill a Medicare carrier or a durable medical equipment carrier with fewer than 10 full-time equivalent employees
- Claims from providers who submit an average of fewer than 10 claims per month
- Medicare roster billing
- Medicare demonstration project billing
- Some Medicare Secondary Payer claims
- Claims submitted by Medicare beneficiaries
- Claims submitted by Medicare managed care plans
- Claims for services/supplies furnished outside of the United States
- When there is a disruption in electricity or communication connections lasting more than 2 days that is outside of a provider's control

TOP OF FORM ◉

Midwest Insurance Company
2515 South O Street
Suite 160
Lincoln NE 68000

HEALTH INSURANCE CLAIM FORM

APPROVED BY NATIONAL UNIFORM CLAIM COMMITTEE (NUCC) 02/12

PICA								PICA

1. MEDICARE (Medicare#) MEDICAID (Medicaid#) TRICARE (ID#/DoD#) CHAMPVA (Member ID#) GROUP HEALTH PLAN [X] (ID#) FECA BLK LUNG (ID#) OTHER (ID#) 1a. INSURED'S I.D. NUMBER (For Program in Item 1) 2984567

2. PATIENT'S NAME (Last Name, First Name, Middle Initial) Mitchell, Caleb, S
3. PATIENT'S BIRTH DATE MM 04 DD 18 YY 1973 SEX M [X] F [ ]
4. INSURED'S NAME (Last Name, First Name, Middle Initial) Mitchell, Caleb, S

Centers for Medicare and Medicaid Services

A black Quick Response (QR) code symbol and the date of the revised CMS-1500 insurance form (02/12) appear in the top left corner. Insert name and address of insurance company in the top right corner of the form with no punctuation. If the third line of the address is not used, leave the line blank and enter the city, state, and ZIP code on the fourth line. Examples follow:

Workbook Exercises: **Use this format to demonstrate that the student knows where to direct the claim even though some carriers (e.g., Medicare) do not follow this guideline.**

- ABC Insurance Company
  123 Anywhere Street
  Suite 99
  Anycity XY 12345
- XYZ Insurance Company
  456 Anywhere Street
  Anytown XY 12345-0000

FIELD 1 Ⓡ TYPE OF HEALTH INSURANCE COVERAGE INDICATOR

HEALTH INSURANCE CLAIM FORM

APPROVED BY NATIONAL UNIFORM CLAIM COMMITTEE (NUCC) 02/12

Midwest Insurance Company
2515 South O Street
Suite 160
Lincoln NE 68000

CARRIER

PICA								PICA
1. MEDICARE	MEDICAID	TRICARE	CHAMPVA	GROUP HEALTH PLAN	FECA BLK LUNG	OTHER	1a. INSURED'S I.D. NUMBER	(For Program in Item 1)
(Medicare#)	(Medicaid#)	(ID#/DoD#)	(Member ID#)	X (ID#)	(ID#)	(ID#)	2984567	

2. PATIENT'S NAME (Last Name, First Name, Middle Initial)	3. PATIENT'S BIRTH DATE MM DD YY	SEX	4. INSURED'S NAME (Last Name, First Name, Middle Initial)
Mitchell, Caleb, S	04 18 1973	M X F	Mitchell, Caleb, S

Centers for Medicare and Medicaid Services

COMMERCIAL PAYERS: Indicate the type of health insurance coverage applicable to this claim by placing an X in the appropriate box. *Note: Some payer instructions state to mark only the box for the primary insurance plan and include the secondary insurance information in the correct location on the claim form.*

> *Workbook Exercises:* Mark both boxes to indicate primary and secondary insurance plans if the patient has secondary coverage.

Group Health Plan: Mark this box for those covered under any group contract insurance (e.g., insurance obtained through employment), as well as for patients who receive services paid by managed care programs (e.g., HMOs, PPOs, IPAs).

> *Workbook Exercises:* If the insured is employed, assume the insurance is through the employer and mark "Group" insurance; otherwise, assume it is an individual policy and mark "Other."

Other: Mark "Other" for an individual health plan covered under an individual insurance policy.

MEDICARE: Mark this box for patients who receive Medicare benefits.

Medicare/Medicaid: Mark "Medicare" and "Medicaid" if the patient is covered under both Medicare and Medicaid programs.

Medicare/Medigap: Mark "Medicare" and, if the patient has supplemental federal Medigap coverage, also mark "Group."

MSP: Mark "Group" or "Other" (depending on the type of health plan) and "Medicare" when a Medicare patient has other insurance primary to Medicare coverage.

TRICARE: Mark "TRICARE" for individuals receiving TRICARE benefits.

FIELD 1A Ⓡ INSURED'S ID NUMBER

HEALTH INSURANCE CLAIM FORM

APPROVED BY NATIONAL UNIFORM CLAIM COMMITTEE (NUCC) 02/12

Midwest Insurance Company
2515 South O Street
Suite 160
Lincoln NE 68000

CARRIER

PICA								PICA
1. MEDICARE	MEDICAID	TRICARE	CHAMPVA	GROUP HEALTH PLAN	FECA BLK LUNG	OTHER	1a. INSURED'S I.D. NUMBER	(For Program in Item 1)
(Medicare#)	(Medicaid#)	(ID#/DoD#)	(Member ID#)	X (ID#)	(ID#)	(ID#)	2984567	

2. PATIENT'S NAME (Last Name, First Name, Middle Initial)	3. PATIENT'S BIRTH DATE MM DD YY	SEX	4. INSURED'S NAME (Last Name, First Name, Middle Initial)
Mitchell, Caleb, S	04 18 1973	M X F	Mitchell, Caleb, S

Centers for Medicare and Medicaid Services

FIELD 1A Ⓡ Continued

COMMERCIAL PAYERS: Insert the insured's policy (identification or certificate) number in the left portion of this field as it appears on the insurance card, *without spacing or punctuation*.

MEDICARE: Insert the patient's Medicare Health Insurance Claim Number (HICN) from the patient's Medicare card in the left portion of this field, regardless of whether Medicare is the primary or secondary payer (e.g., Medicare/Medigap, Medicare/Medicaid, MSP).

TRICARE: Insert the 10-digit Department of Defense (DOD) Benefit Number as shown on the back of the insured's ID card in the left portion of this field. Then, if the patient is a NATO beneficiary, add "NATO" or, if the sponsor is a security agent, add "SECURITY."

FIELD 2 Ⓡ PATIENT'S NAME

Midwest Insurance Company
2515 South O Street
Suite 160
Lincoln NE 68000

HEALTH INSURANCE CLAIM FORM
APPROVED BY NATIONAL UNIFORM CLAIM COMMITTEE (NUCC) 02/12

PICA						PICA
1. MEDICARE (Medicare#)	MEDICAID (Medicaid#)	TRICARE (ID#/DoD#)	CHAMPVA (Member ID#)	GROUP HEALTH PLAN [X] (ID#)	FECA BLK LUNG (ID#)	OTHER (ID#)	1a. INSURED'S I.D. NUMBER (For Program in Item 1) 2984567

2. PATIENT'S NAME (Last Name, First Name, Middle Initial)	3. PATIENT'S BIRTH DATE	SEX	4. INSURED'S NAME (Last Name, First Name, Middle Initial)
Mitchell, Caleb, S	MM 04 DD 18 YY 1973	M [X] F [ ]	Mitchell, Caleb, S

Centers for Medicare and Medicaid Services

THIRD-PARTY PAYERS: Insert the last name, first name, and middle initial of the patient—in that order—as shown on the patient's identification card, even if it is misspelled. Do not use nicknames, abbreviations, titles (e.g., Dr.), or professional suffixes (e.g., MD). If the patient uses a last name suffix such as "Jr.," enter it after the last name and before the first name. Use commas to separate the last name, first name, and middle initial. If a name is hyphenated, a hyphen may be used. Do not use periods within the name. Some examples follow:

- Hyphenated name: Mary Jones-Brown = Jones-Brown, Mary
- Prefixed name: Cynthia B. McDougall = McDougall, Cynthia, B.
- Last name with suffix: Robert Allen Brown Sr. = Brown Sr., Robert, Allen
- Seniority name with numeric suffix: James N. Peri, III = Peri III, James, N.

FIELD 3 Ⓡ PATIENT'S DATE OF BIRTH AND SEX

Midwest Insurance Company
2515 South O Street
Suite 160
Lincoln NE 68000

HEALTH INSURANCE CLAIM FORM
APPROVED BY NATIONAL UNIFORM CLAIM COMMITTEE (NUCC) 02/12

PICA						PICA
1. MEDICARE (Medicare#)	MEDICAID (Medicaid#)	TRICARE (ID#/DoD#)	CHAMPVA (Member ID#)	GROUP HEALTH PLAN [X] (ID#)	FECA BLK LUNG (ID#)	OTHER (ID#)	1a. INSURED'S I.D. NUMBER (For Program in Item 1) 2984567

2. PATIENT'S NAME (Last Name, First Name, Middle Initial)	3. PATIENT'S BIRTH DATE	SEX	4. INSURED'S NAME (Last Name, First Name, Middle Initial)
Mitchell, Caleb, S	MM 04 DD 18 YY 1973	M [X] F [ ]	Mitchell, Caleb, S

Centers for Medicare and Medicaid Services

FIELD 3 ® Continued

THIRD-PARTY PAYERS: Insert the patient's birth date using eight digits (020920XX). The patient's age must be as follows to correlate with the diagnosis in Field 21:

- Birth: Newborn diagnosis
- Birth to 17 years: Pediatric diagnosis

- 12 to 55 years: Maternity diagnosis
- 15 to 124 years: Adult diagnosis

Mark an "X" in the appropriate box to indicate the patient's gender. If the sex is unknown, leave blank.

FIELD 4 ® INSURED'S NAME

Midwest Insurance Company
2515 South O Street
Suite 160
Lincoln NE 68000

HEALTH INSURANCE CLAIM FORM
APPROVED BY NATIONAL UNIFORM CLAIM COMMITTEE (NUCC) 02/12

| 1. MEDICARE (Medicare#) | MEDICAID (Medicaid#) | TRICARE (ID#/DoD#) | CHAMPVA (Member ID#) | GROUP HEALTH PLAN (ID#) [X] | FECA BLK LUNG (ID#) | OTHER (ID#) | 1a. INSURED'S I.D. NUMBER 2984567 | (For Program in Item 1) |

2. PATIENT'S NAME (Last Name, First Name, Middle Initial)	3. PATIENT'S BIRTH DATE	SEX	4. INSURED'S NAME (Last Name, First Name, Middle Initial)
Mitchell, Caleb, S	MM 04 DD 18 YY 1973	M [X] F [ ]	Mitchell, Caleb, S

Centers for Medicare and Medicaid Services

THIRD-PARTY PAYERS: Insert the insured's full last name, first name, and middle initial. Follow the same format protocol as described in Field 2 regarding nicknames, abbreviations, titles, suffixes, hyphenated names, commas, and periods.

MEDICARE: If the insured is also the patient, leave blank. If the insured is other than the patient, list the name of the insured.

MSP: If there is insurance primary to Medicare, list the name of the insured. If the insured and patient are the same, enter the word "SAME."

TRICARE: Insert the sponsor's last name, first name, and middle initial. Leave blank if the patient is the insured and "Self" is checked in Field 6.

FIELD 5 ® PATIENT'S ADDRESS

5. PATIENT'S ADDRESS (No., Street) 444 Sheridan Way	6. PATIENT RELATIONSHIP TO INSURED Self [X] Spouse [ ] Child [ ] Other [ ]	7. INSURED'S ADDRESS (No., Street) 444 Sheridan Way	
CITY Woodland Hills	STATE XY	8. RESERVED FOR NUCC USE	CITY Woodland Hills	STATE XY
ZIP CODE 12345	TELEPHONE (Include Area Code) (555) 4862233		ZIP CODE 12345	TELEPHONE (Include Area Code) (555) 4862233

Centers for Medicare and Medicaid Services

THIRD-PARTY PAYERS: Insert the patient's mailing address—on the first line, enter the street address; on the second line, the city and two-character state code (e.g., CO = Colorado); and on the third line, enter the ZIP code. *Optional:* If the patient is the same as the insured, it is not necessary to enter the address. *Optional:* The telephone number does not need to be reported. Punctuation is not necessary, except when using a nine-digit ZIP code, then enter a hyphen between the first five digits and the last four digits. Some examples follow:

- St. Charles = no period after St
- Nine-digit ZIP code = 12345-6789

Workbook Exercises: Insert the patient's name and telephone number, even if it is the same as the insured.

TRICARE: Insert the patient's mailing address and residential telephone number. Provide the actual place of residence; do not enter a Post Office box number. If the address contains a rural route box number, list that, too. Use an APO/FPO address if the person is residing overseas.

FIELD 6 C PATIENT'S RELATIONSHIP TO INSURED

5. PATIENT'S ADDRESS (No., Street)		6. PATIENT RELATIONSHIP TO INSURED	7. INSURED'S ADDRESS (No., Street)	
444 Sheridan Way		Self [X] Spouse [ ] Child [ ] Other [ ]	444 Sheridan Way	
CITY	STATE	8. RESERVED FOR NUCC USE	CITY	STATE
Woodland Hills	XY		Woodland Hills	XY
ZIP CODE	TELEPHONE (Include Area Code)		ZIP CODE	TELEPHONE (Include Area Code)
12345	(555) 4862233		12345	(555) 4862233

Centers for Medicare and Medicaid Services

THIRD-PARTY PAYERS: Indicate the patient's relationship to the insured. Descriptions follow:

- Self = insured is the patient, or if the insured is someone else and the patient has a unique Member Identification Number and the payer requires the identification number be reported on the claim
- Spouse = patient is husband, wife, or qualified partner of insured as described by the plan
- Child = patient is minor dependent of insured

- Other = patient is "other" than self, spouse, or child, which may include employee, ward, dependent, or domestic partner as defined by the insured's plan

TRICARE: Indicate the patient's relationship to the sponsor. If patient is the sponsor, mark "Self" (e.g., retiree). If the patient is a child or stepchild, mark the box for child. If "Other" is marked, indicate how the patient is related to the sponsor in Field 19 or on an attachment (e.g., former spouse).

FIELD 7 C INSURED'S ADDRESS

5. PATIENT'S ADDRESS (No., Street)		6. PATIENT RELATIONSHIP TO INSURED	7. INSURED'S ADDRESS (No., Street)	
444 Sheridan Way		Self [X] Spouse [ ] Child [ ] Other [ ]	444 Sheridan Way	
CITY	STATE	8. RESERVED FOR NUCC USE	CITY	STATE
Woodland Hills	XY		Woodland Hills	XY
ZIP CODE	TELEPHONE (Include Area Code)		ZIP CODE	TELEPHONE (Include Area Code)
12345	(555) 4862233		12345	(555) 4862233

Centers for Medicare and Medicaid Services

THIRD-PARTY PAYERS: Insert the insured's permanent address and telephone number following the same format as in Field 5. *Note: The insured's address may be different from the patient's address in Field 5.*

MEDICARE: Do not complete if Field 4 is blank. Insert "SAME" if Field 4 is filled in and the address is identical

to that listed in Field 5. Insert address if different from that listed in Field 5.

TRICARE: Insert "SAME" if address is the same as that of the patient's address listed in Field 5. Insert the sponsor's address (e.g., an APO/FPO address or active duty sponsor's duty station or the retiree's mailing address) if different from the patient's address.

FIELD 8 N / A RESERVED FOR NUCC USE

5. PATIENT'S ADDRESS (No., Street)		6. PATIENT RELATIONSHIP TO INSURED	7. INSURED'S ADDRESS (No., Street)	
444 Sheridan Way		Self [X] Spouse [ ] Child [ ] Other [ ]	444 Sheridan Way	
CITY	STATE	8. RESERVED FOR NUCC USE	CITY	STATE
Woodland Hills	XY		Woodland Hills	XY
ZIP CODE	TELEPHONE (Include Area Code)		ZIP CODE	TELEPHONE (Include Area Code)
12345	(555) 4862233		12345	(555) 4862233

Centers for Medicare and Medicaid Services

THIRD-PARTY PAYERS: Field reserved for NUCC use.

FIELD 9 Ⓒ OTHER INSURED'S NAME

9. OTHER INSURED'S NAME (Last Name, First Name, Middle Initial)	10. IS PATIENT'S CONDITION RELATED TO:	11. INSURED'S POLICY GROUP OR FECA NUMBER
		F23
a. OTHER INSURED'S POLICY OR GROUP NUMBER	a. EMPLOYMENT? (Current or Previous) [ ] YES [X] NO	a. INSURED'S DATE OF BIRTH MM DD YY SEX M [ ] F [ ]
b. RESERVED FOR NUCC USE	b. AUTO ACCIDENT? PLACE (State) [ ] YES [X] NO	b. OTHER CLAIM ID (Designated by NUCC)
c. RESERVED FOR NUCC USE	c. OTHER ACCIDENT? [ ] YES [X] NO	c. INSURANCE PLAN NAME OR PROGRAM NAME Midwest Insurance Company
d. INSURANCE PLAN NAME OR PROGRAM NAME	10d. CLAIM CODES (Designated by NUCC)	d. IS THERE ANOTHER HEALTH BENEFIT PLAN? [ ] YES [X] NO *If yes,* complete items 9, 9a, and 9d.

Centers for Medicare and Medicaid Services

THIRD-PARTY PAYERS: When additional group health coverage exists, enter other insured's full last name, first name, and middle initial that are enrolled in another health plan, *if it is different from that shown in Field 2.* Follow the same protocol as described in Field 2 regarding nicknames, abbreviations, titles, suffixes, hyphenated names, commas, and periods. For primary insurance submission, do not fill in.

MEDICARE: Do not complete for primary insurance. Do not list Medicare supplemental coverage, other than Medigap on the primary Medicare claim. Other claims are forwarded automatically if a contract exists—if not, a separate claim needs to be filed.

Medicare/Medicaid: Insert Medicaid patient's full name in last name, first name, and middle initial, in that sequence. Follow the same protocol as described in Field 2 regarding nicknames, abbreviations, titles, suffixes, hyphenated names, commas, and periods.

Medicare/Medigap: Enter the last name, first name, and middle initial of the Medigap enrollee if it differs from that in Field 2; otherwise, insert "SAME." Follow the same protocol as described in Field 2 regarding nicknames, abbreviations, titles, suffixes, hyphenated names, commas, and periods. Only Medicare participating physicians and suppliers should complete Field 9 and its subdivisions, and only when the beneficiary wishes to assign his or her benefits under a Medigap policy to the participating physician or supplier. Do not complete if no Medigap benefits are assigned.

MSP: Do not fill in.

TRICARE: Do not fill in for primary insurance. For secondary insurance held by someone other than the patient, insert the name of the insured. Fields 11a–d should be used to report other health insurance held by the patient.

FIELD 9A Ⓒ OTHER INSURED'S POLICY OR GROUP NUMBER

COMMERCIAL PAYERS: Insert the policy and/or group number of the other (secondary) insured's insurance coverage. Do not use punctuation or a space to separate digits within the number.

MEDICARE: Follow appropriate secondary coverage guidelines.

Medicare/Medicaid: Insert Medicaid policy number. Check with your local fiscal intermediary for individual state guidelines.

Medicare/Medigap: Insert the policy and/or group number of the Medigap enrollee preceded by the word

"MEDIGAP," "MG," or "MGAP." If a patient has a third insurance (i.e., employer supplemental), all information for the third insurance should be submitted on an attachment.

Workbook Exercises: **Enter the word "MEDIGAP."**

MSP: Leave blank.

TRICARE: Insert the policy or group number of the other insured's secondary insurance policy.

FIELD 9B ©RESERVED TO NUCC USES

THIRD-PARTY PAYERS: Field reserved for NUCC use.

FIELD 9C © RESERVED FOR NUCC USE

COMMERCIAL PAYERS: Field reserved for NUCC use.

MEDICARE: Follow appropriate secondary coverage guidelines.

Medicare/Medicaid: Do not fill in.

Medicare/Medigap: Insert the Medigap insurer's claim processing address. Abbreviate the street address, delete the city name, and use the two-letter state postal code and ZIP code. *Note: If a carrier-assigned unique identifier (sometimes called "Other Carrier Name and Address," or OCNA) for a*

Medigap insurer is known, insert it in Field 9d, and leave Field 9c blank. An address example follows:

- 264 Oak Drive, Santa Barbara, California 93105 = 264 Oak Dr CA 93105

MSP: Do not fill in.

TRICARE: For secondary coverage held by someone other than the patient, insert the name of the other insured's employer or name of school.

FIELD 9D ©INSURANCE PLAN OR PROGRAM NAME

COMMERCIAL PAYERS: Insert name of secondary insurance plan or program.

MEDICARE: Follow appropriate secondary coverage guidelines.

Medicare/Medicaid: Do not fill in.

Medicare/Medigap: Insert the Medigap insurer's nine-digit alphanumeric PAYERID number if known (often called the OCNA key), and Field 9c may be left blank. If not known, insert the name of the Medigap enrollee's insurance company. For participating providers, all of the information in Fields 9 through 9d must be complete and correct or the Medicare carrier cannot

electronically forward the claim information to the Medigap insurer.

MSP: Do not fill in.

TRICARE: For secondary coverage held by someone other than the patient, enter name of insured's other health insurance program. On an attached sheet, provide a complete mailing address for all other insurance information and insert the word "ATTACHMENT" in Field 10d. If the patient is covered by a health maintenance organization, attach a copy of the document indicating that the service is not covered by the HMO.

FIELD 10A ®PATIENT'S CONDITION RELATED TO EMPLOYMENT

9. OTHER INSURED'S NAME (Last Name, First Name, Middle Initial)	10. IS PATIENT'S CONDITION RELATED TO:	11. INSURED'S POLICY GROUP OR FECA NUMBER
		F23
a. OTHER INSURED'S POLICY OR GROUP NUMBER	a. EMPLOYMENT? (Current or Previous) □YES ☒NO	a. INSURED'S DATE OF BIRTH SEX MM DD YY M☐ F☐
b. RESERVED FOR NUCC USE	b. AUTO ACCIDENT? PLACE (State) □YES ☒NO	b. OTHER CLAIM ID (Designated by NUCC)
c. RESERVED FOR NUCC USE	c. OTHER ACCIDENT? □YES ☒NO	c. INSURANCE PLAN NAME OR PROGRAM NAME Midwest Insurance Company
d. INSURANCE PLAN NAME OR PROGRAM NAME	10d. CLAIM CODES (Designated by NUCC)	d. IS THERE ANOTHER HEALTH BENEFIT PLAN? □YES ☒NO *If yes,* complete items 9, 9a, and 9d.

Centers for Medicare and Medicaid Services

THIRD-PARTY PAYERS: Mark "YES" or "NO" to indicate whether patient's diagnosis described by the code

in Field 21 is the result of an accident or injury that occurred on the job or an industrial illness.

FIELD 10B ® PATIENT'S CONDITION CAUSED BY AUTO ACCIDENT

THIRD-PARTY PAYERS: Mark "YES" in Field 10b to indicate a third-party liability case and file the claim with the other liability insurance or automobile insurance company. Enter the abbreviation of the state in which the accident took place (e.g., VA for Virginia).

TRICARE: Mark "YES" or "NO" to indicate whether automobile liability applies to one or more of the

services described in Field 24. If "YES," provide information concerning potential third-party liability. If a third party is involved in the accident, the beneficiary must complete Form DD 2527 (Statement of Personal Injury—Possible Third-Party Liability) and attach it to the claim.

FIELD 10C ® PATIENT'S CONDITION CAUSED BY OTHER TYPE OF ACCIDENT

THIRD-PARTY PAYERS: Mark "YES" or "NO" to indicate whether the patient's condition is related to an accident other than automobile or employment. Verify primary insurance.

TRICARE: Mark "YES" or "NO" to indicate whether another accident (not automobile or work related)

applies to one or more of the services described in Field 24. If so, provide information concerning potential third-party liability. If third party is involved in the accident, the beneficiary must complete Form DD 2527 (Statement of Personal Injury—Possible Third-Party Liability) and attach it to the claim.

FIELD 10D © CLAIM OR CONDITION CODES DESIGNATED BY NUCC

THIRD-PARTY PAYERS: Generally, do not complete. However, if required to provide a Claim Code or a subset of Condition Code* to indicate such things as employment status, same-day transfer, or a pregnancy indicator (e.g., AA 5 abortion performed due to rape), enter code in this field. When reporting more than one code, enter three blank spaces and then the next code.

MEDICARE: Do not complete.

Medicare/Medicaid: Insert the patient's Medicaid (MCD) number preceded by the abbreviation "MCD."

Workbook Exercises: Leave blank.

FIELD 11 © INSURED'S POLICY OR GROUP NUMBER

9. OTHER INSURED'S NAME (Last Name, First Name, Middle Initial)	10. IS PATIENT'S CONDITION RELATED TO:	11. INSURED'S POLICY GROUP OR FECA NUMBER F23
a. OTHER INSURED'S POLICY OR GROUP NUMBER	a. EMPLOYMENT? (Current or Previous) ☐ YES ☒ NO	a. INSURED'S DATE OF BIRTH MM DD YY SEX M ☐ F ☐
b. RESERVED FOR NUCC USE	b. AUTO ACCIDENT? PLACE (State) ☐ YES ☒ NO	b. OTHER CLAIM ID (Designated by NUCC)
c. RESERVED FOR NUCC USE	c. OTHER ACCIDENT? ☐ YES ☒ NO	c. INSURANCE PLAN NAME OR PROGRAM NAME Midwest Insurance Company
d. INSURANCE PLAN NAME OR PROGRAM NAME	10d. CLAIM CODES (Designated by NUCC)	d. IS THERE ANOTHER HEALTH BENEFIT PLAN? ☐ YES ☒ NO *If yes*, complete items 9, 9a, and 9d.

PATIENT AND INSURED INF

Centers for Medicare and Medicaid Services

COMMERCIAL PAYERS: There are several options to consider when completing this field: (1) When the insured's name, listed in Field 4, is not the same as the patient listed in Field 2, insert the insured's policy

number here. (2) When the insured is not the patient, and the insurance plan issues a separate ID number to the patient, insert the patient's ID number in Field 1a and the insured's ID number in Field 11. (3) If the

---

*Condition codes may be found at the National Uniform Claim Committee website: http://www.nucc.org (see "Code Sets").

FIELD 11 © Continued

insurance plan has a group number, insert the group number in Field 11. Do not use a hyphen or space to separate digits.

MEDICARE: Enter "NONE" if other insurance is not primary to Medicare and go to Field 12. Field 11 must be completed by the physician/supplier to acknowledge that a good faith effort has been made to determine whether Medicare is the primary or secondary payer.

Medicare/Medicaid: Follow Medicare guidelines.

Medicare/Medigap: Follow Medicare guidelines.

MSP: Enter the insured's policy and/or group number only when insurance is primary to Medicare and complete Fields 11a through 11c.

TRICARE: Do not complete.

FIELD 11A © INSURED'S DATE OF BIRTH AND SEX

THIRD-PARTY PAYERS: Insert the insured's eight-digit date of birth (020920XX) and gender if different from that listed in Field 3; otherwise, leave blank.

FIELD 11B ® OTHER CLAIM ID DESIGNED BY NUCC AND MISCELLANEOUS DATA

COMMERCIAL PAYERS: Enter the "Other Claim ID," which is designed by NUCC. Enter the qualifier to the left of the vertical dotted line—enter the identifier number to the right of the vertical dotted line.

MEDICARE: If there is a change in the insured's insurance status (e.g., retired), enter the six- or eight-digit date of retirement preceded by the word "RETIRED" to the right of the vertical dotted line.

MSP: Insert the employer's name of primary insurance, if applicable. Submit paper claims with a copy of the primary payer's Remittance Advice (RA) document to be considered for Medicare Secondary Payer benefits. Instances when Medicare may be secondary include the following:

1. Group coverage
   - Disability (large group health plan)
   - End-stage renal disease
   - Working aged
2. Liability coverage
   - Automobile
   - Commercial
   - Homeowner
3. Work-related illness/injury
   - Black lung
   - Veterans' benefits
   - Workers' compensation

TRICARE: Insert sponsor's branch of service, using abbreviations (e.g., United States Air Force 5 USAF).

FIELD 11C © INSURANCE PLAN OR PROGRAM NAME

COMMERCIAL PAYERS: Insert the name of the insurance plan or program. *Note: Some payers require the primary insurer's identification number rather than the name in this field.*

MSP: Enter the nine-digit insurance-assigned PAYRID number or, if not available, insert the complete name of

the insurance plan or program that is *primary to Medicare.* Include the primary payer's claim processing address and telephone number directly on the EOB if it is not already listed.

TRICARE: Insert "TRICARE."

FIELD 11D Ⓒ OTHER HEALTH BENEFIT PLAN INDICATION

THIRD-PARTY PAYERS: Mark "YES" or "NO" to indicate whether there is another health plan. If "YES," Fields 9, 9a, and 9d must be completed.

MEDICARE: Leave blank.

FIELD 12 Ⓡ PATIENT'S OR AUTHORIZED PERSON'S SIGNATURE

READ BACK OF FORM BEFORE COMPLETING & SIGNING THIS FORM. 12. PATIENT'S OR AUTHORIZED PERSON'S SIGNATURE I authorize the release of any medical or other information necessary to process this claim. I also request payment of government benefits either to myself or to the party who accepts assignment below.	13. INSURED'S OR AUTHORIZED PERSON'S SIGNATURE I authorize payment of medical benefits to the undersigned physician or supplier for services described below.
SIGNED *Caleb S. Mitchell* DATE 03/20/20XX	SIGNED *Caleb S. Mitchell*

or

READ BACK OF FORM BEFORE COMPLETING & SIGNING THIS FORM. 12. PATIENT'S OR AUTHORIZED PERSON'S SIGNATURE I authorize the release of any medical or other information necessary to process this claim. I also request payment of government benefits either to myself or to the party who accepts assignment below.	13. INSURED'S OR AUTHORIZED PERSON'S SIGNATURE I authorize payment of medical benefits to the undersigned physician or supplier for services described below.
SIGNED Signature on file DATE	SIGNED Signature on file

Centers for Medicare and Medicaid Services

THIRD-PARTY PAYERS: Release of medical information for claims processing is indicated by a signature here; *this is not mandated by HIPAA.* If there is no signature, leave blank. For medical practices that wish to obtain the patient's signature indicating consent to release information, have the patient or the authorized representative sign and date this field. If the patient has signed a consent form, "Signature on File" can be entered here. Some carriers accept the acronym "SOF." The consent form must be current, may be lifetime, and must be in the physician's file. When the patient's representative signs, the relationship to the patient must be indicated. If the signature is indicated by a mark (X), a witness must sign his or her name and insert the address next to the mark.

> *Workbook Exercises:* **The abbreviation "SOF" can be used.**

MEDICARE: Payment of benefits to the physician (if the physician accepts assignment) *and* release of medical information for claims processing is indicated by a signature here. Have the patient or the authorized representative sign and date this field. If the patient has signed a consent form, "Signature on File" or the abbreviation "SOF" can be inserted. The form must be current, may be lifetime, and must be in the physician's file. When the patient's representative signs, the relationship to the patient *must* be indicated. If the signature is by a mark (X), a witness must sign his or her name and enter the address next to the mark.

TRICARE: Authorization of payment of benefits to the physician (if the physician accepts assignment) and release of medical information for claims processing is indicated by a signature here. Have the patient or the authorized representative sign and date this field. "Signature on File" may be used if a consent form has been signed.

> *Workbook Exercises:* **"Signature on file" or the abbreviation "SOF" can be used.**

FIELD 13 Ⓒ INSURED'S OR AUTHORIZED PERSON'S SIGNATURE

READ BACK OF FORM BEFORE COMPLETING & SIGNING THIS FORM. 12. PATIENT'S OR AUTHORIZED PERSON'S SIGNATURE I authorize the release of any medical or other information necessary to process this claim. I also request payment of government benefits either to myself or to the party who accepts assignment below.	13. INSURED'S OR AUTHORIZED PERSON'S SIGNATURE I authorize payment of medical benefits to the undersigned physician or supplier for services described below.
SIGNED *Caleb S. Mitchell* DATE 03/20/20XX	SIGNED *Caleb S. Mitchell*

or

READ BACK OF FORM BEFORE COMPLETING & SIGNING THIS FORM. 12. PATIENT'S OR AUTHORIZED PERSON'S SIGNATURE I authorize the release of any medical or other information necessary to process this claim. I also request payment of government benefits either to myself or to the party who accepts assignment below.	13. INSURED'S OR AUTHORIZED PERSON'S SIGNATURE I authorize payment of medical benefits to the undersigned physician or supplier for services described below.
SIGNED Signature on file DATE	SIGNED Signature on file

Centers for Medicare and Medicaid Services

FIELD 13 ⒸContinued

COMMERCIAL PAYERS: Insert patient's signature when benefits are assigned. The abbreviation "SOF" may be used if the patient's signature is on file.

MEDICARE: Do not complete.

Medicare/Medicaid: Do not complete.

Medicare/Medigap: Participating providers should obtain a signature to authorize payment of "mandated" Medigap benefits when required. Insert the signature of

the patient or authorized representative, or insert "Signature on File" if the signature is on file as a separate Medigap authorization.

MSP: The signature of the patient or authorized representative should appear in this block or insert "SOF" if the signature is on file for benefits assigned from the primary carrier.

TRICARE: Do not complete.

FIELD 14 ⒸDATE OF CURRENT ILLNESS, INJURY, OR LAST MENSTRUAL PERIOD IF PREGNANT

14. DATE OF CURRENT ILLNESS, INJURY, or PREGNANCY (LMP) MM DD YY 02 16 20XX QUAL. 431	15. OTHER DATE QUAL. 444	MM DD YY 03 24 20XX	16. DATES PATIENT UNABLE TO WORK IN CURRENT OCCUPATION MM DD YY MM DD YY FROM 03 24 20XX TO 04 07 20XX
17. NAME OF REFERRING PROVIDER OR OTHER SOURCE DN Thomas Rothschild MD	17a. 17b. NPI 23345678XX		18. HOSPITALIZATION DATES RELATED TO CURRENT SERVICES MM DD YY MM DD YY FROM 03 24 20XX TO 03 30 20XX
19. ADDITIONAL CLAIM INFORMATION (Designated by NUCC)			20. OUTSIDE LAB? YES X NO $ CHARGES

Centers for Medicare and Medicaid Services

THIRD-PARTY PAYERS: Insert the eight-digit date the patient's first symptoms occurred from the current illness, if stated in the medical record; date of injury or accident; or for pregnancy, first day of last menstrual period (LMP). For chiropractic treatment, enter the eight-digit date that treatment began. In the right portion of the field, enter the applicable qualifier to identify which date is being reported. Examples follow:

- 431   Onset of current symptoms or illness
- 484   Last menstrual period

MEDICARE: Insert the eight-digit date the patient's first symptoms occurred from the current illness, if stated in the medical record; date of injury or accident; or for pregnancy, first day of last menstrual period. For chiropractic treatment, enter the eight-digit date that treatment began. *Do not enter a qualifier; Medicare does not use this information.*

FIELD 15 ⒸOTHER DATE RELATED TO PATIENT'S CONDITION OR TREATMENT

14. DATE OF CURRENT ILLNESS, INJURY, or PREGNANCY (LMP) MM DD YY 02 16 20XX QUAL. 431	15. OTHER DATE QUAL. 444	MM DD YY 03 24 20XX	16. DATES PATIENT UNABLE TO WORK IN CURRENT OCCUPATION MM DD YY MM DD YY FROM 03 24 20XX TO 04 07 20XX
17. NAME OF REFERRING PROVIDER OR OTHER SOURCE DN Thomas Rothschild MD	17a. 17b. NPI 23345678XX		18. HOSPITALIZATION DATES RELATED TO CURRENT SERVICES MM DD YY MM DD YY FROM 03 24 20XX TO 03 30 20XX
19. ADDITIONAL CLAIM INFORMATION (Designated by NUCC)			20. OUTSIDE LAB? YES X NO $ CHARGES

Centers for Medicare and Medicaid Services

COMMERCIAL PAYERS: Insert another eight-digit date related to the patient's condition or treatment. Enter the appropriate qualifier between the left-hand set of vertical, dotted lines to identify which date is being reported. Examples follow:

- 304   Latest visit or consultation
- 444   First visit or consultation
- 439   Accident

- 453   Acute manifestation of a chronic condition
- 454   Initial treatment
- 455   Last x-ray
- 471   Prescription

MEDICARE: Do not complete.

TRICARE: Insert eight-digit date when patient had same or similar illness, if applicable, and documented in the medical record.

FIELD 16 ⓒ DATES PATIENT UNABLE TO WORK IN CURRENT OCCUPATION

14. DATE OF CURRENT ILLNESS, INJURY, or PREGNANCY (LMP)	15. OTHER DATE	16. DATES PATIENT UNABLE TO WORK IN CURRENT OCCUPATION
MM 02 DD 16 YY 20XX QUAL. 431	QUAL. 444 MM 03 DD 24 YY 20XX	FROM MM 03 DD 24 YY 20XX TO MM 04 DD 07 YY 20XX
17. NAME OF REFERRING PROVIDER OR OTHER SOURCE	17a.	18. HOSPITALIZATION DATES RELATED TO CURRENT SERVICES
DN Thomas Rothschild MD	17b. NPI 23345678XX	FROM MM 03 DD 24 YY 20XX TO MM 03 DD 30 YY 20XX
19. ADDITIONAL CLAIM INFORMATION (Designated by NUCC)		20. OUTSIDE LAB? ☐ YES ☒ NO $ CHARGES

Centers for Medicare and Medicaid Services

THIRD-PARTY PAYERS: Insert eight-digit dates patient is employed but cannot work in current occupation. *FROM:* Enter first *full* day patient was unable to perform job duties. *TO:* Enter last day patient was disabled before returning to work. An entry in this field may indicate employment-related insurance coverage.

FIELD 17 ⓒ NAME OF REFERRING OR ORDERING PROVIDER

14. DATE OF CURRENT ILLNESS, INJURY, or PREGNANCY (LMP)	15. OTHER DATE	16. DATES PATIENT UNABLE TO WORK IN CURRENT OCCUPATION
MM 02 DD 16 YY 20XX QUAL. 431	QUAL. 444 MM 03 DD 24 YY 20XX	FROM MM 03 DD 24 YY 20XX TO MM 04 DD 07 YY 20XX
17. NAME OF REFERRING PROVIDER OR OTHER SOURCE	17a.	18. HOSPITALIZATION DATES RELATED TO CURRENT SERVICES
DN Thomas Rothschild MD	17b. NPI 23345678XX	FROM MM 03 DD 24 YY 20XX TO MM 03 DD 30 YY 20XX
19. ADDITIONAL CLAIM INFORMATION (Designated by NUCC)		20. OUTSIDE LAB? ☐ YES ☒ NO $ CHARGES

Centers for Medicare and Medicaid Services

COMMERCIAL PAYERS: Insert complete name and degree of the physician who referred or ordered the services reported on this claim. Do not list other referrals (i.e., friends or family). Enter applicable qualifier to the left of the vertical, dotted line to identify which provider is being reported. Qualifier examples follow:

- DN   Referring provider
- DK   Ordering provider
- DQ   Supervising provider

If multiple providers are involved, enter one provider using the following priority order:

1. Referring provider
2. Ordering provider
3. Supervising provider

MEDICARE: Insert the name and degree of referring or ordering physician on all claims for Medicare-covered services and items resulting from a physician's order or referral. Enter applicable qualifier (listed under Commercial Carriers) to the left of the vertical, dotted line to identify which provider is being reported. Use a separate claim form for each referring and/or ordering physician.

Surgeon: All surgeons must complete this field for Medicare claims. Insert the primary surgeon's name on an assistant surgeon's claim and in situations when the patient has not been referred.

Referring Physician: When a physician refers a patient to another physician for a service, insert the referring physician's name.

Supervising Physician: When a physician extender (e.g., nurse practitioner) refers a patient for a consultation, enter the name of the physician supervising the physician extender.

Ordering Physician: A physician who orders non-physician services for the patient, such as diagnostic radiology, laboratory, and pathology tests; pharmaceutical services; durable medical equipment (DME); parenteral and enteral nutrition; and immunosuppressive drugs.

When the ordering physician is also the performing physician (e.g., the physician who actually performs the in-office laboratory tests), the performing physician's name and assigned NPI number must appear in Field 17 and the taxonomy number* in Field 17b.

---

*Taxonomy codes identify the provider type classification, and/or area of specialization and may also be entered in Field 19, 24I, 24J, and the shaded portion of 32b and/or 33b according to provider guidelines.

FIELD 17 ⓒ Continued

When a patient is referred to a physician who also orders and performs a diagnostic service, a *separate claim* form is required for the diagnostic service.

- Insert the original referring physician's name and NPI in Fields 17 and 17b of the first claim form.
- Insert the ordering (performing) physician's name and NPI in Fields 17 and 17b of the second claim form.

TRICARE: Insert name, degree, and address (optional) of referring provider for all consultation claims. If the patient was referred from a military treatment facility (MTF), insert the name of the MTF and attach DD Form 2161 or SF 513, "Referral for Civilian Medical Care."

FIELD 17A ⓒ ID NUMBER OTHER THAN NPI

14. DATE OF CURRENT ILLNESS, INJURY, or PREGNANCY (LMP) MM DD YY	15. OTHER DATE MM DD YY	16. DATES PATIENT UNABLE TO WORK IN CURRENT OCCUPATION MM DD YY TO MM DD YY
02 16 20XX QUAL. 431	QUAL. 444 03 24 20XX	FROM 03 24 20XX TO 04 07 20XX
17. NAME OF REFERRING PROVIDER OR OTHER SOURCE DN Thomas Rothschild MD	17a.	18. HOSPITALIZATION DATES RELATED TO CURRENT SERVICES MM DD YY MM DD YY
	17b. NPI 23345678XX	FROM 03 24 20XX TO 03 30 20XX
19. ADDITIONAL CLAIM INFORMATION (Designated by NUCC)		20. OUTSIDE LAB? ☐ YES ☒ NO $ CHARGES

Centers for Medicare and Medicaid Services

THIRD-PARTY PAYERS: Insert ID qualifiers in the box immediately to the right of 17a and the referring, ordering, or supervising provider numbers (other than NPI) in the larger area when required by local carriers. Examples of Qualifiers approved by the National Uniform Claim Committee (NUCC) are:

- OB   State license number
- 1G   Provider UPIN number
- G2   Provider commercial number
- LU   Location number for supervising provider

MEDICARE: Leave blank.

FIELD 17B ⓒ NPI NUMBER

14. DATE OF CURRENT ILLNESS, INJURY, or PREGNANCY (LMP) MM DD YY	15. OTHER DATE MM DD YY	16. DATES PATIENT UNABLE TO WORK IN CURRENT OCCUPATION MM DD YY TO MM DD YY
02 16 20XX QUAL. 431	QUAL. 444 03 24 20XX	FROM 03 24 20XX TO 04 07 20XX
17. NAME OF REFERRING PROVIDER OR OTHER SOURCE DN Thomas Rothschild MD	17a.	18. HOSPITALIZATION DATES RELATED TO CURRENT SERVICES MM DD YY MM DD YY
	17b. NPI 23345678XX	FROM 03 24 20XX TO 03 30 20XX
19. ADDITIONAL CLAIM INFORMATION (Designated by NUCC)		20. OUTSIDE LAB? ☐ YES ☒ NO $ CHARGES

Centers for Medicare and Medicaid Services

THIRD-PARTY PAYERS: Insert the NPI number when a service was ordered or referred by a physician, or when supervising a physician extender.

FIELD 18 ⓒ HOSPITALIZATION DATES RELATED TO CURRENT SERVICES

14. DATE OF CURRENT ILLNESS, INJURY, or PREGNANCY (LMP) MM DD YY	15. OTHER DATE MM DD YY	16. DATES PATIENT UNABLE TO WORK IN CURRENT OCCUPATION MM DD YY TO MM DD YY
02 16 20XX QUAL. 431	QUAL. 444 03 24 20XX	FROM 03 24 20XX TO 04 07 20XX
17. NAME OF REFERRING PROVIDER OR OTHER SOURCE DN Thomas Rothschild MD	17a.	18. HOSPITALIZATION DATES RELATED TO CURRENT SERVICES MM DD YY MM DD YY
	17b. NPI 23345678XX	FROM 03 24 20XX TO 03 30 20XX
19. ADDITIONAL CLAIM INFORMATION (Designated by NUCC)		20. OUTSIDE LAB? ☐ YES ☒ NO $ CHARGES

Centers for Medicare and Medicaid Services

FIELD 18 © Continued

THIRD-PARTY PAYERS: Insert six- or eight-digit admitting and discharge dates in this field when a medical service is furnished as a result of, or subsequent to, a related (inpatient) hospitalization, skilled nursing facility, or nursing home visit. Do not complete for outpatient hospital services, ambulatory surgery, or emergency department services. If the patient is still hospitalized at the time of the billing, leave the discharge date blank.

FIELD 19 © ADDITIONAL CLAIM INFORMATION

14. DATE OF CURRENT ILLNESS, INJURY, or PREGNANCY (LMP)		15. OTHER DATE				16. DATES PATIENT UNABLE TO WORK IN CURRENT OCCUPATION			
MM DD YY		QUAL.	MM DD YY			MM DD YY		MM DD YY	
02 16 20XX QUAL. 431		444	03 24 20XX			FROM 03 24 20XX		TO 04 07 20XX	
17. NAME OF REFERRING PROVIDER OR OTHER SOURCE		17a.				18. HOSPITALIZATION DATES RELATED TO CURRENT SERVICES			
DN Thomas Rothschild MD		17b. NPI	23345678XX			MM DD YY		MM DD YY	
						FROM 03 24 20XX		TO 03 30 20XX	
19. ADDITIONAL CLAIM INFORMATION (Designated by NUCC)						20. OUTSIDE LAB? $ CHARGES			
						☐ YES ☒ NO			

Centers for Medicare and Medicaid Services

COMMERCIAL PAYERS: Depending on commercial carrier guidelines, this field may be completed in a number of different ways. If reporting more than one item of data, enter three blank spaces in between. Some examples are:

- Insert the word "ATTACHMENT" when an operative report, discharge summary, invoice, or other attachment is included. Do not attach documents smaller than 8½" by 11".
- Insert an explanation regarding unusual services or unlisted services.
- Insert all applicable modifiers when modifier -99 is used in Field 24D. If -99 appears with more than one procedure code, list the line number (24-1, 2, 3, etc.) for each -99 listed.
- Insert the drug name and dosage when submitting a claim for not otherwise (NOC) classified drugs. Enter the word "ATTACHMENT" and attach the invoice.
- List the supply when the code 99070 is used.
- NUCC-approved ID qualifiers and numbers may be reported (e.g., OB—state license number, 1G—provider UPIN number, ZZ—provider taxonomy code).
- Enter the phrase "FAXED DOCUMENTATION" when faxing a report.

MEDICARE: CMS guidelines state this field may be completed in a number of different ways depending on the circumstances of the services provided to the patient. This field can only contain up to three conditions per claim. Some common uses are:

- When submitting a claim for *not otherwise classified (NOC) drugs,* enter the drug's name and dosage with the word "ATTACHMENT" and include a copy of the invoice.
- When submitting a claim for a physical or occupational therapist, psychotherapist, chiropractor, or podiatrist, enter the attending physician's NPI and taxonomy number and either the six-digit or eight-digit date of the patient's latest visit pertaining to the claim.
- For *unlisted procedures,* include a concise description. If there is not sufficient room in this field, send an attachment.
- When *modifier -99* is used in Field 24D (e.g., 99–80 51), enter all applicable modifiers. If -99 appears with more than one procedure code, list the line number (1, 2, 3, etc.) for each -99 listed.
- When an independent laboratory renders an electrocardiogram or collects a specimen from a *patient who is homebound or institutionalized,* enter, "Homebound."
- When a *Medicare beneficiary refuses to assign benefits* to a participating provider, enter the statement "Patient refuses to assign benefits." No payment to the physician will be made on the claim in this case.
- When submitting a claim to obtain an intentional denial from Medicare as the primary payer for *hearing aid testing* and a secondary payer is involved, enter "Testing for hearing aid."

FIELD 19 C Continued

- When *providers share postoperative care* for global surgery claims, enter either a six- or eight-digit assumed and relinquished dates of care for each provider.
- When an examination is done prior to dental surgery, enter the type of dental surgery to be performed.
- When a physician gives service to a *hospice patient* but the hospice in which the patient resides does

not employ the physician, enter the statement "Attending physician, not hospice employee."
- When a *purchased interpretation of a diagnostic test* is performed, enter the NPI of the performing physician.

TRICARE: This block is typically reserved for local use (e.g., to indicate a referral authorization number or enter an x-ray date for chiropractic treatment).

FIELD 20 C OUTSIDE LABORATORY CHARGES BEING BILLED

14. DATE OF CURRENT ILLNESS, INJURY, or PREGNANCY (LMP)		15. OTHER DATE					16. DATES PATIENT UNABLE TO WORK IN CURRENT OCCUPATION						
MM 02	DD 16	YY 20XX QUAL. 431	QUAL. 444	MM 03	DD 24	YY 20XX	FROM	MM 03	DD 24	YY 20XX	TO	MM 04	DD 07	YY 20XX

17. NAME OF REFERRING PROVIDER OR OTHER SOURCE	17a.		18. HOSPITALIZATION DATES RELATED TO CURRENT SERVICES						
DN Thomas Rothschild MD	17b. NPI 23345678XX		FROM MM 03 DD 24 YY 20XX			TO MM 03 DD 30 YY 20XX			

19. ADDITIONAL CLAIM INFORMATION (Designated by NUCC)	20. OUTSIDE LAB? ☐ YES ☒ NO	$ CHARGES

Centers for Medicare and Medicaid Services

THIRD-PARTY PAYERS: Insert "YES" when billing for diagnostic laboratory tests that were performed *outside* the physician's office. Typically "NO" is marked, which means the tests were performed by the billing physician in the office laboratory. If "YES," enter purchase price of the test in the Charges portion of this field and complete Field 32.

MEDICARE: Follow Third-Party Payer guidelines. *Note: All clinical laboratory services must be billed to Medicare on an assigned basis.*

FIELD 21 R DIAGNOSIS, SYMPTOM, OR SIGN OF ILLNESS OR INJURY

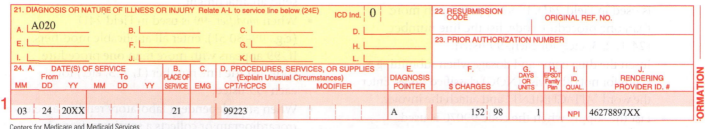

Centers for Medicare and Medicaid Services

ALL THIRD-PARTY PAYERS: Insert the applicable ICD indicator to the left of the vertical, dotted lines in the upper right-hand portion of this field to identify which version of ICD codes are being reported:

- 9 *ICD-9-CM*
- 0 *ICD-10-CM*

Insert up to 12 diagnostic codes in priority order (A–L), with the primary diagnosis in the first position (A).

Codes must be carried out to their highest degree of specificity. Enter the codes, left-justified on each line and do not use decimal points, spaces, or add any code narratives. Code only the conditions or problems that the physician is actively treating and that relate directly to the services billed.

FIELD 22 ⓒ RESUBMISSION AND/OR ORIGINAL CLAIM REFERENCE NUMBER

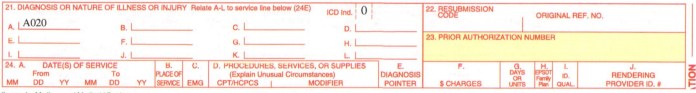

Centers for Medicare and Medicaid Services

THIRD-PARTY PAYERS: When *resubmitting a claim*, enter the appropriate reference number or bill frequency code, left justified in the left-hand side of the field. Refer to the most current payer instructions regarding this field. Examples follow:

- 7   Replacement of prior claim
- 8   Void/cancel of prior claim

MEDICARE: Leave blank.

TRICARE: Leave blank.

FIELD 23 ⓒ PRIOR AUTHORIZATION NUMBER

Centers for Medicare and Medicaid Services

COMMERCIAL PAYERS: Insert any of the following assigned by the payer for current services: Prior authorization number, referral number, mammography pre-certification number, or Clinical Laboratory Improvement Amendments (CLIA) number.

MEDICARE: CMS guidelines state this field may be completed in a number of different ways depending on the circumstances of the services provided to the patient. Only one condition may be reported per claim and when submitting multiple page claims, list only the diagnosis from the first page on subsequent pages. Some common uses are:

- Insert the 10-digit Quality Improvement Organization (QIO) prior authorization or precertification number for procedures requiring prior approval.
- Insert the investigational device exemption (IDE) number if billing for an investigational device.

- Insert the 10-digit CLIA (Clinical Laboratory Improvement Amendments) federal certification number when billing for laboratory services billed by a physician office laboratory.
- Insert the NPI number of the skilled nursing facility (SNF) when the physician provides services to an SNF patient outside of the facility.
- Insert the NPI of the hospice or home health agency (HHA) when billing for care plan oversight services.

TRICARE: Insert the professional (peer) review organization (PRO) 10-digit prior authorization or precertification number for procedures requiring PRO prior approval. Enter the IDE number when billing for an investigational device. Attach a copy of the authorization.

FIELDS 24A THROUGH 24J LINES OF BILLED SERVICE

Each of the six lines in **Fields 24A through J** has been divided horizontally to accommodate supplemental information in the *top portion* (shaded area) to support billed services. Providers must verify these requirements with each payer. Enter the qualifier, then the information, and do enter a space or hyphen between or within the code number and information. Following are examples of qualifiers used to submit supplemental information.

- CTR   Contract rate
- JO   Dentistry designation system for tooth and areas of the oral cavity
- JP   Universal/National tooth designation system
- N4   National Drug Codes (NDC)
- ZZ   Narrative description of unspecified code

Use the bottom portion of Field 24 to enter data, that is, dates of service, place of service, *CPT* codes, and so forth, for each line of service—a total of six. The shaded areas may not be used to bill 12 lines of service if the case requires more than six detail lines. Claims cannot be "continued" from one to another, so additional information must be entered on a separate claim form; treat it as an independent claim, totaling all charges on each claim. Do not list a procedure on the claim form for which there is no charge. When reporting multiple page claims, only the diagnoses listed on the first page may be used on subsequent pages.

FIELD 24A ® DATE(S) OF SERVICE

24. A. DATE(S) OF SERVICE From MM DD YY	To MM DD YY	B. PLACE OF SERVICE	C. EMG	D. PROCEDURES, SERVICES, OR SUPPLIES (Explain Unusual Circumstances) CPT/HCPCS	MODIFIER	E. DIAGNOSIS POINTER	F. $ CHARGES	G. DAYS OR UNITS	H. EPSDT Family Plan	I. ID. QUAL.	J. RENDERING PROVIDER ID. #
1	03 24 20XX		21		99223		A	152 98	1		NPI	46278897XX
2	03 25 20XX		21		99233		A	76 97	1		NPI	46278897XX
3	03 26 20XX	03 28 20XX	21		99232		A	166 68	3		NPI	46278897XX
4	03 29 20XX		21		99231		A	37 74	1		NPI	46278897XX
5	03 30 20XX		21		99238		A	65 26	1		NPI	46278897XX
6										NPI	

25. FEDERAL TAX I.D. NUMBER	SSN EIN	26. PATIENT'S ACCOUNT NO.	27. ACCEPT ASSIGNMENT? (For govt. claims, see back)	28. TOTAL CHARGE	29. AMOUNT PAID	30. Rsvd for NUCC Use
208765432	X	MIT123	X YES NO	$ 499 63	$ 10 00	

Centers for Medicare and Medicaid Services

THIRD-PARTY PAYERS: In the "From" date, insert the month, day, and year (eight digits with no spaces) for each procedure, service, or supply reported in Field 24D. Make sure the dates shown are no earlier than the date of the current illness if listed in Field 14. If the "From" and "To" dates are the same, enter only the "From" date. *Note: Some payers may use different*

date formats and require that both the "From" and "To" dates be filled in.

Enter the "To" date when reporting a consecutive range of dates for the same procedure code; the number of days or units will be reported in Field 24G. Use a separate line for each month and a separate claim form for a different year.

FIELD 24B Ⓡ PLACE OF SERVICE

24. A.	DATE(S) OF SERVICE From			To		B. PLACE OF SERVICE	C. EMG	D. PROCEDURES, SERVICES, OR SUPPLIES (Explain Unusual Circumstances) CPT/HCPCS	MODIFIER	E. DIAGNOSIS POINTER	F. $ CHARGES		G. DAYS OR UNITS	H. EPSDT Family Plan	I. ID. QUAL.	J. RENDERING PROVIDER ID. #
	MM	DD	YY	MM	DD	YY											
1	03	24	20XX				21		99223		A	152	98	1		NPI	46278897XX

Centers for Medicare and Medicaid Services

THIRD-PARTY PAYERS: Insert the appropriate "Place of Service" code shown in Figure A-2. Identify by location where the service was performed or an item was used. Use the inpatient hospital code (21) only when a service is provided to a patient admitted to the hospital for an overnight stay. Enter the name, address, and provider number of the hospital in Field 32.

11	Doctor's office	26	Military treatment facility
12	Patient's home	31	Skilled nursing facility (swing bed visits)
21	Inpatient hospital	32	Nursing facility (intermediate/long-term care facilities)
22	Outpatient hospital or urgent care center		
23	Emergency department—hospital	33	Custodial care facility (domiciliary or rest home services)
24	Ambulatory surgical center		
25	Birthing center	81	Independent laboratory

FIGURE A-2 Partial list of place of service codes

FIELD 24C Ⓒ EMERGENCY

24. A.	DATE(S) OF SERVICE From			To		B. PLACE OF SERVICE	C. EMG	D. PROCEDURES, SERVICES, OR SUPPLIES (Explain Unusual Circumstances) CPT/HCPCS	MODIFIER	E. DIAGNOSIS POINTER	F. $ CHARGES		G. DAYS OR UNITS	H. EPSDT Family Plan	I. ID. QUAL.	J. RENDERING PROVIDER ID. #
	MM	DD	YY	MM	DD	YY											
1	03	24	20XX				21		99223		A	152	98	1		NPI	46278897XX

Centers for Medicare and Medicaid Services

COMMERCIAL PAYERS: Check with payers to determine if this emergency indicator is required. If "Yes" enter "Y," if "No," leave blank.

MEDICARE: Do not complete.

TRICARE: Insert "Y" (yes) in the bottom unshaded area of this field to indicate the service was provided in a hospital emergency department; leave blank if it does not apply.

FIELD 24D ®️ PROCEDURE, SERVICE, OR SUPPLY *CPT* CODE

24. A. DATE(S) OF SERVICE From MM DD YY	To MM DD YY	B. PLACE OF SERVICE	C. EMG	D. PROCEDURES, SERVICES, OR SUPPLIES (Explain Unusual Circumstances) CPT/HCPCS	MODIFIER	E. DIAGNOSIS POINTER	F. $ CHARGES	G. DAYS OR UNITS	H. EPSDT Family Plan	I. ID. QUAL.	J. RENDERING PROVIDER ID. #
1	03 24 20XX		21		99223		A	152 98	1		NPI	46278897XX
2	03 25 20XX		21		99233		A	76 97	1		NPI	46278897XX
3	03 26 20XX	03 28 20XX	21		99232		A	166 68	3		NPI	46278897XX
4	03 29 20XX		21		99231		A	37 74	1		NPI	46278897XX
5	03 30 20XX		21		99238		A	65 26	1		NPI	46278897XX
6										NPI	

25. FEDERAL TAX I.D. NUMBER	SSN EIN	26. PATIENT'S ACCOUNT NO.	27. ACCEPT ASSIGNMENT? (For govt. claims, see back)	28. TOTAL CHARGE	29. AMOUNT PAID	30. Rsvd for NUCC Use
208765432	☐ ☒ X	MIT123	☒ X YES ☐ NO	$ 499 63	$ 10 00	

Centers for Medicare and Medicaid Services

PHYSICIAN OR SUPPLIER INFORMATION

COMMERCIAL PAYERS: Insert the appropriate *CPT* or *HCPCS* code for each procedure, service, or supply and applicable modifier without a hyphen. Up to four modifiers may be placed per line of service. Some carriers may still accept use of multiple modifier -99 with the modifiers listed in Field 19.

MEDICARE: Insert one *CPT* or *HCPCS* code and applicable modifiers (up to four) for each line of service representing a procedure, service, or supply. Do not include a

hyphen or narrative description. When procedure codes do not require modifiers, leave modifier area blank. For multiple surgical procedures, list the procedure with the highest fee first. For unlisted procedure codes or a "not otherwise classified" (NOC) code, include a narrative description in Field 19. If information does not fit in this area, include an attachment. Submit an operative note as a claim attachment when inserting an unlisted surgery code.

TRICARE: Follow Medicare guidelines.

FIELD 24E ®️ DIAGNOSTIC CODE REFERENCE LETTER INDICATOR (POINTER)

21. DIAGNOSIS OR NATURE OF ILLNESS OR INJURY Relate A-L to service line below (24E) ICD Ind. 0		22. RESUBMISSION CODE ORIGINAL REF. NO.
A. A020 B. C. D.		
E. F. G. H.		23. PRIOR AUTHORIZATION NUMBER
I. J. K. L.		

24. A. DATE(S) OF SERVICE From MM DD YY	To MM DD YY	B. PLACE OF SERVICE	C. EMG	D. PROCEDURES, SERVICES, OR SUPPLIES (Explain Unusual Circumstances) CPT/HCPCS	MODIFIER	E. DIAGNOSIS POINTER	F. $ CHARGES	G. DAYS OR UNITS	H. EPSDT Family Plan	I. ID. QUAL.	J. RENDERING PROVIDER ID. #
1	03 24 20XX		21		99223		A	152 98	1		NPI	46278897XX
2	03 25 20XX		21		99233		A	76 97	1		NPI	46278897XX
3	03 26 20XX	03 28 20XX	21		99232		A	166 68	3		NPI	46278897XX
4	03 29 20XX		21		99231		A	37 74	1		NPI	46278897XX
5	03 30 20XX		21		99238		A	65 26	1		NPI	46278897XX
6										NPI	

25. FEDERAL TAX I.D. NUMBER	SSN EIN	26. PATIENT'S ACCOUNT NO.	27. ACCEPT ASSIGNMENT? (For govt. claims, see back)	28. TOTAL CHARGE	29. AMOUNT PAID	30. Rsvd for NUCC Use
208765432	☐ ☒ X	MIT123	☒ X YES ☐ NO	$ 499 63	$ 10 00	

Centers for Medicare and Medicaid Services

PHYSICIAN OR SUPPLIER INFORMATION

FIELD 24E Ⓒ Continued

THIRD-PARTY PAYERS: Insert the diagnostic code reference letter (A–L) as shown in Field 21 to relate the procedures performed on that date of service to the primary diagnosis. When multiple services are performed, link first the primary reference letter for each service; other applicable diagnoses reference letters may follow. Enter the letters, left-justified—without commas or spaces in between. DO NOT USE ACTUAL *ICD-10-CM* CODES IN THIS FIELD.

MEDICARE: Insert only one diagnostic code reference letter per line item linking the diagnostic code listed in Field 21 to the *CPT* code listed. When multiple services are performed, insert one primary diagnostic reference number for each service.

FIELD 24F Ⓡ CHARGES

24. A. DATE(S) OF SERVICE From MM DD YY	To MM DD YY	B. PLACE OF SERVICE	C. EMG	D. PROCEDURES, SERVICES, OR SUPPLIES (Explain Unusual Circumstances) CPT/HCPCS | MODIFIER	E. DIAGNOSIS POINTER	F. $ CHARGES	G. DAYS OR UNITS	H. EPSDT Family Plan	I. ID. QUAL.	J. RENDERING PROVIDER ID. #
1	03 24 20XX		21		99223	A	152 98	1		NPI	46278897XX
2	03 25 20XX		21		99233	A	76 97	1		NPI	46278897XX
3	03 26 20XX	03 28 20XX	21		99232	A	166 68	3		NPI	46278897XX
4	03 29 20XX		21		99231	A	37 74	1		NPI	46278897XX
5	03 30 20XX		21		99238	A	65 26	1		NPI	46278897XX
6										NPI	

25. FEDERAL TAX I.D. NUMBER	SSN EIN	26. PATIENT'S ACCOUNT NO.	27. ACCEPT ASSIGNMENT? (For govt. claims, see back)	28. TOTAL CHARGE	29. AMOUNT PAID	30. Rsvd for NUCC Use
208765432	☐ ☒ X	MIT123	☒ X YES ☐ NO	$ 499 63	$ 10 00	

PHYSICIAN OR SUPPLIER INFORMATION

Centers for Medicare and Medicaid Services

THIRD-PARTY PAYERS: Insert the charge for each listed service from the appropriate fee schedule. Enter the dollar amount, right-justified in Field 24F and the cent amount left-justified after the dotted line. *Do not use commas when reporting dollar amount or enter dollar signs or decimal points. Always include cents and enter 00 if the amount is a whole number.* If the same service is performed on consecutive days (see Field 24, line 3), multiply the fee for a single service by the number of times it was performed (noted in days or units) and enter the total for this line of service (e.g., 55.56 × 3 = 166.68). *Note: Some third-party payer computer systems may automatically multiply the fee for consecutive days, in which case the single fee should be listed.*

Workbook Exercises: For private commercial carriers and TRICARE cases, use the Mock Fees. For Medicare participating provider cases, use the Participating fees. For Medicare nonparticipating provider cases, use the Limiting Charge.

FIELD 24G ® NUMBER OF DAYS OR UNITS

24. A. DATE(S) OF SERVICE From MM DD YY	To MM DD YY	B. PLACE OF SERVICE	C. EMG	D. PROCEDURES, SERVICES, OR SUPPLIES (Explain Unusual Circumstances) CPT/HCPCS	MODIFIER	E. DIAGNOSIS POINTER	F. $ CHARGES	G. DAYS OR UNITS	H. EPSDT Family Plan	I. ID. QUAL.	J. RENDERING PROVIDER ID. #
1	03 24 20XX		21		99223		A	152 98	1		NPI	46278897XX
2	03 25 20XX		21		99233		A	76 97	1		NPI	46278897XX
3	03 26 20XX	03 28 20XX	21		99232		A	166 68	3		NPI	46278897XX
4	03 29 20XX		21		99231		A	37 74	1		NPI	46278897XX
5	03 30 20XX		21		99238		A	65 26	1		NPI	46278897XX
6										NPI	

25. FEDERAL TAX I.D. NUMBER	SSN EIN	26. PATIENT'S ACCOUNT NO.	27. ACCEPT ASSIGNMENT? (For govt. claims, see back)	28. TOTAL CHARGE	29. AMOUNT PAID	30. Rsvd for NUCC Use
208765432	☐ ☒ X	MIT123	☒ YES ☐ NO	$ 499 63	$ 10 00	

Centers for Medicare and Medicaid Services

THIRD-PARTY PAYERS: Insert the number of days or units that apply to each line of service. Most commonly, a service is performed only one time; enter the numeral 1. This field is important for calculating multiple visits, number of miles, units of supplies, drugs, anesthesia minutes, or oxygen volume. If reporting fraction of a unit, use the decimal point. For example, when a physician reports consecutive hospital care services using *CPT* code number 99232 on March 26, 27, and 28, it would be listed and totaled as shown in line 3 of the claim form example.

FIELD 24H © EARLY AND PERIODIC SCREENING, DIAGNOSIS, AND TREATMENT

24. A. DATE(S) OF SERVICE From MM DD YY	To MM DD YY	B. PLACE OF SERVICE	C. EMG	D. PROCEDURES, SERVICES, OR SUPPLIES (Explain Unusual Circumstances) CPT/HCPCS	MODIFIER	E. DIAGNOSIS POINTER	F. $ CHARGES	G. DAYS OR UNITS	H. EPSDT Family Plan	I. ID. QUAL.	J. RENDERING PROVIDER ID. #
1	03 24 20XX		21		99223		A	152 98	1		NPI	46278897XX

Centers for Medicare and Medicaid Services

THIRD-PARTY PAYERS: This field is most commonly used for Medicaid "Early & Periodic Screening, Diagnosis, and Treatment" related services. If there is no requirement to report a "reason code," enter "Y" for "Yes" or "N" for "No" in the bottom portion of the field. If there is a payer requirement to report a reason code, enter the code, right-justified in the top shaded area of the field. Common reason codes examples follow:

- S2 Under treatment
- ST New service requested

MEDICARE: Do not complete.

FIELD 24I ⊙ ID QUALIFIER

24. A. DATE(S) OF SERVICE						B. PLACE OF SERVICE	C. EMG	D. PROCEDURES, SERVICES, OR SUPPLIES (Explain Unusual Circumstances)		E. DIAGNOSIS POINTER	F. $ CHARGES		G. DAYS OR UNITS	H. EPSDT Family Plan	I. ID. QUAL.	J. RENDERING PROVIDER ID. #	
From			To					CPT/HCPCS	MODIFIER								
MM	DD	YY	MM	DD	YY												
03	24	20XX				21		99223		A	152	98	1		NPI	46278897XX	

Centers for Medicare and Medicaid Services

THIRD-PARTY PAYERS: Generally, leave blank. If the provider does not have an NPI number, enter the ID qualifier in the shaded portion of the field. NUCC-approved ID qualifier examples follow:

- OB State license number
- 1B Blue Shield provider number
- 1C Medicare provider number

- 1D Medicaid provider number
- 1G Provider UPIN number
- ZZ Provider taxonomy

MEDICARE: Generally, leave blank. If the provider does not have an NPI number, enter the ID qualifier "IC" in the shaded portion of the field.

FIELD 24J ⊙ RENDERING PROVIDER ID

24. A. DATE(S) OF SERVICE						B. PLACE OF SERVICE	C. EMG	D. PROCEDURES, SERVICES, OR SUPPLIES (Explain Unusual Circumstances)		E. DIAGNOSIS POINTER	F. $ CHARGES		G. DAYS OR UNITS	H. EPSDT Family Plan	I. ID. QUAL.	J. RENDERING PROVIDER ID. #
From			To					CPT/HCPCS	MODIFIER							
MM	DD	YY	MM	DD	YY											
03	24	20XX				21		99223		A	152	98	1		NPI	46278897XX
03	25	20XX				21		99233		A	76	97	1		NPI	46278897XX
03	26	20XX	03	28	20XX	21		99232		A	166	68	3		NPI	46278897XX
03	29	20XX				21		99231		A	37	74	1		NPI	46278897XX
03	30	20XX				21		99238		A	65	26	1		NPI	46278897XX
															NPI	

Centers for Medicare and Medicaid Services

THIRD-PARTY PAYERS: Insert the rendering provider's NPI number in the *lower, unshaded portion*. For "incident to" services, if the provider who ordered the service is not supervising the physician extender (e.g., nurse practitioner), insert the NPI of the supervisor. If the rendering physician does not have an NPI identification number, enter the non-NPI number in the top shaded area of the field.

TRICARE: Insert the attending physician's state license number in the lower, unshaded portion of the field. The state license number is an alpha character followed by six numeric digits. If there are not six digits, enter the appropriate number of zero(s) after the alpha character to make six digits (i.e., Z9876 would be Z009876).

FIELD 25 ® FEDERAL TAX ID NUMBER

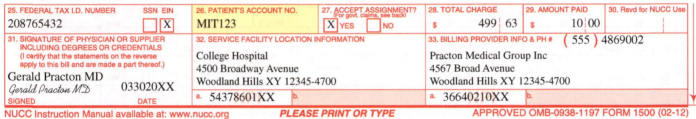

THIRD-PARTY PAYERS: For physicians employed by and billing as a *group*, insert the medical group's federal tax ID number (EIN or Social Security) and mark the corresponding box. For physicians who are *independent contractors* (not employees), insert their individual federal tax ID number. Left-justify the entry and do not enter spaces or hyphens. *Note: Some third-party payers may not require the completion of this field.*

Workbook Exercises: Enter the Practon Medical Group, Inc., tax ID number and mark "EIN."

FIELD 26 © PATIENT'S ACCOUNT NUMBER

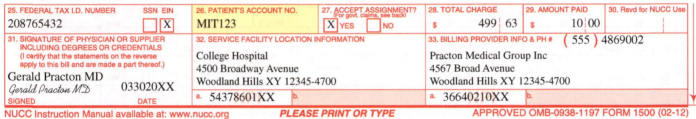

THIRD-PARTY PAYERS: Insert the patient's account number assigned by the physician's computer system. Do not use spaces or punctuation. Completion of this field is required when Medicare is billed electronically.

Workbook Exercises: List the patient account number when provided.

FIELD 27 ® ACCEPT ASSIGNMENT INDICATOR

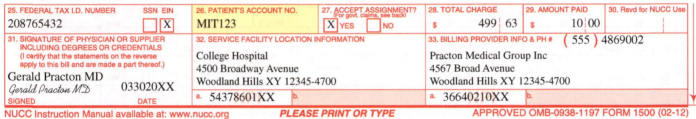

COMMERCIAL PAYERS: Mark "YES" or "NO" to indicate whether the physician accepts assignment of benefits. If yes, then the physician agrees to accept the allowed amount paid by the third party as payment in full plus any copayment and/or deductible.

Workbook Exercises: Mark "YES."

FIELD 27 Ⓡ Continued

MEDICARE: Mark "YES" or "NO" to indicate whether the physician accepts assignment of Medicare benefits. If this field is left blank, "NO" is assumed, and a participating physician's claim will be denied. The following provider/supplier must file claims on an *assignment basis:*

- Clinical diagnostic laboratory services performed in physician's office.

    Physicians may accept assignment on clinical laboratory services but not other services and should submit two separate claims, one "assigned" for laboratory and one "nonassigned" for other services. Submit all charges on a nonassigned claim, indicating "NO" in Field 27, and write "I accept assignment for the clinical laboratory tests" in the shaded portion of Field 24.

- Participating physician and supplier services.
- Services of physician assistants, nurse practitioners, clinical nurse specialists, nurse midwives, certified registered nurse anesthetists, clinical psychologists, and clinical social workers.
- Ambulatory surgical center services.

- Home dialysis supplies and equipment paid under Method II (monthly capitation payment).
- Ambulance services
- Drugs and biologicals
- Simplified billing roster for influenza virus and pneumococcal vaccines

Medicare/Medicaid: Mark "YES." Claims for services to individuals dually entitled to Medicare and Medicaid can only be paid on an assignment basis.

Medicare/Medigap: If Medigap is indicated in Field 9 and Medigap payment authorization is indicated in Field 13, the provider shall also be a participating provider and accept assignment of Medicare and Medigap benefits for all covered charges. Mark "YES."

MSP: Mark "YES" or "NO" to indicate whether the physician accepts assignment of benefits for primary insurance and Medicare.

Workbook Exercises: Mark "YES."

TRICARE: Follow Commercial Payer guidelines. *Note: Participation in TRICARE may be made on a case-by-case basis.*

FIELD 28 Ⓡ TOTAL CHARGE

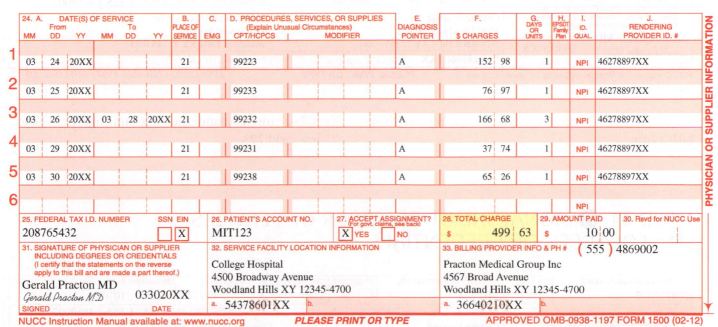

THIRD-PARTY PAYERS: Insert total charges, including cents, for services listed in Field(s) 24F. If more than one unit is listed in Field 24G, multiply the number of units by the charge and list the total amount in 24F. Do not enter dollar signs, commas, or decimal points. Enter 00 in the cents area if the amount is a whole number.

FIELD 29 © AMOUNT PAID

25. FEDERAL TAX I.D. NUMBER	SSN EIN	26. PATIENT'S ACCOUNT NO.	27. ACCEPT ASSIGNMENT? (For govt. claims, see back)	28. TOTAL CHARGE	29. AMOUNT PAID	30. Rsvd for NUCC Use
208765432	☐ ☒	MIT123	☒ YES ☐ NO	$ 499 ¦ 63	$ 10 ¦ 00	
31. SIGNATURE OF PHYSICIAN OR SUPPLIER INCLUDING DEGREES OR CREDENTIALS (I certify that the statements on the reverse apply to this bill and are made a part thereof.) Gerald Practon MD *Gerald Practon MD* 033020XX SIGNED DATE		32. SERVICE FACILITY LOCATION INFORMATION College Hospital 4500 Broadway Avenue Woodland Hills XY 12345-4700 a. 54378601XX b.			33. BILLING PROVIDER INFO & PH # (555) 4869002 Practon Medical Group Inc 4567 Broad Avenue Woodland Hills XY 12345-4700 a. 36640210XX b.	

NUCC Instruction Manual available at: www.nucc.org   *PLEASE PRINT OR TYPE*   APPROVED OMB-0938-1197 FORM 1500 (02-12)
Centers for Medicare and Medicaid Services

COMMERCIAL PAYERS: Insert only the amount paid for the charges listed on the claim.

MEDICARE: Follow Commercial Payer guidelines.

MSP: Insert only the amount paid for charges listed on the claim. It is mandatory to enter amount paid by the primary carrier and send electronically or attach an explanation of benefits document when billing Medicare as the secondary payer.

TRICARE: If payment is made by any other health insurances, the amount must be entered and the other health insurance explanation of benefits, other documents, or denial showing the amounts paid must accompany the claim. Payment from the beneficiary should not be included.

FIELD 30 © BALANCE ON CLAIM/ RESERVED FOR NUCC USE

25. FEDERAL TAX I.D. NUMBER	SSN EIN	26. PATIENT'S ACCOUNT NO.	27. ACCEPT ASSIGNMENT? (For govt. claims, see back)	28. TOTAL CHARGE	29. AMOUNT PAID	30. Rsvd for NUCC Use
208765432	☐ ☒	MIT123	☒ YES ☐ NO	$ 499 ¦ 63	$ 10 ¦ 00	
31. SIGNATURE OF PHYSICIAN OR SUPPLIER INCLUDING DEGREES OR CREDENTIALS (I certify that the statements on the reverse apply to this bill and are made a part thereof.) Gerald Practon MD *Gerald Practon MD* 033020XX SIGNED DATE		32. SERVICE FACILITY LOCATION INFORMATION College Hospital 4500 Broadway Avenue Woodland Hills XY 12345-4700 a. 54378601XX b.			33. BILLING PROVIDER INFO & PH # (555) 4869002 Practon Medical Group Inc 4567 Broad Avenue Woodland Hills XY 12345-4700 a. 36640210XX b.	

NUCC Instruction Manual available at: www.nucc.org   *PLEASE PRINT OR TYPE*   APPROVED OMB-0938-1197 FORM 1500 (02-12)
Centers for Medicare and Medicaid Services

THIRD-PARTY PAYERS: Leave blank; reserved for NUCC use.

TRICARE: Insert balance due on claim (figures in Field 28 less Field 29).

FIELD 31 ® SIGNATURE OF PROVIDER OF SERVICES WITH DEGREES OR CREDENTIALS

25. FEDERAL TAX I.D. NUMBER	SSN EIN	26. PATIENT'S ACCOUNT NO.	27. ACCEPT ASSIGNMENT? (For govt. claims, see back)	28. TOTAL CHARGE	29. AMOUNT PAID	30. Rsvd for NUCC Use
208765432	☐ ☒	MIT123	☐ YES ☒ NO	$ 499 ¦ 63	$ 10 ¦ 00	
31. SIGNATURE OF PHYSICIAN OR SUPPLIER INCLUDING DEGREES OR CREDENTIALS (I certify that the statements on the reverse apply to this bill and are made a part thereof.) Gerald Practon MD *Gerald Practon MD* 033020XX SIGNED DATE		32. SERVICE FACILITY LOCATION INFORMATION College Hospital 4500 Broadway Avenue Woodland Hills XY 12345-4700 a. 54378601XX b.			33. BILLING PROVIDER INFO & PH # (555) 4869002 Practon Medical Group Inc 4567 Broad Avenue Woodland Hills XY 12345-4700 a. 36640210XX b.	

NUCC Instruction Manual available at: www.nucc.org   *PLEASE PRINT OR TYPE*   APPROVED OMB-0938-1197 FORM 1500 (02-12)
Centers for Medicare and Medicaid Services

FIELD 31 Ⓡ Continued

THIRD-PARTY PAYERS: Insert the provider's name including degrees or credentials and show the signature of the physician or the physician's representative above or below the name. Do not enter the name of the association or corporation. Enter the six- or eight-digit date the form was prepared; do not use spacing or punctuation (082720XX). Some insurance carriers will accept a stamped signature, but the stamp must be completely inside the field . A signature on file may be accepted by some carriers. *Note: In a computerized environment, the signed participating contract with the third-party payer (e.g., Medicare, Medicaid,* *Blue Plans) signed by the physician allows the physician's signature to be printed in this field where it would normally be signed.*

MEDICARE: If the physician, supplier, or authorized person's signature is missing, but the signature is on file, or if any authorization is attached to the claim, or if the signature field has "Signature on file" and/or a computer-generated signature, Medicare will accept the claim. Guidelines for nonphysician practitioners may vary. See Medicare's website, http://www.cms.gov, for detailed Medicare requirements.

FIELD 32 Ⓒ FACILITY LOCATION INFORMATION

25. FEDERAL TAX I.D. NUMBER	SSN EIN	26. PATIENT'S ACCOUNT NO.	27. ACCEPT ASSIGNMENT? (For govt. claims, see back)	28. TOTAL CHARGE	29. AMOUNT PAID	30. Rsvd for NUCC Use
208765432	☐ ☒	MIT123	☒ YES ☐ NO	$ 499 ¦ 63	$ 10 ¦ 00	
31. SIGNATURE OF PHYSICIAN OR SUPPLIER INCLUDING DEGREES OR CREDENTIALS (I certify that the statements on the reverse apply to this bill and are made a part thereof.) Gerald Practon MD *Gerald Practon MD* 033020XX SIGNED DATE		32. SERVICE FACILITY LOCATION INFORMATION College Hospital 4500 Broadway Avenue Woodland Hills XY 12345-4700 a. 54378601XX b.		33. BILLING PROVIDER INFO & PH # (555) 4869002 Practon Medical Group Inc 4567 Broad Avenue Woodland Hills XY 12345-4700 a. 36640210XX b.		

NUCC Instruction Manual available at: www.nucc.org **PLEASE PRINT OR TYPE** APPROVED OMB-0938-1197 FORM 1500 (02-12)

Centers for Medicare and Medicaid Services

THIRD-PARTY PAYERS: Do not complete if the facility furnishing services is the same as that of the biller listed in Field 33. If the place of service is *other* than the patient's home (POS 12) or the doctor's office (POS 11), enter the name of the facility on the first line; street address on the second line; and the city, two-digit state code, and ZIP code (including a hyphen if using a nine-digit code) on the third line. Do not use punctuation in the address. Leave one space between the city and state code, and one space between the state and ZIP code. For example, if services are performed in a hospital, enter the hospital's name and address. For durable medical equipment, enter the *location* where the *order is taken.* When billing for purchased diagnostic tests performed outside the physician's office but billed by the physician, insert the facility's name, address, and ZIP code. Format examples follow:

- 555 S. Center Street, #100 = 555 S Center Street 100
- 123 North Broadway Avenue = 123 N Broadway Avenue

TRICARE: Indicate the name of the military treatment facility, or other facility where services were rendered.

FIELD 32A Ⓒ NPI NUMBER

25. FEDERAL TAX I.D. NUMBER	SSN EIN	26. PATIENT'S ACCOUNT NO.	27. ACCEPT ASSIGNMENT? (For govt. claims, see back)	28. TOTAL CHARGE	29. AMOUNT PAID	30. Rsvd for NUCC Use
208765432	☐ ☒	MIT123	☒ YES ☐ NO	$ 499 ¦ 63	$ 10 ¦ 00	
31. SIGNATURE OF PHYSICIAN OR SUPPLIER INCLUDING DEGREES OR CREDENTIALS (I certify that the statements on the reverse apply to this bill and are made a part thereof.) Gerald Practon MD *Gerald Practon MD* 033020XX SIGNED DATE		32. SERVICE FACILITY LOCATION INFORMATION College Hospital 4500 Broadway Avenue Woodland Hills XY 12345-4700 a. 54378601XX b.		33. BILLING PROVIDER INFO & PH # (555) 4869002 Practon Medical Group Inc 4567 Broad Avenue Woodland Hills XY 12345-4700 a. 36640210XX b.		

NUCC Instruction Manual available at: www.nucc.org **PLEASE PRINT OR TYPE** APPROVED OMB-0938-1197 FORM 1500 (02-12)

Centers for Medicare and Medicaid Services

THIRD-PARTY PAYERS: If a service facility is listed in Field 32, insert the NPI of the facility.

FIELD 32B Ⓒ OTHER ID NUMBER

THIRD-PARTY PAYERS: Enter the two-digit NUCC-approved ID qualifier and number to indicate the type of non-NPI payer-assigned unique identifier listed in Field 32A. For purchased diagnostic tests, insert the supplier's PIN. For certified mammography screening centers, insert the six-digit FDA-approved certification number. For durable medical, orthotic, and prosthetic claims, insert the PIN of the location where the order was

accepted if the name and address were not provided in Field 32. Examples follow:

- OB   State license number
- G2   Provider commercial number
- LU   Location number

MEDICARE: Leave blank.

FIELD 33 Ⓡ BILLING PROVIDER INFORMATION

25. FEDERAL TAX I.D. NUMBER	SSN EIN	26. PATIENT'S ACCOUNT NO.	27. ACCEPT ASSIGNMENT? (For govt. claims, see back)	28. TOTAL CHARGE	29. AMOUNT PAID	30. Rsvd for NUCC Use
208765432	☐ ☒	MIT123	☒ YES ☐ NO	$ 499 63	$ 10 00	
31. SIGNATURE OF PHYSICIAN OR SUPPLIER INCLUDING DEGREES OR CREDENTIALS (I certify that the statements on the reverse apply to this bill and are made a part thereof.)		32. SERVICE FACILITY LOCATION INFORMATION		33. BILLING PROVIDER INFO & PH # (555) 4869002		
Gerald Practon MD		College Hospital		Practon Medical Group Inc		
Gerald Practon MD 033020XX		4500 Broadway Avenue		4567 Broad Avenue		
SIGNED DATE		Woodland Hills XY 12345-4700		Woodland Hills XY 12345-4700		
		a. 54378601XX	b.	a. 36640210XX	b.	

NUCC Instruction Manual available at: www.nucc.org   **PLEASE PRINT OR TYPE**   APPROVED OMB-0938-1197 FORM 1500 (02-12)

Centers for Medicare and Medicaid Services

THIRD-PARTY PAYERS: Insert the name of the provider or supplier billing for services on the first line; street address on the second line; and the city, two-digit state code, and ZIP code (including a hyphen if using a nine-digit code) on the third line. Do not use

punctuation in the address. Insert one space between the city and state code, and one space between the state and ZIP code. Insert the telephone number with area code to the right of the field title; do not use a hyphen or space as a separator within the telephone number.

FIELD 33A Ⓡ BILLING PROVIDER NPI NUMBER

25. FEDERAL TAX I.D. NUMBER	SSN EIN	26. PATIENT'S ACCOUNT NO.	27. ACCEPT ASSIGNMENT? (For govt. claims, see back)	28. TOTAL CHARGE	29. AMOUNT PAID	30. Rsvd for NUCC Use
208765432	☐ ☒	MIT123	☒ YES ☐ NO	$ 499 63	$ 10 00	
31. SIGNATURE OF PHYSICIAN OR SUPPLIER INCLUDING DEGREES OR CREDENTIALS (I certify that the statements on the reverse apply to this bill and are made a part thereof.)		32. SERVICE FACILITY LOCATION INFORMATION		33. BILLING PROVIDER INFO & PH # (555) 4869002		
Gerald Practon MD		College Hospital		Practon Medical Group Inc		
Gerald Practon MD 033020XX		4500 Broadway Avenue		4567 Broad Avenue		
SIGNED DATE		Woodland Hills XY 12345-4700		Woodland Hills XY 12345-4700		
		a. 54378601XX	b.	a. 36640210XX	b.	

NUCC Instruction Manual available at: www.nucc.org   **PLEASE PRINT OR TYPE**   APPROVED OMB-0938-1197 FORM 1500 (02-12)

Centers for Medicare and Medicaid Services

THIRD-PARTY PAYERS: Enter the NPI of the billing provider.

TRICARE: Insert the physician or group's tax ID number.

FIELD 33B BILLING PROVIDER OTHER ID NUMBER

THIRD-PARTY PAYERS: Insert the two-digit NUCC qualifier identifying the non-NPI number followed by the ID number. Do not enter a space, hyphen, or other separator between the qualifier and number. Examples follow:

- OB   State license number
- B2   Provider commercial number
- ZZ   Provider taxonomy

MEDICARE: Leave blank.

BOTTOM OF FORM

Enter insurance billing specialist's reference initials in lower left corner of the insurance claim form.

APPENDIX B

MEDICAL ASSISTING TASK LIST AND COMPETENCY TABLES REFERENCING CHAPTERS, PROCEDURES, AND JOB SKILLS TO EACH COMPETENCY

- AMT Medical Assisting Task List for the RMA (Table B-1)
- CAAHEP Educational Competencies (Table B-2)
- ABHES Curriculum Competencies (Table B-3)
- CMA (AAMA) Certification Examination Content (Table B-4)
- RMA (AMT) Certification Examination Competencies (Table B-5)
- CMAS (AMT) Examination Specifications (Table B-6)

AMT MEDICAL ASSISTING TASK LIST FOR THE RMA*

The American Medical Technologists developed the Medical Assisting Task List (2015) that includes various tasks that medical assistants perform but are not necessarily limited to. It represents an inventory of the Registered Medical Assistant's (RMA) job role** with respect to contemporary health care.

TABLE B-1 **Medical Assisting Task List for the Registered Medical Assistant, Developed by the American Medical Technologists, 05/2015**

AMT Medical Assisting Task List

I. GENERAL MEDICAL ASSISTING KNOWLEDGE

A. Anatomy and Physiology
 1. Body systems
 2. Disorders and diseases
 3. Wellness and nutrition

B. Medical Terminology
 1. Word parts
 2. Definitions
 3. Common abbreviations and symbols
 4. Spelling

C. Medical Law
 1. Medical Law
 2. Licensure, certification, and registration
 3. Terminology

D. Medical Ethics
 1. Principles of medical ethics

E. Human Relations
 1. Patient relations
 2. Interpersonal skills

F. Patient Education
 1. Patient instruction
 2. Patient resource materials
 3. Documentation

II. ADMINISTRATIVE MEDICAL ASSISTING

A. Insurance
 1. Terminology
 2. Plans
 3. Claims
 4. Coding
 5. Insurance finance applications

B. Financial Bookkeeping
 1. Terminology
 2. Patient billing
 3. Collections
 4. Fundamental medical office accounting procedures
 5. Banking procedures
 6. Employee payroll
 7. Financial mathematics

C. Medical Receptionist/Secretarial/Clerical
 1. Terminology
 2. Reception
 3. Scheduling
 4. Oral and written communications
 5. Records and chart management
 6. Transcription and dictation
 7. Supplies and equipment management
 8. Computer applications
 9. Office safety

AMT
American Medical Technologists
Certifying Excellence in Allied Health

10700 W. Higgins Road Suite 150
Rosemont, Illinois 60018
Phone: (847) 823-5169
Fax: (847) 823-0458
www.amt1.com

The task list is reprinted with permission from the American Medical Technologists.
**Only general and administrative skills are listed.*

CAAHEP EDUCATIONAL COMPETENCIES*

The Commission on Accreditation and Allied Health Education Programs (CAAHEP) has developed standards and guidelines for medical assisting educational programs. These curriculum standards have been adopted by the American Association of Medical Assistants (AAMA) and used by the Medical Assisting Education Review Board (MAERB) in the accreditation process for programs who train individuals to enter the medical assisting profession. Following are the 2015 core curriculum requirements, which identify three areas that have been determined to be entry-level competencies for medical assistants:** (1) knowledge (cognitive), (2) skills (psychomotor), and (3) behavior (affective). Chapters, procedures, and job skills are cross-referenced to each competency to help locate them in the *Administrative Medical Assisting* textbook and *Workbook*.

TABLE B-2 Commission on Accreditation of Allied Health Education Programs (CAAHEP) Standards and Guidelines for Medical Assisting Educational Programs, 2015

CAAHEP Standards and Guidelines					
CONTENT AREA I: Anatomy & Physiology					
COGNITIVE (KNOWLEDGE)		PSYCHOMOTOR (SKILLS)		AFFECTIVE (BEHAVIOR)	
I.C. Anatomy & Physiology	Reference	I.P. Anatomy & Physiology	Reference	I.A. Anatomy & Physiology	Reference
1. Describe structural organization of the human body	JS 1-5	1. Measure and record (clinical tasks—included)		1. Incorporate critical thinking skills when performing patient assessment	Pro 6-5, 6; JS 6-4; Ch 7
2. Identify body systems	JS 1-5	2. Perform (clinically-related tasks—not included)		2. Patient care (clinically-related tasks—not included)	
3. Describe: (a) body planes, (b) directional terms, (c) quadrants, and (d) body cavities	JS 1-5	3. Perform patient screening using established protocols	Pro 6-5; JS 6-1	3. Show awareness of a patient's concerns related to the procedure being performed	Ch 3; Pro 7-4, 5
4. List major organs in each body system	JS 1-5	4. Verify rules of medication administration (clinical tasks—not included)			
5. Identify the anatomical location of major organs in each body system	JS 1-5	5. Administering medication (clinical tasks—not included)			
6. thru 10. (clinically-related tasks—not included)		6. thru 10. (clinically-related tasks—not included)			
11. Identify the classifications of medications including: (a) indications for use, (b) desired effects, (c) side effects, and (d) adverse reactions	Online student resources for Chapter 10	11. Obtain specimens (clinical tasks—not included)			
12. thru 14. (clinically-related tasks—not included)		12. thru 14. (clinically-realted tasks—not included)			

(*continues*)

* *2015 Standards and Guidelines for the Accreditation of Educational Programs in Medical Assisting, Appendix B, Core Curriculum for Medical Assistants, Medical Assisting Education Review Board (MAERB). Inclusion of this Core Curriculum does not constitute any form of endorsement of this textbook by MAERB or CAAHEP. 2016 print date.*
** *Only those clinical competencies that apply to this text are listed.*

TABLE B-2 (continued)

CAAHEP Standards and Guidelines					
CONTENT AREA I: Anatomy & Physiology					
COGNITIVE (KNOWLEDGE)		PSYCHOMOTOR (SKILLS)		AFFECTIVE (BEHAVIOR)	
CONTENT AREA II: Applied Mathematics					
II.C. Applied Mathematics	Reference	II.P. Applied Mathematics	Reference	II.A. Applied Mathematics	Reference
1. Demonstrate knowledge of basic math computations	Pro 13-1 thru 13-3; JS 13-2, 3, 6; JS 14-1, 2, 5; JS 15-1, 3, 5, 6, 8, 9, 15-11 thru 15-13; JS 18-2, 3, 4; JS 19-4 thru 19-9; JS 20-1 thru 20-6, 10	3. Maintain lab test results using flow sheets	Fig 9-3; Ex 9-3; JS 9-6	1. Reassure a patient of the accuracy of the test result	JS 9-6
2. Apply mathematical computations to solve equations	JS 19-4 thru 19-9				
5. Identify both abbreviations and symbols used in calculating medication dosages	Table 10-4, JS 10-4, 5, 8				
6. Analyze health care results as reported in graphs and tables	Fig 9-2, 9-3; 9-10; Ex 9-3; Job Skill 9-6				
CONTENT AREA III: Infection Control					
III.C. Infection Control	Reference	III.P. Infection Control	Reference	III.A. Infection Control	Reference
5. Define the principles of standard precautions	Ch 5	1. Participate in bloodborne pathogen training	Ch 5	1. Recognize the implications for failure to comply with Center for Disease Control (CDC) regulations in health care settings	Ch 5, 10
6. Define personal protective equipment for all body fluids, secretions, and excretions; blood; nonintact skin; mucous membranes	Ch 5				
7. Identify Center for Disease Control (CDC) regulations that impact health care practices	Ch 5, 10	10. Demonstrate proper disposal of biohazardous material (sharps, regulated wastes)	Ch 5		

(continues)

TABLE B-2 (*continued*)

CAAHEP Standards and Guidelines					
CONTENT AREA IV: Nutrition					
COGNITIVE (KNOWLEDGE)		PSYCHOMOTOR (SKILLS)		AFFECTIVE (BEHAVIOR)	
IV.C. Nutrition		IV.P. Nutrition		IV.A. Nutrition	
1. thru 3. Dietary nutrients and functions (clinically-related skills—not included)		1. Dietary needs (clinically-related skills—not included)		1. Dietary change (clinically-related skills—not included)	
CONTENT AREA V: Concepts of Effective Communication					
V.C. Concepts of Effective Communication	Reference	V.P. Concepts of Effective Communication	Reference	V.A. Concepts of Effective Communication	Reference
1. Identify styles and types of verbal communication	Pro 4-2 thru 4-11	1. Use feedback techniques to obtain patient information including: (a) reflection, (b) restatement, and (c) clarification	Pro 4-1; JS 4-3, 4	1. Demonstrate: (a) empathy, (b) active listening, and (c) nonverbal communication	Pro 4-1; JS 4-1, 2, 4-10 thru 13; Ch 5, 18, 21
2. Identify types of non-verbal communication	Ch 4	2. Respond to nonverbal communication	JS 4-1; Ch 21	2. Demonstrate the principles of self-boundaries	Pro 4-1, 8; JS 4-10, 11
3. Recognize barriers to communication	Pro 4-2 thru 4-10; JS 4-6 thru 4-11	3. Use medical terminology correctly and pronounce accurately to communicate information to providers and patients	JS 1-1 and "Abbreviation and Spelling Review" in each chapter of WB; JS 9-1, 3, 4, 5, 6; JS 11-1 thru 11-10	3. Demonstrate respect for individual diversity including: (a) gender, (b) race, (c) religion, (d) age, (e) economic status, and (f) appearance	Ch 4; JS 4-3 thru 4-9, 11, 12, 13
4. Identify techniques for overcoming communication barriers	Pro 4-2 thru 4-10	4. Coach patients regarding: (a) office policies, (b) health maintenance, (c) disease prevention, and (d) treatment plan	Ch 1, 3, 5, 6; JS 2-2, 3; Pro 5-5	4. Explain to a patient the rationale for performance of a procedure	Ch 3
5. Recognize the elements of oral communication using a sender-receiver process	Pro 4-2 thru 4-11	5. Coach patients appropriately considering: (a) cultural diversity, (b) developmental life stage, and (c) communication barriers	Pro 4-2, 3 JS 4-3 thru 4-13		
6. Define coaching a patient as it relates to: (a) health maintenance, (b) disease prevention, (c) compliance with treatment plan, (d) community resources, and (e) adaptations relevant to individual patient needs	JS 2-2, 3; Ch 3; JS 5-2, 3	6. Demonstrate professional telephone techniques	Ch 3; Pro 6-1 thru 6-7; JS 6-1, 4		

(*continues*)

TABLE B-2 (*continued*)

CAAHEP Standards and Guidelines					
CONTENT AREA V: Concepts of Effective Communication					
COGNITIVE (KNOWLEDGE)		PSYCHOMOTOR (SKILLS)		AFFECTIVE (BEHAVIOR)	
V.C. Concepts of Effective Communication	Reference	V.P. Concepts of Effective Communication	Reference	V.A. Concepts of Effective Communication	Reference
7. Recognize elements of fundamental writing skills	JS 3-4; JS 7-6; Pro 11-1, 2, 3; JS 11-1 thru 11-10; JS 12-6, 7, 8	7. Document telephone messages accurately	JS 6-2		
8. Discuss applications of electronic technology in professional communication	Ch 1, 4, 6	8. Compose professional correspondence utilizing electronic technology	JS 1-6; JS 9-5; Pro 11-1, 2, 3; JS 11-2, 11-4 thru 11-10; JS 12-6, 7, 8; JS 21-2, 3, 4		
9. Identify medical terms labeling the word parts		9. Develop a current list of community resources related to patients' health care needs	Pro 5-4; JS 5-3		
10. Define medical terms and abbreviations related to all body systems	JS 1-1 and "Abbreviation and Spelling Review" in each chapter of WB; Online Ch 21	10. Facilitate referrals to community resources in the role of a patient navigator	Pro 5-4; JS 5-3		
11. Define the principles of self-boundaries	Ch 4	11. Report relevant information concisely and accurately	JS 1-6; Pro 6-1, 2; JS 6-2, 3; JS 9-1, 2, 3, 5, 6; JS 11-2 thru 11-10; JS 19-1, 2; JS 21-2, 3, 4		
12. Define patient navigator	Ch 1				
13. Describe the role of the medical assistant as a patient navigator	Ch 1, 3				
14. Relate the following behaviors to professional communication: (a) assertive, (b) aggressive, and (c) passive	Ch 1				
15. Differentiate between adaptive and nonadaptive coping mechanisms	Ch 1				
16. Differentiate between subjective and objective information	Ch 4				

(*continues*)

TABLE B-2 (*continued*)

CAAHEP Standards and Guidelines					
CONTENT AREA V: Concepts of Effective Communication					
COGNITIVE (KNOWLEDGE)		PSYCHOMOTOR (SKILLS)		AFFECTIVE (BEHAVIOR)	
V.C. Concepts of Effective Communication	Reference	V.P. Concepts of Effective Communication	Reference	V.A. Concepts of Effective Communication	Reference
17. Discuss the theories of: (a) Maslow, (b) Erikson, and (c) Kubler-Ross	Ch 1, 4				
18. Discuss examples of (a) cultural, (b) social, and (c) ethnic diversity	Ch 4				
CONTENT AREA VI: Administrative Functions					
VI.C. Administrative Functions	Reference	VI.P. Administrative Functions	Reference	VI.A. Administrative Functions	Reference
1. Identify different types of appointment scheduling methods	Ch 7	1. Manage appointment scheduling using established priorities	JS 7-1 thru 7-4	1. Display sensitivity when managing appointments	Pro 6-5, 6; JS 6-1 thru 6-4; Ch 7
2. Identify advantages and disadvantages of the following appointment systems: (a) manual and (b) electronic	Ch 7	2. Schedule a patient procedure	Pro 7-6, 7; JS 7-5, 7		
3. Identify critical information required for scheduling patient procedures	Ch 5, 6, 9; Pro 7-4; JS 7-5, 6, 9	3. Create a patient's medical record	JS 5-1; Pro 8-6; JS 8-4, 5; JS 9-1, 2, 5		
4. Define types of information contained in the patient's medical record	Ch 5, 6, 7, 8, 9	4. Organize a patient's medical record	Pro 8-6; Ch 9		
5. Identify methods of organizing the patient's medical record based on: (a) problem-oriented medical record (POMR), (b) source-oriented medical record (SOMR)	Ch 8, 9	5. File patient medical records	JS 8-1 thru 8-5		
6. Identify equipment and supplies needed for medical records in order to: (a) create, (b) maintain, and (c) store	Ch 8, 9	6. Utilize an EMR			
7. Describe filing indexing rules	Ch 8	7. Input patient data utilizing a practice management system	Ch 6, 7, 8, 9		
8. Differentiate between electronic medical records (EMR) and a practice management system	Ch 9	8. Perform routine maintenance of administrative or clinical equipment	JS 19-4		

(*continues*)

TABLE B-2 (*continued*)

CAAHEP Standards and Guidelines					
CONTENT AREA VI: Administrative Functions					
COGNITIVE (KNOWLEDGE)		**PSYCHOMOTOR (SKILLS)**		**AFFECTIVE (BEHAVIOR)**	
VI.C. Administrative Functions	**Reference**	**VI.P. Administrative Functions**	**Reference**	**VI.A. Administrative Functions**	**Reference**
9. Explain the purpose of routine maintenance of administrative and clinical equipment	JS 19-4	9. Perform an inventory with documentation	JS 19-4		
10. List steps involved in completing an inventory	JS 19-4				
11. Explain the importance of data back-up	Ch 8, 9				
12. Explain meaningful use as it applies to EMR	Ch 3, 8, 9, 10				
CONTENT AREA VII: Basic Practice Finances					
VII.C. Basic Practice Finances	**Reference**	**VII.P. Basic Practice Finances**	**Reference**	**VII.A. Basic Practice Finances**	**Reference**
1. Define the following bookkeeping terms: (a) charges, (b) payments, (c) accounts receivable, (d) accounts payable, and (e) adjustments	Ch 13, 15, 20	1. Perform accounts receivable procedures to patient accounts including posting: (a) charges, (b) payments, and (c) adjustments	JS 13-2, 5, 6; Pro 15-1; JS 15-1; JS 15-1, 3, 5, 8, 11; JS 18-2, 3, 4	1. Demonstrate professionalism when discussing patient's billing record	Pro 13-1, 3, 4; JS 13-4, 5, 6
2. Describe banking procedures as related to the ambulatory care setting	Ch 14, 20	2. Prepare a bank deposit	Pro 14-1; JS 14-1; JS 20-1 thru 4	2. Display sensitivity when requesting payment for services rendered	Ch 14
3. Identify precautions for accepting the following types of payments: (a) cash, (b) check, (c) credit card, and (d) debit card	Ch 13, 14, 15; Pro 13-3, 4, 5; JS 13-4, 6, 7	3. Obtain accurate patient billing information	Pro 5-2; JS 5-1; Pro 13-3, 4; JS 13-4		
4. Describe types of adjustments made to patient accounts including: (a) nonsufficient funds (NSF) check, (b) collection agency transaction, (c) credit balance, and (d) third party	Ch 13; JS 15-1, 3, 5, 8, 11	4. Inform a patient of financial obligations for services provided	Pro 13-3, 4; JS 13-4, 5		
5. Identify types of information contained in the patient's billing record	Pro 13-1; JS 15-2				
6. Explain patient financial obligations for services rendered	Pro 13-1; JS 13-4, 5, 6				

TABLE B-2 (*continued*)

CAAHEP Standards and Guidelines					
CONTENT AREA VIII: Third-Party Reimbursement					
COGNITIVE (KNOWLEDGE)		PSYCHOMOTOR (SKILLS)		AFFECTIVE (BEHAVIOR)	
VIII.C. Third-Party Reimbursement	Reference	VIII.P. Third-Party Reimbursement	Reference	VIII.A. Third-Party Reimbursement	Reference
1. Identify (a) types of third-party plans, (b) information to file a third-party claim, and (c) the steps for filing a third-party claim	Ch 2, 18, App A	1. Interpret information on an insurance card	Ch 18	1. Interact professionally with third-party representatives	Ch 18
2. Outline managed care requirements for patient referral	Ch 2, 18	2. Verify eligibility for services including documentation	JS 18-1	2. Display tactful behavior when communicating with medical providers regarding third-party requirements	Ch 18
3. Describe processes for: (a) verification of eligibility for services, (b) precertification, and (c) preauthorization	Ch 2, 18	3. Obtain precertification or preauthorization including documentation	Ch 2; JS 18-1	3. Show sensitivity when communicating with patients regarding third-party requirements	Ch 13, 18
4. Define patient-centered medical home (PCMH)	Ch 2	4. Complete an insurance claim	JS 18-2, 3, 4		
5. Differentiate between fraud and abuse	Ch 18				
CONTENT AREA IX: Procedure and Diagnostic Coding					
IX.C. Procedural and Diagnostic Coding	Reference	IX.P. Procedural and Diagnostic Coding	Reference	IX.A. Procedural and Diagnostic Coding	Reference
1. Describe how to use the most current procedural coding system	Ch 16	1. Perform procedural coding	Pro 16-1, 2; JS 16-2 thru 16-6	1. Utilize tactful communication skills with medical providers to ensure accurate code selection	Ch 13, 16, 17
2. Describe how to use the most current diagnostic coding classification system	Ch 17	2. Perform diagnostic coding	Pro 17-1, 2; JS 17-1 thru 17-5		
3. Describe how to use the most current HCPCS level II coding system	Ch 16	3. Utilize medical necessity guidelines	Ch 9, 17		
4. Discuss the effects of: (a) upcoding and (b) downcoding	Ch 16, 17				
5. Define medical necessity as it applies to procedural and diagnostic coding	Ch 2, 17, 18				

TABLE B-2 (*continued*)

CAAHEP Standards and Guidelines					
CONTENT AREA X: Legal Implications					
COGNITIVE (KNOWLEDGE)		PSYCHOMOTOR (SKILLS)		AFFECTIVE (BEHAVIOR)	
X.C. Legal Implications	Reference	X.P. Legal Implications	Reference	X.A. Legal Implications	Reference
1. Differentiate between scope of practice and standards of care for medical assistants	Ch 3	1. Locate a state's legal scope of practice for medical assistants	JS 3-3	1. Demonstrate sensitivity to patient rights	JS 3-6, 7; JS 5-1
2. Compare and contrast provider and medical assistant roles in terms of standard of care	Ch 3	2. Apply HIPAA rules in regard to: (a) privacy and (b) release of information	JS 3-2; Ch 5	2. Protect the integrity of the medical record	JS 3-2; JS 5-1; Ch 10, 16, 17
3. Describe the components of the Health Information Portability & Accountability Act (HIPAA)	Ch 3, 5, 8, 9, 10, 17, 18	3. Document patient care accurately in the medical record	JS 9-1, 2, 3, 5, 6; JS 10-5, 6, 7, 8; Ch 16, 17		
4. Summarize the Patient Bill of Rights	JS 3-6	4. Apply the Patient's Bill of Rights as it relates to: (a) choice of treatment, (b) consent for treatment, and (c) refusal of treatment	JS 3-6		
5. Discuss licensure and certification as they apply to health care providers	Ch 1, 2, 3, 21	5. Perform compliance reporting based on public health statutes	Ch 16, 17, 18		
6. Compare civil and criminal law as they apply to the practicing medical assistant	Ch 3	6. Report an illegal activity in the health care setting following proper protocol	JS 3-5		
7. Define: (a) negligence, (b) malpractice, (c) statute of limitations, (d) Good Samaritan Act, (e) Uniform Anatomical Gift Act, (f) living will/advance directives, (g) medical durable power of attorney, (h) Patient Self-Determination Act (PSDA), and (i) risk management	Ch 1, 3, 5	7. Complete an incident report to an error in patient care	Pro 19-5		
8. Describe the following types of insurance: (a) liability, (b) professional (malpractice), and (c) personal injury	Ch 3				
9. List and discuss legal and illegal applicant interview questions	Ch 19, 21				

(*continues*)

TABLE B-2 (*continued*)

CAAHEP Standards and Guidelines					
CONTENT AREA X: Legal Implications					
COGNITIVE (KNOWLEDGE)		PSYCHOMOTOR (SKILLS)		AFFECTIVE (BEHAVIOR)	
X.C. Legal Implications	Reference	X.P. Legal Implications	Reference	X.A. Legal Implications	Reference
10. Identify: (a) Health Information Technology for Economic and Clinical Health (HITECH) Act, (b) Genetic Information Nondiscrimination Act of 2008 (GINA), and (c) Americans with Disabilities Act Amendments Act (ADAAA)	a) Ch 3, 19				
11. Describe the process in compliance reporting: (a) unsafe activities, (b) errors in patient care, (c) conflicts of interest, and (d) incident reports	Ch 3, 19				
12. Describe compliance with public health statutes: (a) communicable diseases, (b) abuse, neglect, and exploitation, and (c) wounds of violence	Ch 3				
13. Define the following medical legal terms: (a) informed consent, (b) implied consent, (c) expressed consent, (d) patient incompetence, (e) emancipated minor, (f) mature minor, (g) subpoena duces tecum, (h) respondeat superior, (i) res ipsa loquitur, (j) locum tenens, (k) defendant-plaintiff, (l) deposition, (m) arbitration-mediation, and (n) Good Samaritan laws	Ch 3				

(*continues*)

TABLE B-2 (*continued*)

CAAHEP Standards and Guidelines					
CONTENT AREA XI: Ethical Considerations					
COGNITIVE (KNOWLEDGE)		PSYCHOMOTOR (SKILLS)		AFFECTIVE (BEHAVIOR)	
XI.C. Ethical Considerations	Reference	XI.P. Ethical Considerations	Reference	XI.A. Ethical Considerations	Reference
1. Define (a) ethics and (b) morals	Ch 3	1. Develop a plan for separation of personal and professional ethics	JS 3-1	1. Recognize the impact personal ethics and morals have on the delivery of health care	JS 3-1
2. Differentiate between personal and professional ethics	JS 3-1	2. Demonstrate appropriate responses to ethical issues	Ch 3		
3. Identify the effect of personal morals on professional performance	Ch 3				
CONTENT AREA XII: Protective Practices					
XII.C. Protective Practices	Reference	XII.P. Protective Practices	Reference	XII.A. Protective Practices	Reference
1. Identify: (a) safety signs, (b) symbols, and (c) labels	Ch 5	1. Comply with: (a) safety signs, (b) symbols, and (c) labels	Ch 5; Fig 5-17; Table 5-1	1. Recognize the physical and emotional effects on persons involved in an emergency situation	JS 5-9; Pro 6-6; JS 6-4; Ch 7
2. Identify safety techniques that can be used in responding to accidental exposure to: (a) blood, (b) other body fluids, (c) needle sticks, and (d) chemicals	Ch 5	2. Demonstrate proper use of: (a) eyewash equipment, (b) fire extinguishers, and (c) sharps disposal containers	Pro 5-7, 8; JS 5-7 Ch 5	2. Demonstrate self-awareness in responding to an emergency situation	JS 5-9
3. Discuss fire safety issues in an ambulatory health care environment	Ch 5	3. Use proper body mechanics	JS 5-4		
4. Describe fundamental principles for evacuation of a health care setting	Pro 5-9	4. Participate in a mock exposure event with documentation of specific steps	Pro 5-9; JS 5-8, 9		
5. Describe the purpose of Safety Data Sheets (SDS) in a health care setting	Ch 5	5. Evaluate the work environment to identify unsafe working conditions	JS 5-5		
6. Discuss protocols for disposal of biological chemical materials	Ch 5, 10				
7. Identify principles of: (a) body mechanics, and (b) ergonomics	Fig 5-13, 14, 15, 16; Pro 5-6; JS 5-4				
8. Identify critical elements of an emergency plan for response to a natural disaster or other emergency	Pro 5-9; JS 5-9				

ABHES CURRICULUM COMPETENCIES*

The Accrediting Bureau of Health Education Schools (ABHES) is a nationally recognized, independent, non-profit accrediting agency of institutions and educational programs that predominantly provide allied health education. Policies, procedures, and standards have been developed for the accreditation of medical assisting programs and the 2017 entry-level competencies required for successful completion are outlined as follows.* Chapters, procedures, and job skills are cross-referenced to each competency to help locate them in the *Administrative Medical Assisting* textbook and *Workbook*.

TABLE B-3 Accrediting Bureau of Health Education Schools (ABHES) Competencies for Medical Assisting Programs, 2017

ACCREDITING BUREAU OF HEALTH EDUCATION SCHOOLS (ABHES) Programmatic Evaluation Standards for Medical Assisting (Chapter VII, Section A) 2017	
1. GENERAL ORIENTATION: Graduates will be able to:	**Reference**
a. Describe the current employment outlook for the medical assistant	Ch 1, 2, 21
b. Compare and contrast the allied health professions and understand their relation to medical assisting	Table 1-2
c. Describe medical assistant credentialing requirements and the process to obtain the credential and comprehend the importance of credentialing	JS 1-4
d. List the general responsibilities and skills of the medical assistant	Ch 1, 21; JS 1-3: JS 2-5
2. ANATOMY AND PHYSIOLOGY: Graduates will be able to:	**Reference**
a. List all body systems, their structure and functions	JS 1-5; Ch 11
d. Apply a system of diet and nutrition: 1. Explain the importance of diet and nutrition 2. Educate patients regarding proper diet and nutrition guidelines 3. Identify categories of patients that require special diets or diet modifications	Ch 5
3. MEDICAL TERMINOLOGY: Graduates will be able to:	**Reference**
a. Define and use entire basic structure of medical words and be able to accurately identify in the correct context, that is, root, prefix, suffix, combinations, spelling, and definitions	WB: Ch 1-21; JS 1-1, 5
b. Build and dissect medical terms from roots/suffixes to understand the word element combinations that create medical terminology	WB: Ch 1-21; JS 1-1, 5
c. Apply various medical terms for each specialty	Tables: 2-3, 4; JS 1-5; 2-3, 4
d. Define and use medical abbreviations when appropriate and acceptable	WB: Ch 1-21 JS 1-1; JS 2-4; JS 10-4 thru 10-8; Ch 11; JS 13-2; JS 15-2
4. MEDICAL LAW AND ETHICS: Graduates will be able to:	**Reference**
a. Follow documentation guidelines	Pro 9-2, 3; JS 9-1 thru 9-6; JS 10-5, 6, 8; Ch 11
b. Institute federal and state guidelines when: 1. Releasing medical records or information 2. Entering orders in and utilizing electronic health records	JS 3-2, 4; JS 10-4 thru 10-8 Table 9-1; Pro 7-4; Pro 9-1 thru 9-4; JS 9-1 thru 9-6; JS 11-4 thru 11-10

(continues)

---

* Only those clinical competencies that apply to this text are listed.

TABLE B-3 (*continued*)

ACCREDITING BUREAU OF HEALTH EDUCATION SCHOOLS (ABHES) Programmatic Evaluation Standards for Medical Assisting (Chapter VII, Section A) 2017	
4. MEDICAL LAW AND ETHICS: Graduates will be able to:	**Reference**
c. Follow established policies when initiating or terminating medical treatment	JS 3-4
d. Distinguish between employer and personal liability coverage	Ch 3
e. Perform risk management procedures	Ch 3
f. Comply with federal, state, and local health laws and regulations as they relate to health care settings:	JS 3-5; JS 9-3; Ch10; JS 13-4, 5, 6; Ch 16, 18, 19, 20, 21
1. Define scope of practice for the medical assistant within the state that the medical assistant is employed	JS 3-3
2. Describe what procedures can and cannot be delegated to the medical assistant and by whom within various employment settings	JS 3-3; Ch 10
3. Comply with meaningful use regulations	Ch 2, 3, 8, 9, 10, 11
g. Display compliance with Code of Ethics of the profession	Ch 1 thru 21; JS 3-1
h. Demonstrate compliance with HIPAA guidelines, the ADA Amendments Act, and the Health Information Technology for Economic and Clinical Health (HITECH) Act	Ch 3, 18, 19
5. HUMAN RELATIONS: Graduates will be able to:	**Reference**
a. Respond appropriately to patients with abnormal behavior patterns	Ch 4
b. Provide support for terminally ill patients:	Ch 1
1. Use empathy when communicating with terminally ill patients	Ch 1
2. Identify common stages that terminally ill patients experience	Ch 1
3. List organizations/support groups that can assist patients and family members of patients experiencing terminal illnesses	Ch 1
c. Intervene on behalf of the patient regarding issues/concerns that may arise, that is, insurance policy information, medical bills, physician/provider orders, etc.	Ch 1, 2, 4, 13
d. Discuss developmental stages of life	Ch 4
e. Analyze the effect of hereditary, cultural, and environmental influences on behavior	JS 4-5
f. Demonstrate an understanding of the core competencies for Interprofessional Collaborative Practice (i.e., values/ethics, roles/responsibilities, interprofessional communication, and teamwork)	Ch 1, 2, 3, 19; JS 4-1, 3, 4, and 4-6 thru 4-13
g. Partner with health care teams to attain optimal patient health outcomes	Ch 2; JS 3-6
h. Display effective interpersonal skills with patients and health care team members	Ch 2; Pro 4-11
i. Demonstrate cultural awareness	JS 4-5
6. PHARMACOLOGY: Graduates will be able to:	**Reference**
a. Identify drug classification, usual dose, side effects, and contraindications of the most commonly used medications	JS 10-3
c. Prescriptions:	JS 10-1 thru 10-8
1. Identify parts of prescriptions	JS 10-4 thru 10-6
2. Identify appropriate abbreviations that are accepted in prescription writing	JS 10-4 thru 10-8
3. Comply with legal aspects of creating prescriptions including federal and state laws	JS 10-4 thru 10-6

(*continues*)

TABLE B-3 (*continued*)

ACCREDITING BUREAU OF HEALTH EDUCATION SCHOOLS (ABHES)	
Programmatic Evaluation Standards for Medical Assisting (Chapter VII, Section A) 2017	
6. PHARMACOLOGY: Graduates will be able to:	**Reference**
d. Properly use *Physician's Desk Reference (PDR)*, drug handbook and other drug references to identify a drug's classification, usual dosage, usual side effects, and contraindications	JS 10-1, 2, 3
7. ADMINISTRATIVE PROCEDURES: Graduates will be able to:	**Reference**
a. Gather and process documents	JS 6-2, 3; Pro 8-2, 3, 6; JS 8-1 thru 8-5; JS 9-1, 2, 5, 6; JS 12-1, 2, 4, and 6 thru 9; JS 13-2; JS 14-2, 3, 4; Ch 15; JS 18-1; JS 19-1, 3, 9; JS 20-10
b. Navigate electronic health records systems and practice management software	WB: Ch 5, 8, 9, 11; JS 11-2 thru 11-10; Ch 15, 19
c. Perform billing and collection procedures	Pro 13-1 thru 13-8; JS 13-1, 2, 5; JS 14-2, 3, 4; Pro 15-1; JS 15-1 thru 15-13; Ch 16, 17; JS 18-1
d. Process insurance claims	JS 16-1 thru 16-6; JS 17-1 thru 17-6; JS 18-2 thru 18-4
e. Apply scheduling principles	Pro 7-1 thru 7-7; JS 7-1 thru 7-7
f. Maintain inventory of equipment and supplies	JS 19-4, 5, 6, 8
g. Display professionalism through written and verbal communication	JS 2-1; Pro 4-1 thru 4-11; JS 4-1 thru 4:13; Pro 6-1 thru 6-7; JS 6-2 thru 6-4; JS 7-6; JS 9-4, 5; Pro 11-1; JS 11-2 thru 11-10; JS 12-1, 2, 4, 6 thru 9; JS 13-5; JS 19-2: 21-1 thru 21-4
h. Perform basic computer skills	JS 2-1; JS 11-2 thru 11-10; Ch 15, 16, 19
8. CLINICAL PROCEDURES: Graduates will be able to:	**Reference**
b. Obtain vital signs, patient history, and formulate chief complaint	JS 6-1, 4
g. Recognize and respond to medical office emergencies	JS 5-5 thru 5-9; JS 6-4
h. Teach self-examination disease management and health promotion	Pro 5-5
i. Identify community resources and Complementary and Alternative Medicine (CAM) practices	Ch 1; Pro 5-4; JS 5-3; Ch 16
j. Make adaptations with patients with special needs	JS 4-6 thru 4-11, Ch 7
k. Make adaptations to care for patients across their lifespan	Ch 1
9. MEDICAL LABORATORY PROCEDURES: Graduates will be able to:	**Reference**
c. Dispose of biohazardous materials	Ch 10
10. CAREER DEVELOPMENT: Graduates will be able to:	**Reference**
a. Perform the essential requirements of employment such as resume writing, effective interviewing, dressing professionally, time management, and following up appropriately	Pro 21-1 thru 21-6; JS 21-1 thru 21-4
b. Demonstrate professional behavior	Ch 1 thru 21
c. Explain what continuing education is and how it is acquired	Ch 1

CMA (AAMA) CERTIFICATION EXAMINATION* CONTENT

The American Association of Medical Assistants (AAMA) has developed a content outline for the Certified Medical Assistant (CMA [AAMA]) certification examination

as follows.** Chapters are cross-referenced to each competency to help locate them in the *Administrative Medical Assisting* textbook and *Workbook*.

TABLE B-4 American Association of Medical Assistants (AAMA) Certified Medical Assistant (CMA [AAMA]) Examination Content Outline (09/2014)

CMA (AAMA) Competencies	Textbook and Workbook References
I. A-G GENERAL	
A. Psychology	**Reference**
1. Understanding Human Behavior	**Ch 4**
a. Behavioral theories	Ch 4
(1) Maslow	Ch 4
(2) Erikson	Ch 4
b. Defense mechanisms	Ch 1
(1) Common types	Ch 1
(2) Recognition and management	Ch 1
2. Human Growth and Development	**Ch 4**
a. Normal developmental patterns/milestones	Ch 4
3. Death and Dying	**Ch 1**
B. Communication	**Reference**
1. Therapeutic/Adaptive Responses to Diverse Populations	**Ch 4**
a. Visually impaired	Ch 4
b. Hearing impaired	Ch 4
c. Age specific	Ch 4
(1) Geriatric	Ch 4
(2) Pediatric/adolescent	Ch 4
d. Seriously/terminally ill	Ch 1
e. Intellectual disability	Ch 4
f. Illiterate	Ch 4
g. Non-English speaking	Ch 4
h. Anxious/angry/distraught	Ch 4
i. Socially/culturally/ethnically diverse	Ch 4

(continues)

* Printed with permission by the American Association of Medical Assistants.
** Only those competencies that apply to administrative skills are listed.

TABLE B-4 (*continued*)

CMA (AAMA) Competencies	Textbook and Workbook References
2. Nonverbal Communication	**Ch 4**
a. Body language	Ch 4
(1) Posture	Ch 4
(2) Position	Ch 4
(3) Facial expression	Ch 4
(4) Territoriality/physical boundaries	Ch 4
(5) Gestures	Ch 4
(6) Touch	Ch 4
(7) Mannerisms	Ch 4
(8) Eye contact	Ch 4
3. Communication Cycle	**Ch 4**
a. Sender-message-receiver-feedback	Ch 4
b. Listening skills	Ch 4
(1) Active/therapeutic	Ch 4
c. Assess patient level of understanding	Ch 2
(1) Reflection	Ch 4
(2) Restatement	Ch 4
(3) Clarification	Ch 4
(4) Feedback	Ch 4
d. Barriers to communication	Ch 4
(1) Internal distractions	Ch 4
(a) Pain	Ch 4
(b) Hunger	Ch 4
(c) Anger	Ch 4
(2) External/environmental distractions	Ch 4
(a) Temperature	Ch 4
(b) Noise	Ch 4
4. Collection of Data	**Ch 4**
a. Types of questions	Ch 4
(1) Exploratory	Ch 4
(2) Open-ended	Ch 4
(3) Closed/Direct	Ch 4

TABLE B-4 (*continued*)

CMA (AAMA) Competencies	Textbook and Workbook References
5. Telephone Techniques	**Ch 6**
a. Call management	Ch 6
(1) Screening/gathering data	Ch 6
(2) Emergency/urgent situations	Ch 6
b. Messages	Ch 6
(1) Taking messages	Ch 6
(2) Leaving messages	Ch 6
6. Interpersonal Skills	**Ch 1, 4**
a. Displaying impartial conduct without regard to race, religion, age, gender, sexual orientation, socioeconomic status, physical challenges, special needs, lifestyle choices	Ch 4
b. Recognizing stereotypes and biases	Ch 4
c. Demonstrating empathy/sympathy/compassion	Ch 1, 4
C. Professionalism	**Reference**
1. Professional Behavior	**Ch 1, 19, 21**
a. Professional situations	Ch 1, 19, 21
(1) Displaying tact, diplomacy, courtesy, respect, dignity	Ch 1, 19, 21
(2) Demonstrating responsibility, integrity/honesty	Ch 1, 19, 21
(3) Responding to criticism	Ch 1, 19, 21
b. Professional image	Ch 1, 19, 21
2. Performing as a Team Member	**Ch 1, 19, 21**
a. Principles of health care team dynamics	Ch 1, 19, 21
(1) Cooperation for optimal outcomes	Ch 1, 19, 21
(2) Identification of the roles and credentials of health care team members	Ch 1, 19, 21
b. Time management principles	Ch 1, 19
(1) Prioritizing responsibilities	1, 19
D. Medical Law/Regulatory Guidelines	**Reference**
1. Advance Directives	**Ch 3**
a. Living will	Ch 3
b. Medical durable power of attorney	Ch 3
c. Patient Self-Determination Act (PSDA)	Ch 3
2. Uniform Anatomical Gift Act	**Ch 3**
3. Occupational Safety and Health (OSH) Act	**Ch 5**
4. Food and Drug Administration (FDA)	**Ch 10**
5. Clinical Laboratory Improvement Act (CLIA '88)	**N/A**
6. Americans with Disabilities Act Amendments Act (ADAAA)	**Ch 19**

(continues)

TABLE B-4 (*continued*)

CMA (AAMA) Competencies	Textbook and Workbook References
7. Health Insurance Portability and Accountability Act (HIPAA)	**Ch 3, 5, 8, 9, 17, 18**
a. Health insurance portability access and renewal without preexisting conditions	Ch 18
b. Coordination of care to prevent duplication of services	Ch 18
8. Health Information Technology for Economic and Clinical Health (HITECH) Act	**Ch 3**
a. Patient's right to inspect, amend, and restrict access to his/her medical record	Ch 5, 9
9. Drug Enforcement Agency (DEA)	**Ch 10**
a. Controlled Substances Act of 1970	Ch 10
10. Medical Assistant Scope of Practice	**Ch 3, 10**
a. Consequences of failing to operate within scope	Ch 3
11. Genetic Information Nondiscrimination Act of 2008	**Ch 18, 19**
12. Centers for Disease Control and Prevention (CDC)	**Ch 5, 10**
13. Consumer Protection Acts	**Ch 13**
a. Fair Debt Collection Practices Act	Ch 13
b. Truth in Lending Act of 1968 (Regulation Z)	Ch 13
14. Public Health and Welfare Disclosure	**Ch 3, 9**
a. Public health statutes	Ch 3, 9
(1) Communicable diseases	Ch 3, 9
(2) Vital statistics	Ch 3, 9
(3) Abuse/neglect/exploitation against child/elder	Ch 3, 9
(a) Domestic abuse	Ch 3, 9
(4) Wounds of violence	Ch 3, 9
15. Confidentiality	**Ch 3, 5, 6, 7, 9, 10**
a. Electronic access audit/activity log	Ch 9
b. Use and disclosure of protected health information (PHI)	Ch 5, 6, 7, 9
(1) Consent/authorization to release	Ch 3
(2) Drug and alcohol treatment records	Ch 9, 10
(3) HIV-related information	Ch 3, 9
(4) Mental health	Ch 3, 9
16. Health Care Rights and Responsibilities	**Ch 3**
a. Patients' Bill of Rights/Patient Care Partnership	Ch 3
b. Professional liability	Ch 3
(1) Current standard of care	Ch 3
(2) Standards of conduct	Ch 3
(3) Malpractice coverage	Ch 3

TABLE B-4 (*continued*)

CMA (AAMA) Competencies	Textbook and Workbook References
c. Consent to treat	Ch 3
(1) Informed consent	Ch 3
(2) Implied consent	Ch 3
(3) Expressed consent	Ch 3
(4) Patient incompetence	Ch 3
(5) Emancipated minor	Ch 3
(6) Mature minor	Ch 3
17. Medicolegal Terms and Doctrines	**Ch 3**
a. Subpoena duces tecum	Ch 3
b. Subpoena	Ch 3
c. Respondeat superior	Ch 3
d. Res ipsa loquitor	Ch 3
e. Locum tenens	Ch 3
f. Defendant-plaintiff	Ch 3
g. Deposition	Ch 3
h. Arbitration-mediation	Ch 3
i. Good Samaritan laws	Ch 3
18. Categories of Law	**Ch 3**
a. Criminal law	Ch 3
(1) Felony/misdemeanor	Ch 3
b. Civil law	Ch 3
(1) Contracts (physician–patient relationships)	Ch 3
(a) Legal obligations to the patient	Ch 3
(b) Consequences for patient noncompliance	Ch 3
(c) Termination of medical care	Ch 3
(i) Elements/behaviors for withdrawal of care	Ch 3
(ii) Patient notification and documentation	Ch 3
(d) Ownership of medical records	Ch 3, 9
(2) Torts	Ch 3
(a) Invasion of privacy	Ch 3
(b) Negligence	Ch 3
(c) Intentional torts	Ch 3
(i) Battery	Ch 3
(ii) Assault	Ch 3

(*continues*)

TABLE B-4 (*continued*)

CMA (AAMA) Competencies	Textbook and Workbook References
(iii) Slander	Ch 3
(iv) Libel	Ch 3
c. Statutory law	Ch 3
(1) Medical practice acts	Ch 3
d. Common law (legal precedents)	Ch 3
E. Medical Ethics	**Reference**
1. Ethical Standards	**Ch 1, 3**
2. Factors Affecting Ethical Decisions	**Ch 3**
a. Legal	Ch 3
b. Moral	Ch 3
F. Risk Management, Quality Assurance, and Safety	**Reference**
1. Workplace Accident Prevention	**Ch 5**
a. Slips/trips/falls	Ch 5
2. Safety Signs, Symbols, Labels	**Ch 5**
3. Environmental Safety	**Ch 5**
a. Ergonomics	Ch 5
b. Electrical safety	Ch 5
c. Fire prevention/extinguisher use/regulations	Ch 5
4. Compliance Reporting	**Ch 5**
a. Reporting unsafe activities and behaviors	Ch 5, 19
b. Disclosing errors in patient care	Ch 5, 19
c. Insurance fraud, waste, and abuse	Ch 18
d. Conflicts of interest	Ch 1
e. Incident reports	Ch 5, 19
G. Medical Terminology	**Reference**
1. Word Parts	**WB Ch 1-21**
2. Definitions/Medical Terminology	**WB Ch 1-21**
a. Medical specialties	Table 2-4, 2-5
II. H-M ADMINISTRATIVE	
H. Medical Reception	**Reference**
1. Medical Record Preparation	**Ch 5, 9**
2. Demographic Data Review	**Ch 5, 18**
a. Identity theft prevention	Ch 5
b. Insurance eligibility verification	Ch 18

TABLE B-4 (*continued*)

CMA (AAMA) Competencies	Textbook and Workbook References
3. Handling Vendors/Business Associates	**Ch 5**
4. Reception Room Environment	**Ch 5**
a. Comfort	Ch 5
b. Safety	Ch 5
c. Sanitation	Ch 5
5. Practice Information Packet	**Ch 5**
a. Office policies	Ch 5, 19
b. Patient financial responsibilities	Ch 5, 13
I. Patient Navigator Advocate	**Reference**
1. Resource Information	**Ch 2, 5**
a. Provide information about community resources	Ch 5
b. Facilitate referrals to community resources	Ch 5
c. Referral follow-up	Ch 2, 5
J. Medical Business Practices	**Reference**
1. Written Communication	**Ch 9, 11**
a. Letters	Ch 9, 11
b. Memos/interoffice communications	Ch 11
c. Reports	Ch 9, 11
2. Business Equipment	**Ch 19**
a. Routine maintenance	Ch 19
b. Safety precautions	Ch 5
3. Office Supply Inventory	**Ch 19**
a. Inventory control/recordkeeping	Ch 19
4. Electronic Applications	**Ch 1, 3, 8, 9, 10, 11, 12, 18, 19, 21**
a. Medical management systems	Ch 9, 11
(1) Database reports	Ch 9
(2) Meaningful use regulations	Ch 3, 8, 9, 10
b. Spreadsheets, graphs	Ch 9
c. Electronic mail	Ch 12
d. Security	Ch 5
(1) Password/screen saver	Ch 8, 9
(2) Encryption	Ch 8
(3) Firewall	Ch 8

(*continues*)

TABLE B-4 (*continued*)

CMA (AAMA) Competencies	Textbook and Workbook References
e. Transmission of information	Ch 8, 9, 21
(1) Facsimile/scanner	Ch 5, 9, 12
(2) Patient portal to health data	Ch 3, 5, 7
f. Social media	Ch 4
K. Establish Patient Medical Record	**Reference**
1. Recognize and Interpret Data	**Ch 9, 11**
a. History and physical	Ch 9
b. Discharge summary	Ch 9
c. Operative note	Ch 9
d. Diagnostic test/lab report	Ch 9
e. Clinic progress note	Ch 9, 11
f. Consultation report	Ch 9, 11
g. Correspondence	Ch 9, 11
h. Charts, graphs, tables	Ch 9
i. Flow sheet	Ch 9
2. Charting Systems	**Ch 9**
a. Problem-oriented medical record (POMR)	Ch 9
b. Source-oriented medical record (SOMR)	Ch 9
L. Scheduling Appointments	**Reference**
1. Scheduling Guidelines	Ch 7
a. Appointment matrix	Ch 7
b. New patient appointments	Ch 7
(1) Identify required information	Ch 7
c. Established patient appointments	Ch 7
(1) Routine	Ch 7
(2) Urgent/emergency	Ch 7
d. Patient flow	Ch 7
(1) Patient needs/preference	Ch 7
(2) Physician preference	Ch 7
(3) Facility/equipment requirements	Ch 7
e. Outside services (e.g., lab, x-ray, surgery, outpatient procedures, hospital admissions)	Ch 7
2. Appointment Protocols	**Ch 7**
a. Legal aspects	Ch 7
b. Physician referrals	Ch 7
c. Cancellations/no-shows	Ch 7
d. Physician delay/unavailability	Ch 7

TABLE B-4 (*continued*)

CMA (AAMA) Competencies	Textbook and Workbook References
e. Reminders/recall systems	Ch 7
(1) Appointment cards	Ch 7
(2) Phone calls/text messages/email notifications	Ch 7
(3) Tickler file	Ch 7
M. Practice Finances	**Reference**
1. Financial Terminology	**Ch 13, 15, 20**
a. Accounts receivable	Ch 13, 15, 20
b. Accounts payable	Ch 13, 15, 20
c. Assets	Ch 15, 20
d. Liabilities	Ch 15, 20
e. Aging of accounts	Ch 15, 20
f. Debits	Ch 15
g. Credits	Ch 15
h. Diagnosis-Related Groups (DRGs)	Ch 13
i. Relative Value Studies (RVSs)	Ch 13
2. Financial Procedures	**Ch 13, 15, 18, 20**
a. Payment receipts	Ch 13, 20
(1) Copays	Ch 13, 15
b. Data entry	Ch 15
(1) Post charges	Ch 15, 18
(2) Post payments	Ch 15
(3) Post adjustments	Ch 15
c. Manage petty cash accounts	Ch 15
d. Financial calculations	Ch 15, 18
e. Billing procedures	Ch 13
(1) Itemized statements	Ch 13
(2) Billing cycles	Ch 13
f. Collection procedures	Ch 13
(1) Aging of accounts	Ch 13, 15, 20
(2) Preplanned payment options	Ch 13
(3) Credit arrangements	Ch 13
(4) Use of collection agencies	Ch 13
3. Diagnostic and Procedural Coding Applications	**Ch 16, 17, 18**
a. *Current Procedural Terminology (CPT)*	Ch 16
(1) Modifiers	Ch 16

(*continues*)

TABLE B-4 (*continued*)

CMA (AAMA) Competencies	Textbook and Workbook References
(2) Upcoding	Ch 16
(3) Bundling of charges	Ch 16
b. *International Classification of Diseases, Clinical Modification (ICD-CM)* (Current schedule)	Ch 17
c. Linking procedure and diagnosis codes	Ch 17, 18
d. *Healthcare Common Procedure Coding System (HCPCS Level II)*	Ch 16
4. Third-Party Payers/Insurance	**Ch 2, 13, 16, 18**
a. Types of plans	Ch 2, 18
(1) Commercial	Ch 2, 18
(2) Government	Ch 2, 18
(a) Medicare	Ch 2, 19
(i) Advanced Beneficiary Notice (ABN)	Ch 18
(b) Medicaid	Ch 18
(c) TRICARE/CHAMPVA	Ch 18
(3) Managed care organizations (MCOs)	Ch 2, 18
(a) Managed care requirements	Ch 2, 18
(i) Care referrals	Ch 2, 18
(ii) Precertification	Ch 2
[a] Diagnostic and surgical procedures	Ch 16
(iii) Prior authorization	Ch 2
[a] Medications	Ch 10
(4) Workers' compensation	Ch 18
b. Insurance claims	Ch 18
(1) Submission	Ch 18
(2) Appeals/denials	Ch 18
(3) Explanation of benefits (EOB)	Ch 13
III. N-V CLINICAL	
N. Anatomy and Physiology	**Reference**
1. Body as a Whole	**WB Ch 1-21**
a. Structural units	WB Ch 1-21
O. Infection Control	**Reference**
7. Standard Precautions/Blood-Borne Pathogen Standards	**Ch 5**
d. Blood	Ch 5
(1) HIV-HBV-HCV	Ch 5

TABLE B-4 (*continued*)

CMA (AAMA) Competencies	Textbook and Workbook References
f. Personal protective equipment (PPE)	Ch 5
(1) Gowns	Ch 5
(2) Gloves	Ch 5
(3) Masks	Ch 5
(4) Caps	Ch 5
(5) Eye protection	Ch 5
g. Post-exposure plan	Ch 5
8. Biohazard Disposal/Regulated Waste	**Ch 5**
a. Sharps	Ch 5
b. Blood and body fluids	Ch 5
c. Safety data sheets (SDS)	Ch 5
d. Spill kit	Ch 5
P. Patient Intake and Documentation of Care	**Reference**
1. Medical Record Documentation	**Ch 9**
a. Subjective data	Ch 9
(1) Chief complaint	Ch 9
(2) Present illness	Ch 9
(3) Past medical history	Ch 9
(4) Family history	Ch 9
(5) Social and occupational history	Ch 9
(6) Review of systems	Ch 9
b. Objective data	Ch 9
c. Making corrections	Ch 9
d. Treatment/compliance	Ch 9
Q. Patient Preparation and Assisting the Provider	**Reference**
3. Examinations	**Ch 9**
a. Methods	Ch 9
(1) Auscultation	Ch 9
(2) Palpation	Ch 9
(3) Percussion	Ch 9
(4) Mensuration	Ch 9
(5) Manipulation	Ch 9
(6) Inspection	Ch 9
4. Procedures	**Ch 5**
a. Procedure explanation and patient instructions	Ch 5

(*continues*)

TABLE B-4 (*continued*)

CMA (AAMA) Competencies	Textbook and Workbook References
5. Patient Education/Health Coach	Ch 1-7, 9, 10, 12, 13, 14, 16, 18, 19, 20
a. Health maintenance and disease prevention	Ch 5
b. Alternative medicine	Ch 1, 16
6. Wellness/Prevention Care	**Ch 5**
a. Cancer screening	Ch 5
b. Sexually transmitted disease prevention	Ch 5
g. Domestic violence screening and detection	Ch 5
R. Nutrition	**Reference**
1. Basic Principles	**Ch 5**
2. Special Dietary Needs	**Ch 5**
U. Pharmacology	**Reference**
For the 50 most commonly used medications, see the "Top 200 Drugs" at http://www.rxlist.com	Ch 10
1. Medications	**Ch 10**
a. Classes of drugs	Ch 10
b. Drug actions/desired effects	Ch 10
c. Adverse reactions	Ch 10
d. Physician's Desk Reference (PDR)	Ch 10
e. Storage of drugs	Ch 10
2. Preparing and Administering Oral and Parenteral Medications	**Ch 10**
d. Routes of administration	Ch 10
3. Prescriptions	**Ch 10**
a. E-prescribing	Ch 10
b. Controlled substances	Ch 10
4. Medication Recordkeeping	**Ch 10**
a. Reporting/documenting errors	Ch 10
5. Immunizations	**Ch 10**
a. Recordkeeping	Ch 10
(1) Vaccine information statement (VIS)	Ch 10
V. Emergency Management/Basic First Aid	**Reference**
1. Assessment and Screening	**Ch 5**
2. Identification and Response to Emergencies	**Ch 5**
3. Office Emergency Readiness	**Ch 5**
b. Emergency response plan	Ch 5
(1) Evacuation plan	Ch 5

RMA CERTIFICATION EXAMINATION* COMPETENCIES

The American Medical Technologists (AMT) has established (2009) competencies and construction parameters for the Registered Medical Assistant (RMA)

certification examination as follows.** Chapters are cross-referenced to each competency to help locate them in the *Administrative Medical Assisting* textbook and *Workbook*.

TABLE B-5 American Medical Technologists (AMT) Competencies and Construction Parameters for the Registered Medical Assistant (RMA) Certification Examination 2009

RMA (AMT) Competencies	Textbook and Workbook References
I. GENERAL MEDICAL ASSISTING KNOWLEDGE	
A. Anatomy and Physiology	**Reference**
1. Body systems—Identify the structure and function of the following systems:	**JS 1-5; Ch 9**
a. Skeletal	Ch 9
b. Muscular	Ch 9
c. Endocrine	Ch 9
d. Urinary	Ch 9
e. Reproductive	Ch 9
f. Gastrointestinal	Ch 9
g. Nervous	Ch 9
h. Respiratory	Ch 9
i. Cardiovascular/Circulatory	Ch 9
j. Integumentary	Ch 9
k. Special senses	Ch 9
3. Wellness	**Ch 1, 4**
a. Identify nutritional factors that are required for, or influence wellness	Ch 1
b. Identify factors associated with exercise that are required for, or influence, wellness	Ch 1
c. Identify factors associated with lifestyle choices that are required for, or influence, wellness	Ch 1, 4
B. Medical Terminology	**Reference**
1. Word parts	**WB Ch 1-21**
2. Definitions	**WB Ch 1-21**
3. Common abbreviations and symbols	**WB Ch 1-21; Table 2-4; Table 7-1; Ch 9; Table 10-3, 4; Table 12-3, 4; Table 13-2; Table 15-2**
a. Identify and understand utilization of medical abbreviations and symbols	WB Ch 1-21

(*continues*)

* *RMA competencies are reprinted with permission from the American Medical Technologists.*
** *Only those clinical competencies that apply to administrative skills are listed.*

TABLE B-5 (*continued*)

RMA (AMT) Competencies	Textbook and Workbook References
4. Spelling	**WB Ch 1-21**
a. Spell medical terms accurately	WB Ch 1-21
C. Medical Law	**Reference**
1. Identify and understand the application of:	**Ch 3, 9, 16, 17, 18, 19, 21**
a. Types of consent used in medical practice	Ch 3
b. Disclosure laws and regulations (including HIPAA Security and Privacy Acts, state and federal laws)	Ch 3, 5, 8, 9, 10, 17, 18
c. Laws, regulations, and acts pertaining to the practice of medicine	Ch 3, 9, 16, 17, 18, 19, 21
d. Scope of practice acts regarding medical assisting	Ch 3
e. Patient Bill of Rights legislation	Ch 1, 3
2. Licensure, certification, and registration	**Ch 1**
a. Identify credentialing requirements of medical professionals	Ch 1
3. Terminology	**Ch 3**
a. Define terminology associated with medical law	Ch 3
D. Medical Ethics	**Reference**
1. Principles of medical ethics and ethical conduct	**Ch 1, 3**
a. Identify and employ proper ethics in practice as a medical assistant	Ch 3
b. Identify the principles of ethics established by the American Medical Association	Ch 3
c. Identify and understand the application of the AMA Patient Bill of Rights	Ch 3
d. Recognize unethical practices and identify the proper response	Ch 3
e. Recognize the importance of professional development through continuing education	Ch 1
E. Human Relations	**Reference**
1. Patient relations	**Ch 1, 4, 19**
a. Identify age-group specific responses and support	Ch 4
b. Identify and employ professional conduct in all aspects of patient care	Ch 1, 4
c. Understand and properly apply communication methods	Ch 4, 19
d. Identify and respect cultural and ethnic differences	Ch 4
e. Respect and care for patients without regard for age, gender, sexual orientation, or socioeconomic level	Ch 4
2. Interpersonal relations	**Ch 1, 4, 19, 21**
a. Employ appropriate interpersonal skills with:	
(1) employer/administration	Ch 1, 4, 19, 21
(2) coworkers	Ch 1, 4, 19, 21
(3) vendors	Ch 1, 4, 19, 21
(4) business associates	Ch 1, 4, 19, 21
b. Observe and respect cultural diversity in the workplace	Ch 4

TABLE B-5 (*continued*)

RMA (AMT) Competencies	Textbook and Workbook References
F. Patient Education	**Reference**
1. Patient instruction—Identify and apply proper written and verbal communication to instruct patients in:	**Ch 1-7, 5, 9, 10, 12, 13, 14, 18, 19, 20**
a. health and wellness	Ch 1
b. nutrition	Ch 1, 5
c. hygiene	Ch 1, 5
d. treatment and medications	Ch 5
e. pre- and postoperative care	Ch 5
f. body mechanics	Ch 5
g. personal and physical safety	Ch 5
2. Patient resource materials	**Ch 5**
a. Develop, assemble, and maintain appropriate patient brochures and informational materials	Ch 5
3. Documentation	**Ch 9, 16, 17, 18**
a. Understand and utilize proper documentation of patient encounters and instruction	Ch 9, 16, 17, 18
II. ADMINISTRATIVE MEDICAL ASSISTING	
A. Insurance	**Reference**
1. Terminology	**Ch 2, 18**
a. Identify and define terminology associated with various insurance types in the medical office	Ch 2, 18
2. Plans	**Ch 2, 18**
a. Identify and understand the application of government, medical, disability, and accident insurance plans	Ch 2, 18
b. Identify and appropriately apply plan policies and regulations for programs including:	
(1) HMO, PPO, EPO, indemnity, open, etc.	Ch 2, 18
(2) short-term and long-term disability	Ch 18
(3) Family Medical Leave Act (FMLA)	Ch 19
(4) workers' compensation	Ch 18
(a) complete first reports	Ch 18
(b) complete follow-up reports	Ch 18
(5) Medicare (including Advance Beneficiary Notice [ABN])	Ch 18
(6) Medicaid	Ch 18
(7) CHAMPUS/TRICARE and CHAMPVA	Ch 18
3. Claims	**Ch 3, 13, 18**
a. Complete and file insurance claims	Ch 18
(1) File claims for paper and Electronic Data Interchange	Ch 18
(2) Understand and adhere to HIPAA Security and Uniformity Regulations	Ch 3, 18

(continues)

TABLE B-5 (*continued*)

RMA (AMT) Competencies	Textbook and Workbook References
b. Evaluate claims response	Ch 18
(1) Understand and evaluate explanation of benefits	Ch 13
(2) Evaluate claims rejection and utilize proper follow-up procedures	Ch 18
4. Coding	**Ch 16, 17, 18**
a. Identify HIPAA-mandated coding systems and references	Ch 16, 17
(1) *ICD-10-CM*	Ch 17
(2) *CPT*	Ch 16
(3) *HCPCS*	Ch 16
b. Properly apply diagnosis and procedure codes to insurance claims	Ch 18
5. Insurance finance applications	**Ch 13, 15, 18, 19, 20**
a. Identify and comply with contractual requirements of insurance plans	Ch 13, 15, 18, 20
b. Process insurance payments and contractual write-off amounts	Ch 13, 15, 18
c. Track unpaid claims	Ch 18
d. Generate aging reports	Ch 15, 19
B. Financial Bookkeeping	**Reference**
1. Terminology	**Ch 15, 20**
a. Understand terminology associated with medical financial bookkeeping	Ch 15, 20
2. Patient billing	**Ch 13, 15, 18**
a. Maintain and explain physician's fee schedules	Ch 13, 15, 18
b. Collect and post payments	Ch 13, 15, 18
c. Manage patient ledgers and accounts	Ch 13, 15, 18
d. Understand and prepare Truth in Lending Statements	Ch 13
e. Prepare and mail itemized statements	Ch 13, 15
f. Understand and employ available billing methods	Ch 13, 15
g. Understand and employ billing cycles	Ch 13
3. Collections	**Ch 13, 18, 20**
a. Prepare aging reports and identify delinquent accounts	Ch 13, 18, 20
b. Perform skip tracing	Ch 13, 18
c. Understand application of the Fair Debt Collection Practices Act	Ch 13, 18
d. Identify and understand bankruptcy and small claims procedures	Ch 13
e. Understand and perform appropriate collection procedures	Ch 13
4. Fundamental medical office accounting procedures	**Ch 15, 20**
a. Employ appropriate accounting procedures	Ch 15, 20
(1) pegboard/double entry	Ch 15
(2) computerized	Ch 15

TABLE B-5 (*continued*)

RMA (AMT) Competencies	Textbook and Workbook References
b. Perform daily balancing procedures	Ch 15, 20
c. Prepare monthly trial balance	Ch 15, 20
d. Apply accounts receivable and payable principles	Ch 15, 20
5. Banking procedures	**Ch 14, 15, 20**
a. Understand and manage petty cash account	Ch 15, 20
b. Prepare and make bank deposits	Ch 14, 15, 20
c. Maintain checking accounts	Ch 20
d. Reconcile bank statements	Ch 14, 20
e. Understand check-processing procedures and requirements	Ch 14
(1) nonsufficient funds (NSF)	Ch 14, 15
(2) endorsements	Ch 14
f. Process payables and practice obligations	Ch 20
g. Understand and maintain disbursement accounts	Ch 20
6. Employee payroll	**Ch 20**
a. Prepare employee payroll	Ch 20
(1) understand hourly and salary payroll procedures	Ch 20
(2) understand and apply payroll withholding and deductions	Ch 20
b. Understand and maintain payroll records	Ch 20
(1) prepare and maintain payroll tax deduction/withholding records	Ch 20
(2) prepare employee tax forms	Ch 20
(3) prepare quarterly tax forms and deposits	Ch 20
c. Understand terminology pertaining to payroll and payroll tax	Ch 20
7. Financial mathematics	**Ch 13, 15, 19, 20**
a. Understand and perform appropriate calculations related to patient and practice accounts	Ch 13, 15, 20
C. Medical Receptionist/Secretarial/Clerical	**Reference**
1. Terminology	**Ch 5, 11**
a. Understand and correctly apply terminology associated with medical receptionist and secretarial duties	Ch 5, 11
2. Reception	**Ch 4, 5, 9**
a. Employ appropriate communication skills when receiving and greeting patients	Ch 4, 5
b. Understand basic emergency triage in coordinating patient arrivals	Ch 5
c. Screen visitors and sales persons arriving at the office	Ch 5
d. Obtain patient demographics and information	Ch 5
e. Understand and maintain patient confidentiality during check-in procedures	Ch 5

(*continues*)

TABLE B-5 (*continued*)

RMA (AMT) Competencies	Textbook and Workbook References
f. Prepare patient record	Ch 5, 9
g. Assist patients into examination rooms	Ch 5
3. Scheduling	**Ch 7**
a. Employ appointment scheduling system	Ch 7
(1) identify and employ various scheduling styles (wave, open, etc.)	Ch 7
b. Employ proper procedures for cancellations and missed appointments	Ch 7
c. Understand referral and authorization process	Ch 2, 7, 18
d. Understand and manage patient recall system	Ch 7
e. Schedule nonoffice appointments (hospital admissions, diagnostic tests, surgeries)	Ch 7
4. Oral and written communication	**Ch 1, 4, 6, 8, 11, 12**
a. Employ appropriate telephone etiquette	Ch 6
b. Perform appropriate telephone technique	Ch 6
c. Instruct patients via telephone	Ch 6
d. Inform patients of test results per physician instruction	Ch 6
e. Receive, process, and document results received from outside provider	Ch 8
f. Compose correspondence employing acceptable business format	Ch 11, 12
g. Employ effective written communication skills adhering to ethics and laws of confidentiality	Ch 11, 12
h. Employ active listening skills	Ch 1, 4, 6
5. Records and chart management	**Ch 3, 8, 9**
a. Manage patient medical record system	Ch 8, 9
b. Record diagnostic test results in patient chart	Ch 9
c. File patient and physician communication in chart	Ch 8
d. File materials according to proper system	Ch 8
(1) chronological	Ch 8
(2) alphabetical	Ch 8
(3) problem-oriented medical records (POMR)	Ch 9
(4) subject	Ch 8
e. Protect, store, and retain medical records according to proper conventions and HIPAA privacy regulations	Ch 8
f. Prepare and release private health information as required, adhering to state and federal guidelines	Ch 3, 9
g. Identify and employ proper documentation procedures adhering to standard charting guidelines	Ch 9
6. Transcription and dictation	**Ch 11**
a. Transcribe notes from dictation system	Ch 11
b. Transcribe letter or notes from direct dictation	Ch 11

TABLE B-5 (*continued*)

RMA (AMT) Competencies	Textbook and Workbook References
7. Supplies and equipment management	**Ch 19**
a. Maintain inventory of medical/office supplies and equipment	Ch 19
b. Coordinate maintenance and repair of office equipment	Ch 19
c. Maintain equipment maintenance logs according to OSHA regulations	Ch 19
8. Computer applications	**Ch 3, 9, 11, 12, 15**
a. Identify and understand hardware components	
b. Identify and understand application of basic software and operating systems	Ch 9, 11, 12, 15
c. Recognize software application for patient record maintenance, bookkeeping, and patient accounting system	Ch 9, 15
d. Employ procedures for integrity of information and compliance with HIPAA Security and Privacy regulations	Ch 3, 9
9. Office safety	**Ch 3, 5, 10, 19**
a. Maintain office sanitation and comfort	Ch 5
b. Develop and maintain office safety manual	Ch 5
c. Develop emergency procedures and policies	Ch 5
d. Employ procedures in compliance with Occupational Safety and Health Administration (OSHA) guidelines and regulations	Ch 5, 19
(1) hazard communication	Ch 5, 19
(2) engineering and work practice controls	Ch 19
(3) employee training program	Ch 3, 5, 19
(4) standard precautions	Ch 3, 5
e. Maintain records of biohazardous waste and chemical disposal	Ch 5, 10
III. CLINICAL MEDICAL ASSISTING	
E. Physical Examinations	**Reference**
1. Medical history	**Ch 4, 9**
a. Obtain patient history employing appropriate terminology and abbreviations	Ch 9
b. Differentiate between subjective and objective information	Ch 4, 9
c. Understand and employ SOAP and POMR Charting systems for recording information	Ch 9
F. Clinical Pharmacology	**Reference**
1. Terminology	**Ch 10**
a. Define terminology associated with pharmacology	Ch 10
b. Identify and define common prescription abbreviations	Ch 10
3. Prescriptions	**Ch 10**
a. Identify and define drug schedules and legal prescription requirements	Ch 10
b. Understand procedures for completing prescriptions and authorization of medical refills	Ch 10
c. Identify and perform proper documentation of medication transactions	Ch 10

(*continues*)

TABLE B-5 (*continued*)

RMA (AMT) Competencies	Textbook and Workbook References
4. Drugs	**Ch 10**
a. Identify Drug Enforcement Agency regulations for ordering, dispensing, prescribing, storing, and documenting regulated drugs	Ch 10
b. Identify and define drug categories	Ch 10
c. Identify commonly used drugs	Ch 10
d. Identify and describe routes of medication administration	Ch 10
(1) parenteral	Table 10-3
(2) rectal	Table 10-3
(3) topical	Table 10-3
(4) vaginal	Table 10-3
(5) sublingual	Table 10-3
(6) oral	Table 10-3
(7) inhalation	Table 10-3
(8) instillation	Table 10-3
e. Demonstrate ability to use drug references (*Physician's Desk Reference*)	Ch 10
K. First Aid and Emergency Response	**Reference**
2. Legal responsibilities	**Ch 3**
a. Understand protection and limits of the Good Samaritan Act	Ch 3
b. Understand scope of practice when providing first aid	Ch 3
c. Understand mandatory reporting guidelines and procedures	Ch 3

CMAS EXAMINATION SPECIFICATIONS*

The American Medical Technologists (AMT) has developed (2008) competencies and examination specifications for the Certified Medical Administrative Specialist

(CMAS) as follows. Chapters are cross-referenced to each competency in to help locate them in the *Administrative Medical Assisting* textbook and *Workbook*.

TABLE B-6 American Medical Technologists (AMT) Competencies and Examination Specifications for the Certified Medical Administrative Specialist (CMAS) Examination 2008

CMAS (AMT) Competencies	Textbook and Workbook References
I. MEDICAL ASSISTING FOUNDATIONS	
A. Medical Terminology	**Reference**
1. Use and spell basic medical terms appropriately	WB Ch 1-21
2. Identify root words, prefixes, and suffixes	
3. Define basic medical terms	WB Ch 1-21
B. Anatomy and Physiology	**Reference**
1. Know basic structures and functions of body systems	Ch 9
2. Know various disorders of the body (diseases, conditions, syndromes)	
C. Legal and Ethical Considerations	**Reference**
1. Apply principles of medical law and ethics to the health care setting	Ch 3
2. Recognize legal responsibilities of, and know scope of practice for the medical administrative specialist	Ch 3
3. Know basic laws pertaining to medical practice	Ch 3, 16, 17, 18, 19
4. Know and observe disclosure laws (patient privacy, minors, confidentiality)	Ch 3
5. Know the principles of medical ethics established by the AMA	Ch 1, 3
6. Recognize unethical practices and identify ethical responses for situations in the medical office	Ch 3
D. Professionalism	**Reference**
1. Employ human relations skills appropriate to the health care setting	Ch 1, 4
2. Display behaviors of a professional medical administrative specialist	Ch 1, 2, 4
3. Participate in appropriate continuing education	Ch 1 thru 7, 9, 10, 12, 13, 14, 18, 19, 20
II. BASIC CLINICAL MEDICAL OFFICE ASSISTING*	
A. Basic Health History Interview	**Reference**
1. Obtain preliminary health histories from patients	Ch 9

(continues)

---

* The CMAS Competencies and Examination Specifications are reprinted with permission from the American Medical Technologists.
* Not all clinical competencies are listed.

TABLE B-6 (*continued*)

CMAS (AMT) Competencies	Textbook and Workbook References
E. Basic Charting	**Reference**
1. Chart patient information	Ch 9, 10
III. MEDICAL OFFICE CLERICAL ASSISTING	
A. Appointment Management and Scheduling	**Reference**
1. Schedule and monitor patient and visitor appointments	Ch 7
2. Address cancellations and missed appointments	Ch 7
3. Prepare information for referrals and preauthorizations	Ch 2, 18
4. Arrange hospital admissions and surgery, and schedule patients for outpatient diagnostic tests	Ch 7
5. Manage recall system and file	Ch 7, 8
B. Reception	**Reference**
1. Receive and process patients and visitors	Ch 5
2. Screen visitors and vendors requesting to see physician	Ch 5
3. Coordinate patient flow into examining rooms	Ch 5
C. Communication	**Reference**
1. Employ effective written and oral communication	Ch 4, 6 11, 12, 19, 21
2. Address and process incoming telephone calls from outside providers, pharmacies, and vendors	Ch 6, 10
3. Employ appropriate telephone etiquette when screening patient calls and addressing office business	Ch 6
4. Recognize and employ proper protocols for telephone emergencies	Ch 6
5. Format business documents and correspondence appropriately	Ch 11, 12
6. Process incoming and outgoing mail	Ch 12
D. Patient Information and Community Resources	**Reference**
1. Order and organize patient informational materials	Ch 5
2. Maintain list of community referral resources	Ch 5
IV. MEDICAL RECORDS MANAGEMENT	
A. Systems	**Reference**
1. Demonstrate knowledge of, and manage patient medical records systems	Ch 9, 10
2. Manage documents and patient charts using paper methods	Ch 8, 9, 10
3. Manage documents and patient charts using computerized methods	Ch 9
B. Procedures	**Reference**
1. File records alphabetically, numerically, by subject, and by color	Ch 8
2. Employ rules of indexing	Ch 8
3. Arrange contents of patient charts in appropriate order	Ch 8, 9, 10
4. Document and file laboratory results and patient communication in charts	Ch 8, 9

TABLE B-6 (*continued*)

CMAS (AMT) Competencies	Textbook and Workbook References
5. Perform corrections and additions to records	Ch 9, 11
6. Store, protect, retain, and destroy records appropriately	Ch 8, 9, 10
7. Transfer files	Ch 3, 9
8. Perform daily chart management	Ch 8, 9, 10
9. Prepare charts for external review and audits	Ch 9
C. Confidentiality	**Reference**
1. Observe and maintain confidentiality of records, charts, and test results	Ch 3, 8, 9, 11
2. Observe special regulations regarding the confidentiality of protected information	Ch 3, 9
V. HEALTH CARE INSURANCE PROCESSING, CODING, AND BILLING	
A. Insurance Processing	**Reference**
1. Understand private/commercial health care insurance plans (PPO, HMO, traditional indemnity)	Ch 2, 18
2. Understand government health care insurance plans (Medicare, Medicaid, Veteran's Administration, CHAMPUS, TRICARE, use of Advance Beneficiary Notices)	Ch 2, 18
3. Process patient claims using appropriate forms (including superbills) and time frames	Ch 18
4. Process Workers' Compensation/disability reports and forms	Ch 18
5. Submit claims for third-party reimbursements including the use of electronic transmission methods	Ch 18
B. Coding	**Reference**
1. Understand procedure and diagnosis coding	Ch 16, 17, 18
2. Employ *Current Procedural Terminology (CPT)* and Evaluation and Management codes appropriately	Ch 16
3. Employ *International Classification of Diseases (ICD-CM)* codes appropriately	Ch 17
4. Employ *Health Care Financing Administration Common Procedure Coding System (HCPCS)* codes appropriately	Ch 16
C. Insurance Billing and Finances	**Reference**
1. Understand health care insurance terminology (deductible, copayment, preauthorization, capitation, coinsurance)	Ch 18
2. Understand billing requirements for health care insurance plans	Ch 13, 18
3. Process insurance payments	Ch 13
4. Track unpaid claims, and file and track appeals	Ch 18
5. Understand fraud and abuse regulations	Ch 18
VI. MEDICAL OFFICE FINANCIAL MANAGEMENT	
A. Fundamental Financial Management	**Reference**
1. Understand basic principles of accounting	Ch 20
2. Perform bookkeeping procedures including balancing accounts	Ch 15, 18, 20

(*continues*)

TABLE B-6 (*continued*)

CMAS (AMT) Competencies	Textbook and Workbook References
3. Perform financial computations	Ch 13, 15, 18, 20
4. Manage accounts payable	Ch 20
5. Manage accounts receivable	Ch 13, 15, 18, 20
6. Prepare monthly trial balance (reports)	Ch 20
7. Understand basic audit controls	Ch 15, 20
8. Understand professional fee structures	Ch 13, 15, 16, 18
9. Understand physician/practice owner compensation provisions	Ch 13
10. Understand credit arrangements	Ch 13
11. Manage other financial aspects of office management	Ch 20
B. Patient Accounts	**Reference**
1. Manage patient accounts/ledgers	Ch 13, 15, 18
2. Manage patient billing (methods, cycle billing procedures)	Ch 13, 15, 18
3. Manage collections in compliance with state and federal regulations	Ch 13, 15
C. Banking	**Reference**
1. Understand banking services and procedures (accounts, lines of credit, checking endorsements, deposits, reconciliation, and statements)	Ch 14, 15, 20
2. Manage petty cash	Ch 15, 20
D. Payroll	**Reference**
1. Prepare employee payroll and reports	Ch 20
2. Maintain payroll tax deduction procedures and records	Ch 20
VII. MEDICAL OFFICE INFORMATION PROCESSING	
A. Fundamentals of Computing	**Reference**
1. Possess fundamental knowledge of computing in the medical office including keyboarding, data entry, and retrieval	Ch 11, 15
2. Possess fundamental knowledge of PC-based environment	Ch 11
3. Possess fundamental knowledge of word processing, spreadsheet, database, and presentation graphics applications	Ch 11
4. Employ procedures for ensuring the integrity and confidentiality of computer-stored information	Ch 11, 12
B. Medical Office Applications	**Reference**
1. Employ medical office software applications	
2. Use computer for billing and financial transactions	
3. Employ email applications	Ch 12

TABLE B-6 *(continued)*

CMAS (AMT) Competencies	Textbook and Workbook References
VIII. MEDICAL OFFICE MANAGEMENT*	
A. Office Communications*	Reference
1. Facilitate staff meetings and in-service, and ensure communication of essential information to staff	Ch 19
B. Business Organization Management*	Reference
1. Manage medical office business functions	Ch 19
2. Manage office mailing and shipping services	Ch 12
3. Manage outside vendors and supplies	Ch 5, 6, 19
4. Manage contracts and relationships with associated health care providers	Ch 2, 18
5. Comply with licensure and accreditation requirements	Ch 2, 19
C. Human resources*	Reference
1. Manage/supervise medical office staff	Ch 19
2. Conduct performance reviews and disciplinary action	Ch 19
3. Maintain office policy manual	Ch 19
4. Manage staff payroll and scheduling	Ch 20
5. Manage staff recruiting in compliance with state and federal laws	Ch 19
6. Orient and train new staff	Ch 19
7. Manage employee benefits	Ch 19
D. Safety	Reference
1. Maintain office safety, maintain office safety manual, and post emergency instructions	Ch 5
2. Observe emergency safety requirements	Ch 5
3. Maintain records of biohazard waste, hazardous chemicals (Material Safety Data Sheets), and safety conditions	Ch 5
4. Comply with Occupational Safety and Health Act (OSHA) guidelines and regulations	Ch 5
E. Supplies and Equipment	Reference
1. Manage medical and office supply inventories and order supplies	Ch 19
2. Maintain office equipment and arrange for (and maintain records of) equipment maintenance and repair	Ch 19
F. Physical Office Plant	Reference
1. Maintain office facilities and environment	Ch 5, 19
G. Risk Management and Quality Assurance	Reference
1. Understand and employ risk management and quality assurance concepts	Ch 3

* "Asterisked (*) areas addressed by the Medical Office Management job function may or may not be performed by the Certified Medical Administrative Specialist at entry-level practice. Nevertheless, the competent specialist should have sound knowledge of these management functions at certification level." (AMT)

GLOSSARY

The number in parentheses after each term is the chapter in which the term is discussed in depth.

A

ABA routing number (14)   Coding system developed by the American Bankers Association and used on checks to identify the location of the bank; also called *bank number* or *transit*

abstract (9)   In the context of handling a medical record, to extract, or take out, specific information, or to summarize from documentation in a patient's chart; often done for insurance purposes

account (15)   Formal record of all transactions made on an individual's financial record, listing debits, credits, and balance; may be computerized. In a medical practice using a manual bookkeeping system, this term is referred to as a ledger or ledger card.

accounting (15)   A system of recording and summarizing business and financial transactions and analyzing, verifying, and reporting the results

accounts payable (20)   Amount of money due to a creditor on an account

accounts payable (A/P) ledger (15)   Record book that lists detailed amounts owed to creditors for the operation of a business, such as supplies and equipment, services rendered, or facility expenses

accounts receivable (A/R) (13)   Total amount of money owed for services rendered by all parties

accounts receivable control (15)   Daily summary of dollar amounts that remain unpaid on all accounts

accounts receivable (A/R) ledger (15)   Record book (log) that lists all patients' outstanding accounts showing how much each one owes for services rendered

accreditation (1)   Process of meeting a state standard or being evaluated and recognized by a national organization as meeting predetermined standards

active listening (4)   Giving the speaker your undivided attention, resisting urges to respond verbally, mentally focusing and concentrating on the message being relayed

add-on codes (16)   *CPT* five-digit codes, indicated by a plus symbol (+), that have been designed to be used with primary procedure codes; descriptions usually start with "each additional," "list separately," or "second lesion"

adjudicate (18)   To settle judicially as in a determination of payment for an insurance claim

adjuster (18)   Employee of an insurance carrier to whom a case is assigned and who follows the case until it is adjusted, or settled; grants verbal authorization in workers' compensation cases for testing, procedures, surgeries, and referrals

adjustment (15)   Credit entry made on an account or ledger to decrease a balance that may be due to professional discounts, courtesy adjustments (write-offs), disallowances by insurance companies, or to correct bookkeeping errors

administrative law (3)   Law that governs the activities of government agencies such as the Internal Revenue Service, Medicare, and Medicaid

administrative medical assistant (1)   Office personnel whose responsibilities include a variety of secretarial and clerical duties. In a physician's office, works in the front office and may perform managerial and supervisory functions, manage office personnel, and participate in service activities aimed at improving the health of the community.

Advance Beneficiary Notice (ABN) (18)   Waiver of liability form provided by the physician's office and given to Medicare beneficiaries to be signed prior to services being rendered that may be deemed not medically necessary and therefore not paid by Medicare

advance directive (3)   Document stating an individual's preference about treatment if the person becomes incompetent or unable to communicate with medical personnel. It may instruct physicians to withhold or withdraw life-sustaining procedures, or it may contain a request to receive all available treatment. Two types of advance directives are a living will and health care (durable) power of attorney.

agenda (18)   List of items to be discussed at a staff meeting

aggressive (1)   One whose behavior is belligerent, confrontational, pushy, forward, or overbearing

aging accounts (13)   Analysis of accounts receivable indicating 30-, 60-, 90-, and 120-day delinquency

alphabetical filing (8)   Arrangement of names in alphabetical sequence according to filing units

American Association of Medical Assistants (AAMA) (1)   National association of medical assistants, medical assisting students, and medical assisting educators with both state and local chapters; recognized by the American Medical Association (AMA)

American Medical Technologists (AMT) (1) Association that features a registered medical assistant (RMA) and certified medical administrative specialist (CMAS) program and examination for certification as well as student membership

annotate (12) To make explanatory notations in the margins of correspondence so that actions can be taken

answering service (6) Business that specializes in taking and relaying telephone messages when offices are closed

appointment abbreviations (7) Shortened words or coded numbers indicating types of appointments, types of patients, types of insurance, and reasons for appointments

appointment block (7) Segment of time set aside in the appointment schedule for a specific patient type or procedure

appointment book (7) Set of sheets used to schedule and record time set aside for patients to see health care practitioners for procedures and services

appointment card (7) Small card preprinted with the physician's name, address, and telephone number showing the day, date, and time of an appointment; given to the patient to serve as a reminder

appointment schedule (7) List designating chronological fixed times for patients to meet with the physician and/or receive medical services

assertive (1) One who appears confident and is self-assured

assets (15) Any possessions, either physical objects (tangible) or resources (intangible), having money value. Tangible assets include cash, inventory, furniture, fixtures, and equipment; intangible assets may be a service, trademark, or goodwill.

assignment (13, 18) Agreement by which a patient assigns to another party (e.g., a physician) the right to receive payment from a third party (e.g., insurance plan or program) for the service the patient has received

associate practice (2) Two or more physicians operating as solo practitioners billing under separate tax identification numbers, sharing office expenses, employees, and the on-call schedule

Association of Records Managers and Administrators, Inc. (ARMA International) (8) Nonprofit records management association organized to promote research and provide standardized filing guidelines

attending physician (9) Medical staff member who is legally responsible for the care and treatment given to a patient

audit (9) Periodic examination or review of patient records to verify recordkeeping, documentation for level of service billed, and proper medical care

authorization form (3) Document for use and disclosure of protected health information not included in a consent form that delineates the purpose for which the health care information is to be used and disclosed

automated appointment reminder system (7) Computer-generated system that retrieves appointment data from the computer's scheduling system and supports integrated phone, email, text, and mobile app messaging

automated teller machine (ATM) (14) Computerized terminal that enables a customer to deposit, withdraw, or transfer funds, or obtain other bank services

automatic transfer of funds (14) Withdrawal of funds from one account and transfer to another, in specific amounts, at specified times, and according to a prior written agreement

B

back ordered (B/O) (18) Invoice notation indicating that an ordered item will be sent as soon as it is made available to the supplier

backup (8) Duplicate data file; equipment designed to complete or redo an operation if primary equipment fails

balance (15) Amount owed on a credit transaction after payments and adjustments have been recorded; also known as *outstanding*, *running*, or *unpaid balance*

balance sheet (20) Systematic statement of the assets, liabilities, and capital of a business on a specified date

bank statement (14) Monthly itemization of all transactions of a checking account, showing checks paid, deposits made, service charges, and beginning and ending balances; may be accompanied by canceled checks, photocopies of checks, or recorded on microfiche; contains a *bank reconciliation* form to be completed by the payer

bankruptcy (13) State of being legally unable to pay one's debts

bar code sorter (BCS) (12) Code imprinted on first-class mail to speed sorting and delivery

bearer (14) Person delivering an item for payment

beneficiary (18) One who qualifies for health insurance to receive medical benefits

benefit list (18) List of benefits, that is, services and procedures that are covered under the insurance plan or program

benign (17) Neoplasms (growths) that are noninvasive and do not *metastasize* (spread to other tissue); noncancerous

bias (4) To prejudge or have a one-sided opinion that influences your judgment negatively

bill (13) Statement of fees owed for services rendered

binder file folder (8) Document container with clamps for securing data

bioethics (3) Branch of ethics concerning moral issues, questions, and problems that arise in the practice of medicine and in biomedical research

biohazard (5) Material that is potentially harmful to humans, such as body fluid

birthday rule (18) Informal procedure adopted by the health industry, which is used to determine the primary insurance plan when both parents cover a child. The health plan of the person whose birthday (month and day, *not year*) falls earlier in the calendar year will pay first, and the plan of the other person covering the dependent will be the secondary payer.

blind letter (21)   Communication expressing an interest in a job should one become available

body language (4)   Body movements, sending a message without words; referred to as nonverbal communication

bonding (3)   Obligation of an insurance company or bonding agency to protect an employer against financial loss caused by the acts or omissions of employees

bookkeeping (15)   Process used for analyzing and recording business transactions for the purpose of collecting amounts due and reporting the financial condition of the business at a future date

brand name (10)   Proprietary or trade name of a drug as copyrighted by the manufacturer

bundled code (16)   Code that contains a grouping of one or more services that are related to a procedure; coding and billing for these individual services should not be done

burnout (1)   Condition of severe or chronic mental, physical, and/or emotional stress characterized by a specific set of symptoms, which is brought on by working too long and too hard

C

caduceus (2)   Symbol of the medical profession. The winged, snake-entwined staff carried by Mercury depicting Hermes, the Greek god of science, commerce, eloquence, invention, cunning, and guide of departed souls to Hades

callbacks (6)   Term indicating that a return telephone call is necessary

capital (15)   Physician's share in a business plus operating profit; also known as *owner's equity* or *net worth*

capitation (2, 13)   Method of payment for health services by which a health group is prepaid a fixed, per capita amount for each patient served, without considering the actual amount of service provided to each patient

caption (8)   Name or number used in a filing system under which records are filed

case history (9)   Past and current information used in the evaluation process by the physician; part of the medical record

cellular telephone (6)   Wireless telephone that communicates through cell sites (antenna towers) placed in sections of a city. The caller/receiver is automatically transferred from cell to cell as he or she moves around.

certification (1)   Statement issued by a board or association that verifies that a person meets professional standards

Certified Clinical Medical Assistant (CCMA) (1)   Title received after appropriate training in clinical procedures and passing a certification examination administered by the Healthcareers Association (HCA)

Certified Mail (12)   Service of the U.S. Postal Service that provides, for a fee, a receipt to the sender of first-class mail and a record of its delivery

Certified Medical Administrative Assistant (CMAA) (1)   Title received after appropriate training in administrative procedures and passing a certification examination administered by the Healthcareers Association (HCA)

Certified Medical Administrative Specialist (CMAS) (1)   Title received after appropriate training in administrative procedures and passing a certification examination administered by the American Medical Technologists (AMT)

Certified Medical Assistant (CMA [AAMA]) (1)   Title received after appropriate training in administrative and clinical procedures and passing a certification examination administered by the American Association of Medical Assistants (AAMA)

charge (13, 15, 18)   Amount billed (price) for professional services rendered; "fees" is the preferred term in current usage; a debit to an account

charge-out system (8)   Procedure in a filing system provided to account for items removed from the files

check (CK) (14)   Order to pay; a common form of money exchange

checking account (14)   Account on which interest may be paid depending on the balance. Monies are deposited into the account, and the bank will accept valid orders (e.g., checks) to pay funds to designated recipients

CHEDDAR (9)   Abbreviation for *chief complaint, history, examination, details of complaints, drugs* and *dosage, assessment,* and *return visit;* used as a format for charting

chemical name (10)   Name, usually long and often complicated, describing the main chemical content of a drug

chronological résumé (21)   Data sheet that outlines experience and education by dates

civil law (3)   Statute that enforces private rights and liabilities, as differentiated from criminal law

claim (18)   Request for payment under an insurance contract or bond

clearinghouse (18)   Centralized location where claims are received, edited, and distributed electronically to insurance companies

clinic (2)   Establishment where patients undergo physical examination and treatment by a group of health care professionals practicing medicine together; may include several physicians of the same or different specialties; is sometimes limited to serving poor or public patients; and is sometimes limited to facilities for graduate or undergraduate medical education

clinical medical assistant (1)   Back-office medical assistant who performs clinical and laboratory duties

cloaning (9)   Documentation that is worded exactly or similar to previous entries or encounters; also called "cut-and-paste" documentation

closed fracture (16)   Broken bone that has not penetrated the skin

clustering (7)   Act of scheduling patients with similar ailments in group sequence

code linkage (17)   Connecting the diagnostic code to the procedure code on the insurance claim so that the procedure or service is justified

coding compliance program (16)   Program designed to ensure that national coding guidelines and standards are adhered to

coinsurance (13, 16)   Cost-sharing requirement under a health insurance policy that stipulates the insured assumes a percentage of the costs of covered services

collection ratio (13)   Proportion of money owed to money collected on accounts receivable

colloquialisms (4)   Slang or informal language

combination code (17)   Single diagnostic code used to classify (1) two diagnoses, (2) a diagnosis with a secondary process, or (3) a diagnosis with an association complication

combination résumé (21)   Data sheet that combines specific dates of work experience with education and skills

commercial filing system (8)   Customized guides and folders manufactured for professional office use

communicate (4)   Transfer information from one party to another

communication cycle (4)   Basic elements needed to communicate: (1) *sender*, person who has an idea or information and wants to convey it; (2) *message*, content that needs to be communicated; (3) *channel*, method of sending the message to the receiver; (4) *receiver*, recipient getting the message and interpreting it; and (5) *feedback*, response from the receiver used to decide if clarification is necessary

community resources (5)   National, state, county, city, and private agency information and programs made available at the local level, such as Alcoholics Anonymous, hospice care, or the Multiple Sclerosis Society

comorbidity (17)   Coexisting medical conditions

complaint (3)   Formal, legal document that outlines facts and legal reasons to support a claim by the plaintiff in a civil case

complementary and alternative medicine (CAM) (16) Medical treatments used in conjunction with conventional medical treatments in the United States or in place of existing therapies or products

compliance plan (3)   Written protocol outlining practice standards that include office policies and procedures, HIPAA law, and federal and state mandates

computer-assisted coding (CAC) (16)   Software program that uses natural language processing software that automatically assigns codes to clinical procedures and services

computer program (7)   See *software*

computerized provider order entry (CPOE) (9, 10) Entry of data into a computerized health record system by an authorized medical professional

concurrent care (16)   The provision of similar services (e.g., hospital visits) to the same patient by more than one physician on the same day

conference call (6)   Telephone call linking several persons at different geographic locations in one conversation; teleconferencing

consent form (3)   One-time signed document used to disclose personally identifiable health information for treatment, payment, or routine health care operations; not required by law

consultation (16)   Second opinion rendered by a physician in a home, office, hospital, or extended care facility regarding a condition or need for surgery and may initiate diagnostic or therapeutic services; the service must be requested, recorded, and reported

consulting physician (9)   Provider whose opinion or advice regarding evaluation or management of a specific problem is requested by another physician

consumer-directed health plan (CDHP) (2)   An alternative to traditional and managed care plans, CDHPs offer a tiered benefit structure with low premiums, high-deductible catastrophic insurance, and a number of different types of prespending tax-savings accounts in which money may be rolled-over from year to year. It provides a built-in incentive, which allows patients more freedom in decision making and motivates savings of health care dollars.

continuing education units (CEUs) (1)   Credit for course hours that an individual receives for attending or taking part in an educational program. State and organization requirements vary when renewing a professional license or certification; also known as *continuing education credit (CEC)*; documented in time (e.g., 1.0 CEU = 10 hours).

contract law (3)   Agreements that are legally enforceable by law between two or more parties; requires an offer, acceptance of the offer, and promise to perform

conversion privilege (18)   Clause in a group insurance policy that allows the insured to continue the same or lesser coverage under an individual policy

coordination of benefits (COB) (18)   Provisions and procedures used by insurers to avoid duplicate payment for losses insured under more than one insurance policy

copayment (copay) (13, 16)   Type of cost-sharing whereby the insured pays a specified amount per unit of service and the insurer pays the rest of the cost; in managed care, flat fee that is owed prior to receiving services

counseling (16)   Discussion with the patient or family member regarding diagnostic results, impressions, and recommended diagnostic studies; prognosis; risks and benefits of treatment options; instructions for treatment and/or follow-up; compliance with treatment options; risk factor reduction; and patient and family education

cover letter (21)   In job seeking, a letter of introduction prepared to accompany a résumé

covered entities (3)   Those who provide health care and/or send data electronically that is protected under HIPAA law such as health care professionals, health plans, health care clearinghouses, and hospitals

credit (13)   From the Latin *credere*, "to believe" or "to trust"; trust in regard to financial obligations; in banking, a deposit or addition to a bank account

credits (15)   Bookkeeping entries reflecting a decrease in the account balance; include payments by debtors (patients) of a sum received on their account or an adjustment (write-off)

criminal law (3)   Laws (felonies and misdemeanors) made to protect the public against the harmful acts of others and regulate crimes against the state such as arson, burglary, rape, robbery, and murder

critical care (16)   Care of an unstable, acutely ill or injured patient requiring constant bedside attention by a physician requiring high-complexity decision making; most commonly rendered in a critical care area (e.g., coronary care unit, intensive care unit, respiratory care unit) or emergency care facility

currency (14)   Paper money in circulation, issued by the government through an act of law

cut (8)   Term used in filing to describe the size of the tab on the back of a file folder; usually expressed as a fraction, for example, *one-half cut*

cycle billing (13)   Sending itemized statements to portions of the accounts receivable at certain times of the month; can be divided by alphabet, account number, insurance type, or by calendar day of first visit

D

databases (8)   Collection of data (information) stored electronically

daysheet (15)   Register for recording all daily business transactions; also known as *daybook, daily journal sheet, daily record sheet*, or *general ledger*

debit (15)   Basic bookkeeping term used to describe an increase in assets; a fee or charge added to the balance of a patient account

debit card (13)   Card used by bank customers to either withdraw cash from an affiliated automated teller machine (ATM) or make electronic transfers of cash from a customer's bank account to a merchant's account; also called a *bank card*

debits (15)   Bookkeeping entries reflecting money owed (charges); the increase of a patient account balance, an asset, or a business expense, or the decrease of a liability of an owner's equity

deductible (deduc) (18)   Amount the insured must pay in a calendar or fiscal year before policy benefits begin

deductions (20)   Amounts withheld from an employee's gross income for income tax purposes

defendant (3)   Person sued (defending or denying action); usually the physician in a malpractice case

defensive (4)   A response to protect oneself from a perceived threat; usually unconscious. The threat may stem from anxiety, guilt, loss of self-esteem, or an injured ego.

demeanor (4)   How a person appears; his or her expressions and body language

dependents (18)   Under an insurance contract, the spouse and children of the insured; in some cases, domestic partners

deposit record (14)   Printed receipt for a deposit issued by the bank

deposit slip (14)   Form, also known as a *deposit ticket*, provided by banks to itemize monies placed in a savings or checking account

deposits (14)   Funds given to a bank to be credited to an account

DHL Worldwide Express (12)   National and international letter and package delivery service

diagnosis (9, 16, 17, 18)   Determination of the nature of a disease or injury

diagnostic file (8)   Information based on the characteristics of a disease or illness learned from patient case histories and filed for reference

diplomate (21)   Physician certified by a medical board in a field of specialization

direct deposit service (14)   Process by which a check's issuer transmits the check directly to the payee's program or service bank for credit to the latter's account

disaster (5)   Sudden event (calamity or tragedy) that results in great damage such as a threat to health or loss of property or life and may ultimately affect society and/or the environment

disbursement record (20)   Chronological register of monthly business expenditures and yearly totals

discrimination (4)   To unfairly treat an individual or group based on age, culture, gender, race, religion, lifestyle, or sexual orientation

displaced anger (4)   Anger that is completely unrelated to the event that is presently occurring; it may be built up or held in from another event and released at an inappropriate time

domestic mail (12)   Mail delivered in the United States and U.S. territories

double-entry accounting (15)   Bookkeeping system of financial records used in business, whereby equal accounting debits and credits are recorded for each transaction

downcoding (16)   Submitted procedure code changed to a lower level by a computer system

download (8)   Process of transferring data (file or program) from a central computer to a remote computer

downtime (8)   Period during which a computer is malfunctioning or not operating correctly

Drug Enforcement Administration (DEA) (10) Federal agency whose mission is to enforce the controlled substance laws and regulations of the United States and to bring to justice those organizations involved in the growing, manufacturing, or distributing of controlled substances; issues narcotic and hypnotic licenses to physicians

dun (13)   Message or phrase used on the billing statement to remind a person about a delinquent payment

E

edit (11)   Revisions, alterations, and refinements made to documents before final printing

electronic files (8)   Collection of related data stored under a single title in a computerized system

electronic funds transfer system (EFTS) (14)
Paperless computerized system that enables funds to be debited, credited, or transferred. For paying bills, a claim is made by electronic notification and a transfer of funds is simultaneously effected; in other words, one computer transfers information to another computer, eliminating the need for personal handling of bills, checks, or similar documents.

electronic health record (EHR) (9)   Computerized medical record system that has the capability to capture and store data in electronic form and to be transmitted within one medical practice or health care organization

electronic health record (EHR) practice management system (6, 7, 8, 9)   Comprehensive computerized system that manages all aspects of the health record and the medical practice (e.g., appointment scheduler, accounts receivable, accounts payable, patient billing, health insurance claim submission, patients' medical records) and has the capability of transmitting and receiving electronic data from providers outside the medial practice; also referred to as *total practice management system (TPMS)*

electronic job search (21)   Locate and investigate job sites and employment opportunities by using the Internet

electronic mail (email) (12)   Process of sending, receiving, storing, and forwarding messages and memos in digital form over the Internet

electronic medical record (9)   Digital electronic version of all entries in patient charts

electronic messaging system (6)   A computerized approach used in total practice management systems (TPMS) that allows secure messages to be sent via the computer to members of the health care team and received as "tasks" to be acted upon

emancipated minors (3)   Children of any age who fall outside the jurisdiction and custody of their parents or guardians and who may make financial and medical decisions

emergency care (6, 16)   Medical care given for a serious medical condition resulting from injury or illness that if not given immediately puts a person's life in danger

empathy (1)   Pertaining to projection of one's own consciousness into another person's situation

employee handbook (18)   Written procedures for general personnel policies

employee's earning record (20)   Payroll record kept for each employee that shows demographic information and rate of pay, marital status, number of exemptions, hours worked, total earnings, amounts deducted from gross income, and net income

Employee's Withholding Allowance Certificate (Form W-4) (20)   Document completed yearly by new and existing employees to indicate exemptions claimed for tax withholding purposes

employer identification number (EIN) (20)   Nine-digit number issued by the Internal Revenue Service to identify tax accounts of employers; also called *tax identification number (TIN)*

Employer's Quarterly Federal Tax Return (20)
Schedule of financial information (Form 841) required four times a year by governmental bodies

employment agencies (21)   Business organizations that contract with employers to locate, test, and refer qualified job applicants to potential employers

enclosure (enc) (12)   Supplemental item contained in an envelope with a written communication

encoder (16, 17)   Computerized or Web-based software program used to search for, locate, and verify code selections

encryption (8)   Encoding of computer data for security purposes, making data appear like gibberish to unauthorized computer users

endorsement (14)   Approval signature on the reverse side of a check that indicates liability for payment of funds disbursed in the case of default or nonpayment; on an item payable to the order of the endorser, it acknowledges receipt of the funds

enunciate (4)   Vocalize, speak, pronounce, articulate

e-prescribing (10)   Using computerized software to create and authorize prescriptions including the filling of new prescriptions, refill authorizations, changes in requests, cancelled prescriptions, and verification of filled prescriptions

ergonomics (5)   Science and technology that seek to fit the anatomical and physical needs of the worker to the workplace

established patient (7)   Individual who has received professional health care services from the physician or another physician of the same specialty who belongs to the same group practice within the past 3 years

ethics (3)   Standards of conduct generally accepted as a moral guide for behavior

ethnic (4)   A group of society defined by origin or race

etiology/manifestation (17)   The underlying cause (etiology) of a disease or condition and the characteristics, signs, or symptoms (manifestation) associated with that disease/condition that occur due to the underlying condition

etiquette (3)   Customary code of conduct, courtesy, and manners

exclusions (18)   Specific hazards, perils, or conditions listed in an insurance policy for which the policy will not pay

exclusive provider organization (EPO) (2)   Managed care plan operating with a limited network of physicians and a designated primary care physician for each subscriber; governed by state health insurance laws

exemptions (20)   Deductions from gross income allowed a taxpayer that reduce the amount of income on which the individual is taxed

expert testimony (3)   Statement given concerning a scientific, technical, or professional matter by a person with authority regarding the matter, such as a physician

explanation of benefits (EOB) (13)   Recap sheet that accompanies an insurance check from a private or federal insurance plan, showing the breakdown of payment determination on a claim. In the Medicare program, this document is called a Remittance Advice (RA) for physicians and a

Medicare Summary Notice (MSN) for patients; in the Medicaid program, this document is called a Remittance Advice (RA); and in the TRICARE program, this document is called a Summary Payment Voucher.

extend (15)   To carry forward the balance of an individual account or ledger

F

face sheet (5)   Portion of hospital intake record that provides identifying data

facsimile (fax) communication (12)   Electronic process for transmitting written communications over telecommunication lines

Federal Express (FedEx) (12)   National and international letter and package delivery service

Federal Insurance Contributions Act (FICA) (20)   Law that sets amounts for Social Security taxes and benefits; most frequently termed *Social Security tax*

Federal Unemployment Tax Act (FUTA) (20)   Law that provides for taxes to be collected at the federal level to help subsidize individual states' administration of their unemployment compensation programs

federal withholding tax (FWT) (20)   Deduction from an employee's gross income determined by the number of withholding exemptions and amount earned for a pay period; also referred to as *federal income tax deduction*

fee-for-service (FFS) (2, 13, 18)   Method of payment; the patient or insurance company pays the physician for professional services according to a specific schedule of fees

fee schedule (13)   List of medical procedures and services with amounts charged

feedback (4)   Oral or nonverbal response such as repeating, restatement, paraphrasing, examples, questions, or summaries

file folder (8)   Folded cover or container that holds records; typically 8½″ × 11″

file guide (8)   Pressboard sheet or metal divider used in a filing system to guide the eye to a section of a file and to provide support for records

file label (8)   Sticker used in filing that attaches to the file folder tab or other part of a folder; it may carry a caption or color code

file tab (8)   Projection above the body of a folder or guide; used for labeling

first-listed condition (17)   The condition, problem, or other reason for the health encounter that is chiefly responsible for the services provided; also referred to as the primary diagnosis

fiscal intermediary (18)   Contractor that processes and pays provider claims on behalf of state or federal agencies or insurance companies; also called *fiscal agent*

fixed interval (7)   See *stream schedule*

flextime (1)   System that allows employees to choose their own times for starting and finishing work within a broad range of available hours

flow sheet (9)   One-page lists, charts, and graphs that allow the physician to quickly find medical information and perform comparative evaluations; used for medical data that are hard to track in narrative progress notes

Food and Drug Administration (FDA) (10)   Federal agency that approves new drugs and determines if they are to be sold as a prescription drug or over the counter, processes new drug applications, regulates package inserts and advertising, issues recalls, and enforces all drug legislation

forgery (14)   Fraudulent signature on document

form letter (11)   Standardized communication that may be personalized by the insertion of variable information

format (11, 21)   General composition or style (e.g., shape, size, spacing) of a letter, report, or document

full block letter style (11)   Typed communication, also known as *block style*, formatted with all lines flush with the left margin

functional résumé (21)   Data sheet that highlights qualifications and skills

G

garnishment (13)   To attach a debtor's property or wages for payment of a debt

general ledger (15)   Record that contains all of the financial transactions of all accounts; it has equal debits and credits as evidenced by a trial balance; see *daysheet*

generic name (10)   Name assigned to a drug by the United States Adopted Name (USAN) Council for each pharmaceutical company that manufactures the drug after the patent has run out for the original manufacturer of the drug; the name is usually not capitalized

given name (8)   Individual's first name

grace period (18)   Specified time interval after a premium payment is due in which the policyholder may make such payment and during which the protection of the policy continues

grievance committee (3)   Impartial panel established to listen to and investigate patients' complaints about medical care or excessive fees

gross income (20)   Revenues before deductions

group practice (2)   Three or more physicians sharing office space, expenses, employees, and income; using one tax identification number; and billing claims under a group name

H

hazardous waste (5)   A substance that is dangerous and potentially damaging to humans and the environment

HCPCS Level II codes **(16)**   A second-level coding system used to code those services, products, supplies, drugs, and procedures that are generally not fully listed in the *CPT* codebook

health care power of attorney (3) Document that names another individual as a decision maker when a patient becomes terminally ill or comatose. It may be used for medical decisions including life-prolonging treatment; also known as *durable power of attorney for health care.*

health information management (HIM) (9) (1) A profession that concentrates on health care data and the management of health care information; (2) department of a hospital or large clinic that stores and manages medical records; previously called *medical records department;* (3) health care professional who collects, integrates, analyzes, and codes health care data

Health Information Technology for Economic and Clinical Health Act (HITECH) (3) Promotes the adoption of meaningful use of health information technology by offering financial incentives to providers who demonstrate *meaningful use* of electronic health record systems; also imposes new breach notification requirements

Health Insurance Portability and Accountability Act (HIPAA) (3) Provides a standardized framework within which all insurance companies and providers work to enhance the portability of health care coverage; increase accuracy of data; protect private health information and the rights of patients; reduce fraud, abuse, and waste in the health care delivery system; upgrade efficiency and financial management; expedite claim processing; lower administrative costs and simplify implementation; promote Medical Saving Accounts; provide better access to long-term care coverage; and improve customer satisfaction to restore trust in the health care system

health maintenance organization (HMO) (2, 18) Managed care plan offering prepaid health care for a fixed fee to subscribers in a designated geographic area; enrollees receive benefits when they obtain services provided or authorized by selected providers, generally with a primary care physician (gatekeeper)

hospice (1) National program that offers medical care and support to patients and family members dealing with a terminal illness and the loss of a loved one

hospital (2) Facility that provides 24-hour acute care and treatment for the sick and injured

human resource department (21) Organizational unit in a business that has the functional responsibility to ensure that personnel policies are implemented legally and proactively, and to recruit, screen, test, hire, train, counsel, and promote workers; synonymous with *personnel department*

human resource management (18) Division of the management team that focuses on recruiting, hiring, training, and staff development

I

implied contract (3) Agreement derived as a result of implication or the situation, general language, or conduct of the patient

independent practice association (IPA) (2) Group of individual health care providers who contract with managed care plans to provide care at a discounted rate in their own office setting

indexing unit (8) Parts of a patient's name that has been separated into components (units) to be considered when filing

infectious waste (5) Something that has come in contact with body fluids that can potentially transmit infection

inscription (10) Section appearing on a prescription showing the name of the drug, quantity of ingredients, and dose strength

insurance agent (18) Representative of an insurance company licensed by the state who solicits, negotiates, or effects contracts of insurance and services the policyholder for the insurer

insurance application (18) Signed statement of facts requested by an insurance company on the basis of which it decides whether or not to issue an insurance policy; it becomes part of the health insurance contract if a policy is issued

insured (18) Individual or organization who contracts for a policy of insurance and is protected in case of loss of property, life, or health under the terms of the insurance policy

interoffice memorandum (11) Written informal communication circulated within an organization or office

interpersonal skills (1) Exemplary personality characteristics that relate to the interactions between individuals, for example, dedication, commitment, integrity, consideration, respect, friendliness, openness, sensitivity, positive attitude, responsibility, and displaying a sense of warmth and genuineness

inventory cards (19) Forms that indicate pertinent data about a specific item to facilitate reordering

invoice (19) Itemized statement of merchandise ordered from a supplier stating quantity, shipping date, price, and other charges

itinerary (19) Detailed outline for a trip

J

job descriptions (19) Written statements outlining work requirements for a particular position

justification (11) In word processing, the spacing of words on each line of text so that the text is centered or the ends of the lines are flush at the right and left margins

L

laboratory (2) Facility where research, experimentation, and the physical and clinical analysis of specimens are performed

laboratory report (9) Clinical record of the findings of physical and chemical analysis of specimens

lateral file (8) Cabinet in which records are stored perpendicular to the opening of the file; also called *vertical file*

ledger card (13, 15) Individual financial record indicating charges, payments, adjustments, and balances owed

letter template (11)   Document formatted with each component of a letter (i.e., letterhead, date line, inside address) used to eliminate setting up various components of a letter, saving time and keystrokes

liabilities (15)   Legal obligations of one person to another; debts

licensure (1)   Credentialing sanctioned by state legislature (the government), which passes laws making it illegal for an individual who is not licensed to engage in the activities of a licensed occupation

limitations (18)   Provision of an insurance policy that lists exceptions or reductions to specific coverage

limiting charge (13)   Highest amount a physician who does not have a contract with Medicare (nonparticipating physician) can charge a Medicare patient

litigation (3)   Lawsuit

living will (3)   Document, not legally binding, stating the desires of an individual should he or she become incompetent because of injury or illness when death is imminent

M

mail merge (11)   Software program used to create, address, sort, and print letters; typically used for form letters with the same text but may have different greetings sent to patients at various addresses

mail classifications (12)   Categories of mail service determined by size, contents, weight, frequency of mailing, destination, and speed of delivery

major medical (18)   Insurance policy especially designed to offset heavy medical expenses resulting from catastrophic or prolonged illness or injury

malignant (17)   Harmful neoplasm (new growth) that has the capability of spreading and invading other tissue; often called *cancer*

managed care organization (MCO) (2)   Health care delivery plan that strives to manage the cost, quality, and delivery of health care by emphasizing preventive medicine, reviewing the utilization of services, and contracting with a network of providers; payment is by capitation with some fee-for-service

manipulate (16)   Joint mobilization technique; realigning a fractured long bone using manual pressure, traction, or angulation; also called *reduction*

Material Safety Data Sheets (MSDS) (5)   Pages of information provided for each chemical by its manufacturer listing 16 criteria as outlined by OSHA's Hazard Communication Standards

matrix (7)   Template indicating times to establish an appointment schedule including times allocated for new patients, established patients, brief visits, in-office surgery, specific conditions, and times blocked off when the physician is out of the office

meaningful use (9)   Electronic health record technology used in a meaningful way for the purpose of electronic exchange of health information, electronic prescribing, and submission of information on clinical quality measures

medical assistant (2)   Multiskilled allied health professional whose practitioners work primarily in ambulatory settings such as medical offices and clinics. Medical assistants function as members of the health care delivery team and perform administrative and clinical procedures.

medical center (2)   Facility offering medical services at sites other than a hospital setting

medical identity theft (5)   Illegally using another person's name or insurance information to falsely obtain medical services or products

medical necessity (2, 17, 18)   Health care services or products that a prudent physician provides to a patient for the purpose of preventing, diagnosing, or treating an illness, injury, disease or its symptoms. It must be provided in a manner that is in accordance with generally accepted standards of medical practice, performed at the proper level, and provided in an appropriate setting.

medical record (9)   Written or graphic information documenting facts and events during the rendering of patient care

medical report (9)   Permanent, legal document in letter or report format formally stating the elements performed and results of an examination and treatment of a patient

Medicare Administrative Contractor (MAC) (18)   Insurance carriers who contract to pay Medicare Part B claims; formerly called *fiscal agents*

Medicare Remittance Advice (RA) (16)   See *explanation of benefits*

Medicare Summary Notice (MSN) (16)   See *explanation of benefits*

minimum necessary standard (3)   To make a reasonable effort to limit the disclosure of protected health information to the minimum necessary to accomplish the intended purpose of the use, disclosure, or request

MinuteClinic (2)   Offers a limited range of basic tests and treatments at a lower cost than most doctor's offices; found in small-scale chain stores and generally staffed by physician assistants or nurse practitioners

mixed punctuation (11)   Style of letter punctuation in which a colon or a comma is placed after the salutation and complimentary close

modified block format (11)   Typed communication with a balanced appearance, formatted with date, closing, and writer's information aligned starting at the center; all other lines are flush with the left margin

modified wave (7)   System used to schedule appointments in which patients are allocated appointment times in the first half of each hour, with the second half of each hour left open for work-ins and emergencies

money order (14)   Instrument (similar to a check) purchased for face value (plus a fee) at a bank, post office, or other place of business; it is signed by and issued according to the purchaser's instructions

morbidity (17)   Diseased condition or state; number of sick people in relation to a population

mortality (17)   Cause of death

multipurpose billing form (13) All-encompassing tracking device typically containing procedures and services, diagnoses, fees, next appointment, and other information; also called *charge slip, communicator, encounter form, fee ticket, patient service slip, routing form, superbill,* and *transaction slip;* it may be used when a patient submits an insurance claim or to extract information for insurance billing

multiskilled health practitioner (MSHP)* (1) Persons cross-trained to provide more than one function, often in more than one discipline. These combined functions can be found in a broad spectrum of health-related jobs, ranging in complexity from the nonprofessional to the professional level, including both clinical and administrative functions. The additional functions (skills) added to the original health care worker's job may be of a higher, lower, or parallel level. The terms *multiskilled, multicompetent,* and *cross-trained* can be used interchangeably.

multispecialty practice (2) Group of physicians at the same location, each specializing in a different field of medicine

N

National Center for Competency Testing (NCCT) (1) An independent certifying agency that validates the competence of a person's knowledge in different areas of the medical profession through examination

National Certified Medical Assistant (NCMA) (1) One who is a high school graduate or equivalent, a graduate of an approved course of study in the area of certification, or who has 2 years of work experience, and passes a competency examination in the administrative and clinical areas

National Certified Medical Office Assistant (NCMOA) (1) One who is a high school graduate or equivalent, a graduate of an approved course of study in the area of certification, or who has 1 year of work experience, and passes a competency examination in the administrative area

National Correct Coding Initiative (NCCI) (16) Coding edits developed via federal legislation that relate to *CPT* and *HCPCS* codes for outpatient and physician services; used by Medicare carriers to process professional claims and curtail improper coding practices, detect incorrect reporting of codes, eliminate unbundling of services, and prevent payments from being made due to inappropriate code assignments

National Healthcareer Association (NHA) (1) Association that offers a number of certification examinations for several allied health care areas including Certified Medical Administrative Assistant (CMAA) and Certified Clinical Medical Assistant (CCMA)

National Provider Identifier (NPI) (18) Ten-digit number, mandated by HIPAA and issued on a lifetime basis as a standard unique health identifier for health care providers, clearinghouses, and plans who conduct electronic transactions (may be used on paper claims); used by Medicare, Medicaid, TRICARE, CHAMPVA, and may be adopted by private insurance carriers

---

* *This definition was adopted by the National Multiskilled Health Practitioner Clearinghouse (NMHPC) advisory panel*

natural language processing (NLP) (16) Software program used for transcribing medical records that has artificial intelligence technology built in; it scans a document the physician has input using free-text and singles out key terms, converting them into procedure codes

neoplasm (17) Spontaneous new growth or formation of tissue; often referred to as a *tumor*

net income (20) Employee's income after deductions have been made

network (21) To form links and interconnect with other people

new patient (7) Individual who has not received any professional services from the physician or another physician of the same specialty who belongs to the same group practice within the past 3 years

noncompliant (4) In a medical setting, refusing to obey the doctor's treatment plan

nonparticipating fee (13) Set amount paid to physicians who do not have a Medicare contract

nonparticipating physician (nonpar) (13) Physician who decides not to accept the determined allowable charge from an insurance plan as the full fee for professional services rendered; in the Medicare program, a nonparticipating provider is one who does not accept assignment—payment goes directly to the patient, and the patient is responsible for paying the bill in full. However, a nonparticipating physician has two options of either not accepting assignment for all services or accepting assignment for some services and not accepting assignment for others.

nonsufficient funds (NSF) (14) Term indicating a check drawn against an account is in excess of the account balance, in which case, the check is marked with the notation "NSF" or "refer to maker" and returned, unpaid, to the presenter; sometimes referred to as a *bounced check*. The customer's account is assessed a fee of several dollars for each NSF check regardless of whether the bank pays it or not.

nonverbal communication (4) Communication without words, expressed through body posture, hand movements, manner of walking, and facial expressions; also called *body language*

no-show (7) Patient who does not keep a scheduled appointment and does not notify the office to cancel

numerical filing (8) Arrangement of records in number sequence

O

objective information (4, 9) In a medical context, facts that are apparent to the observer; descriptive of findings that can be seen, heard, felt, or measured such as swelling, bleeding, blood pressure, heart sounds, a lump, or laboratory test values

Occupational Safety and Health Administration (OSHA) (5) Division of the U.S. Department of Labor that sets standards according to the Occupational Safety and Health Act on safe and healthful working conditions

office manager (OM) (18)   Individual who has administrative responsibilities for the control or direction of employees

office policies and procedures manual (18)   Written guide describing office routines and practices

open access (7)   Appointment scheduling system that allows patients to call and come in the same day; also referred to as *same-day scheduling, same-day access,* and *advanced access*

open accounts (13, 15)   Accounts that are open to charges made from time to time; physicians' patient accounts are usually called *open-book accounts*. Record of business transactions on the books that represents an unsecured account receivable where credit has been extended without a formal written contract; payment is expected within a specified period.

open fracture (16)   Broken bone in which the bone has penetrated the skin; also referred to as a *compound fracture*

open punctuation (11)   Style of letter punctuation in which no punctuation mark is placed after the salutation or complimentary close

open-ended questions (4)   Questions that allow a person to formulate a response and elaborate

open-shelf files (8)   Cabinets with horizontal shelves for record storage

optical character recognition (OCR) (12)   Computer device that can read printed or typed characters and then digitally convert them into text or numerical data

ordering physician (9)   Physician requesting nonphysician services for a patient (e.g., diagnostic laboratory tests, pharmaceutical drugs, or durable medical equipment)

outguide (8)   Manila sheet or folder inserted when a file is taken from a file drawer or cabinet to signal that it has been removed from the file; a substitution card

overdraft (14)   Charge against an account in excess of the account balance

P

packing slip (19)   Statement included in a package, indicating the contents

pandemic emergency (5)   New infectious virus, capable of being transmitted from human to human and affecting a large population over a wide geographic area to which the world population will have no or little immunity

partial disability (18)   Illness or injury that prevents a person from performing one or more of the functions of a regular job; may be temporary or permanent

participating fee (13)   Amount paid to physicians who have contracts with Medicare

participating physician (par) (13)   A physician who agrees to accept an insurance plan's preestablished fee or reasonable charge as the maximum amount collected for services rendered, also called *member physician*; in the Medicare program, a participating provider is one who accepts assignment, agrees to the approved amount based on the Medicare fee schedule as the full charge for services rendered, and receives the payment check. Patients must pay a cost share and/or deductible or both for services rendered.

partnership (2)   Two or more physicians associated in the practice of medicine under a legal partnership agreement

password (8)   Secret word, phrase, code, or symbol input for security purposes to identify the authorized computer user who wishes to gain access to the computer system

patient advocate (2)   One who promotes and supports the interests of the patient

patient-centered medical home (PCMH) (2)   An approach to care (model of care) for children, youth, and adults in which a primary care physician (PCP) heads up a team of medical professionals who deliver comprehensive care

patient instruction form (5)   Checklist of topics and fill-in sheet used by the physician that summarizes a patient's office visit and outlines instructions and a treatment plan

patient navigator (1)   Health care professionals, who provide emotional support and help, coordinate patient care by connecting patients with resources and guiding them through the healthcare system so that timely care is provided; frequently used when chronic diseases are present so that informed medical decisions are made and the treatment plan is understood and followed

patient status (16)   Determination of whether somebody is a new or established patient

payee (14)   Person named on a draft or check as the recipient of the amount shown; also known as *bearer*

payer (14)   Party responsible for payment of the amount owed as shown on a check or note

payroll (20)   Wages or salary paid in return for goods or services; list of employees and their compensation

payroll tax (20)   Charge levied by government authority on salaries and wages

perceptions (4)   Assumptions that people make based on their awareness; individual discernment

performance evaluation (21)   Summary of an employee's work habits, behaviors, efficiency, and effectiveness on the job

permanent disability (PD) (18)   Illness or injury that is not resolved and prevents an insured person from performing all the functions of a regular job

petty cash fund (15)   Small amount of monies readily available for minor office expenses

pharmaceutical (10)   Relating to pharmacy, drugs, and medicine

pharmaceutical representative (10)   Professional salesperson who represents a pharmaceutical firm and offers information on drugs and other products; called a "detail rep" or "detail person"

pharmacist (10)   Person with degree who is skilled in the art or practice of preparing, preserving, compounding, and dispensing drugs; a druggist; an apothecary

photocopy (11)   Term designating all the processes employed in producing multiple copies

photocopy machine (11)   Duplicating machine that reproduces graphic matter onto paper in a few seconds

physician's fee profile (13)   Compilation kept by each insurance carrier of a physician's charges and payments made through the years for each professional service rendered to a patient; as charges are increased, so are payments, and the profile is then updated through the use of computer data

Physicians' Desk Reference (PDR) **(10)**   Reference book used by physicians and medical assistants to find information about prescription drugs; it contains those drugs submitted to the publisher by drug companies

place of service (16, 18, App A)   Location where a medical service is taking place

placeholder (17)   The character (x) used as a fourth, fifth, or sixth digit in diagnostic coding with certain seven-digit codes to allow for future expansion of the *ICD-10-CM* codebook; if it exists, it must be used or the code is invalid

plaintiff (3)   One who institutes a lawsuit or action

point-of-service (POS) plan (2)   Managed care plan that contracts with independent providers at a discounted rate. Members have the choice at the time services are needed (i.e., at the point-of-service) of receiving services from an HMO, PPO, or fee-for-service plan; sometimes referred to as *open-ended HMOs, swing-out HMOs, self-referral options, flex plans,* or *multiple option plans.* A patient can self-refer himself or herself to a specialist or see a nonnetwork provider for a higher coinsurance payment.

portability (3)   The transferability of an insurance benefit from one source (e.g., job) to another when the worker loses or changes jobs

portfolio (21)   Compilation of items that represents a job applicant's skills and accomplishments

post (15)   To record or transfer financial entries, debits or credits, to an account, for example, daysheet, computerized account or ledger, bank deposit slip, check register, or journal

postdated check (14)   Check dated for deposit at a future date; cannot be considered valid or payable until that date

practice information brochure (19)   Pamphlet that describes medical office policies and procedures is designed as an instrument for communication to answer frequently asked questions and improve the physician/patient relationship; also used as a marketing tool

preauthorization (2, 18)   Process of requesting permission to render a service/procedure to the patient in which the insurance plan determines the medical necessity and appropriateness of the service; also called *prior authorization* or *prior approval*

precertification (2, 18)   To determine whether services (surgery, tests, hospitalization) are covered under a patient's health insurance policy

predetermination (2, 18)   Finding out the maximum dollar amount that will be paid for specific services and procedures; also called *preestimate of cost* or *pretreatment estimate*

preexisting condition (18)   An injury that occurred, a disease that was contracted, or a physical condition that existed before the issuance of a health insurance policy

preferred provider organization (PPO) (2, 18)   Type of health program in which enrollees receive the highest level of benefits when obtaining services from a physician, hospital, or other health care provider called "preferred providers"; enrollees may receive substantial but reduced benefits when obtaining care from a provider of their own choice that is not a "preferred provider"

prejudice (4)   Judgment formed prior to gathering all facts

premium (18)   Payment made on a regular schedule to keep an insurance policy in force

prescriptions (10)   Medical preparations compounded according to directions written by a physician to a pharmacist and consisting of four parts: *superscription, inscription, subscription,* and *signature*

primary care physician (PCP) (2)   Physician who assumes the ongoing responsibility for the overall treatment of a patient; usually a general or family practitioner, internist, gynecologist, or pediatrician; also referred to as *gatekeepers* in managed care plans

primary diagnosis (17)   Condition, problem, or other reason for the health encounter that is chiefly responsible for services; also referred to as the first-listed condition

principal diagnosis (17)   Condition established after study that prompted the hospitalization; used only in an inpatient setting

privileged information (3)   Data or confidential exchange between a professional (e.g., physician, attorney) and a client or patient, related to the treatment and progress of the patient, that may be released or disclosed only when written authorization of the patient or guardian is obtained

problem-oriented medical record (POMR) (9) Medical recordkeeping organizational system that contains data lists of the patients' permanent and temporary problems, each numbered and dated. Other lists are included, for example, medications, blood pressures, lab results, and surgeries.

professional corporation (2)   Entity unto itself with a legal and business status that is independent of its shareholders

professional courtesy (13)   Discount or discharge of a debt granted to certain individuals at the discretion of the physician rendering the service

professionalism (1)   Conduct, aspirations, and qualities characteristic of a profession

prognosis (9)   Forecast of the outcome of a disease or injury

progress report (9)   Written observations made at examinations of a patient subsequent to an initial examination

proofreading (11)   Locating and marking the corrections as needed while reading a document

proprietorship (15)   Owner's net worth; that is, that which is equal to the assets of the business minus the liabilities of the business; also known as *owner's equity* or *capital*

protected health information (PHI) (3)   Information about the patient's past, present, or future health condition that contains personal identifying data

protocol (6)   Set of instructions used for reference that prescribes strict adherence to correct etiquette and preference

provider (18)   Person or institution that gives medical care

purchase order (19)   Written authorization to a merchant to deliver merchandise, materials, or services at an agreed-on price

purge (8)   Procedure used in filing to remove outdated files or items from files, folders, or computer disks

Q

qualified diagnoses (17)   Final medical impression made by a physician using the terms *rule-out, suspected, suspicion of, questionable, likely, probably,* or *possible,* as if they existed or were established but have not been; also called *working diagnosis*

qualitative analysis (16)   Laboratory test that determines the presence of an agent within the body

quantitative analysis (16)   Laboratory test that measures how much of an agent is within the body

quantum merit **(13)**   Latin for "as much as he deserves"; a common-law principle that means the patient promises to pay the physician as much as he or she deserves for labor

R

reception area (5)   Outer office provided for patients who are awaiting appointments

recertification (1)   Process, outlined by a certifying board by which a medical professional is reassessed to renew certification; test or continuing education to ensure that professional competencies are updated and current

reconciliation (14)   Act of proving the accuracy of all transactions that have occurred on a checking account by performing mathematical computations and comparing the bank's records with those of the customer

recycle (8)   Using saved material (e.g., wastepaper) and processing it for reuse

Red Flags Rule (5)   Rule from Section 114 of the Fair and Accurate Credit Transactions Act that states all those who act as "creditors" need to have a written prevention and detection program for identity theft that includes policies and procedures to verify a patient's identity and targets areas (red flags) where identity theft may occur; the Red Flags Program Clarification Act was subsequently passed that excludes doctor offices

referral (2, 7, 16, 18)   Procedure followed when a primary care physician recommends and sends the patient to another physician for further medical treatment

referring physician (9)   Physician sending a patient to another physician for the transfer of total or partial medical care. This term is also used loosely for a physician who sends a patient to a specialist for a consultation or for a diagnostic test.

reflective listening (4)   To think about, dwell on, mull over, and study or weigh what has been said

Registered Mail (12)   First-class mail service that provides, for a fee, a record that mail has been delivered and guarantees an indemnity if it is not received

Registered Medical Assistant (RMA) (1)   Title received after appropriate training in administrative and clinical areas and passing a certification examination administered by the American Medical Technologists (AMT)

registration (1)   Statement issued by a state or national board or association that verifies that a person meets professional standards

registration form (5)   Questionnaire designed to provide identifying data

registration kiosk (5)   Stand-alone structure providing information and services; offers self-serve computer system to register patients, update demographic information, and process payments in a medical office

Remittance Advice (RA) (13, 18)   See *Medicare Remittance Advice*

remote coder (16, 17)   Coders who work at locations other than in the physician's office (e.g., home or billing service)

respondeat superior **(3)**   Latin for "let the master answer." A physician's responsibility for any actions performed by his or her employees in the course of their work, including ones that may injure or harm another individual; also known as *vicarious liability.*

results-oriented résumé (21)   Summary of work experience that focuses on results, not characteristics. This type of résumé helps prospective employers reduce the risks that are associated with hiring because it shows what the job seeker has accomplished as well as his or her attitude toward work.

résumé (21)   Summary of education, skills, and work experience, usually in outline form

revenue cycle (13)   Life of the patient account from creation to payment

risk management (3)   Identifying problem practices or behaviors, then taking action to control or eliminate them

S

savings account (14)   Money deposited in a bank or similar institution where it earns interest and has been set aside for future use

scope of practice (3)   The range of education, training, ability, and skills a health care professional is expected to have and operate within according to the law and within the standard of care

scores (8)   Creases along the lower front flap of a file folder that unfold to allow the folder to expand

screening (6)   Process of asking good questions to evaluate and determine the action to be taken on a telephone call or to determine the person who should receive the telephone call

scribe (17) Medical assistant who follows (shadows) the physician into treatment rooms and records, according to the direction of the physician, all the elements of the history, physical examination, and medical decision-making process that are needed for evaluation and management services, as well as details about tests, surgical procedures, and diagnoses

separate procedure (16) *CPT* five-digit procedure code that, if not performed separately, is an integral part of another procedure; often bundled into other procedures

service charges (14) Fees assessed on a bank account for processing transactions and for account maintenance

service endorsement (12) Notification to the U.S. Postal Service on the envelope stating what is to be done with undelivered mail

sharps containers (5) Medical waste containers to dispose of sharp objects (e.g., needles) made of rigid puncture-resistant material that, when sealed, are leak resistant and cannot be reopened without great difficulty

shelf life (10) Length of time a drug may be kept before it begins to deteriorate

sign (9) Indication of the presence or existence of a disease or body function disorder; objective evidence or observable physical phenomenon typically associated with a given condition

signature (10) Section of a prescription that gives instructions to the patient on how to take or apply the medication; also known as *transcription*

signature card (14) Document required by banks to identify those authorized to act on (sign) an account or safe deposit box; signing indicates acknowledgment to handle the account according to existing bank laws

simplified letter style (11) Written communication typed without a salutation or complimentary close

single-entry accounting (15) Type of accounting where each transaction is entered only once in the account books. It is not self-balancing; in other words, it does not rely on equal debits or credits.

skip (13) Debtor who has moved and left no forwarding address

SOAP (9) Abbreviation for *subjective* complaints, *objective* findings, *assessment* of status to obtain diagnosis and implement a treatment *plan*; a method of structuring progress or chart notes

Social Security (FICA) taxes (20) Charges levied by the federal government on employers and employees that provide funds to pay retired people or their survivors who are entitled to receive such payments, either because they paid Social Security taxes themselves or because Congress declared them eligible

software (7) Computer instructions permanently stored in or temporarily programmed into hardware

solo physician practice (2) One physician working alone whose charges are based on a fee-for-service arrangement

source-oriented record (SOR) (9) Common paper-based medical record management system that arranges documents according to sections

speakerphone (6) Telephone with a microphone designed for hands-free communication

specialized care center (2) Facility where a team of specialists treats patients who have similar medical conditions

staff meetings (18) Scheduled gatherings of office personnel for the purpose of informing, training, problem solving, and exchanging of ideas

stale check (14) Check that is previously dated and so old when presented for payment that it is no longer valid; time limit can vary from 90 days to 6 months, and such information is noted on the face of the check; also called a *stale dated check*

standard precautions (5) Minimum infection prevention practices that apply to all patient care, regardless of suspected or confirmed infection status

State Disability Insurance (SDI) (20) Insurance program that covers off-the-job injury or illness and is paid for by deductions from employee paychecks; similar programs are Temporary Disability Insurance and Unemployment Compensation Disability

state withholding tax (20) Charge levied by a state government on employers and employees that provides funds for state use; amounts determined by individual states

stereotype (4) Generalized or oversimplified conception concerning an individual, group, or form of behavior

stop payment orders (14) Written orders by a signer on the account revoking a check before the bank issues payment. A fee may be assessed for stop payment requests, which are typically carried out if there is loss of a check, a disagreement about a purchase, or a disagreement about a payment; it may not be instituted if a check guarantee card was used in the money transaction.

stream (7) System of advance appointment scheduling in which patients are allocated specific periods of time for office visits and procedures; also called *fixed interval*

stress (1) Natural reaction of the body to any physical, psychological, or emotional demand (pleasant or unpleasant) placed on it either internally or externally

subject filing (8) Alphabetical arrangement of records filed by topic or grouped under a main theme

subjective information (4, 9) In a medical context, any information that the patient provides to the physician describing symptoms that exist in the mind but cannot be seen, heard, felt, or measured such as pain, light-headedness, or nausea

subpoena (3) Latin for "under penalty"; a writ that commands a witness to appear at a trial or other proceeding and give testimony, the disobedience to which may be punishable as a contempt of court

subpoena duces tecum (3) Latin for "under penalty in his possession"; a subpoena that requires a witness to appear in court with his or her records, although the judge may permit mailing of records so that the physician is not required to appear in court, which is the typical scenario experienced in many medical practices

subscription (10) Section of a prescription giving directions to the pharmacist on the total quantity of the drug to be given and the form of the medication (e.g., capsules, tablets)

superscription (10) First element imprinted on a prescription; shown as a symbol (Rx), which stands for the word *recipe* (Latin for "take")

surgical approach (16) Entry point into interior parts of the body that is used by physicians performing surgical procedures, for example, open incision, scope, approaching through a body orifice (ear, nose, vagina)

surname (8) Individual's last name

sympathy (1) Pertaining to concern for another person's feelings, thoughts, and experiences

symptom (9) Any indication of disease or disorder that is perceived or experienced by the patient; usually described in subjective terms, for example, depressed, confused, experiencing pain, or tired

T

telecommunication (6) Transmission of voice or data over a distance

telemedicine (2) Wireless transfer of medical information via electronic technology to provide health care when there is a separation between the health care professional and the patient

telephone log (6) Written, dated record of all incoming telephone calls noting the reason for the call and action taken

telephone reference aid (6) Alphabetical list of frequently called telephone numbers

telephone routing decision grid (6) Record of various types of incoming calls identifying who the call should be forwarded (routed) to

template (7) A preset format or pattern, used as a guide which designates various time frames for specific appointment types

temporary disability (TD) (18) Illness or injury that temporarily prevents an injured person from performing the functions of a regular job

thesaurus (11) Reference book of alphabetized words with their synonyms and antonyms; also found in word processing software

third-party payer (18) Party (insurance carrier or medical assistance program) other than the physician or patient who intervenes to pay hospital or medical expenses; also known as *third-party carrier*

tickler file (8) Chronological file system that calls attention to future dates of appointments or business matters; a follow-up file that "tickles" the memory

time limit (18) Period of time in which a notice of claim or proof of loss must be filed

time zones (6) The contiguous United States is divided from east to west into four time zones, Eastern, Central, Mountain, and Pacific, each being 1 hour earlier than the next. Most of the United States observes daylight savings time during the summer months, except Arizona and Hawaii.

timecard (20) Record of days and hours worked for each pay period

tort (3) Wrongful act or injury to a person that is grounds for legal civil action

total disability (18) Illness or injury that prevents a person from performing the duties of his or her occupation or from engaging in any other type of work for remuneration

total practice management system (TPMS) (6, 7, 8, 9) See *electronic health record practice management system*

transcription (10) See *signature*

transcriptionist (11) Person who converts voice-recorded dictation to hardcopy

treating or performing physician (9) Provider who renders a service to a patient or completes a test

triage (6) System of decision making in which patients are selected for allocation of treatment according to the seriousness of their ailment

true wave (7) System of appointment scheduling that allows for variables and flexibility and assumes the time allowed for appointments will average out each hour

type of service (TOS) (16) Kind of service or procedure provided by a medical doctor (e.g., office visit, laboratory test, surgery)

U

Unbundling (16) Breaking down a procedure into separate billable codes with charges to increase reimbursement; also known as *fragmentation, exploding,* or *à la carte medicine*

Unemployment Compensation Disability (UCD) (20) Insurance program that covers off-the-job injury and illness and is paid for by deductions from employee paychecks; similar programs are State Disability Insurance and Temporary Disability Insurance (TDI)

United Parcel Service (UPS) (12) National and international letter and package delivery service

United States Postal Service (USPS) (12) Domestic and international mail delivery service

upcoding (16) Practice of coding and billing a health plan for a procedure that reimburses the physician at a higher rate than the procedure actually done; also known as *code creep, overcoding,* or *overbilling*

urgent care (6) Treatment of injuries or conditions that need prompt medical attention within 24 hours to prevent serious deterioration of a patient's health, but is not life threatening; also known as *after-hours care*

urgent care center (2) Private, for-profit facility offering extended hours that employ salaried physicians who provide primary and urgent care; also known as *freestanding emergency centers* or *ambulatory centers*

usual, customary, and reasonable (UCR) (13)   A usual fee is one that an individual physician normally charges for a given professional service to a private patient; a customary fee is in the range of usual fees charged by providers of similar training and experience in a geographic area; a reasonable fee meets the two previous criteria or is justifiable by responsible medical opinion considering the special circumstances of the case

utilization review (2)   Evaluation process performed by qualified health care professionals to determine the quality, appropriateness, and medical necessity of medical care

V

verbal communication (4)   The use of language or spoken words to transmit messages

veteran (18)   One who has served in the United States Armed Forces and has received an honorable discharge

virus (8)   Hidden program that enters a computer by means of an outside source, such as software, CD, or online services; can be harmless (flashing an on-screen message) or harmful (replicating itself throughout CD and memory, using up or wiping out data or memory and eventually causing the system to crash)

voice mail (6)   Storing and forwarding of one-way messages combining elements of the telephone, the computer, and a recording device

voucher (13, 14, 15)   (1) Receipt stating details (as evidence) of a disbursement of cash. (2) Part of the check that has no negotiable value and that remains in the checkbook after a check is written and removed. It is used to itemize or to specify the purpose for which a check is drawn; also called a *check stub* or *check register*. (3) In insurance, a payment check.

W

Wage and Tax Statement (Form W-2) (20)   Tax form identifying employer and employee that shows gross earnings and deductions for federal, state, FICA, Medicare, and local income taxes. Form is sent by the employer to the IRS and to each employee annually; a copy is attached by the employee to his or her tax return.

wage base (20)   Annual maximum amount of monies earned on which certain taxes are levied

waiting period (w/p) (18)   Time that must elapse before a benefit is paid; also known as *excepted period*

waiver (18)   Attachment to an insurance policy that excludes certain illnesses or disabilities that would otherwise be covered

warrant (14)   Check that is not considered negotiable but can be converted into a negotiable instrument or cash

withdrawal (14)   Removal of funds from a checking account by writing a check or using an ATM; from a savings account, a withdrawal slip may be completed or an ATM may be used

word processing (11)   Communications system using computerized and text-editing equipment to produce printed letters, reports, and other office documents; includes memory

word processing log (11)   Record of incoming and outgoing word processing documents used for accessing written communications quickly and easily

X

x-ray report (9)   Written findings of an examination of a radiographic study on film

Z

zone improvement plan (ZIP + 4) (12)   Numerical codes, which consist of five or nine digits, written or keyed on envelopes to facilitate the sorting and delivery of mail

INDEX

Page numbers in *italics* indicate figures and tables. Page numbers followed by *(onl.)* indicate references from Chapter 21 available online only.